ADVANC
RECONSTRUCTION
Hip 2

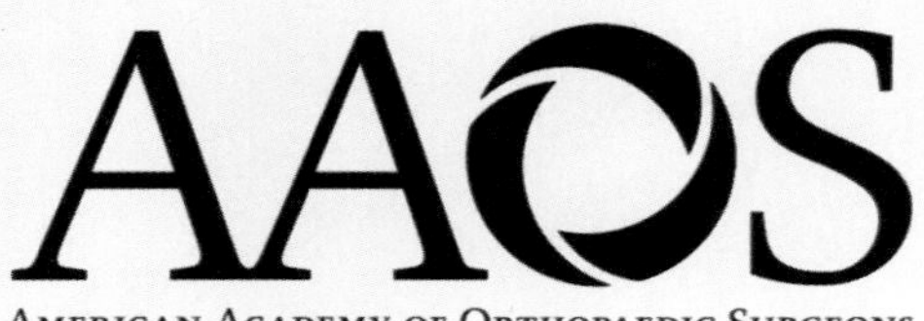

ADVANCED RECONSTRUCTION
Hip 2

Edited by

Jay R. Lieberman, MD
Professor and Chairman
Department of Orthopaedic Surgery
Keck School of Medicine of USC
Professor of Biomedical Engineering
Viterbi School of Engineering of USC
University of Southern California
Los Angeles, California

Daniel J. Berry, MD
L.Z. Gund Professor of Orthopedic Surgery
Consultant
Department of Orthopedic Surgery
Mayo Clinic
Rochester, Minnesota

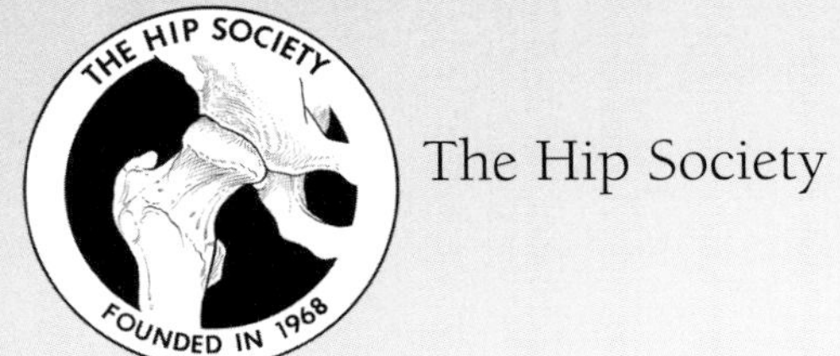

The Hip Society

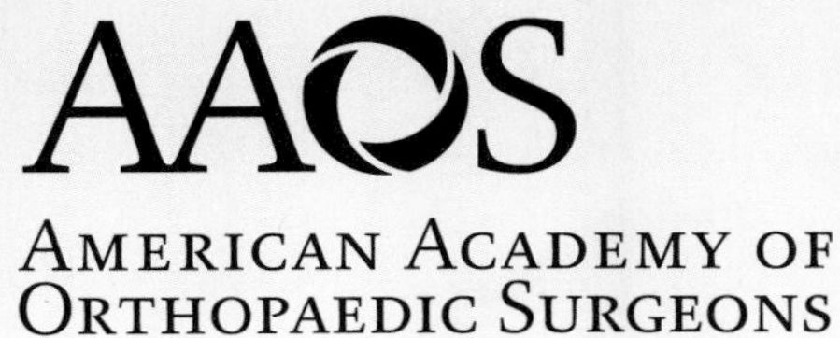

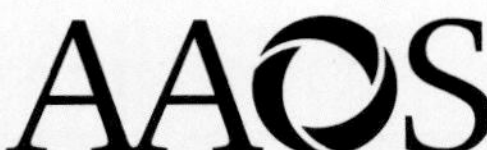

AMERICAN ACADEMY OF ORTHOPAEDIC SURGEONS

Staff

Ellen C. Moore, *Chief Education Officer*

Hans Koelsch, PhD, *Director, Department of Publications*

Lisa Claxton Moore, *Senior Manager, Book Program*

Laura Goetz, *Managing Editor*

Kathleen Anderson, *Senior Editor*

Steven Kellert, *Senior Editor*

Michelle Wild, *Associate Senior Editor*

Courtney Dunker, *Editorial Production Manager*

Abram Fassler, *Publishing Systems Manager*

Suzanne O'Reilly, *Graphic Designer*

Susan Morritz Baim, *Production Coordinator*

Karen Danca, *Permissions Coordinator*

Charlie Baldwin, *Digital and Print Production Specialist*

Hollie Muir, *Digital and Print Production Specialist*

Emily Douglas, *Page Production Assistant*

Genevieve Charet, *Editorial Coordinator*

Rachel Winokur, *Editorial Coordinator/Copy Editor*

Brian Moore, *Manager, Electronic Media Programs*

Katie Hovany, *Digital Media Specialist*

Library of Congress Control Number:

Published 2017 by the
American Academy of Orthopaedic Surgeons
9400 West Higgins Road
Rosemont, IL 60018

ISBN 978-1-62552-557-4
Printed in the USA

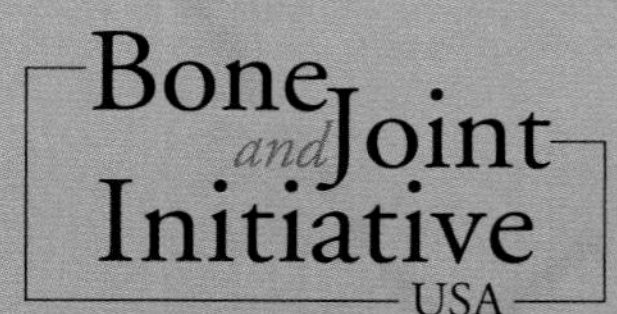

Acknowledgments

Explore the full portfolio of AAOS educational programs and publications across the orthopaedic spectrum for every stage of an orthopaedic surgeon's career, at www.aaos.org. The AAOS, in partnership with Jones & Bartlett Learning, also offers a comprehensive collection of educational and training resources for emergency medical providers, from first responders to critical care transport paramedics. Learn more at www.aaos.org/ems.

Contributors

Matthew P. Abdel, MD
Associate Professor of Orthopedic Surgery, Mayo Clinic College of Medicine
Senior Associate Consultant, Department of Orthopedic Surgery
Mayo Clinic
Rochester, Minnesota

Derek F. Amanatullah, MD, PhD
Assistant Professor
Department of Orthopaedic Surgery
Stanford University
Redwood City, California

David Backstein, MD, MEd, FRCSC
Associate Professor, Surgery
Head, Granovsky Gluskin Division of Orthopaedics
Mount Sinai Health System
University of Toronto
Toronto, Ontario, Canada

Rishi Balkissoon, MD, MPH
Assistant Professor
Adult Reconstructive Orthopaedic Surgery
University of Rochester Medical Center
Rochester, New York

William P. Barrett, MD
Director, Center for Joint Replacement
Proliance Orthopedic Associates
Renton, Washington

Paul E. Beaulé, MD, FRCSC
Professor of Surgery
Head, Division of Orthopedics
The Ottawa Hospital/University of Ottawa
Ottawa, Ontario, Canada

Asheesh Bedi, MD
Harold and Helen W. Gehring Professor
Division Chief, Sports Medicine and Shoulder Surgery
Department of Orthopaedic Surgery
University of Michigan
Ann Arbor, Michigan

Michael E. Berend, MD
Midwest Center for Joint Replacement - Midwest Specialty Surgery Center
Joint Replacement Surgeons of Indiana Research Foundation
Indianapolis, Indiana

Jonathan L. Berliner, MD
Department of Orthopaedic Surgery
University of California, San Francisco
San Francisco, California

Daniel J. Berry, MD
L.Z. Gund Professor of Orthopedic Surgery
Consultant
Department of Orthopedic Surgery
Mayo Clinic
Rochester, Minnesota

Michael Bolognesi, MD
Chief, Division of Adult Reconstruction
Department of Orthopaedic Surgery
Duke University Medical Center
Durham, North Carolina

Barrett Steven Boody, MD
Department of Orthopaedic Surgery
Northwestern Memorial Hospital
Chicago, Illinois

Mathias P. G. Bostrom, MD
Attending Orthopaedic Surgeon
Adult Reconstruction & Joint Replacement Division
Hospital for Special Surgery
New York, New York

Kevin J. Bozic, MD, MBA
Chair of Surgery and Perioperative Care
Dell Medical School, University of Texas at Austin
Austin, Texas

Adam C. Brekke, MD
Department of Orthopaedic Surgery
Vanderbilt Orthopaedics and Rehabilitation
Nashville, Tennessee

Timothy S. Brown, MD
Department of Orthopaedic Surgery
University of Texas Southwestern Medical Center
Dallas, Texas

James A. Browne, MD
Associate Professor of Orthopaedic Surgery
Division Head of Adult Reconstruction
University of Virginia
Charlottesville, Virginia

Miguel E. Cabanela, MD
Professor of Orthopedics
Department of Orthopedic Surgery
Mayo Clinic
Rochester, Minnesota

John J. Callaghan, MD
Professor
Department of Orthopaedics
University of Iowa
Iowa City, Iowa

Hugh U. Cameron, MBChB, FRCSC
Orthopaedic Surgeon
Sunnybrook Hospital
Toronto, Ontario, Canada

Joshua L. Carter, MD
Midwest Center for Joint Replacement
Indianapolis, Indiana

John C. Clohisy, MD
Daniel C. and Betty B. Viehmann Distinguished Professor
Department of Orthopaedic Surgery
Washington University School of Medicine
St. Louis, Missouri

David F. Dalury, MD
Clinical Professor of Orthopedics
University of Maryland
Chief of Orthopedic Surgery
University of Maryland St. Joseph Medical Center
Towson, Maryland

Craig J. Della Valle, MD
Chief, Division of Adult Reconstruction
Professor of Orthopaedic Surgery
Department of Orthopaedic Surgery
Rush University Medical Center
Chicago, Illinois

Douglas A. Dennis, MD
Surgeon
Colorado Joint Replacement
Denver, Colorado

Ajit Deshmukh, MD
Assistant Professor
Adult Reconstructive Orthopaedic Surgery
NYU Langone Medical Center/VA New York Harbor Healthcare System
New York, New York

Michael J. Dunbar, MD, FRCSC, PhD
Professor of Surgery
Dalhousie University
Halifax, Nova Scotia, Canada

Clive P. Duncan, MD, MSc, FRCSC
Professor and Emeritus Chair
Department of Orthopaedics
University of British Columbia
Vancouver, British Columbia, Canada

Randa Elmallah, MD
Orthopaedic Surgery
University of Mississippi Medical Center
Jackson, Mississippi

Mohammad Ali Enayatollahi, MD
Postdoctoral Research Fellow
Rothman Institute at Thomas Jefferson University
Philadelphia, Pennsylvania

C. Anderson Engh, Jr, MD
Orthopaedic Surgeon
Anderson Orthopaedic Research Institute
Alexandria, Virginia

Keith A. Fehring, MD
Hip and Knee Reconstruction Fellow
Department of Orthopedic Surgery
Mayo Clinic
Rochester, Minnesota

Thomas K. Fehring, MD
Co-Director, OrthoCarolina
Hip and Knee Center
OrthoCarolina
Charlotte, North Carolina

Bryan Flynn, MD, FRCSC
Arthroplasty Fellow
Division of Orthopaedics
Dalhousie University
Halifax, Nova Scotia, Canada

Donald S. Garbuz, MD, FRCSC
Professor and Head
Division of Lower Limb Reconstruction & Oncology
Department of Orthopaedics
University of British Columbia
Vancouver, British Columbia, Canada

Jean W. M. Gardeniers, MD, PhD, DTHM
Consultant Orthopaedic Surgeon
Department of Orthopaedics
Radboud University Medical Center
Nijmegen, Netherlands

Kevin L. Garvin, MD
Professor and Chair
Department of Orthopaedic Surgery and Rehabilitation
University of Nebraska Medical Center
Omaha, Nebraska

Jeremy M. Gililland, MD
Orthopaedic Surgeon
Department of Orthopaedics
University of Utah
Salt Lake City, Utah

Francis B. Gonzales, MD
Assistant Clinical Professor
Fellowship Program Director
Department of Orthopaedic Surgery
University of California, San Diego
San Diego, California

Stuart B. Goodman, MD, PhD, FRCSC, FACS
Robert L. and Mary Ellenburg Professor of Surgery
Professor, Department of Orthopaedic Surgery and (by courtesy) Bioengineering
Department of Orthopaedic Surgery
Stanford University
Stanford, California

Christopher Grayson, MD
Adult Reconstruction and Arthritis Surgery
Florida Orthopaedic Institute
Tampa, Florida

Allan E. Gross, MD, FRCSC, O.Ont
Professor of Surgery
Division of Orthopaedic Surgery
Mount Sinai Hospital, University of Toronto
Toronto, Ontario, Canada

George J. Haidukewych, MD
Academic Chairman of Orthopedic Surgery
Level One Orthopedics
Orlando Health
Orlando, Florida

Rhett K. Hallows, MD
Orthopedic Surgeon
Duke Orthopedics
Duke University Medical Center
Durham, North Carolina

William G. Hamilton, MD
Orthopaedic Surgeon
Anderson Orthopaedic Research Institute
Alexandria, Virginia

Arlen D. Hanssen, MD
Professor
Department of Orthopedic Surgery
Mayo Clinic
Rochester, Minnesota

Curtis W. Hartman, MD
Associate Professor
Department of Orthopaedic Surgery and Rehabilitation
University of Nebraska Medical Center
Omaha, Nebraska

Nathanael Heckmann, MD
Orthopaedic Surgery
Keck School of Medicine
University of Southern California
Los Angeles, California

Patrick K. Horst, MD
Department of Orthopaedic Surgery
University of California, San Francisco
San Francisco, California

James L. Howard, MD, MSc, FRCSC
Program Director and Assistant Professor
Division of Orthopaedic Surgery
Western University, London Health Sciences Centre
London, Ontario, Canada

Jonathan R. Howell, MBBS, MSc, FRCS (Tr & Orth)
Consultant Orthopaedic Surgeon
Princess Elizabeth Orthopaedic Centre
Royal Devon and Exeter NHS Foundation Trust
Exeter, England, United Kingdom

William Hozack, MD
Walter Annenberg Professor of Joint Replacement
Sidney Kimmel Medical School
Thomas Jefferson University
Rothman Institute Orthopedics
Philadelphia, Pennsylvania

Der-Chen Timothy Huang, MD
Orthopedic Fellow
Joint Replacement Institute
St. Vincent Medical Center
Los Angeles, California

Michael H. Huo, MD
Professor
Department of Orthopaedic Surgery
University of Texas Southwestern Medical Center
Dallas, Texas

Cathy Huynh, BS
Project Director
Anderson Orthopaedic Research Institute
Alexandria, Virginia

Richard Iorio, MD
Chief of Adult Reconstruction
William and Susan Jaffe Professor of Orthopaedic Surgery
Department of Orthopaedic Surgery
NYU Langone Medical Center
Hospital for Joint Diseases
New York, New York

Joshua J. Jacobs, MD
Professor and Chairman
Department of Orthopaedic Surgery
Rush University Medical Center
Associate Provost for Research
Rush University
Vice Dean for Research
Rush Medical College
Chicago, Illinois

Jason M. Jennings, MD, DPT
Orthopaedic Surgeon
Colorado Joint Replacement, Porter Adventist Hospital
Denver, Colorado

William A. Jiranek, MD
Professor and Chief of Adult Reconstruction
Alison and Abbott Byrd Chair in Orthopaedic Surgery
Department of Orthopedic Surgery
Virginia Commonwealth University School of Medicine
Richmond, Virginia

Robert B. Jones, MD
Adult Reconstruction Fellow
Department of Orthopaedic Surgery
University of Utah
Salt Lake City, Utah

Y. Julia Kao, MD
Adult Reconstruction and Joint Replacement
Resurgens Orthopaedics
Atlanta, Georgia

Erdan Kayupov, MSE
Research Fellow
Department of Orthopaedic Surgery
Rush University Medical Center
Chicago, Illinois

James A. Keeney, MD
Chief, Adult Hip & Knee Reconstruction Service
Associate Professor
Department of Orthopaedic Surgery
University of Missouri
Columbia, Missouri

Scott S. Kelley, MD
Professor
Department of Orthopedic Surgery
Duke University
Durham, North Carolina

Bryan T. Kelly, MD
Chief, Sports Medicine and Shoulder Service
Hospital for Special Surgery
New York, New York

Raymond H. Kim, MD
Surgeon
Colorado Joint Replacement
Denver, Colorado

Kevin Koo, MD, FRCSC
Clinical Associate
Division of Orthopaedics
University of Toronto
Toronto, Ontario, Canada

Paul Kuzyk, MD, MASc, FRCSC
Assistant Professor, Orthopaedic Surgeon
Department of Orthopaedic Surgery
Mount Sinai Hospital, University of Toronto
Toronto, Ontario, Canada

Paul F. Lachiewicz, MD
Consulting Professor
Department of Orthopaedics
Duke University Medical Center
Durham, North Carolina

Matthew Landrum, MD
Department of Orthopaedic Surgery
University of Texas Southwestern Medical Center
Dallas, Texas

Christopher M. Larson, MD
Twin Cities Orthopedics
Edina, Minnesota

Nicholas J. Lash, MBChB, FRACS
Clinical Fellow
Department of Orthopaedics, Lower Limb Reconstruction & Oncology
University of British Columbia
Vancouver, British Columbia, Canada

Cameron K. Ledford, MD
Assistant Professor
Department of Orthopedic Surgery
University of Kansas Medical Center
Kansas City, Kansas

Brett R. Levine, MD, MS
Associate Professor
Department of Orthopedic Surgery
Rush University Medical Center
Chicago, Illinois

David G. Lewallen, MD
Professor of Orthopedic Surgery
Department of Orthopedic Surgery
Mayo Clinic
Rochester, Minnesota

Jay R. Lieberman, MD
Professor and Chairman
Department of Orthopaedic Surgery
Keck School of Medicine of USC
Professor of Biomedical Engineering
Viterbi School of Engineering of USC
University of Southern California
Los Angeles, California

Steve S. Liu, MD
Associate Research Scientist
Department of Orthopaedics
University of Iowa
Iowa City, Iowa

Adolph V. Lombardi, Jr, MD, FACS
President
Joint Implant Surgeons, Inc
New Albany, Ohio

Tad M. Mabry, MD
Assistant Professor of Orthopedics
Department of Orthopedic Surgery
Mayo Clinic
Rochester, Minnesota

Steven J. MacDonald, MD, FRCSC
Professor of Orthopedic Surgery and Department Chair
Department of Orthopedic Surgery
London Health Sciences Centre
London, Ontario, Canada

Rami Madanat, MD, PhD, FEBOT
Attending Orthopaedic Surgeon
Department of Orthopaedics and Traumatology
Helsinki University Hospital
Helsinki, Finland

Tatu J. Mäkinen, MD, PhD, FEBOT
Arthroplasty Clinical Fellow
Division of Orthopaedic Surgery
Mount Sinai Hospital, University of Toronto
Toronto, Ontario, Canada

Henrik Malchau, MD, PhD
Professor
Department of Orthopedics
Massachusetts General Hospital, Harvard Medical School
Boston, Massachusetts

William J. Maloney, MD
Chairman
Department of Orthopaedic Surgery
Stanford University
Redwood City, California

Thomas Marceau-Cote, MD, FRCSC
Arthroplasty Fellow
Division of Orthopaedics
Dalhousie University
Halifax, Nova Scotia, Canada

Cody L. Martin, MD
Department of Orthopaedic Surgery
University of Florida College of Medicine Jacksonville
Jacksonville, Florida

Bassam A. Masri, MD, FRCSC
Professor and Head
Department of Orthopaedics
University of British Columbia
Vancouver, British Columbia, Canada

R. Michael Meneghini, MD
Associate Professor
Department of Orthopedics
Indiana University School of Medicine
Indianapolis, Indiana

Ryan A. Mlynarek, MD
Department of Orthopaedic Surgery
University of Michigan
Ann Arbor, Michigan

Michael Mont, MD
Chairman
Department of Orthopedics
Cleveland Clinic
Cleveland, Ohio

Charles L. Nelson, MD
Chief of Adult Reconstruction and Associate Professor of Orthopaedic Surgery
University of Pennsylvania
Philadelphia, Pennsylvania

Matthew C. Niesen, MD
Adult Reconstruction Fellow
Department of Orthopedic Surgery
Mayo Clinic
Phoenix, Arizona

Daniel A. Oakes, MD
Associate Professor of Clinical Orthopaedic Surgery
Director, USC Joint Replacement Program
Department of Orthopaedic Surgery
Keck School of Medicine of USC
University of Southern California
Los Angeles, California

Mary I. O'Connor, MD
Director and Professor
Center for Musculoskeletal Care at Yale Medicine and Yale New Haven Health
Professor
Department of Orthopaedics and Rehabilitation
Yale School of Medicine
New Haven, Connecticut

Liza Osagie-Clouard, MBBS
Royal National Orthopaedic Hospital
London, England, United Kingdom

Alex Pagé, MD, FRCSC
Adult Reconstruction Fellow
The Ottawa Hospital
Ottawa, Ontario, Canada

Wayne G. Paprosky, MD
Professor
Department of Orthopaedic Surgery
Rush University Medical Center
Winfield, Illinois

Javad Parvizi, MD, FRCS
James Edwards Professor of Orthopaedic Surgery
Rothman Institute at Thomas Jefferson University
Philadelphia, Pennsylvania

Christopher E. Pelt, MD
Assistant Professor
Department of Orthopaedics
University of Utah
Salt Lake City, Utah

Kevin I. Perry, MD
Assistant Professor
Department of Orthopedic Surgery
Mayo Clinic
Rochester, Minnesota

Christopher L. Peters, MD
Professor and Chief, Adult Reconstruction and Hip Preservation
Department of Orthopaedics
University of Utah
Salt Lake City, Utah

Gregory G. Polkowski, MD, MSc
Assistant Professor
Department of Orthopaedic Surgery
Vanderbilt Orthopaedic Institute
Nashville, Tennessee

Christopher Pomeroy, MD
OrthoIndy
Indianapolis, Indiana

Peter Pyrko, MD, PhD
Assistant Professor of Orthopedic Surgery
Adult Reconstruction
Department of Orthopedics
Loma Linda University
Loma Linda, California

Amar S. Ranawat, MD
Associate Professor of Orthopaedic Surgery
Hospital for Special Surgery
New York, New York

Chitranjan S. Ranawat, MD
Professor of Orthopaedic Surgery
Weill Cornell Medical College
Attending Orthopaedic Surgeon
Hospital for Special Surgery
New York, New York

Michael D. Ries, MD
Arthroplasty Fellowship Co-Director
Reno Orthopaedic Clinic
Reno, Nevada

Wim H. C. Rijnen, MD, PhD
Orthopaedic Surgeon
Department of Orthopaedics
Radboud University Medical Center
Nijmegen, Netherlands

Ola Rolfson, MD, PhD
Attending Orthopaedic Surgeon
Department of Orthopaedics
Sahlgrenska University Hospital
Mölndal, Sweden

Aaron G. Rosenberg, MD
Director of Adult Reconstruction
Department of Orthopedic Surgery
Rush University Medical Center
Chicago, Illinois

Brett D. Rosenthal, MD
Department of Orthopaedic Surgery
Northwestern University
Chicago, Illinois

James R. Ross, MD
Orthopedic Surgeon
Boca Care Orthopedics
Boca Raton, Florida

Oleg A. Safir, MD, MEd, FRCSC
Associate Professor of Surgery
Gluskin Granovsky Division of Orthopaedics
D.H. Gales Director U of T Surgical Skills Centre
Sinai Health System
University of Toronto
Toronto, Ontario, Canada

Nemandra A. Sandiford, MSc, FRCS (Tr & Orth)
Adult Reconstruction and Oncology Fellow
Department of Orthopaedics
University of British Columbia
Vancouver, British Columbia, Canada

Richard F. Santore, MD
Director, Sharp Hip Preservation Center
Department of Orthopaedic Surgery
Sharp Memorial Hospital
San Diego, California

Adam A. Sassoon, MD, MS
Assistant Professor
Department of Orthopaedics and Sports Medicine
University of Washington
Seattle, Washington

Thomas P. Schmalzried, MD
Fellowship Director
Joint Replacement Institute
St. Vincent Medical Center
Los Angeles, California

B. Willem Schreurs, MD, PhD
Orthopaedic Surgeon
Department of Orthopaedics
Radboud University Medical Center
Nijmegen, Netherlands

Joseph M. Schwab, MD
Assistant Professor
Department of Orthopaedic Surgery
Medical College of Wisconsin
Milwaukee, Wisconsin

Peter K. Sculco, MD
Orthopedic Hip and Knee Reconstruction Fellow
Department of Orthopedic Surgery
Mayo Clinic
Rochester, Minnesota

Thorsten M. Seyler, MD, PhD
Assistant Professor
Division of Adult Reconstruction
Department of Orthopaedic Surgery
Duke University
Durham, North Carolina

Courtney E. Sherman, MD
Orthopedic Oncologist and Assistant Professor
Department of Orthopedic Surgery
Mayo Clinic
Jacksonville, Florida

Neil Sheth, MD
Assistant Professor
Department of Orthopaedic Surgery
University of Pennsylvania
Philadelphia, Pennsylvania

Rafael J. Sierra, MD
Professor
Department of Orthopedic Surgery
Mayo Clinic
Rochester, Minnesota

Tom J. J. H. Slooff, MD, PhD
Orthopaedic Surgeon
Department of Orthopaedics
Radboud University Medical Center
Nijmegen, Netherlands

David H. So, MD
Assistant Clinical Professor
Department of Orthopedic Surgery
University of California, Irvine
Orange, California

Mark J. Spangehl, MD
Associate Professor of Orthopaedics
Department of Orthopaedics
Mayo Clinic Arizona
Phoenix, Arizona

Andrew I. Spitzer, MD
Chief, Implant Service
Cedars-Sinai Orthopaedic Center
Cedars-Sinai Medical Center
Los Angeles, California

Scott M. Sporer, MD
Associate Professor
Department of Orthopedic Surgery
Rush University Medical Center
Medical Director Joint Replacement Institute, Central DuPage Hospital
Winfield, Illinois

Bryan D. Springer, MD
Fellowship Director
Adult Reconstruction of the Hip and Knee
OrthoCarolina Hip & Knee Center
Charlotte, North Carolina

Michael D. Stefl, MD
Physician
Department of Orthopaedic Surgery
Los Angeles County and University of Southern California
Los Angeles, California

Rebecca M. Stone, MS, ATC
Twin Cities Orthopedics
Edina, Minnesota

Bernard N. Stulberg, MD
Staff Surgeon
Spine & Orthopaedic Institute
St. Vincent Charity Medical Center
Cleveland, Ohio

Dylan Tanzer, BSc
Faculty of Medicine
Sackler University
Tel Aviv, Israel

Michael Tanzer, MD, FRCSC
Professor and Jo Miller Chair
Division of Orthopaedic Surgery
McGill University
Montreal, Quebec, Canada

Michael J. Taunton, MD
Assistant Professor
Department of Orthopedic Surgery
Mayo Clinic
Rochester, Minnesota

A. J. Timperley, MBChB, FRCS, DPhil (Oxon)
Orthopaedic Surgeon
Princess Elizabeth Orthopaedic Centre
Royal Devon Exeter NHS Foundation Trust
Exeter, England, United Kingdom

Robert T. Trousdale, MD
Professor
Department of Orthopedic Surgery
Mayo Clinic
Rochester, Minnesota

Thomas P. Vail, MD
James L. Young Professor and Chairman
Department of Orthopaedic Surgery
University of California, San Francisco
San Francisco, California

Alexander R. Vap, MD
Assistant Professor
Department of Orthopaedic Surgery
Virginia Commonwealth University
Richmond, Virginia

Andrew Waligora, MD
Adult Reconstruction Fellow
Department of Orthopedic Surgery
Virginian Commonwealth University Medical Center
Richmond, Virginia

Sharon Walton, MD
Orthopedic Surgery Fellow
Department of Orthopedic Surgery
New York University
New York, New York

Zachary D. Weidner, MD
Orthopaedic Surgeon
The Centers for Advanced Orthopaedics
Prince William Orthopaedics
Manassas, Virginia

Stuart L. Weinstein, MD
Ignacio V. Ponseti Chair and Professor of Orthopaedic Surgery
Professor of Pediatrics
Department of Orthopaedic Surgery
University of Iowa Hospitals & Clinics
Iowa City, Iowa

Preface

We are excited to present you with the second edition of *Advanced Reconstruction: Hip*. The first edition, which was published in 2005, was extremely popular and well received by the orthopaedic community, so the American Academy of Orthopaedic Surgeons and The Hip Society decided that it was time to develop a second edition. We are honored to be the editors of both the first and second editions of this text. We believe that this text has been popular because it is used by surgeons to enhance their ability to plan and carry out a specific surgical technique or manage a difficult clinical problem.

The chapters in this book are organized to allow the surgeon to prepare quickly for a particular surgical procedure. Each chapter contains photographs, illustrations, diagrams, and radiographs that highlight critical aspects of the surgical technique or management strategies. Surgical videos are presented with some chapters. Because the book is really a surgical guide, it has not been heavily referenced. The book is divided into five sections: Primary Total Hip Arthroplasty; Complex Total Hip Arthroplasty; Complications After Total Hip Arthroplasty; Revision Total Hip Arthroplasty; and Alternative Reconstruction Procedures.

We are quite fortunate to have experts in the field contribute the 70 chapters in this book. These chapters allow for a rapid review of a surgical technique or for more detailed study of a specific problem related to hip disease. The authors review the indications, contraindications, and surgical technique when confronted with a specific hip problem or when using a particular implant. Hip surgery has changed since the publication of the first edition. We have added a number of new chapters, including: anterior approach to the hip both with and without a specialized surgical table, treatment of failed metal-on-metal total hip arthroplasties, and the management of taper corrosion.

We want to thank the authors for dedicating their time and expertise to help us create this text. The chapters contain truly outstanding photographs, illustrations, and radiographs, all of which required extra effort to identify and include in this book. We also want to thank Laura Goetz, Managing Editor, and Lisa Claxton Moore, Senior Manager, Book Program, for their hard work and editorial expertise. This book could never been published without their significant commitment to this project. Finally, we want to thank both the American Academy of Orthopaedic Surgeons and The Hip Society for their support of this project. Our hope is that surgeons will use this text to enhance the care of their patients with hip disease.

Jay R. Lieberman, MD
Daniel J. Berry, MD
Editors

Table of Contents

SECTION 1
Primary Total Hip Arthroplasty
Daniel J. Berry, MD

Chapter 1
Primary Total Hip Arthroplasty: Posterolateral Approach and Extensile Methods

Matthew P. Abdel, MD

Indications

The posterolateral approach to the hip is commonly used because of its simplicity, the ease of dissection in internervous planes, the preservation of the abductor musculature, the potential to extend the approach, and the ability to accommodate trochanteric osteotomies (Charnley osteotomy, trochanteric slide osteotomy, and extended trochanteric osteotomy [ETO]). The posterolateral approach can be used for primary and revision total hip arthroplasty (THA), hemiarthroplasty, resurfacing procedures, resection arthroplasty, drainage of a septic hip, open reduction and internal fixation (ORIF) of fractures of the posterior column or posterior wall of the acetabulum, osteochondral grafting, and removal of loose bodies. In patients requiring arthroplasty, the posterolateral approach is particularly helpful in those with developmental dysplasia of the hip who may require a femoral shortening osteotomy. The posterolateral approach is also used for patients in whom primary THA is difficult and who may require a trochanteric osteotomy, such as patients with ankylosis, protrusio acetabuli, or extensive heterotopic ossification.

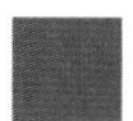

Contraindications

There are few contraindications to the posterior approach. The primary relative contraindication is the need to preserve vascularity of the femoral head because of disruption of the posterior blood supply from branches of the medial femoral circumflex artery. This scenario most often occurs in patients requiring procedures other than arthroplasty, such as in young patients requiring ORIF of anterior fractures of the femoral head or fractures of the femoral neck, patients requiring loose body removal, or patients with sepsis of the hip requiring drainage. However, the vascularity of the femoral head can be preserved with the use of a limited posterolateral approach in which the obturator externus muscle, the quadratus femoris muscle, and thus the posterior blood supply are preserved.

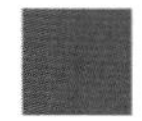

Alternative Treatments

Alternative approaches to the hip include the direct anterior (Smith-Petersen), anterolateral (Watson-Jones), direct lateral (Hardinge), and transtrochanteric. The major advantage of these alternative approaches is that they preserve the posterior blood supply, which is particularly important in young patients undergoing ORIF of anterior fractures of the femoral head or any fracture of the femoral neck. Specific disadvantages of the direct anterior approach include a risk to the lateral femoral cutaneous and femoral nerves. The concern with the anterolateral and direct lateral approaches includes disruption of the abductors, with a possible resultant limp. Currently, transtrochanteric osteotomies are reserved for hip preservation procedures that require surgical hip dislocation.

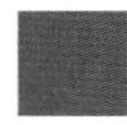

Results

The posterolateral approach has been in use since the 1970s and is the most common approach used for THA in the United States. Proponents of the posterolateral approach cite the unobstructed view of the acetabulum and femur, decreased surgical time, reduced blood loss, faster recovery, lack of postoperative limp and abductor weakness, and decreased risk of heterotopic ossification compared with other approaches. Postoperative dislocations have been a concern with the posterolateral approach. Reported rates of dislocation in patients who have undergone THA using the posterolateral approach have historically ranged from

Dr. Abdel or an immediate family member serves as a board member, owner, officer, or committee member of the Minnesota Orthopaedic Society.

Table 1 Results of Total Hip Arthroplasty Using the Posterolateral Approach

Authors (Year)	Number of Hips	Implant Type	Procedure or Approach (Hips)	Mean Patient Age in Years (Range)	Mean Follow-up in Months (Range)	Success Rate (%)[a]	Results
Robinson et al (1980)	160	Cemented	No repair	63 (29-85)	7.6 (1-23)	92.5	The posterior approach provided a shorter surgical time, required fewer blood transfusions, and resulted in a shorter hospital stay compared with a control cohort of 160 lateral transtrochanteric approaches
Woo and Morrey (1982)	735	Varied	Piriformis repair	62.1 (13-95)	37.2 (12-125)	94.2	Historical series that found an increased risk of dislocation in patients with previous surgery In addition, one-third of patients underwent an additional procedure for instability
Pellicci et al (1998)	1,074	Hybrid	Repair of SER only (395 for one surgeon; 160 for the other surgeon) or repair of SER, capsule, quadratus femoris, and gluteus maximus tendon (395 for one surgeon; 124 for the other surgeon)	NR (NR)	12 (NR)	Repair of SER only: 96 Repair of SER, capsule, quadratus femoris, and gluteus maximus tendon: 100	Two different surgeons at two different institutions reporting their results in a combined series
White et al (2001)	1,515	Varied	No repair (1,078) or repair of SER and capsule (437)	NR (NR)	6 (NR)	No repair: 95.2 Repair: 99.3	Avulsion fracture of the greater trochanter developed in 4 of 437 hips managed with capsular repair (0.9%)
Weeden et al (2003)	945	Noncemented	Repair of SER, capsule, and gluteus maximus tendon	62.3 (36-86)	76.8 (24-112)	99.2	Of 8 dislocations, 3 occurred within the first postoperative year and were treated nonsurgically, 3 required revision surgery and placement of a constrained liner, and 2 dislocated after trauma and were managed nonsurgically
Suh et al (2004)	346	Varied	No repair (250) or repair of SER and capsule (96)	No repair: 53.5 ±10.4[b] Repair: 53.3 ± 10.8[b]	12 (NR)	No repair: 93.6 Repair: 99	28-mm femoral heads were used in all patients
Berry et al (2005)	3,646	Varied	No repair	64 (12-97)	126 (0-378)	93.1	Larger femoral head diameter was associated with a lower long-term cumulative risk of dislocation, particularly with use of the posterolateral approach
Kim et al (2008)	670	Varied	Preservation of SER (220), repair of SER (282), or no repair (168)	Preservation: 45.6 ± 14.6[b] (17-77) Repair: 47.6 ± 13.8[b] (21-79) No repair: 49.2 ± 15.1[b] (20-78)	Preservation: 22.8 (12-34) Repair: 50.4 (34.8-72) No repair: 90 (72-106)	Preservation: 100 Repair: 96.1 No repair: 94.7	Evolution of technique over time with variable length of follow-up, which may influence dislocation rates
Ji et al (2012)	99	Noncemented	Repair of SER and capsule	51 (18-78)	39 (24-54)	100	Randomized clinical trial compared with 97 direct lateral hips (3% dislocation rate)
Kumar et al (2014)	512	Cemented	Repair of SER and capsule	67 (35-89)	33.6 (6-79)	99.2	22-mm femoral heads were used

NR = not reported, SER = short external rotators.
[a] Success is defined as the absence of dislocation.
[b] Data are mean ± standard deviation.

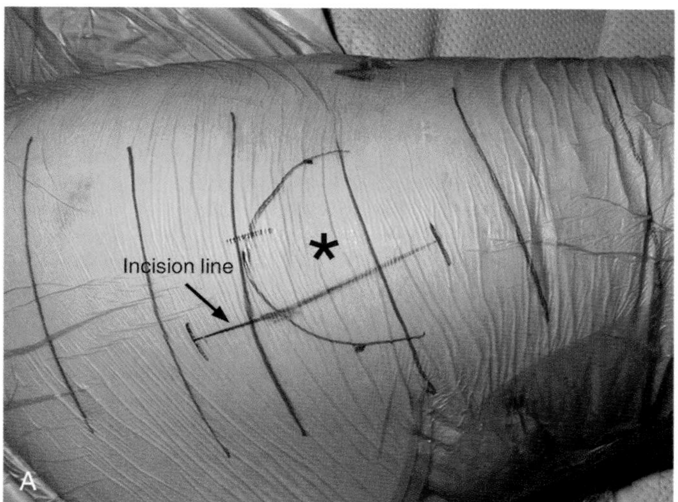

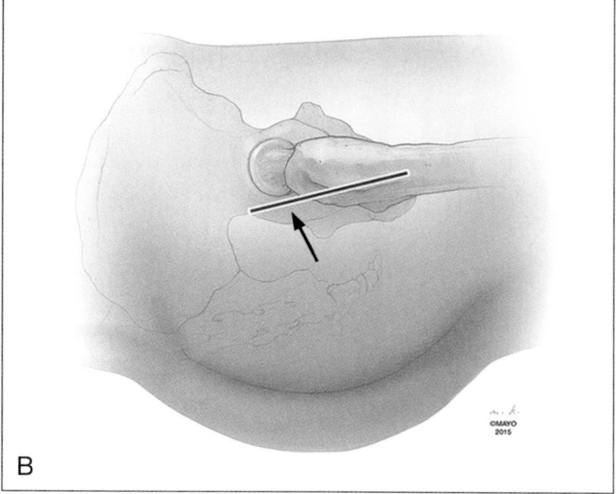

Figure 1 Lateral-view intraoperative photograph (**A**) and illustration (**B**) of a right hip show the incision (arrow) centered over the posterolateral corner of the greater trochanter (asterisk), with one-third of the incision proximal and two-thirds of the incision distal to the tip of the greater trochanter. The incision (**B**, arrow) terminates at the center of the femur. (Panel B reproduced with permission from the Mayo Foundation for Medical Education and Research, Rochester, MN.)

4% to 8% (**Table 1**). However, because of increased understanding of the role of the posterior structures in providing a soft-tissue restraint to dislocation, most surgeons now repair the short external rotators and capsule. Several studies in which this contemporary method was used have reported dramatically reduced dislocation rates (<1%; **Table 1**).

Techniques

Setup/Exposure

- The patient is placed in the lateral decubitus position with the pelvis level. If the pelvis is tilted or rotated or if the patient is not adequately secured, the position of the acetabular implant will be affected.
- The dependent arm and the underside of the fibular head and lateral malleolus of the dependent leg are cushioned.
- The superior, posterior, and anterior borders of the greater trochanter are palpated and marked.
- The posterolateral corner of the greater trochanter is marked by dividing the trochanter into thirds.
- The incision is centered over the posterolateral corner of the greater trochanter, with one-third of the incision proximal and two-thirds of the incision distal to the tip of the greater trochanter (**Figure 1**).
- The length of the incision is typically 12 to 15 cm and depends on the patient's body habitus and the complexity of the procedure.
- The incision may be straight or curvilinear, with the proximal limb angled posteriorly to facilitate later placement of the femoral implant.
- The distal portion of the incision terminates at the center of the femur, usually anterior to the bony insertion of the gluteus maximus tendon.
- After bony landmarks have been identified, the skin is incised sharply through the subcutaneous tissue down to the level of the fascia.
- The fascia is sharply incised distally in line with the incision (**Figure 2**).
- Proximally, only the thin fascia of the gluteus maximus muscle belly is sharply incised in a slightly posterior direction.
- The leg is abducted, and the gluteus maximus muscle belly fibers are separated bluntly to the level of the proximal incision. Care is taken to split the fascia in line with the incision. If the split is too posterior, the gluteus maximus will obscure the exposure.
- With the leg still abducted, a Charnley self-retaining retractor is placed at the level of the greater trochanter to retract the gluteus maximus and fascia.
- Takedown of the gluteus maximus tendon at its bony insertion is rarely required during primary THA.

Instruments/Equipment/Implants Required

- A curved C-retractor is used.
- An Aufranc retractor is used.
- A Cobb elevator is used.
- A large Steinmann pin is used.
- A bent Hohmann retractor is used.

Procedure

ARTHROTOMY

- The affected hip is internally rotated to optimize the exposure of the posterior structures.

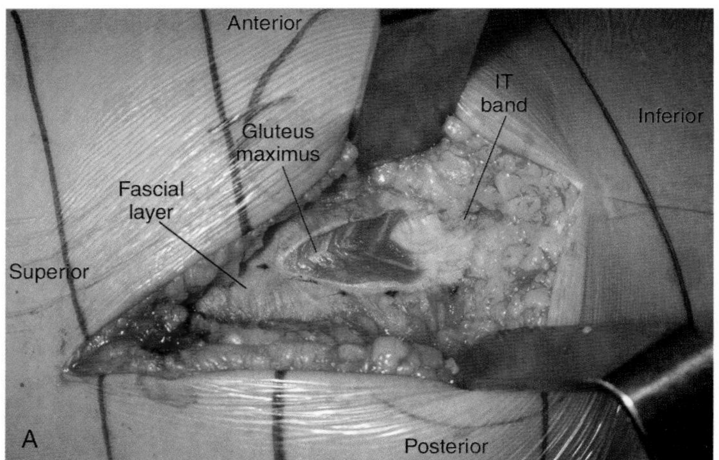

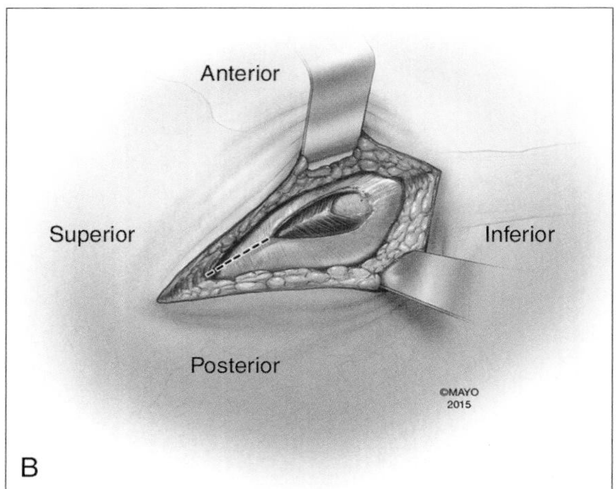

Figure 2 Intraoperative photograph (**A**) and illustration (**B**) of a right hip show sharp incision of the fascia distally in line with the incision. The thin fascia of the gluteus maximus muscle belly is incised proximally in a slightly posterior direction, and the gluteus maximus muscle belly fibers are separated bluntly. IT = iliotibial. (Panel B reproduced with permission from the Mayo Foundation for Medical Education and Research, Rochester, MN.)

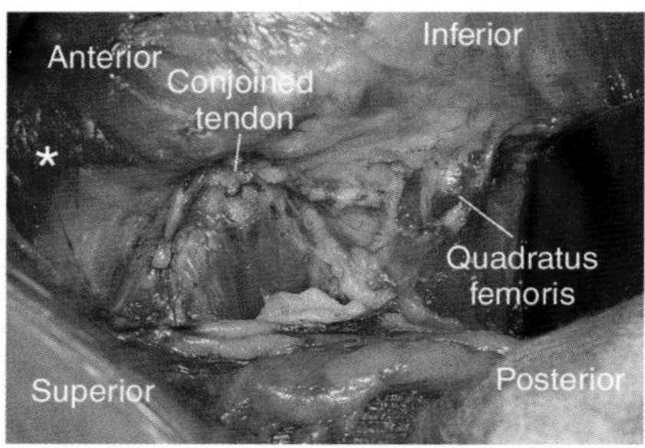

Figure 3 Intraoperative photograph of a right hip shows the fat plane between the gluteus medius (asterisk) and the piriformis tendon. The conjoined tendon and the quadratus femoris muscle also are visible.

- The fat plane between the gluteus medius and the piriformis tendon is identified with gentle palpation (**Figure 3**).
- A curved C-retractor is placed deep to the gluteus medius, superficial to the gluteus minimus, and superior to the piriformis tendon (**Figure 4**).
- An Aufranc retractor is placed at the level of the inferior femoral neck and quadratus femoris muscle.
- The gluteus minimus muscle is elevated from the hip capsule with the use of a narrow Cobb elevator, and the curved C-retractor is placed deep to the gluteus minimus and superior to the piriformis tendon (**Figure 5**).
- The piriformis tendon and the conjoined tendon (superior gemellus, inferior gemellus, and obturator internus) are divided as close to their insertions as possible. Each is tagged with a nonabsorbable suture of medium length for later repair (**Figure 6**).
- The piriformis tendon and the conjoined tendon are reflected posteriorly to protect the sciatic nerve.
- Although the superior retractor typically does not need to be adjusted, it may be necessary to divide a portion of the obturator externus at the level of the femoral neck, with subsequent repositioning of the inferior retractor just inferiorly on the femoral neck.
- A capsulotomy is performed from the posterosuperior acetabulum to the tip of the trochanter, in line with the posterior border of the abductors. The length of the capsule is preserved to facilitate later closure.
- The capsulotomy is continued inferiorly along the femoral neck, from deep to superficial, to the level of the lesser trochanter.
- When completed correctly, the capsulotomy forms a trapezoidal shape (**Figure 7**).
- The superior and inferior limbs of the capsule are each tagged with a nonabsorbable suture (of longer length than the sutures marking the short external rotators) for later repair.
- The quadratus femoris is not routinely taken down.

ACETABULAR EXPOSURE

- After the capsulotomy has been completed, the hip is gently dislocated with a combination of flexion, adduction, and internal rotation.
- The hip is brought to a position of neutral flexion-extension and 90° of internal rotation so that the femoral neck cut can be made parallel to the ground.
- The level of resection of the femoral neck is determined on the basis of careful preoperative templating and is marked intraoperatively.
- A trial prosthesis is used to determine the angle of resection.
- The femoral neck cut is completed with a saw, allowing unobstructed access to the acetabulum.

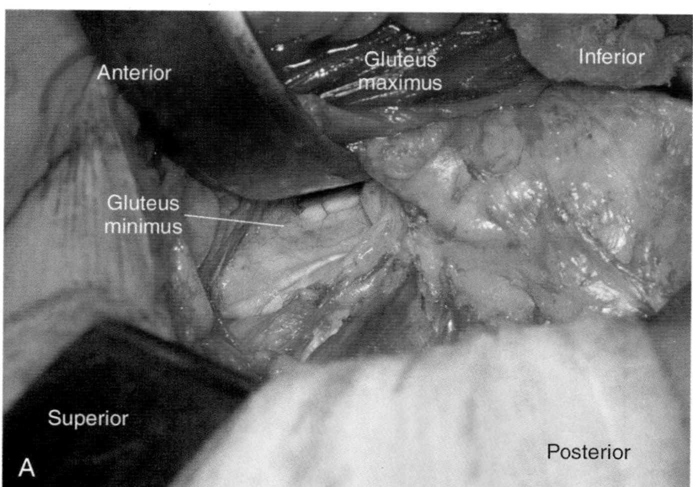

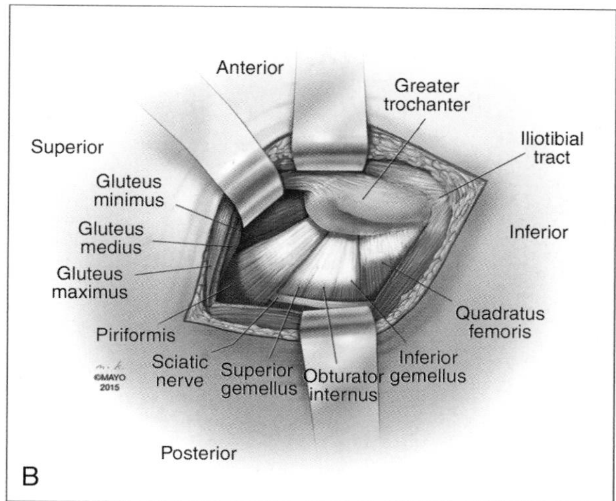

Figure 4 Intraoperative photograph (**A**) and illustration (**B**) of a right hip show placement of a curved C-retractor deep to the gluteus medius, superficial to the gluteus minimus, and superior to the piriformis tendon. (Panel B reproduced with permission from the Mayo Foundation for Medical Education and Research, Rochester, MN.)

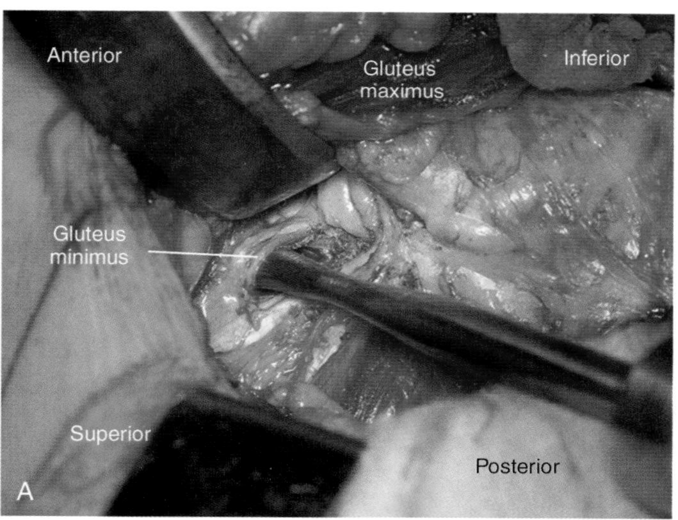

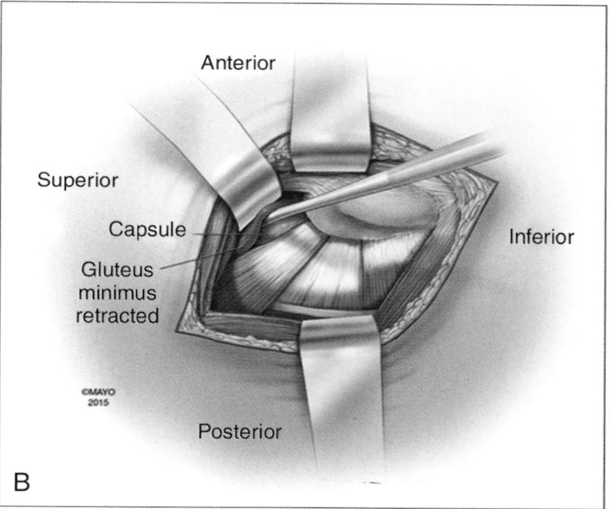

Figure 5 Intraoperative photograph (**A**) and illustration (**B**) of a right hip show the use of a narrow Cobb elevator to elevate the gluteus minimus muscle from the hip capsule, with the curved C-retractor still between the gluteus medius and the gluteus minimus. (Panel B reproduced with permission from the Mayo Foundation for Medical Education and Research, Rochester, MN.)

- With the leg in approximately 15° of internal rotation and slight flexion, the curved C-retractor is placed anteriorly at approximately the 2 o'clock position in a right hip or the 10 o'clock position in a left hip (**Figure 8**).
- The retractor is placed in the acetabulum and is gently extended over the anterior rim of the acetabulum in an extralabral manner to allow for safe retraction of the proximal femur.
- Occasionally, it is necessary to release the reflected head of the rectus femoris muscle from the supra-acetabular region to allow for more excursion of the femur.
- A large Steinmann pin is placed in the ilium to retract the abductors.
- A small capsulotomy is made inferiorly to allow placement of a curved cobra retractor deep to the transverse acetabular ligament.
- A bent Hohmann retractor is placed posteriorly (extralabrally, but intracapsularly) with the limb extended to minimize tension on the sciatic nerve. To avoid injury to the sciatic nerve, care is taken

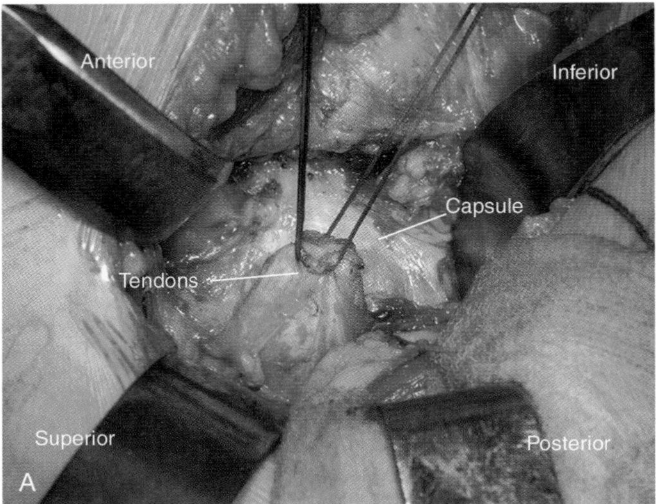

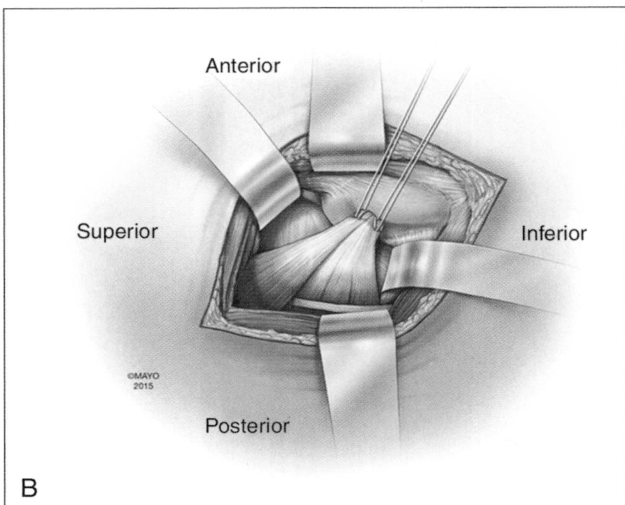

Figure 6 Intraoperative photograph (**A**) and illustration (**B**) of a right hip show division of the piriformis tendon and the conjoined tendon as close to their insertions as possible. Each tendon is tagged with a nonabsorbable suture for later repair. (Panel B reproduced with permission from the Mayo Foundation for Medical Education and Research, Rochester, MN.)

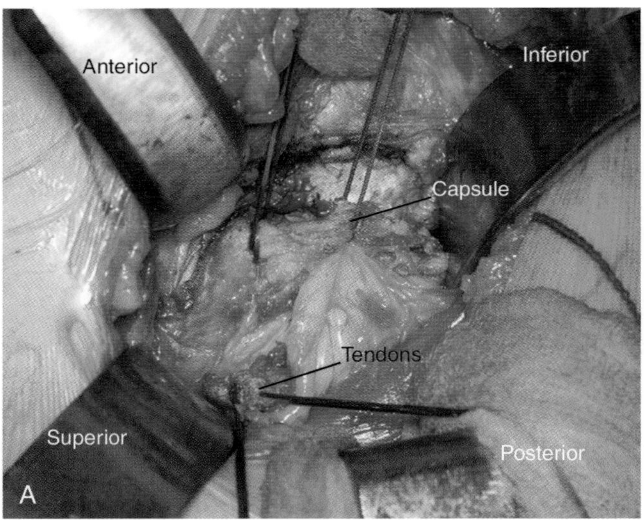

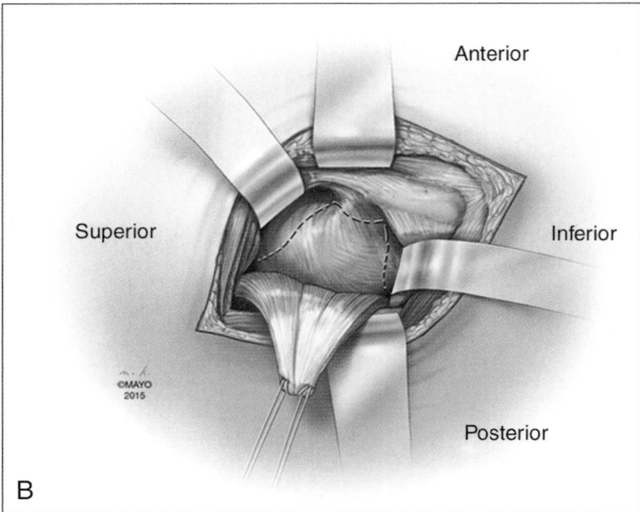

Figure 7 Intraoperative photograph (**A**) and illustration (**B**) of a right hip show the capsulotomy, which results in a trapezoidal shape (**B**, dashed line). The superior and inferior limbs of the capsule are tagged with nonabsorbable sutures. (Panel B reproduced with permission from the Mayo Foundation for Medical Education and Research, Rochester, MN.)

to place this retractor against the posterior wall.

- After the acetabular retractors are placed, any remaining labrum is excised.
- The tissue in the cotyloid fossa is removed to expose the medial wall and teardrop.
- The acetabulum is prepared with hemispheric reamers.
- An acetabular implant (press-fit or cemented) is inserted.

FEMORAL EXPOSURE

- After the acetabular implant is inserted, the leg is brought to neutral flexion-extension and internally rotated 90°.
- A femoral elevator is placed underneath the medial femoral neck, an Aufranc retractor is placed underneath the lesser trochanter, and the curved C-retractor is placed laterally to protect the abductors (**Figure 9**).
- The hip is flexed to approximately 70°, and the 90° of internal rotation is maintained.
- The femoral canal is prepared for insertion of a noncemented or cemented stem.

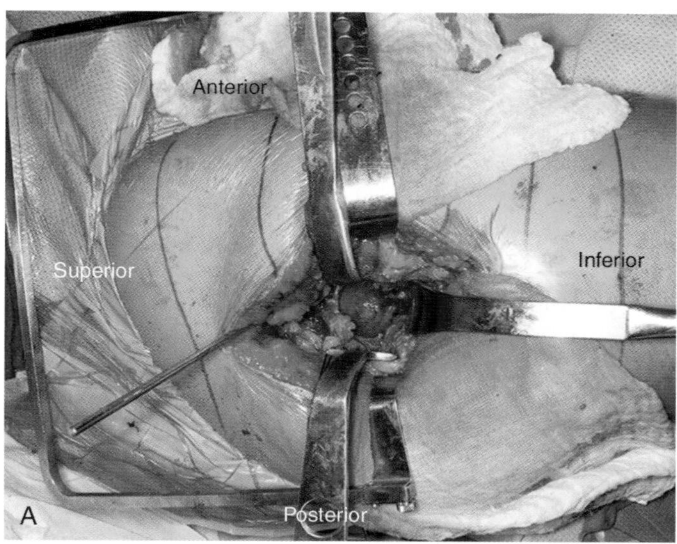

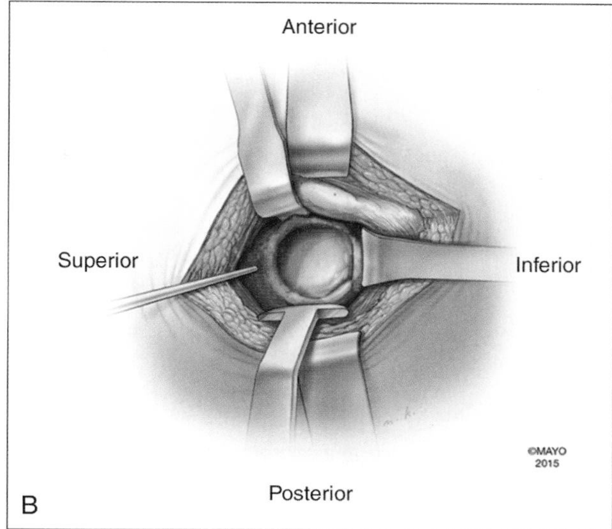

Figure 8 Intraoperative photograph (**A**) and illustration (**B**) of a right hip show exposure of the acetabulum with a curved C-retractor placed anteriorly, a Steinmann pin placed superiorly, a bent Hohmann retractor placed posteriorly, and an Aufranc retractor placed inferiorly. (Panel B reproduced with permission from the Mayo Foundation for Medical Education and Research, Rochester, MN.)

EXTENSILE APPROACHES

- An extensile approach is rarely required during primary THA and occasionally is required during revision THA.
- If necessary, the posterolateral approach can be extended to achieve further exposure of both the acetabulum and the femur in sequence.
- To allow additional excursion of the femur, the gluteus maximus tendon can be taken down at its bony insertion, and the reflected head of the rectus femoris muscle can be released from the supra-acetabular region.
- If a more extensile approach is required, a trochanteric osteotomy (Charnley standard, trochanteric slide, or ETO) can be done.
- Although the trochanteric slide osteotomy and the ETO incorporate the origin of the vastus lateralis muscle, the Charnley standard osteotomy does not (**Figure 10**).

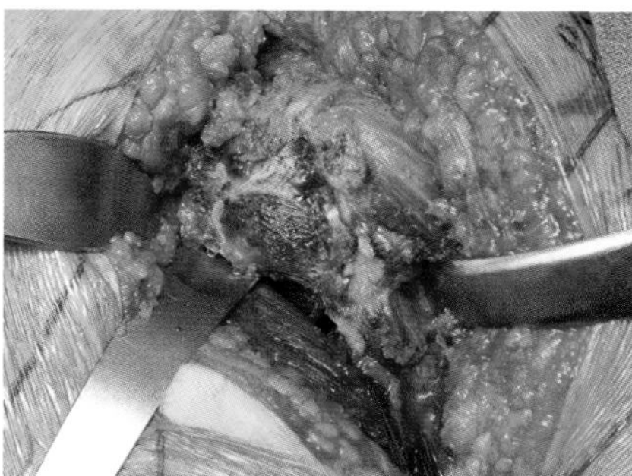

Figure 9 Intraoperative photograph of a right hip shows exposure of the femur with a femoral elevator placed underneath the medial femoral neck, an Aufranc retractor placed underneath the lesser trochanter, and a curved C-retractor placed laterally.

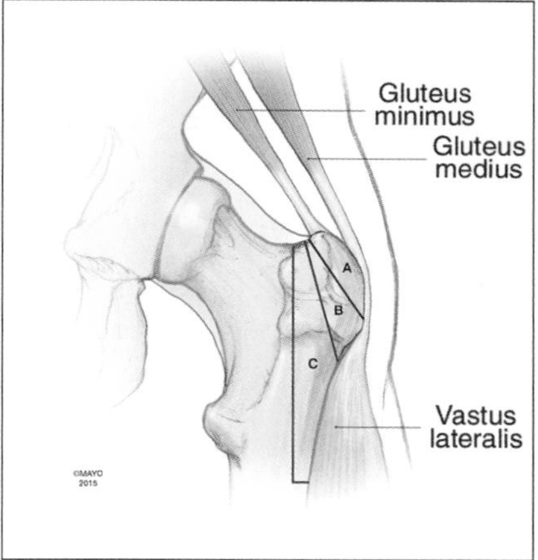

Figure 10 Illustration shows the levels of the Charnley standard osteotomy (A), the trochanteric slide osteotomy (B), and the extended trochanteric osteotomy (C). (Reproduced with permission from the Mayo Foundation for Medical Education and Research, Rochester, MN.)

EXTENDED TROCHANTERIC OSTEOTOMY

- The ETO is useful in revision THA because it facilitates extraction and reimplantation of the femoral implant and enhances acetabular exposure.
- The ETO is planned preoperatively to allow 5 cm of isthmic diaphyseal cortex for revision implant fixation if possible.
- The osteotomy is typically located 12 to 15 cm from the tip of the greater trochanter and can be done before or after stem removal.
- If dislocation is difficult because of stiffness, the ETO can aid with exposure.
- The osteotomy is initiated along the posterior aspect of the proximal femur.
- The linea aspera is exposed by partial elevation of the vastus lateralis muscle and release of the gluteus

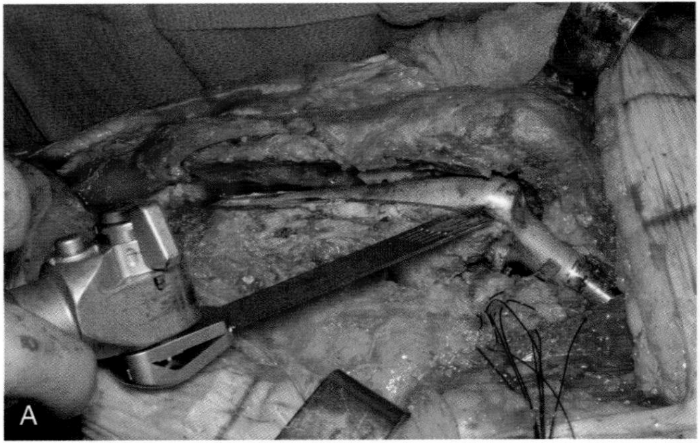

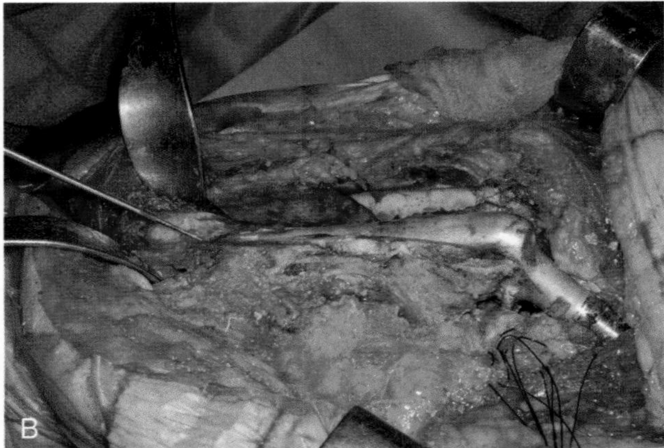

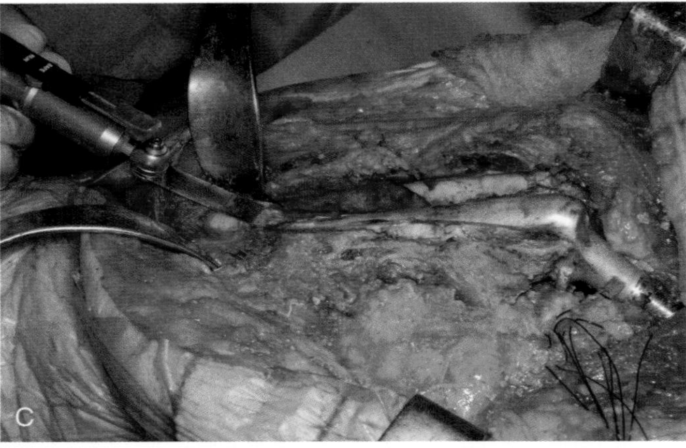

Figure 11 Intraoperative photographs of a left hip show steps in extended trochanteric osteotomy (ETO) in a patient undergoing primary total hip arthroplasty. **A,** The ETO is completed with the use of a thin oscillating saw from the posterior aspect of the greater trochanter to the distal aspect of the posterior femur. **B,** A high-speed pencil-tip burr is used approximately 1 cm short of the distal extent of the ETO to round the corners of the osteotomy and reduce the stress risers. **C,** A small, thin oscillating blade is used to complete the distal extent of the ETO at a 45° angle approximately 1 to 2 cm distal to the intended site of the transverse osteotomy.

maximus insertion subperiosteally.

- The distal aspect of the osteotomy is marked.
- The author of this chapter prefers to use a thin oscillating saw from the posterior aspect of the greater trochanter to the distal aspect of the posterior femur (**Figure 11, A**).
- Approximately 1 cm proximal to the previously identified distal extent of the osteotomy, a high-speed pencil-tip burr is used to round the corners of the osteotomy and reduce stress risers (**Figure 11, B**).
- A smaller thin oscillating blade is used to complete the distal extent of the osteotomy at a 45° angle approximately 1 to 2 cm distal to the intended site of the transverse osteotomy (**Figure 11, C**).
- Before the osteotomy is opened, the proximal portion of the anterior limb of the osteotomy is completed, either by cutting from posterior to anterior over the shoulder of the implant or by cutting along the anterior femur from within the hip joint with a saw or burr, and the anterior extension of the osteotomy is scored from distal to proximal with either a straight osteotome (deep to the vastus lateralis) or series of drill holes (through the musculature).
- A series of curved osteotomes are inserted in the posterior limb of the osteotomy, carefully elevating the osteotomy limb.
- To decrease the risk of subsequent fracture, the tethering anterior proximal soft tissue and the remaining capsule from the osteotomy fragment are released. This step allows unobstructed views of the acetabulum and the femur.
- Relative approximation of the osteotomy fragments is usually accomplished with two to four wires or cables passed around the diaphysis and the trochanteric fragment. The process is aided by abducting and internally rotating the leg.

REPAIR OF THE POSTERIOR CAPSULE AND SHORT EXTERNAL ROTATORS

- As discussed previously, posterior repair is essential because it markedly decreases the rate of postoperative instability in patients treated with the posterior approach.
- After the hip is reduced, two holes are drilled through the posterior trochanter.
- A suture passer is placed through the proximal hole, and the nonabsorbable sutures from the proximal capsule and piriformis tendon are

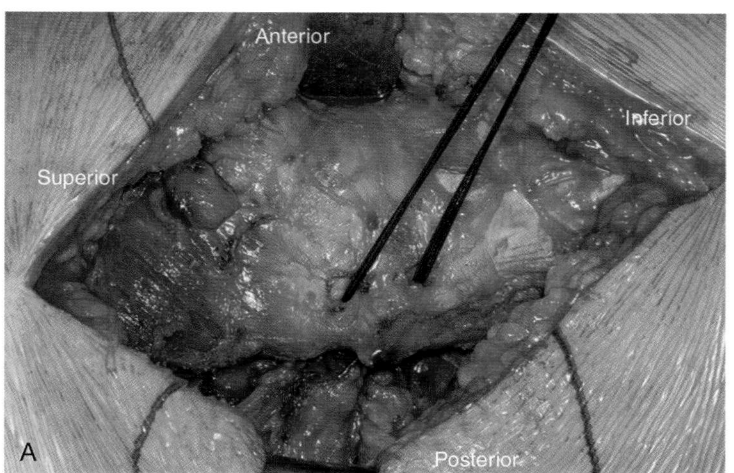

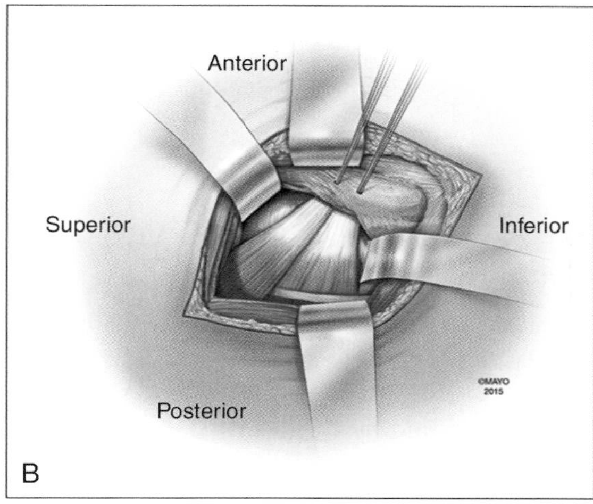

Figure 12 Intraoperative photograph (**A**) and illustration (**B**) of a right hip show the completion of primary total hip arthroplasty using a posterior approach. Two holes are drilled through the posterior trochanter, a suture passer is placed through the proximal hole, and the nonabsorbable sutures from the proximal capsule and piriformis tendon are pulled through the hole. A similar process is completed through the inferior hole. The appropriate sutures are tied together with the leg in abduction, slight extension, and external rotation. (Panel B reproduced with permission from the Mayo Foundation for Medical Education and Research, Rochester, MN.)

pulled through the hole (**Figure 12**).

- Similarly, the nonabsorbable sutures from the distal capsule and conjoined tendon are pulled through the distal hole.
- With the leg in abduction, slight extension, and external rotation, the longer proximal sutures and the distal sutures of the capsule are tied together.
- The medium-length proximal and distal sutures of the piriformis and conjoined tendons are tied together.
- If the quadratus femoris or gluteus maximus tendon were released, they are reapproximated with figure-of-8 bioabsorbable sutures.

Wound Closure

- After the posterior repair has been completed, the fascia is closed with multiple interrupted bioabsorbable sutures.
- In patients with substantial subcutaneous tissue, an additional layer of interrupted bioabsorbable sutures is placed.
- The subcutaneous layer is closed with interrupted monofilament bioabsorbable sutures.
- The skin is closed with a running monofilament bioabsorbable suture.

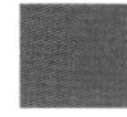

Postoperative Regimen

The postoperative regimen includes in-hospital physical therapy to assist with mobilization. Barring any complications, the patient is allowed to bear weight as tolerated immediately after surgery and to complete stair activities on postoperative day 1. While the patient is at rest, the hip is maintained in an abducted position with the use of an abduction pillow. Gait aids are used for approximately 3 to 6 weeks postoperatively depending on patient factors. To reduce the risk of hip dislocation, hip flexion should be limited to 90° and internal rotation and/or adduction should be avoided for 6 weeks postoperatively. In addition, the patient should sit only in high-backed chairs, should use raised toilet seats, and should sleep with a pillow between the legs for 6 weeks postoperatively. At 6 weeks postoperatively, the precautions are gradually relaxed.

Avoiding Pitfalls and Complications

Although multiple complications can occur with the posterolateral approach, most are not exclusive to the approach. These complications include sciatic and femoral nerve injuries, heterotopic ossification, and instability. Because of its proximity to the acetabulum, the sciatic nerve may be injured intraoperatively with any approach to the hip. If the posterolateral approach is used, the sciatic nerve should be gently palpated throughout the entire procedure. The incision should be long enough to avoid undue tension on the nerve with posterior retraction. If a bent Hohmann retractor is placed posteriorly for acetabular exposure, the leg should be extended and the retractor should be carefully placed extralabrally but through the capsule and directly against the posterior wall. Similarly, the femoral nerve is at risk during placement of the anterior acetabular retractor. The retractor should be placed in the acetabulum and then gently extended over the anterior rim of the acetabulum. Heterotopic ossification occurs less often with the posterolateral approach than with other approaches. However, all marrow contents should be suctioned during femoral preparation, and soft tissues should be irrigated frequently. The risk of postoperative instability is decreased with meticulous posterior repair of the capsule and short external rotators (**Table 1**).

Bibliography

Archibeck MJ, Rosenberg AG, Berger RA, Silverton CD: Trochanteric osteotomy and fixation during total hip arthroplasty. *J Am Acad Orthop Surg* 2003;11(3):163-173.

Berry DJ, von Knoch M, Schleck CD, Harmsen WS: Effect of femoral head diameter and operative approach on risk of dislocation after primary total hip arthroplasty. *J Bone Joint Surg Am* 2005;87(11):2456-2463.

Ji HM, Kim KC, Lee YK, Ha YC, Koo KH: Dislocation after total hip arthroplasty: A randomized clinical trial of a posterior approach and a modified lateral approach. *J Arthroplasty* 2012;27(3):378-385.

Kim YS, Kwon SY, Sun DH, Han SK, Maloney WJ: Modified posterior approach to total hip arthroplasty to enhance joint stability. *Clin Orthop Relat Res* 2008;466(2):294-299.

Kumar V, Sharma S, James J, Hodgkinson JP, Hemmady MV: Total hip replacement through a posterior approach using a 22 mm diameter femoral head: The role of the transverse acetabular ligament and capsular repair in reducing the rate of dislocation. *Bone Joint J* 2014;96-B(9):1202-1206.

Pätiälä H, Lehto K, Rokkanen P, Paavolainen P: Posterior approach for total hip arthroplasty: A study of postoperative course, early results and early complications in 131 cases. *Arch Orthop Trauma Surg* 1984;102(4):225-229.

Pellicci PM, Bostrom M, Poss R: Posterior approach to total hip replacement using enhanced posterior soft tissue repair. *Clin Orthop Relat Res* 1998;(355):224-228.

Robinson RP, Robinson HJ Jr, Salvati EA: Comparison of the transtrochanteric and posterior approaches for total hip replacement. *Clin Orthop Relat Res* 1980;(147):143-147.

Suh KT, Park BG, Choi YJ: A posterior approach to primary total hip arthroplasty with soft tissue repair. *Clin Orthop Relat Res* 2004;(418):162-167.

Weeden SH, Paprosky WG, Bowling JW: The early dislocation rate in primary total hip arthroplasty following the posterior approach with posterior soft-tissue repair. *J Arthroplasty* 2003;18(6):709-713.

White RE Jr, Forness TJ, Allman JK, Junick DW: Effect of posterior capsular repair on early dislocation in primary total hip replacement. *Clin Orthop Relat Res* 2001;(393):163-167.

Woo RY, Morrey BF: Dislocations after total hip arthroplasty. *J Bone Joint Surg Am* 1982;64(9):1295-1306.

Chapter 2

Primary Total Hip Arthroplasty: Anterolateral and Direct Lateral Approaches

Tad M. Mabry, MD
David G. Lewallen, MD

Indications

The two transgluteal approaches—anterolateral and direct lateral—may be used for a variety of hip reconstructive procedures. The common features of these approaches include direct splitting of the gluteus medius and minimus musculature proximally; anterior capsulotomy; and preservation of the posterior soft-tissue sleeve, including the posterior capsule and the external rotator musculature. The essential difference between a direct lateral and an anterolateral approach is the handling of the soft tissues at the distal extent of the muscle split. In the direct lateral approach, the vastus lateralis is elevated in continuity with the gluteal flap, and in the anterolateral approach the vastus lateralis is not elevated.

The main indications for the transgluteal approaches include primary and revision total hip arthroplasty (THA). The use of these approaches has been associated with a low risk for prosthetic hip dislocation because of the preservation of the posterior soft-tissue envelope. Many surgeons will selectively use a transgluteal approach rather than the posterolateral approach when treating a patient who is at elevated risk for hip dislocation. Patient-related factors associated with a high risk for postoperative hip dislocation include prior hip surgery; neurologic disorders such as Parkinson disease, seizure disorders, and spasticity; cognitive impairment, such as dementia and alcoholism; and hip fracture. Secondary indications for the transgluteal approaches include joint-preserving procedures in which femoral head viability must be preserved, such as open reduction and internal fixation of a displaced femoral neck fracture and open irrigation of septic arthritis of a native hip. Extensile modifications of these transgluteal approaches allow for increased access to the femur for revision procedures by way of extended osteotomy.

Contraindications

There are few true contraindications to transgluteal approaches. Rather, there are patients in whom other approaches might be used more effectively. For example, the posterolateral approach might be more effective in patients in whom direct access to the posterior column is needed for plating, implant removal, bone grafting, and/or excision of heterotopic bone. Proximal dissection may be necessary in patients who have a very high hip center (for example, Crowe type IV hip dysplasia) or in whom an acetabular component has failed and substantial proximal migration has occurred. The necessary proximal dissection might violate the superior gluteal nerve, which exits the pelvis through the greater sciatic notch superior to the piriformis muscle, runs anteriorly deep to the gluteus medius, and innervates the abductors (gluteus medius and minimus muscles) and the tensor fascia latae. The safe zone for the superior gluteal nerve lies within 4 to 5 cm of the superior aspect of the greater trochanter. Dissection should be restricted to this area to avoid injury to the nerve. No such safe zone exists for a trochanter that has substantially migrated superiorly relative to the pelvis.

Dr. Lewallen or an immediate family member has received royalties from Mako/Stryker, Pipeline Biomedical Holdings, and Zimmer Biomet; is a member of a speakers' bureau or has made paid presentations on behalf of Zimmer Biomet; serves as a paid consultant to Pipeline Biomedical Holdings and Zimmer Biomet; serves as an unpaid consultant to and has stock or stock options held in Ketai Medical; and serves as a board member, owner, officer, or committee member of the American Joint Replacement Registry and the Orthopaedic Research and Education Foundation. Neither Dr. Mabry nor any immediate family member has received anything of value from or has stock or stock options held in a commercial company or institution related directly or indirectly to the subject of this chapter.

Table 1 Dislocation Rates for Total Hip Arthroplasty

Authors (Year)	Number of Hips	Procedure or Approach	Mean Patient Age in Years (Range)	Mean Follow-up (Range)	Dislocation Rate (%)
Woo and Morrey (1982)	770	Direct lateral	62 (13-95)	3.1 yr (1-10.4 yr)	2.3
Frndak et al (1993)	50	Direct lateral	70 (NR)	2.8 yr (1-4 yr)	2
Moskal and Mann (1996)	421	Modified direct lateral: primary, 306; revision, 115	66 (27-95)	≥2 yr	Primary: 0 Revision: 2.6
Mulliken et al (1998)	712	Modified direct lateral	64.3 (19-87)	3.6 yr (2-6.5 yr)	0.3
Masonis and Bourne (2002)	10,245	Anterolateral: 826 Direct lateral: 3,438 Posterolateral (with repair): 2,262 Posterolateral (without repair): 3,719	N/A	N/A	Anterolateral: 2.2 Direct lateral: 0.6 Posterolateral (with repair): 2 Posterolateral (without repair): 4
Berry et al (2005)[a]	12,801	Anterolateral: 9,155 Posterolateral: 3,646	64 (12-97)	10.5 yr (0-31.5 yr)	Anterolateral: 3.1 Posterolateral: 6.9
Queen et al (2011)	35	Direct lateral: 8 Posterior: 12 Anterolateral: 15	Direct lateral: 58 ± 7[b] Posterior: 55 ± 8[b] Anterior: 55 ± 11[b]	6 wk	None

N/A = not available, NR = not reported.

[a] Transtrochanteric approach used in 8,246 patients. Mean patient age is based on the full cohort of 21,047 primary THAs.

[b] Data reported are mean ± standard deviation.

Alternative Treatments

The main alternatives to the transgluteal approaches for hip arthroplasty are the posterolateral approach and the direct anterior approach. Compared with the posterolateral approach, the transgluteal approaches afford equal exposure of the femur and acetabulum for proper component preparation and implantation, as well as a lower risk for postoperative dislocation. However, the potential for failed repair of the abductor muscles may increase the risk for a postoperative limp and/or a slower recovery of ambulation without walking aids. Compared with the direct anterior approach, the transgluteal approaches may be used to manage a wider variety of hip conditions while affording better exposure. However, the preservation of the posterior soft tissues with the direct anterior approach allows for a very low dislocation risk without the danger of the abductor muscle split that is common to the transgluteal approaches.

The Watson-Jones and Smith-Petersen anterior approaches are well-established alternatives to the transgluteal approaches for joint-preserving procedures, such as open reduction and internal fixation of femoral neck fractures and open irrigation of sepsis of a native hip. These alternative approaches provide sufficient joint exposure and preserve the femoral head blood supply while minimizing or avoiding splitting of the abductor muscles.

Results

Multiple studies have reported the results of the transgluteal approaches, with special attention to the excellent stability provided by the preservation of the posterior soft-tissue envelope (**Table 1**). One study reported on the effects of femoral head diameter and surgical approach on the risk for dislocation after 12,801 primary THAs performed via an anterolateral or posterolateral approach at one institution. When an anterolateral approach was performed, the 10-year cumulative dislocation rate was 3.8% for 22-mm femoral heads, 3.0% for 28-mm heads, and 2.4% for 32-mm heads. The risk was significantly higher when the posterolateral approach was performed: 12.1% for 22-mm femoral heads, 6.9% for 28-mm heads, and 3.8% for 32-mm heads. A different study reviewed 712 primary THAs performed via a modified direct lateral approach and followed for a minimum of 2 years. The risk for dislocation during the follow-up period was 0.3%; however, the authors of that study noted a moderate-to-severe limp in 10% of patients. An earlier study described a similar direct lateral approach in 50 consecutive THAs followed for a mean of 2.8 years. There was only one dislocation and seven patients with a limp at last follow-up. A comprehensive review of the literature noted a lower risk for dislocation but a higher risk for postoperative limp when comparing the transgluteal approaches with the posterolateral approach. Unlike the three previously discussed studies, which noted an increased risk for limping after transgluteal approaches, a recent study did not show any difference in the gait mechanics of patients analyzed 6 weeks after primary THA performed via a posterolateral or a transgluteal approach. These findings underscore the importance of careful soft-tissue handling and repair whenever these approaches are used.

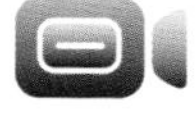

Video 2.1 Difficult Exposures From the Anterolateral Approach. Tad M. Mabry, MD (7 min)

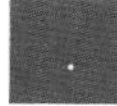

Techniques

Setup/Exposure

- The patient is placed in the lateral decubitus position with the entire hip and lower extremity prepared and draped to allow for free range of motion.
- This position allows the extremity to be situated over the side of the table into a sterile pocket on the abdominal side of the patient during femoral preparation.

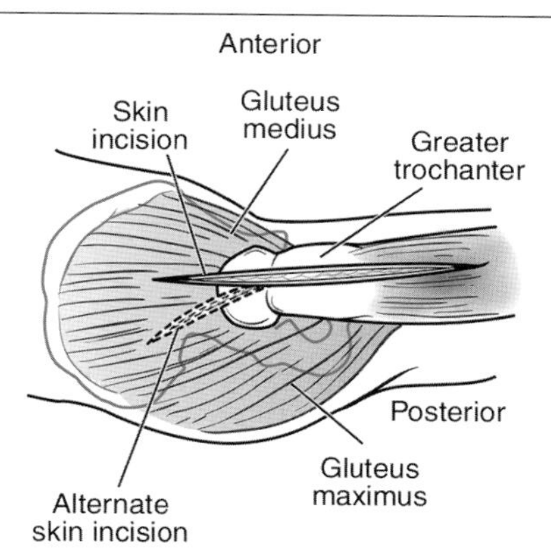

Figure 1 Illustration of a right hip shows two options for skin incision. The incision may be straight and centered over the femoral shaft (skin incision) or have a gentle proximal posterior curve to facilitate exposure of the femoral canal (alternate skin incision). (Reproduced from Lewallen DG: Primary total hip arthroplasty: Anterolateral and direct lateral approaches, in Lieberman JR, Berry DJ, eds: *Advanced Reconstruction: Hip.* Rosemont, IL, American Academy of Orthopaedic Surgeons, 2005, pp 11-16.)

- The incision is centered over the trochanter and extends in line with the femur distally.
- Proximally, the incision curves slightly posteriorly, which will facilitate femoral preparation (**Figure 1**).
- The subcutaneous tissues and fascia are divided in line with the skin incision.
- If necessary, hypertrophic bursal tissue is débrided to allow for direct visualization of the gluteus medius.
- The most anterior portion of the gluteus medius inserts obliquely onto the greater trochanter, and the central and posterior portions are oriented more vertically in line with the femoral shaft. Degenerative tearing of these muscles is a common finding (**Figure 2**).

Instruments/Equipment/Implants Required

- The transgluteal approaches may be successfully performed with a wide variety of instruments and implants.
- The authors of this chapter use a combination of sharp (Meyerding) and blunt (Deaver) handheld retractors during the initial exposure. Often, a Charnley-type self-retaining retractor is useful during some or all of the exposure.
- After hip dislocation, the neck osteotomy may be made with either a reciprocating or an oscillating saw.
- Acetabular exposure is obtained using a combination of the following: large bone hook, Meyerding retractor, Deaver retractor, Hohmann retractor, and cobra retractor. Femoral exposure is obtained using these same instruments.
- The excellent exposure provided by the approaches described in this chapter will allow the surgeon to use all available acetabular and femoral implants according to a patient's unique anatomy and the surgeon's discretion.

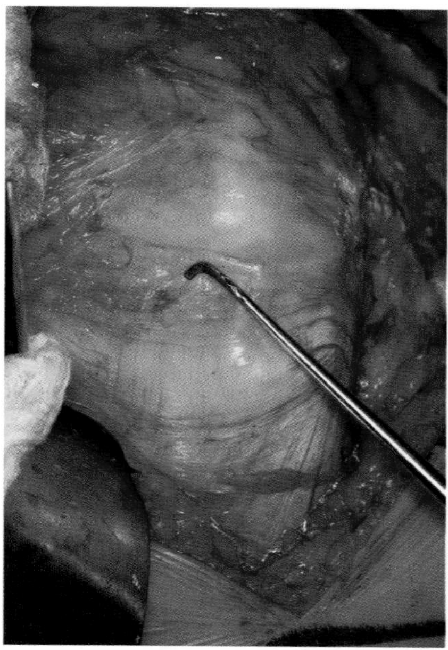

Figure 2 Intraoperative photograph of a hip shows degenerative tearing or attenuation of the tendinous abductor insertion onto the greater trochanter.

Procedure

ANTEROLATERAL APPROACH

- A curved, J-shaped incision is made to detach the anterior portion of the gluteus medius directly off the greater trochanter. This allows proximal and anterior retraction of the obliquely oriented anterior portion of the muscle (**Figure 3**).
- For most primary THAs, approximately 40% of the muscle is mobilized while leaving the more robust and vertically oriented central and posterior attachments intact.
- Muscle splitting must not extend more than 5 cm proximal to the tip of the greater trochanter to avoid injury to the superior gluteal nerve.
- The gluteus minimus is identified and divided from its attachment to the trochanter, allowing for visualization of the anterior hip capsule, after which an arthrotomy may be performed with either subtotal capsulectomy or T-shaped capsular flaps, based on surgeon preference (**Figure 4**).

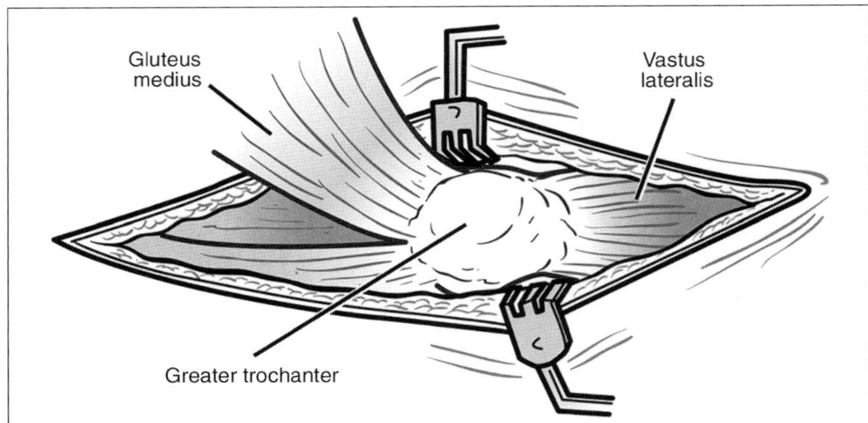

Figure 3 Illustration of a right hip shows retraction of the skin, subcutaneous tissue, and fascia with a Charnley self-retaining retractor. The anterior portion of the gluteus medius is released from the anterior portion of the greater trochanter. The split is extended proximally through the substance of the muscle. The split should not extend more than 5 cm proximal to the tip of the greater trochanter to protect the superior gluteal nerve. (Reproduced from Lewallen DG: Primary total hip arthroplasty: Anterolateral and direct lateral approaches, in Lieberman JR, Berry DJ, eds: *Advanced Reconstruction: Hip.* Rosemont, IL, American Academy of Orthopaedic Surgeons, 2005, pp 11-16.)

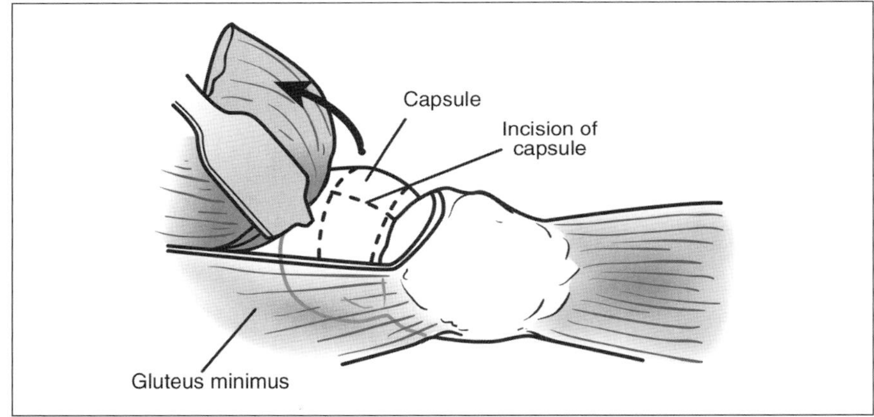

Figure 4 Illustration of a right hip shows the gluteal muscles retracted superiorly and proximally. The anterior and lateral portions of the capsule are incised or excised. (Reproduced from Lewallen DG: Primary total hip arthroplasty: Anterolateral and direct lateral approaches, in Lieberman JR, Berry DJ, eds: *Advanced Reconstruction: Hip.* Rosemont, IL, American Academy of Orthopaedic Surgeons, 2005, pp 11-16.)

DIRECT LATERAL APPROACH

- The anterior portion of the vastus lateralis is elevated in continuity with the anterior portion of the gluteus medius. Many surgeons find this tissue to be especially beneficial at the time of wound closure in patients in whom degenerative abductor muscle tears have developed (**Figure 5**).
- Variations of this approach involve changes in the amount of abductor or vastus lateralis muscles released as the musculotendinous sleeve.
- Another variation elevates a thin wafer of trochanter with the intact muscle insertion rather than muscle alone.
- Regardless of the technique used, excessive splitting or proximal dissection must be avoided to protect the superior gluteal nerve.
- Arthrotomy is performed as described previously for the anterolateral approach.

DISLOCATION

- After arthrotomy is performed, the hip is gradually brought into a position of flexion, adduction, and external rotation.
- The inferior capsular attachments around the base of the femoral neck are released. This is a critical step that allows safe anterior dislocation of the hip without excessive force.
- The extremity is placed into a sterile pocket (**Figure 6**), and the femoral neck osteotomy is performed according to the preoperative plan for femoral reconstruction.

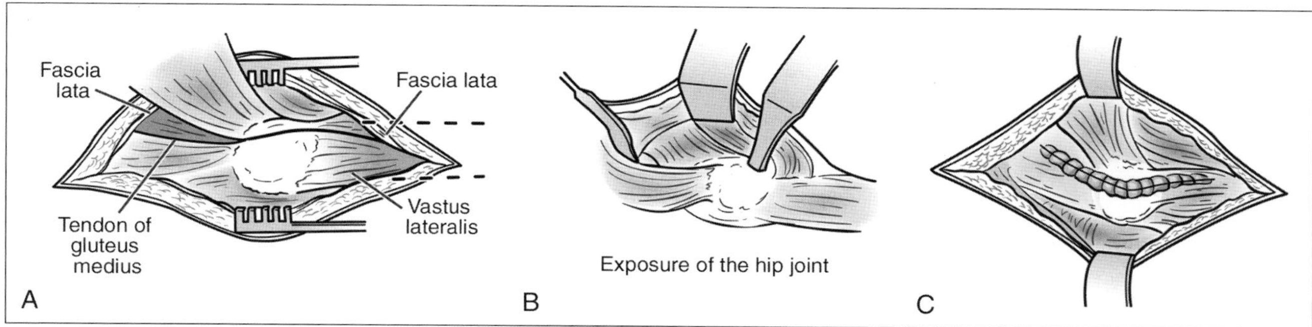

Figure 5 Illustrations of a right hip show the direct lateral approach. **A,** The insertion of the gluteus medius is elevated from the anterior portion of the greater trochanter and extended proximally into the substance of the gluteus medius and minimus muscles. The abductor muscle split should not extend more than 5 cm proximal to the tip of the greater trochanter. The vastus lateralis is split distally in continuity with the gluteus muscles. **B,** The vastus lateralis is subperiosteally elevated, and the entire myofascial unit is retracted anteriorly to expose the hip capsule. **C,** The myofascial unit is repaired side-to-side with multiple interrupted sutures that provide a secure attachment. (Reproduced from Lewallen DG: Primary total hip arthroplasty: Anterolateral and direct lateral approaches, in Lieberman JR, Berry DJ, eds: *Advanced Reconstruction: Hip.* Rosemont, IL, American Academy of Orthopaedic Surgeons, 2005, pp 11-16.)

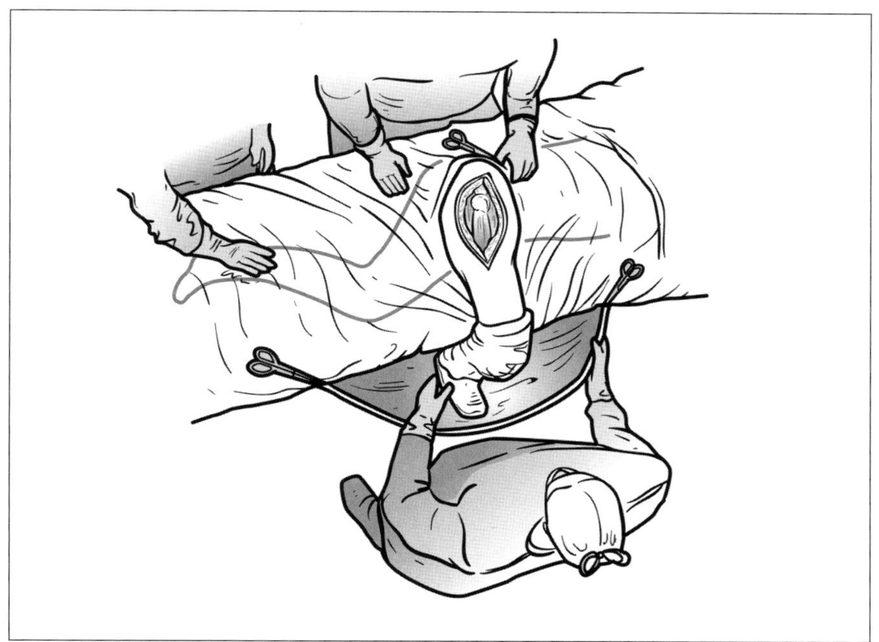

Figure 6 Illustration shows placement of the surgical foot and lower leg placed into the sterile pocket after dislocation of the hip by adduction, external rotation, and longitudinal traction. Positioning of the surgical leg perpendicular to the floor allows the surgeon to assess the rotational alignment of the femoral prosthesis in a clinically reproducible manner. (Reproduced from Lewallen DG: Primary total hip arthroplasty: Anterolateral and direct lateral approaches, in Lieberman JR, Berry DJ, eds: *Advanced Reconstruction: Hip.* Rosemont, IL, American Academy of Orthopaedic Surgeons, 2005, pp 11-16.)

ACETABULAR EXPOSURE

- Acetabular exposure is facilitated by deliberate positioning of the femur and multiple retractors (**Figure 7**).
- The affected limb is placed into a position of slight hip flexion, with the knee extended and the foot just inside the sterile pocket.
- The femur is retracted posteriorly with a large bone hook until a curved retractor can be placed over the posterior wall or into the ischium. This maneuver provides exposure of the posterior one-half of the socket in most patients, but it can be supplemented with posterosuperior placement of another curved retractor if necessary.
- The anterior one-half of the socket is exposed with two separate curved retractors. The first retractor is inserted into the anterior column, which will retract the bulk of the abductor muscles released during the exposure, and the second retractor is placed over the anteroinferior rim of the acetabulum to retract the remaining soft tissues.
- This reproducible technique allows circumferential visualization of the socket and facilitates safe and accurate component preparation.

FEMORAL EXPOSURE

- The femur is again brought into a position of flexion, adduction, and external rotation, with the surgical limb placed into a sterile pocket. The femur can be exposed with multiple retractors to allow for safe preparation.

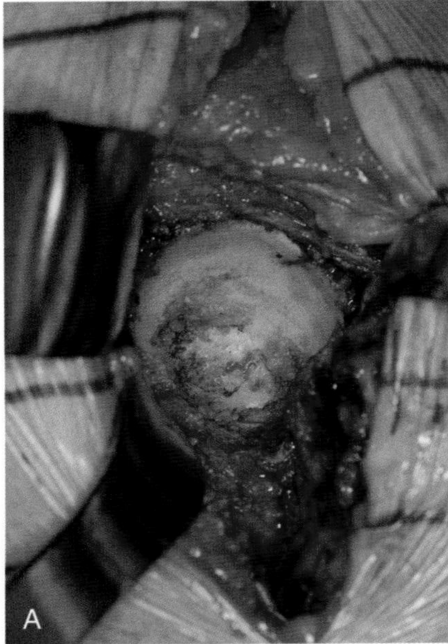

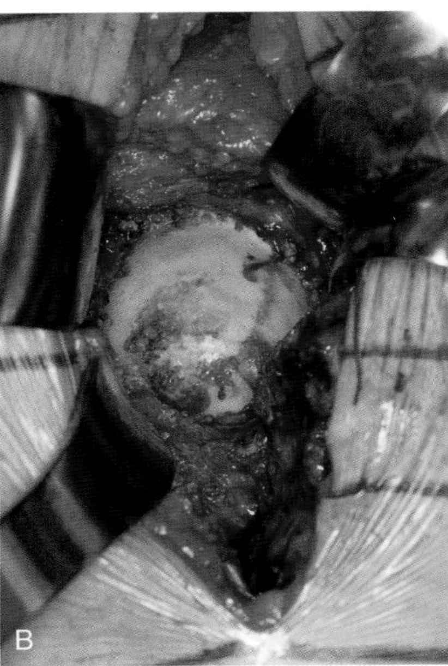

Figure 7 Intraoperative photographs show the excellent acetabular exposure obtained with three (**A**) or four (**B**) retractors. The femur is retracted posteriorly and inferiorly (to the right). The anterior soft tissues (left side of photographs) are retracted with two separate retractors, each exposing a separate quadrant of the socket. The fourth retractor, placed posterosuperior, is most useful in patients who have bulky posterior abductor attachments.

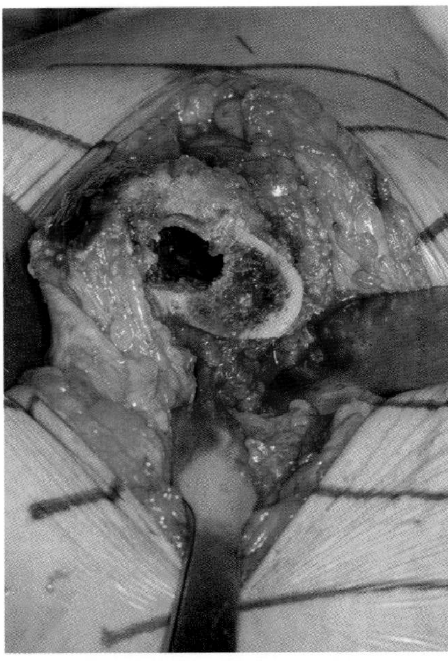

Figure 8 Intraoperative photograph of a left hip shows the elevated femur as well as three retractors placed to protect the remaining abductor muscle attachments during femoral preparation. Note the excellent exposure of the trochanter and the entire calcar femorale without overhanging muscle.

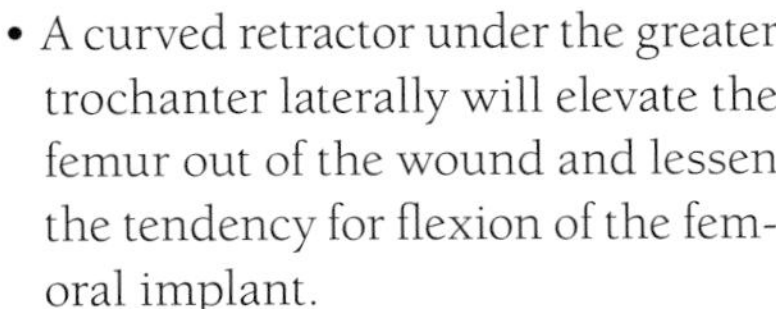

- A curved retractor under the greater trochanter laterally will elevate the femur out of the wound and lessen the tendency for flexion of the femoral implant.
- A different curved retractor is placed medially over the calcar femorale to further elevate the femur and expose the bone for instrumentation.
- A third retractor, if necessary, is placed in line with the femoral shaft over the posterior abductors and under the posterior bone of the femoral neck to elevate the femur and depress the muscle, protecting both structures from unintended damage (**Figure 8**).

EXTENSILE MODIFICATIONS

- If greater access to the femur is required, most often during revision procedures, well-described modifications to the previously described approaches may facilitate the final reconstruction.
- One extensile option is a laterally based extended osteotomy that can be performed either before or after hip dislocation following exposure via a modified direct lateral approach. The lateral one-third of the femoral shaft, including the entire greater trochanter and remaining posterior abductor attachments, can be elevated from front-to-back using this technique.
- One disadvantage of the laterally based extensile osteotomy compared with a posterior extensile osteotomy is the substantially greater soft-tissue stripping from the osteotomized fragment related to the initial elevation of the abductors. However, retention of the posterior soft-tissue envelope using the laterally based extensile technique is believed to confer greater stability.
- Another extensile option is the anteriorly based extended trochanteric osteotomy (**Figure 9**). This technique must be used before hip dislocation, and it could be considered a transosseous direct lateral approach. Rather than elevating the gluteus medius and vastus lateralis from the bone, the anterior one-half of the trochanter is osteotomized in continuity with the anterior portion of the femoral shaft distally. The osteotomized anterior segment is retracted anteriorly with abductors attached proximally and the vastus lateralis attached distally. The extended trochanteric osteotomy allows excellent access into the distal portion of the femur, effectively bypassing the deforming force of the anterior femoral bow, and facilitates proper preparation

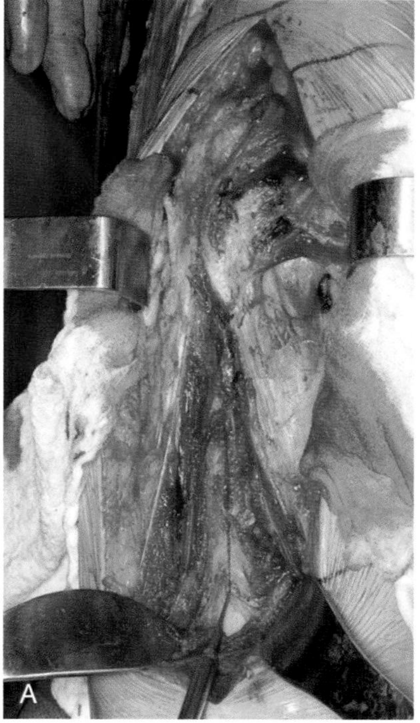

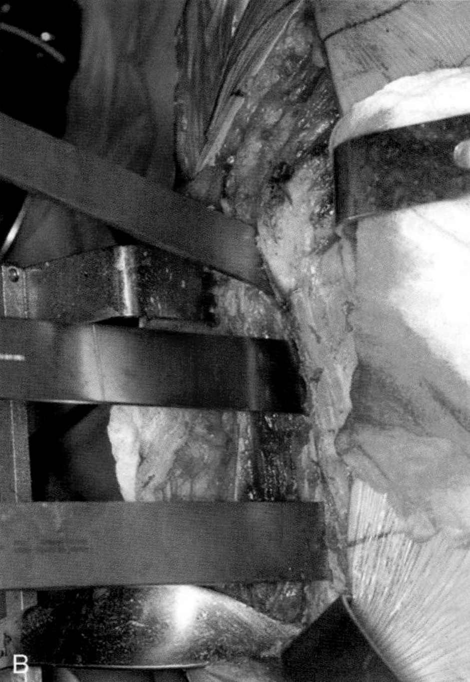

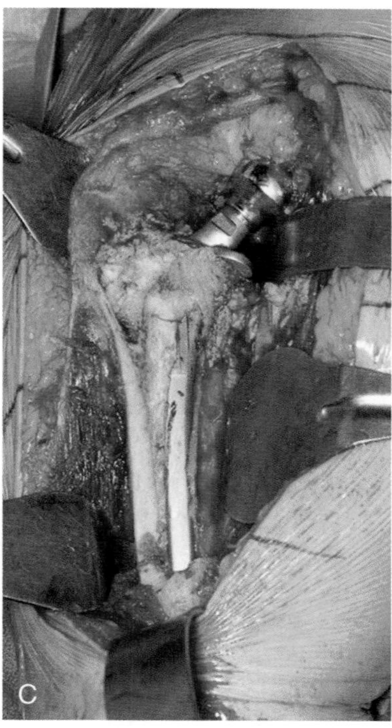

Figure 9 Intraoperative photographs of a right hip show the anteriorly based extended trochanteric osteotomy. **A,** The vastus lateralis is split in continuity with the abductor muscles as in the direct lateral approach. **B,** The tissues are not lifted off the bone. Instead, the anterior trochanter and a portion of the proximal shaft are osteotomized and elevated anteriorly. Care is taken to maintain the vascularity of the anterior fragment by way of its muscle attachments. After the osteotomy and retraction of the anterior fragment, the remaining femur is externally rotated. **C,** Excellent exposure is obtained for femoral component removal and/or implantation.

and implantation of distally fixed noncemented implants.

- After either type of extensile osteotomy, the fragment typically is reduced and repaired with wire or cable cerclage fixation based on bone quality and surgeon preference.

Wound Closure

- After the reconstructive procedure is complete, the hip is reduced and stability confirmed.
- The anterior musculotendinous sleeve is repaired using nonabsorbable sutures passed through bone in the anterior trochanter. This closure can be supplemented with additional side-to-side soft-tissue repair.
- Meticulous attention to the abductors throughout the procedure is critical to minimize the potential for long-term issues related to pain, weakness, or a limp.

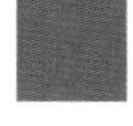

Postoperative Regimen

After a transgluteal approach to the hip, most patients are allowed to bear weight as tolerated immediately postoperatively using walking aids for support as needed. Usually, abduction strengthening exercises are not begun until 8 to 12 weeks postoperatively to allow healing of the muscle-tendon attachments. If an extensile modification is used, patients typically are prescribed protected weight bearing for 6 to 12 weeks postoperatively. The duration of protected weight bearing is based on healing of the osteotomy and the nature of the femoral reconstruction.

Avoiding Pitfalls and Complications

The main disadvantages of the transgluteal approaches include abductor weakness and limping resulting from either superior gluteal nerve injury, which can occur with excessive proximal splitting of the gluteus medius, or failed repair of the musculotendinous unit to the trochanter; slower recovery of abductor power compared with the direct anterior or posterolateral approaches; and lack of visualization or access to the femoral shaft distally. Additional disadvantages include the potential for femoral stem malposition or trochanteric fracture as a result of trochanteric impingement during prosthesis insertion.

To minimize these risks, careful attention to surgical technique is essential. In general, it is better to carefully release and repair a larger proportion of the abductors rather than to minimize the anterior release and then inadvertently damage the muscle beyond repair. Strategic retractor placement will facilitate acetabular and femoral preparation and will minimize this risk for muscle injury. If used appropriately, the transgluteal approaches can facilitate both simple and complex reconstructions of the acetabulum and femur with a low risk for postoperative dislocation.

Bibliography

Berry DJ: Anterior extended greater trochanteric osteotomy. *Seminars in Arthroplasty* 2004;15:126-129.

Berry DJ, von Knoch M, Schleck CD, Harmsen WS: Effect of femoral head diameter and operative approach on risk of dislocation after primary total hip arthroplasty. *J Bone Joint Surg Am* 2005;87(11):2456-2463.

Frndak PA, Mallory TH, Lombardi AV Jr: Translateral surgical approach to the hip: The abductor muscle "split". *Clin Orthop Relat Res* 1993;(295):135-141.

MacDonald SJ, Cole C, Guerin J, Rorabeck CH, Bourne RB, McCalden RW: Extended trochanteric osteotomy via the direct lateral approach in revision hip arthroplasty. *Clin Orthop Relat Res* 2003;(417):210-216.

Masonis JL, Bourne RB: Surgical approach, abductor function, and total hip arthroplasty dislocation. *Clin Orthop Relat Res* 2002;(405):46-53.

Moskal JT, Mann JW III: A modified direct lateral approach for primary and revision total hip arthroplasty: A prospective analysis of 453 cases. *J Arthroplasty* 1996;11(3):255-266.

Mulliken BD, Rorabeck CH, Bourne RB, Nayak N: A modified direct lateral approach in total hip arthroplasty: A comprehensive review. *J Arthroplasty* 1998;13(7):737-747.

Queen RM, Butler RJ, Watters TS, Kelley SS, Attarian DE, Bolognesi MP: The effect of total hip arthroplasty surgical approach on postoperative gait mechanics. *J Arthroplasty* 2011;26(6 suppl):66-71.

Ramesh M, O'Byrne JM, McCarthy N, Jarvis A, Mahalingham K, Cashman WF: Damage to the superior gluteal nerve after the Hardinge approach to the hip. *J Bone Joint Surg Br* 1996;78(6):903-906.

Woo RY, Morrey BF: Dislocations after total hip arthroplasty. *J Bone Joint Surg Am* 1982;64(9):1295-1306.

Video Reference

Mabry TM: Video. ***Difficult Exposures From the Anterolateral Approach***. Rochester, MN, 2014.

Chapter 3
Total Hip Arthroplasty: The Modern Posterior Approach

Thomas P. Vail, MD
Jonathan L. Berliner, MD
Patrick K. Horst, MD

Indications

Evolution of the posterior approach to total hip arthroplasty (THA) has resulted in accelerated postoperative recovery times and decreased complication rates. Advancements in the understanding of hip joint anatomy and efforts to protect muscle and repair the hip capsule have resulted in improved tissue preservation with the posterior approach. These changes have addressed risks historically associated with the posterior approach, including a higher rate of dislocation or muscle injury that can lengthen or complicate rehabilitation. Recent research has focused on the hip capsule, the gluteal muscles, and the short external rotators. Careful protection of the ischiofemoral ligament during exposure, combined with a strong capsular repair, results in dislocation rates comparable with or superior to those of other exposures. Recognition of the surgical anatomy, including the fiber orientation and pennate structure of the gluteal muscles, allows access to the joint to be achieved with minimal damage to the soft tissues and associated innervation. Improvements in bearing function have allowed the appropriate use of larger-diameter articulations commensurate with the acetabular size, further contributing to joint stability and function. As a result of these advances, the posterior approach has become a highly functional, predictable, and reliable approach for THA.

Adaptations of the posterior exposure, such as the posterolateral, dorsal, and Southern approaches, similarly enter the hip joint through the gluteus maximus muscle and behind the gluteus medius muscle. These approaches were designed to meet certain goals in the context of the knowledge and devices of the era in which they were used. The use of minimally invasive approaches has waned owing to the recognition of unique complications associated with a narrow focus on incision length and the limited data to support their use. However, the goals of minimal tissue injury, brief hospitalization or outpatient surgery, and rapid return to full function are of the highest priority and can be achieved with the modern posterior approach to THA (**Table 1**).

The Moore posterior approach, which was originally described as a technique for inserting a bulky, monoblock proximal femoral hemiarthroplasty prosthesis, became the standard exposure for both primary and revision THA. The Moore approach was widely adopted in an era in which broad exposure was desired and quick recovery and shorter length of stay were not emphasized. Surgical theory at the time supported exposure of structures such as the sciatic nerve in an effort to minimize the risk of injury and complete excision of the hip capsule to facilitate acetabular exposure. The classic Moore approach included optional release of the short external rotators, the quadratus femoris muscle, and the distal insertion of the gluteus maximus. Because of the broad exposure, variations of the technique were used to gain access to the sciatic nerve, the posterior column, the lateral rim of the acetabulum, the proximal hamstring muscles, the hip joint, the labrum, and the piriformis tendon.

Modern versions of the posterior approach reflect improved understanding of the surgical anatomy and allow surgeons to perform THA with minimal tissue trauma and optimal implant position. As a surgeon becomes familiar with the principles of THA using this

Dr. Vail or an immediate family member has received royalties from and serves as a paid consultant to DePuy Synthes; has stock or stock options held in Biomimedica; and serves as a board member, owner, officer, or committee member of the American Association of Hip and Knee Surgeons, the American Board of Orthopaedic Surgery, the Hip Society, and the Knee Society. Dr. Horst or an immediate family member is an employee of Arthrex. Neither Dr. Berliner nor any immediate family member has received anything of value from or has stock or stock options held in a commercial company or institution related directly or indirectly to the subject of this chapter.

Table 1 Results of Total Hip Arthroplasty Using the Posterior Approach

Authors (Year)	Number of Hips Treated	Procedure or Approach	Mean Patient Age in Years (Range)	Mean Follow-up in Months (Range)	Dislocation Rate (%)	Results
Woolson et al (2004)	135	MPA or posterior	MPA: 60 (20-81) Posterior: 63 (35-91)	≥6 (NA)	MPA: 0 Posterior: 1.2	Retrospective cohort study No differences in surgical time, estimated blood loss, postoperative transfusion rates, LOS, or discharge disposition MPA group had significantly higher rates of wound complications, implant malpositioning, and intraoperative fracture
Ogonda et al (2005)	219	MPA or posterior	MPA: 67 (NR) Posterior: 66 (NR)	1.5 (1.5-3)	MPA: 0.9 Posterior: 0.9	RCT No significant difference in patient-reported outcome scores, transfusion rates, pain scores, analgesic use, LOS, early walking ability, or implant position Early discharge was associated with patient age and preoperative hemoglobin level
Palan et al (2009)	1,089	Posterior or antero-lateral	Posterior: 67 (NR) Anterolateral: 68 (NR)	≤60 (3-60)[a]	Posterior: 2.3 Anterolateral: 2.1	Prospective nonrandomized multicenter study Posterior approach group had higher OHS and OHS change scores at 3 mo and 1 yr No differences in OHS or OHS change scores at 5 yr No difference in dislocation or revision rates
Hailer et al (2012)	78,098	MPA, posterior, or direct lateral	NA[b]	32.4 (0-72)	NR[c]	Retrospective registry study Revision for dislocation occurred at a higher rate in the posterior approach group compared with the lateral approach group (adjusted relative risk, 1.3) Revision for dislocation occurred at a higher rate in the MPA group compared with the lateral approach group (adjusted relative risk, 4.2)
Ji et al (2012)	196	Posterior or direct lateral	51 (18-78)	37.9 (24-57)	Posterior: 0 Direct lateral: 3.1	RCT Lateral group had higher rate of limping at 6-mo follow-up No difference in Harris hip score or gait mechanics between groups at final follow-up No difference in postoperative transfusion rates or implant position between groups
Barrett et al (2013)	87	Posterior or DAA	Posterior: 63 (NR) DAA: 61 (NR)	12	Posterior: 2.3[d] DAA: 0	RCT DAA group had improved function and patient-reported outcomes at 6 wk and 3 mo At 6 mo, no significant functional differences or differences in PROM scores between groups DAA group had significantly shorter LOS (2.28 vs 3.02 d) No significant differences in implant position or dislocation rate

DAA = direct anterior approach, EQ-5D = EuroQol Five Dimension, LOS = length of stay, MPA = mini-incision posterior approach, NA = not applicable, NR = not reported, OHS = Oxford hip score, PROM = patient-reported outcome measure, RCT = randomized controlled trial.

[a] 73% had 5-yr follow-up.

[b] Four covariate age groups: <50 yr (3% of the study cohort), 50-59 yr (11%), 60-75 yr (55%), >75 yr (30%).

[c] 0.5% of all hips included in the study were revised for dislocation.

[d] The acetabular component was noted to be positioned at 59° inclination and 58° anteversion.

[e] Mean follow-up reported for 6 of 16 studies included in the meta-analysis.

[f] Dislocations reported in 13 of 16 studies included in the meta-analysis.

[g] PROM data were available for 4,962 patients at 6 yr.

Table 1 Results of Total Hip Arthroplasty Using the Posterior Approach (*continued*)

Authors (Year)	Number of Hips Treated	Procedure or Approach	Mean Patient Age in Years (Range)	Mean Follow-up in Months (Range)	Dislocation Rate (%)	Results
Berstock et al (2014)	1,498	MPA or posterior	MPA: 66 (61-73) Posterior: 67 (58-73)	31.3 (12-60)[e]	MPA: 1.2 Posterior: 1.0[f]	Systematic review of 12 RCTs and 4 nonrandomized trials No difference in dislocation rates, postoperative PROMs (Harris hip score, Western Ontario and McMaster Universities Osteoarthritis Index score, Medical Outcomes Study 12-Item Short Form score), or complications (intraoperative fracture, nerve injury, infection, thromboembolic events, limb-length discrepancy)
Jameson et al (2014)	37,593	Posterior or direct lateral	69 (18-106)	All hips, PROM data: 7 All hips, complication data: 12	NR	Retrospective registry study No difference in complications (bleeding, wound complications, readmission, dislocation) or all-cause revisions Posterior approach group had higher OHS and EQ-5D score in multivariate analysis Revision rate for dislocation was equal for both the posterior and direct lateral approach groups (0.15%)
Lindgren et al (2014)	42,233	Posterior or direct lateral	Posterior: 69 (NR) Direct lateral: 69 (NR)	All patients: 12[g]	NR	Retrospective registry study Better mean EQ-5D score with the posterior approach than with the direct lateral approach (76 and 75, respectively) Better mean satisfaction score with the posterior approach than with the direct lateral approach (18 and 15, respectively) Better mean pain score with the posterior approach than with the direct lateral approach (13 and 15, respectively) Although statistically significant, these reported differences are small
Rodriguez et al (2014)	120	Posterior or DAA	Posterior: 59 (NR) DAA: 60 (NR)	Functional outcomes: 3 PROMs: 12	Posterior: 1.7 DAA: 0	Prospective nonrandomized study No differences in functional milestones after 6 wk No differences in PROMs, surgical time, complications, or implant alignment at any time point Posterior approach group had 1 dislocation; DAA group had none

DAA = direct anterior approach, EQ-5D = EuroQol Five Dimension, LOS = length of stay, MPA = mini-incision posterior approach, NA = not applicable, NR = not reported, OHS = Oxford hip score, PROM = patient-reported outcome measure, RCT = randomized controlled trial.

[a] 73% had 5-yr follow-up.

[b] Four covariate age groups: <50 yr (3% of the study cohort), 50-59 yr (11%), 60-75 yr (55%), >75 yr (30%).

[c] 0.5% of all hips included in the study were revised for dislocation.

[d] The acetabular component was noted to be positioned at 59° inclination and 58° anteversion.

[e] Mean follow-up reported for 6 of 16 studies included in the meta-analysis.

[f] Dislocations reported in 13 of 16 studies included in the meta-analysis.

[g] PROM data were available for 4,962 patients at 6 yr.

approach, the extent of soft-tissue dissection and the length of the incision can be progressively limited. However, the posterior approach can be extended into a broader exposure, if indicated, to accommodate patient size, joint stiffness, or other factors. The goal of a less invasive posterior approach is not simply to reduce the incision size but to achieve a highly functional hip arthroplasty with reduced pain, faster recovery, and improved patient satisfaction.

Contraindications

Contraindications to the posterior approach are limited due to its versatile nature and the option to convert to an extensile exposure. The posterior approach can accommodate most surgical procedures of the hip and can be used by surgeons with a broad range of experience. If the posterior approach is used in femoral head–sparing procedures such as drainage of a pyarthrosis, resurfacing, or femoral neck débridement, the blood supply to the femoral head may be at risk. Depending on the extent of the exposure or the need to dislocate the femoral head, the integrity of the branches of the medial femoral circumflex artery may be compromised, limiting blood supply to the femoral head. If preservation of the femoral head is necessary, dissection should be limited to preserve the quadratus femoris and the extension of the medial femoral circumflex vessels coursing posteriorly into the Weitbrecht retinacula, which supplies blood to varying amounts of epiphyseal bone. An inherent risk of the approach is the proximity of the sciatic nerve on the posterior column. However, the rate of sciatic nerve injury is very low in most published series of THA using a posterior approach.

In patients who are at increased risk for dislocation, such as those who have a neurodegenerative or cognitive disorder, or in patients in whom capsular repair is not possible, the posterior approach may carry a slightly higher risk of instability compared with an anterior or anterolateral approach. However, the posterior approach may still be indicated in patients at risk for dislocation if the alternative would be an approach with which the surgeon has less experience.

All surgical approaches to the hip may be more complicated in obese or very muscular patients or in patients with stiff joints, acetabular protrusion, or retained hardware. The posterior approach is not specifically contraindicated in these patients. However, particular emphasis on a small skin incision should be avoided because an excessively small incision can increase the risk of soft-tissue damage or intraoperative fracture; compromise accurate bone preparation, leading to undesired outcomes such as eccentric reaming of the acetabulum; or result in improper positioning and sizing of the femoral implant. The degree and nature of the hip pathology should be considered as well. Patients with severe dysplasia resulting in superior displacement of the femoral head require wider exposures. Limited surgical approaches are difficult in patients who have a history of previous hip procedures, such as osteotomy, or who are undergoing a revision arthroplasty procedure.

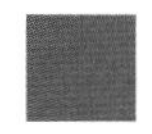

Alternative Treatments

Many alternative approaches to the hip are available. Each has advantages and potential shortcomings. The classic surgical exposures for THA include the extended posterior (Moore) approach, the anterior (Smith-Petersen) approach with or without a specialized surgical table, the direct lateral (Hardinge) approach, and the anterolateral (Watson-Jones) approach. Modifications of each exposure have been described in an effort to limit the incision size and soft-tissue dissection. The anterior approach can provide excellent acetabular exposure, but the difficulty of access to the femoral shaft may result in increased rates of fracture. The direct lateral and anterolateral approaches have been associated with altered postoperative gait mechanics as well as reduced patient-reported outcomes because of incomplete healing after detachment of a portion of the abductor mechanism as a part of the exposure.

Because indications for each approach overlap, no definitive algorithm exists for selecting an approach. The choice of exposure is often influenced by the surgeon's training or the patient's specific needs and desires.

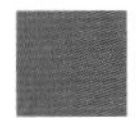

Results

The short- and long-term success of THA via the posterior approach has been validated in numerous large registry-based outcome studies demonstrating excellent long-term survival, and in case series showing early return to function and reduced hospital length of stay. Reflecting the increased interest in rapid recovery, recent comparative analyses have evaluated the outcomes of modern variations of the posterior approach (**Table 1**). The literature does not provide sufficient evidence to confirm an advantage of one approach over another when comparing length of stay, return to function, risk of complications, markers of muscle injury, or long-term implant performance.

Numerous large retrospective studies using registry data have not consistently demonstrated a difference between the posterior and direct lateral approaches in terms of postoperative complications or long-term implant survival. Similarly, most studies do not demonstrate a notable difference in the postoperative dislocation rate when comparing the modern posterior approach with other approaches. The historical concern of dislocation related to the posterior approach has become less relevant because current techniques include careful capsular and soft-tissue repairs. Improved patient-reported outcome scores documented in several reports comparing the posterior approach with a lateral approach may be related to the preservation of the abductor attachments.

Comparison of the current posterior approach with the direct anterior approach is of greatest interest because both approaches avoid detachment of the abductors. The direct anterior approach has grown in popularity because of the focus on less invasive surgical procedures for the purpose of rapid recovery and rehabilitation. For example, although the posterior approach remains the most common approach, the direct anterior approach is used in approximately 20% of the procedures performed by surgeons who are members of the American Association of Hip and Knee Surgeons. Several prospective studies have compared the posterior approach with the direct anterior approach. In a recent randomized controlled trial, improved functional measures noted 6 weeks postoperatively in patients treated with the anterior approach had disappeared at 6-month follow-up. Furthermore, no statistically significant differences were found between the groups in terms of patient-reported outcome measure scores or complications. Numerous small prospective series have demonstrated more rapid recovery and improved early postoperative functional measures with the anterior approach compared with other surgical exposures. However, some researchers have questioned whether these observed improvements in postoperative recovery are the consequence of patient selection or recent advances in pain management, rehabilitation protocols, regional anesthesia, and preoperative patient education.

The focus on so-called minimally invasive or mini-incision approaches to the hip has waned because the preponderance of evidence has suggested that a smaller surgical incision offers little clinical benefit and increases the potential for complications. Specifically, studies of mini-incision approaches consistently have not demonstrated superior outcomes in terms of intraoperative blood loss, rates of postoperative transfusion or dislocation, and patient-reported outcome measure scores and satisfaction.

Technique

Setup/Exposure

- The patient is placed in the lateral decubitus position.
- All downside pressure points are padded.
- An axillary roll is placed under the thorax for additional protection of the shoulder and the brachial plexus.
- The pelvis is stabilized with a pelvic positioning device. Generally, the pelvis is biased toward the side of the table closer to the pubis. Moving the pelvis forward toward the edge of the table facilitates placement of the affected leg off of the front of the table intraoperatively to improve access to the proximal femur.
- The pelvis is stably fixed in a methodic manner to facilitate positioning and alignment of the acetabular implant. The anterior superior iliac spines are positioned perpendicular to the floor, and the gluteal cleft is positioned parallel to the floor.
- The dependent leg is positioned to accommodate later intraoperative assessment of leg lengths.
- The affected extremity is prepped and draped in sterile fashion.
- An adhesive, bacteriostatic covering is applied over the surgical site.
- To limit the risk of contamination of the incision with skin flora, hands and instruments are prevented from touching the uncovered skin.
- The skin incision is directed obliquely and passes directly over the acetabulum.
- The incision is perpendicular to the transverse acetabular ligament and is in line with the expected position of the handle of the acetabular reamer that will be used later in the procedure.
- The proximal-to-distal and anterior-to-posterior position of the skin incision is determined on the basis of palpation of the greater trochanter.
- With the patient's leg in neutral rotation on the surgical table, the incision is positioned at the junction of the anterior two-thirds and posterior one-third of the greater trochanter. The incision is placed approximately parallel to the femoral shaft with the hip flexed at 40° to 50° (**Figure 1**).
- Placement of the incision from proximal to distal is influenced by the patient's femoral neck-shaft angle. The incision is placed slightly more distal in a varus hip and slightly more proximal in a valgus hip. Typically, one-half of the incision is proximal to the tip of the trochanter and one-half is distal to the tip of the trochanter.
- When the patient's hip is flexed, the properly placed skin incision will be positioned to provide access to the femur. Likewise, when the hip is in a more neutral or extended position, the same position of the incision provides a better view of the acetabulum. Proper placement of the incision combined with strategic movement of the femur during the procedure creates a mobile window to the relevant structures as visualization is needed. In other words, the skin incision and the femur move with the retractors to allow visualization of the bone structures, with the limb positioned as needed to facilitate visualization.
- The length of the incision also depends on the size of the patient, the depth of the subcutaneous fat, and the compliance of the soft tissues.
- A longer incision is required in larger, more muscular, and stiffer patients to allow proper preparation of the femur and acetabulum without placing excess stress on

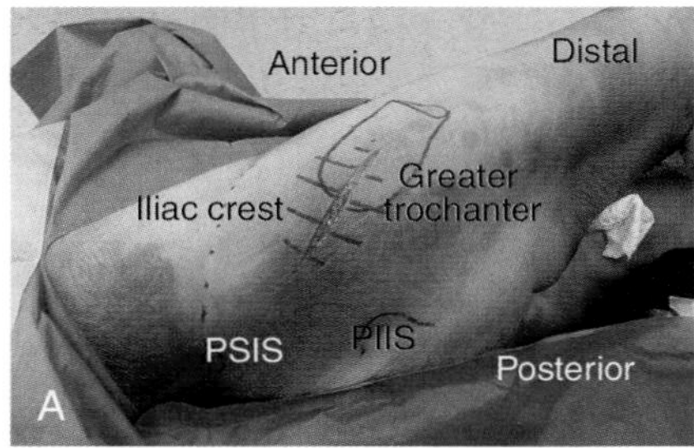

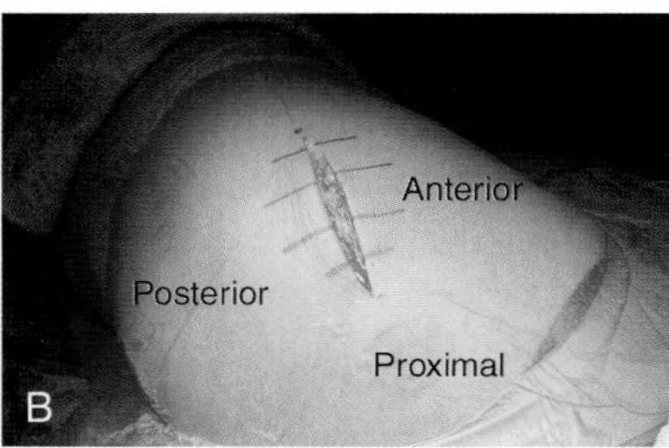

Figure 1 **A,** Photograph of the right hip from a cadaver specimen shows the modern posterior approach hip incision in relationship to the posterior superior iliac spine (PSIS), posterior inferior iliac spine (PIIS), greater trochanter, and iliac crest. **B,** Intraoperative photograph of a left hip shows the posterior incision.

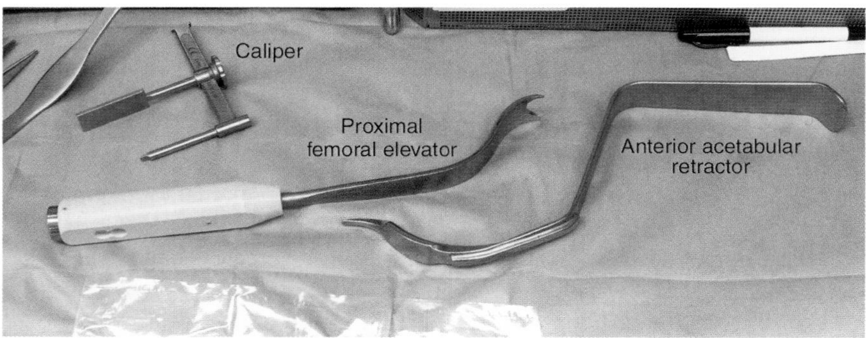

Figure 2 Photograph shows an anterior acetabular retractor and a proximal femoral elevator, which are used to obtain adequate exposure of the acetabulum and proximal femur while minimizing soft-tissue injury. A caliper is shown as well; it is used to measure the length and offset of the femoral neck.

the retractors. The incision length may be increased at any point in the procedure.

Instruments/Equipment/ Implants Required

- To aid in exposure, slender and lower-profile instruments are used, the number of retractors is limited, and lighted retractors, in-line broach handles, and offset reamers are used.
- An anterior acetabular retractor, a proximal femoral elevator, and a caliper are useful (**Figure 2**).
- The anterior acetabular retractor should have a sharp tip and a light, allowing it to be securely placed under direct visualization into the anterior column to illuminate the acetabulum.
- Angled reamers and cup inserters are helpful to accommodate smaller-sized incisions. Modified curved or S-shaped acetabular reamers and cup inserters help to avoid excessive tension on the skin and soft tissues during reaming and cup insertion. However, if incision placement is optimized, angled instruments and special lighting are not required.
- A pulsatile lavage device is used for copious mechanical irrigation of the wound, particularly after the use of broaches, reamers, and other surgical instruments. The lavage is primarily directed at removing debris from the bone and implant surfaces. Care is taken not to damage the soft tissues with overly aggressive pressurized lavage.

Procedure

- After the skin is incised, the subcutaneous tissue is sharply divided down to the fascia of the gluteus maximus posteriorly and proximally and to the fascia lata anteriorly and distally.
- The thin investing fascia of the gluteus maximus muscle is incised in line with the skin incision.
- After the fascia lata is reached, the incision is angled slightly distally in line with the femoral shaft.
- The fascial incision extends distally to the musculotendinous junction of the tensor fascia lata muscle and does not extend into the tensor fasciae unless required.
- The fascia over the gluteus maximus is carefully separated without cutting the muscle fibers (**Figure 3**).
- Careful handling of the gluteus maximus muscle is necessary. The gluteus maximus muscle is separated in line with the muscle fibers near the middle and posterior thirds of its pennate structure.
- The gluteus maximus muscle is separated proximally until the posterior border of the gluteus medius is visible deep to the gluteus maximus. Careful separation of the fibers is necessary to avoid injury to the muscle and its nerve supply.
- A self-retaining retractor, such as a Charnley retractor, is placed carefully underneath the gluteus maximus muscle under low tension to hold open the wound and facilitate deeper dissection. Care is taken to avoid damage to the underlying gluteus medius when this retractor is placed.
- Dissection below the gluteus maximus begins with incision of the trochanteric bursa with Metzenbaum scissors.
- The trochanteric bursa is sharply incised along the posterior edge of the gluteus medius muscle

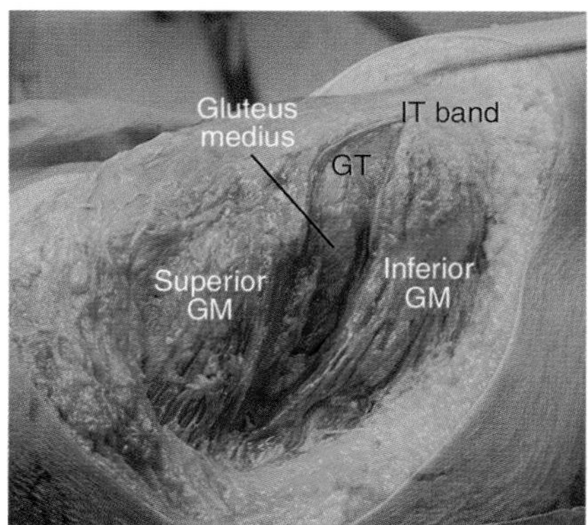

Figure 3 Photograph of the right hip from a cadaver specimen shows the separation of the gluteus maximus (GM) in the raphe between the middle and posterior thirds of its pennate structure. After the muscle is split along the length of the fibers, the greater trochanter (GT) and the underlying gluteus medius are visualized. IT = iliotibial.

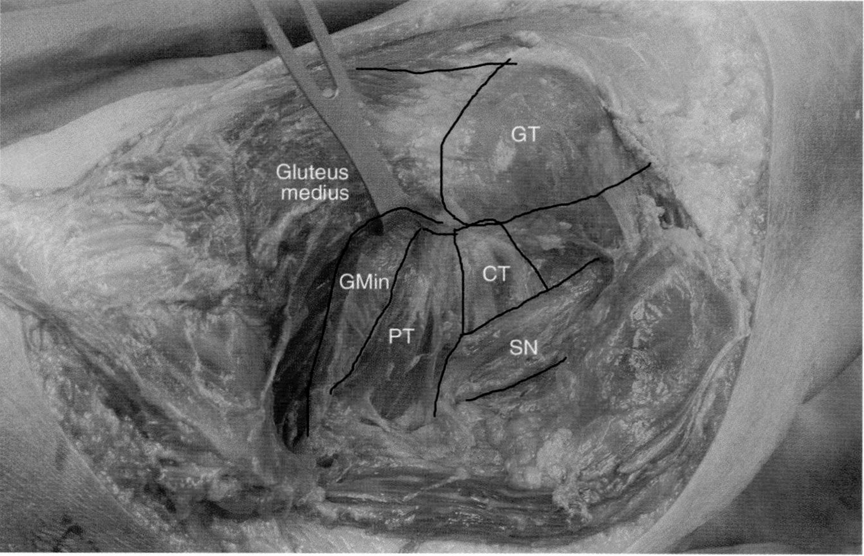

Figure 4 Photograph of the right hip from a cadaver specimen with the gluteus maximus reflected shows the anatomic relationship of the sciatic nerve (SN) to the piriformis tendon (PT) and conjoined tendon (CT). Placement of a retractor under the gluteus medius at its insertion onto the greater trochanter (GT) reveals the junction of the underlying gluteus minimus (GMin) and PT.

beginning just above its trochanteric insertion. The incision is carried distally to the proximal aspect of the quadratus femoris muscle.

- The bursa is reflected posteriorly with a sponge to expose the posterior border of the gluteus medius muscle and the short external rotator muscles.
- Hemostasis is carefully maintained with cautery during this part of the procedure because the bursa is well vascularized and large veins often overlie the piriformis tendon and the short external rotators.
- The sciatic nerve is palpated as it exits from underneath the piriformis and courses distally over the short external rotators and the ischial tuberosity (**Figure 4**). Exposure of the sciatic nerve is not necessary.
- The piriformis tendon is identified just deep to the posterior edge of the gluteus medius muscle.
- To enable better visualization of the piriformis muscle and the conjoined tendon (composed of the obturator externus, superior gemellus, obturator internus, and inferior gemellus), a blunt Hohmann retractor is placed underneath the gluteus medius muscle, over the piriformis and gluteus minimus muscles, and around the anterior femoral neck onto the anterior hip capsule (**Figure 4**).
- The interval between the gluteus medius and the piriformis is opened. Sharp dissection with a knife blade or electrocautery is sometimes required to open this interval.
- The posterior border of the gluteus medius is retracted gently to expose the interval between the superior edge of the piriformis tendon and the inferior edge of the gluteus minimus. Gentle retraction is necessary to avoid excessive tension on the superior gluteal neurovascular pedicle.
- The short external rotators and the posterior capsular incision are mobilized. The gluteus minimus is protected and left undisturbed.
- The ischiofemoral ligament, which contributes substantially to posterior hip stability, is preserved for later repair.
- An approximately L-shaped incision is made, creating a flap consisting of the piriformis and short external rotators in a single capsulotendinous layer or in separate layers. The authors of this chapter prefer to create the flap in two layers to facilitate later repair of both structures independently.
- The flap is tagged to facilitate anatomic repair at the time of wound closure.
- The incision begins at the acetabular rim and courses along the superior border of the piriformis tendon distally to the insertion of the piriformis muscle at the piriformis fossa near the greater trochanter. The lower limb of the incision extends distally along the intertrochanteric line to the superior

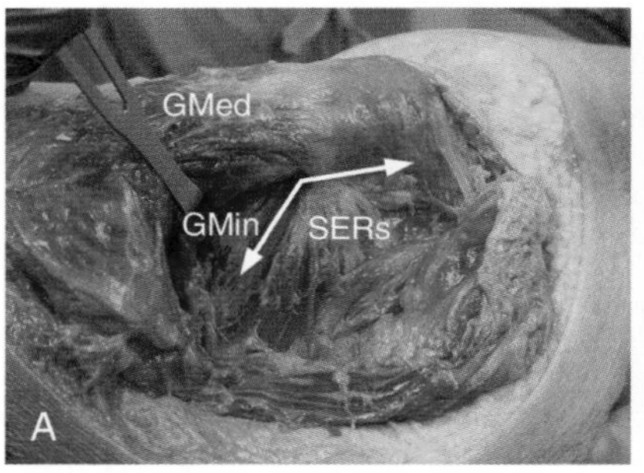

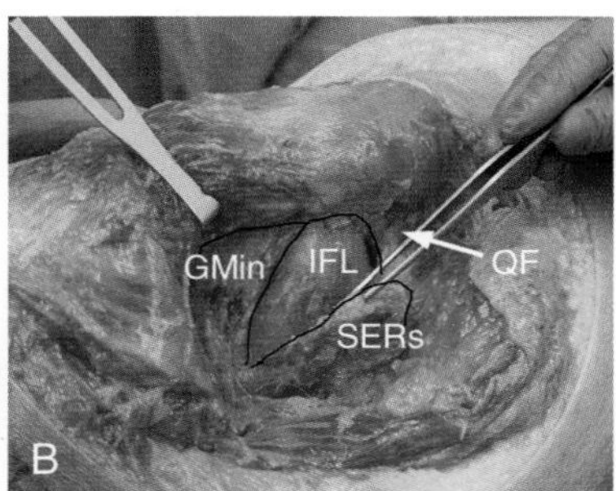

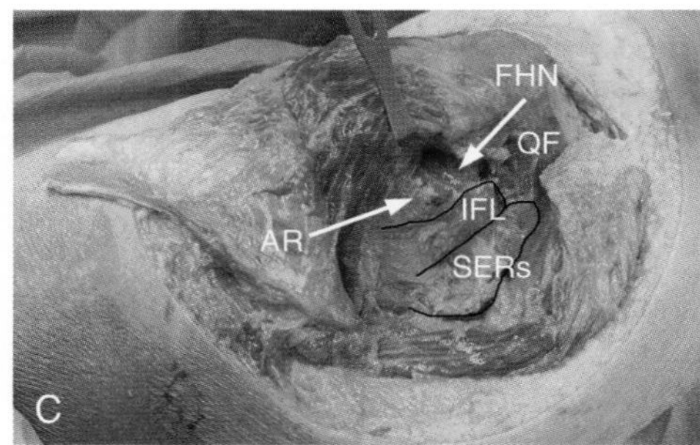

Figure 5 Photographs of the right hip from a cadaver specimen with the gluteus maximus reflected. **A,** The appearance of the approximately L-shaped incision (arrows) between the gluteus minimus (GMin) and the piriformis tendon. The incision extends distally through the short external rotators (SERs). **B,** The creation of the capsulotendinous flap in two layers (black lines). In the first layer, the SERs are reflected to expose the underlying ischiofemoral ligament (IFL). **C,** The reflection of the IFL and the SERs (black lines) to expose the underlying acetabular rim (AR) and femoral head and neck (FHN). The incision extends distally to the superior margin of the quadratus femoris (QF). After the incision is made, the hip can be dislocated posteriorly. GMed = gluteus medius.

border of the quadratus femoris (**Figure 5, A**).

- The shape of the incision preserves the entirety of the ischiofemoral ligament, which is incorporated into the repair of the posterior flap at the end of the procedure (**Figure 5, B**).
- The capsulotendinous flap is reflected posteriorly with the use of the previously placed suture, protecting the sciatic nerve and exposing the hip joint (**Figure 5, C**).
- The femoral head is dislocated posteriorly by means of flexion and internal rotation of the hip. The knee is kept flexed during this step to minimize tension on the sciatic nerve.
- The offset and length of the femoral neck are measured so that these dimensions can be compared with the preoperative plan (**Figure 6**).
- Careful measurement is critical to success in order to achieve the desired goal of either changing the offset and length or maintaining the offset and length as desired and planned.
- The measurements can be confirmed by means of intraoperative imaging.
- A femoral neck osteotomy is done with a sagittal saw at a level determined preoperatively by templating or intraoperatively in relation to the lesser trochanter.
- Care is taken to avoid notching of the greater trochanter, which would result in a stress riser that could lead to greater trochanter fracture.

ACETABULAR PREPARATION AND EXPOSURE

- The posterior approach affords excellent visualization of the acetabulum when the femur is translated forward through a combination of leg positioning and anterior capsular elevation.
- Optimal leg positioning is achieved by placing the hip in 45° of flexion and 10° of adduction, thereby relaxing the anterior hip capsule.
- To allow further translation of the femur, the anterior fibers of the hip capsule are elevated off the rim of the acetabulum with the use of electrocautery or sharp dissection.
- The anterior acetabular retractor is placed with direct visualization underneath the femoral neck and over the anterior lip of the acetabulum.
- The femur is retracted anteriorly to provide an unobstructed view of the acetabulum (**Figure 7, A**).
- If visualization is not adequate, the inferior capsule is palpated to assess tension. Inadequate visualization is likely the result of a tight inferior capsule. If necessary, the inferior capsule is divided radially at the 6-o'clock position with electrocautery. An inferior acetabular retractor is placed, if necessary, to aid in acetabular exposure (**Figure 7, A**). Electrocautery is preferable to the use of a knife blade because branches of the obturator artery may be present in this location.
- After the inferior capsule is mobilized, the transverse acetabular ligament is visible. This ligament does not attach to the femur and does not need to be excised or divided unless it obstructs the view of osteophytes at the inferior border of the acetabulum.
- With the femur retracted anteriorly, the degenerative labrum is excised, marginal osteophytes are removed, and acetabular reaming begins.
- To facilitate reaming of the acetabulum and placement of the acetabular implant, the Charnley retractor may be removed. Visualization of the entire acetabulum can be achieved with the use of only the anterior acetabular retractor and a Hibbs or Hohmann retractor posteriorly (**Figure 7, B**).
- Forceful posterior retraction is

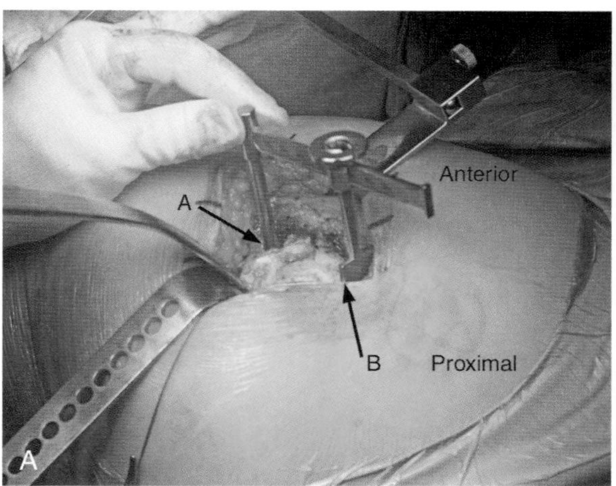

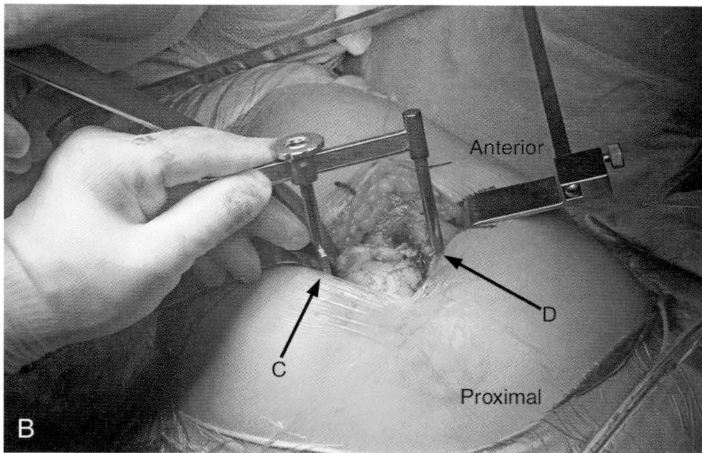

Figure 6 Intraoperative photographs of a left hip. **A,** Measurement of the femoral neck length with the use of a caliper extending from the neck cut and superior margin of the quadratus femoris (A) to the most superior point on the femoral head (B). **B,** Measurement of femoral offset with the use of a caliper extending from the most medial portion of the femoral head (C) to the posterior aspect of the greater trochanter (D). These measurements are recorded and are measured again when the trial implants are placed, using the same landmarks and taking into account the size of the acetabular cup and polyethylene liner.

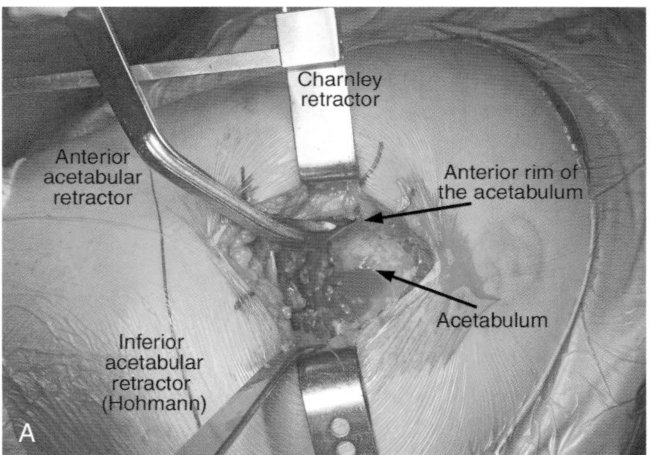

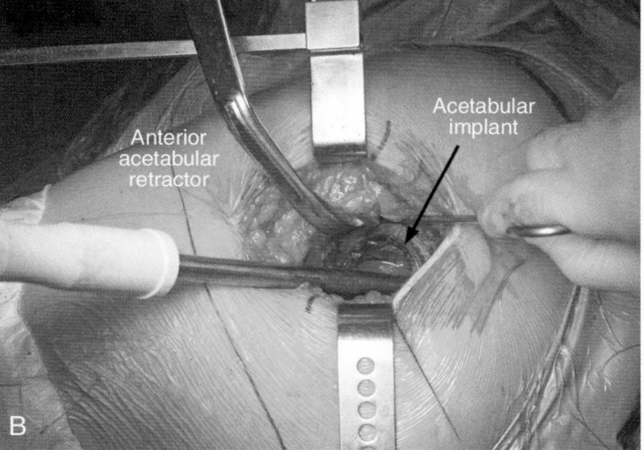

Figure 7 **A,** Intraoperative photograph of a left hip shows retractor placement for acetabular exposure. An anterior acetabular retractor is placed along the anterior rim of the acetabulum, translating the femur anteriorly. An inferior acetabular retractor is used along the posteroinferior rim of the acetabulum if necessary. **B,** Intraoperative photograph of the same hip shows reaming. The inferior retractor has been removed to avoid obstruction of the reamer.

limited to avoid pressure on the sciatic nerve.

- Successful acetabular reaming requires creation of a spheric socket shape and avoidance of asymmetric or misdirected reaming.
- Care is taken to ensure that the femur does not push the reamer posteriorly into the posterior column and that the skin and soft tissue at the inferior aspect of the wound do not raise the reamer into the lateral rim of the acetabulum.

FEMORAL PREPARATION AND EXPOSURE

- Femoral preparation is typically done after placement of the acetabular implant to minimize bleeding from the femoral canal during preparation of the acetabulum.
- The hip is flexed so that the femoral shaft aligns with the skin incision, and the limb is internally rotated to 90° or more.
- A narrow retractor is placed beneath the femoral neck to elevate and expose the proximal femur and protect the posterior soft tissues.

- A sponge is placed underneath the retractor to better distribute pressure and protect the skin edge and posterior soft tissues. A second retractor, such as a sharp Hohmann retractor, is placed medial to the calcar femorale, if necessary.
- The combination of limb positioning and retractor placement allows sufficient visualization to ensure proper lateralization and anteversion of the femoral broaches and reaming devices.
- Careful movements of the proximal femoral elevator and the leg permit better visualization of the piriformis fossa or calcar femorale to optimize implant fit and position while reducing the risk of a calcar split or other intraoperative femur fracture.
- Trial reduction is performed to ensure implant fit, limb length, joint stability, soft-tissue tensioning, and motion without impingement.
- Intraoperative radiography can be useful to assess implant position size, limb length, and restoration of offset.
- Generally, the anteversion of the femoral implant re-creates the natural femoral anteversion, and the acetabular cup is positioned parallel to the transverse acetabular ligament. This strategy re-creates the combined natural anteversion of the patient's hip instead of using an arbitrary target as a guide.

PROSTHESIS IMPLANTATION

- When the femoral and acetabular implants are placed, they are carefully passed through the wound to avoid contamination by the skin edges or obstruction of the porous surface of the implant by soft tissue.
- The previously discussed principles of soft-tissue management, including movement of the limb and retractors to avoid excess skin tension, are followed during implantation of the prosthesis.
- Irrigation of the bone bed helps to avoid inadvertent contamination of the wound.
- During placement of the acetabular implant, the femur is retracted forward to avoid the risk of retroversion or vertical socket placement resulting from bone or soft-tissue obstruction.
- The proximal femur is exposed by means of limb positioning and retractor placement, and the final femoral implant is placed.

Wound Closure

- The wound is cleansed with the use of a mechanical lavage system.
- If any devitalized tissue is present, it is sharply débrided.
- Skin edges are carefully inspected. Any edges that appear macerated or damaged are débrided. Removal of damaged tissue minimizes the risk of wound dehiscence, infection, or hematoma.
- Hemostasis is ensured before closure. Particular attention is directed to the inferior capsular branches of the obturator vessels and the branches of the medial femoral circumflex vessels running in the quadratus femoris muscle and on the posterior aspect of the femoral neck.
- Suction drains typically are not used but are placed if desired.
- Intravenous tranexamic acid (10 mg/kg) is administered.
- Anatomic wound closure is performed to restore the normal tissue relationships.
- Meticulous closure of the posterior hip capsule is necessary to reduce the risk of postoperative posterior hip dislocation. Several clinical studies support repair of the hip capsule because it is associated with a lower rate of posterior hip dislocation.
- The apex of the triangular capsulotendinous posterior flap, including the piriformis tendon, is pulled beneath the posterior border of the gluteus medius tendon toward the piriformis fossa. The suture is passed through the gluteus medius tendon or trochanteric drill holes (**Figure 8**).
- The flap is sutured to the gluteus medius tendon to maintain compliance of the repair.
- The upper portion of the repair can be strengthened by placing sutures directly into the hip capsule.
- The remainder of the wound is closed in layers, starting with the fascia of the gluteus maximus and any part of the tensor fasciae that was incised, proceeding to the subcutaneous layer, and finishing with nylon skin sutures or skin adhesive.
- A small, moisture-proof dressing is applied.

Postoperative Regimen

Preoperative patient education, accelerated postoperative rehabilitation, and multimodal analgesia with limited use of narcotics have been shown to result in shorter postoperative hospital stays and quicker return to function. Rapid recovery protocols have been augmented with the use of regional anesthesia and intraoperative periarticular local injections. Patients on a rapid rehabilitation protocol typically are mobilized to full weight bearing on the day of the procedure and are targeted for discharge within 24 to 48 hours if medically stable.

Several studies have assessed the benefit of capsular repair after THA performed via the posterior approach. Overall, capsular repair has been shown to be effective, with rates of dislocation often less than 1% and multiple studies reporting no instances of dislocation. Postoperative hip precautions are therefore at the discretion of the surgeon. One of the authors of this chapter does not

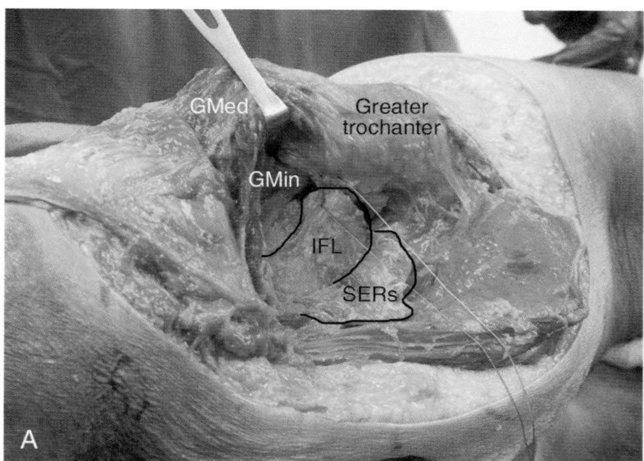

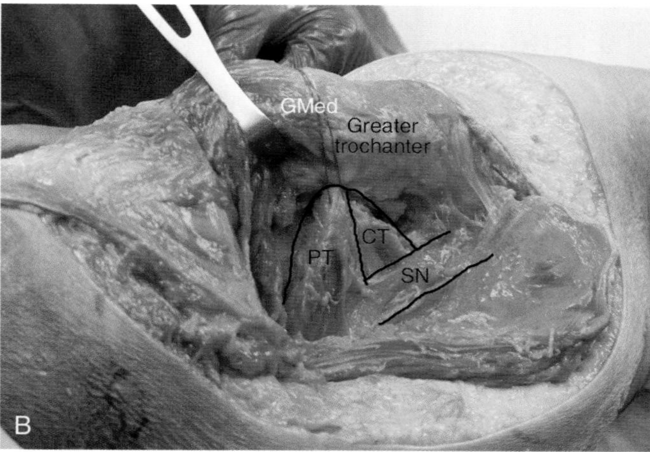

Figure 8 Photographs of the right hip from a cadaver specimen show closure of the posterior capsulotendinous structures. **A,** After the final implants are placed, the ischiofemoral ligament (IFL) can be reapproximated, strengthening the posterior capsular closure. **B,** After the IFL is closed, the short external rotators (SERs), including the piriformis tendon (PT) and conjoined tendon (CT; bounded by the black arc), are sutured to the tendinous insertion of the gluteus medius (GMed) on the greater trochanter. The relationship of the tendons to the sciatic nerve (SN) (indicated by parallel black lines) is demonstrated. GMin = gluteus minimus.

impose any posterior hip precautions postoperatively (T.P.V.). Patients are mobilized to full weight bearing using crutches or a walker on the day of the procedure and are instructed to discontinue use of the crutches or walker when desired, generally within days after surgery.

Preoperative strategies to facilitate patient satisfaction and timely recovery include patient education and the use of preemptive multimodal analgesia. Preoperative patient education can help prepare patients and their families for the procedure and expedite postoperative rehabilitation.

Avoiding Pitfalls and Complications

A major advantage of the posterior approach is the ease with which the surgeon can extend the incision to improve visualization and exposure. With experience and an improved understanding of the relevant anatomy, the surgeon can progressively limit the extent of the incision and soft-tissue dissection by using retraction maneuvers and limb-positioning adjustments to take advantage of skin, fat, fascia, and muscle compliance at each layer of the exposure. The prolonged use of self-retaining retractors should be avoided because they can damage soft tissues and compromise soft-tissue healing. The amount of exposure ultimately depends on the surgeon's judgment. A successful outcome is more important than the length of the incision. Poor visualization can result in soft-tissue injury, inaccurate reaming, and suboptimal implant placement. To avoid these pitfalls, the surgeon should lengthen the incision if the procedure becomes difficult or if placement of instruments in the wound would require excess pressure on soft tissues.

To minimize the risk of postoperative dislocation, care must be taken to perform meticulous dissection, preservation, and repair of the short external rotators and the capsule. This attention to detail will facilitate a robust capsular repair during closure. To ensure accurate acetabular implant placement, sufficient mobilization of the femur anterior to the acetabulum is necessary. Poor mobilization of the femur can result in misdirection of the acetabular reamers or the acetabular implant. Similarly, poor visualization of the proximal femur can result in varus positioning or undersizing of the femoral implant. Intraoperative radiography with trial implants is helpful to ensure correct implant positioning.

Bibliography

Barrett WP, Turner SE, Leopold JP: Prospective randomized study of direct anterior vs postero-lateral approach for total hip arthroplasty. *J Arthroplasty* 2013;28(9):1634-1638.

Bergin PF, Doppelt JD, Kephart CJ, et al: Comparison of minimally invasive direct anterior versus posterior total hip arthroplasty based on inflammation and muscle damage markers. *J Bone Joint Surg Am* 2011;93(15):1392-1398.

Berstock JR, Blom AW, Beswick AD: A systematic review and meta-analysis of the standard versus mini-incision posterior approach to total hip arthroplasty. *J Arthroplasty* 2014;29(10):1970-1982.

Chiu FY, Chen CM, Chung TY, Lo WH, Chen TH: The effect of posterior capsulorrhaphy in primary total hip arthroplasty: A prospective randomized study. *J Arthroplasty* 2000;15(2):194-199.

Hailer NP, Weiss RJ, Stark A, Kärrholm J: The risk of revision due to dislocation after total hip arthroplasty depends on surgical approach, femoral head size, sex, and primary diagnosis: An analysis of 78,098 operations in the Swedish Hip Arthroplasty Register. *Acta Orthop* 2012;83(5):442-448.

Hewitt JD, Glisson RR, Guilak F, Vail TP: The mechanical properties of the human hip capsule ligaments. *J Arthroplasty* 2002;17(1):82-89.

Jameson SS, Mason J, Baker P, et al: A comparison of surgical approaches for primary hip arthroplasty: A cohort study of patient reported outcome measures (PROMs) and early revision using linked national databases. *J Arthroplasty* 2014;29(6):1248-1255.e1.

Jewett BA, Collis DK: High complication rate with anterior total hip arthroplasties on a fracture table. *Clin Orthop Relat Res* 2011;469(2):503-507.

Ji HM, Kim KC, Lee YK, Ha YC, Koo KH: Dislocation after total hip arthroplasty: A randomized clinical trial of a posterior approach and a modified lateral approach. *J Arthroplasty* 2012;27(3):378-385.

Lindgren JV, Wretenberg P, Kärrholm J, Garellick G, Rolfson O: Patient-reported outcome is influenced by surgical approach in total hip replacement: A study of the Swedish Hip Arthroplasty Register including 42,233 patients. *Bone Joint J* 2014;96-B(5):590-596.

Ogonda L, Wilson R, Archbold P, et al: A minimal-incision technique in total hip arthroplasty does not improve early postoperative outcomes: A prospective, randomized, controlled trial. *J Bone Joint Surg Am* 2005;87(4):701-710.

Palan J, Beard DJ, Murray DW, Andrew JG, Nolan J: Which approach for total hip arthroplasty: Anterolateral or posterior? *Clin Orthop Relat Res* 2009;467(2):473-477.

Pour AE, Parvizi J, Sharkey PF, Hozack WJ, Rothman RH: Minimally invasive hip arthroplasty: What role does patient preconditioning play? *J Bone Joint Surg Am* 2007;89(9):1920-1927.

Rodriguez JA, Deshmukh AJ, Rathod PA, et al: Does the direct anterior approach in THA offer faster rehabilitation and comparable safety to the posterior approach? *Clin Orthop Relat Res* 2014;472(2):455-463.

White RE Jr, Forness TJ, Allman JK, Junick DW: Effect of posterior capsular repair on early dislocation in primary total hip replacement. *Clin Orthop Relat Res* 2001;(393):163-167.

Woolson ST, Mow CS, Syquia JF, Lannin JV, Schurman DJ: Comparison of primary total hip replacements performed with a standard incision or a mini-incision. *J Bone Joint Surg Am* 2004;86(7):1353-1358.

Chapter 4
Primary Total Hip Arthroplasty Through the Direct Anterior Approach on a Standard Surgical Table

Peter Pyrko, MD, PhD
William Hozack, MD

Indications

Since the 1970s, total hip arthroplasty (THA) has most often been performed through the direct lateral approach or the posterior approach to the hip. More recently, surgeons have used several new approaches, often called minimally invasive, with the goals of improving outcomes and minimizing damage to the structures surrounding the hip. Among these approaches, the direct anterior approach (DAA) has achieved popularity surpassing that of other new approaches.

The DAA uses the Hueter interval, an anterior approach to the hip that was first described in 1881 and is also known as the Smith-Petersen approach because of its description in 1917 in the United States. It uses the intermuscular and internervous interval between the sartorius muscle, which is innervated by the femoral nerve, and the tensor fascia lata muscle (TFL), which is innervated by the superior gluteal nerve. Its proponents posit that less muscular damage occurs with this approach than with other approaches, resulting in quicker recovery and decreased postoperative pain; however, this claim requires more thorough investigation.

Hip arthroplasty using the DAA was first described in the 1950s, with acceptable outcomes. However, the training of early arthroplasty surgeons emphasized a transtrochanteric approach, and orthopaedic residents typically were instructed in the use of the DAA primarily for the management of pediatric hip infections. The modern American experience with the DAA dates to 1980, when a series of 104 procedures performed with the approach was published. The authors of the study reported a mean procedure length of 65 minutes and substantial blood loss requiring transfusions. One of the authors of the study subsequently modified and improved the original technique. In particular, that author advocated approaching the joint through the fascial sleeve that envelopes the TFL, instead of performing an incision medial to the TFL (a key difference between the modern DAA and the Smith-Petersen approach). This method has substantially influenced modern DAA procedures.

Dr. Hozack or an immediate family member has received royalties from, serves as a paid consultant to, and has received research or institutional support from Stryker and serves as a board member, owner, officer, or committee member of The Hip Society. Neither Dr. Pyrko nor any immediate family member has received anything of value from or has stock or stock options held in a commercial company or institution related directly or indirectly to the subject of this chapter.

Although more surgeons are now learning the DAA during their training, knowledge of the approach in general is limited. Most surgeons who use the DAA learned it after completion of formal orthopaedic training. When trauma surgeons began performing hip arthroplasty, the use of a trauma table and intraoperative fluoroscopy became more prevalent. Interest in the approach also has given rise to the development of new surgical tables, retractors, and instrumentation (**Figure 1**).

Because the area just medial to the Hueter interval contains multiple vital structures, including the femoral artery and nerve, a thorough understanding of anatomy of the anterior thigh is required to use the DAA successfully. The most prominent landmark is the anterior superior iliac spine (ASIS), which can be easily palpated in the lower, lateral area of the abdomen, superior to the pubis. The sartorius and the inguinal ligament insert on the ASIS, and the TFL and gluteus medius attach just lateral to it. The lateral femoral cutaneous nerve (LFCN) emerges beneath the inguinal ligament and courses laterally over the belly of the sartorius muscle, in the area of the incision and the TFL distally. The femoral nerve, artery, and vein are located medial to the sartorius. The rectus femoris muscle, which divides proximally into direct (originating from the anterior

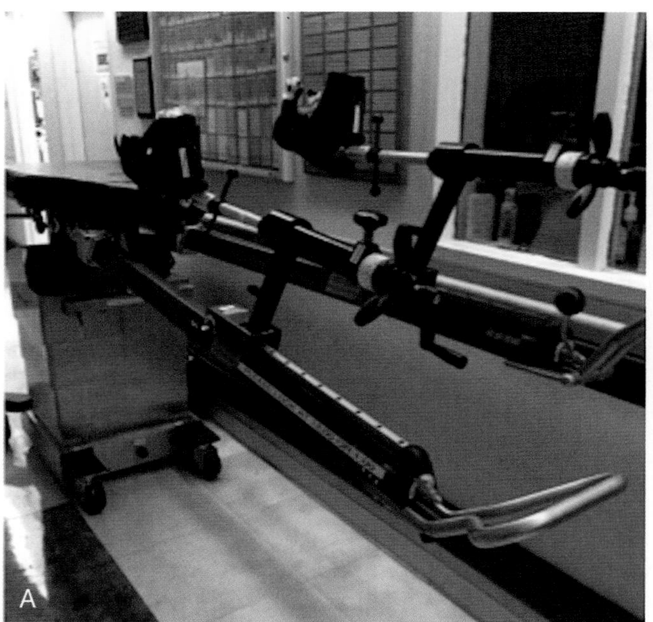

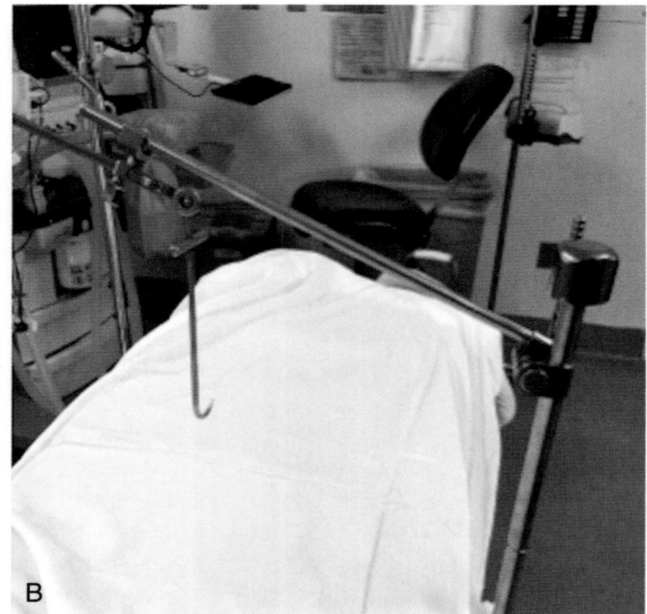

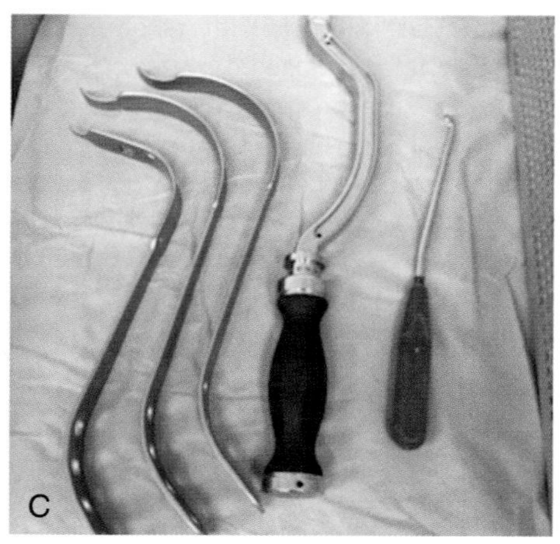

Figure 1 Photographs show a surgical table (**A**), table attachment (**B**), and retractors and instrumentation (**C**) that have been developed for use in total hip arthroplasty through the direct anterior approach.

inferior iliac spine) and reflected (originating from the anterior lip of the acetabulum) heads, runs deep to the sartorius. The gluteus medius and minimus (the abductor complex) originate from the iliac wing, run deep to the TFL, and insert on the lateral aspect of the greater trochanter. The origins of the vastus lateralis and the vastus intermedius are located deeper, on the anterior aspect of the femur at the intertrochanteric line. The iliopsoas muscle and tendon emerge under the inguinal ligament, pass over the hip capsule, and descend posteriorly to attach to the lesser trochanter.

Indications for THA are the same regardless of the approach used. Although the selection of the approach is usually dictated by the surgeon's preference, aspects of each approach can make the procedure more or less difficult in particular patient groups.

Contraindications

Although the DAA has no true contraindications, the approach may be more difficult in some patients than in others. As with other approaches, obesity and muscular body habitus can make the DAA more difficult. Although the adipose tissue overlying the anterior thigh is usually less prominent than the adipose tissue in the lateral or posterior gluteal region and may not hinder the approach, the presence of a substantial panniculus exposes the DAA wound to a moist environment that may promote chronic skin irritation, wound complications such as fungal infections (many obese patients have preexisting fungal infection in that area), or even small areas of dehiscence. These patients require additional wound care and preoperative screening for fungal panniculitis. Some surgeons advocate the use of an abdominal binder to keep the panniculus away from the incision to avoid wound complications, or use of an alternative surgical approach.

Conversion to THA through the DAA can also present a challenge to the surgeon. It is impossible to remove lateral plates through a direct anterior incision. However, additional small incisions can be made to remove screws or smaller plates.

Despite misconceptions to the contrary, both proximal and distal extensions to the DAA are possible; however, they may be difficult for a surgeon who has limited experience with this approach. In patients undergoing complicated procedures that would require substantial distal or proximal dissection, such as periprosthetic femur fracture fixation or THA requiring shortening osteotomy, a surgeon who has limited experience with the DAA may consider a different approach for the procedure. However, experienced surgeons can perform some complicated procedures, including revisions, through the DAA.

Alternative Treatments

As noted, any of the other approaches to the hip can be used for THA, with the choice depending primarily on the surgeon's preference and familiarity with each approach. When the DAA is used, the authors of this chapter prefer to use a standard surgical table that occasionally is flexed to facilitate femoral exposure. Alternatives include the use of a specialized surgical table with or without intraoperative fluoroscopy, or the use of a standard surgical table with special attachments.

The use of a specialized surgical table facilitates manipulation of the affected extremity. The patient is positioned on a radiolucent pedestal that ends at the level of the ischium, with the pubis rested on the post placed between the thighs (**Figure 1, A**). The patient's feet are placed in supportive boots. Femoral exposure is achieved by flexion, adduction, and external rotation and can be held in place with the use of a locking mechanism that is part of the table. Traction can be applied, and dislocation is possible without an in situ femoral neck cut. A fluoroscopic C-arm can be placed under the table to evaluate the positioning of the acetabular and femoral implants. Because the feet are in the boots, limb lengths are often assessed radiographically as well. These special tables are expensive, and specific complications have been associated with their use. Pudendal nerve palsy can result from pressure of the post on the pudendal nerve. Fractures of the ankle resulting from manipulation of the feet have been reported. When fluoroscopy is used, protective gear must be worn by the entire surgical team. Additionally, patient positioning requires extra surgical time, especially early in the team's learning curve.

Some surgeons use a hook-and-arm mechanism that can be attached in a sterile manner to a standard surgical table (**Figure 1, B**). Acetabular exposure is achieved in a standard manner. When femoral exposure begins, the table is flexed, the attachment is affixed to the table, the hook is placed under the femur, and the femur is elevated. After adequate exposure is achieved, the mechanism is locked. This method can be awkward because the hook must be re-placed each time the hip is reduced for trialing.

Results

Proponents of minimally invasive approaches to the hip have often postulated that their patients have better outcomes. Surgeons who frequently use the DAA report that their patients have decreased muscle damage and pain, faster recovery, and improved gait mechanics. The authors of one recent article described more rapid cessation of walking aids with the DAA than with other approaches. However, most of the existing studies lack the necessary design characteristics or power to validate these claims. Studies of gait patterns after use of the DAA exemplify this problem. The authors of one study of gait patterns after THA using the DAA described the patients as having better stride time and cadence speed at 6 weeks postoperatively. Another study compared patients who underwent THA through the DAA or direct lateral approach with normal control subjects. Both groups had abnormal gait, but the gait patterns of DAA patients resembled those of normal subjects more closely. The authors of a different study described less stiffness in DAA patients than in other patients, but the difference disappeared at 6 months postoperatively. Although recovery in the first few postoperative weeks may be more rapid with this approach, substantial improvement in long-term outcomes has not been demonstrated in appropriately powered randomized trials (**Table 1**). In addition, the DAA carries the risk of complications specific to the approach, which are discussed later in this chapter.

Techniques

Setup/Exposure

- Primary and revision THA can be performed through the DAA with the patient in the supine position on a standard orthopaedic surgical table (**Figure 2, A**). The use of a standard surgical table with the affected leg unconstrained facilitates intraoperative assessment of limb length and stability. Supine positioning improves assessment of limb lengths intraoperatively because it reduces the influence of pelvic obliquity.

Table 1 Studies of Total Hip Arthroplasty Comparing the Direct Anterior Approach With Other Approaches

Authors (Year)	Number of Patients	Approach (Patients)	Mean Patient Age in Years	Follow-up	Results
Bergin et al (2011)	57	DAA (29) or posterior (28)	68 (DAA group) 65 (posterior approach group)	2 d	Inflammatory markers were slightly decreased in the DAA group compared with the posterior approach group
Bremer et al (2011)	50	DAA (25) or transgluteal (25)	NR	1 yr	Detachment of the abductor insertion, partial tears and tendinitis, bursal fluid, and fatty atrophy of the abductors was less common on MRI in the DAA group than in the transgluteal approach group
Barrett et al (2013)	77	DAA (43) or posterolateral (44)	NR	6 wk, 3 mo, 6 mo, and 12 mo	More patients in the DAA group than in the posterolateral approach group climbed stairs normally and walked without assistance at 6 wk postoperatively There was a difference only at the 6-wk follow-up; results were similar between the groups at 3-, 6-, and 12-mo follow-up
Taunton et al (2014)	54	DAA (27) or mini-posterior (27)	NR	Mean, 6 mo	Time to unassisted ambulation was 22 d in the DAA group and 28 d in the mini-posterior approach group

DAA = direct anterior approach, NR = not reported.

- The patient is positioned on a bump that is centered on the ASIS. The most distal aspect of the bump should be in line with the most distal aspect of the ischium, which can be palpated when the hip is flexed.
- If the surgical plan requires hyperflexion of the table, the ASIS and the bump should be placed at the flexion point of the table. Flexion of the hip aids in femoral exposure by providing an easier angle for broaching and insertion of the femoral stem.
- The patient is positioned with the flank of the affected side in line with the edge of the table. An arm board placed on the contralateral side of the table provides extra space for abduction of the nonoperated leg during femoral preparation.
- Limb length is assessed before draping to ensure that the patient's shoulders, hips, and ankles are aligned to allow proper intraoperative assessment of limb length.
- The patient is prepped and draped in the usual manner (**Figure 2, B**).
- Depending on the surgeon's preference, both legs can be sterilely draped to allow easy assessment of limb length, or the nonoperated leg can be palpated through the drape (**Figure 2, C**).

Instruments/Equipment/ Implants Required

- The DAA can be performed with standard orthopaedic hip instrumentation.
- At the institution of the authors of this chapter, retractors, the surgical table, and the hip bump are used in the direct lateral approach to the hip as well.

Procedures

STANDARD DAA

- The incision begins 2 cm distal and lateral to the ASIS (**Figure 3, A**) and extends up to 10 cm toward the lateral aspect of the knee in line with the TFL.
- The surgeon can use the hip flexion crease to help identify the proximal position of the incision.
- The TFL is identified by the muscular fibers coursing laterally from the ASIS and by perforating vessels that enter anteriorly into the muscle belly.
- The fascia of the TFL is incised approximately 1 cm lateral to the interval with cautery, and the muscle is swept laterally off its posteromedial fascia (**Figure 3, B**).
- The superior neck of the femur is identified by palpation.
- A blunt Hohmann retractor is placed on the superior neck of the femur.
- A sharp Hohmann retractor is placed on the lateral aspect of the greater trochanter, retracting the TFL laterally.
- Another retractor is used to pull the sartorius medially.
- The branches of the lateral circumflex femoral artery exposed by the placement of these retractors are carefully cauterized and transected (**Figure 3, C**).
- The remainder of the posterior fascia of the TFL is incised to expose the anterior hip capsule (**Figure 3, D**).

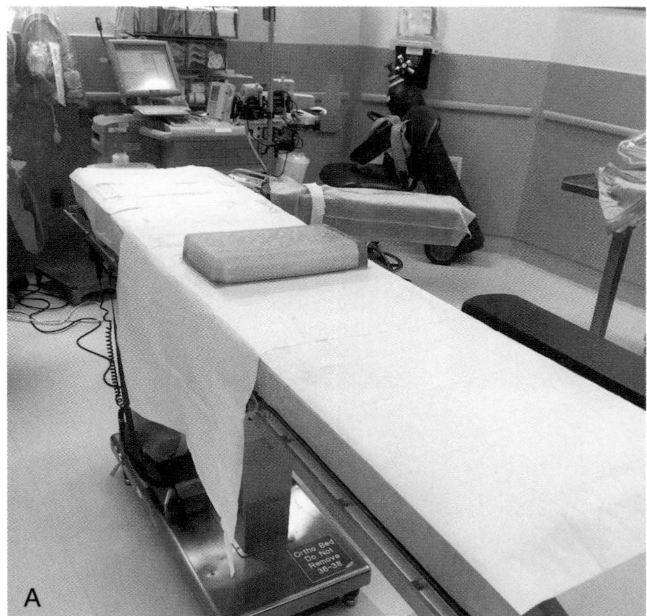

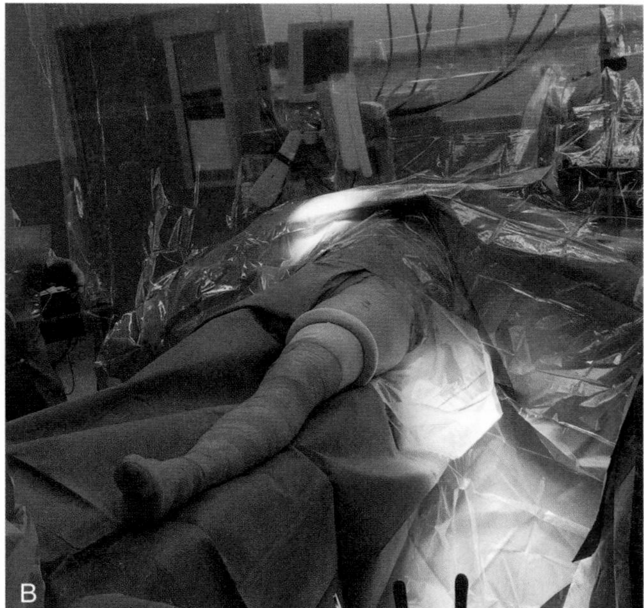

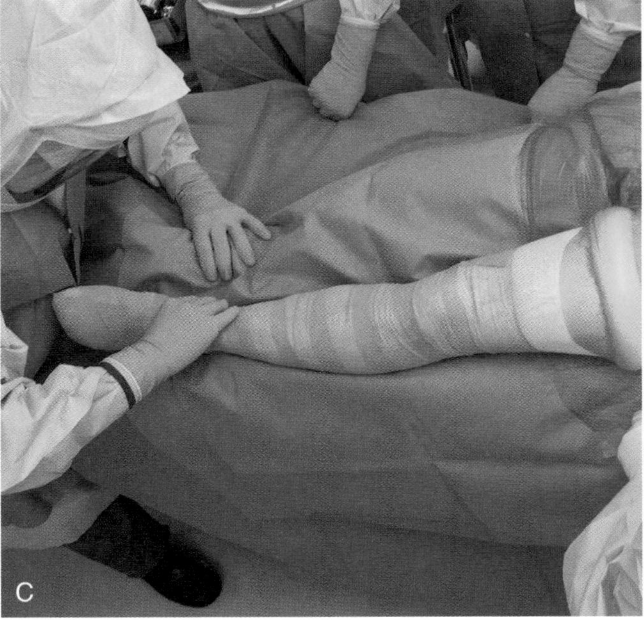

Figure 2 Photographs show setup and positioning for total hip arthroplasty through the direct anterior approach on a standard surgical table. The patient is positioned on a bump (**A**) and prepped and draped in the usual manner (**B**). **C,** Even with the contralateral limb draped out of the surgical field, the surgeon can still compare the limb lengths.

- The inferior femoral neck is identified, and a blunt Hohmann retractor is placed on its surface, with care taken to place the retractor proximally and not distally. Care is taken to stay proximal to the quadriceps muscle to avoid unnecessary bleeding.
- A space between the capsule and a reflected head of the rectus muscle is developed with a Cobb retractor and a sharp Hohmann retractor. A light source is placed into this space on the anterior column.
- The anterior capsule is excised.
- A double osteotomy of the femoral neck is performed (**Figure 4, A**).
- The femoral head is removed (**Figure 4, B**). A benefit of this approach is that it avoids the need for dislocation of the femoral head.
- The acetabulum is exposed with three retractors. First, a narrow sharp Hohmann retractor is placed on the posterior acetabulum. Second, the retractor over the anterior column is repositioned directly onto

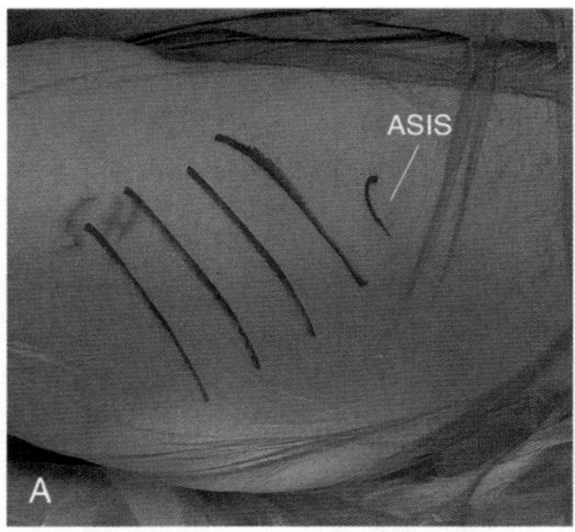

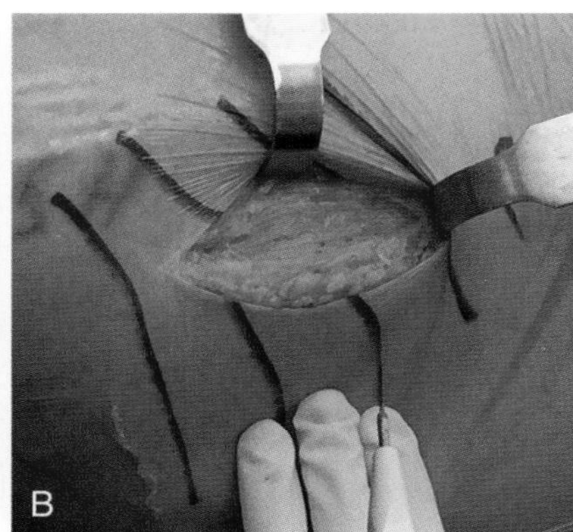

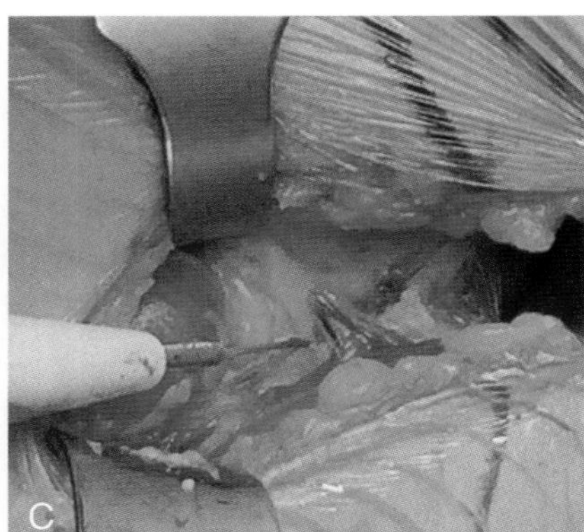

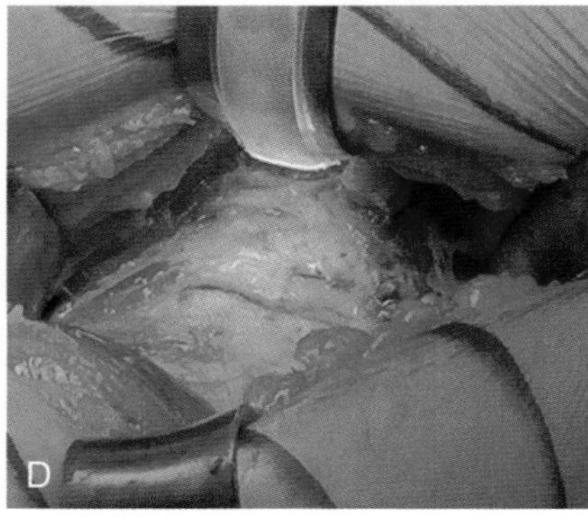

Figure 3 Intraoperative photographs show the initial exposure for total hip arthroplasty through the direct anterior approach on a standard surgical table. The incision begins 2 cm distal and lateral to the anterior superior iliac spine (**A**) and is carried down to the fascia of the tensor fascia lata muscle (**B**). **C,** The vessels crossing the surgical field are identified and cauterized. **D,** The anterior hip capsule is exposed.

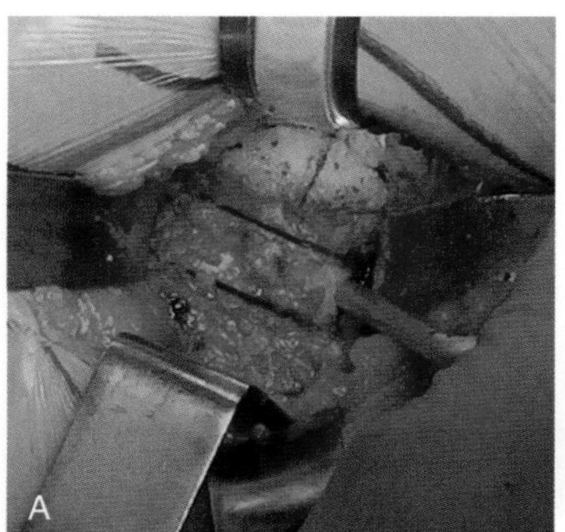

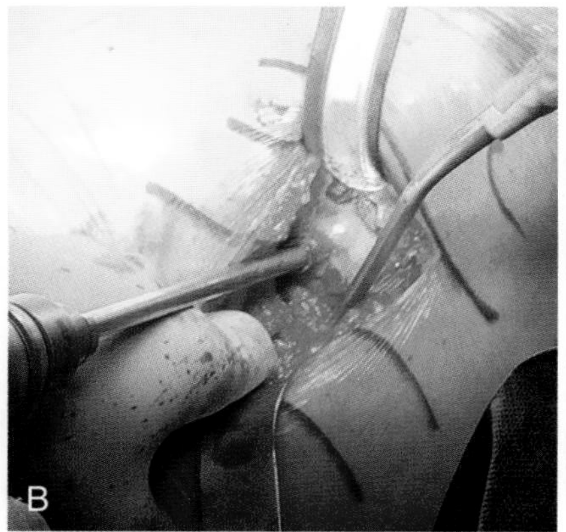

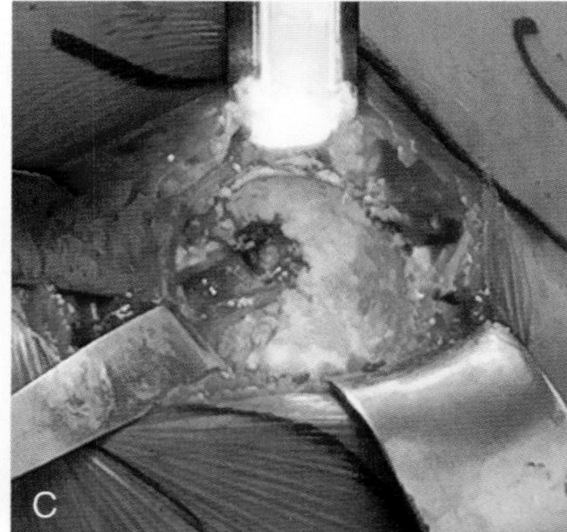

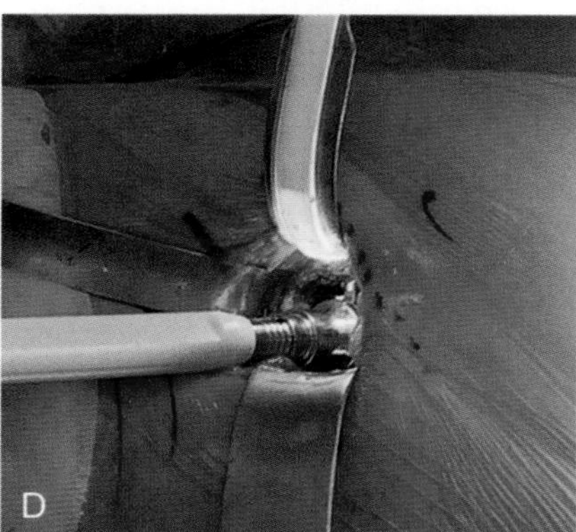

Figure 4 Intraoperative photographs show acetabular exposure and reaming. **A,** A double femoral neck osteotomy is performed. **B,** The intervening section between the femoral neck and the femoral head is removed. **C,** After removal of the femoral neck, the acetabulum is exposed. **D,** Reaming of the acetabulum is performed.

bone. Finally, a blunt Hohmann retractor is placed into the teardrop through an incision in the inferior capsule (**Figure 4, C**).

- The acetabulum is prepared in standard fashion (**Figure 4, D**). A noncemented hemispheric acetabular implant is placed.
- Attention is turned to femoral exposure. The contralateral limb is abducted, and the ipsilateral limb is placed in a figure-of-4 position (**Figure 5, A**). This position places the femur in 90° of external rotation and facilitates exposure of the proximal femur.
- Retractors are placed laterally and medially to expose the osteotomized femoral neck.
- A triangular part of the capsule between the abductors and the posterosuperior acetabulum is identified and excised (**Figure 5, B**).
- The superior capsule is incised down to the inner aspect of the greater trochanter in line with the lateral aspect of the femoral neck cut.
- A two-pronged retractor is placed into the space that was created. It should extend over the tip of the greater trochanter between the greater trochanter and the gluteus medius muscle.
- A vertical capsular release in the superior capsule is performed in line with this retractor down to the femoral neck, at which point it curves medially toward the piriformis fossa (**Figure 5, C**).
- Release of the piriformis muscle usually is not necessary.
- A bone hook is placed into the femoral neck and is used to gently raise the femur over and above the posterior acetabular rim (**Figure 5, D**). This move should not require much force.
- After the femur is elevated, the leg is positioned in adduction and external rotation to allow access to the femoral canal.

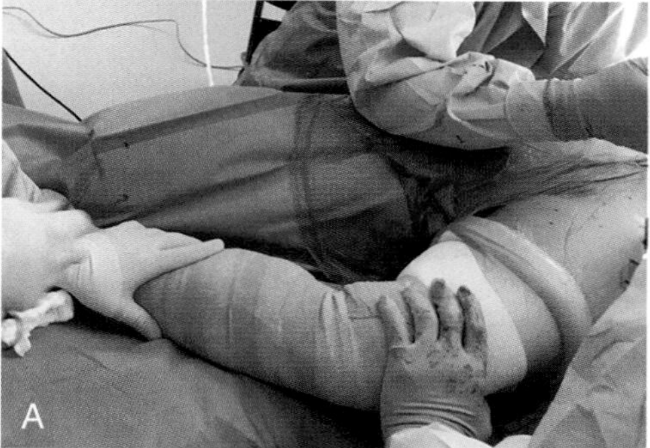

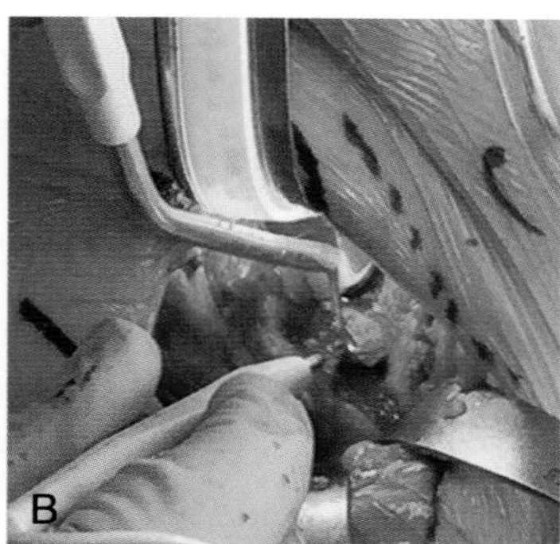

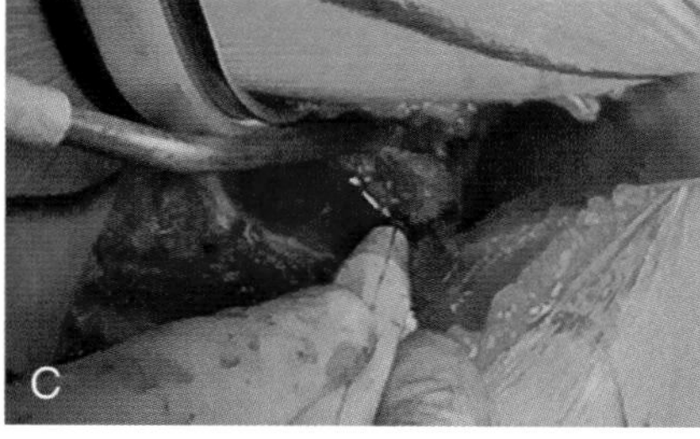

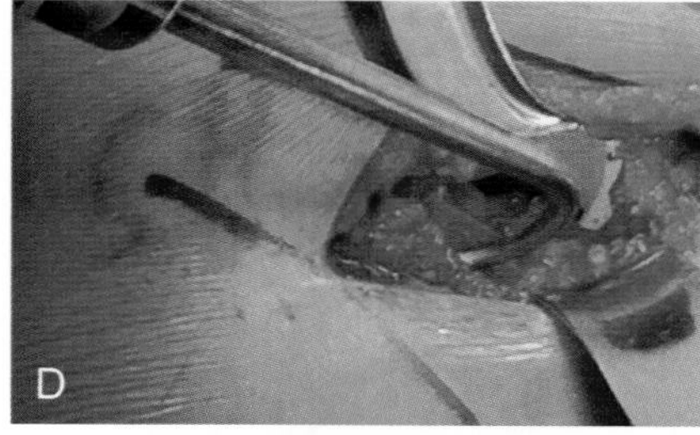

Figure 5 Intraoperative photographs show femoral exposure. **A,** The affected limb is placed in a figure-of-4 position. **B,** The posteromedial capsule is excised. **C,** The superolateral capsule is released. **D,** The femur is elevated.

- Femoral retractors are repositioned as needed.
- The femoral neck cut is checked, then revised if necessary. It is important to ensure sufficient femoral exposure and deliverance of the femur from under the posterior acetabular rim into the incision. Easy access to the femoral canal is necessary for correct insertion of a tapered stem. Inadequate femoral exposure can result in medial fractures of the femoral neck, perforation of the femoral canal, varus positioning of the stem within the canal, undersizing of the stem, and increased damage to the TFL and skin at the proximal aspect of the wound.
- Insertion of the tapered stem requires a precise sequence of steps to avoid common intraoperative complications. First, after the proximal femur is exposed, the remnant of the lateral femoral neck is removed with the use of a box osteotome or large, angled rongeurs or nibblers (**Figure 6, A**). This step removes a small amount of bone at the base of the piriformis fossa that might otherwise divert the path of the stem during broaching and force the stem into varus.
- With the use of a curved, blunt curet, the canal is opened and its direction is determined (**Figure 6, B**). Care must be taken not to perforate the femoral cortex, particularly in obese patients and patients with osteoporosis or femoral deformity. With the DAA, a posterior perforation is most common.
- Sequential broaches are used to contour the femur in both the mediolateral and AP dimensions (**Figure 6, C**). The trajectory of the broaches must follow the initial path of the curved curet. The surgeon must take care to minimize the number of blows with the mallet, frequently retract the mallet, and occasionally pause between blows to prevent fracture by reducing hoop stresses on the femur.

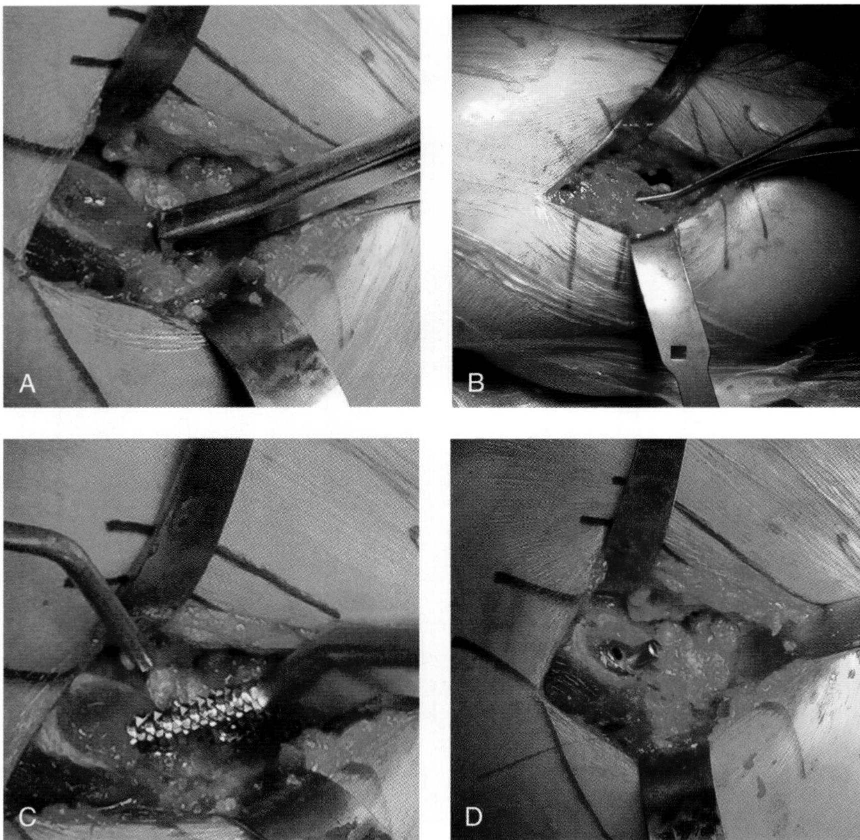

Figure 6 Intraoperative photographs show femoral preparation. **A,** The lateral femoral neck cortex is removed with a box osteotome. **B,** The direction of the femoral canal is determined with the use of a curved, blunt curet. **C,** The broaching begins. **D,** The final broach is seated in the femoral canal.

- In the process of malleting, the surgeon should ensure that some force is directed laterally to achieve lateralization of the broach and avoid varus positioning of the stem. Some surgeons use a specially designed first broach to ensure lateralization.
- Anteversion is determined by palpation of the knee epicondyles and should be carefully controlled to ensure that it remains constant throughout femoral preparation. Alteration of the anteversion after femoral broaching has been performed can compromise the rotational stability of the implant.
- Broaching continues until the final broach size, which was predicted by means of preoperative templating, is reached.
- Several clues help the surgeon determine that the final broach has been reached. First, this broach will seat firmly on the medial femoral neck cut (**Figure 6, D**). At this time, the sound that accompanies the broaching will change to a higher, sharper metallic pitch. Second, gentle malleting at this point will not result in advancement of the broach. Third, torsional force applied to the broach handle at this time should not result in rotational movement of the broach. Vigilant attention must be paid to these clues because vigorous malleting after the final broach size has been reached can result in fracture.
- Trial reduction is performed with the broach and a standard femoral neck segment.
- Stability is assessed in adduction and external rotation, in abduction and external rotation, and in flexion and external and internal rotation (**Figure 7, A** through **C**). Testing the hip in adduction and external rotation is important to assess for anterior dislocation.
- On the basis of the preoperative radiographs and intraoperative assessment, the surgeon should determine whether additional offset or length is required to ensure satisfactory soft-tissue tension and stability.
- Assessment of limb lengths is performed with the use of the patient's medial malleoli as reference points (**Figure 7, D**). The surgeon must ensure that the lower extremities are aligned with the patient's torso because abduction and adduction will result in apparent change in limb lengths.
- After stability and limb lengths are assessed and found to be satisfactory, the hip is dislocated and the broach is removed.
- The femoral prosthesis is gently introduced into the canal by hand in the space created by the broaching (**Figure 8, A**). The use of a stem insertion device may increase the risk of fracture because the insertion device can encounter the greater trochanter or can be pushed anteriorly by the proximal aspect of the wound, thereby forcing the stem into varus and resulting in fracture.
- After the stem has been partially advanced by hand, a stem insertion device may be used to impact the stem into place (**Figure 8, B**). Short, repeated taps with occasional pauses are used to reduce hoop stresses, and the surgeon should listen for a

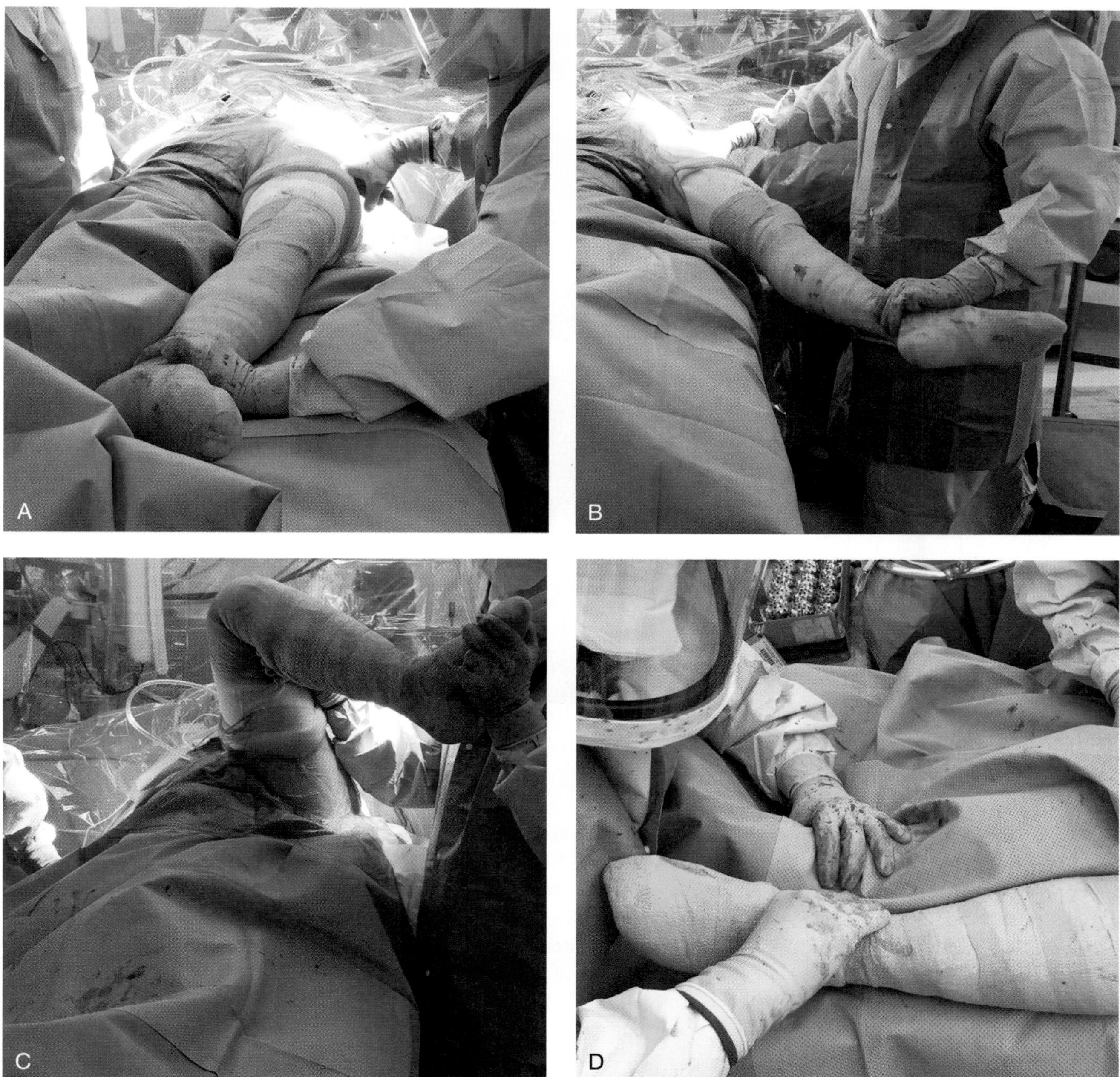

Figure 7 Intraoperative photographs show assessment of hip stability in adduction and external rotation (**A**), in abduction and external rotation (**B**), and in flexion and external rotation (**C**) as well as comparison of limb lengths (**D**). Stability is also assessed in flexion and internal rotation.

change in the pitch of the sound that accompanies insertion.

- If the prosthesis fails to advance to a position similar to that attained by the broach, it should be removed because this scenario indicates that the prosthesis is likely placed in the wrong position. Attempts at forceful advancement likely will result in a fracture.
- Because of the porous coating, the final prosthesis is larger than the broach of the same size; therefore, it will usually advance approximately 2 mm less than the final broach did.
- Care must be taken to avoid using the shortest trial femoral neck on

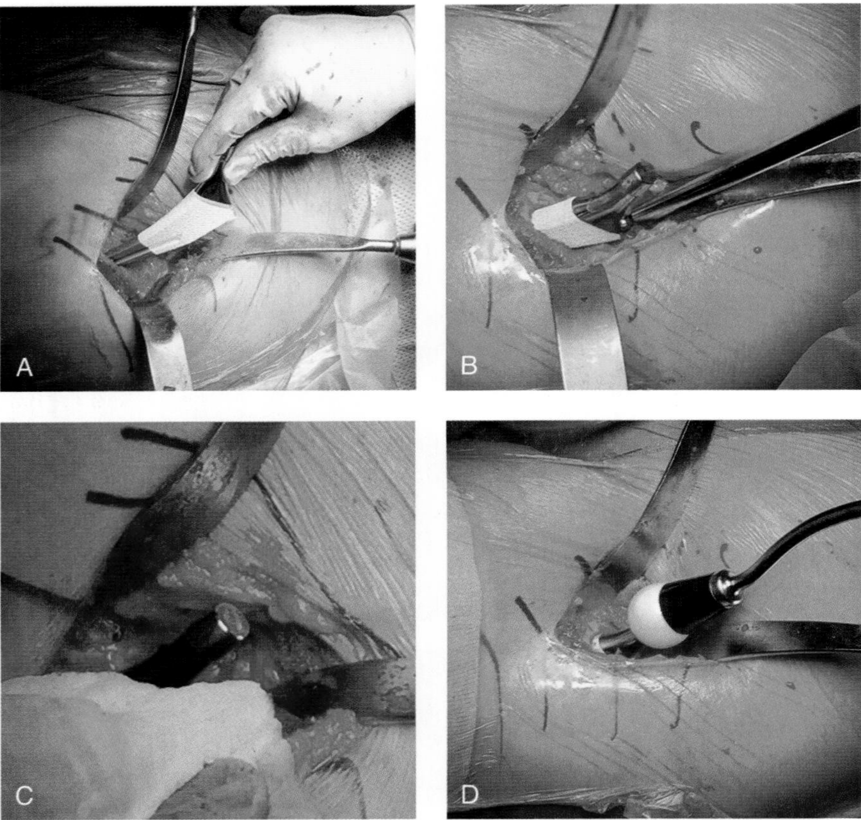

Figure 8 Intraoperative photographs show placement of the definitive implant. The prosthesis is placed by hand (**A**) and advanced with the stem insertion device (**B**). **C,** The trunnion is thoroughly cleaned. **D,** The final femoral head is impacted.

the broach, to allow for shortening of the femoral neck if the definitive prosthesis seats higher than the final broach did.

- After insertion of the definitive prosthesis and placement of the trial femoral head, a final assessment of leg lengths and stability is performed.
- After lavage is performed, the interior of the acetabulum is carefully inspected for debris.
- The taper trunnion is carefully cleaned and dried (**Figure 8, C**) to ensure that no debris is left on the taper that could lead to corrosion after the final femoral head is impacted.
- The definitive femoral head is applied onto the clean trunnion (**Figure 8, D**).
- Reduction is performed.

DISTAL OR PROXIMAL EXTENSION OF THE DAA

- A common complaint about the DAA is that distal extension of the approach is difficult or impossible. The authors of a recent cadaver study of the DAA attempted distal extension of the approach and claimed that it results in nerve damage and that passage of cerclage cables around the femur inevitably causes muscle damage.
- However, the authors of this chapter find that cerclage cables can easily be passed around the femur beneath the vastus musculature if care is taken to stay as close to the bone as possible.
- Additionally, although following the interval distally between the muscular structures can damage the neurovascular structures crossing the field and supplying the vastus lateralis muscle, extension of the exposure does not require this technique.
- Instead, the surgeon can perform a split in the vastus lateralis muscle starting lateral to the intertrochanteric line, in a fashion similar to the extension of the extended iliofemoral approach to the acetabulum. In fact, the DAA can be considered a portion of the iliofemoral approach to the acetabulum, the distal extension of which is commonly used in trauma surgery.
- In the technique used by the authors of this chapter, the initial anterior incision is carried laterally, the tensor fascia is transected and later repaired, and the approach connects to the standard lateral approach to the femur. The denervation resulting from this technique is similar to the denervation that occurs during the split of the vastus lateralis muscle in the lateral approach to the hip.
- Proximal extension of the DAA is possible when the iliofemoral approach is used. An osteotomy of the ASIS is performed, and the TFL is detached from the ilium. Distally, this approach is the same as the DAA. In fact, surgeons sometimes perform THA through an anterior approach when a periacetabular osteotomy is abandoned because of severe arthritis in the hip joint discovered intraoperatively.

Wound Closure

- The wound is irrigated.
- The fascia of the TFL is closed with a continuous stitch, with care taken to work in small increments medially to protect the LFCN, which runs just medial to the fascial incision.
- The subcutaneous tissue is closed in layers, including closure of the

Scarpa fascia if it is present, closure of the dermis, and finally running subcuticular closure.
- Topical skin adhesive is applied.
- After the topical skin adhesive is dry, a waterproof dressing is applied.

Postoperative Regimen

Many patients younger than age 65 years can be discharged on the day of surgery after meeting the discharge requirements set by the physical therapist. Most patients are released on postoperative day 1. No outpatient physical therapy is required. Patients are asked to ambulate to perform activities of daily living.

Avoiding Pitfalls and Complications

The literature clearly demonstrates that the DAA to the hip is not easy to learn. Studies have shown that a surgeon must perform approximately 100 procedures before the complication rate decreases from the initial level. Because performing this many procedures may take substantial time, the transition to this approach can be very difficult. Ideally, a surgeon would learn this approach during residency or fellowship training, much as other approaches for THA are learned. Some studies suggest that when THA is performed through the DAA by a surgeon well versed in the approach, the complication rate is similar to that of other common approaches. With larger femoral heads, the use of which has coincided with the increased popularity of the DAA, the dislocation rate is low (studies have reported rates of 0.96% and 1.5%), but it is not lower than that of other approaches as proponents of the DAA originally claimed it would be.

Certain complications are specific to the DAA. These complications include damage to the LFCN, which may manifest as numbness in the nerve distribution area on the lateral thigh or as painful meralgia paresthetica, which can be distressing to the patient. The incidence of these problems ranges from 1% to 67%. Because numbness on the lateral thigh may not be immediately obvious to the patient, the wide range of reported rates of LFCN-related complications may depend on how carefully the surgeon was looking for them in the postoperative period. Regardless of the incidence, the risk of this specific complication should be discussed preoperatively with patients who will undergo surgery through the DAA, as part of the consent process. Most of these issues resolve without intervention within several months postoperatively. Understanding the anatomy and staying lateral to the Smith-Petersen approach as described earlier in this chapter prevents direct damage to the nerve. Gentle retraction and respect for the soft tissue will help minimize stretch injury to the nerve.

Because of the proximity of the groin and the presence of a panniculus that can overlie the incision in the early postoperative period, the DAA carries a well-documented increased risk of wound complications. Some surgeons advocate the use of an abdominal binder to keep the incision dry and away from the panniculus and preoperative screening for fungal infection in the groin and panniculus area. Most wound complications can be managed with wound care alone and do not require additional surgical management. The use of a specialized surgical table for the DAA, which is not described in detail in this chapter, can result in ankle fractures, nerve traction injuries, and pudendal nerve injury.

Fractures of the greater trochanter or the calcar and perforations of the femoral canal resulting from suboptimal femoral exposure have been reported. Although the incidence of these complications clearly decreases with the number of procedures performed by the surgeon, they still occur even when the procedure is performed by a highly experienced surgeon. Understanding the process of femoral release as described earlier, finding the direction of the canal with a curved curet, and obtaining good femoral exposure can minimize the occurrence of this complication.

Bibliography

Barrett WP, Turner SE, Leopold JP: Prospective randomized study of direct anterior vs postero-lateral approach for total hip arthroplasty. *J Arthroplasty* 2013;28(9):1634-1638.

Berend KR, Lombardi AV Jr, Seng BE, Adams JB: Enhanced early outcomes with the anterior supine intermuscular approach in primary total hip arthroplasty. *J Bone Joint Surg Am* 2009;91(suppl 6):107-120.

Bergin PF, Doppelt JD, Kephart CJ, et al: Comparison of minimally invasive direct anterior versus posterior total hip arthroplasty based on inflammation and muscle damage markers. *J Bone Joint Surg Am* 2011;93(15):1392-1398.

Bhandari M, Matta JM, Dodgin D, et al; Anterior Total Hip Arthroplasty Collaborative Investigators: Outcomes following the single-incision anterior approach to total hip arthroplasty: A multicenter observational study. *Orthop Clin North Am* 2009;40(3):329-342.

Bhargava T, Goytia RN, Jones LC, Hungerford MW: Lateral femoral cutaneous nerve impairment after direct anterior approach for total hip arthroplasty. *Orthopedics* 2010;33(7):472.

Bremer AK, Kalberer F, Pfirrmann CW, Dora C: Soft-tissue changes in hip abductor muscles and tendons after total hip replacement: Comparison between the direct anterior and the transgluteal approaches. *J Bone Joint Surg Br* 2011;93(7):886-889.

Ganz R, Klaue K, Vinh TS, Mast JW: A new periacetabular osteotomy for the treatment of hip dysplasias: Technique and preliminary results. 1988. *Clin Orthop Relat Res* 2004;(418):3-8.

Goulding K, Beaulé PE, Kim PR, Fazekas A: Incidence of lateral femoral cutaneous nerve neuropraxia after anterior approach hip arthroplasty. *Clin Orthop Relat Res* 2010;468(9):2397-2404.

Grob K, Monahan R, Gilbey H, Yap F, Filgueira L, Kuster M: Distal extension of the direct anterior approach to the hip poses risk to neurovascular structures: An anatomical study. *J Bone Joint Surg Am* 2015;97(2):126-132.

Jewett BA, Collis DK: High complication rate with anterior total hip arthroplasties on a fracture table. *Clin Orthop Relat Res* 2011;469(2):503-507.

Kennon RE, Keggi JM, Wetmore RS, Zatorski LE, Huo MH, Keggi KJ: Total hip arthroplasty through a minimally invasive anterior surgical approach. *J Bone Joint Surg Am* 2003;85(suppl 4):39-48.

Maffiuletti NA, Impellizzeri FM, Widler K, et al: Spatiotemporal parameters of gait after total hip replacement: Anterior versus posterior approach. *Orthop Clin North Am* 2009;40(3):407-415.

Martin CT, Pugely AJ, Gao Y, Clark CR: A comparison of hospital length of stay and short-term morbidity between the anterior and the posterior approaches to total hip arthroplasty. *J Arthroplasty* 2013;28(5):849-854.

Masonis J, Thompson C, Odum S: Safe and accurate: Learning the direct anterior total hip arthroplasty. *Orthopedics* 2008;31(12 suppl 2).

Matta JM, Shahrdar C, Ferguson T: Single-incision anterior approach for total hip arthroplasty on an orthopaedic table. *Clin Orthop Relat Res* 2005;(441):115-124.

Mayr E, Nogler M, Benedetti MG, et al: A prospective randomized assessment of earlier functional recovery in THA patients treated by minimally invasive direct anterior approach: A gait analysis study. *Clin Biomech (Bristol, Avon)* 2009;24(10):812-818.

Meneghini RM, Pagnano MW, Trousdale RT, Hozack WJ: Muscle damage during MIS total hip arthroplasty: Smith-Petersen versus posterior approach. *Clin Orthop Relat Res* 2006;(453):293-298.

Nakata K, Nishikawa M, Yamamoto K, Hirota S, Yoshikawa H: A clinical comparative study of the direct anterior with mini-posterior approach: Two consecutive series. *J Arthroplasty* 2009;24(5):698-704.

Sariali E, Leonard P, Mamoudy P: Dislocation after total hip arthroplasty using Hueter anterior approach. *J Arthroplasty* 2008;23(2):266-272.

Seng BE, Berend KR, Ajluni AF, Lombardi AV Jr: Anterior-supine minimally invasive total hip arthroplasty: Defining the learning curve. *Orthop Clin North Am* 2009;40(3):343-350.

Siguier T, Siguier M, Brumpt B: Mini-incision anterior approach does not increase dislocation rate: A study of 1037 total hip replacements. *Clin Orthop Relat Res* 2004;(426):164-173.

Taunton MJ, Mason JB, Odum SM, Springer BD: Direct anterior total hip arthroplasty yields more rapid voluntary cessation of all walking aids: A prospective, randomized clinical trial. *J Arthroplasty* 2014;29(9 suppl):169-172.

Varin D, Lamontagne M, Beaulé PE: Does the anterior approach for THA provide closer-to-normal lower-limb motion? *J Arthroplasty* 2013;28(8):1401-1407.

Chapter 5

Primary Total Hip Arthroplasty Through the Direct Anterior Approach With the Use of a Specialized Surgical Table

William G. Hamilton, MD
Zachary D. Weidner, MD
Francis B. Gonzales, MD

Indications

The direct anterior approach (DAA) for primary total hip arthroplasty (THA) is an intermuscular and internervous approach that preserves the abductor muscles. The use of the approach has increased as the result of the availability of training courses and facilities, improved surgical instruments, published data supporting the approach, and patient demand. Proponents of the DAA suggest that it is less invasive and results in less pain, earlier mobilization, and faster recovery compared with other approaches. Emerging clinical data will help determine whether these claims are supported. The modern DAA uses the interval between the rectus femoris and tensor fasciae latae (TFL) muscles for access to the hip.

An advantage of the DAA is that it spares the major soft-tissue structures that stabilize the hip and allows normal gait. Unlike the posterior approach, the DAA preserves the gluteus maximus, posterior capsule, and short external rotator muscle groups, potentially reducing the risk of posterior instability. Because the gluteus medius and gluteus minimus muscles are not detached in the DAA approach, the risk of abductor weakness and Trendelenburg gait is reduced. In addition, the gluteus maximus and TFL muscles, which collectively abduct and stabilize the hip joint, are preserved. These differences may explain why some studies of THA report faster recovery times with the DAA than with other approaches.

The use of a specialized table to facilitate anterior access to the hip was first described in the United States in 1996. Subsequent refinements made the procedure safer and easier. Available variations include a stand-alone surgical table, leg positioners that can be attached to a standard surgical table, and a manual or hydraulic hook to elevate the femur.

Although THA can be performed through the DAA with or without the use of a specialized surgical table, the use of a specialized table has advantages. The specialized table is well padded, allowing the patient to lie comfortably in a flat, level position. A padded groin post secures the patient in the center of the table and prevents the patient from sliding when traction is applied. Although acetabular exposure is routine and typically is not affected by the choice of table, the specialized table greatly facilitates femoral exposure. The foot is fixed in a surgical boot and attached to a leg spar, allowing for rotation, free abduction/adduction, flexion, and extension of the leg. Femoral exposure requires controlled hyperextension, external rotation, and adduction of the affected leg. A femoral bone hook placed around the proximal femur is attached to a manual or hydraulic lift that elevates and supports the femur to provide maximal exposure, facilitating femoral broaching and stem insertion. These features of the specialized surgical table decrease the physical difficulty of maximizing visualization while performing the procedure on a patient with large body size. Because the femoral bone hook and leg spar replicate the role that would otherwise be played by a surgical assistant, the number of surgical personnel required for the procedure is reduced. The table also helps to avoid awkward torqueing of the lower extremity and minimizes soft-tissue trauma.

A specialized surgical table also has the advantage of allowing unobstructed

Dr. Hamilton or an immediate family member serves as a paid consultant to and is a member of a speakers' bureau or has made paid presentations on behalf of DePuy Synthes; and has received research or institutional support from Zimmer Biomet, DePuy Synthes, and Inova Health System. Dr. Weidner or an immediate family member has stock or stock options held in Johnson & Johnson. Dr. Gonzales or an immediate family member serves as a paid consultant to and has received research or institutional support from Zimmer Biomet.

access for intraoperative fluoroscopy to guide accurate bone preparation, implant positioning and sizing, and measurement of leg lengths (**Figure 1**). The pelvis can shift during the procedure, and minor rotational adjustments of the fluoroscopic camera allow the surgeon to replicate the view. During acetabular preparation, fluoroscopy can be used to guide reaming, but it is primarily used to determine the position of the acetabular cup and confirm placement of the cup on reamed bone (**Figure 2**). During femoral preparation, fluoroscopy is used to check the level of the femoral neck cut, ensure appropriate femoral stem size, and reestablish native femoral offset and leg lengths. By superimposing the final intraoperative AP fluoroscopic image of the hip over an AP fluoroscopic image (flipped horizontally, from left to right) of the nonoperated hip, the surgeon can confirm appropriate femoral offset and leg lengths (**Figure 3**).

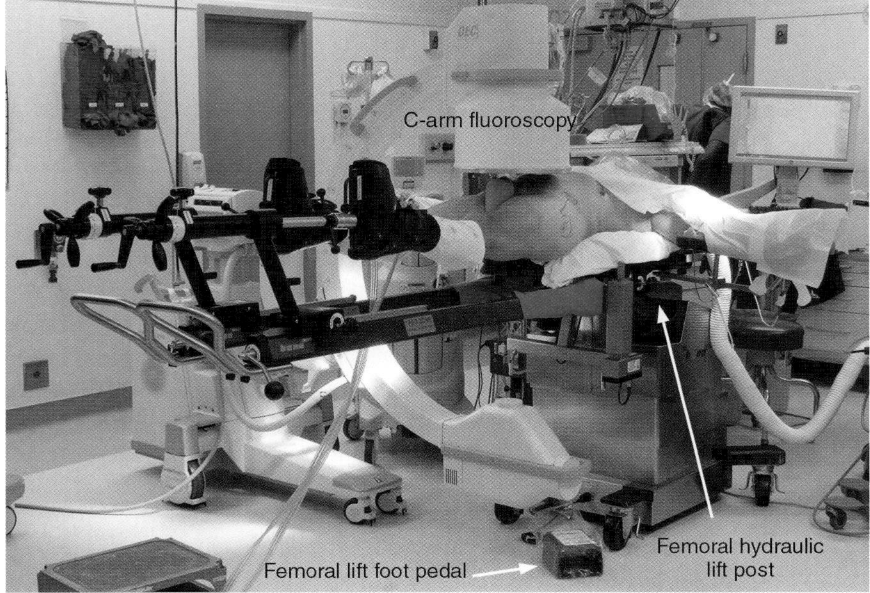

Figure 1 Photograph shows a specialized table used for total hip arthroplasty through the direct anterior approach. A femoral hydraulic lift post and leg spars enable simple, precise, and free control of the affected leg. The specialized table allows easy access for intraoperative fluoroscopy to guide implant placement.

Disadvantages of the use of a specialized surgical table for the DAA include the high initial cost of the table and the required training. The surgeon must become an expert in the use of the table and train surgical staff on proper manipulation of the leg spar during the procedure. Although the table reduces the number of assistants required for the procedure, one assistant must take on the responsibility of maneuvering the leg. If a surgeon performs a variety of procedures in 1 day, the table must be replaced with a standard surgical table for other procedures, which can take additional time. Although early versions of the table were shown to cause ankle injuries, modern refinements such as the use of a padded boot to hold the foot have nearly eliminated this complication.

Most patients who meet the classic indications for primary THA are candidates to undergo the procedure via a DAA. Preoperative templating is necessary to determine the expected implant size and position. The femoral neck osteotomy should be planned in relation to bony landmarks. The so-called saddle of the femoral neck, which is the low point of the lateral femoral neck adjacent to the greater trochanter, is directly visualized intraoperatively and serves as a consistent bony landmark for the osteotomy. Although any type of femoral stem can be used, the use of long, straight

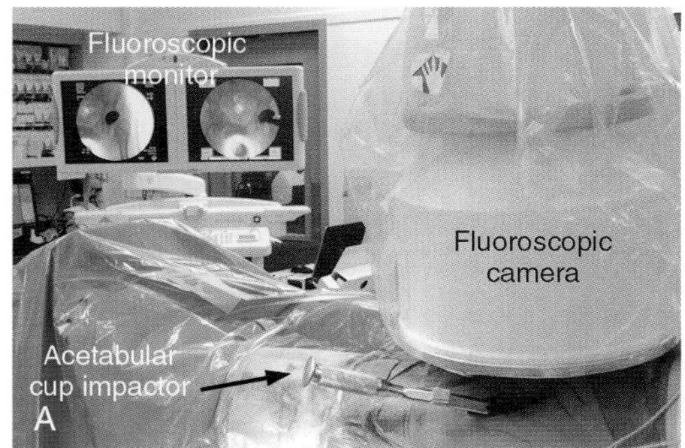

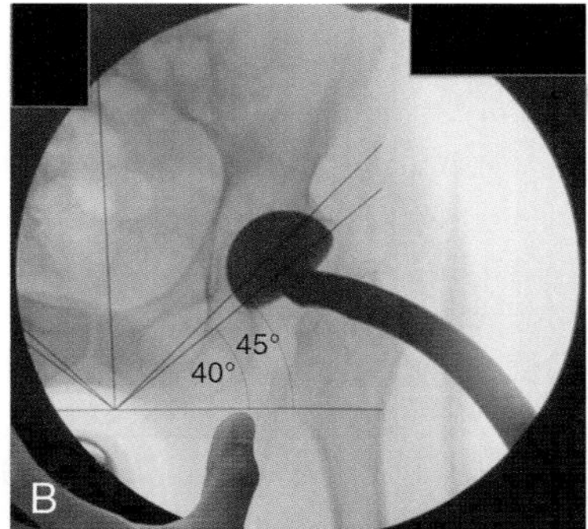

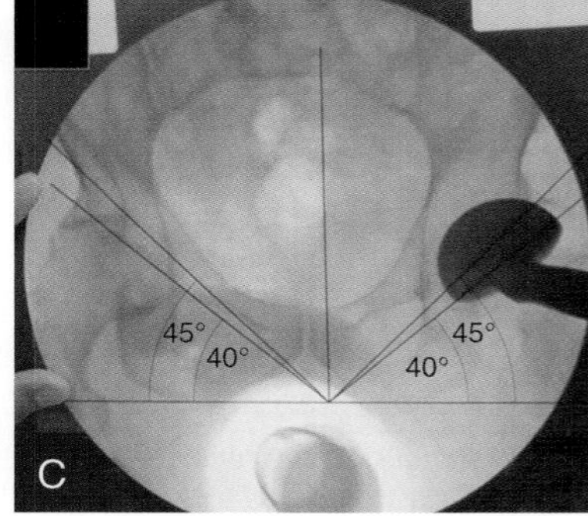

Figure 2 **A,** Intraoperative photograph shows the use of fluoroscopy to guide placement of the acetabular cup. AP fluoroscopic images of a left hip (**B**) and the pelvis (**C**) are used in confirming accurate acetabular cup placement, with a labeled transparency placed over each image.

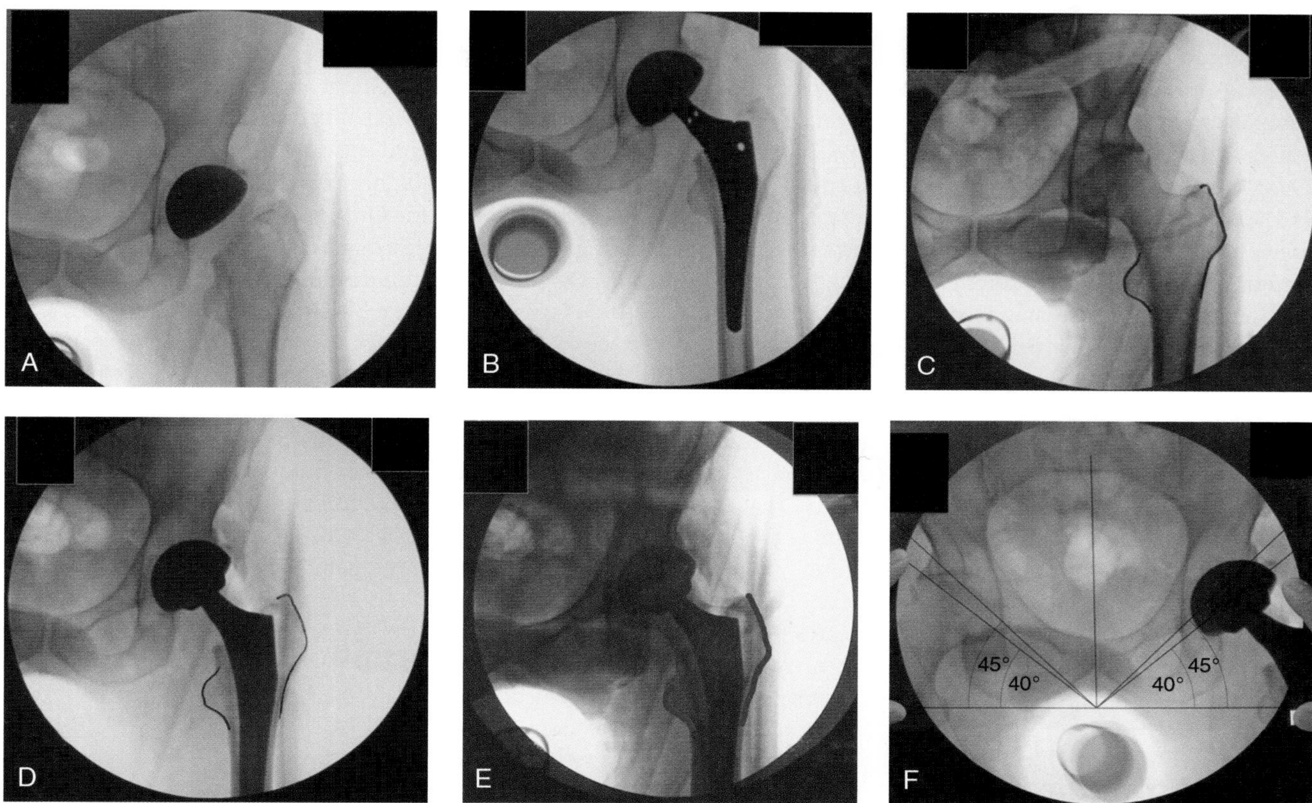

Figure 3 AP fluoroscopic images of a left hip after femoral neck osteotomy (**A**) and with a trial femoral stem in place (**B**) demonstrate appropriate level of femoral neck osteotomy and correct implant size based on femoral canal fill. **C** through **E,** Images of the overlay technique. **C,** AP fluoroscopic image of the nonoperated hip flipped horizontally from left to right. **D,** AP fluoroscopic image of the affected hip demonstrates the final implants in place. The greater and lesser trochanter are outlined in blue. **E,** Image of the AP fluoroscopic view of the nonoperated hip (flipped horizontally) superimposed over the AP fluoroscopic view of the affected hip after THA demonstrates that the two images exhibit shared greater and lesser trochanter bony outlines (in blue). The overlay technique is used to confirm restoration of femoral offset and leg lengths, with the greater and lesser trochanter, respectively, serving as bony landmarks. **F,** AP fluoroscopic image of the pelvis with final implants in place in the left hip demonstrates accurate acetabular cup position and equal leg lengths.

stems or stems that require reaming of the canal is more challenging because of the increased exposure needed for straight reaming. As a result, proximally coated stems that require only broaching are preferred. Stems that are shorter and have a cutout on the lateral shoulder of the stem are more easily inserted with the DAA than are longer stems. Retractors that are specially designed to optimize exposure and minimize soft-tissue damage are available. Straight instrumentation can be used, particularly when instrumenting the acetabulum; however, the use of an offset broach handle, reamer, and impactor designed for this approach facilitates accurate placement of implants (**Figure 4**).

During the preoperative evaluation, anatomic features of the patient that may make the DAA more technically demanding than in most patients should be noted. Often, factors that contribute to a challenging DAA would complicate the procedure with any approach. The presence of a muscular thigh and a large, firm belly can make femoral access and preparation more difficult. Although THA can be technically demanding in obese patients with any approach, the procedure may not be substantially more challenging with the DAA than

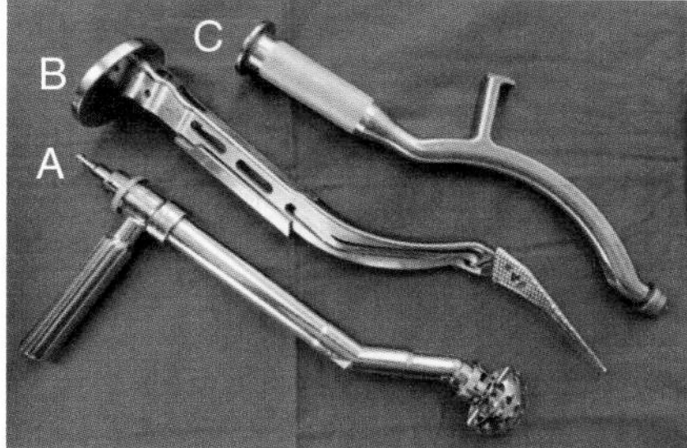

Figure 4 Photograph shows an offset reamer (**A**), a broach handle (**B**), and an acetabular cup impactor (**C**) designed to help the surgeon avoid soft-tissue impingement and ensure correct implant placement during the direct anterior approach to total hip arthroplasty.

with other approaches. Obese patients typically have less adipose tissue around the anterior hip than in the lateral and posterior aspect of the thigh. However, a large anterior pannus is a concern because it may overhang on the incision and lead to wound-healing complications. In patients with a large anterior pannus, the use of a postoperative girdle or a sterile occlusive dressing placed at the time of closure may help to avoid these wound-healing complications. Exposure for femoral preparation can be difficult in patients with wide iliac wings or short femoral necks, whereas exposure is easier in patients with greater femoral offset. Surgeons who are inexperienced with the DAA may find it helpful to perform it only in thinner, less muscular patients with good bone quality and higher femoral offset until they gain proficiency.

Contraindications

Relative contraindications to the use of the DAA include proximal femoral deformity, which can make access to the femoral canal challenging. Patients with Crowe type III or IV hip dysplasia, which requires a subtrochanteric shortening osteotomy of the femur, may best be treated with a different approach. Any acetabular deficiency that requires augmentation or grafting of the posterior wall or column can be difficult to manage via the DAA. Preexisting hardware requiring removal through a separate incision may dictate an alternative approach; alternatively, the hardware can be removed through an accessory incision before the DAA is used.

Alternative Treatments

Alternative approaches used in THA that allow equal exposure to the hip include the posterolateral (Moore-Southern), anterolateral (Watson-Jones), direct lateral (Hardinge), and transtrochanteric approaches. The alternative to performing the DAA with the patient placed on a specialized surgical table is performing it on a standard surgical table. However, a specialized table has notable advantages that make performing surgery via the DAA easier for the authors of this chapter.

Although the advantages of the anterior approach have been described, the authors of this chapter think that the approach itself is not the most important aspect of performing a successful THA. Factors that can lead to a successful result, regardless of approach, include preservation of critical soft-tissue and neurovascular structures, component fixation and position, restoration of leg lengths and offset, hemostasis, and proper perioperative management. For any surgeon deciding to adopt a new approach, it is important to implement appropriate training and patient selection to avoid catastrophic complications.

Results

The largest series published in approximately the past decade in which a specialized surgical table was used for THA are listed in **Table 1**. A few reports have compared the results of the DAA with the results of other surgical approaches for THA (**Table 2**). In a prospective, randomized study of 100 patients who underwent THA with either the DAA or with a direct lateral approach, researchers found statistically significantly better Harris hip scores, Medical Outcomes Study 36-Item Short Form scores, and Western Ontario and McMaster Universities Index scores in the DAA group at 6 weeks, 6 months, and 1 year postoperatively. However, the results equalized between the groups at a 2-year follow-up. In a prospective, randomized study of 87 patients who underwent THA via direct anterior or posterolateral approaches, statistically significant findings included earlier discharge, a greater percentage of patients able to walk without limitation and use stairs normally at 6 weeks, and higher Hip Disability and Osteoarthritis Outcome Scores at 3 months in the DAA group. No statistically significant differences between the two groups were found beyond 3 months. One prospective, randomized gait analysis study comparing the DAA with an anterolateral approach for THA reported statistically significant improvement in a larger number of gait parameters in the DAA group than in the anterolateral approach group at 6 and 12 weeks postoperatively.

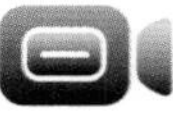

Video 5.1 Anterior Approach with a Leg-holding Traction Device. Gregory W. Brick, MD (24 min)

Techniques

Setup/Exposure

- The patient is placed in the supine position on the specialized surgical table and is secured with a groin post and foot boots attached to leg spars (**Figure 5**).
- The affected hip is prepped and draped.
- The handle that supports the femoral hook is placed over sterile draping onto the femoral lift attached to the table (**Figure 6**).
- The anterior superior iliac spine (ASIS) and the greater trochanter are palpated and identified.
- An incision is made directly over the TFL, starting approximately 3 cm lateral and 1 cm distal to the ASIS, and ending 2 to 3 cm anterior to the greater trochanter (**Figure 7, A**). Staying lateral to the ASIS will prevent injury to the lateral femoral cutaneous nerve (LFCN). The average incision length is 8 to 12 cm.

Table 1 Results of Total Hip Arthroplasty With the Use of a Specialized Surgical Table

Authors (Year)	Number of Hips	Approach	Mean Patient Age in Years (Range)	Mean Follow-up in Months (Range)	Success Rate (%)[a]	Results
Siguier et al (2004)	1,037	Mini-incision anterior	67.8 (23-93)	NR	99.2	10 dislocations No intraoperative fractures 5 deep infections 8 hips underwent revision
Matta et al (2005)	494	Single-incision anterior	64 (27-91)	NR	100	3 dislocations 12 intraoperative fractures 1 deep infection
Sariali et al (2008)	1,764	Hueter anterior	69.2 (22-94)	12 (NR)	99.9	27 dislocations 2 hips underwent revision All hips were evaluated at 3-mo follow-up, but only 73% were available for 12-mo follow-up
Bhandari et al (2009)	1,277	Single-incision anterior	65 (NR)	NR	97.3	8 dislocations 9 intraoperative fractures 3 deep infections 35 hips underwent revision
Woolson et al (2009)	247	Anterior	67.7 (36-90)	8.4 (0.5-29)	NR	No dislocations 18 intraoperative fractures 2 deep infections
Jewett and Collis (2011)	800	Anterior	62.5 (23-91)	21.6 (0-60)	99	7 dislocations 24 intraoperative fractures 7 deep infections 8 hips underwent revision
De Geest et al (2013)	300	Direct anterior[b]	69.8 (34-95)	12 (NR)	96.3	2 dislocations 13 intraoperative fractures 6 deep infections 11 hips underwent revision

NR = not reported.
[a] Success is defined as procedures not requiring revision.
[b] Intraoperative fluoroscopy was not used.

- The incision should not cross the inguinal crease. If extension of the incision is necessary, the proximal part of the incision is curved laterally in an attempt to keep the incision out of the abdominal crease.
- To avoid skin necrosis, the incision is extended as needed to ensure sufficient exposure and prevent undue traction on the skin at the edges of the incision.

Instruments/Equipment/Implants Required

- A specialized table that allows the legs to freely rotate and move into full extension and adduction is used. Boots applied to the feet facilitate traction. A hook that can elevate the femur for femoral exposure is helpful. The bed should allow the free use of fluoroscopy.
- A C-arm fluoroscopy unit is used, preferably one with the larger (12-in) tube.
- A shower curtain drape is used.
- Retractors designed specifically for the anterior approach are used (although there is considerable overlap with retractors used between approaches).
- Angled or offset acetabular reamers and impactors may be used.
- Angled and/or offset broach handles

Table 2 Results of Studies of Total Hip Arthroplasty Comparing the Direct Anterior Approach With Other Approaches

Authors (Year)	Number of Hips	Approach	Mean Patient Age in Years (Range)	Mean Follow-up in Months (Range)	Success Rate (%)[a]	Results
Nakata et al (2009)[b]	195	DAA or MPA	64.3 (38-88)	NR	100	DAA group had less need for assistive devices at 3 wk postoperatively and better walking scores at 2 mo postoperatively Total Merle d'Aubigné score was equal between the groups at 2 and 6 mo 1 dislocation (MPA) 5 intraoperative fractures (2 DAA, 3 MPA) No deep infections
Restrepo et al (2010)[c]	100	DAA or direct lateral	DAA: 62 (35-84.5) Direct lateral: 60 (40.1-76.1)	24	100	Harris hip, WOMAC, and SF-36 scores were better in DAA group at 6 wk, 6 mo, and 1 yr postoperatively Results were equal at 2 yr postoperatively No dislocations, intraoperative fractures, or deep infections
Barrett et al (2013)[c]	87	DAA or PA	DAA: 61.4 (NR) PA: 63.2 (NR)	12 (NR)	98.9	DAA group had shorter LOS, better ambulatory ability, and better stair climbing ability at 6 wk postoperatively Results were equal between the groups at 6 mo postoperatively 1 dislocation (PA) 1 intraoperative fracture (PA) No deep infections 1 revision required after PA
Martin et al (2013)[b]	88	DAA or PA	DAA: 63 (NR) PA: 57 (NR)	NR	100	DAA group had shorter LOS No difference in postoperative SF-36 or WOMAC scores between the groups 4 dislocations (1 DAA, 3 PA) 1 intraoperative fracture (DAA) No deep infections
Poehling-Monaghan et al (2015)[b]	222	DAA or MPA	64 (29-91)	2	NR	No difference in LOS between the groups MPA group had less reliance on gait aids at 2 wk postoperatively DAA group had higher Harris hip score but lower rate of return to work at 2 mo postoperatively

DAA = direct anterior approach, LOS = length of stay, MPA = mini-incision posterior approach, NR = not reported, PA = posterior approach, SF-36 = Medical Outcomes Study 36-Item Short Form, WOMAC = Western Ontario and McMaster Universities Osteoarthritis Index.

[a] Success is defined as procedures not requiring revision.

[b] Retrospective study.

[c] Prospective randomized study.

for femoral instrumentation are used.
- Femoral implant design features that facilitate the approach described in this chapter are shorter length, cutout/relief of the shoulder of the prosthesis, and broach only (or flexible type reamers).

Procedure

- The subcutaneous tissue is divided, and the fascia directly over the TFL is incised in line with the incision (**Figure 7, B**).
- With a gentle motion of the surgeon's index finger, the medial border of the TFL muscle is peeled from the fascia that separates the TFL and the sartorius muscle (**Figure 7, C**).
- When the interval between the TFL and sartorius muscles is opened posteriorly, a mobile window is visible proximal to the saddle, the bony landmark where the inside of the greater trochanter connects to the distal lateral femoral neck. A blunt cobra retractor is placed in this window to retract the TFL (superficial) and the gluteus medius (deep) laterally, exposing the superolateral capsule overlying the lateral femoral neck.
- A retractor is used to retract the rectus femoris muscle medially, exposing an adjacent fascia. Release of this fascia mobilizes the rectus femoris muscle, allowing access to the anterior capsule.
- Medial retraction of the rectus femoris muscle allows visualization of the ascending branches of the lateral femoral circumflex vessels traversing the field (**Figure 8**). Because these vessels tend to bleed intermittently, hemostasis must be obtained throughout the procedure.
- An aponeurosis is released in the distal and lateral direction, exposing the vastus lateralis muscle and further mobilizing the femur.

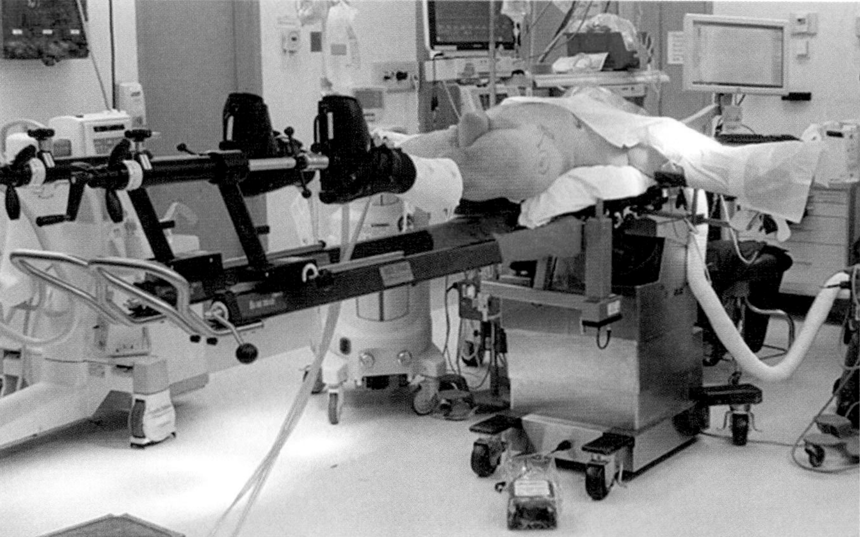

Figure 5 Photograph shows a patient secured in a supine position on a specialized surgical table for total hip arthroplasty through the direct anterior approach. A groin post is between the patient's legs, and the patient's feet are secured in boots attached to the leg spars.

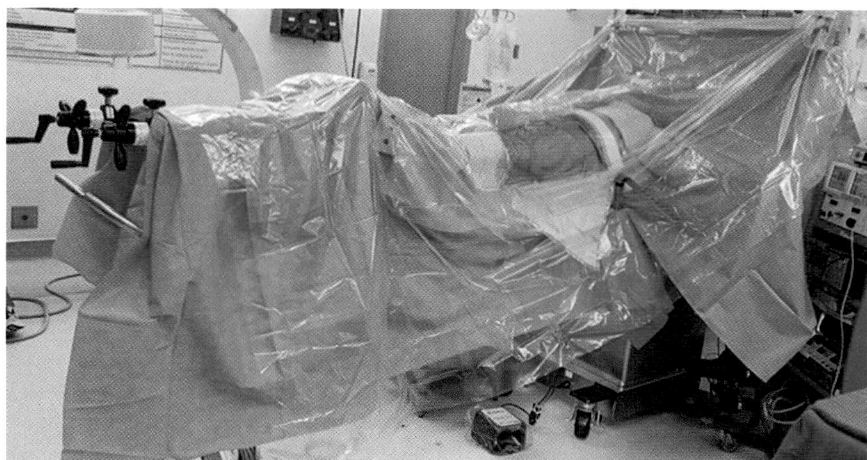

Figure 6 Intraoperative photograph shows draping of a patient on a specialized surgical table in preparation for total hip arthroplasty. The support handle of the femoral hook is secured in sterile fashion onto the femoral lift on the table.

- Proximally, a periosteal elevator is used medially to elevate the reflected head of the rectus femoris muscle off the anterior capsule and anterolateral acetabular groove.
- Release of the reflected head of the rectus femoris muscle can help to improve visualization, but is not required.
- A retractor is placed over the capsule anteriorly to retract the rectus femoris muscle medially and provide direct access to the entire anterior capsule.

CAPSULAR RELEASE

- Knowledge of the anatomy of the hip capsule, specifically its attachment

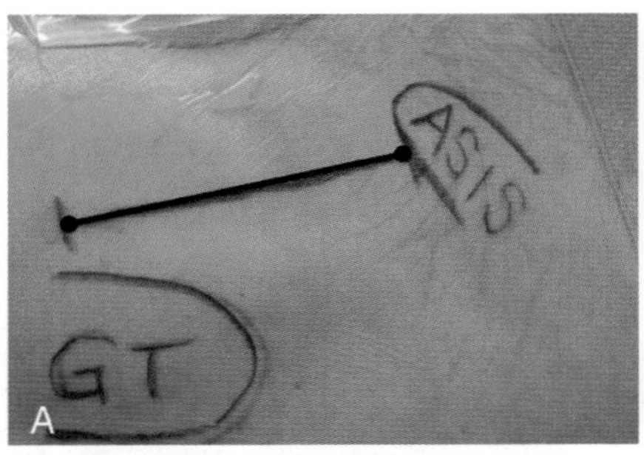

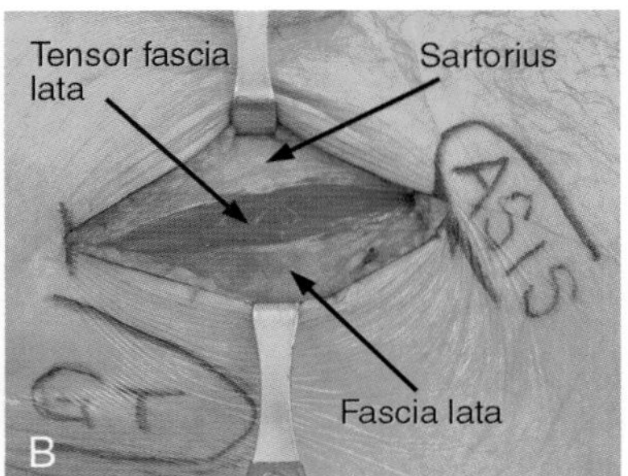

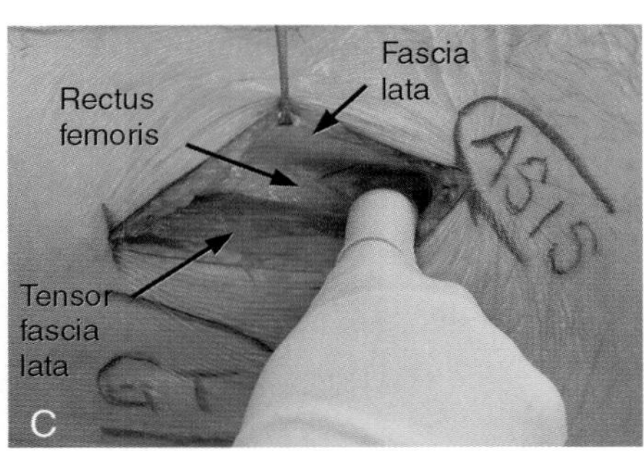

Figure 7 Intraoperative photographs of a left hip. **A,** The incision is marked approximately 2 to 3 cm lateral and 1 cm distal to the anterior superior iliac spine (ASIS) and extending to a point 2 to 3 cm anterior to the greater trochanter (GT). Staying lateral to the ASIS reduces the risk of injury to the lateral femoral cutaneous nerve. **B,** The incision of the fascia lata is made directly over the tensor fascia lata lateral to the interval between the tensor fascia lata and the sartorius. **C,** The interval between the tensor fascia lata and the rectus femoris is shown. The tensor fascia lata muscle is retracted laterally, exposing the rectus femoris (deep) medially.

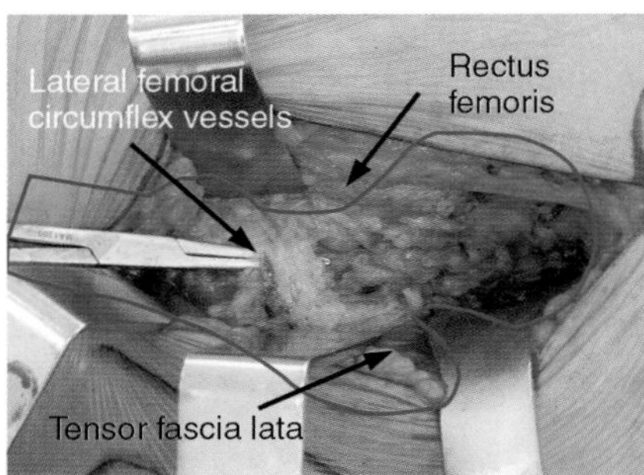

Figure 8 Intraoperative photograph of a left hip shows the ascending branches of the lateral femoral circumflex vessels, which traverse the field with the tensor fascia lata lateral and the rectus femoris medial. Blue outline indicates the position of the femoral head and neck.

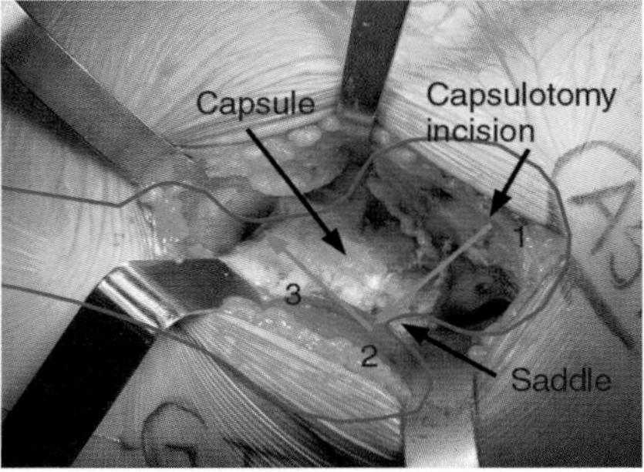

Figure 9 Intraoperative photograph of a left hip shows the anterior capsule incision (green arrows), which begins at the anterolateral acetabular rim (1) at the origin of the reflected head of the rectus femoris. The incision extends toward the so-called saddle (2), the bony landmark at which the inside of the greater trochanter connects to the distal lateral femoral neck. The incision is carried distally along the intertrochanteric line (3). Blue outline indicates the position of the femoral head and neck.

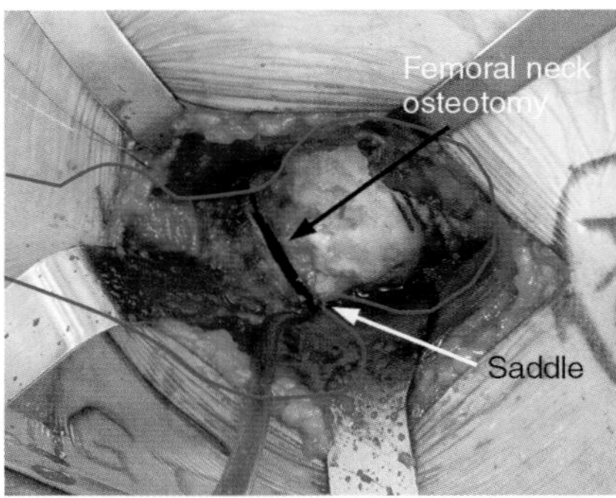

Figure 10 Intraoperative photograph of a left hip shows the femoral neck osteotomy. The blue outline indicates the position of the femoral head and neck. The saddle is used as a bony landmark to guide the osteotomy.

around the proximal femur, enables the surgeon to perform the necessary capsular releases to expose the acetabulum and mobilize the femur. Anterior capsulotomy or capsulectomy can be performed.

- The capsular incision is begun at the anterolateral acetabular rim just lateral to the reflected head of the rectus femoris muscle and directed toward the saddle.
- The capsular incision is continued distally along the intertrochanteric line, releasing the capsule from the bone (**Figure 9**).
- Tag sutures are placed at each end of the capsule to facilitate retraction for later acetabular exposure. These sutures can be used later to reapproximate the capsule if capsular closure is performed.
- With the capsule open, retractors are placed within the capsule around the medial and lateral aspect of the femoral neck.
- Medial and lateral capsular releases from the proximal femur are crucial to enable acetabular preparation and mobilization of the femur for femoral preparation.
- The medial capsule is released distally and medially directly from the femur at the calcar.
- The lateral capsule is released just inside the greater trochanter at the saddle.

FEMORAL NECK OSTEOTOMY

- For the femoral neck osteotomy, the lower leg is placed in slight traction and external rotation.
- The saddle is used as a bony landmark to guide the level of femoral neck resection determined on the basis of preoperative templating. The cut is made in situ with direct visualization of the saddle (**Figure 10**).
- The osteotomy is begun with the saw blade pointed medial and posterior at the femoral neck.

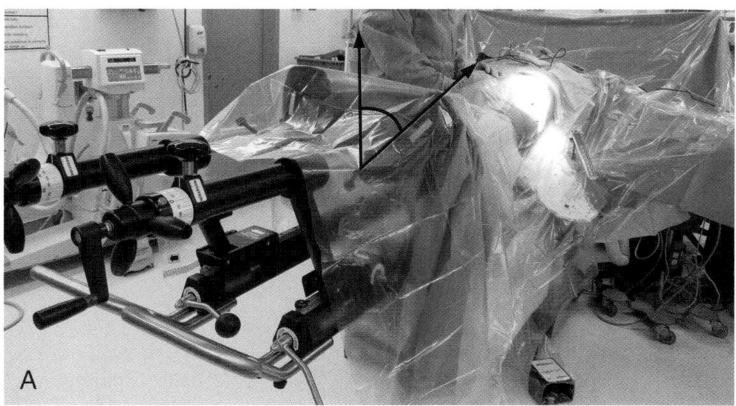

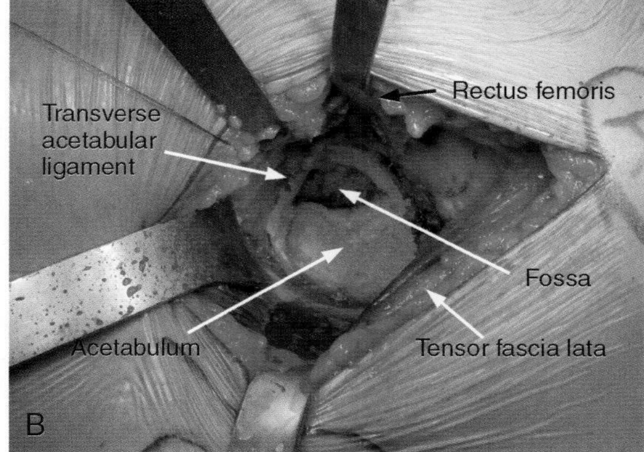

Figure 11 **A,** Intraoperative photograph of a left hip shows patient positioning for acetabular preparation with the leg in slight traction and 30° to 45° of external rotation (angle between black arrows). **B,** Intraoperative photograph shows exposure of the acetabulum, which is easily achieved via the direct anterior approach.

- An osteotome is used laterally in a vertical direction to complete the osteotomy and avoid fracture of the greater trochanter.
- A corkscrew is placed into the femoral head for removal.
- The femoral head is rotated several times inside the acetabulum to ensure that the ligamentum teres is severed.
- During removal of the femoral head, care is taken to ensure that the sharp edges of the femoral neck at the site of the osteotomy do not injure the TFL.
- If desired, or if necessary to remove the femoral head, a segmental cut of the femoral neck (napkin ring technique), consisting of a 2-cm proximal subcapital cut made after and parallel to the existing femoral neck osteotomy, can be used. Removal of this wedge of femoral neck facilitates removal of the femoral head.

ACETABULAR PREPARATION

- The operated leg is positioned in slight traction and 30° to 45° of external rotation, and retractors are placed to expose the acetabulum (**Figure 11**).
- A retractor is placed at the midposterior acetabular rim just inside the capsule and outside the labrum.
- A second retractor is placed just proximal to the transverse acetabular ligament.
- Optionally, a retractor can be placed anterosuperiorly under the reflected head of the rectus femoris muscle to improve visualization.
- A release of the prominent inferior band of capsule can improve access to the acetabulum and allow further shifting of the femur posteriorly.
- The labrum and osteophytes are excised. Removal of the pulvinar, ligamentum teres, and medial osteophytes exposes the fovea, which guides the amount of medialization during reaming.
- Before reaming, the surgeon may find it helpful to become oriented to the view of the acetabulum.
- The reamer is typically positioned with the surgeon's hand slightly raised from a line parallel to the floor for anteversion.
- To ensure appropriate reaming orientation, the reamer handle is held low toward the floor and toward the patient's body to avoid impingement of soft tissue both posteriorly and inferiorly, respectively (**Figure 12, A**).
- Care is taken to maintain an inferior and posterior position of the reamer. The femur and soft tissues of the thigh can push the reamer anteriorly and superiorly and cause eccentric reaming of the acetabulum.
- Fluoroscopy can be used to check the position and progress of the reamer but usually is not necessary.
- The final implant is inserted.
- Fluoroscopy is used to assess for cup abduction and anteversion (**Figure 2, B** and **C**).
- Any necessary changes in cup position are made as the cup is impacted into its final position.
- Internal anatomic landmarks such as the transverse acetabular ligament are used to confirm appropriate cup positioning (**Figure 12, B**).
- Screws are placed if desired.
- The final liner is inserted.

FEMORAL PREPARATION

- The operated leg is brought to neutral rotation to allow placement of the femoral bone hook inside the TFL around the proximal femur, slightly distal to the vastus ridge.
- With the femur in maximum external rotation, a retractor is placed on the posteromedial femoral neck, and a long curved retractor is placed around the tip of the greater trochanter and inside the abductor muscles.

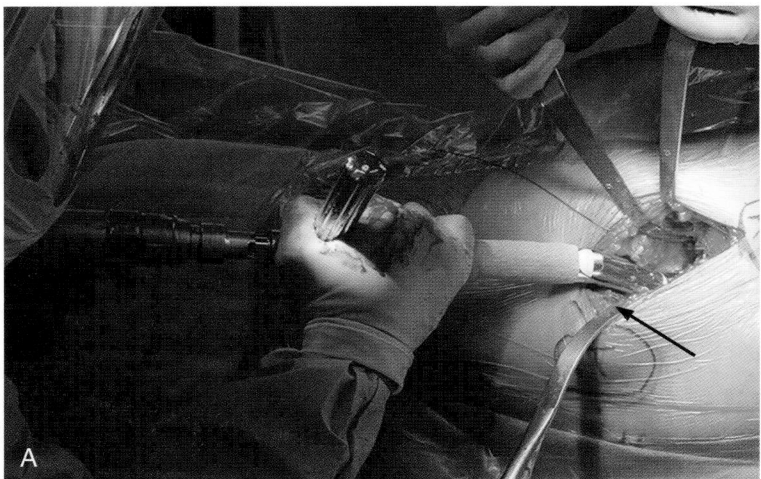

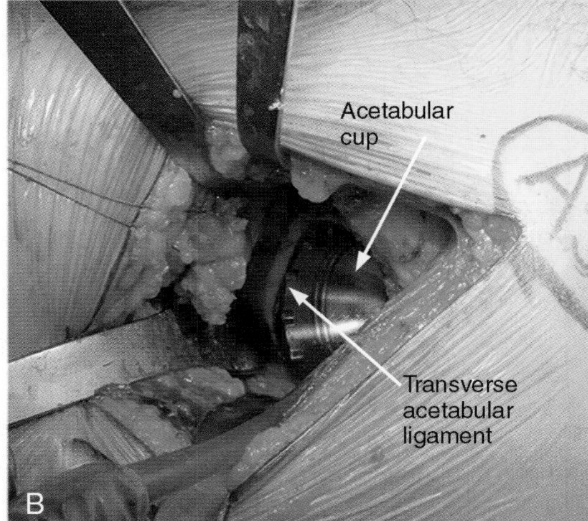

Figure 12 **A,** Intraoperative photograph of a left hip shows acetabular preparation. The surgeon should aim for 12° to 15° of anteversion by raising the hand slightly above the plane of the floor in 40° to 45° of abduction. The use of offset instruments helps to avoid soft-tissue impingement both posteriorly and inferiorly. The arrow indicates the offset acetabular reamer. **B,** Intraoperative photograph shows the acetabular cup positioned in 5° to 10° less anteversion compared with the transverse acetabular ligament, which is appropriate for the direct anterior approach.

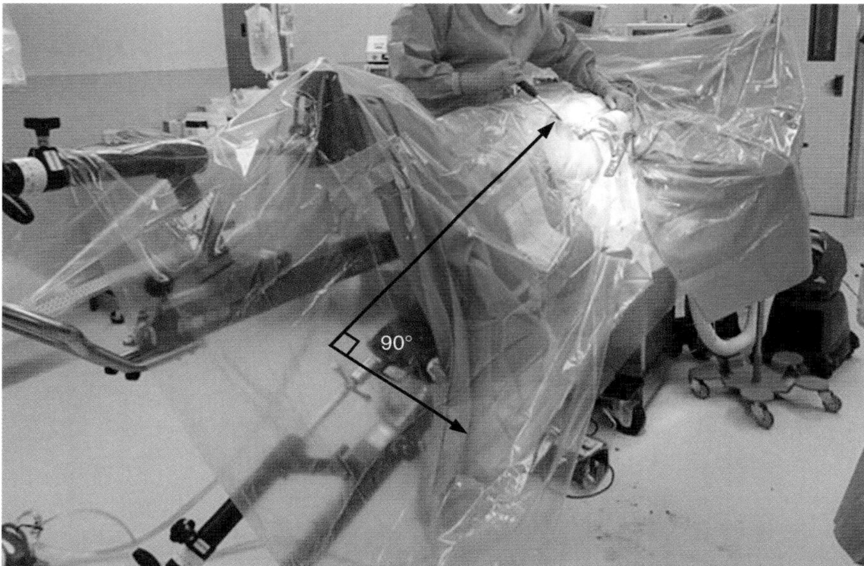

Figure 13 Intraoperative photograph of a left hip shows femoral preparation, which is simplified with the use of the specialized table. The femoral bone hook attached to the hydraulic lift and leg spar allows precise positioning of the affected leg in hyperextension and adduction with 90° of external rotation.

- A portion of the visualized posterior capsule is released to improve femoral mobilization.
- Traction on the leg is released.
- The leg is lowered toward the floor into hyperextension and adduction, delivering the proximal femur for preparation (**Figure 13**).
- The femoral bone hook is placed into the support handle attached to the surgical table.
- If direct access to the femoral canal is not obtained with the patient in this position, additional capsular releases are performed.
- The inferomedial capsule is sufficiently released off the calcar.
- The posterolateral capsule is released progressively until the bed of the greater trochanter is completely exposed and delivered anteriorly (**Figure 14**).
- The long curved retractor should be positioned outside the greater trochanter to retract the abductor muscles and elevate the femur.
- Inadequate posterolateral release of the capsule from inside the greater trochanter may result in small trochanteric avulsion fractures.
- In patients with severely contracted hips, the short external rotator muscles can be sequentially released to improve access to the femoral canal. The conjoined tendon (obturator internus and superior and inferior gemellus muscles) inside the greater trochanter just outside the lateral capsule is released first. The piriformis tendon at the inside tip of the greater trochanter is released for additional exposure.

- The obturator externus muscle, which inserts distal to the obturator internus muscle adjacent to the cut femoral neck, functions as a hip stabilizer and should not be released (**Figure 14**).
- After adequate access to the femur is achieved, standard sequential broaching techniques are used.
- The lower leg is placed in external rotation, hyperextension, and adduction.
- Care is taken to guide the broach handle laterally (toward the floor) and posteriorly (toward the patient's body) to avoid lateral and posterior perforation (**Figure 15, A**). Offset broach handles can help avoid soft-tissue impingement (**Figure 15, B**).
- The femoral stem should be parallel to the posterior cortex of the proximal femur to ensure the appropriate amount of anteversion.
- Holding the broach handle firmly with an internal rotational force will help ensure accurate anteversion (**Figure 15**).
- After the final broach is firmly seated without advancement, the appropriate trial femoral neck and head, determined on the basis of preoperative templating, are attached.
- Final implants are placed in a manner similar to that used for the placement of the trial implants (**Figure 16**).

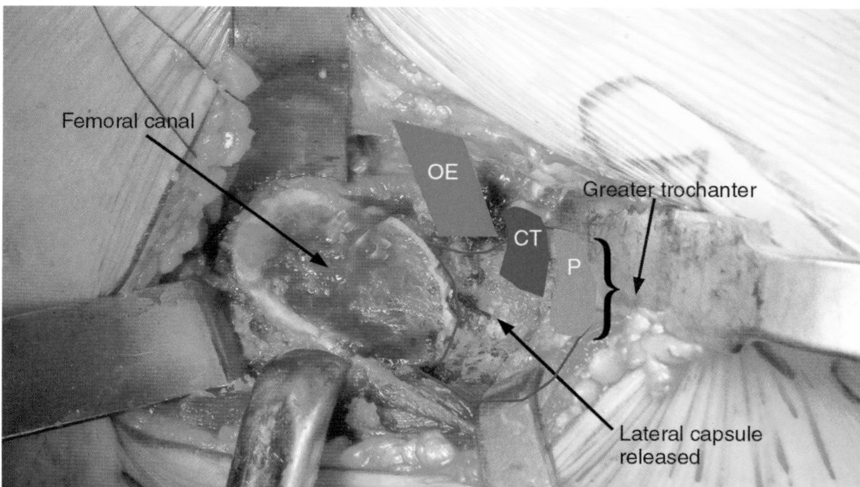

Figure 14 Intraoperative photograph of a left hip shows release of the lateral capsule from the inside of the greater trochanter (outlined in blue). The proximal femur is delivered anteriorly until direct access to the femoral canal is achieved. The locations of the short external rotators are labeled: conjoined tendon (obturator internus, superior gemellus, and inferior gemellus; blue [CT]), piriformis tendon (purple [P]), and obturator externus tendon (green [OE]).

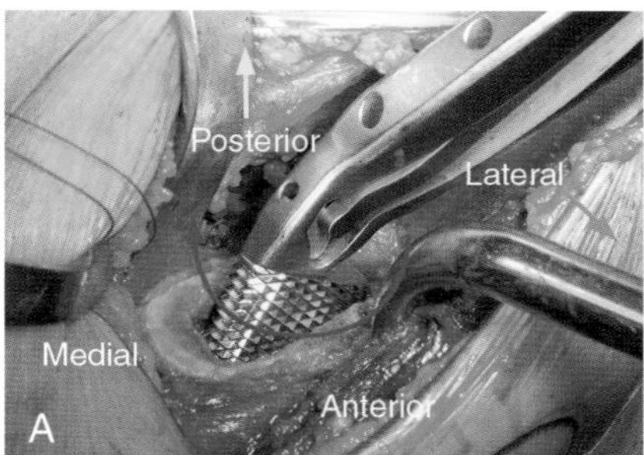

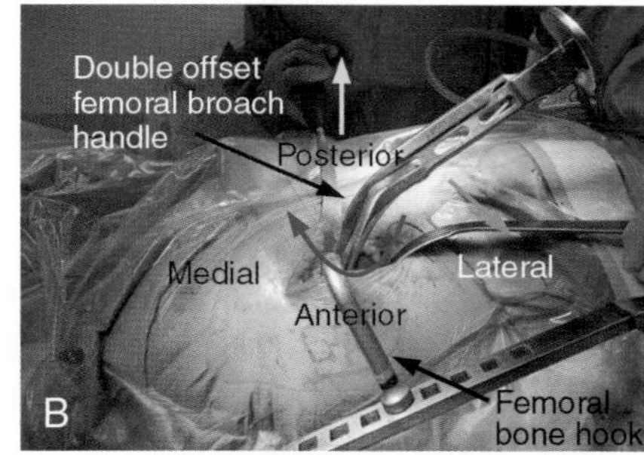

Figure 15 Intraoperative photographs of a left hip show femoral broaching (**A**) with an offset handle (**B**). Before femoral broaching is performed, the lower leg is placed in 90° of external rotation, hyperextension, and adduction. Care is taken to guide the broach handle laterally (green arrow pointing toward the floor) to avoid lateral perforation and posteriorly (yellow arrow pointing toward the patient's torso) to avoid perforation posterior to the proximal femur. The presence of soft tissue can result in excessive anteversion of the femoral stem. A firm grip on the broach handle with an internal rotational force helps to ensure accurate anteversion (blue arrow).

REDUCTION

- The circulating assistant lifts the patient's leg off the floor out of hyperextension and adduction and returns the leg to the neutral horizontal position in which it was situated at the beginning of the procedure.
- Traction and internal rotation are applied to the leg spar to reduce the hip.
- The tension of the abductor muscles and hip stability are checked.
- Routine checking of hip range of motion during the procedure is not necessary, but it can be done if desired.
- To evaluate for posterior impingement and anterior dislocation, the operated leg is placed in 70° to 90° of external rotation with 45° of hyperextension.
- To test for anterior impingement and posterior dislocation, the foot boot is released from the table spar and the leg is placed in flexion, adduction, and internal rotation.
- Fluoroscopy can be used at this point in the procedure to check the size and position of the femoral prosthesis as well as restoration of leg lengths and offset. The relative

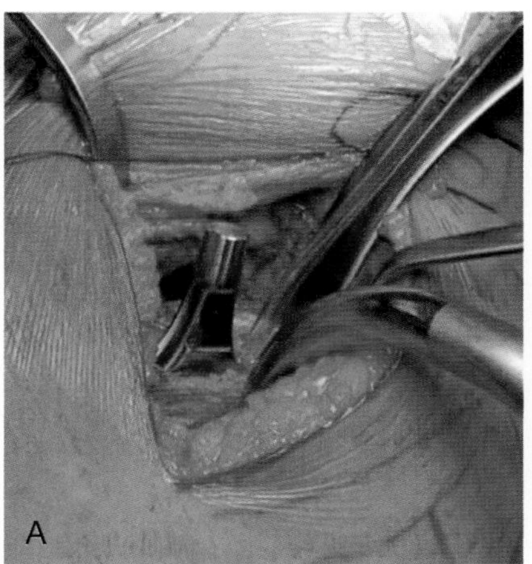

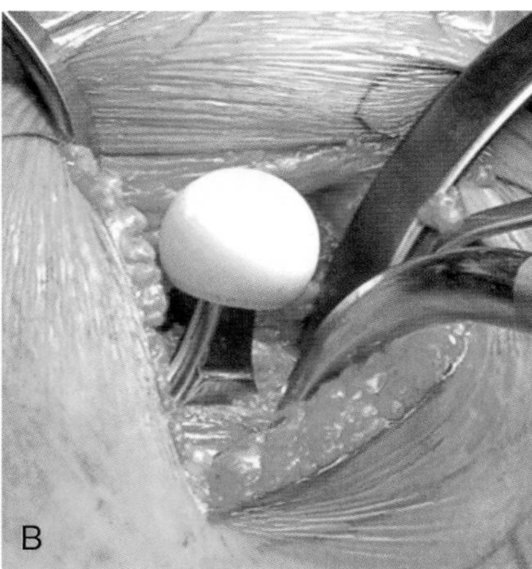

Figure 16 Intraoperative photographs of a left hip show placement of the final femoral stem (**A**) and the final femoral head (**B**).

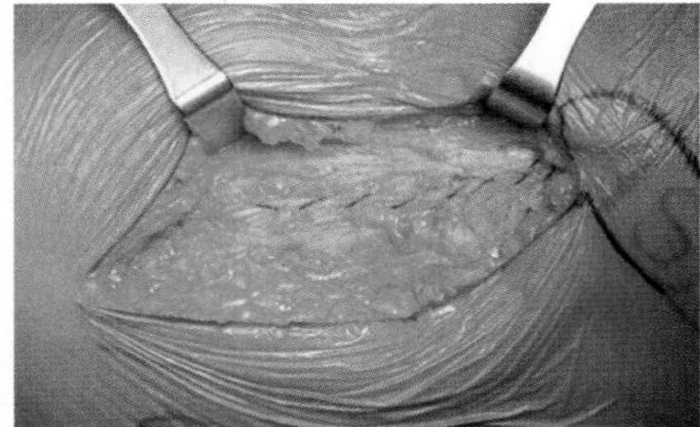

Figure 17 Intraoperative photograph of a left hip shows closure of the fascia over the tensor fascia lata.

position of the lesser trochanters can be checked and/or the preoperative and postoperative length and offset can be compared using the overlay technique (**Figure 3, B** through **F**).

Wound Closure

- Before the wound is closed, care is taken to check for residual bleeding, specifically from the ascending branches of the lateral femoral circumflex vessels and near the capsule. It is important to coagulate any significant bleeding to prevent hematoma or wound complications caused by excessive bleeding. Surgical ties, electrocautery, or bipolar electrocautery can be used to achieve coagulation.
- Closure of the capsule is optional.
- The fascia over the TFL is closed (**Figure 17**).
- The skin is closed in the surgeon's preferred fashion.

Postoperative Regimen

Standard wound management procedures are appropriate in most patients. However, when the patient's abdomen rests on the incision, careful management of the incision and pannus in the early postoperative period is important to keep the incision clean and dry and to minimize the risk of infection. Covering the incision with a sterile occlusive dressing for 10 to 14 days postoperatively can be helpful. A girdle worn in the postoperative period can lift a pendulous abdomen away from the incision.

Rehabilitation protocols vary depending on patient needs and surgeon preferences. Typically, the patient is allowed to mobilize on the day of the procedure, bear weight as tolerated, and advance activity as tolerated. The patient is encouraged to perform abductor and hip flexor strengthening exercises postoperatively. Most surgeons impose few, if any, postoperative restrictions on the movement or position of the operated limb. From the patient's perspective, the lack of restrictions on hip movement or position is a substantial advantage of the DAA and may improve perceived outcomes of the procedure. The patient is allowed to resume full activity without limitation at 6 to 12 weeks postoperatively.

Avoiding Pitfalls and Complications

Femoral exposure is the most technically challenging aspect of the DAA for primary THA. The learning curve is substantial, and complications have been shown to decrease after a surgeon's first 30 to 200 cases. Early in a surgeon's experience with the DAA, surgical time and blood loss are greater than would occur with a posterior approach. Therefore, a surgeon learning this technique should attend training courses, practice on cadaver models, observe procedures performed by other surgeons, and initially perform the procedure only on patients whose anatomy is favorable for this approach.

The LFCN is at risk in the DAA because of its proximity to the interval between the sartorius and TFL muscles. The reported incidence of injury to the LFCN with this approach varies from zero to 67%. Patients typically report paresthesia, numbness, or a burning sensation on the anterolateral thigh. These symptoms typically decrease over time, although the reported rate of improvement has varied widely, ranging from 6% of patients who experience complete resolution of symptoms at 1 year postoperatively to 83% having complete resolution at 2 years postoperatively. Despite the frequency of this adverse event, multiple studies have shown that LFCN injury does not appear to affect the patient's functional outcome. Intraoperatively, working inside the fascia of the TFL muscle can help reduce the frequency of LFCN damage. Additionally, to protect the LFCN, care should be taken to avoid working medial to the interval between the sartorius and TFL muscles. Patients should be educated preoperatively about the possibility of postoperative sensory abnormalities of the anterolateral thigh.

Femoral perforation most commonly occurs laterally and posteriorly. This complication can be avoided by ensuring that the femoral canal finder is appropriately advanced down the femoral canal. The broach handle must be held down toward the floor and in toward the patient's body. If femoral perforation is suspected, it can be confirmed fluoroscopically. Perforation can be managed by redirecting the broach and placing the stem into the intended position. In patients in whom femoral perforation occurs, weight bearing should be protected postoperatively.

Trochanteric fractures have been reported, and they can be easily avoided with appropriate technique. The most common cause of intraoperative trochanter fracture is attempted elevation of the femur prior to adequate capsular release. Such elevation typically causes an avulsion of the posterior lip of the trochanter. The surgeon should confirm that adequate release of the capsule has been achieved before lifting the femur, and then watch the trochanter as the femur is lifted and pulled laterally to ensure that the trochanter elevates safely. Forceful lifting of the femur, either with a retractor or with the hydraulic lift, should be avoided. Small avulsion fractures typically do not require treatment or any change in the postoperative rehabilitation protocol. When making the femoral neck osteotomy, the surgeon must take care to avoid injury to the greater trochanter. At the time of the femoral neck osteotomy, the greater trochanter is located posteriorly, requiring the saw blade to be directed in a posteromedial direction rather than straight up and down. Injury to the greater trochanter with involvement of the abductor insertion should be treated intraoperatively.

Bibliography

Barrett WP, Turner SE, Leopold JP: Prospective randomized study of direct anterior vs postero-lateral approach for total hip arthroplasty. *J Arthroplasty* 2013;28(9):1634-1638.

Bhandari M, Matta JM, Dodgin D, et al; Anterior Total Hip Arthroplasty Collaborative Investigators: Outcomes following the single-incision anterior approach to total hip arthroplasty: A multicenter observational study. *Orthop Clin North Am* 2009;40(3):329-342.

De Geest T, Vansintjan P, De Loore G: Direct anterior total hip arthroplasty: Complications and early outcome in a series of 300 cases. *Acta Orthop Belg* 2013;79(2):166-173.

Goulding K, Beaulé PE, Kim PR, Fazekas A: Incidence of lateral femoral cutaneous nerve neuropraxia after anterior approach hip arthroplasty. *Clin Orthop Relat Res* 2010;468(9):2397-2404.

Jewett BA, Collis DK: High complication rate with anterior total hip arthroplasties on a fracture table. *Clin Orthop Relat Res* 2011;469(2):503-507.

Kennon RE, Keggi JM, Wetmore RS, Zatorski LE, Huo MH, Keggi KJ: Total hip arthroplasty through a minimally invasive anterior surgical approach. *J Bone Joint Surg Am* 2003;85(suppl 4):39-48.

Light TR, Keggi KJ: Anterior approach to hip arthroplasty. *Clin Orthop Relat Res* 1980;(152):255-260.

Martin CT, Pugely AJ, Gao Y, Clark CR: A comparison of hospital length of stay and short-term morbidity between the anterior and the posterior approaches to total hip arthroplasty. *J Arthroplasty* 2013;28(5):849-854.

Masonis J, Thompson C, Odum S: Safe and accurate: Learning the direct anterior total hip arthroplasty. *Orthopedics* 2008;31(12 suppl 2).

Matta JM, Shahrdar C, Ferguson T: Single-incision anterior approach for total hip arthroplasty on an orthopaedic table. *Clin Orthop Relat Res* 2005;(441):115-124.

Mayr E, Nogler M, Benedetti MG, et al: A prospective randomized assessment of earlier functional recovery in THA patients treated by minimally invasive direct anterior approach: A gait analysis study. *Clin Biomech (Bristol, Avon)* 2009;24(10):812-818.

Mirza AJ, Lombardi AV Jr, Morris MJ, Berend KR: A mini-anterior approach to the hip for total joint replacement: Optimising results. Improving hip joint replacement outcomes. *Bone Joint J* 2014;96-B(11 suppl A):32-35.

Nakata K, Nishikawa M, Yamamoto K, Hirota S, Yoshikawa H: A clinical comparative study of the direct anterior with mini-posterior approach: Two consecutive series. *J Arthroplasty* 2009;24(5):698-704.

Poehling-Monaghan KL, Kamath AF, Taunton MJ, Pagnano MW: Direct anterior versus miniposterior THA with the same advanced perioperative protocols: Surprising early clinical results. *Clin Orthop Relat Res* 2015;473(2):623-631.

Post ZD, Orozco F, Diaz-Ledezma C, Hozack WJ, Ong A: Direct anterior approach for total hip arthroplasty: Indications, technique, and results. *J Am Acad Orthop Surg* 2014;22(9):595-603.

Restrepo C, Parvizi J, Pour AE, Hozack WJ: Prospective randomized study of two surgical approaches for total hip arthroplasty. *J Arthroplasty* 2010;25(5):671-679.e1.

Sariali E, Leonard P, Mamoudy P: Dislocation after total hip arthroplasty using Hueter anterior approach. *J Arthroplasty* 2008;23(2):266-272.

Siguier T, Siguier M, Brumpt B: Mini-incision anterior approach does not increase dislocation rate: A study of 1037 total hip replacements. *Clin Orthop Relat Res* 2004;(426):164-173.

Woolson ST, Pouliot MA, Huddleston JI: Primary total hip arthroplasty using an anterior approach and a fracture table: Short-term results from a community hospital. *J Arthroplasty* 2009;24(7):999-1005.

Video Reference

Brick GW: Anterior approach with a leg-holding traction device, in Schwarzkopf R, ed: *Surgical Techniques in Orthopaedics: Total Hip Arthroplasty* [Blu-Ray]. Rosemont, IL, American Academy of Orthopaedic Surgeons, 2014.

Chapter 6

Primary Total Hip Arthroplasty Through the Anterior-Based Muscle-Sparing Approach on a Standard Surgical Table

Scott S. Kelley, MD

Thorsten M. Seyler, MD, PhD

Rhett K. Hallows, MD

Indications

Comparison of surgical approaches to the hip is difficult because of the lack of standard terminology or a classification system. Numerous anterior approaches have been described for total hip arthroplasty (THA), including the direct anterior (Smith-Petersen), Hueter, Watson-Jones, Rottinger, Bauer, Dall, Hardinge, Ganz, and Levine approaches. To further complicate terminology, many of these approaches have descriptors such as modified, mini, minimally invasive, or muscle-sparing. Many surgical approaches to the hip require specialized implants, retractors, surgical tables, and/or surgical navigation systems or intraoperative fluoroscopy.

In comparing surgical approaches to the hip, the role of muscle detachment is more important than that of the muscle interval used for dissection. The surgical approach is defined by its relationship to the greater trochanter (posterior, posterior-superior, anterior, or transtrochanteric) and the specific muscles detached. Other considerations include body or leg position (supine versus lateral, flexion versus extension), the type of surgical table required, and the need for fluoroscopy or computer-assisted navigation. The authors of this chapter suggest that the surgical approaches to the hip should be classified simply as posterior, posterior-superior, transtrochanteric, anterolateral, anterior-based muscle-sparing (ABMS), and direct anterior (anterior to the tensor fascia lata).

Although multiple terms have been used to describe the ABMS approach, it is inaccurate to characterize it as either an anterolateral or a modified Watson-Jones approach because both of those approaches involve detachment of the abductor muscles. Moreover, the Watson-Jones approach was originally described as an interval for exposure of fractures of the femoral neck rather than as a surgical approach to the hip joint. As first described in 2004, the ABMS approach used the Watson-Jones interval but did not include detachment of the abductors. The ABMS approach is similar to the direct anterior approach (DAA) but uses a standard surgical table. To facilitate leg position during the approach, the authors of this chapter recommend a split lower extremity table drop or a split leg pegboard attachment (an inexpensive attachment for a standard surgical table). The extremity is prepped free, allowing intraoperative assessment of range of motion (ROM) and stability. Because the patient is positioned laterally, dissection can be done through an extensile or a so-called minimally invasive approach, resulting in the versatility of this approach for both primary and revision scenarios. The ABMS approach does not put the femoral cutaneous nerve at risk, and it facilitates faster recovery because it does not violate the abductor muscles. Although any femoral implant design can be accommodated, the authors of this chapter prefer to use a tapered femoral implant that requires reaming. This type of implant is easily placed via the ABMS approach.

Variations of the ABMS approach for THA used in Europe are often referred to as anterolateral minimally invasive. This designation erroneously implies that the abductor muscles are detached because historically, the term lateral has been associated with detachment of a portion of the abductor muscles. Also, the term minimally invasive detracts from the more important concept of muscle sparing. Muscle detachment or damage is of

Dr. Kelley or an immediate family member is a member of a speakers' bureau or has made paid presentations on behalf of Smith & Nephew. Dr. Seyler or an immediate family member serves as an unpaid consultant to Heraeus Medical. Dr. Hallows or an immediate family member serves as a paid consultant to Total Joint Orthopedics.

Table 1 Comparison of the Direct Anterior Approach and the Anterior-Based Muscle-Sparing Approach in Total Hip Arthroplasty

Factor	Direct Anterior Approach	Anterior-Based Muscle-Sparing Approach
Surgical table	Specialized surgical table or specialized femur elevator/hook setup	Standard surgical table
Patient position	Supine	Lateral decubitus or supine
Exposure	Substantial learning curve	Familiar anatomic exposure
Visualization	Limited visualization of the acetabulum Often requires indirect visualization using fluoroscopy Limited access to femur	Extensile approach possible to allow access to the proximal femur
Intraoperative testing of stability and range of motion	Limited	Standard
Instrumentation	Offset	Standard in-line
Implant selection	Short stems required	Unlimited implant options and stem compatibility: standard length, straight reaming, cemented, revision
Femoral preparation	Broach-only systems	Broach-only and ream-and-broach systems
Patient selection	Limited by body mass index and body habitus Use of a specialized surgical table contraindicated in patients who have undergone amputation	Unlimited
Revision options	Acetabular revision, simple femoral implant exchange, calcar wiring	Acetabular revision, femoral implant revision, calcar wiring, claw plate fixation, extended trochanteric osteotomy, trochanteric slide osteotomy, abductor muscle advancement, open reduction and internal fixation of periprosthetic fracture
Complications	Lateral cutaneous femoral nerve injury, femoral fractures, ankle fractures, injury to the femoral nerve, bleeding from the lateral circumflex femoral artery	Femoral fractures, heterotopic ossification, rare femoral nerve injury, bleeding from the lateral circumflex femoral artery

greater consequence than the length of the incision. The muscle-sparing nature of the ABMS makes it an attractive alternative in patients who are at increased risk for dislocation (neuromuscular and cognitive disorders including cerebral palsy, muscular dystrophy, psychosis, dementia, Parkinson disease, cervical myelopathy, and alcoholism).

Contraindications

The ABMS approach has few contraindications. Because this approach is technically demanding, the most important contraindication is insufficient surgical training or lack of familiarity with the relevant anatomy. The need for access to the posterior acetabular wall for hardware removal or bone grafting is a relative contraindication to the ABMS approach. This approach has no limitations related to patient body mass index (BMI) because it avoids the potential for wound complications that can result when a pendulous abdomen rests on a more anteriorly based incision.

Alternative Treatments

The DAA with the use of a specialized surgical table is a muscle-sparing approach that serves as an alternative to the ABMS approach. Comparison of the DAA and the ABMS approach is provided in **Table 1**. In recent years, the DAA has gained popularity. However, this approach has unique challenges. Distal extension of the approach, if required to gain exposure to the hip, poses a substantial risk to neurovascular structures. The development and increased use of short implants has been largely driven by these anatomic challenges and the difficulty of placing standard implants through the DAA. Short implants are experimental, and although they have been termed bone preserving, in reality they are canal preserving at best.

If the DAA is performed with the use of a specialized table or a modified fracture table, factors beyond the cost of the table itself must be considered, such as the expense of fluoroscopy and the patient's and surgeon's radiation exposure resulting from the use of fluoroscopy. On average, the surgeon and patient are exposed to 2.97 mGy of ionized radiation during a fluoroscopically assisted procedure using the DAA. According to the Radiation Effects Research Foundation, the upper limit to avoid radiation-induced cataract formation is 800 mGy, which corresponds to a threshold of 269 procedures if a surgeon does not wear eye protection. This limit is similar to the recommendations of the National Council on Radiation Protection and Measurements.

Femoral exposure is more difficult with the DAA, and bone hooks are needed to mobilize the femur. The use of bone hooks, combined with the use of shorter implants, places the patient at higher risk of intraoperative fracture. An intraoperative fracture is further complicated if the patient is positioned supine on a specialized table because this position often necessitates a second incision and/or patient repositioning for fracture management. The use of a specialized table may make intraoperative assessment of stability and ROM difficult. Patients with a high BMI and a pendulous abdomen are at higher risk of wound healing complications with the DAA than with the ABMS approach.

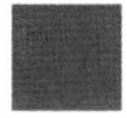

Results

Anterior-based approaches to the hip are associated with a decreased risk of postoperative dislocation and provide excellent exposure to the acetabulum and femur for prosthesis implantation. However, clinical outcomes using different surgical approaches to the hip are comparable after recovery from the initial surgical trauma, and surgeons often modify previously described techniques on the basis of their own experience. Most of the relatively few studies that have reported on outcomes of the ABMS approach are small and report on early outcomes and the learning curve associated with the surgical technique. Proponents of the ABMS approach highlight the unobstructed access to the proximal femur and acetabulum that it provides. Other reported advantages of the ABMS approach include faster recovery, less muscle damage, reliable implant positioning, low dislocation rates, and decreased postoperative pain and narcotic requirement. Prospective randomized trials with greater numbers of patients are needed to determine long-term outcomes of the approach. In 2011, the authors of this chapter described the ABMS approach, reviewed the literature on anterior approaches, and reported initial results. **Table 2** summarizes the results of the available studies. The confusion regarding terminology is illustrated in the approach names listed in **Table 2** itself: minimally invasive anterolateral, anterolateral tissue-sparing, minimally invasive Watson-Jones, and modified Watson-Jones.

Video 6.1 ABMS: Anterior-Based, Muscle-Sparing Approach to the Hip. Johannes F. Plate, MD, PhD; Thorsten M. Seyler, MD, PhD; James Messersmith, PA-C; Rhett K. Hallows, MD; Scott S. Kelley, MD (10 min)

Techniques

Setup/Exposure

- A surgical table that allows a split leg extension option can be used. Alternatively, a peg board with a cutout of leg support section is affixed to the table (**Figure 1**).
- The patient is placed in the lateral decubitus position. Alternatively, the supine position can be used.
- The surgeon stands in front of the surgical table, facing the patient.
- The entire leg is prepped and draped into the surgical field to allow assessment of full ROM and hip stability after placement of trial and final implants.

Instruments/Equipment/Implants Required

- A sharp, narrow width, 90° bent Hohmann retractor is needed.
- Standard width blunt-tipped curved cobra retractors are used.
- Double-curved sharp cobra (side-specific for right and left) are required.
- A two-pronged femoral elevator is used.
- A blunt-tipped, long, narrow width, straight Hohmann retractor is optional.

Procedure

EXPOSURE

- The anterior superior iliac spine and the trochanteric portion of the proximal femur serve as landmarks for the incision. The midpoint of the incision should be on a line between the anterior superior iliac spine and the center of the greater trochanter.
- An anterior, slightly curvilinear incision is made in the skin along the anterior border of the proximal femur, with half of the incision proximal to the proximal femur and half of the incision distal to the proximal femur.
- A longitudinal incision is made in the fascia, parallel and approximately 1 cm anterior to the proximal femur (**Figure 2**).
- The muscular plane between the gluteus medius (posterior) and the tensor fascia lata (anterior) is bluntly dissected.
- Curved cobra retractors are placed over the superior and inferior femoral neck (**Figure 3, A**).
- The rectus femoris is dissected from the capsule with an elevator.
- The medial cobra retractor is placed

Table 2 Results of Total Hip Arthroplasty With the Use of an Anterior-Based Muscle-Sparing Approach

Author(s) (Year)	Number of Patients	Approach	Mean Patient Age in Years (Range)	Follow-up in Months	Success Rate (%)[a]	Results
Rottinger (2006)	47	ABMS[b]	66 (28-86)	Final: 3	100	Mean HHS was 92 at 3- and 6-mo follow-up Mean cup inclination was 44° as demonstrated on radiographs No intraoperative or perioperative complications
Wohlrab et al (2008)	40	ABMS[c] (20) or Bauer (20)	ABMS: 60 (42-71) Bauer: 64 (47-73)	Final: 3	100	No significant difference in visual analog pain scale scores between the two approaches ABMS showed advantages in HHS, range of motion, and muscle damage (measured by CPK and myoglobinemia levels) compared with the transgluteal Bauer approach at 6 and 12 wk postoperatively
D'Arrigo et al (2009)	209	ABMS[d] (20), direct anterior (20), minimally invasive Hardinge (20), or standard Hardinge (149)	ABMS: 66.3 (38-74) Direct anterior: 64 (47-74) Minimally invasive Hardinge: 66 (46-71) Standard Hardinge: 65 (46-71)	NA	NA	No difference in mean HHS was detected between groups at 6-wk follow-up Muscle-sparing approaches (direct anterior and ABMS) demonstrated early functional outcomes better than those of other approaches Study authors concluded that the ABMS was safer and less technically demanding than the other minimally invasive approaches studied and was suitable for use with different stems because of the good femoral and acetabular exposure
Bernasek et al (2010)	92	ABMS[c] (47) or Hardinge (45)	NA	Minimum: 12	100	No significant differences were found between the groups with regard to mean surgical time, HHS, EBL, and LOS Mean radiographic femoral implant alignment and mean radiographic postoperative abduction angle of the acetabular cup were similar in both groups
Martin et al (2011)	83	ABMS[b] (42) or Hardinge (41)	ABMS: 66.7 ± 10.1[e] Hardinge: 63.1 ± 10.2[e]	Final: 12	100	Significantly longer surgical time (P = 0.000078) and less EBL in the ABMS group (P = 0.008) No difference between groups in LOS Mean HHS, Merle d'Aubigné and Postel, and Medical Outcomes Study 36-Item Short Form scores were similar between the groups at final follow-up Gait analysis revealed similar results between the groups CT analysis revealed no significant difference in implant position, heterotopic ossification, or loosening

ABMS = anterior-based muscle-sparing, CPK = creatine phosphokinase, EBL = estimated blood loss, HHS = Harris hip score, LOS = length of stay, NA = not available, UCLA = University of California-Los Angeles.
[a] Success is defined as procedures not requiring revision.
[b] Study authors used the term minimally invasive anterolateral approach.
[c] Study authors used the term minimally invasive Watson-Jones approach.
[d] Study authors used the term anterolateral tissue-sparing approach.
[e] Data reported are mean ± standard deviation.
[f] Study authors used the term modified Watson-Jones approach.

Table 2 Results of Total Hip Arthroplasty With the Use of an Anterior-Based Muscle-Sparing Approach (*continued*)

Author(s) (Year)	Number of Patients	Approach	Mean Patient Age in Years (Range)	Follow-up in Months	Success Rate (%)[a]	Results
Müller et al (2011)	37	ABMS[b] (21) or Hardinge (16)	NA	Final: 12	NA	A higher serum of myoglobin concentration was measured at 6 and 24 h postoperatively in the Hardinge group compared with ABMS group Study authors concluded that abductor muscle and tendon damage occurred with both approaches, but the ABMS approach more successfully spared the gluteus medius muscle and resulted in better clinical outcomes
Mandereau et al (2012)	103	ABMS[b]	67 ± 11[e] (35-96)	Final: 12	NA	CT analysis demonstrated mean cup inclination of 44.7° ± 4.6[e], cup anteversion of 9.2° ± 9.2°[e], and femoral anteversion of 23.5° ± 9.4°[e] Mean total CPK was 390.9 ± 252[e] µg/L at 24 h and 319 ± 256[e] µg/L at 48 h postoperatively Mean morphine consumption was 2 ± 7.5[e] mg over the first 24 h 6 patients experienced approach-related complications Study authors concluded that the ABMS approach provides rapid functional recovery with reliable and reproducible acetabular implant position but greater variability of femoral implant position
Chen and Berger (2013)	113	ABMS[f] (87 outpatient, 26 inpatient)	56 (38-73)	Final: 12	99	1 complication (deep infection), which occurred 3 wk postoperatively Study authors concluded that total hip arthroplasty can be successfully performed on an outpatient basis using the ABMS approach
Queen et al (2013)	30	ABMS[f] (10), posterior (10), or Hardinge (10)	ABMS: 57.6 Posterior: 57 Hardinge: 60	Final: 12	100	No significant difference in HHS, UCLA activity score, or gait was found between approaches at 1 yr postoperatively
Repantis et al (2015)	90	ABMS[b] (45) or Watson-Jones with partial detachment (45)	ABMS: 66.2 (NA) Watson-Jones: 68.3 (NA)	Mean: 48	100	No significant difference in Medical Outcomes Study 36-Item Short Form scores between the two groups ABMS approach was associated with lower visual analog pain scale scores at 2 wk, but no significant difference was detected at final follow-up No significant difference was found between approaches in terms of EBL, transfusion rate, heterotopic ossification, or walking endurance

ABMS = anterior-based muscle-sparing, CPK = creatine phosphokinase, EBL = estimated blood loss, HHS = Harris hip score, LOS = length of stay, NA = not available, UCLA = University of California-Los Angeles.
[a] Success is defined as procedures not requiring revision.
[b] Study authors used the term minimally invasive anterolateral approach.
[c] Study authors used the term minimally invasive Watson-Jones approach.
[d] Study authors used the term anterolateral tissue-sparing approach.
[e] Data reported are mean ± standard deviation.
[f] Study authors used the term modified Watson-Jones approach.

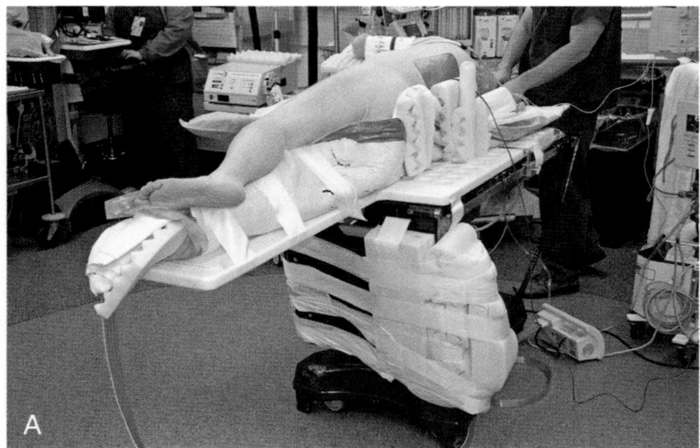

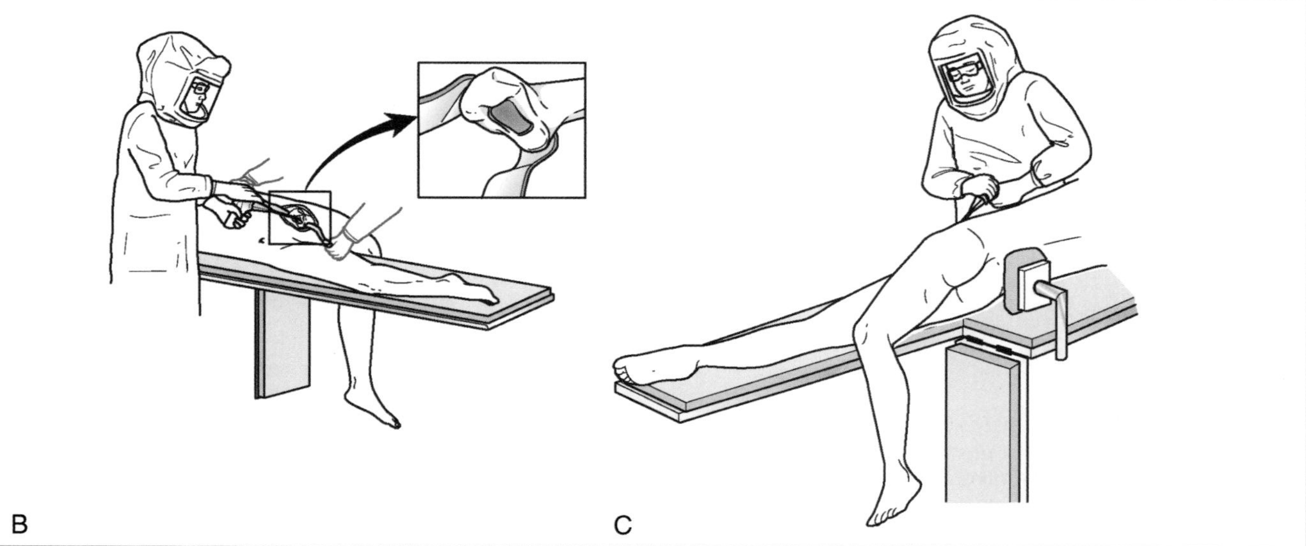

Figure 1 **A,** Photograph shows a patient positioned on a standard surgical table with the entire leg support lowered and a modified peg board affixed to the table. The peg board converts the lower half of the surgical table into a split table. **B,** Illustration depicts the surgical table, which supports the contralateral leg and allows the affected leg to be extended, adducted, and externally rotated for femoral preparation. Inset shows exposure of the proximal femur for canal preparation. **C,** Illustration depicts the surgeon standing in front of the surgical table and facing the patient.

under the rectus femoris muscle to allow visualization of the capsule as far medial as possible.

- A capsulotomy is performed parallel to the superior border of the femoral neck and is extended distally to the junction of the femoral neck and the greater trochanter (**Figure 3, B**).
- A heavy tag stitch is placed in the superolateral corner of the capsular flap to facilitate retraction and exposure.
- When using a standard surgical table with split leg extension, the posterior leg extension drop-down allows improved placement of the affected extremity in extension, adduction, and external rotation for femoral preparation.
- Although the hip can be dislocated with extension and external rotation, a safer option is to perform a femoral neck osteotomy and remove the femoral head when the acetabulum is fully exposed. The initial osteotomy cut is made at the junction of the femoral head and neck. The femur is mobilized away from the femoral head, and the definitive cut is made. The so-called saddle (the low point of the lateral femoral neck adjacent to the greater trochanter) can be used as a reference. Alternatively, the lesser trochanter can serve as a reference when the leg is placed in a slight figure-of-4 position.
- Femoral mobilization is crucial

because it provides exposure of both the acetabulum and the proximal femur. The methods of dissection and mobilization can be adjusted depending on patient characteristics (BMI, severity of disease, degree of femoral neck varus, muscle mass). The required releases typically include stripping of the capsule and obturator externus and skeletonization of the piriformis fossa (**Figure 4**).

- After the femur is fully mobilized, the leg is extended and the femur is retracted posteriorly.

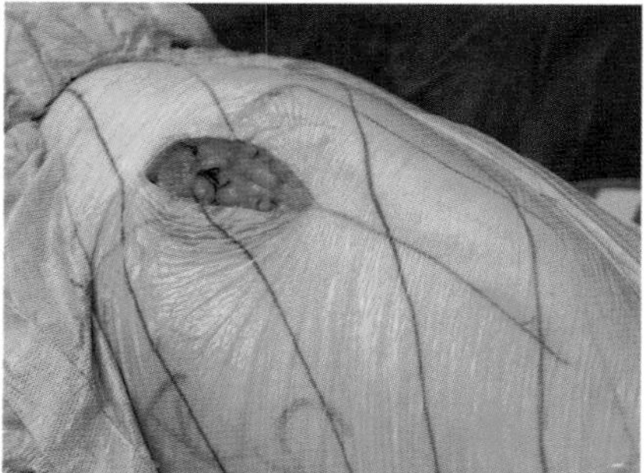

Figure 2 Intraoperative photograph of a left hip shows the location of the anterior incision along the anterior border of the proximal femur. The incision can be small or extended to facilitate access to the proximal femur for revision procedures.

- The femoral head is removed.
- Anterior and posterior cobra retractors are placed, after which a Steinmann pin is placed in the ilium at the 12-o'clock position to retract the capsule and abductor muscles superiorly and posteriorly for acetabular exposure (**Figure 5**). An inferior blunt-tipped straight Hohmann retractor can be placed to assess transverse acetabular ligament and acetabular orientation prior to reaming.

BONE PREPARATION

- The acetabulum is reamed. The choice of reamer depends on surgeon preference. Exposure is usually sufficient to allow the use of straight reamers.
- Acetabular implants are placed.
- The affected leg is placed in extension, adduction, and external rotation to expose the femur.
- A specialized modified cobra retractor is placed over the greater trochanter to retract the abductor muscles.
- A two-pronged retractor is placed under the medial compression buttress (that is, the calcar) medially to expose the cut surface of the proximal femoral neck.
- Femoral reaming and broaching is performed (**Figure 6**).
- The appropriately sized broach is selected, and the trial implants are placed in the femoral head and neck.
- The hip is reduced. With the leg free, full hip ROM is performed to evaluate stability and check for implant impingement (**Figure 7**).
- The final implants are placed. Any stem design, including stems that require straight reaming (**Figure 6**) or cemented stems (**Figure 8**), can be used with this approach.

Wound Closure

- The capsule is reapproximated with a nonabsorbable suture. However, hip stability does not depend on closure of this layer because the approach does not violate the abductor muscles (**Figure 9**).
- The fascia is repaired with synthetic absorbable suture, followed by approximation of subcutaneous tissue and skin closure.
- The subcutaneous and subcuticular layer is closed with interrupted 2-0 and running 3-0 absorbable suture (or staples).

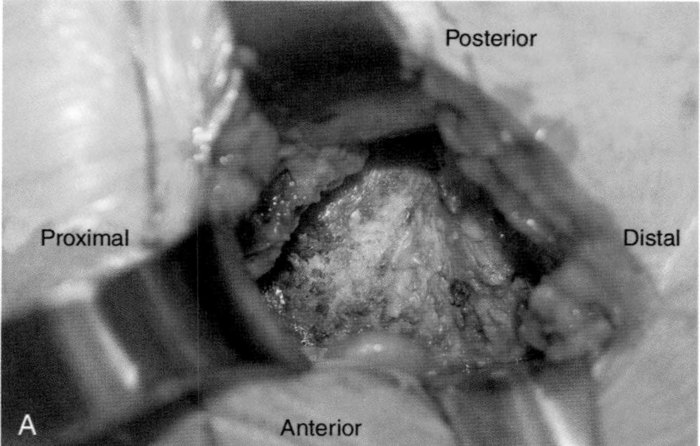

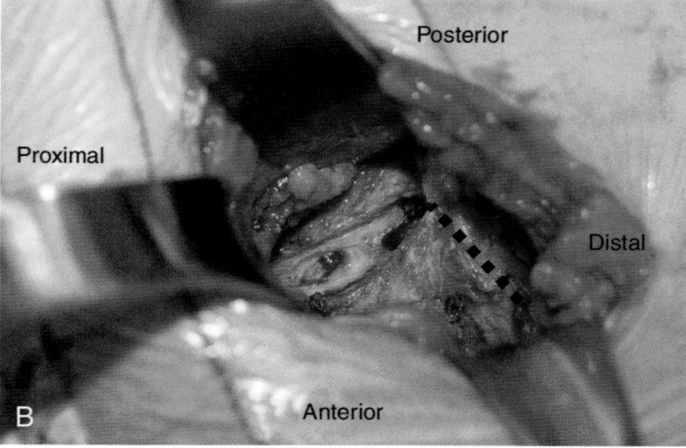

Figure 3 **A,** Intraoperative photograph of a left hip shows curved retractors placed over the superior and inferior femoral neck. **B,** A cobra retractor is placed under the rectus femoris muscle to allow visualization of the capsule. A capsulotomy (dotted line) is performed parallel to the superior border of the femoral neck and is extended distally to the junction of the femoral neck and the greater trochanter.

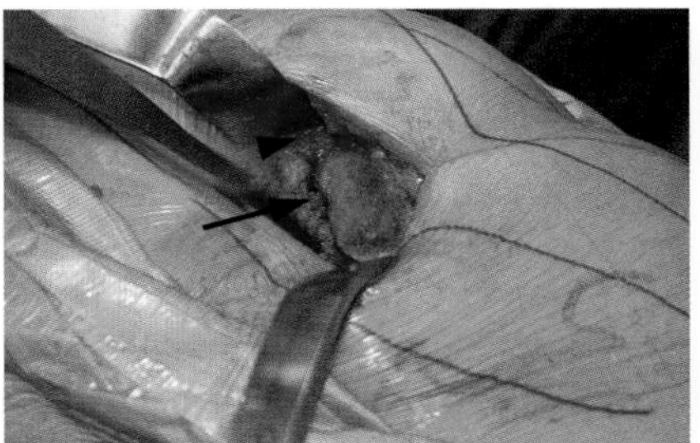

Figure 4 Intraoperative photograph of a left hip shows the femoral neck osteotomy after stripping of the posterior capsule and obturator externus, and the skeletonization of the piriformis fossa (arrow). The arrowhead indicates the greater trochanter.

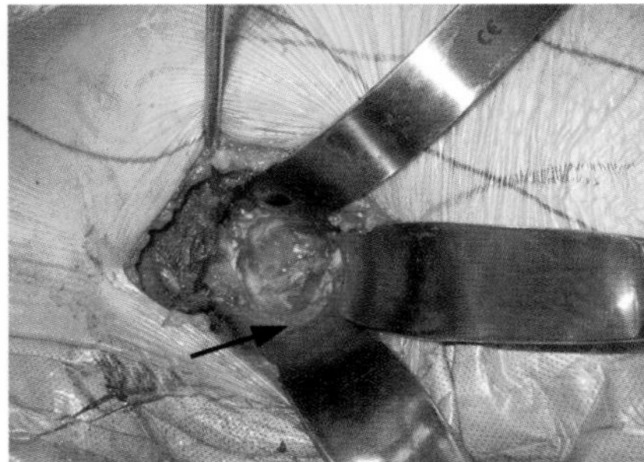

Figure 5 Intraoperative photograph of a left hip shows placement of anterior, inferior, and posterior cobra retractors and placement of a Steinmann pin in the ilium at the 12-o'clock position to retract the capsule and abductor muscles superiorly and posteriorly for acetabular exposure. The arrow indicates the transverse acetabular ligament.

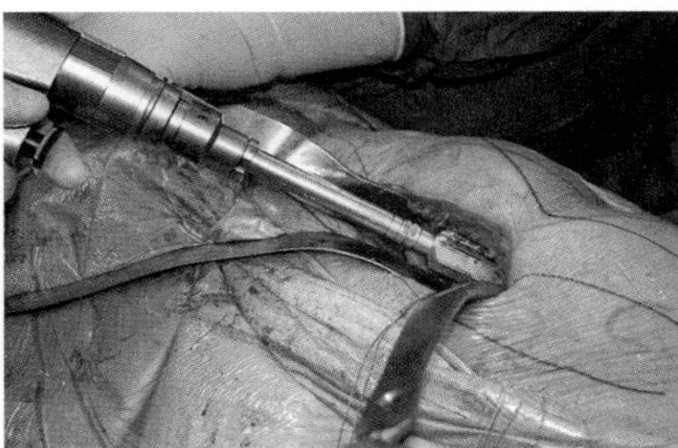

Figure 6 Intraoperative photograph of a left hip shows preparation of the femoral canal with the use of a straight in-line reamer. Access to the proximal femur is unobstructed.

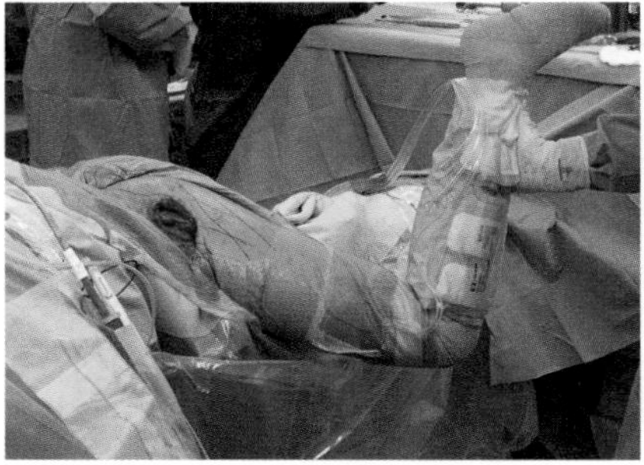

Figure 7 Intraoperative photograph of a left hip and lower extremity shows testing of hip stability and range of motion after placement of trial implants.

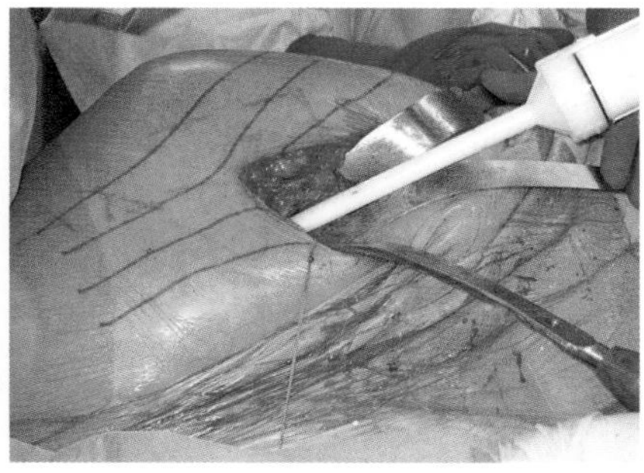

Figure 8 Intraoperative photograph of a right hip shows cement pressurization, which is facilitated with the use of the anterior-based muscle-sparing approach.

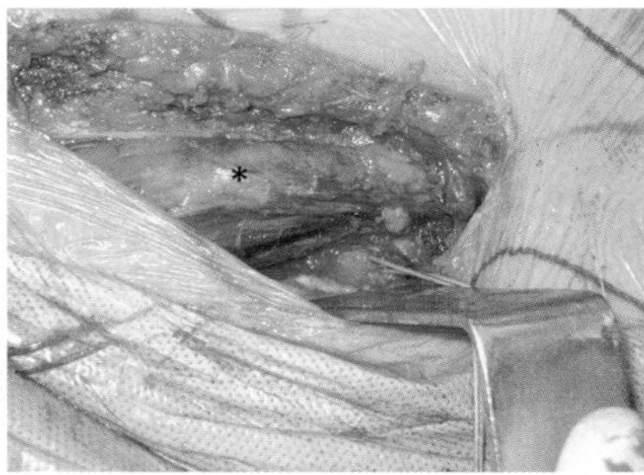

Figure 9 Intraoperative photograph of a left hip shows the abductor muscles (asterisk) before closure of the capsular flaps. A tag stitch is placed in the capsular flap. Because the adductor muscles are preserved, damage (contusion) is minimal, enabling faster recovery.

- No drain is used.
- In larger patients, a negative-pressure dressing is applied on the incision.

Postoperative Regimen

Patients typically are mobilized with physical therapy the day of the procedure and without postoperative hip precautions. Patients are instructed to use a forearm (Lofstrand) crutch for ambulatory assistance as needed. Most patients discontinue use of ambulatory assistive devices before the 2-week postoperative follow-up examination.

The average length of stay in the hospital after THA is 1 to 2 days, and the procedure has been performed on an outpatient basis. The risk of deep vein thrombosis (DVT) is assessed during the preoperative examination on the basis of patient-specific factors. Patients at low risk of DVT are given 325 mg of aspirin twice daily for 30 days postoperatively, whereas patients at high risk for DVT are given low-molecular-weight heparin. Follow-up examinations are conducted at 2 weeks, 6 weeks, and 1 year postoperatively. Routine clinical and radiographic surveillance is performed every 2 to 3 years thereafter.

Avoiding Pitfalls and Complications

The ABMS approach has a substantial learning curve. The surgeon should practice the approach on cadaver specimens before implementing it in a clinical scenario. Although new surgical approaches often require the use of new implant designs that can lead to implant-specific complications and that have their own learning curve, the ABMS approach allows the surgeon to use any implant system, including long stems that require reaming and cemented implants. Two of the authors of this chapter (T.M.S., R.K.H.), having used both the DAA and the ABMS approach, finds the ABMS approach to be easier because the patient is positioned in the standard lateral decubitus position and the surgeon's preferred implant system can be used.

Failure to adequately mobilize the femur increases the risk of femoral fracture and may compromise femoral fixation. Sequential stripping of the posterior capsule and obturator externus, as well as skeletonization of the piriformis fossa, is necessary to allow adequate exposure and mobilization of the femur and reduce the risk of intraoperative fracture of the proximal femur. Adequate femoral mobilization also requires careful attention to the angle of the leg during each step of the procedure.

Inadequate soft-tissue releases, incorrect retractor positioning, and inappropriate leg positioning can result in eccentric reaming during preparation of both the femoral canal and the acetabulum. Intraoperative radiography can be used to check acetabular implant version and reduce the risk of complications resulting from eccentric reaming (varus femoral implant position and penetration or fracture of the femoral canal). The use of intraoperative radiography or fluoroscopy can help the surgeon adapt to the ABMS approach and avoid common pitfalls.

Bibliography

Anterior Total Hip Arthroplasty Collaborative Investigators, Bhandari M, Matta JM, Dodgin D, et al: Outcomes following the single-incision anterior approach to total hip arthroplasty: A multicenter observational study. *Orthop Clin North Am* 2009;40(3):329-342.

Bauer R, Kerschbaumer F, Poisel S, Oberthaler W: The transgluteal approach to the hip joint. *Arch Orthop Trauma Surg* 1979;95(1-2):47-49.

Beaulé PE, Griffin DB, Matta JM: The Levine anterior approach for total hip replacement as the treatment for an acute acetabular fracture. *J Orthop Trauma* 2004;18(9):623-629.

Bernasek TL, Lee WS, Lee HJ, Lee JS, Kim KH, Yang JJ: Minimally invasive primary THA: Anterolateral intermuscular approach versus lateral transmuscular approach. *Arch Orthop Trauma Surg* 2010;130(11):1349-1354.

Bertin KC, Röttinger H: Anterolateral mini-incision hip replacement surgery: A modified Watson-Jones approach. *Clin Orthop Relat Res* 2004;(429):248-255.

Chen D, Berger RA: Outpatient minimally invasive total hip arthroplasty via a modified Watson-Jones approach: Technique and results. *Instr Course Lect* 2013;62:229-236.

Chow J, Penenberg B, Murphy S: Modified micro-superior percutaneously-assisted total hip: Early experiences & case reports. *Curr Rev Musculoskelet Med* 2011;4(3):146-150.

Curtin BM, Armstrong LC, Bucker BT, Odum SM, Jiranek WA: Patient Radiation Exposure During Fluoro-Assisted Direct Anterior Approach Total Hip Arthroplasty. *J Arthroplasty* 2016;31(6):1218-1221.

Dall D: Exposure of the hip by anterior osteotomy of the greater trochanter: A modified anterolateral approach. *J Bone Joint Surg Br* 1986;68(3):382-386.

D'Arrigo C, Speranza A, Monaco E, Carcangiu A, Ferretti A: Learning curve in tissue sparing total hip replacement: Comparison between different approaches. *J Orthop Traumatol* 2009;10(1):47-54.

Ganz R, Gill TJ, Gautier E, Ganz K, Krügel N, Berlemann U: Surgical dislocation of the adult hip: A technique with full access to the femoral head and acetabulum without the risk of avascular necrosis. *J Bone Joint Surg Br* 2001;83(8):1119-1124.

Gibson A: Posterior exposure of the hip joint. *J Bone Joint Surg Br* 1950;32(2):183-186.

Greidanus NV, Chihab S, Garbuz DS, et al: Outcomes of minimally invasive anterolateral THA are not superior to those of minimally invasive direct lateral and posterolateral THA. *Clin Orthop Relat Res* 2013;471(2):463-471.

Grob K, Monahan R, Gilbey H, Yap F, Filgueira L, Kuster M: Distal extension of the direct anterior approach to the hip poses risk to neurovascular structures: An anatomical study. *J Bone Joint Surg Am* 2015;97(2):126-132.

Hansen BJ, Hallows RK, Kelley SS: The Rottinger approach for total hip arthroplasty: Technique and review of the literature. *Curr Rev Musculoskelet Med* 2011;4(3):132-138.

Hardinge K: The direct lateral approach to the hip. *J Bone Joint Surg Br* 1982;64(1):17-19.

Hueter C: Die Verletzungen und Krankheiten des Hüftgelenksgegend (einschliesslich der Hüftgelenks und der oberen Hälfte des Oberschenkels), in Hueter C, ed: *Grundriss der Chirurgie.* Leipzig, Germany, F. C. W. Vogel, 1882, pp 870-945.

Hunter SC: Southern hip exposure. *Orthopedics* 1986;9(10):1425-1428.

Khanuja HS, Banerjee S, Jain D, Pivec R, Mont MA: Short bone-conserving stems in cementless hip arthroplasty. *J Bone Joint Surg Am* 2014;96(20):1742-1752.

Kocher T: Resection coxae, in Kocher T, ed: *Chirurgische Operationslehre.* Jena, Germany, Gustav Fischer, 1902, pp 523-530.

Langenbeck B: Ueber die Schussverletzungen des Hueftgelenks. *Arch Klin Chir* 1874;16:263-338.

Mandereau C, Brzakala V, Matsoukis J: Functional recovery, complications and CT positioning of total hip replacement performed through a Röttinger anterolateral mini-incision: Review of a continuous series of 103 cases. *Orthop Traumatol Surg Res* 2012;98(1):8-16.

Martin R, Clayson PE, Troussel S, Fraser BP, Docquier PL: Anterolateral minimally invasive total hip arthroplasty: A prospective randomized controlled study with a follow-up of 1 year. *J Arthroplasty* 2011;26(8):1362-1372.

Matta JM, Shahrdar C, Ferguson T: Single-incision anterior approach for total hip arthroplasty on an orthopaedic table. *Clin Orthop Relat Res* 2005;(441):115-124.

McBryde CW, Revell MP, Thomas AM, Treacy RB, Pynsent PB: The influence of surgical approach on outcome in Birmingham hip resurfacing. *Clin Orthop Relat Res* 2008;466(4):920-926.

Moore AT: The self-locking metal hip prosthesis. *J Bone Joint Surg Am* 1957;39(4):811-827.

Müller M, Tohtz S, Springer I, Dewey M, Perka C: Randomized controlled trial of abductor muscle damage in relation to the surgical approach for primary total hip replacement: Minimally invasive anterolateral versus modified direct lateral approach. *Arch Orthop Trauma Surg* 2011;131(2):179-189.

National Council on Radiation Protection and Measurements (NCRP): Limitation of Exposure to Ionizing Radiation: Recommendations of the National Council on Radiation Protection and Measurements. Bethesda, MD, NCRP (Report No. 116), 1993.

Palan J, Beard DJ, Murray DW, Andrew JG, Nolan J: Which approach for total hip arthroplasty: Anterolateral or posterior? *Clin Orthop Relat Res* 2009;467(2):473-477.

Queen RM, Schaeffer JF, Butler RJ, et al: Does surgical approach during total hip arthroplasty alter gait recovery during the first year following surgery? *J Arthroplasty* 2013;28(9):1639-1643.

Repantis T, Bouras T, Korovessis P: Comparison of minimally invasive approach versus conventional anterolateral approach for total hip arthroplasty: A randomized controlled trial. *Eur J Orthop Surg Traumatol* 2015;25(1):111-116.

Restrepo C, Mortazavi SM, Brothers J, Parvizi J, Rothman RH: Hip dislocation: Are hip precautions necessary in anterior approaches? *Clin Orthop Relat Res* 2011;469(2):417-422.

Rottinger H: Minimally invasive anterolateral surgical approach for total hip arthroplasty: Early clinical results. *Hip Int* 2006;16(suppl 4):42-47.

Schaffer JL, Bozic KJ, Dorr LD, Miller DA, Nepola JV: AOA symposium: Direct-to-consumer marketing in orthopaedic surgery. Boon or boondoggle? *J Bone Joint Surg Am* 2008;90(11):2534-2543.

Smith-Petersen MN: A new supra-articular subperiosteal approach to the hip joint. *Am J Orthop Surg* 1917;15:592-595.

Watson-Jones R: Fractures of the neck of the femur. *Br J Surg* 1936;23:787-808.

Wohlrab D, Droege JW, Mendel T, et al: Minimally invasive vs. transgluteal total hip replacement: A 3-month follow-up of a prospective randomized clinical study [German]. *Orthopade* 2008;37(11):1121-1126.

Video Reference

Plate JF, Seyler TM, Messersmith J, Hallows RK, Kelley SS: Video: *ABMS: Anterior-Based, Muscle-Sparing Approach to the Hip*. Durham, NC, 2017.

Chapter 7
Preoperative Planning and Templating in Total Hip Arthroplasty

Kevin L. Garvin, MD
Curtis W. Hartman, MD

Introduction

The primary goals of total hip arthroplasty (THA) are pain relief and improved function. Achievement of these goals is highly dependent on the precision of the surgical procedure. Templating improves the surgeon's ability to restore leg length and offset and to place the components accurately, and it ensures proper implant selection based on the patient's anatomy.

Preoperative Planning and Hip Biomechanics

Comprehensive preoperative planning is critically important to a successful outcome after THA. A comprehensive patient history and physical examination, including radiographs of the affected limb, are essential in evaluating a patient with hip pathology because they may reveal medical diagnoses that dictate further evaluation by the patient's internist or other specialists. Often, these specialists assist with the perioperative management of the patient. Templating of the hip is done after the patient's health is determined to be acceptable for anesthesia and surgery.

Reconstruction of leg length and offset are necessary to restore hip biomechanics, and restoration of normal hip biomechanics is imperative to excellent outcomes after THA. Better postoperative function is increasingly important because younger patients are undergoing surgery. With widespread use of more durable materials, longevity of implant systems is taken for granted. However, even today, durability can be negatively affected by failure to restore length and offset. Lengthening of the affected leg is a contributing factor in aseptic loosening. Data indicate that a leg-length inequality of 10 mm results in an asymmetric increase in muscle group activity, with a lateral imbalance when standing. The lumbar spine is subjected to sagittal and rotational stresses, and the hip of the long leg is subjected to increased stresses at the articulating surfaces; this imbalance is thought to cause chondral damage and unilateral arthrosis.

Limb-length discrepancy (LLD) is among the easiest of parameters by which to quantify the quality of a THA. There were 14,979 total orthopaedic claims in the United States from 1985 to 1998, the highest percentage of which involved joint procedures (29%). Patient dissatisfaction resulting from unequal limbs is the type of postoperative imperfection that can yield itself to exaggeration as "improper performance of surgery," and result in legal action. LLD after THA can have substantial effects on patient satisfaction, limp, and pain relief.

True LLD is an absolute difference in limb length as measured by scanogram or, more typically, from the anterior superior iliac spine to the medial malleolus. The use of standing blocks placed under the foot is another technique to measure limb inequality. Functional (apparent) LLD is caused by soft-tissue contracture, primarily of the adductors, or a fixed obliquity between the pelvis and the lumbosacral spine.

Femoral offset is the distance along the medial-lateral direction from the center of the femoral head to a line bisecting the long axis of the femur (**Figure 1**). Femoral stem offset is the distance along the medial-lateral direction from the center of rotation of the prosthetic femoral head to a line bisecting the long axis of the stem. Increasing offset reduces the risk for dislocation by two distinct mechanisms. First, increased offset results in decreased risk for bone-on-bone impingement. Second,

Dr. Garvin or an immediate family member serves as an unpaid consultant to Trak Surgical, and serves as a board member, owner, officer, or committee member of the American Academy of Orthopaedic Surgeons, the American Orthopaedic Association, The Hip Society, and The Knee Society. Dr. Hartman or an immediate family member is a member of a speakers' bureau or has made paid presentations on behalf of and serves as a paid consultant to Smith & Nephew, has stock or stock options held in Trak Surgical, and has received research or institutional support from Pfizer and Smith & Nephew.

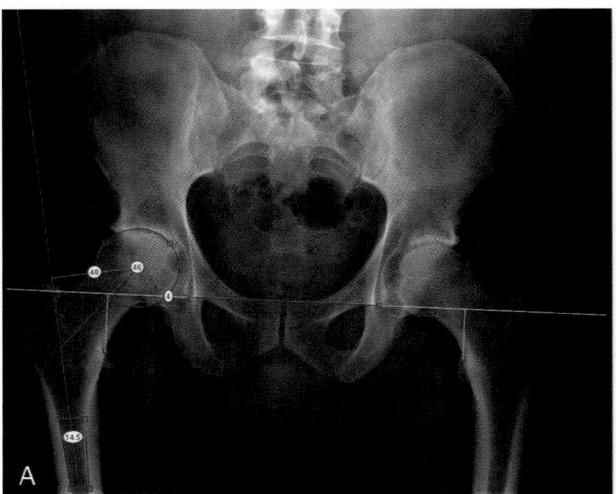

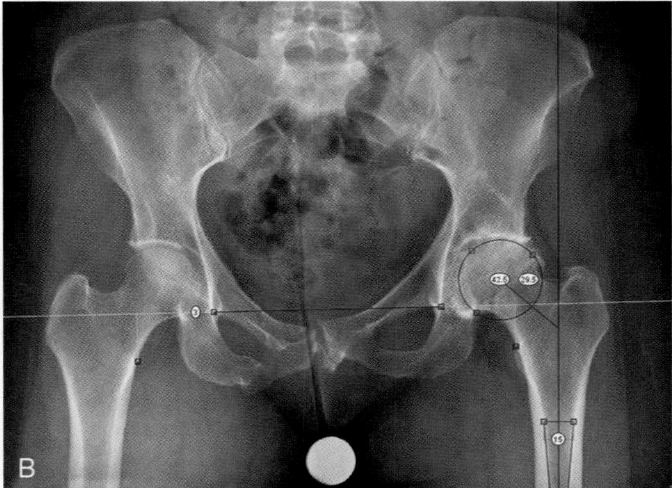

Figure 1 AP pelvic radiographs demonstrate femoral offset, leg length difference, femoral head diameter, and endosteal diameter determined via digital templating. **A,** The femoral offset of the right hip is 48 mm, femoral head diameter is 46 mm, the right hip is 4 mm longer than the left hip, and the endosteal diameter is 14.5 mm. **B,** The femoral offset of the left hip is 29.5 mm, femoral head diameter is 42.5 mm, the left hip is 3 mm shorter than the right hip, and the endosteal diameter is 15 mm.

increasing offset increases soft-tissue tension. Increased offset improves leverage and thus reduces the abductor muscle force required, thereby improving abductor efficiency and gait. The effect of reduced abductor muscle force in turn results in reduced joint reactive force across the hip joint, reduced stresses in the articulating surfaces, and ultimate improvement in wear of the prosthesis.

Templating the Hip

Templating is one of the final necessary steps in preparing for a THA. Templating for THA has several purposes. First, it facilitates implant selection. The implant selected for a large-boned elderly patient who has osteopenia may be different from the implant selected for a young patient who has congenital or developmental dysplasia of the hip. Second, templating helps determine optimal placement of the acetabular and femoral implants to restore leg length and offset. Finally, templating helps the surgeon prepare for both expected and unexpected problems. A patient with a varus femoral neck angle will require a femoral implant that can be used to restore offset. Templating for the acetabular implant may reveal that a dysplastic hip will require an autogenous femoral head graft to provide adequate stability for the acetabulum. Problems associated with hardware removal also will be identified.

Imaging

The essential tools for templating include appropriate radiographs of the hip, a full range of templates, and radiograph-marking pencils. Most digital radiography packages include digital templating software. Digital templating is more accurate than standard onlay templating. The hip should be templated with adequate time remaining before the procedure to obtain the necessary implants and instruments required for surgical reconstruction.

The radiographs should include an AP view of the entire pelvis and a lateral view of the femur. If the hip cannot be internally rotated, then the patient should be placed prone with the affected limb in slight external rotation (15° to 20°) to mimic an anatomic position. The preferred lateral radiograph is a modification of the frog-lateral or the table down (Lowenstein lateral) view. It also is useful to template the contralateral hip. Typically, templates are magnified 20% to match the radiographic magnification, and the surgeon must know the amount of magnification before using templates. If the radiographs are digitized, the surgeon should communicate with the radiology technician to determine the amount of magnification. A radiographic marker of known size can be used at the level of the greater trochanter to control for magnification. With most digital templating packages, this type of marker can be used to more accurately determine the magnification. The surgeon must take care to ensure that the marker is appropriately placed at the level of the joint. Incorrect placement of the marker can result in sizing errors up to 26%. A marker placed inaccurately on the table will appear undersized, whereas a marker placed on the anterior surface of the hip will be magnified. These errors are compounded in larger patients. A mathematical method has been developed to assess the vertical and horizontal position of the radiographic marker.

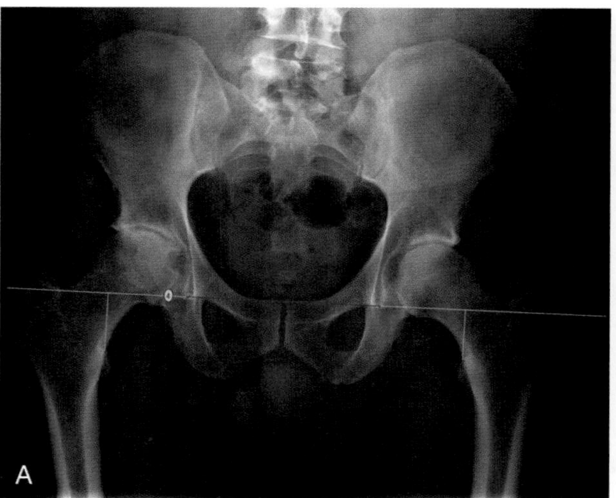

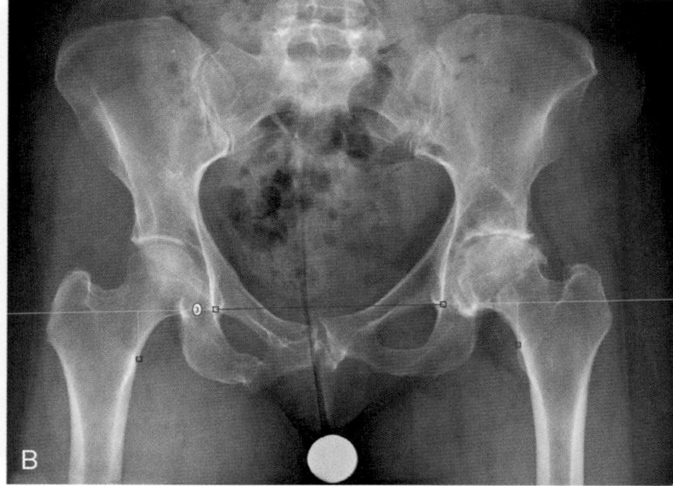

Figure 2 AP pelvic radiographs demonstrate limb-length discrepancy measurements using the acetabular teardrops as the horizontal reference. **A,** The right hip is 4 mm longer than the left hip. **B,** The left hip is 3 mm shorter than the right hip. The vertical lines represent the distance from the horizontal to the top of the lesser trochanter. The difference in length between the two lines is calculated by the software and represents the limb-length discrepancy.

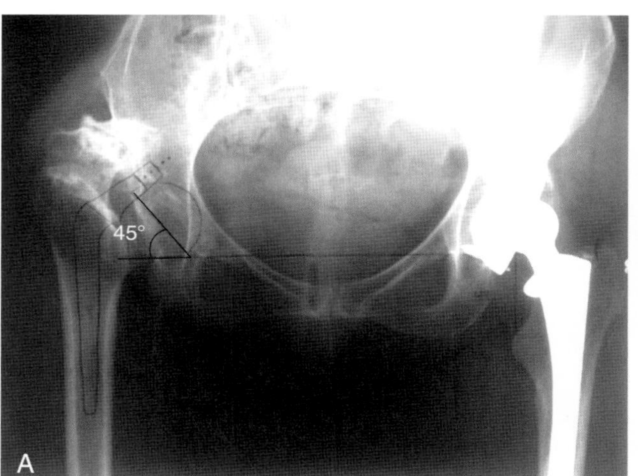

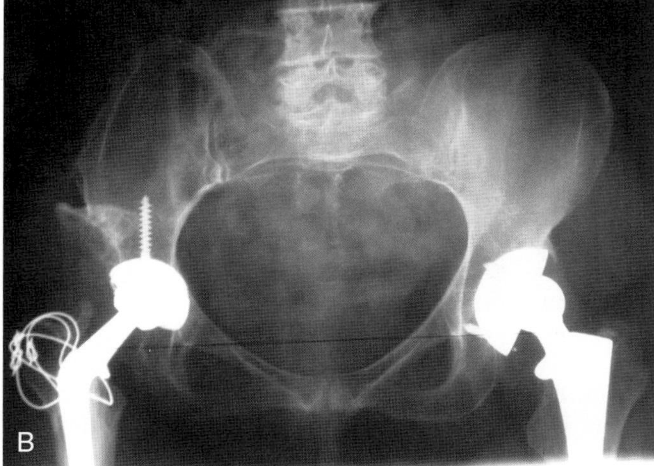

Figure 3 **A,** Preoperative AP pelvic radiograph demonstrates Crowe type IV dysplasia of the right hip, which is templated for reconstructing an anatomic center of rotation. **B,** Postoperative AP radiograph demonstrates acetabular reconstruction with a small implant to restore anatomic position. (Reproduced from Garvin KL: Primary total hip arthroplasty: Preoperative planning and templating, from Lieberman JR, Berry DJ, eds: *Advanced Reconstruction: Hip*. Rosemont, IL, American Academy of Orthopaedic Surgeons, 2005, pp 41-46.)

Technique

Preoperative templating should be done to reconstruct the limb to an anatomic length if possible. The patient history and physical examination, along with radiographs, determine the amount of LLD. Before the template is placed on the radiographs, several landmarks should be identified. One of the most reliable radiographic landmarks is the acetabular teardrop, which is the landmark of the inferomedial acetabulum. A line connecting the teardrops of the two hips serves as the horizontal reference from which the center of hip rotation can be measured (**Figure 2**). The line also helps determine the acetabular and femoral measurements. Acetabular implant placement is normally at the lateral edge of the teardrop, with abduction inclination of 45° as drawn on the radiograph (**Figure 3, A**). In the ideal patient, the lateral aspect of the acetabular implant on the template will extend to the lateral rim of the acetabulum. Implant placement may vary from this anatomic position, depending on the requirements for reconstruction and the patient's anatomy. The implants also should be placed to maximize bony containment and the surface area of contact.

In the example of the templating process described in this chapter, the

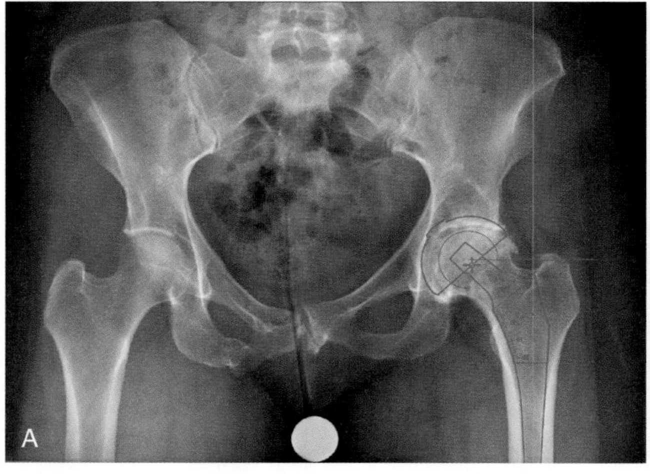

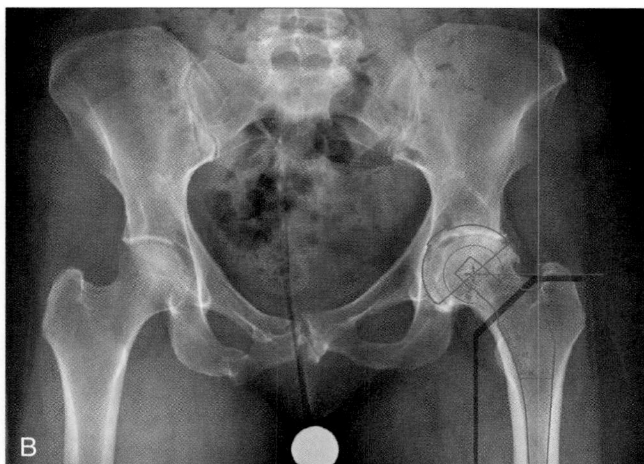

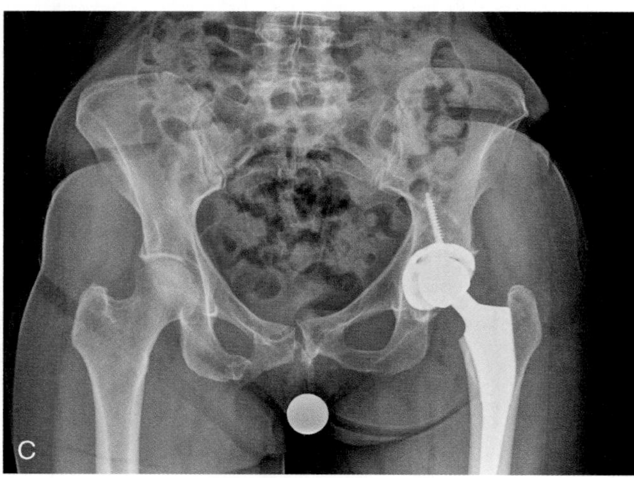

Figure 4 **A,** AP pelvic radiograph with a templated left hip demonstrates inferomedial placement of the acetabular implant relative to the anatomic center of rotation. **B,** AP pelvic radiograph demonstrates that the proposed reconstruction will add slight length and offset to anatomically restore the hip biomechanics. **C,** Postoperative AP pelvic radiograph demonstrates reconstruction of limb length and offset as predicted by the preoperative template.

acetabular template is placed medial and inferior to the center of rotation, and the template shows that the proposed reconstruction will affect limb length and offset (**Figure 4**). The difference in lengths and offset of the acetabulum are added to the femoral implant measurements and accounted for to restore the patient's anatomy. The offset of the femoral implant should include the anatomic offset of the patient's proximal femur as well as any difference that might be measured from the medial or lateral position of the acetabular implant. Next, the femoral implant that will restore leg length and offset is chosen. Most implants have dual offset (standard and high) options to accommodate anatomic variability. The postoperative radiograph demonstrates the reconstructed hip (**Figure 4, C**). The acetabular implant is well positioned, and the femoral implant has been placed to reconstruct the hip and restore length and offset.

Depending on the severity of the disease in patients with developmental dysplasia of the hip, the hip anatomic position may be relatively normal or may be severely shortened and dislocated. Patients with mild dysplasia have nearly normal anatomy, and anatomic reconstruction of the acetabulum usually is possible in these patients. Patients with moderate involvement or a high-riding hip may require cephalad acetabular implant placement or augmentation of the bone and/or implant to achieve anatomic positioning. Patients who have severe dysplasia frequently require small components, which can be placed in the anatomic position (**Figure 3**). To compensate for the anatomic position of the acetabular implant, it may be necessary to shorten the femur.

Patients who have posttraumatic arthrosis require special attention during preoperative planning and templating. It may be necessary to remove the retained hardware if it interferes with implant placement (**Figure 5**). Necessary equipment, including a full complement of screwdrivers; a broken screw removal set; and a high-speed, metal-cutting burr, should be readily available at the time of surgery. Additionally, the surgeon should know from preoperative planning how removal of

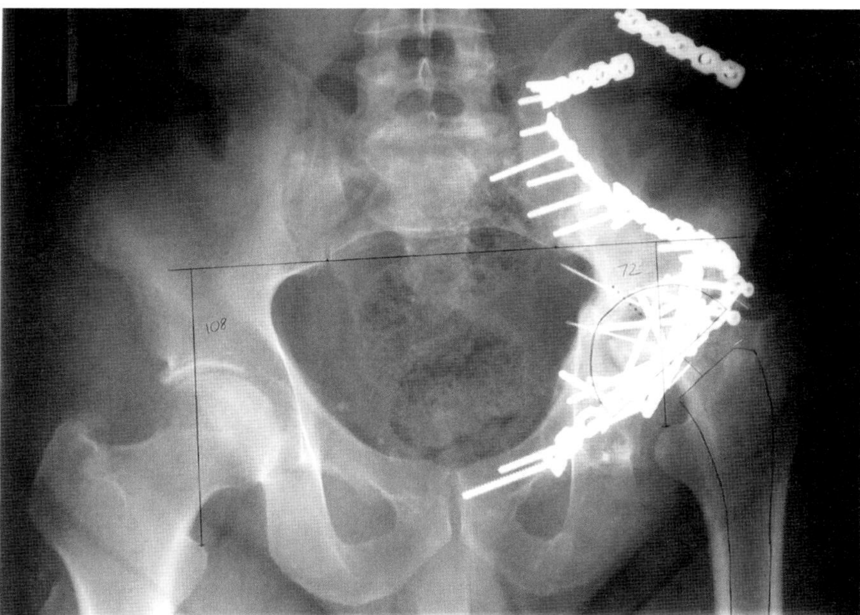

Figure 5 AP pelvic radiograph of a 39-year-old man who had an acetabular fracture 8 years prior. Traumatic arthritis and a 36-mm limb-length discrepancy developed on the left side. The sacroiliac joint was used for referencing because of alteration of the patient's anatomy. (Reproduced from Garvin KL: Primary total hip arthroplasty: Preoperative planning and templating, from Lieberman JR, Berry DJ, eds: *Advanced Reconstruction: Hip*. Rosemont, IL, American Academy of Orthopaedic Surgeons, 2005, pp 41-46.)

the retained hardware will affect the integrity of the bone; whether the acetabular fracture has been anatomically reconstructed and, if not, whether it will require augmentation; and whether the femur is anatomically reconstructed and, if not, whether an osteotomy will be necessary.

Results

The authors of this chapter performed a retrospective analysis of several consecutive patients who had a history of THA and from whom a digital pelvic radiograph was obtained. All measurements were calculated using preoperative planning and templating software. Two measurements were obtained: for the first one, the radiograph was calibrated with a radiographic marker of known diameter. For the second measurement, the magnification factor was arbitrarily set at 120%. The diameter of the prosthetic femoral head was measured and compared with the known diameter. Intraclass correlation coefficients (ICCs) were calculated to evaluate the level of agreement between the measured head diameter and the known head diameter. Stratified analyses were used to evaluate the effects of sex, age, and body mass index on the level of agreement between the measured and known head diameter. The authors of this chapter calculated the ideal magnification factor for each hip.

The overall ICC for the first measurement was 0.910 (95% confidence interval [CI]: 0.871-0.938). The overall ICC for the second measurement was 0.952 (95% CI: 0.924-0.969). This difference was not significant. When controlling for sex, the ICC in women was 0.791 (95% CI: 0.680-0.871) for the first measurement and 0.943 (95% CI: 0.888-0.968) for the second measurement. This difference was significant. In men, the ICC was 0.919 (95% CI: 0.852-0.955) for the first measurement and 0.936 (95% CI: 0.885-0.964) for the second measurement. This difference was not significant. The mean ideal magnification factor was 119%.

These results suggest that female sex is a risk factor for inaccurate calibration of digital radiographs when attempting to use a digital marker. The surgeon should take care in calibrating radiographs of females with a digital marker. If there is a question about the placement of the radiographic marker, the authors of this chapter default to a calibration of 119%.

Summary

Failure to restore leg length is a common cause of litigation after THA. The process of preoperative planning and templating is essential to minimize this error in patients undergoing THA. Additionally, patients should be counseled preoperatively that it is not always possible to achieve equal limb length and that mild to moderate LLD may be unavoidable. However, careful preoperative planning and templating along with appropriate implant selection and meticulous surgical technique helps restore optimal hip biomechanics, hip stability, and limb length.

Bibliography

Archibeck MJ, Cummins T, Tripuraneni KR, et al: Inaccuracies in the use of magnification markers in digital hip radiographs. *Clin Orthop Relat Res* 2016;474(8):1812-1817.

Boese CK, Bredow J, Dargel J, Eysel P, Geiges H, Lechler P: Calibration marker position in digital templating of total hip arthroplasty. *J Arthroplasty* 2016;31(4):883-887.

Committee on Professional Liability: *Managing Orthopaedic Malpractice Risk.* Rosemont, IL, American Academy of Orthopaedic Surgeons, 2000.

Gamble P, de Beer J, Petruccelli D, Winemaker M: The accuracy of digital templating in uncemented total hip arthroplasty. *J Arthroplasty* 2010;25(4):529-532.

Gurney B: Leg length discrepancy. *Gait Posture* 2002;15(2):195-206.

Röder C, Vogel R, Burri L, Dietrich D, Staub LP: Total hip arthroplasty: Leg length inequality impairs functional outcomes and patient satisfaction. *BMC Musculoskelet Disord* 2012;13:95.

Sinclair VF, Wilson J, Jain NP, Knowles D: Assessment of accuracy of marker ball placement in pre-operative templating for total hip arthroplasty. *J Arthroplasty* 2014;29(8):1658-1660.

Visuri T, Lindholm TS, Antti-Poika I, Koskenvuo M: The role of overlength of the leg in aseptic loosening after total hip arthroplasty. *Ital J Orthop Traumatol* 1993;19(1):107-111.

Chapter 8
Primary Total Hip Arthroplasty With a Cemented Acetabular Implant

Chitranjan S. Ranawat, MD
Amar S. Ranawat, MD
Y. Julia Kao, MD

Indications

In the United States, the use of cemented all-polyethylene acetabular implants for primary total hip arthroplasty (THA) has become less common because of the increased use of noncemented fixation. Cemented acetabular fixation is commonly performed in other countries because of its durability, reproducibility, cost-effectiveness, and modest wear rates. In the United States today, acetabular cement is most commonly used for fixation of a liner into a noncemented cup during revision or as part of a cement-in-cement revision procedure. However, some surgeons continue to use cemented, all-polyethylene acetabular implants in all patients undergoing primary THA.

The authors of this chapter recommend cement fixation in patients who have undergone pelvic irradiation because biologic ingrowth is unlikely to occur in these patients. The use of a cemented all-polyethylene acetabular implant and a noncemented femoral implant (so-called reverse hybrid THA) has shown excellent short-term and midterm results in younger (age range, 55 to 64 years), active patients in recent studies based on Swedish and Norwegian registry data. The reverse hybrid technique was developed in response to the finding of better long-term (>10 years) results of noncemented femoral implants compared with cemented femoral implants in patients younger than 60 years and the theory that the use of cross-linked polyethylene results in improved long-term survival of cemented acetabular implants. In addition, the use of cement fixation in primary THA procedures can be advantageous in revision scenarios because failure of a cemented implant results in sclerosis of the underlying bone, whereas failure of a noncemented acetabular implant results in massive osteolysis.

Contraindications

Cemented fixation is contraindicated in patients with extensive cyst formation, excessive bleeding at the acetabulum that cannot be controlled with hypotensive analgesia, and/or weak cancellous bone, which is seen in patients with inflammatory arthropathy, dysplasia, or protrusio acetabuli. Cemented fixation should be avoided in patients with severe cardiopulmonary disease because embolic events can occur when cement is pressurized.

Alternative Treatments

The use of noncemented acetabular cups is an alternative to the use of cemented all-polyethylene acetabular implants.

Dr. C. Ranawat or an immediate family member has received royalties from ConforMIS, DePuy Synthes, and Stryker; is a member of a speakers' bureau or has made paid presentations on behalf of Mitek Sports Medicine and Stryker; serves as a paid consultant to Mitek Sports Medicine and Stryker; has stock or stock options held in ConforMIS; has received research or institutional support from CeramTec; and serves as a board member, owner, officer, or committee member of the Eastern Orthopaedic Educational Foundation and the Hip Society. Dr. A. Ranawat or an immediate family member has received royalties from ConforMIS, DePuy Synthes, Pipeline, and Stryker; is a member of a speakers' bureau or has made paid presentations on behalf of ConvaTec, DePuy Synthes, and Stryker; serves as a paid consultant to CeramTec and DePuy Synthes; has stock or stock options held in ConforMIS and Strathspey Crown; has received research or institutional support from CeramTec, DePuy Synthes, and Stryker; has received nonincome support (such as equipment or services), commercially derived honoraria, or other non–research-related funding (such as paid travel) from DePuy Synthes and Stryker; and serves as a board member, owner, officer, or committee member of the American Academy of Orthopaedic Surgeons, the American Association of Hip and Knee Surgeons, the Eastern Orthopaedic Association, The Hip Society, and The Knee Society. Neither Dr. Kao nor any immediate family member has received anything of value from or has stock or stock options held in a commercial company or institution related directly or indirectly to the subject of this chapter.

Table 1 Results of Total Hip Arthroplasty With a Cemented Acetabular Implant

Author(s) (Year)	Number of Hips	Implant Type	Mean Patient Age in Years (Range)	Minimum Follow-up (Years)	Success Rate (%)[a]	Results
DeLee and Charnley (1976)	141	Charnley	NR	10	100	98 (69.5%) showed demarcation of the cement from the bone of the acetabulum, of which 13 showed various degrees of migration of the cemented socket
Stauffer (1982)	231	Charnley	63.6 (39-84)	10	97	7 were revised for loosening of the acetabular implant
Brick and Poss (1988)	267	Mixed	60.33 (28-82)	11	96.9	24% had mechanical loosening of the acetabular and femoral implant
Ritter et al (1992)	238	Charnley	67-68 (NR)	10	95.4	Increased failure rates were affected by patient age at time of surgery and metal backing of the acetabular implant
Wroblewski and Siney (1993)	193	Charnley	47 (23.58-68.08)	18	97	Socket wear is the factor most likely to negatively affect survival of low-friction arthroplasty
Kavanagh et al (1994)	112	Charnley	65 (38-85)	20	84	The probability of 20-yr survival without implant revision was 84%
Ranawat et al (1995)	236	Mixed	61 (NR)	5	99.2	The state of the bone-cement interface as seen on the early postoperative radiograph can predict the longevity of a cemented socket with a high degree of probability
Mulroy et al (1995)	105	Harris-II (Stryker Howmedica Osteonics) with the use of computer-assisted design	61 (21-85)	10	95	Second-generation cementing techniques were used in this study
Callaghan et al (2004)	27	Charnley	54.4 (35-69)	30	88	88% of implants remained intact at final follow-up or patient death
Della Valle et al (2004)	40	Charnley	53 (23-83)	20	77	77.3% survivorship at 21-yr follow-up, with revision for aseptic loosening or radiographic evidence of loosening as the endpoint

NR = not reported.
[a] Success is defined as procedures not requiring revision.
Adapted from Ranawat CS, Ranawat AS: Primary total hip arthroplasty: Cemented acetabulum, in Lieberman JR, Berry DJ: *Advanced Reconstruction: Hip*. Rosemont, IL, American Academy of Orthopaedic Surgeons, 2005, pp 47-53.

Results

In patients with cemented acetabular implants, rates of revision for osteoarthritis at 10- to 20-year follow-up range from 2% to 14% (**Table 1**). Similarly, rates of radiographic loosening at 10- to 20-year follow-up range from 3% to 24%.

Techniques

Setup/Exposure

- Pain is managed with the use of preemptive analgesia prior to surgery

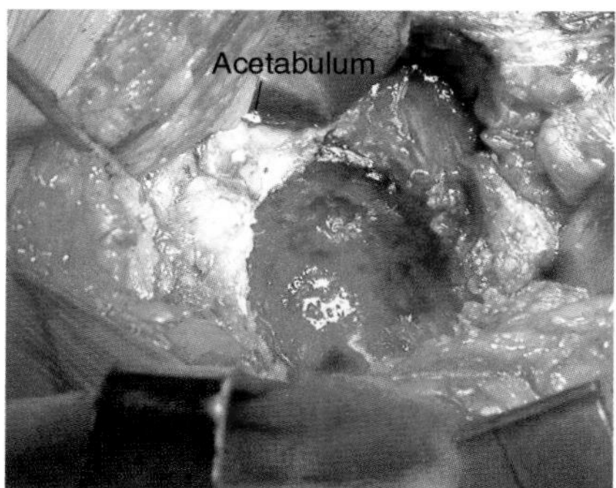

Figure 1 Intraoperative photograph shows acetabular exposure with a Steinmann pin superiorly, an Aufranc retractor inferiorly, a C-retractor anteriorly, and a 90° bent Hohmann retractor posteriorly. (Reproduced from Ranawat CS, Ranawat AS: Primary total hip arthroplasty: Cemented acetabulum, in Lieberman JR, Berry DJ: *Advanced Reconstruction: Hip.* Rosemont, IL, American Academy of Orthopaedic Surgeons, 2005, pp 47-53.)

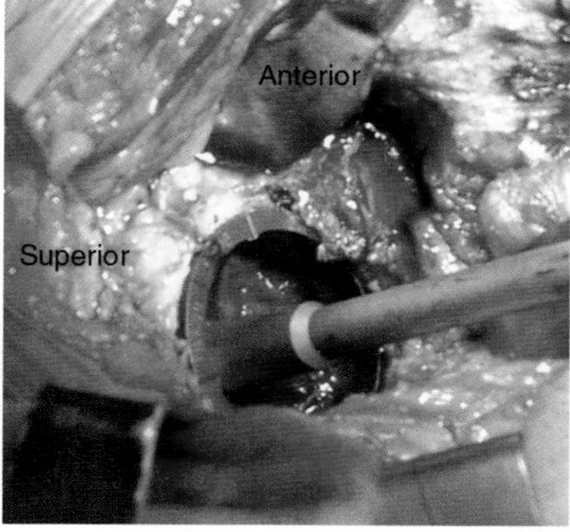

Figure 2 Intraoperative photograph shows the trial acetabular implant, which should spin easily between two fingers. (Reproduced from Ranawat CS, Ranawat AS: Primary total hip arthroplasty: Cemented acetabulum, in Lieberman JR, Berry DJ: *Advanced Reconstruction: Hip.* Rosemont, IL, American Academy of Orthopaedic Surgeons, 2005, pp 47-53.)

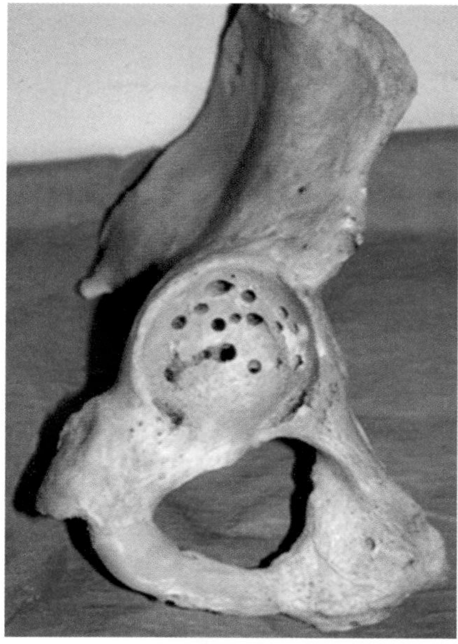

Figure 3 Photograph of a bone model shows drill holes for fixation in the pubis, ischium, and ilium. (Reproduced from Ranawat CS, Ranawat AS: Primary total hip arthroplasty: Cemented acetabulum, in Lieberman JR, Berry DJ: *Advanced Reconstruction: Hip.* Rosemont, IL, American Academy of Orthopaedic Surgeons, 2005, pp 47-53.)

as well as with a postoperative multimodal protocol.

- Hypotensive, regional anesthesia is used. The mean arterial pressure should be kept between 50 and 55 mm Hg.
- The surgeon's preferred patient position and surgical approach may be used. Sufficient acetabular exposure is required.
- The authors of this chapter typically use the posterior approach.
- Anterior femoral mobilization is enhanced by partial release of the gluteus maximus tendon at its insertion, releasing the rectus femoris reflected head, and excision of the labrum.
- The transverse ligament is preserved to aid in the containment and pressurization of the cement.

Procedure

BONE PREPARATION

- After sufficient exposure is achieved, the acetabulum is reamed circumferentially.
- The direction of reaming is guided by the desired final position of the implant.
- Reaming continues until cancellous bleeding bone is encountered in both the anterior and posterior columns where the pubis and ischial tuberosity meet the pelvis.
- Care is taken to preserve the medial wall of the acetabulum and maintain cancellous bone medially (**Figure 1**).
- The appropriate size and position of the acetabular implant are determined.
- A hemispheric trial implant is inserted.
- The surgeon should be able to spin the trial implant easily between two fingers to allow a sufficient gap for cement fixation (**Figure 2**). Typically, 1 mm of overreaming is required.
- With the use of a high-speed burr, holes are drilled in the ilium, ischium, and pubis for additional fixation (**Figure 3**).
- Pulsatile lavage is used to remove blood and fat debris.

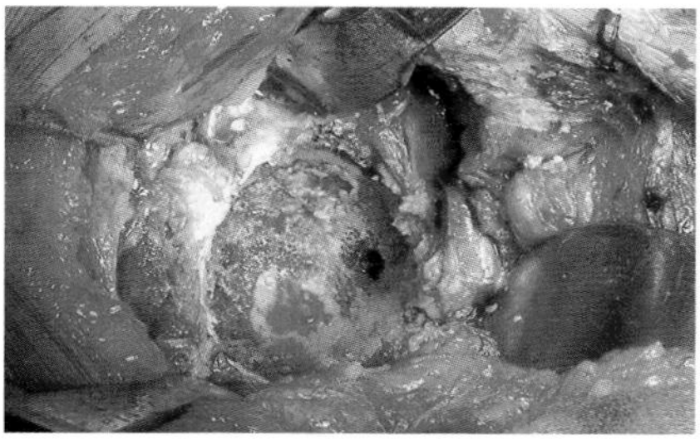

Figure 4 Intraoperative photograph shows the dry cancellous acetabular bone bed after preparation. (Reproduced from Ranawat CS, Ranawat AS: Primary total hip arthroplasty: Cemented acetabulum, in Lieberman JR, Berry DJ: *Advanced Reconstruction: Hip.* Rosemont, IL, American Academy of Orthopaedic Surgeons, 2005, pp 47-53.)

- The bone is dried (**Figure 4**).

PROSTHESIS IMPLANTATION

- The acetabular bed is dried with sponges soaked in epinephrine.

Alternatively, iliac wing suction devices can be used.
- Cement with a doughlike consistency is inserted into the acetabulum. The cement is pressurized with a bulb syringe device for 30 seconds (**Figure 5**).
- Excess cement is removed from the teardrop.
- The insertion device is used to place the implant. The implant should engage inferiorly before being placed in the intended position (**Figure 6**).
- The insertion device is removed.
- During polymerization of the cement, direct pressure is maintained on the acetabular cup to prevent displacement (**Figure 7**).
- Excess cement is removed.
- The version and lateral opening of the implant are adjusted as necessary.
- Anterior bony osteophytes that may result in impingement are removed.
- The femur is prepared, and the femoral implant is placed.

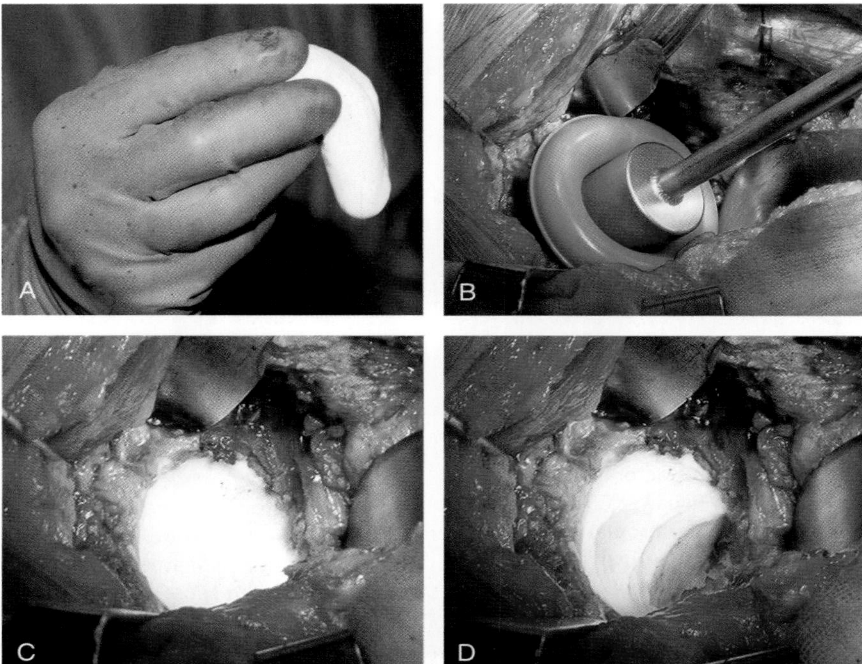

Figure 5 **A,** Photograph shows the doughlike cement before it is inserted into the dry acetabular bed. Intraoperative photographs of a hip show the use of a bulb syringe to pressurize the cement (**B**), the cement after pressurization (**C**), and the removal of cement from the teardrop (**D**). (Reproduced from Ranawat CS, Ranawat AS: Primary total hip arthroplasty: Cemented acetabulum, in Lieberman JR, Berry DJ: *Advanced Reconstruction: Hip*. Rosemont, IL, American Academy of Orthopaedic Surgeons, 2005, pp 47-53.)

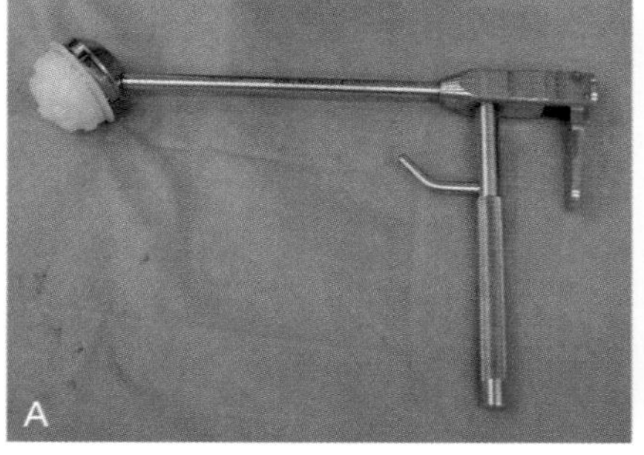

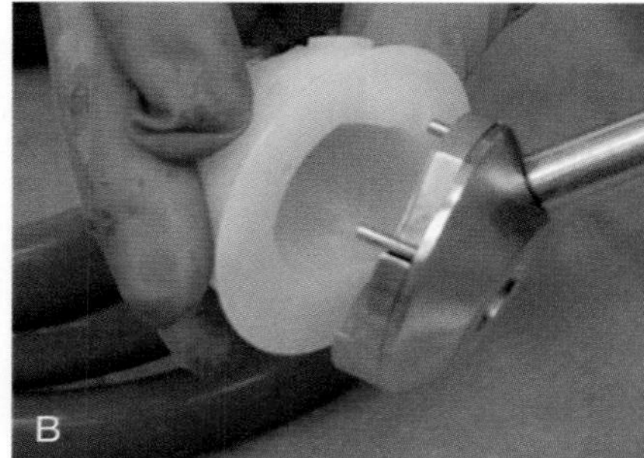

Figure 6 **A,** Photograph shows the highly cross-linked polyethylene implant and cup-holding device. **B,** Close-up photograph of the cup-holding device. (Reproduced from Ranawat CS, Ranawat AS: Primary total hip arthroplasty: Cemented acetabulum, in Lieberman JR, Berry DJ: *Advanced Reconstruction: Hip*. Rosemont, IL, American Academy of Orthopaedic Surgeons, 2005, pp 47-53.)

Wound Closure

- The wound is thoroughly irrigated.
- Intraoperative local injection is performed to assist in pain management.
- The insertions of the gluteus maximus and quadratus femoris tendons are repaired with nonabsorbable sutures.
- The superior capsule is closed with nonabsorbable suture.
- The short external rotators and the posterior capsule are repaired with two nonabsorbable sutures passed through drill holes in the greater trochanter.
- The authors of this chapter typically do not use drains when good hemostasis is achieved.
- The fascia is reapproximated with interrupted bioabsorbable sutures superimposed with a continuous running baseball stitch.
- The subcutaneous tissue is closed with bioabsorbable suture.
- The skin is closed with absorbable monofilament suture.
- A topical skin adhesive is applied.

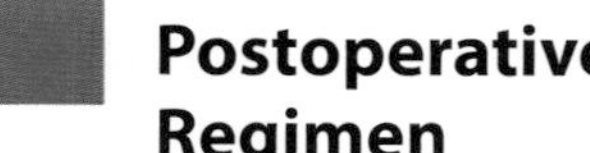

Postoperative Regimen

Patients are allowed to bear weight as tolerated with posterior hip precautions

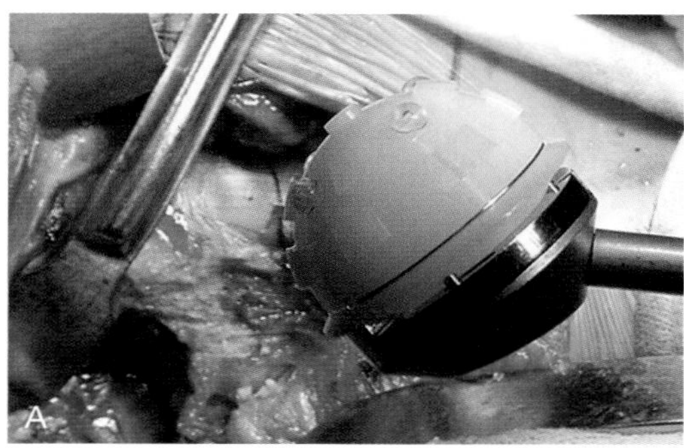
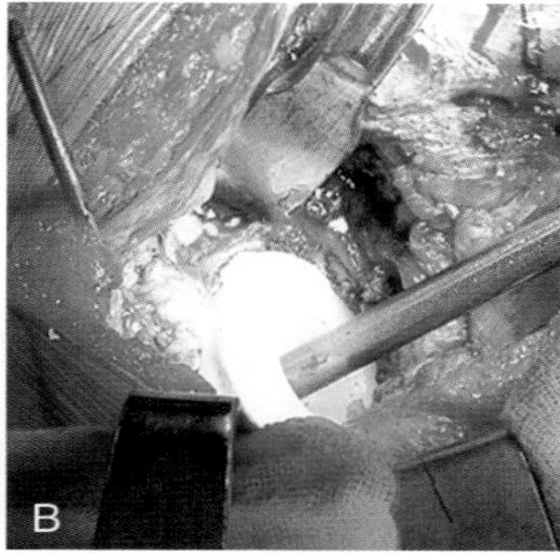

Figure 7 **A,** Intraoperative photograph shows the insertion of the acetabular cup with the cup-holding device. **B,** Intraoperative photograph of a hip shows the cement during the process of polymerization. (Reproduced from Ranawat CS, Ranawat AS: Primary total hip arthroplasty: Cemented acetabulum, in Lieberman JR, Berry DJ: *Advanced Reconstruction: Hip*. Rosemont, IL, American Academy of Orthopaedic Surgeons, 2005, pp 47-53.)

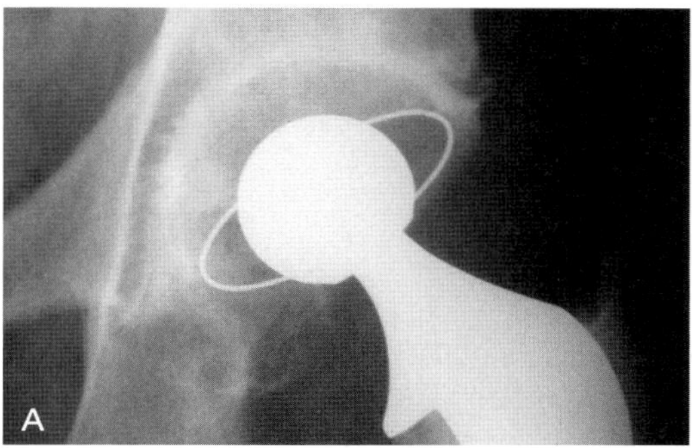
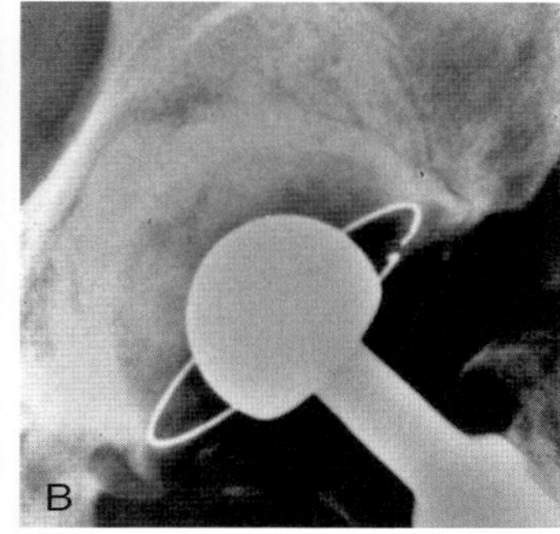

Figure 8 **A,** AP radiograph of a left hip obtained 6 weeks postoperatively demonstrates excellent cement interdigitation in all three DeLee and Charnley zones. **B,** AP radiograph of a left hip obtained 6 weeks postoperatively demonstrates early demarcation in all three DeLee and Charnley zones. (Reproduced from Ranawat CS, Ranawat AS: Primary total hip arthroplasty: Cemented acetabulum, in Lieberman JR, Berry DJ: *Advanced Reconstruction: Hip*. Rosemont, IL, American Academy of Orthopaedic Surgeons, 2005, pp 47-53.)

and continuous nonnarcotic multimodal analgesia.

Avoiding Pitfalls and Complications

Failure of cemented acetabular fixation before 10 years postoperatively is typically the result of insufficient initial microinterlock of cement and bone. Evidence of demarcation at the cement-bone interface on early postoperative radiographs can help predict this complication (**Figure 8**). In the experience of the authors of this chapter, successful microinterlock and macrointerlock can be achieved by selecting patients with adequate initial bone stock and ensuring meticulous surgical technique during cement fixation. Intraoperatively, the use of hypotensive, regional anesthesia is key to optimal results because it minimizes blood loss, decreases the risk of deep vein thrombosis, and reduces postoperative pain. Additionally, hypotensive anesthesia facilitates cement pressurization by minimizing acetabular bleeding, which can hinder penetration of cement into cancellous acetabular bone.

Bibliography

Brick GW, Poss R: Long-term follow-up of cemented total hip replacement for osteoarthritis. *Rheum Dis Clin North Am* 1988;14(3):565-577.

Callaghan JJ, Templeton JE, Liu SS, et al: Results of Charnley total hip arthroplasty at a minimum of thirty years: A concise follow-up of a previous report. *J Bone Joint Surg Am* 2004;86(4):690-695.

Creighton MG, Callaghan JJ, Olejniczak JP, Johnston RC: Total hip arthroplasty with cement in patients who have rheumatoid arthritis: A minimum ten-year follow-up study. *J Bone Joint Surg Am* 1998;80(10):1439-1446.

DeLee JG, Charnley J: Radiological demarcation of cemented sockets in total hip replacement. *Clin Orthop Relat Res* 1976;(121):20-32.

Della Valle CJ, Kaplan K, Jazrawi A, Ahmed S, Jaffe WL: Primary total hip arthroplasty with a flanged, cemented all-polyethylene acetabular component: Evaluation at a minimum of 20 years. *J Arthroplasty* 2004;19(1):23-26.

Hailer NP, Garellick G, Kärrholm J: Uncemented and cemented primary total hip arthroplasty in the Swedish Hip Arthroplasty Register. *Acta Orthop* 2010;81(1):34-41.

Kavanagh BF, Wallrichs S, Dewitz M, et al: Charnley low-friction arthroplasty of the hip: Twenty-year results with cement. *J Arthroplasty* 1994;9(3):229-234.

Lindalen E, Havelin LI, Nordsletten L, et al: Is reverse hybrid hip replacement the solution? *Acta Orthop* 2011;82(6):639-645.

Mäkelä KT, Matilainen M, Pulkkinen P, et al: Failure rate of cemented and uncemented total hip replacements: Register study of combined Nordic database of four nations. *BMJ* 2014;348:f7592.

McCombe P, Williams SA: A comparison of polyethylene wear rates between cemented and cementless cups: A prospective, randomised trial. *J Bone Joint Surg Br* 2004;86(3):344-349.

Morshed S, Bozic KJ, Ries MD, Malchau H, Colford JM Jr: Comparison of cemented and uncemented fixation in total hip replacement: A meta-analysis. *Acta Orthop* 2007;78(3):315-326.

Mulroy WF, Estok DM, Harris WH: Total hip arthroplasty with use of so-called second-generation cementing techniques: A fifteen-year-average follow-up study. *J Bone Joint Surg Am* 1995;77(12):1845-1852.

Ranawat CS, Beaver WB, Sharrock NE, Maynard MJ, Urquhart B, Schneider R: Effect of hypotensive epidural anaesthesia on acetabular cement-bone fixation in total hip arthroplasty. *J Bone Joint Surg Br* 1991;73(5):779-782.

Ranawat CS, Deshmukh RG, Peters LE, Umlas ME: Prediction of the long-term durability of all-polyethylene cemented sockets. *Clin Orthop Relat Res* 1995;(317):89-105.

Ranawat CS, Peters LE, Umlas ME: Fixation of the acetabular component: The case for cement. *Clin Orthop Relat Res* 1997;(344):207-215.

Ritter MA, Faris PM, Keating EM, Brugo G: Influential factors in cemented acetabular cup loosening. *J Arthroplasty* 1992;7(suppl):365-367.

Sochart DH, Porter ML: The long-term results of Charnley low-friction arthroplasty in young patients who have congenital dislocation, degenerative osteoarthrosis, or rheumatoid arthritis. *J Bone Joint Surg Am* 1997;79(11):1599-1617.

Stauffer RN: Ten-year follow-up study of total hip replacement. *J Bone Joint Surg Am* 1982;64(7):983-990.

Veitch SW, Whitehouse SL, Howell JR, Hubble MJ, Gie GA, Timperley AJ: The concentric all-polyethylene Exeter acetabular component in primary total hip replacement. *J Bone Joint Surg Br* 2010;92(10):1351-1355.

Wroblewski BM, Siney PD: Charnley low-friction arthroplasty of the hip: Long-term results. *Clin Orthop Relat Res* 1993;(292):191-201.

Chapter 9

Primary Total Hip Arthroplasty With a Noncemented Acetabular Implant

James A. Keeney, MD

Indications

Noncemented acetabular component fixation can be used in all primary and revision total hip arthroplasty (THA) procedures. Diagnoses commonly include primary osteoarthritis, osteoarthritis secondary to acetabular dysplasia or femoroacetabular impingement, posttraumatic arthritis, osteonecrosis, inflammatory arthritis, protrusio acetabuli, and fracture of the femoral neck. The development of implants with highly porous high-friction materials has allowed use of noncemented implants patients with prior pelvic irradiation, which was previously considered a contraindication to the use of noncemented fixation. The stable fixation afforded by contemporary noncemented acetabular implants and the lower wear rates of highly cross-linked polyethylene have allowed the use of larger-diameter femoral heads (32 to 36 mm) and the increased use of THA in younger and active patients. Recently published studies suggest a substantial reduction in the wear of highly cross-linked polyethylene materials even when used in patients younger than 50 years.

Templating is essential for successful acetabular reconstruction (**Figure 1**). The amount of medialization necessary to ensure contact of at least 80% of the implant surface against the host bone is determined. Preservation of bone around the acetabular implant is desirable to facilitate safe implant removal if future revision surgery is required. However, positioning of the acetabular implant at the level of the medial acetabular wall may be unavoidable in patients with severe acetabular dysplasia. The desired angle of inclination of the acetabular implant should be determined because it affects the amount of the acetabular implant that should be visible when the implant is appropriately positioned. This measurement helps the surgeon ensure intraoperatively that the position of the implant is not excessively

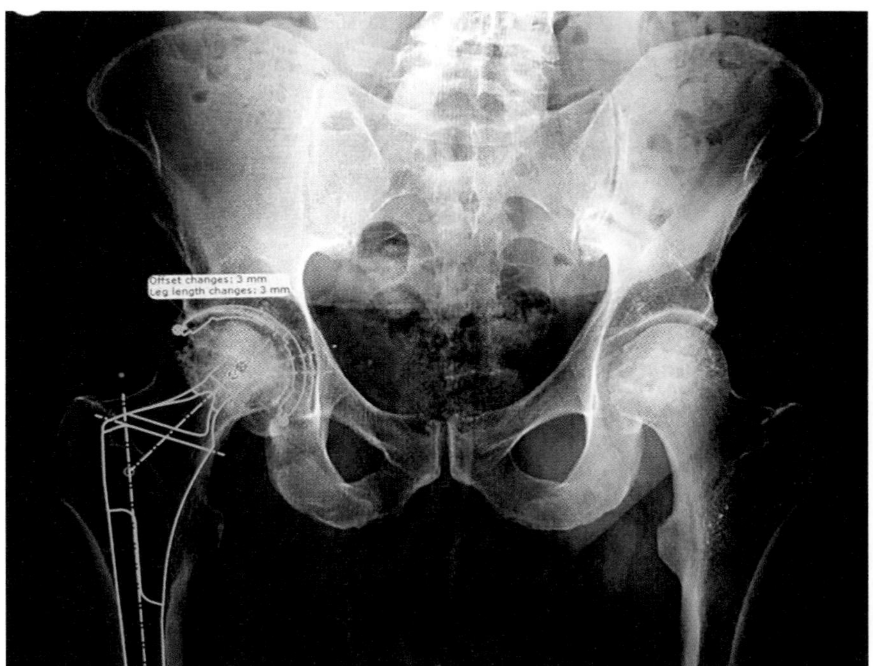

Figure 1 AP pelvic radiograph demonstrates the use of preoperative templating to determine the appropriate position of the acetabular implant and placement of the femoral implant to the desired level of leg length and offset reconstruction.

Dr. Keeney or an immediate family member serves as a paid consultant to OrthoSensor; has received research or institutional support from Stryker; and serves as a board member, owner, officer, or committee member of the Society of Military Orthopaedic Surgeons.

Table 1 Results of Total Hip Arthroplasty With Noncemented Acetabular Implants

Authors (Year)	Number of Hips	Polyethylene Type	Mean Patient Age in Years (Range)	Mean Follow-up in Years (Range)	Success Rate (%)[a]
Kim et al (2003)	118	Conventional	46.8 (21-49)	9.8 (8-11)	100
Hartofilakidis et al (2009)	58	Conventional	39.6 (25-55)	12.4 (10-16)	88
Corten et al (2011)	126	Conventional	64 (NR)	19.5 (17-22)	96
Kim et al (2011)	73	Cross-linked	45 (20-50)	8.5 (7-9)	100
Lachiewicz and Soileau (2012)	118	Conventional	59.3 (22-81)	12 (10-16)	100
Stefl et al (2012)	120	Conventional	59 (55-77)	23.3 (21.7-24.5)	97
Takenaga et al (2012)	115	Conventional	40.1 (17-50)	12 (10-17)	99
Babovic and Trousdale (2013)	124	Cross-linked	38.9 (15-50)	10.5 (10-13)	100

NR = not reported.
[a] Success is defined as survival of the acetabular implant.

horizontal (which would be indicated by exposure of a greater amount of the acetabular cup) or excessively vertical (which in most patients would occur if the acetabular cup is fully seated against the lateral acetabular wall).

Contraindications

The use of noncemented acetabular implants in THA has few absolute contraindications. Active infection is a contraindication to THA, regardless of the method of fixation. Patients with chronic skin colonization in remote sites and patients with unhealed wounds are not appropriate candidates for THA. Staged reconstruction may be considered in patients with a history of infection, but care should be taken to ensure that the infection is resolved before THA is performed. Cemented acetabular implant fixation may be beneficial for patients with limited acetabular bone vascularity or with substantially low-quality bone that will not allow mechanical stability of the prosthesis. Cost considerations may favor the use of cemented fixation, particularly among older patients and low-demand patients or in geographic regions where financial considerations require selection of lower-cost implant materials and techniques.

Alternative Treatments

The main alternative to the use of a noncemented acetabular implant in THA is a cemented acetabular implant.

Results

Studies directly comparing cemented and noncemented acetabular implants at a minimum of 10 years postoperatively have demonstrated more reliable long-term acetabular implant survival with noncemented designs. Historically, failure of noncemented acetabular implants typically involved surface wear of ultra-high–molecular-weight polyethylene bearings and focal osteolytic defects in patients with well-fixed implants. The enhanced material surfaces that have become available since the mid to late 1990s have resulted in more predictable mechanical stability and bony integration. The survivorship rate of implant fixation among second-generation noncemented implants has been reported to be between 96% and 100%.

Analysis of studies of noncemented implants is difficult because of manufacturer-specific differences in acetabular implant design and surface preparation and differences in the type and processing of polyethylene materials, including sterilization techniques. A large, single-institution study comparing 15 noncemented acetabular implant designs in more than 9,500 THAs demonstrated poorer outcomes with smooth beaded or hydroxyapatite-coated implants than with other designs. Implants that included a polyethylene liner with an elevated rim also had higher failure rates than other implants, which could be related to design characteristics or surgical factors. The major factor limiting the long-term durability of both cemented and noncemented implants used in the 20th century was wear of conventional polyethylene and associated periprosthetic osteolysis. The use of cross-linking to improve polyethylene durability has substantially decreased linear polyethylene wear rates up to 10 years after THA, even in patients younger than 50 years who are engaged in a high activity level (**Table 1**).

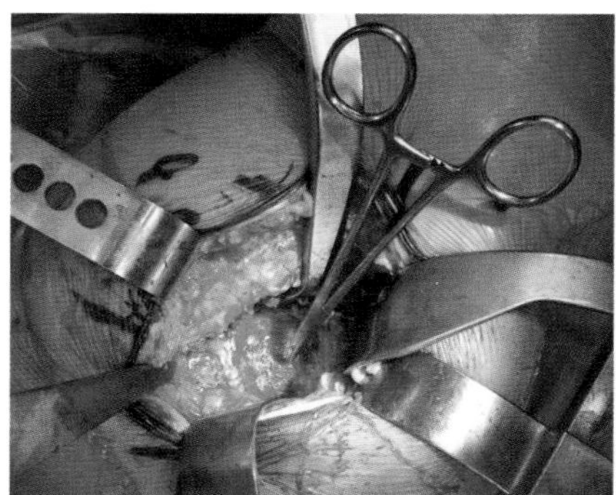

Figure 2 Intraoperative photograph of a hip shows the use of a narrow-tipped clamp to determine the depth of the cotyloid fossa.

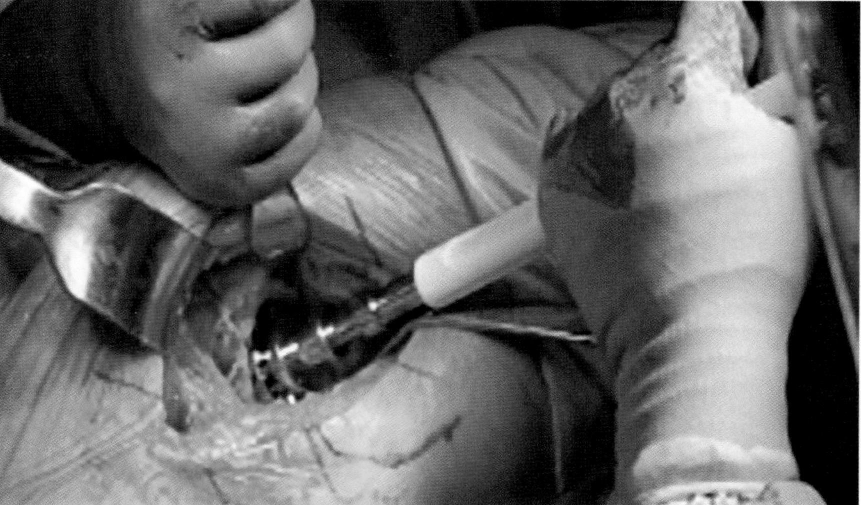

Figure 3 Intraoperative photograph shows initial reaming of the acetabulum to medialize the center of rotation of the hip to the position determined by means of preoperative templating.

Techniques

Setup/Exposure

- Any surgical approach that allows the procedure to be performed safely and effectively can be used.
- Retractors are positioned to allow visualization of the anterior, lateral, posterior, and inferior margins of the acetabulum.

Instruments/Equipment/Implants Required

- The selection of specific retractors and instrumentation depends on the implant system and surgical approach. The author of this chapter performs a posterolateral approach with the following instrumentation.
- A cobra retractor is placed over the anterior acetabular wall. This correlates to a 4-o'clock position for a right THA and an 8-o'clock position for a left THA.
- After the posterior capsule is released directly inferior to the acetabulum (preserving the transverse acetabular ligament and avoiding dissection medial or distal to the capsule), a cobra or elephant-ear–shaped posteroinferior retractor is placed directly inferior to the acetabulum.
- A small Hohmann retractor is placed over the superolateral acetabular wall and engaged with gentle impaction force into the supra-acetabular bone.
- A Meyerding retractor is placed along the margin of the posterior wall to protect the sciatic nerve and posterior soft tissues.
- Acetabular reamers are assembled onto a straight reamer handle.
- An angled impactor is used to facilitate implantation of the acetabular component and to keep the greater trochanter and femur, which are displaced anterior to the acetabulum, from directing the acetabular component into a more retroverted position during component impaction.

Procedure

- The labrum and the remnant of the ligamentum teres are excised to enhance visualization and allow complete assessment of the acetabulum during reaming.
- The location and depth of the cotyloid fossa are determined (**Figure 2**).
- In most patients, reaming will extend approximately to the floor of the native cotyloid fossa.
- A small clamp is used to indicate the depth of reaming and ensure that the planned level of medial reaming is attained and not exceeded.
- An appropriate-size reamer is selected for acetabular preparation. In most patients without acetabular dysplasia, a reamer that is 2 to 3 mm smaller than the size of the patient's native acetabulum is selected.
- In patients with severe dysplasia, the use of a smaller reamer (40 to 44 mm) can help ensure that initial reaming can be performed to a depth that will allow adequate lateral coverage before the acetabular bed is expanded.
- The acetabulum is reamed hemispherically to accommodate the acetabular implant (**Figure 3**).
- In most patients, medialization and expansion of the acetabulum are performed simultaneously.
- The bone obtained during initial reaming (which contains elements of articular cartilage) is saved for later use in cancellous bone grafting if necessary.

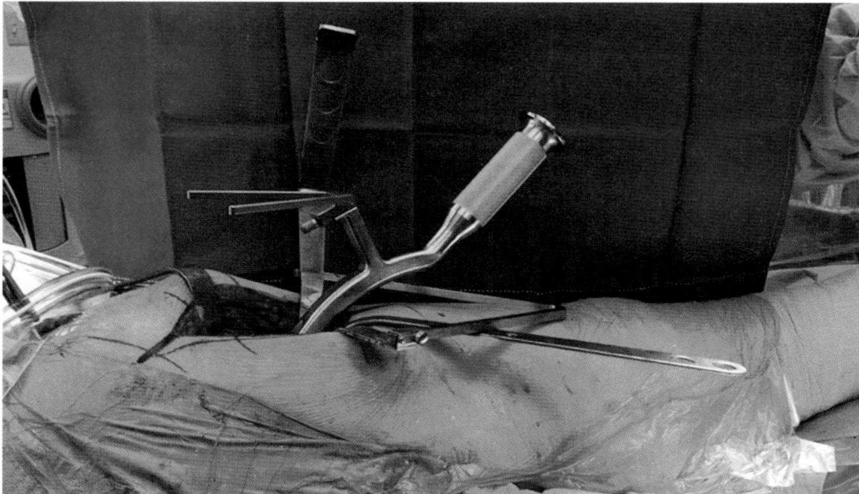

Figure 4 Intraoperative photograph shows placement of an acetabular implant impaction device with an alignment guide.

- Because of small AP pelvic dimensions in some patients with dysplasia, it may be necessary to perform sufficient medialization before expansion of the acetabulum to ensure that lateral coverage can be achieved.
- Care is taken to avoid excessive proximal or medial reaming of the hip socket in advance of expansion because excessive reaming can result in an elliptic rather than a spheric bone bed for implant placement.
- In patients with inadequate bone stock, contained defects are augmented if necessary with cancellous bone graft obtained from the acetabular reamer.
- If a structural bone graft is used in the rare patient with severe acetabular dysplasia, provisional fixation of the bone graft is performed before final reaming of the acetabulum.
- The acetabular bone bed is cleaned and dried thoroughly.
- The patient's position and the alignment of the acetabular cup insertion device are assessed.
- The implant should be positioned with 45° of inclination or less and 10° to 25° of anteversion.
- The use of an alignment guide attached to the cup insertion device can help attain the intended alignment (**Figure 4**).
- The surgical approach may influence the targeted amount of anteversion. A posterior approach may require more anteversion, whereas an anterior approach may require less anteversion.
- Intraoperative radiographic assessment can be used to confirm acetabular implant position.
- Variation in lumbopelvic tilt can affect the patient's position on the surgical table and influence assessment of implant position.
- The acetabular implant is impacted with appropriate force to progressively seat the implant.
- Care is taken not to overimpact an implant that does not readily seat below the acetabular rim. A sclerotic acetabular rim may require an additional 1 mm of reaming to allow peripheral implant seating.
- In addition, care is taken not to overimpact the implant in patients with a thin medial wall or deficient bone.
- After initial seating has been accomplished, the depth of insertion of the implant is assessed.
- If the implant is fully seated and more of the implant is exposed laterally than expected, the position of the implant may be more horizontal (less abducted) than preferred.
- If the implant is fully seated and less of the implant is exposed laterally than expected, the position of the implant may be more vertical (more abducted) than preferred.
- If the implant is not fully seated, it should be inserted to the expected level determined during acetabular preparation. However, up to 2 mm of incomplete seating in the acetabular dome is tolerated if the peripheral cup is in adequate contact with the bone and the implant is stable when subjected to angular and rotational forces.
- The acetabular implant is secured with supplemental screws if desired. Most implants are mechanically stable with primary press-fit fixation according to the manufacturer's specifications.
- The author of this chapter typically uses one supplemental screw in patients with excellent cancellous bone quality and primary press-fit stability of the implant.
- The author of this chapter typically uses two or three supplemental screws in patients with soft cancellous bone, peripheral cup engagement with a dome gap of 1 mm, and implants with more than 15% of the lateral or posterior cup exposed.
- The femoral reconstruction is completed.
- Implant stability is assessed.
- If implant sizing does not match that determined by means of preoperative templating or if optimal implant stability cannot be achieved, intraoperative radiographic assessment is performed.

- The implant may be repositioned using either the cup insertion guide or a rectangular tamp. If the acetabular implant position is changed, screw fixation is strongly recommended to ensure that mechanical stability is maintained after reimpaction of the implant.

Wound Closure

- Deep wound closure restores stability to the posterior surgical window.
- Two drill holes are placed in the greater trochanter, with care taken to ensure that there is more than 1 cm between the superior-most drill hole and the tip of the greater trochanter and that there is more than 1 cm separating the two drill holes.
- Three No. 5 nonabsorbable braided sutures are placed. The first suture is placed through the gluteus medius muscle-tendon junction and sewn into the superior aspect of the posterior capsule. The second suture is placed through the inferior drill hole and sewn into the inferior capsule and short external rotators. The third suture is placed through the gluteus medius muscle-tendon junction and sewn into the piriformis tendon using a modified Kessler suturing technique, in which the suture is passed in a reverse direction back into the gluteus medius tendon, leaving a 1-cm bridge between suture ends.
- After all three sutures have been placed, the first two sutures are passed through the superior drill hole using a suture passer.
- The hip is placed in neutral abduction and rotation.
- The capsule is closed by tying the first two sutures over their respective bone bridges in the greater trochanter.
- The piriformis tendon is tied over the gluteus medius tendon insertion.
- Several acceptable approaches can be used for superficial wound closure. The author of this chapter prefers to use three or four No. 1 synthetic absorbable sutures at evenly spaced intervals in the subcutaneous tissue, using 2-0 monofilament absorbable sutures spaced approximately 7 to 8 mm apart through the remaining subcutaneous/subdermal tissue layer, using either staples or a running subcuticular skin closure with 3-0 monofilament absorbable suture to close the skin, and reinforcing the skin with liquid adhesive (for patients without skin sensitivities) and adhesive strips if a subcuticular closure is used.
- High-quality postoperative radiographs are obtained to assess implant position and stable implant reduction.

Postoperative Rehabilitation

Immediate weight bearing is allowed in most patients. Partial weight bearing may be appropriate or directed in patients with poor bone quality or deficient lateral acetabular coverage. Postoperative hip dislocation precautions are instituted at the surgeon's discretion on the basis of intraoperative assessment. The use of hip precautions after THA is becoming less common because contemporary femoral implant designs have improved the surgeon's ability to adequately restore version, leg length, and offset.

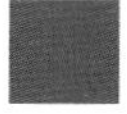

Avoiding Pitfalls and Complications

Preoperative planning is necessary to determine the desired implant position and alignment. The patient's position on the surgical table should be assessed. Intraoperative radiography at the time of implant placement or after assessment of stability can be helpful, especially if the position of the implant relative to the patient's acetabular anatomy does not match the preoperative plan or if prosthetic stability is not achieved with implants placed according to the preoperative plan.

The acetabulum should be prepared hemispherically. Medial and superior reaming should be avoided unless specified in the preoperative plan. Care must be taken when reamers substantially smaller than the templated implant size are used for medialization. Incorrect reaming can contribute to elliptic bone preparation and a gap between the implant and bone at the acetabular dome.

Excessive reaming of the lateral or posterior wall should be avoided. The use of smaller incisions and less invasive surgical approaches can result in decreased visualization of the acetabulum during bone preparation. Inadequate seating of the acetabular reamer can result in eccentric reaming of the lateral acetabular wall during medialization. Holding the reamer in a position of increased anteversion when reaming in a medial and proximal direction can result in eccentric reaming of the posterior wall or column.

Supplemental screw fixation should be considered in patients with poor bone quality, incomplete lateral coverage of the acetabulum (15% to 20%), or medialization beyond the planned center of rotation of the joint.

Bibliography

Babovic N, Trousdale RT: Total hip arthroplasty using highly cross-linked polyethylene in patients younger than 50 years with minimum 10-year follow-up. *J Arthroplasty* 2013;28(5):815-817.

Clohisy JC, Harris WH: Matched-pair analysis of cemented and cementless acetabular reconstruction in primary total hip arthroplasty. *J Arthroplasty* 2001;16(6):697-705.

Corten K, Bourne RB, Charron KD, Au K, Rorabeck CH: What works best, a cemented or cementless primary total hip arthroplasty? Minimum 17-year followup of a randomized controlled trial. *Clin Orthop Relat Res* 2011;469(1):209-217.

Engh CA, Hopper RH Jr, Engh CA Jr: Long-term porous-coated cup survivorship using spikes, screws, and press-fitting for initial fixation. *J Arthroplasty* 2004;19(7 suppl 2):54-60.

García-Rey E, García-Cimbrelo E, Cruz-Pardos A: Cup press fit in uncemented THA depends on sex, acetabular shape, and surgical technique. *Clin Orthop Relat Res* 2012;470(11):3014-3023.

Hallan G, Lie SA, Havelin LI: High wear rates and extensive osteolysis in 3 types of uncemented total hip arthroplasty: A review of the PCA, the Harris Galante and the Profile/Tri-Lock Plus arthroplasties with a minimum of 12 years median follow-up in 96 hips. *Acta Orthop* 2006;77(4):575-584.

Hartofilakidis G, Georgiades G, Babis GC: A comparison of the outcome of cemented all-polyethylene and cementless metal-backed acetabular sockets in primary total hip arthroplasty. *J Arthroplasty* 2009;24(2):217-225.

Howard JL, Kremers HM, Loechler YA, et al: Comparative survival of uncemented acetabular components following primary total hip arthroplasty. *J Bone Joint Surg Am* 2011;93(17):1597-1604.

Joglekar SB, Rose PS, Lewallen DG, Sim FH: Tantalum acetabular cups provide secure fixation in THA after pelvic irradiation at minimum 5-year followup. *Clin Orthop Relat Res* 2012;470(11):3041-3047.

Kim YH, Choi Y, Kim JS: Cementless total hip arthroplasty with alumina-on-highly cross-linked polyethylene bearing in young patients with femoral head osteonecrosis. *J Arthroplasty* 2011;26(2):218-223.

Kim YH, Oh SH, Kim JS: Primary total hip arthroplasty with a second-generation cementless total hip prosthesis in patients younger than fifty years of age. *J Bone Joint Surg Am* 2003;85(1):109-114.

Lachiewicz PF, Soileau ES: Second-generation modular acetabular components provide fixation at 10 to 16 years. *Clin Orthop Relat Res* 2012;470(2):366-372.

Maloney WJ, Galante JO, Anderson M, et al: Fixation, polyethylene wear, and pelvic osteolysis in primary total hip replacement. *Clin Orthop Relat Res* 1999;(369):157-164.

Rorabeck CH, Bourne RB, Mulliken BD, et al: Comparative results of cemented and cementless total hip arthroplasty. *Clin Orthop Relat Res* 1996;(325):330-344.

Stefl MD, Callaghan JJ, Liu SS, Pedersen DR, Goetz DD, Johnston RC: Primary cementless acetabular fixation at a minimum of twenty years of follow-up: A concise update of a previous report. *J Bone Joint Surg Am* 2012;94(3):234-239.

Takenaga RK, Callaghan JJ, Bedard NA, Liu SS, Klaassen AL, Pedersen DR: Cementless total hip arthroplasty in patients fifty years of age or younger: A minimum ten-year follow-up. *J Bone Joint Surg Am* 2012;94(23):2153-2159.

Udomkiat P, Dorr LD, Wan Z: Cementless hemispheric porous-coated sockets implanted with press-fit technique without screws: Average ten-year follow-up. *J Bone Joint Surg Am* 2002;84(7):1195-1200.

Chapter 10
Primary Total Hip Arthroplasty With a Cemented Femoral Implant

Michael J. Dunbar, MD, FRCSC, PhD
Bryan Flynn, MD, FRCSC
Thomas Marceau-Cote, MD, FRCSC

Indications

Femoral implant fixation in total hip arthroplasty (THA) is the subject of debate. Since the advent of low-friction arthroplasty in the early 1960s, the use of polymethyl methacrylate cement has been the preferred method of femoral fixation in THA. Cemented femoral fixation continues to be used for most THA procedures in many European nations, with excellent results. In North America and some European countries, noncemented femoral implants have become more popular than cemented femoral implants. Because of the increased popularity of noncemented fixation in North America, some surgeons consider cemented femoral fixation to be a lost art. Cemented femoral fixation requires careful attention to detail and meticulous technique to obtain reliable long-term outcomes.

Cemented femoral fixation can be used in nearly all THA procedures. It works well regardless of the patient's bone quality and can be used in patients with femoral deformities. It is ideal for use in elderly, sedentary patients with osteopenic and capacious bone (Dorr femur types B and C). Even surgeons who ardently prefer noncemented femoral implants sometimes recommend cemented fixation in patients with a Dorr type C femur. Cemented fixation can prevent bone ingrowth into noncemented implants and is indicated in patients with bone tumors or those who have undergone irradiation. Patients with femoral neck fracture have fewer intraoperative periprosthetic fractures, achieve earlier postoperative weight bearing, and experience better long-term implant survivorship with cemented hemiarthroplasty or THA than with noncemented hemiarthroplasty or THA.

Cemented fixation allows optimization of femoral implant placement. Noncemented femoral implants are designed to accommodate the anatomy of the proximal femur. Numerous styles or designs are manufactured to accommodate variations in femoral morphology, and implant selection requires careful preoperative planning and templating. Because of the large variation in femoral anatomy, optimal positioning of the femoral implant sometimes is not possible. Variation in the local anatomy may dictate aspects of positioning such as the final version of the femoral implant. Attempts to fully seat the implant to optimize leg length can result in intraoperative fracture. In contrast, cementation of the femoral implant inside the broach envelope allows for variation in the position of the final femoral implant to achieve the desired offset, version, and leg length. For these reasons, cemented femoral fixation is useful in patients with abnormal anatomy of the proximal femur, such as patients with developmental dysplasia, patients who have undergone previous osteotomies, and patients who have undergone unsuccessful treatment of a fracture of the proximal femur.

Antimicrobial agents can be added to the cement either by a manufacturer or at the time of the procedure. The ability to use antimicrobial agents with cemented femoral fixation may be particularly valuable when the use of arthroplasty is expanded in medically underserved regions of the world.

Dr. Dunbar or an immediate family member has received royalties from and serves as a paid consultant to Stryker; has received research or institutional support from DePuy Synthes, Emovi, Kinduct Technologies, Stryker, and Zimmer Biomet; and serves as a board member, owner, officer, or committee member of the Arthritis Society of Canada, the Canadian Joint Replacement Registry, the Canadian Orthopaedic Research Society, and the Canadian RSA Network. Neither of the following authors nor any immediate family member has received anything of value from or has stock or stock options held in a commercial company or institution related directly or indirectly to the subject of this chapter: Dr. Flynn and Dr. Marceau-Cote.

Table 1 Results of Total Hip Arthroplasty With a Cemented Femoral Implant

Authors (Year)	Number of Hips	Implant Type	Mean Patient Age in Years (Range)	Follow-up in Years	Success Rate (%)[a]	Results
Kale et al (2000)	132	Spectron (Smith & Nephew)	68 (17-85)	Mean, 10 (range, 5-13)	94	Favorable 10-yr outcomes using a second-generation cementing technique
Wroblewski et al (2007)	22,066	Charnley LFA (DePuy Synthes)	67 (12-93)	Maximum, 31	72.5	Good outcomes reported at ≥30 yr postoperatively
Lewthwaite et al (2008)	130	Exeter Universal (Stryker Howmedica Osteonics)	42 (≤50)	Mean, 12.5 (range, 10-17)	100	99% stem survivorship at 12.5 yr postoperatively in patients aged <50 yr
Callaghan et al (2009)	330	Charnley	65 (29-86)	Minimum, 35	78	Benchmark study for survivorship and natural history of cemented hip replacement in the United States
Ling et al (2009)	433	Original Polished Exeter (Stryker Howmedica Osteonics)	66.8 (30-84)	Mean, 30.6 (range, 5-33)	93.5	Results from the original Exeter series
Aubault et al (2013)	83	Zimmer PF (Zimmer Biomet)	66 (40-82)	Mean, 11 (≥10)	100	Good 10-yr outcomes
Prins et al (2014)	932	Lubinus SP II (Link)	72.3 ± 8.0[b]	Mean, 10 (range, 5-15)	99	10-yr survivorship rate >98% for a specific femoral component
Warth et al (2014)	93	Charnley	42 (18-49)	Mean, 36.9 (range, 35.1-40.8)	82	Study demonstrates durability of cemented total hip arthroplasty in young patients in the United States

LFA = low-friction arthroplasty.
[a] Success is defined as the absence of femoral mechanical failure, expressed as the percentage of stems not revised for aseptic loosening or found to have radiographic evidence of loosening.
[b] Data reported are mean ± standard deviation.

Contraindications

Successful cemented femoral fixation requires adequate quality and quantity of cancellous bone for interdigitation of the cement to create a stable interface. Thus, substantial deficiency of the proximal cancellous bone, such as deficiency resulting from previous intramedullary fixation, is a relative contraindication to cemented femoral fixation.

Cemented femoral fixation in patients with notable cardiopulmonary disease is controversial because of concerns that the pressurization of cement in the femoral canal can increase the embolic load in the cardiopulmonary system. Some authors have reported an increased risk of sudden death in patients undergoing cemented THA, whereas other researchers have found no significant risk related to the use of cement. The exact overall rate of embolic complications is unknown and is estimated to be approximately 0.05% to 0.1%. This concern is a relative contraindication. The surgeon should take the medical status of the patient into consideration and should perform thorough lavage and suction of the femoral canal before cementation to reduce the risk of embolization of marrow contents and fat.

Because cemented femoral fixation requires dry host bone to facilitate successful cement interdigitation, an alternative method of femoral fixation should be considered in patients who require hemodialysis because of renal failure, patients with blood dyscrasia, and patients with bone marrow disorders. These conditions can cause excessive and uncontrollable bleeding in the canal during cementation.

A common argument against the routine use of cemented femoral implants in young or active patients is that the cemented implants do not perform as well as uncemented femoral implants in these patients. However, substantial evidence, including long-term national registry data, refutes this argument (**Table 1**).

Alternative Treatments

Nonsurgical treatment options should be exhausted before surgical intervention is considered in patients with symptomatic hip osteoarthritis. Prolonged nonsurgical treatment should be administered in patients who have unrealistic expectations of surgical treatment because patient satisfaction and outcomes after THA are influenced by preoperative patient expectations. The primary pharmacologic options are oral medications such as acetaminophen, NSAIDs, and narcotics. Radiographically guided intra-articular corticosteroid injections may be considered. Nonpharmacologic management of hip osteoarthritis includes the use of walking aids; a cardiovascular, aquatic, or aerobic exercise program; weight loss in patients with elevated body mass index; and/or psychosocial intervention.

After an appropriate course of nonsurgical management has been attempted without success, surgical options are discussed with the patient. Pelvic osteotomies are an option in young adult patients with hip dysplasia in whom the hip joint may be salvageable. Hip fusion is frequently mentioned as a surgical option for the management of unilateral severe hip osteoarthritis in younger (<20 years), high-demand patients but is rarely used.

The main advantages of hip resurfacing as an alternative to THA with cemented intramedullary femoral fixation are the preservation of femoral bone stock and increased stability. Hip resurfacing enjoyed a resurgence beginning in approximately 2005, but its popularity has decreased because of recent issues associated with metal ions and adverse local soft-tissue reactions.

The main alternative treatment to cemented fixation is noncemented fixation of the femoral implant. Although excellent results have been reported for noncemented femoral fixation, the authors of this chapter prefer cemented fixation because of the advantages previously described.

Results

Long-term outcome series in the United States demonstrate excellent survivorship of cemented femoral implants at 25 years or more. The authors of a systematic review published in 2015 and including 17 studies reported survival rates of 86% to 98% at minimum 20-year follow-up with aseptic loosening as the end point. **Table 1** shows success rates of a variety of cemented implants.

Data from numerous long-standing national joint arthroplasty registries demonstrate excellent long-term outcomes of cemented femoral fixation. In these registries, long-term survivorship of cemented femoral fixation generally demonstrates at least equivalence, if not superiority, compared with noncemented femoral fixation, especially in elderly patients and perhaps even in younger ones.

In Sweden, where the noncemented stem was not widely adopted, the rate of revision is low. A study of data from the Swedish Hip Arthroplasty Register showed that the 10-year survival rate of cemented THA was significantly higher than that of noncemented THA (94% and 85%, respectively). Noncemented fixation had a higher revision rate in the first 2 years postoperatively because of the higher risk of periprosthetic fracture. A study of the Danish Hip Arthroplasty Register demonstrated a similar lower revision rate. The authors of a recent study combining the databases of four nations concluded that the survival of cemented implants for THA was higher than that of noncemented implants in patients age 65 years or older. A study of 62,305 primary cemented THAs from the Norwegian Arthroplasty Register demonstrated a low rate of revision of 5.9% for cemented femoral fixation for aseptic loosening at 18-year follow-up. The New Zealand Joint Registry shows similar results, with THAs with cemented femoral fixation having a higher survival rate when all causes of revision are taken into consideration.

In a 2011 report of data from the National Joint Registry for England and Wales, the revision rate at 5 years for noncemented THA was twice that of cemented THA. For patients younger than 60 years, revision rates of cemented THA and hybrid THA were similar and were lower than that of noncemented THA. The percentage of cemented procedures did not change from 2009 to 2010 after a period of steady decline that began in 2005. The 2014 report showed that the use of cemented fixation was on the rise again. Interestingly, all-cemented THA had the lowest rate of revision, with just 1.4% revision at 10 years. Cemented fixation appeared to have the best implant survivorship, with a 3.2% cumulative probability of revision at 10 years, compared with 7.7% for noncemented fixation. Conversely, the Australian Orthopaedic Association National Joint Replacement Registry showed an increased use of noncemented femoral implants in the past decade, although cemented femoral implants remained the most frequently used. In terms of the best cup/stem combinations, all-cemented THA had the lowest 10-year cumulative percentage of revision, followed by hybrid fixation and then noncemented fixation.

Currently, many surgeons consider cemented femoral fixation to be the preferred method in older patients (≥65 years). The fixation option that should be used in patients younger than 65 years and more active patients is the subject of debate. Concerns related to cemented femoral fixation in young patients have been challenged in multiple studies. In a report on a series of patients younger than 50 years, cemented femoral implants had a 99% survival rate at average 15-year follow-up. The authors of the study concluded that polished, tapered stems perform well even in young patients. In two different studies, researchers reported 93% and 94% survivorship of cemented femoral fixation at 25 and 20 years, respectively, in patients younger than 50 years. The authors of a different study reported 85.2% survivorship of a cemented femoral implant at 22 years. Recent registry studies have shown improved survival of new noncemented implant designs. However, longer follow-up data are needed to confirm these results.

Reports have documented fewer instances of thigh pain with cemented femoral fixation than with noncemented fixation. In one randomized study, the rate of documented thigh pain was more than five times higher in patients with a noncemented implant than in patients with a cemented implant (3% and 17%, respectively). The mechanism of the decrease in thigh pain with cemented fixation is likely related to the transitional modulus of elasticity that the cement provides between the stem and the host bone.

Techniques

Setup/Exposure

- An appropriate intravenous antibiotic is administered 15 to 45 minutes before the skin incision is made.
- Intravenous tranexamic acid and preemptive multimodal analgesia also are administered before the skin incision is made.
- The authors of this chapter use an anterolateral approach to the hip, which is described here. A posterior approach can be used with equal effectiveness.
- The patient is placed in the lateral decubitus position on a surgical frame designed for THA. The pelvis is secured with one post on the sacrum and another on the pubis.
- Care is taken to ensure that the coronal axis of the pelvis is perpendicular to the surgical table and in line with the patient's body.
- The affected leg is prepped from above the iliac crest to the ankle. The leg is draped free with a hip drape, allowing the extremity to be brought across the body into a sterile bag for femoral preparation.
- An iodine-impregnated occlusive dressing is applied at the site of the incision.
- The relative positions of the patella and heel are noted and compared with those of the contralateral leg to facilitate comparison of leg lengths.
- An incision is made directly over the greater trochanter in line with the long axis of the femur, with one-third of the incision proximal to the greater trochanter and two-thirds of the incision distal to the greater trochanter.
- The fascia is split in line with the incision.
- A Charnley retractor is positioned to expose the gluteus medius and the vastus lateralis.
- The trochanteric bursa is excised.
- The leg length and offset are marked with the use of a pin in the iliac wing and a fixed-angle device.
- An arthrotomy is performed, elevating the anterior one-third of the gluteus medius and the vastus lateralis muscles along with the gluteus minimus muscle and hip joint capsule. To facilitate this step, the leg is externally rotated, the Charnley retractor is repositioned deep to the abductors, and Hohmann retractors are placed along the anteroinferior and posterosuperior femoral neck.
- The femoral head is dislocated anteriorly by means of external rotation and adduction.
- Resection of the femoral head is completed on the basis of preoperative templating.

Instruments/Equipment/Implants Required

- Cemented stem broaches and implants are used.
- A closed vacuum mixing system is used.
- A retrograde cement gun with breakaway nozzle is used.
- A canal brush is used.
- Jet lavage irrigation is used.
- Hydrogen peroxide is used.
- A canal suction sponge and canal pressurizer are used.
- A cement restrictor is used.
- A stem centralizer is used.

Procedure

BONE PREPARATION

- Typically, acetabular preparation is performed first.
- The affected leg is brought across the body for femoral preparation.
- The proximal femur is delivered out of the wound and exposed with one Hohmann retractor elevating the femur anteriorly and a second Hohmann retractor placed along the posterior femoral neck to retract the remaining abductors.
- A box osteotome is used to open the femoral canal at the posterolateral femoral neck (**Figure 1, A**), and a T-handled reamer is used to find and reference the anatomic axis of the femur (**Figure 1, B**).

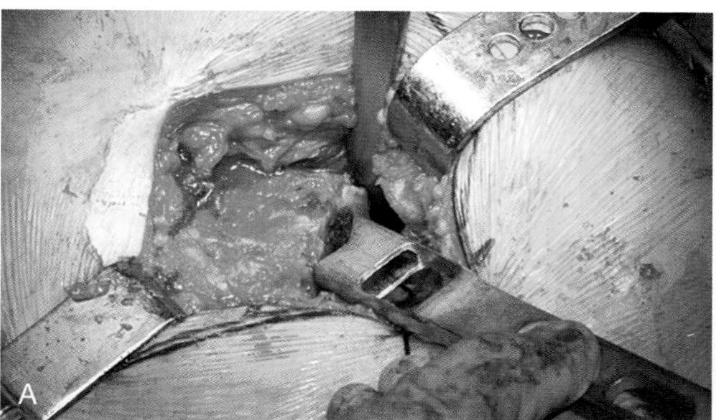

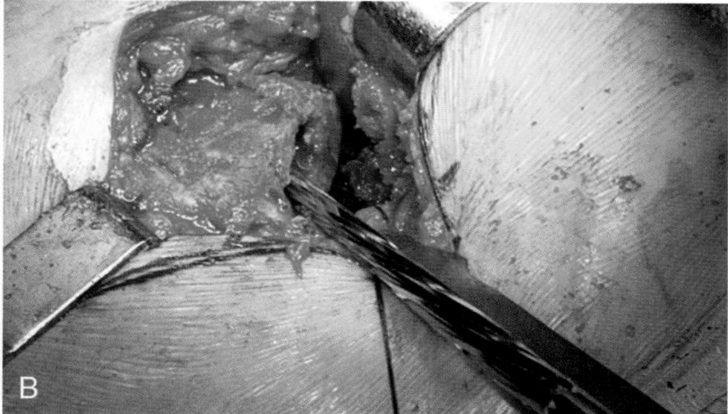

Figure 1 Intraoperative photographs of a left hip. **A,** A box osteotome is used to remove a wedge of posterolateral bone from the proximal femur. **B,** Introduction of a cylindric reamer down the canal to indicate proper varus/valgus alignment of the femur.

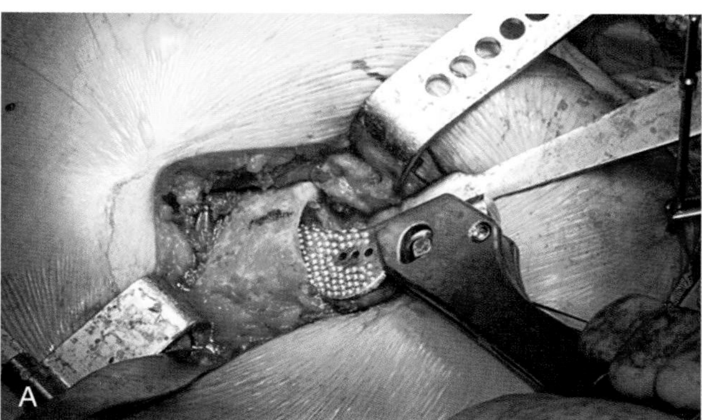

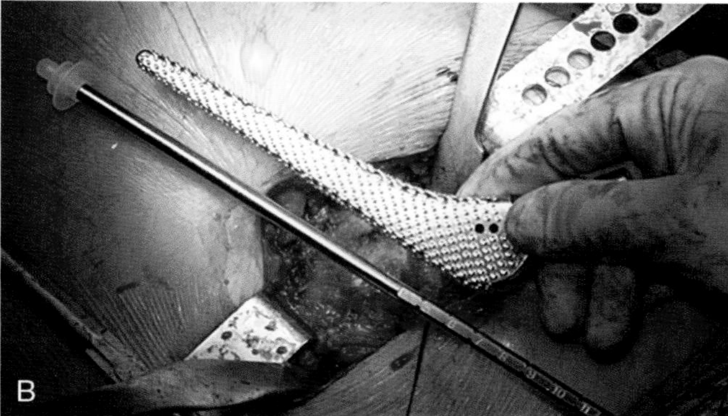

Figure 2 Intraoperative photographs of a left hip. **A,** Broaching of the femur is shown. Circular markings on the broach correspond to the final stem and allow for fine adjustments of stem position within the cement mantle. **B,** The use of the broach as a reference to determine the appropriate level of insertion of the cement restrictor. The level of insertion should allow for 1 to 2 cm of distal cement mantle.

- Broaching is performed (**Figure 2, A**). Although no difference has been found between broach surface finishes, the authors of this chapter routinely use a toothed broach. Broach offset and size initially are selected on the basis of preoperative templating with the goal of re-creating the patient's leg length and offset with a 2-mm cement mantle. Typically, only one or two broaches are required to achieve stability for trial purposes. Overaggressive broaching should be avoided because it removes excess cancellous bone that is necessary for proper cemented fixation.
- The trial implant is inserted.
- Leg length, offset, soft-tissue tension, range of motion, stability, and palpable landmarks are checked.
- Adjustments are made by inserting heads of different length. If necessary, the broach can be exchanged for one with a different range of offset.
- The depth of insertion, varus/valgus orientation, and version of the selected trial broach are marked on the femur with cautery and a surgical marker.
- When the final prosthesis is inserted, fine adjustments can be made by repositioning the implant in the cement mantle relative to these markings.

PROSTHESIS IMPLANTATION

- The broach is removed and is used to measure the desired depth of insertion of the cement restrictor, allowing for 1 to 2 cm of cement mantle distal to the prosthesis (**Figure 2, B**).
- The size of the restrictor is based on the diameter of the femoral canal.
- The restrictor is inserted on a marked handle to confirm position.
- Loose debris is removed with a canal brush (**Figure 3, A**), and blood and fat are cleared from the cancellous bed with copious jet lavage (**Figure 3, B**). Jet lavage is critical to achieving cement penetration because bulb syringe irrigation has

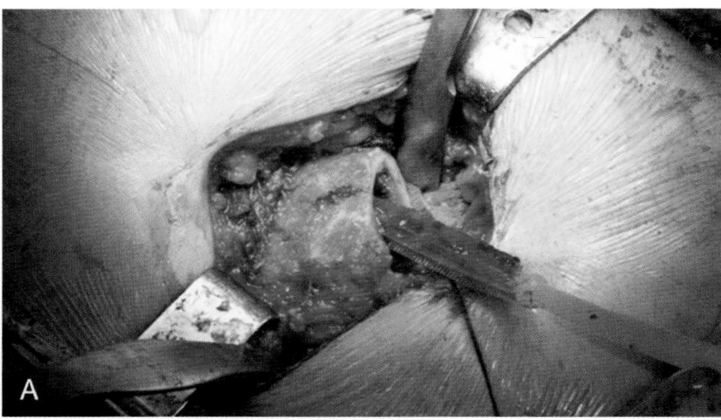

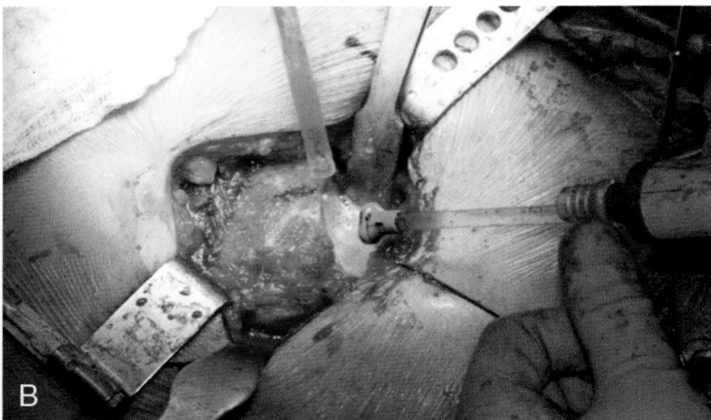

Figure 3 Intraoperative photographs of a left hip. **A,** A canal brush is used to remove loose cancellous bone and debris in preparation for cementation of the femoral implant. **B,** Jet lavage is used to remove blood and fat from the cancellous bone.

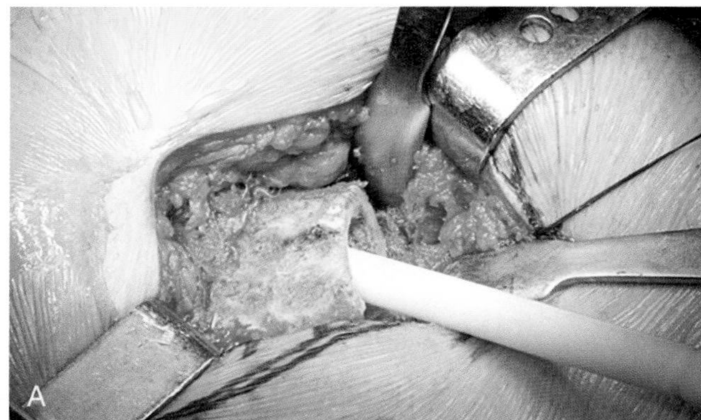

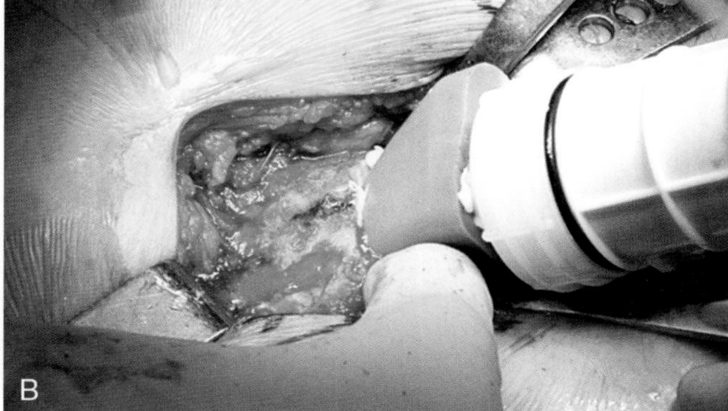

Figure 4 Intraoperative photographs of a left hip. **A,** The introduction of cement into the femoral canal in a retrograde manner with a cement gun. The preserved cancellous bone is clean and dry. **B,** Pressurization of the cement mantle. Extrusion of marrow contents from the exposed femur indicates adequate pressurization.

been shown to be insufficient.

- The canal is cooled with chilled saline to promote hemostasis, prolong working time, reduce the setting temperature of the cement, and improve the cement-prosthesis interface.
- Gauze soaked in hydrogen peroxide is packed into the canal as an additional measure to ensure hemostasis. It is important to vent the femur with suction during this step.
- The gauze is removed, and occlusive suction is maintained to ensure a clean and dry cancellous bed until cementation begins.
- A sponge is packed in the acetabulum to prevent contact with cement.
- Cement is mixed concurrently with femoral preparation. The anesthesiology team is notified that cement will be used in short order. Two 40-g bags of antibiotic-impregnated cement with monomer are added to a closed mixing system under vacuum. Three 40-g bags are used for patients with large femurs. The closed mixing system reduces the porosity of the cement, improving its mechanical properties. The use of a closed mixing system also limits staff exposure to fumes.
- The cement is mixed in the canister, which is then attached to the cement gun.
- The mixing time varies depending on the room temperature, mixing methods, and type of cement but is typically 3 to 3.5 minutes. Mixing is complete when the cement has a doughlike consistency and no longer sticks to surgical gloves.
- Cement is injected in retrograde fashion with the cement gun (**Figure 4, A**).
- Pressure is maintained on the cement with the surgeon's finger while the cement gun is removed and the nozzle is shortened.
- A pressurizer is added to the nozzle, and the femoral canal is occluded while the cement mantle is pressurized (**Figure 4, B**). Extrusion of marrow contents from the exposed femur indicates adequate pressurization.

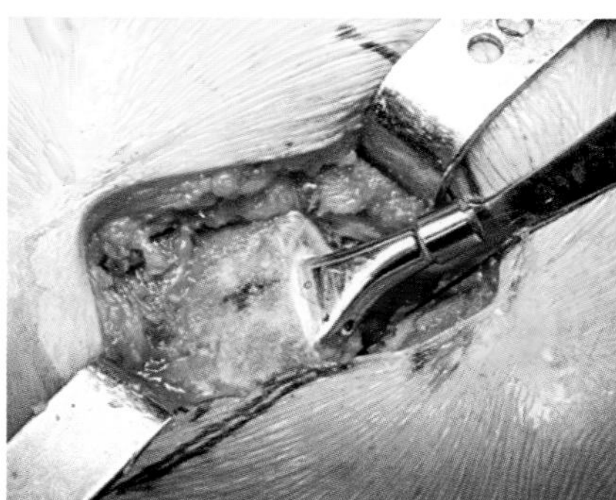

Figure 5 Intraoperative photograph of a left hip shows the final appearance of the cemented femoral stem.

- Pressure is maintained on the cement until nearly the end of its working period to avoid bleeding and achieve maximum additional pressurization from stem insertion. The absence of blood at the cement-bone interface indicates adequate pressurization maintained above perfusion pressure.
- A hollow distal centralizer is applied, and the final stem is inserted along the trajectory of the previous markings from the broach. The medial canal is occluded with a finger during insertion to maximize pressurization. The starting position should be biased posteriorly to avoid a thin cement mantle in Gruen zones 8 and 9. Markings on the stem facilitate its positioning.
- Extruded cement is removed, and the stem is held in position while the cement mantle sets (**Figure 5**).
- Repeat trialing is performed to confirm leg length, offset, range of motion, and stability.
- The final femoral head is applied to a clean and dry taper with a single firm mallet strike and is reduced into the joint.

Wound Closure

- The capsule is closed with a running No. 1 absorbable braided suture.
- A transosseous repair of the abductors is performed with No. 5 braided composite suture and oversewn with absorbable suture.
- The fascia and subcutaneous tissue are closed in standard fashion.
- Subcuticular skin closure is performed.
- Thin adhesive strips are applied.
- The wound is covered with a synthetic dressing.

Postoperative Regimen

The patient is mobilized postoperatively and allowed to bear weight as tolerated. Perioperative antibiotics are continued for 24 hours. Deep vein thrombosis prophylaxis is initiated on postoperative day 1 and continued for 35 days. Multimodal analgesia is administered during the inpatient stay, typically 3 to 5 days. Follow-up examination typically is performed at 6 weeks, 3 months, and 1 year postoperatively, with yearly examinations thereafter.

Avoiding Pitfalls and Complications

Careful templating is necessary to ensure correct leg length and offset. Special consideration is given to the anticipated level of the femoral neck cut. This cut provides an intraoperative reference point to assist in determination of the final depth of insertion of the femoral implant.

The use of cement in femoral fixation requires excellent team communication. The anesthesiology team should be told when cement is about to be used so that they can optimize the patient's oxygenation, fluid status, and blood pressure and be prepared for any complications. Because the cement has a limited working time, the surgeon must be aware of when it is mixed to ensure that adequate time is available to prepare the femoral canal.

Care must be taken to ensure that the femoral canal is dry and that hemostasis is obtained. A canal brush, pressure lavage, cold saline, gauze soaked in hydrogen peroxide, and hypotensive anesthesia all assist in this capacity. Failure to obtain a dry canal can result in poor cement interdigitation into bone or a poor mantle, which can affect survivorship.

Overly aggressive pressurization of cement in the distal canal should be avoided because it can dislodge the cement restrictor and allow cement to penetrate the distal canal. The cement restrictor should be appropriately sized and secured before cement is introduced. In the proximal canal, cement should be pressurized aggressively, with care taken to ensure that the pressurizing gasket makes a good seal between the cement gun and the cut surface of the femoral neck. Pressurizers of various sizes and shapes are available and should be selected on the basis of the size and shape of the cut femoral neck.

The femoral implant should be inserted in a timely manner to ensure that the cement polymerization does not prevent complete seating of the femoral implant. However, the implant should not be inserted too soon because early insertion will result in reduced pressurization. The optimal time for stem insertion depends on the type of cement and the temperature and humidity of the room. Room temperature and humidity should be controlled and standardized to allow more consistent cement working times.

The use of cemented femoral fixation allows variability in the final implant positioning. However, care must be taken to avoid inadvertent valgus positioning of the stem. The final cemented implant can shift into a valgus position more easily than the broach would. The net effect is reduced offset from the trialed implants that can lead to inadvertent instability.

Patience and vigilance are necessary when the femoral implant has been inserted into the cement mantle and the team is waiting for the cement to fully polymerize. An inadvertent movement of the leg by the assistant can affect the final implant position and is more easily correctable if noticed during polymerization than after polymerization is complete.

Bibliography

Aubault M, Druon J, Le Nail L, Rosset P: Outcomes at least 10 years after cemented PF® (Zimmer) total hip arthroplasty: 83 cases. *Orthop Traumatol Surg Res* 2013;99(4 suppl):S235-S239.

Australian Orthopaedic Association: *National Joint Replacement Registry: Hip and Knee Arthroplasty. Annual Report* 2015. Adelaide, South Australia, Australian Orthopaedic Association, 2015. Available at: https://aoanjrr.sahmri.com/documents/10180/217745/Hip%20and%20Knee%20Arthroplasty. Accessed July 22, 2016.

Bedard NA, Callaghan JJ, Stefl MD, Liu SS: Systematic review of literature of cemented femoral components: What is the durability at minimum 20 years followup? *Clin Orthop Relat Res* 2015;473(2):563-571.

Callaghan JJ, Bracha P, Liu SS, Piyaworakhun S, Goetz DD, Johnston RC: Survivorship of a Charnley total hip arthroplasty: A concise follow-up, at a minimum of thirty-five years, of previous reports. *J Bone Joint Surg Am* 2009;91(11):2617-2621.

Garellick G, Kärrholm J, Lindahl H, Malchau H, Rogmark C, Rolfson O; Swedish Hip Arthroplasty Register: *Annual Report 2014.* Gothenburg, Sweden, Swedish Hip Arthroplasty Register, 2015. Available at: http://www.shpr.se/Libraries/Documents/Annual_Report_2014_Eng.sflb.ashx. Accessed July 22, 2016.

Hailer NP, Garellick G, Kärrholm J: Uncemented and cemented primary total hip arthroplasty in the Swedish Hip Arthroplasty Register. *Acta Orthop* 2010;81(1):34-41.

Halley DK, Glassman AH: Twenty- to twenty-six-year radiographic review in patients 50 years of age or younger with cemented Charnley low-friction arthroplasty. *J Arthroplasty* 2003;18(7 suppl 1):79-85.

Jones LC, Hungerford DS: Cement disease. *Clin Orthop Relat Res* 1987;(225):192-206.

Kale AA, Della Valle CJ, Frankel VH, Stuchin SA, Zuckerman JD, Di Cesare PE: Hip arthroplasty with a collared straight cobalt-chrome femoral stem using second-generation cementing technique: A 10-year-average follow-up study. *J Arthroplasty* 2000;15(2):187-193.

Keener JD, Callaghan JJ, Goetz DD, Pederson DR, Sullivan PM, Johnston RC: Twenty-five-year results after Charnley total hip arthroplasty in patients less than fifty years old: A concise follow-up of a previous report. *J Bone Joint Surg Am* 2003;85(6):1066-1072.

Lewthwaite SC, Squires B, Gie GA, Timperley AJ, Ling RS: The Exeter Universal hip in patients 50 years or younger at 10-17 years' followup. *Clin Orthop Relat Res* 2008;466(2):324-331.

Ling RS, Charity J, Lee AJ, Whitehouse SL, Timperley AJ, Gie GA: The long-term results of the original Exeter polished cemented femoral component: A follow-up report. *J Arthroplasty* 2009;24(4):511-517.

Lucht U: The Danish Hip Arthroplasty Register. *Acta Orthop Scand* 2000;71(5):433-439.

Mäkelä KT, Eskelinen A, Pulkkinen P, Paavolainen P, Remes V: Results of 3,668 primary total hip replacements for primary osteoarthritis in patients under the age of 55 years. *Acta Orthop* 2011;82(5):521-529.

Mäkelä KT, Matilainen M, Pulkkinen P, et al: Failure rate of cemented and uncemented total hip replacements: Register study of combined Nordic database of four nations. *BMJ* 2014;348:f7592.

National Joint Registry for England, Wales, and Northern Ireland: *11th Annual Report: 2014.* Hemel Hempstead, England, National Joint Registry, 2014. Available at: http://www.njrcentre.org.uk/njrcentre/Portals/0/Documents/England/Reports/11th_annual_report/NJR%2011th%20Annual%20Report%202014.pdf. Accessed July 22, 2016.

The New Zealand Joint Registry: *Sixteen Year Report: January 1999 to December 2014.* Wellington, New Zealand, New Zealand Orthopaedic Association, 2015. Available at: http://nzoa.org.nz/system/files/Web_DH7657_NZJR2014Report_v4_12Nov15.pdf. Accessed July 22, 2016.

Norwegian National Advisory Unit on Arthroplasty and Hip Fractures: *Report: June 2015.* Bergen, Norway, The Norwegian Arthroplasty Register, 2015. Available at: http://nrlweb.ihelse.net/Rapporter/Report2015_english.pdf. Accessed July 22, 2016.

Prins W, Meijer R, Kollen BJ, Verheyen CC, Ettema HB: Excellent results with the cemented Lubinus SP II 130-mm femoral stem at 10 years of follow-up: 932 hips followed for 5-15 years. *Acta Orthop* 2014;85(3):276-279.

Warth LC, Callaghan JJ, Liu SS, Klaassen AL, Goetz DD, Johnston RC: Thirty-five-year results after Charnley total hip arthroplasty in patients less than fifty years old: A concise follow-up of previous reports. *J Bone Joint Surg Am* 2014;96(21):1814-1819.

Wroblewski BM, Siney PD, Fleming PA: Charnley low-friction arthroplasty: Survival patterns to 38 years. *J Bone Joint Surg Br* 2007;89(8):1015-1018.

Chapter 11

Primary Total Hip Arthroplasty With Extensively Porous-Coated Femoral Implants

C. Anderson Engh, Jr, MD
Cathy Huynh, BS

Indications

A porous-coated, noncemented femoral implant for total hip arthroplasty (THA) was first approved by the FDA in 1983. This porous-coated implant consisted of a straight, nontapered distal cylindric rod and a triangular proximal metaphyseal portion. Studies of this type of implant have demonstrated 98% survivorship of the femoral component at 20 years postoperatively. A porous-coated stem has been used successfully in patients who previously were not considered appropriate candidates for noncemented fixation, such as patients with osteonecrosis, patients with rheumatoid arthritis, and elderly patients with osteoporosis. Many manufacturers now offer extensively porous-coated femoral implants.

At the institution of the authors of this chapter, extensively porous-coated femoral stems were used in all THA procedures for 20 consecutive years, with no difference in mid- to long-term clinical outcomes when comparing patients on the basis of age, sex, diagnosis, or bone quality. Clinical results and bony integration do not differ substantially between patients older than 65 years or those with osteoporosis and younger patients without osteoporosis. Published studies of the extensively porous-coated Anatomic Medullary Locking (AML) stem (DePuy Synthes) femoral implant have demonstrated that the clinical results of THA with extensively porous-coated stems depend primarily on the initial prosthetic fit within the femur, particularly within the diaphysis. This factor is more closely related to the interference fit, or so-called scratch fit, obtained intraoperatively between the femoral porous coating and host bone than it is to patient characteristics.

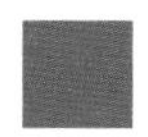

Contraindications

The diameter of the femoral canal can present contraindications to the use of a porous-coated femoral implant. Stems smaller than 10.5 mm are not available; therefore, patients with canals of very small diameter are not good candidates for THA with this type of implant. Patients with canals of very large diameter also are not good candidates for THA with a porous-coated femoral implant because stems larger than 22.5 mm are not available.

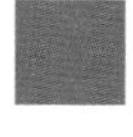

Alternative Treatments

Patients with canals of small diameter can be treated with shorter, distally tapered, proximally coated stems or small-diameter stems with proximal modularity. Patients with large canals can be treated with the use of a cemented stem or a revision-type stem of larger diameter.

Results

In addition to the 20-year 98% femoral survivorship statistic mentioned previously, other retrieval and clinical data are available. An autopsy study of extensively porous-coated stems confirmed the presence of bony ingrowth into the implant surface. On average, bony ingrowth covered 35% of the available porous surface (range, 25% to 43%). The pattern of bony ingrowth was found to be predictable, with the most consistent growth demonstrated at the distal margins of the porous coating. Dual-energy x-ray absorptiometry and videodensitometric research studies have examined

Dr. Engh or an immediate family member has received royalties from, serves as a paid consultant to, and has stock or stock options held in DePuy Synthes; has received research or institutional support from DePuy Synthes and Smith & Nephew; and serves as a board member, owner, officer, or committee member of the American Academy of Orthopaedic Surgeons, the American Association of Hip and Knee Surgeons, and The Hip Society. Neither Ms. Huynh nor any immediate family member has received anything of value from or has stock or stock options held in a commercial company or institution related directly or indirectly to the subject of this chapter.

the effect of bony ingrowth on femoral bone quality. Bone loss resulting from stress shielding occurred on a gradient, with the greatest loss typically adjacent to the proximal third of the implant. The magnitude of the bone loss had a high correlation with the patient's initial bone quality. Patients with preoperative osteopenia or osteoporosis had greater proximal bone loss postoperatively than patients with high initial bone mineral content. Bone loss after THA with an extensively porous-coated stem was not correlated with stem size, duration of implantation, or the patient's weight or age.

Early clinical studies of these stems defined the radiographic appearance of noncemented femoral implants with bony ingrowth, those with fibrous stabilization, and those that were loose. A study from the authors' institution published in 1990 devised a method to grade the radiographic fixation of noncemented femoral implants. In this system, bony ingrowth was indicated by so-called spot welds to endosteal bone at the edge of the porous coating, calcar atrophy, and the lack of migration. Failure of bony ingrowth was indicated by extensive radiolucent lines adjacent to the porous coating, migration of the stem, and a distal pedestal.

Clinical documentation of implant survivorship has been facilitated by the use of autopsy analysis to confirm bony integration and by the development of a clear radiographic definition of bony ingrowth. Most of the relevant publications originate from the institution at which extensively porous-coated stems were developed. However, other centers have duplicated the clinical results (**Table 1**), and some studies have reported greater than 95% survivorship of these stems. Stem survivorship also has been documented in patients with less than optimal bone quality. In a study of 203 patients who were aged 65 years or older at the time of the THA procedure, 97% survivorship of the femoral stem was reported at 12 years postoperatively. A study of 64 patients with rheumatoid arthritis demonstrated 98% survivorship of porous-coated stems at 10 years postoperatively. In a study that included 28 extensively porous-coated stems implanted in young patients who had osteonecrosis and were thought to have altered femoral physiology, no revisions due to aseptic stem loosening were reported at mean 9-year follow-up.

In a study published in 1989 of 1,318 extensively porous-coated stems implanted between 1977 and 1986, 39 insertional fractures were reported (3%); only one-half of the insertional fractures were diagnosed intraoperatively. The rate of proximal fractures was less than that of distal fractures. Proximal fractures were more likely than distal fractures to be diagnosed intraoperatively. Incomplete proximal fractures were managed with protected weight bearing, whereas displaced proximal fractures were managed with cerclage wires. Nondisplaced diaphyseal fissures, the most common type of insertional fracture, were typically diagnosed on postoperative radiographs, were visible on only a single view, and did not involve the posterior femoral cortex.

In a study examining periprosthetic bone loss resulting from stress shielding, clinical and radiographic results of 48 THA procedures in patients with proximal bone loss were compared with the results of 160 THA procedures in patients without proximal bone loss. At a mean of 14 years postoperatively, patients with radiographically observed proximal bone loss as a result of stress shielding were no more likely to have undergone revision surgery, demonstrate particle-induced osteolysis, or experience thigh pain than patients without proximal bone loss.

Thigh pain has been reported in 8% to 14% of patients who have undergone THA with extensively porous-coated stems. However, thigh pain typically does not affect a patient's activity or satisfaction with the procedure. The authors of one study reported thigh pain in 12% of patients, but pain resulted in activity limitation in only 3% of patients. In a different study, researchers assessed the outcomes of 1,545 extensively porous-coated femoral implants. Thigh pain limited activity in 3.6% of patients with the smallest diameter stems (9 to 12.5 mm) and 2.5% of patients with the largest diameter stems (18 to 21 mm). The authors of the study concluded that patients with larger diameter stems were no more likely to have undergone revision, experience implant loosening, or report thigh pain or activity-limiting pain than patients with smaller diameter stems.

Technique

Setup/Exposure

- Any surgical approach to the hip can be used for the placement of an extensively porous-coated femoral implant. However, the 6-inch straight stem design requires moderate retraction of the hip abductors, making these stems more difficult to insert with anterior abductor-sparing approaches.
- The senior author (C.A.E.) of this chapter prefers the posterior approach.
- For the posterior approach, the patient is placed in the lateral decubitus position.

Instruments/Equipment/ Implants Required

- No special instruments are needed other than those supplied by individual manufacturers.

Procedure

- The superficial dissection and the arthrotomy are performed.
- Initial leg length is measured in two ways. First, the surgeon uses a ruler

Table 1 Results of Clinical Studies of Total Hip Arthroplasty With Extensively Porous-Coated (EPC) Stems

Authors (Year)	Number of Hips	EPC Stem Type	Approach	Mean Patient Age in Years (Range)	Mean Follow-up in Years (Range)	Results
Kronick et al (1997)	186	132 Anatomic Medullary Locking (AML; DePuy), 38 Prodigy (DePuy), 4 Solution (DePuy)	Posterior	37.6 (14-50)	8.3 (2-13)	174 hips available at follow-up Femoral revision rate, 1.1%: 1 revision for aseptic loosening and 1 revision in conjunction with an acetabular revision and proximal femoral osteolysis
McAuley et al (1998)	212	AML	Posterior	71 (65-87)	8.5 (5-14)	159 hips available at follow-up Femoral revision rate, 1.3%: 1 revision for aseptic loosening and 1 revision for infection
Jana et al (2001)	65	AML	Posterior	55.1 (24-80)[a]	11.7 (2.2-20.5)	56 hips available at follow-up Femoral revision rate, 1.8%: 1 revision for aseptic loosening
Nercessian et al (2001)	61	AML	Posterior	48.3 (25-64)	10.5 (9-12)	52 hips available at follow-up Femoral revision rate, 5.8%: 1 revision for thigh pain and 2 revisions for proximal femoral osteolysis
Chen et al (2006)	157	Prodigy	Posterior: 126 Lateral: 19	56.2 (20-80)	6.7 (0.1-8.2)	145 hips available at follow-up Femoral revision rate, 0.7%: 1 revision for aseptic loosening
Hartzband et al (2010)	106	Epoch (Zimmer)	Posterior	58 (23-78)	10 (1-14)	101 hips available at follow-up No femoral revisions

[a] Mean age calculated based on total number of hips studied, which includes 17 proximally coated stems.

to measure (at the knees) the difference in femoral lengths between the affected and unaffected extremities (**Figure 1, A**). Second, a threaded Steinmann pin is placed proximal to the affected hip. The pin is bent twice at 90° angles so that the tip touches the greater trochanter. This point is marked with a stitch that will be used to monitor offset and length after placement of the trial implants (**Figure 1, B**). The pin is rotated away from the incision until trial implants are in place, at which time the measurement is repeated.

- The hip is dislocated.
- The femoral head is resected with a provisional osteotomy of the femoral neck on the basis of preoperative templating.
- Either the femur or the acetabulum can be prepared first.
- To perform femoral preparation first, the trial implant is placed at the templated level before the acetabulum is exposed. This method avoids a high initial neck resection, which can make acetabular exposure difficult. Additionally, this method allows determination of the femoral anteversion, which is difficult to change. The position of the acetabulum is easily adjusted and can be determined in combination with the femur to achieve the proper combined anteversion.
- To begin preparation of the femur, straight rigid reamers are used to create a cylindric tube.
- Correct positioning of the pilot hole for the reamer is critical for proper placement of the femoral implant. The pilot hole should be larger than the expected diameter of the femoral stem to reduce the risk of eccentric reaming of the intramedullary canal (**Figure 2**).
- Reaming continues with the use of progressively larger reamers. Care is taken to monitor contact of the reamer with the pilot hole.

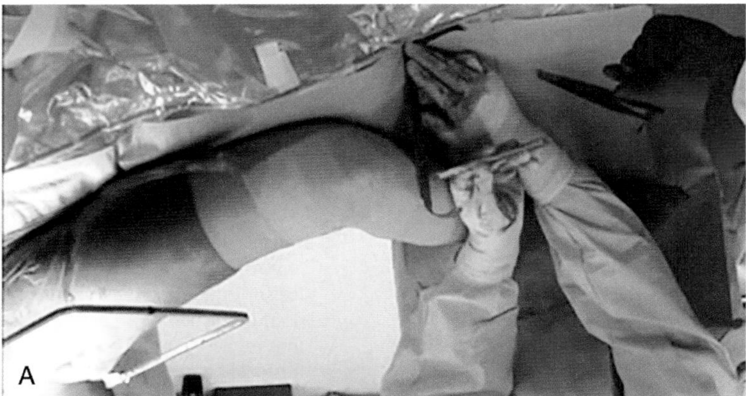

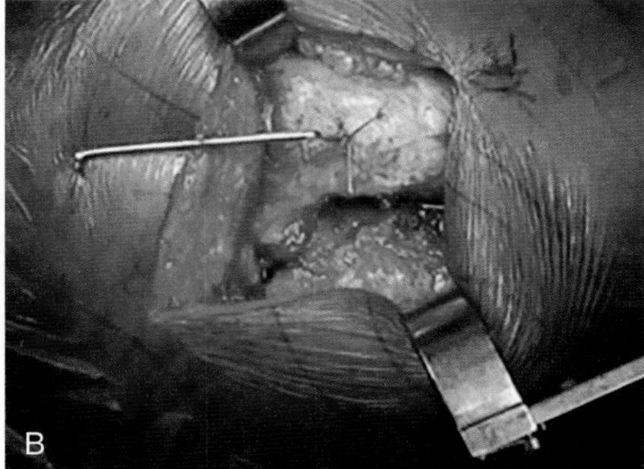

Figure 1 Intraoperative photographs show measurement of leg length. **A,** The relative length of the femurs is measured with the affected hip in the lateral position (in this image, a right hip) and the unaffected (down) knee secured in 90° of flexion. Leg length is measured at the knees. **B,** The same hip shown in panel **A**, viewed from posterior. Hip length and offset are measured with a Steinmann pin in the ilium that is bent to touch the greater trochanter. The location on the greater trochanter is marked with a suture to allow comparison of the position before dislocation and the position after trial reduction.

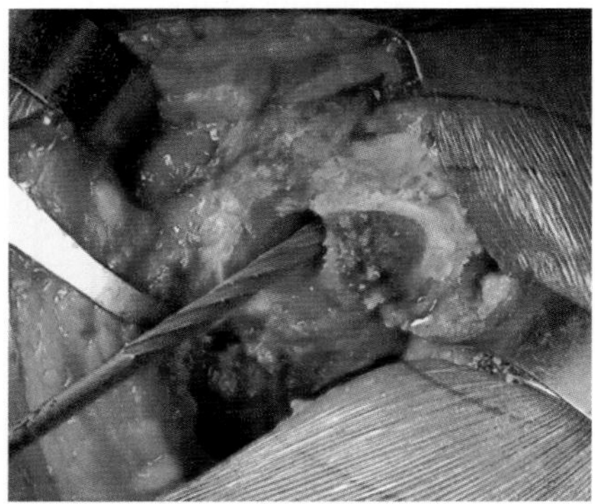

Figure 2 Intraoperative photograph of a right hip addressed via a posterior approach shows the pilot hole in the piriformis fossa. The hole must be sufficiently lateral to prevent impingement of the greater trochanter on the reamers. Any retained superior lateral neck must be removed. As shown here, the medial aspect of the greater trochanter often is removed to allow straight access to the femoral diaphysis.

- To ensure successful distal fixation of the stem, the reamer should be guided by the femoral diaphysis and not by more proximal bone.
- A common error is to place an undersized stem in varus because the direction of reaming was influenced by impingement of the reamer with the greater trochanter. If this impingement is observed, proximolateral bone in the region of the greater trochanter is cleared to allow unobstructed passage of the reamer.
- Reaming continues until audible and tactile feedback indicates that the reamer is in contact with the femoral diaphysis. A reamer of the proper diameter will engage diaphyseal cortical bone for a distance of 3 to 5 cm (**Figure 3, A**). If necessary, an intraoperative radiograph is obtained to verify the alignment of reaming or the amount of cortical contact.
- After preparation of the femoral diaphysis has been completed, the metaphyseal bone is prepared with the use of blunt-tipped proximal reamers and rasps (**Figure 4, A** and **B**). Excessive removal of metaphyseal bone is avoided. Although the stem achieves distal fixation, proximal bone contact and ingrowth are important to ensure long-term fixation and prevent distal migration of wear debris.
- The broach is seated at the templated level (**Figure 5**).
- If metaphyseal cancellous bone remains present when the broach is at the templated level, a larger broach is used if available (**Figure 4, C** and **D**).
- The goal of re-creating femoral anatomy is achieved by adjusting the offset and leg length as required.
- After the desired femoral length and fit are achieved, the acetabulum is prepared if this step was not done before femoral preparation.
- A trial reduction is performed.
- Limb length and offset are assessed during the trial reduction with the use of the previously placed Steinmann pin and by comparing the femoral lengths measured at the knee (**Figure 1**).
- The femoral offset and limb length are adjusted by changing the length of the implant neck, the level at which the implant is seated (which requires recutting the femoral neck to seat the implant more distally), and/or the configuration of the neck of the prosthesis.
- Hip stability is assessed with trial implants in place. For assessment of posterior stability, the hip is placed in flexion, adduction, and internal rotation. In most patients, the hip should be stable in 90° of flexion, 20° of adduction, and at least 50° of internal rotation. Anterior stability

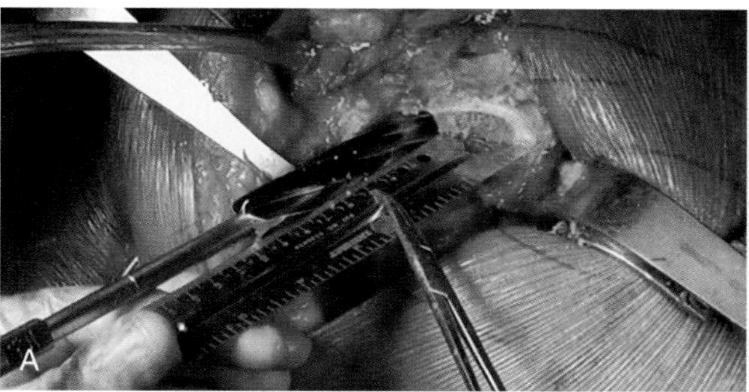

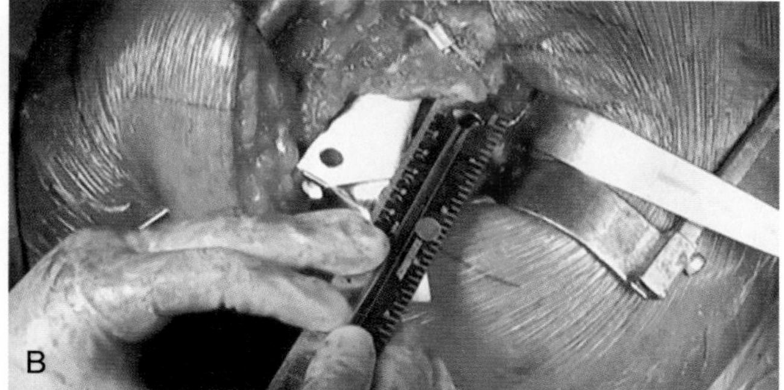

Figure 3 Intraoperative photographs of a right hip show determination of the amount of interference (scratch) fit. **A,** The length of interference fit is measured after the reamer is pushed into the femur until cortical bone is reached. Reamers are increased in diameter until 5 cm of cortical contact is achieved. **B,** The final stem is inserted by hand until the stem reaches cortical bone. The distance between the medial aspect of the implant and the medial femoral resection should be 4 to 6 cm. If the stem sits higher, line-to-line reaming should be performed.

is assessed with the hip in full extension and external rotation.

- After satisfactory leg length, femoral lateralization, and hip stability have been achieved, the trial implants are removed and the final implants are placed.
- The decision is made to either leave the femoral diaphysis underreamed by 0.5 mm or perform line-to-line reaming. To determine the amount of scratch fit, the stem is placed firmly into the canal until it stops. The stem should extend approximately 5 cm above the neck osteotomy (**Figure 3, B**).
- If the stem extends more than 5 cm above the neck osteotomy or seems tight and does not advance as expected on impaction, the stem is removed, and the femoral diaphysis, which was initially underreamed by 0.5 mm, is enlarged to match the diameter of the final stem. The decision to perform line-to-line reaming should be made before the stem is impacted forcefully and becomes stuck. The decision is based on the tightness of the last reamer, the length of tight reaming, and the surgeon's judgment intraoperatively.
- The stem is impacted. It may initially advance 5 mm with each strike of the hammer. As more of the porous-coated surface engages with the bone, the advancement of the stem decreases. In the final 2 cm, the stem may advance only 0.5 mm with each strike of the hammer.

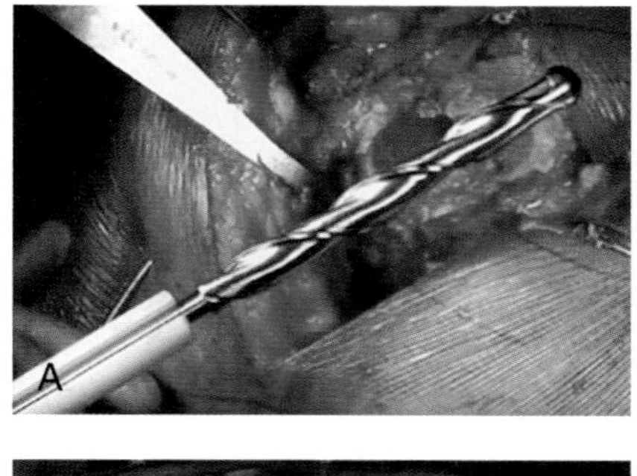

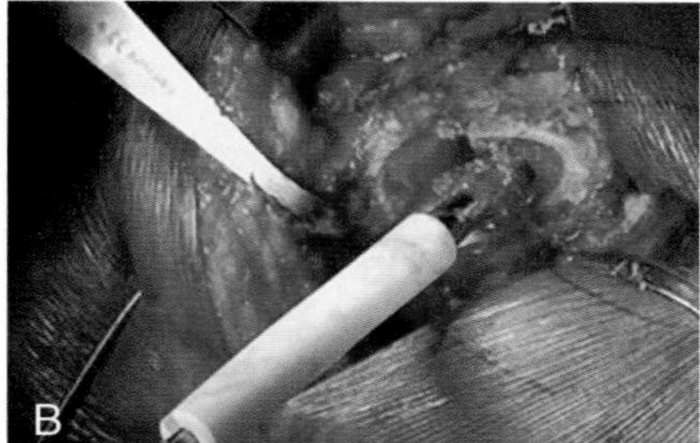

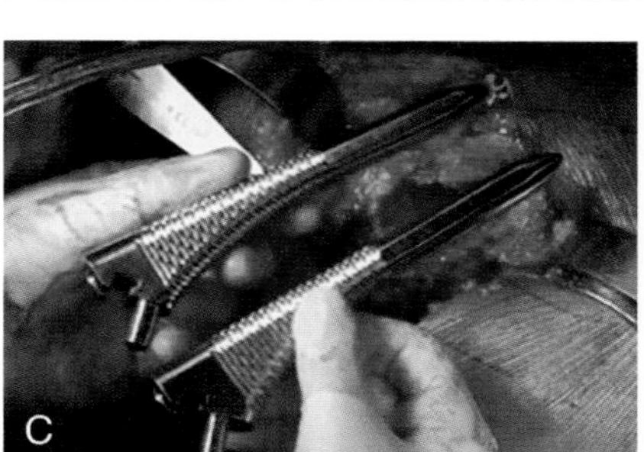

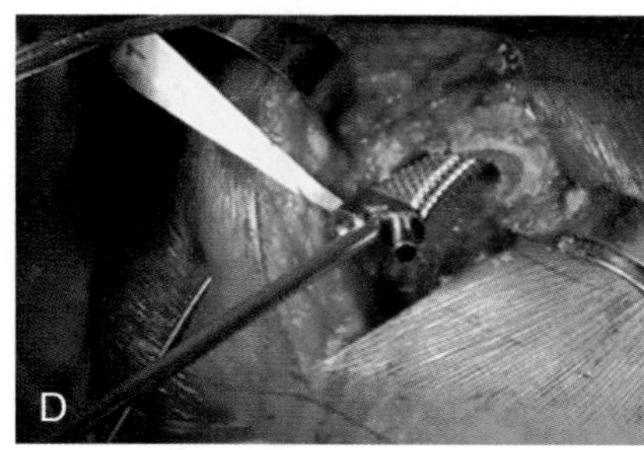

Figure 4 Intraoperative photographs of a right hip show metaphyseal preparation with the use of a blunt-tipped side-cutting reamer and broaches. A blunt-tipped side-cutting reamer (**A**) is moved medially with the blunt tip in contact with endosteal lateral cortex (**B**). The side cutting creates a metaphyseal triangle to match the implant geometry. **C,** The standard-size and large metaphyseal broaches. **D,** Proper initial broach position is shown. As the broach is advanced, metaphyseal bone is removed. Although proximal metaphyseal preparation can be accomplished with broaches alone, side-cutting reamers can be used before broaching to speed the procedure, provided that they are used with care and excessive bone is not removed.

Wound Closure

- The wound is closed in standard fashion.
- The senior author (C.A.E.) prefers a subcuticular stitch for the skin.

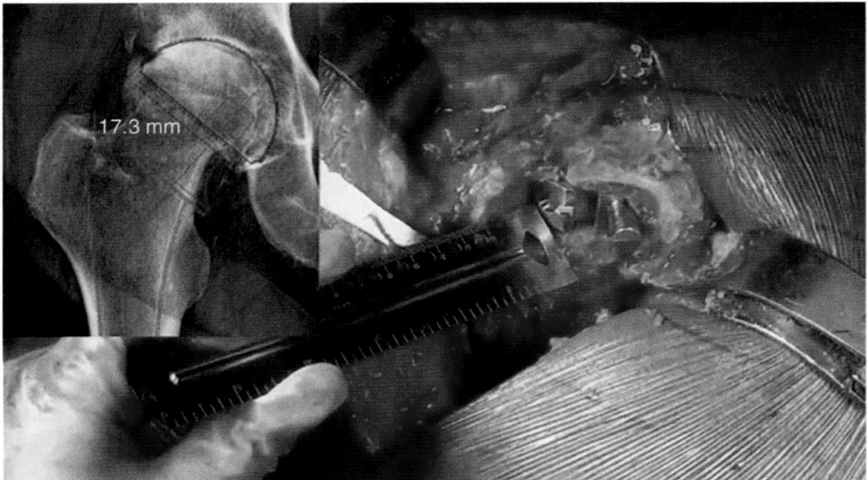

Figure 5 Intraoperative photograph of a right hip shows measurement of the broach seating level. The smaller of the two broaches is seated to a level measured from the tip of the greater trochanter that matches the distance templated on an AP radiograph (inset).

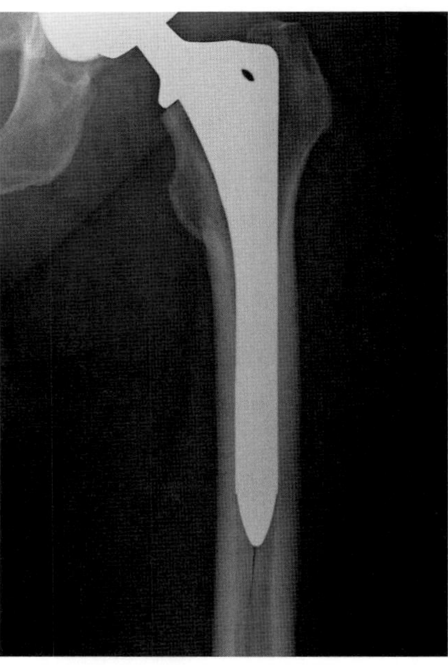

Figure 6 AP radiograph of a left hip obtained 4 weeks after surgery demonstrates a distal insertional fracture.

Postoperative Regimen

Immediate weight bearing is allowed as tolerated. Most patients tolerate full weight bearing. In some patients, weight bearing of 50% or less for 3 to 6 weeks postoperatively is beneficial. The decision to limit weight bearing is typically based on the length of interference fit, the ease of stem insertion, postoperative radiographic evaluation, and the patient's likelihood of falling. Patients with good interference fit obtained intraoperatively and a normal radiograph postoperatively are typically allowed to bear weight as tolerated postoperatively. Weight bearing is limited for 3 to 6 weeks postoperatively in patients in whom the stem was inserted easily, those in whom the stem appears undersized on the postoperative radiograph, or those with a hairline diaphyseal fracture.

Avoiding Pitfalls and Complications

Insertion of extensively porous-coated stems, like that of other noncemented stems, can result in femoral fracture. The stem size must be selected carefully because undersizing the stem can result in a loose implant, whereas oversizing can provide more rigid fixation but can result in an insertional femur fracture. As noted, the most common type of insertional fracture is a nondisplaced diaphyseal fissure (**Figure 6**). Intraoperatively, the surgeon should suspect this type of fracture if a stem that advanced 0.5 to 1 mm with each strike of the hammer suddenly advances 2 mm or more on one strike. This type of fracture can be managed with protected weight bearing for 6 weeks and typically does not affect long-term fixation. Displaced distal fractures are managed with open reduction and internal fixation with the use of a cable screw plate, and with retention of the femoral implant if the stem is stable.

Stem breakage or infection occasionally requires removal of an extensively porous-coated stem. Infection is the most common reason for removal of a stem with bony ingrowth. Stems that need to be revised in the first 4 to 6 weeks after implantation are easy to remove. Stems that have been in vivo for more than 6 months require serial radiographs to determine whether the stem is stable or loose. Loose stems that have migrated are easily removed. Removal of a stable stem is performed through a cortical window or an extended trochanteric slide osteotomy. The stem is sectioned between the proximal triangular portion and distal cylindric portion with a metal-cutting burr. After the metaphyseal portion is removed, the distal portion of the stem is removed with the use of trephines that correspond with the implant diameter. To avoid thermal necrosis of bone, the trephines are irrigated and replaced frequently. When inserting a new stem, the surgeon should bypass the trephined area to avoid the risk of fixation failure resulting from proximal thermal necrosis that may have occurred during removal of the stem.

Bibliography

Belmont PJ Jr, Powers CC, Beykirch SE, Hopper RH Jr, Engh CA Jr, Engh CA: Results of the anatomic medullary locking total hip arthroplasty at a minimum of twenty years: A concise follow-up of previous reports. *J Bone Joint Surg Am* 2008;90(7):1524-1530.

Chen CJ, Xenos JS, McAuley JP, Young A, Engh CA Sr: Second-generation porous-coated cementless total hip arthroplasties have high survival. *Clin Orthop Relat Res* 2006;(451):121-127.

Engh CA, Bobyn JD, Glassman AH: Porous-coated hip replacement: The factors governing bone ingrowth, stress shielding, and clinical results. *J Bone Joint Surg Br* 1987;69(1):45-55.

Engh CA, Hooten JP Jr, Zettl-Schaffer KF, Ghaffarpour M, McGovern TF, Bobyn JD: Evaluation of bone ingrowth in proximally and extensively porous-coated anatomic medullary locking prostheses retrieved at autopsy. *J Bone Joint Surg Am* 1995;77(6):903-910.

Engh CA, Massin P, Suthers KE: Roentgenographic assessment of the biologic fixation of porous-surfaced femoral components. *Clin Orthop Relat Res* 1990;(257):107-128.

Engh CA, McGovern TF, Bobyn JD, Harris WH: A quantitative evaluation of periprosthetic bone-remodeling after cementless total hip arthroplasty. *J Bone Joint Surg Am* 1992;74(7):1009-1020.

Engh CA Jr, Mohan V, Nagowski JP, Sychterz Terefenko CJ, Engh CA Sr: Influence of stem size on clinical outcome of primary total hip arthroplasty with cementless extensively porous-coated femoral components. *J Arthroplasty* 2009;24(4):554-559.

Engh CA Jr, Young AM, Engh CA Sr, Hopper RH Jr: Clinical consequences of stress shielding after porous-coated total hip arthroplasty. *Clin Orthop Relat Res* 2003;(417):157-163.

Glassman AH, Engh CA: The removal of porous-coated femoral hip stems. *Clin Orthop Relat Res* 1992;(285):164-180.

Hartley WT, McAuley JP, Culpepper WJ, Engh CA Jr, Engh CA Sr: Osteonecrosis of the femoral head treated with cementless total hip arthroplasty. *J Bone Joint Surg Am* 2000;82(10):1408-1413.

Hartzband MA, Glassman AH, Goldberg VM, et al: Survivorship of a low-stiffness extensively porous-coated femoral stem at 10 years. *Clin Orthop Relat Res* 2010;468(2):433-440.

Jana AK, Engh CA Jr, Lewandowski PJ, Hopper RH Jr, Engh CA: Total hip arthroplasty using porous-coated femoral components in patients with rheumatoid arthritis. *J Bone Joint Surg Br* 2001;83(5):686-690.

Kronick JL, Barba ML, Paprosky WG: Extensively coated femoral components in young patients. *Clin Orthop Relat Res* 1997;(344):263-274.

Maloney WJ, Sychterz C, Bragdon C, et al: Skeletal response to well fixed femoral components inserted with and without cement. *Clin Orthop Relat Res* 1996;(333):15-26.

McAuley JP, Culpepper WJ, Engh CA: Total hip arthroplasty: Concerns with extensively porous coated femoral components. *Clin Orthop Relat Res* 1998;(355):182-188.

McAuley JP, Moore KD, Culpepper WJ II, Engh CA: Total hip arthroplasty with porous-coated prostheses fixed without cement in patients who are sixty-five years of age or older. *J Bone Joint Surg Am* 1998;80(11):1648-1655.

Nercessian OA, Wu WH, Sarkissian H: Clinical and radiographic results of cementless AML total hip arthroplasty in young patients. *J Arthroplasty* 2001;16(3):312-316.

Schwartz JT Jr, Mayer JG, Engh CA: Femoral fracture during non-cemented total hip arthroplasty. *J Bone Joint Surg Am* 1989;71(8):1135-1142.

Sychterz CJ, Engh CA: The influence of clinical factors on periprosthetic bone remodeling. *Clin Orthop Relat Res* 1996;(322):285-292.

Chapter 12

Primary Total Hip Arthroplasty With Double-Tapered, Noncemented Femoral Stems

David F. Dalury, MD
William A. Jiranek, MD
Andrew Waligora, MD

Indications

Double-tapered noncemented femoral stems can be used for total hip arthroplasty (THA) in almost all patients who have femoral geometry amenable to metaphyseal fixation. Modern double-tapered femoral stems typically are forged from a titanium alloy and have a dual taper, which often is approximately 3°. This taper angle is supported by studies demonstrating that more exaggerated taper angles result in an increased risk of intraoperative and early postoperative periprosthetic fracture. The design and surface coating of the metaphyseal region of each implant is unique and proprietary to the manufacturer. In addition, each stem design has modifications to improve primary stability, including vertical fins, horizontal steps, or a combination of these features.

The designs of contemporary noncemented femoral stems have undergone an evolution driven by clinical results. Despite excellent long-term outcomes of cemented femoral stem fixation in osteoporotic bone, its failure rate in younger patients (younger than 60 years) with more robust bone stock led many researchers to seek other modes of fixation. The use of noncemented femoral stem fixation in THA started to gain attention and support in the late 1970s, when two studies highlighted the importance of osseointegration to provide a long-term anchor for the prosthesis. Initial stability is required to allow the osseointegration needed for long-term success of noncemented femoral implants. Although osseointegration begins 4 to 12 weeks postoperatively, it can continue for up to 3 years after implantation. Studies have demonstrated that the geometry and size of the femoral stem determines initial stability. Despite the ongoing evolution of femoral stem designs, modern double-taper, wedge-shaped stems share characteristics with many earlier implant designs.

The first noncemented femoral implant approved for use in the United States (AML [Anatomic Medullary Locking], DePuy) was cylindric, not tapered. This design, which debuted in the mid 1980s, relied on scratch-fit engagement between its cylindric ingrowth surface and diaphyseal bone. Even with the addition of a proximal collar to transmit forces to the calcar, studies demonstrated substantial proximal stress shielding and activity-limiting thigh pain in some patients.

In the same time period (late 1970s into 1980s), the Karl Zweymüller stem was introduced in Europe. It is considered the first of the classic tapered stems. Its design included 3° tapers in both the coronal and sagittal planes and a rectangular cross-section. The double taper provided axial stability, and the combination of the four-cornered cross-section and compaction broaching provided rotational stability. Despite this design, studies have described substantial proximal stress shielding, indicating an environment of predominately diaphyseal loading. This finding

Dr. Dalury or an immediate family member has received royalties from, is a member of a speakers' bureau or has made paid presentations on behalf of, serves as a paid consultant to, has stock or stock options held in, and has received research or institutional support from DePuy Synthes. Dr. Jiranek or an immediate family member has received royalties from and serves as a paid consultant to DePuy Synthes; has stock or stock options held in Johnson & Johnson; has received research or institutional support from DePuy Synthes and Stryker; and serves as a board member, owner, officer, or committee member of the American Association of Hip and Knee Surgeons, LifeNet Health, and the Orthopaedic Learning Center. Neither Dr. Waligora nor any immediate family member has received anything of value from or has stock or stock options held in a commercial company or institution related directly or indirectly to the subject of this chapter.

is supported by CT scans demonstrating situations in which fewer than all four corners of the stem make proximal contact with the femoral bone. This scenario may result in variable proximal primary and secondary fixation.

The PCA (Porous Coated Anatomic; Howmedica) stem was introduced at approximately the same time as the previous stems. Its design was intended to match the shape of the proximal femur. The stable fixation of this stem relied on three-point fixation that included both metaphyseal loading and a tight diaphyseal fit. Unlike the Zweymüller stem, it required preparation via sequential reaming for diaphyseal engagement. PCA stems had a high prevalence of thigh pain, possibly attributable to the design of the diaphyseal portion of the stem (which was bowed and tended to impinge against the anterior cortex of the femur at the tip and/or modulus of elasticity of the stem).

The HGP (Harris-Galante Porous; Zimmer) and Anatomic Porous Replacement–I (APR-I; Intermedics Orthopaedics) implants were designed to address the shortcomings of their predecessors. The implants were engineered to reduce proximal stress shielding and thigh pain through their proximal geometry, limited porous-coated surface, and use of materials with lower moduli of elasticity. Both stems were made of titanium alloy, were noncircumferentially proximally porous coated, and were implanted with line-to-line diaphyseal reaming in combination with proximal broaching. Follow-up analyses showed that the noncircumferential porous coating of the original HGP stem allowed distal polyethylene particle migration, which resulted in distal osteolysis and thigh pain in some patients.

Second-generation proximally porous-coated stems were developed to address the shortcomings noted previously. These implant designs can be classified primarily into two groups. The first design was a double-tapered wedge implanted with broaching alone used for preparation of the femoral canal. The second design required both diaphyseal reaming and metaphyseal broaching. Both designs were engineered to obtain secure fixation in the proximal femur.

Some early ream-and-broach stems were made of titanium alloys and had a circumferential proximal porous coating of either sintered titanium mesh or titanium beads. Circumferential proximal porous coating was implemented to reduce access of joint fluid and polyethylene debris to the distal bone-implant interface. These implant techniques required distal reaming to allow placement of the cylindrical, non–porous-coated distal portion of the stem. As a result of the circumferential proximal ingrowth, these implant designs reduced the risk of distal osteolysis compared with that of first-generation implants. Additionally, a distal non-ingrowth surface reduced proximal stress shielding.

Current double-tapered noncemented femoral stem designs offer improved torsional stability by following the natural taper of the femoral metaphysis. They offer excellent press-fit fixation in patients with wide variation in proximal femoral anatomy. The self-locking taper design accommodates small amounts of subsidence to increase wedge fixation. Many designs require limited or no distal reaming. These stems have more inherent torsional stability and are less susceptible to surgical error than blade-shaped stems.

Contraindications

Relative contraindications to the use of double-tapered stems include damaged and ectatic proximal femurs. In these patients, diaphyseal or cemented fixation is preferred. Additionally, careful consideration should be given to the use of these stems in patients with proximal femoral deformity with substantial anteversion or retroversion. In these patients, a modular implant may be more appropriate. Similarly, the surgeon should proceed with caution or consider alternative stem designs in patients with atypical anatomy and/or poor bone quality. A cemented femoral implant may be preferable in patients with osteopenic femurs with thin cortices.

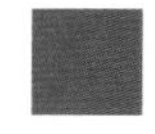

Alternative Treatments

Numerous options are available for the femoral implant, including those that use cemented fixation, extensively coated cylindric stem designs, anatomic stem designs, and modular stems. Certain femoral morphologies may be best managed with an alternative stem design to the double-tapered stem. For instance, even though noncemented fixation can be effective in patients with Dorr type C bone, in some patients, particularly those who have severe osteopenia, cement fixation might be better for such femoral morphology. Additionally, in a patient with a prior subtrochanteric fracture or osteotomy, a stem that uses diaphyseal-like fixation might be advantageous. There also are rare patients in whom, because of an abnormally shaped proximal femur, a double-tapered stem length may preclude fixation and a shorter stem might be the better choice.

Results

Manufacturers have modified implant designs to accommodate minimally invasive and anterior approaches to THA. Despite these trends, double-tapered stems remain popular because of their historical success in patients of all age groups and bone quality types. Results of studies of several implant designs demonstrate excellent midterm and long-term follow-up with highly reliable rates of primary stability, long-term stability, reliable bony ingrowth (**Figure 1**), low rates of thigh pain, acceptable bone remodeling, and low rates of osteolysis (**Table 1**). In the 2013 annual report from the Australian Orthopaedic Association National Joint Replacement Registry, double-tapered noncemented stem designs demonstrated some of the lowest failure rates among all implant designs at 10-year follow-up.

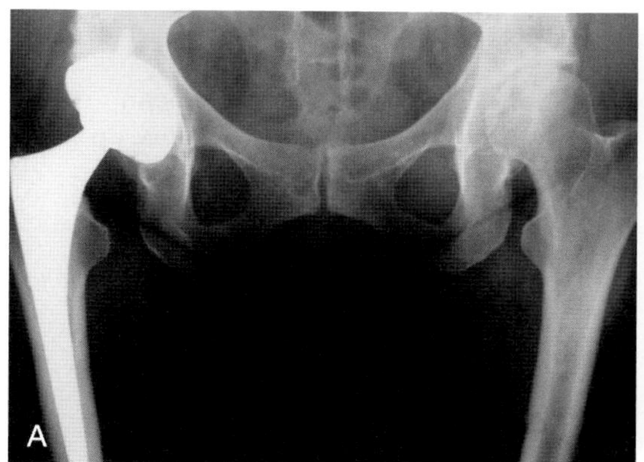

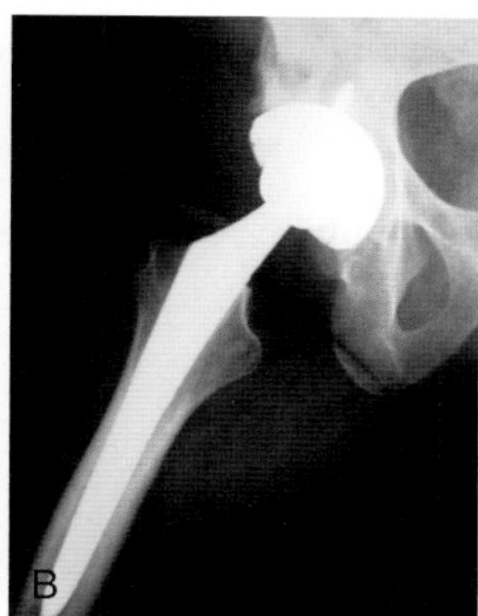

Figure 1 AP pelvic (**A**) and lateral hip (**B**) radiographs demonstrate bony ingrowth 1 year after insertion of a double-tapered stem.

Technique

Setup/Exposure

- Preoperative templating is necessary for estimating implant size; recognizing outliers such as patients with either narrow or capacious femoral canals and patients with prior fractures; identifying characteristics that exclude the use of specific implants; improving the restoration of limb length, offset, and center of rotation; and planning the initial level of resection of the femoral neck (**Figure 2**).
- Tapered stems can be placed via the posterior, anterolateral, or direct anterior approach. The posterior approach is described here.
- An incision of adequate length for the patient's body habitus is placed slightly posterior to the prominence of the greater trochanter. Approximately two-thirds of the incision should be proximal to the greater trochanter.
- A capsule-preserving technique, in which the external rotators are not separated from the capsule, is used. This technique allows repair of the combined tissue at the end of the procedure.
- Adequate exposure can be obtained with the use of three retractors (**Figure 3**). A Mueller-type posterior retractor is used to elevate the femur out of the wound. Two bent Hohmann retractors, one placed medially and the other placed anteriorly and medial to the greater trochanter, are used to provide exposure.

Instruments/Equipment/Implants Required

- Tapered stems can be placed either with a broach-only technique or with the use of reamers and broaches.
- Most surgeons prefer to use reamers because this method allows for proximal lateralization to avoid varus stem alignment and provides guidance on stem size (**Figure 4**).
- Reaming can be done via power or by hand. Most surgeons, including the authors of this chapter, prefer hand reaming. The reamers are used to achieve axial alignment and estimate the appropriate implant size. Reamers are not intended to remove a large amount of bone.
- After reaming is complete, broaching is done with the use of sequential sharp broaches. The broaches initially remove bone and subsequently are used to compact cancellous bone.
- In most modern implant systems, the broach serves as the trial stem for trial reduction (**Figure 5**).

Procedure

- With the femur in the appropriate orientation and the retractors in the appropriate position, the starting point is identified. A box osteotome should be used to ensure a lateral entry point of the stem (**Figure 6**).
- A rasp or a lateralizing reamer may be used to work farther laterally in the greater trochanter to achieve neutral axial alignment (**Figure 7**).
- Handheld or power reamers are progressively used to identify the intramedullary canal. These reamers remove small amounts of cancellous bone but are primarily intended to establish the proper axial alignment of the implant. They are not meant to remove a substantial amount of diaphyseal bone. To allow the broaches to contour the proximal femur, no additional cancellous bone is removed.
- Effective broaching requires a trajectory that will place the tip of the stem in the middle of the medullary canal to prevent flexion or extension of the stem. For example, if the femoral neck is retroverted, the broach path should begin more anteriorly in the femoral neck. In an anteverted femoral neck, the broach should start more posteriorly.

Table 1 Results of Noncemented, Double-Tapered Femoral Stems in Primary Total Hip Arthroplasty

Authors (Year)	Number of Patients (Hips)	Approach	Mean Patient Age in Years (Range)	Mean Follow-up in Years (Range)	Success Rate (%)[a]	Results
Danesh-Clough et al (2007)	193 (210)	Direct lateral	58 (22-85)	6.3 (5-8)	99.5	Mean HHS, 90 All had ingrowth 10% had minor proximal femoral osteolysis 2.8% incidence of thigh pain 3.3% incidence of intraoperative fracture
Incavo et al (2008)	91 (105)	Direct lateral	57 (19-84)	6.7 (5-10.3)	99	Mean HHS, 91 All had ingrowth 3.8% had proximal femoral osteolysis All revisions were unrelated to the femoral implant
Dalury et al (2010)	94 (96)	Posterior	66 (39-92)	5.8 (5-6.3)	100	Mean HHS, 96 All had ingrowth No osteolysis 1% had intraoperative fracture
Goetz et al (2013)	88 (100)	Anterolateral	61.6 (25-92)	5.1 (4-6.6)	100	Mean HHS, 89.5 All but 2 hips had bony ingrowth 1% incidence of thigh pain 2% had severe stress shielding 1% had subsidence
Nishino et al (2013)	41 (50)	Posterior	59 (33-80)	11.2 (10-12.5)	100	Mean Japanese Orthopaedic Association hip score, 91 All had ingrowth 24% had severe stress shielding 56% had proximal osteolysis No patient reported thigh pain
Meding et al (2015)	97 (111)	Posterior	55 (27-72)	22 (20-25)	100	Mean HHS, 87 All had ingrowth 20% had proximal femoral osteolysis 1% had subsidence 1 periprosthetic fracture required revision

HHS = Harris hip score.

[a] Success is defined as implant survival.

- Care is taken to ensure that the soft-tissue envelope does not influence positioning of the broach. Offset broaches may be used to avoid this pitfall. If correct positioning of the broach is in doubt, the length of the incision should be increased.
- The actual orientation of the stem depends on many factors, including the combined anteversion. As a general principle, the surgeon should attempt to attain approximately 45° of combined anteversion, which often requires 15° to 25° of femoral anteversion.
- The orientation of the broach substantially influences hip stability and range of motion (ROM). From the posterior approach, with the assistant holding the knee flexed and the tibia perpendicular to the floor (**Figure 8**), the surgeon can establish the appropriate rotation

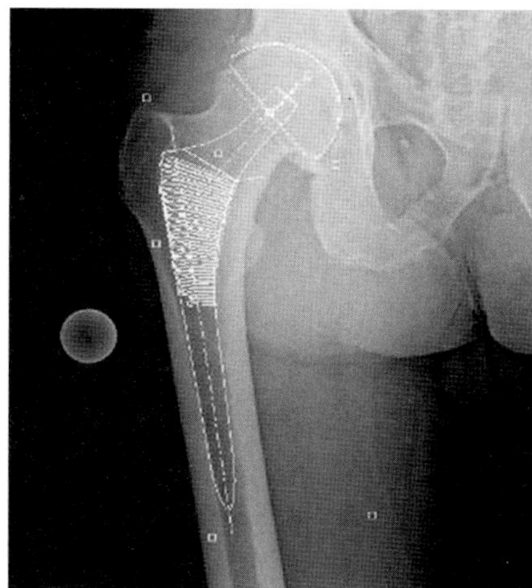

Figure 2 AP radiograph of a right hip demonstrates preoperative templating for total hip arthroplasty with a double-tapered stem.

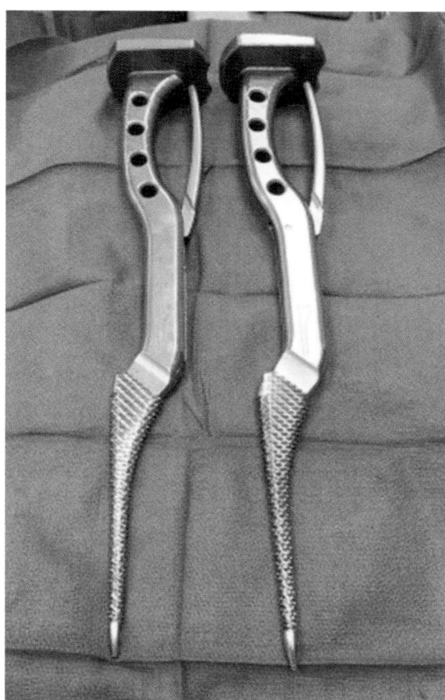

Figure 5 Photograph shows two sequential broaches assembled for use. The sharp edges of these devices remove bone during initial broaching and subsequently aid in impaction of cancellous bone.

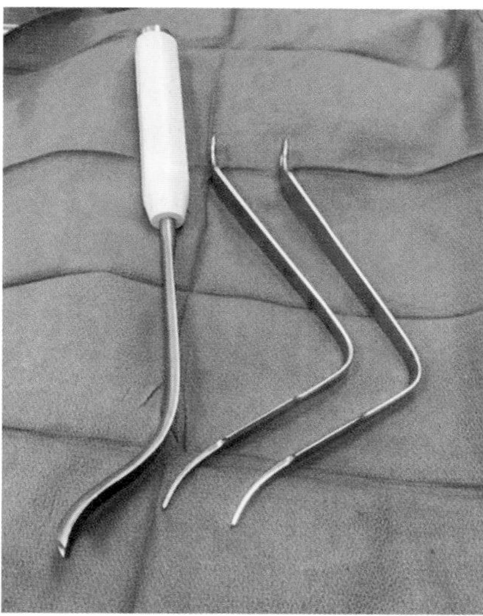

Figure 3 Photograph shows three common retractors used for femoral exposure. The Mueller retractor is on the left. Two bent Hohmann retractors are on the right.

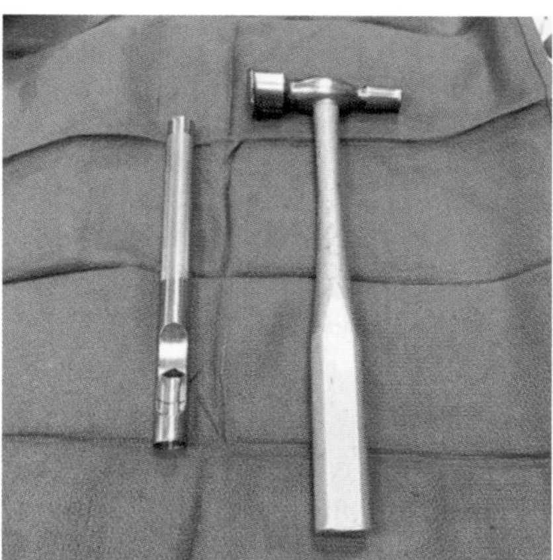

Figure 6 Photograph shows a box osteotome (left) and a mallet (right) used in primary total hip arthroplasty. The osteotome (whether box type or not) is used to both identify the starting point for lateral entry of the femoral stem and remove the remaining lateral femoral neck after the initial cut of the femoral neck. This method helps ensure appropriate lateralization of the femoral implant. A relatively small mallet as shown here is preferred.

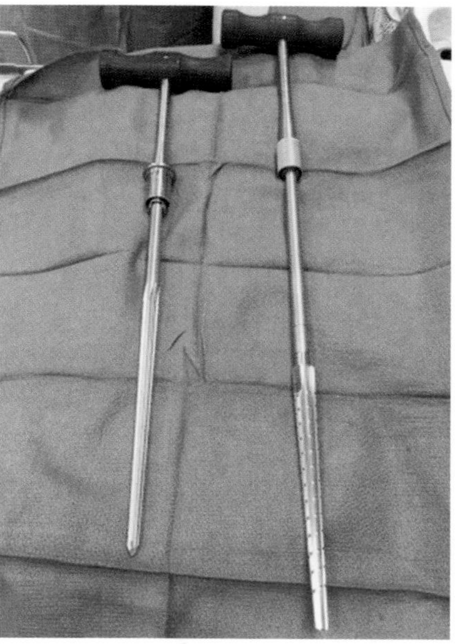

Figure 4 Photograph shows two tapered reamers prepared for hand reaming. Note the attached T-shaped handles. Each reamer corresponds to specific broach and implant sizes. The two laser-etched calibration lines proximal to the cutting surface indicate the appropriate depth for each implant size.

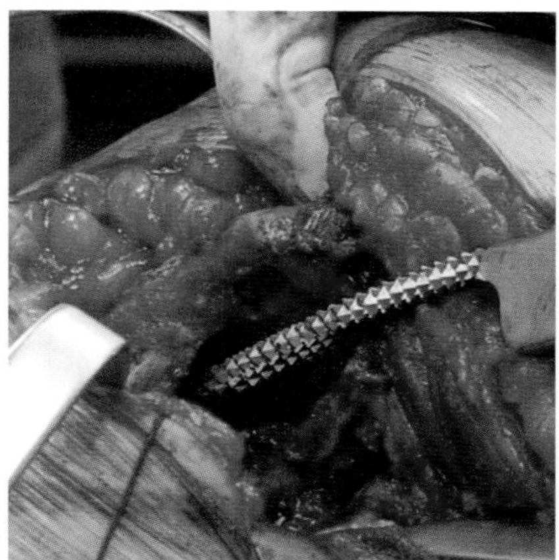

Figure 7 Intraoperative photograph of a left hip shows the use of a rasp to aid in the removal of excess lateral bone.

of the broach (**Figure 9**).

- The broach is seated with the use of a small mallet. The broach should advance with each blow.
- Sequential broaches are used 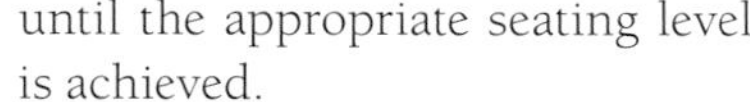 until the appropriate seating level is achieved.
- To decrease the risk of fracture, the surgeon should take care to avoid contact of the medial broach teeth on the medial calcar cortical bone, which can be accomplished by starting the broaching more laterally in the femoral neck.
- A change in the pitch of the sound

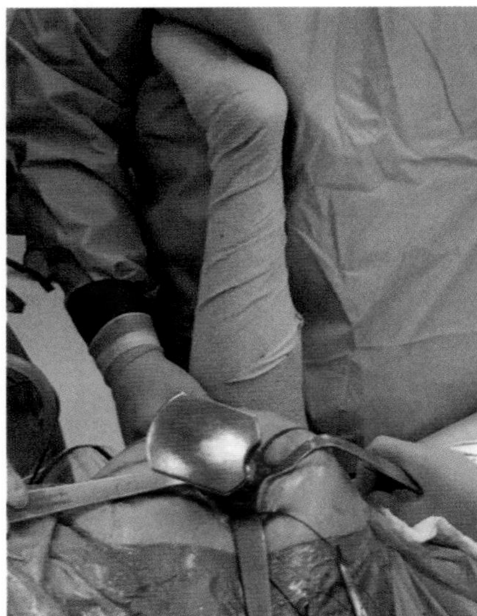

Figure 8 Intraoperative photograph of a right hip shows placement of the knee in flexion with the lower leg perpendicular to the floor, which is an alternative method of estimating the anteversion of the implanted broaches. This technique may be particularly useful in patients in whom the femoral neck is in retroversion. Typically, the goal is to attain 15° to 25° of anteversion.

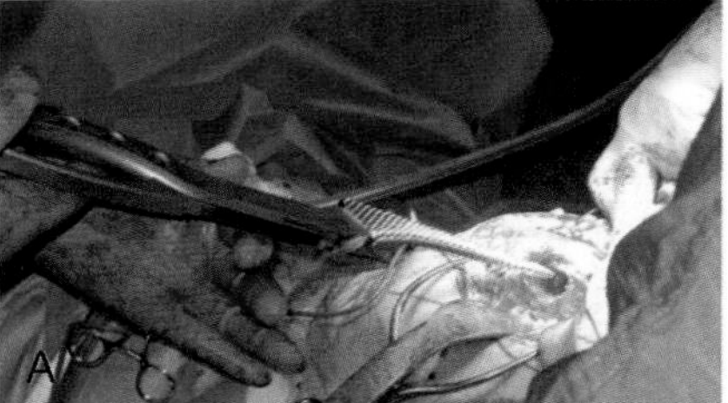

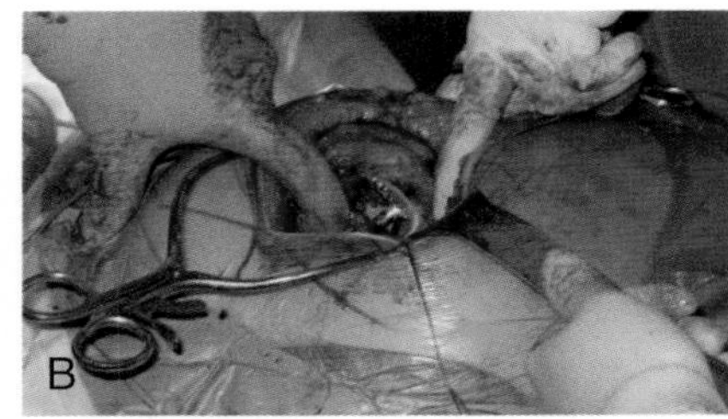

Figure 9 Intraoperative photographs show sequential broaching in a right hip. **A,** Broaching begins with the orientation of each broach in the appropriate version and axis. **B,** The broach is seated.

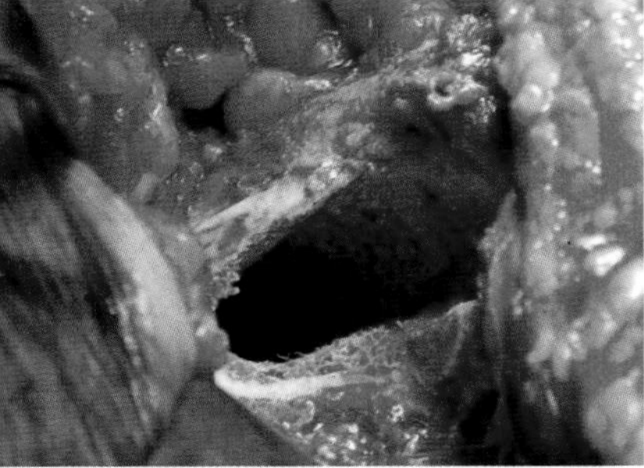

Figure 10 Intraoperative photograph of a left hip shows the femoral canal between steps in the sequential broaching process. In this example, the preparation matches the native version of the proximal femur. The far lateral bone has been removed to ensure the stem follows the appropriate axis.

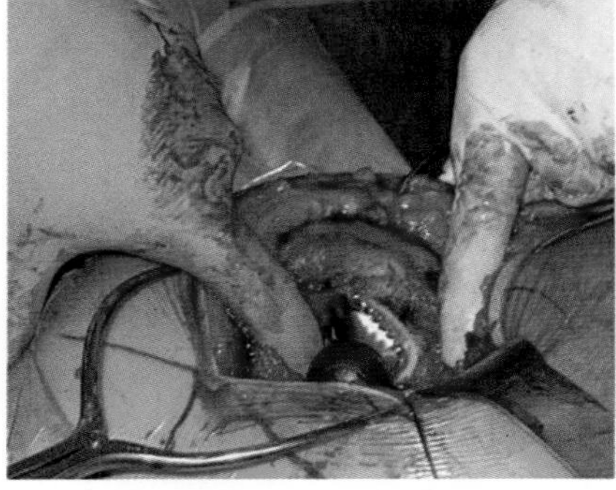

Figure 11 Intraoperative photograph of a right hip shows the use of the final broach to assemble a trial implant. Offset and femoral neck length were individualized to the patient shown here to achieve optimal hip mechanics.

as the broach advances suggests that the hoop stresses are high. Increase in these stresses can result in fracture.

- Completion of broaching may be observed in several ways: the sound changes, as mentioned previously; in the absence of pitch changes, it becomes impossible to sink the broach any farther; or stability (lack of motion of the broach in the surrounding cancellous bone) is observed when the surgeon applies a torsional load (**Figure 10**).
- The depth of seating of the broach will influence the limb length. Reference to the preoperative template or landmarks can help the surgeon ascertain the appropriate depth of seating.
- Most modern stem designs include both standard and high-offset options. The optimal offset is predicted on the basis of preoperative templating. With the broach in place, trial reductions are performed with the use of either the standard or the high-offset option (**Figure 11**).
- After the surgeon is satisfied with the limb length, ROM, stability, and offset (which can be individualized), the broach is removed and the appropriate stem is inserted. Double-tapered stems typically have a porous coating proximally (on the metaphysis) and often have a roughened surface on the diaphysis of the stem. This design allows for bony ingrowth proximally and, in many patients, bony ongrowth distally (**Figure 12**).
- With the broach removed, the canal is irrigated to remove loose bone

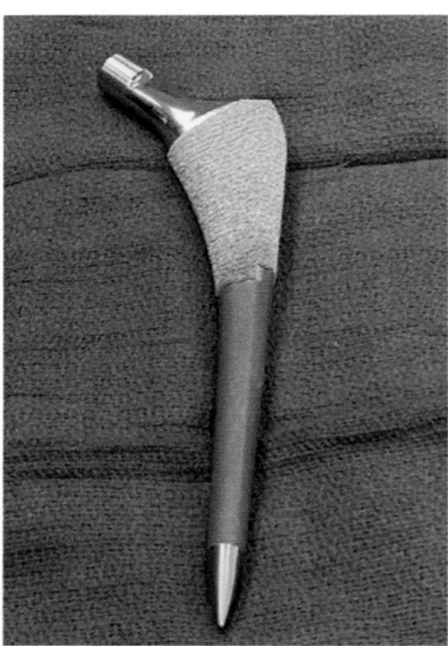

Figure 12 Photograph shows a double-tapered, wedge-shaped implant with a proximal porous coating and a roughened distal surface.

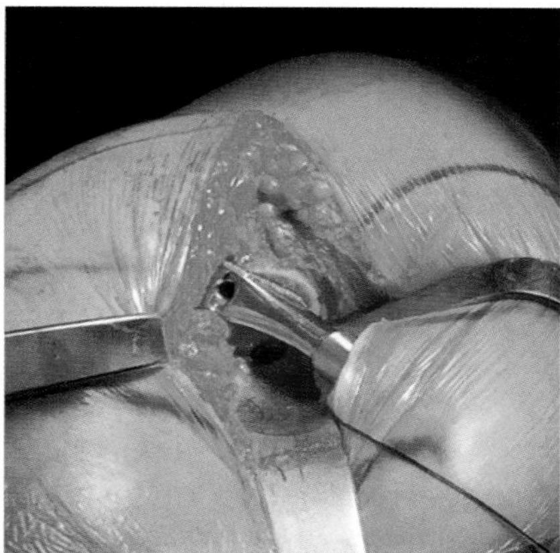

Figure 13 Intraoperative photograph of a right hip shows the final, seated femoral implant.

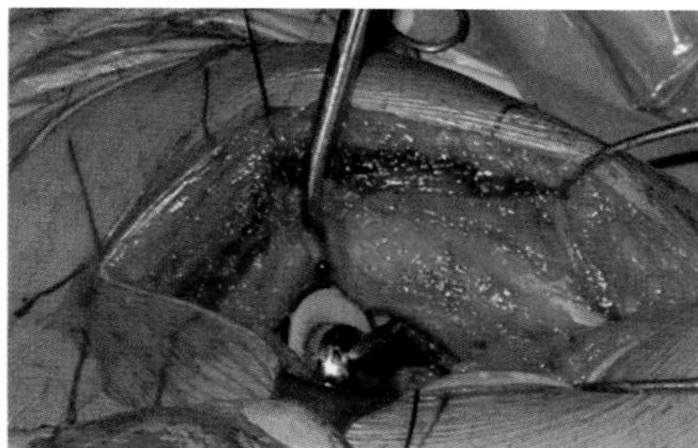

Figure 14 Intraoperative photograph of a right hip shows the final femoral implant. The femoral stem and modular femoral head have been reduced and placed into the position of sleep (20° of flexion and 20° of adduction).

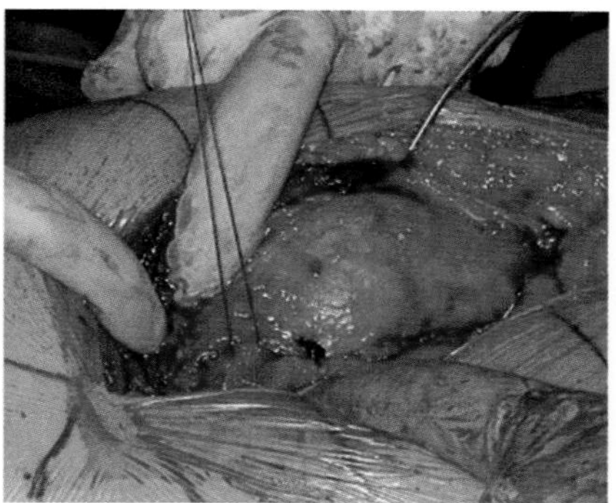

Figure 15 Intraoperative photograph of a right hip shows repair of the posterior capsule and short external rotators to their insertion on the greater trochanter.

fragments that could limit seating of the implant.

- The femur is examined carefully for fracture.
- The stem is inserted initially by hand. Typically, the stem will seat to within approximately one fingerbreadth of the resection level.
- The final seating is done with an insertion device that allows the surgeon to control the orientation of the stem while it is advancing.
- The use of an offset impactor can help provide clearance to the greater trochanter. Care is taken to not wedge the insertion device against the greater trochanter because doing so can result in fracture of the greater trochanter.
- The stem is again impacted with the use of a small mallet with multiple light taps of consistent force. The stem should advance with each tap. Clues suggesting that the implant is fully seated are an increase in the pitch of the sound of impaction and a lack of further advancement of the stem (**Figure 13**).
- Because the porous coating of the final stem is thicker than that of the broach, the final stem will frequently seat more proximally than the broach by 1 to 2 mm. To ensure correct limb length, the broach can be countersunk or a shorter femoral head size used.
- The trunnion taper is cleaned carefully and thoroughly.
- The femoral head is impacted, and the hip is reduced.
- Final ROM is tested, and any impinging bone or soft tissue is removed (**Figure 14**).

Wound Closure

- In the capsule-sparing approach, the capsule and the attached short external rotators are repaired either through drill holes in the greater trochanter or to anchor sutures.
- If the piriformis tendon was taken down, it is repaired if possible (**Figure 15**).
- The fascia, subcutaneous layer, and skin are closed in a standard fashion.

Postoperative Regimen

If the bone quality is adequate and the stem is well seated, a patient is allowed to bear weight as tolerated postoperatively and to progress from the use of a walker to the use of a cane to unassisted ambulation as tolerated. Intraoperative ROM is a good predictor of hip stability and can help the surgeon determine what, if any, activity restrictions are necessary. Most patients can walk unassisted within 4 to 6 weeks postoperatively.

Avoiding Pitfalls and Complications

Thorough preoperative templating is necessary to predict appropriate implant size, implant position, and limb length. In patients with extra-small or extra-large femurs, preoperative planning must include ensuring that appropriate implants are available. Femoral neck-shaft angles vary in patients undergoing THA, and any notable abnormality observed preoperatively must be incorporated into the preoperative plan.

Bone type is an important consideration. In patients with Dorr type A bone, the surgeon may need to ream the diaphysis slightly more aggressively than in other patients to ensure that the planned stem can be seated. Dorr type B bone, the most common type, is the easiest to accommodate. In patients with type C bone, the surgeon may consider using a broach-only technique to improve fixation. Historically, type C bone and osteoporosis were considered relative contraindications to the use of

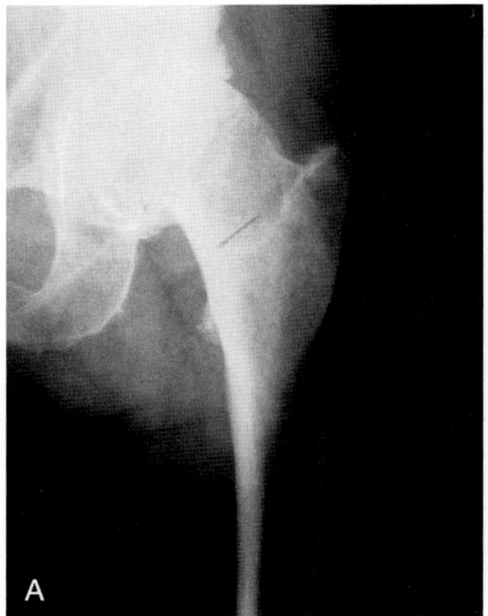

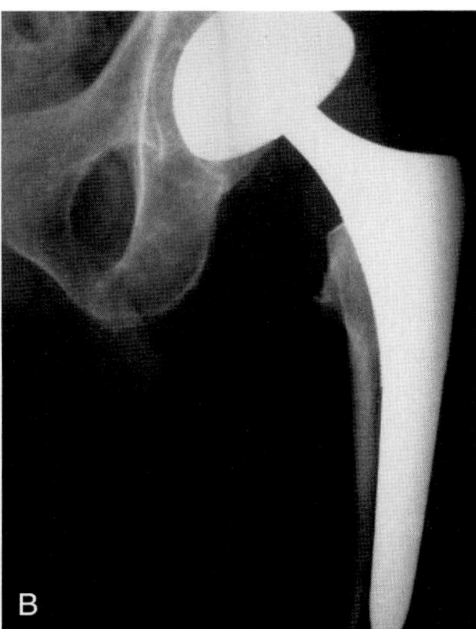

Figure 16 **A,** Preoperative AP radiograph demonstrates a left hip with Dorr type C bone. **B,** AP radiograph obtained 1 year postoperatively demonstrates bony ingrowth into a double-tapered stem in the same patient.

porous-coated stems, but more recent studies have provided good support for noncemented fixation, if carefully performed, in these patients (**Figure 16**).

The use of double-tapered stems presents a particular challenge in patients who have increased femoral neck anteversion as a result of developmental dysplasia of the hip or other causes. Such patients must be identified preoperatively, but these presentations are not strict contraindications for the use of these stems. In many of these patients, the surgeon can establish the appropriate stem orientation with care. However, the surgeon should proceed with caution in these patients because excessive anteversion of the stem may result in placement of a smaller femoral stem than would otherwise be used, and can place the calcar at increased risk of fracture. Some surgeons advocate the use of a prophylactic calcar cerclage cable or wire to prevent recognized and unrecognized fracture propagation.

Intraoperative fractures occur most commonly during femoral preparation, as the surgeon attempts to attain optimal initial stability. Early atraumatic postoperative fractures also can occur as a result of these attempts. Patients with abnormal proximal femoral anatomy and/or poor bone quality are at the highest risk for these injuries. If a fracture remains unidentified, it may continue to propagate and inhibit biologic fixation. Although unidentified fractures may result in early loosening and subsequent failure, implant survivorship in patients with an appropriately managed fracture is similar to that in patients without fracture. In patients with intraoperative fractures of the calcar, the most common and accepted treatment includes removal of the stem and application of cerclage cables or wires both below and around the fracture. The risk of fracture is highest in patients with osteopenia and thinning of the proximal femoral cortex, and in patients with smaller proximal femoral metaphyses.

The risk of intraoperative fracture is increased if the medial aspect of the broach contacts the medial calcar cortical bone before the broach is fully seated. If this contact is observed, the surgeon should ensure that the broach has not been placed with excessive varus, particularly if the broach size is smaller than the templated size. If a calcar crack is observed and the surgeon suspects propagation of the fracture beyond the calcar, an intraoperative AP radiograph should be obtained with the stem removed from the femur. A wire or cable passer can be placed above the lesser trochanter with the lateral aspect of the wire placed distal to the abductor insertion. Care should be taken to avoid passing the wire through or over the psoas tendon sheath, which can cause continued psoas irritation and groin pain. The application of a cerclage cable or wire prevents propagation of the fracture by increasing resistance to hoop stress. Usually, the same stem can then be reinserted with good press-fit stability.

Although extensive literature supports the use of cerclage techniques for the management of identified fractures, little evidence supports the prophylactic use of these techniques. Researchers cite concerns of neurovascular injury, increased surgical time, and increased costs as reasons not to routinely apply cerclage cables or wires.

Bibliography

Archibeck MJ, Berger RA, Jacobs JJ, et al: Second-generation cementless total hip arthroplasty: Eight to eleven-year results. *J Bone Joint Surg Am* 2001;83(11):1666-1673.

Australian Orthopaedic Association National Joint Replacement Registry: *Annual Report.* Adelaide, Australia, Australian Orthopaedic Association, 2013. https://aoanjrr.sahmri.com/documents/10180/127202/Annual%20Report%20 2013?version=1.2&t=1385685288617. Accessed July 20, 2016.

Capello WN, D'Antonio JA, Feinberg JR, Manley MT: Hydroxyapatite-coated total hip femoral components in patients less than fifty years old: Clinical and radiographic results after five to eight years of follow-up. *J Bone Joint Surg Am* 1997;79(7):1023-1029.

Dalury DF, Gonzales RA, Adams MJ: Minimum 5-year results in 96 consecutive hips treated with a tapered titanium stem system. *J Arthroplasty* 2010;25(1):104-107.

Danesh-Clough T, Bourne RB, Rorabeck CH, McCalden R: The mid-term results of a dual offset uncemented stem for total hip arthroplasty. *J Arthroplasty* 2007;22(2):195-203.

Emerson RH Jr, Sanders SB, Head WC, Higgins L: Effect of circumferential plasma-spray porous coating on the rate of femoral osteolysis after total hip arthroplasty. *J Bone Joint Surg Am* 1999;81(9):1291-1298.

Galante J, Rostoker W, Lueck R, Ray RD: Sintered fiber metal composites as a basis for attachment of implants to bone. *J Bone Joint Surg Am* 1971;53(1):101-114.

Goetz DD, Reddy A, Callaghan JJ, Hennessy DW, Bedard NA, Liu SS: Four- to six-year follow-up of primary THA using contemporary titanium tapered stems. *Orthopedics* 2013;36(12):e1521-e1526.

Incavo SJ, Beynnon BD, Coughlin KM: Total hip arthroplasty with the Secur-Fit and Secur-Fit plus femoral stem design: A brief follow-up report at 5 to 10 years. *J Arthroplasty* 2008;23(5):670-676.

Khanuja HS, Vakil JJ, Goddard MS, Mont MA: Cementless femoral fixation in total hip arthroplasty. *J Bone Joint Surg Am* 2011;93(5):500-509.

Kim YH: Titanium and cobalt-chrome cementless femoral stems of identical shape produce equal results. *Clin Orthop Relat Res* 2004;(427):148-156.

Meding JB, Ritter MA, Keating EM, Berend ME: Twenty-year followup of an uncemented stem in primary THA. *Clin Orthop Relat Res* 2015;473(2):543-548.

Nishino T, Mishima H, Kawamura H, Shimizu Y, Miyakawa S, Ochiai N: Follow-up results of 10-12 years after total hip arthroplasty using cementless tapered stem: Frequency of severe stress shielding with Synergy stem in Japanese patients. *J Arthroplasty* 2013;28(10):1736-1740.

Suckel A, Geiger F, Kinzl L, Wulker N, Garbrecht M: Long-term results for the uncemented Zweymuller/Alloclassic hip endoprosthesis: A 15-year minimum follow-up of 320 hip operations. *J Arthroplasty* 2009;24(6):846-853.

Watts CD, Abdel MP, Lewallen DG, Berry DJ, Hanssen AD: Increased risk of periprosthetic femur fractures associated with a unique cementless stem design. *Clin Orthop Relat Res* 2015;473(6):2045-2053.

Xenos JS, Callaghan JJ, Heekin RD, Hopkinson WJ, Savory CG, Moore MS: The porous-coated anatomic total hip prosthesis, inserted without cement: A prospective study with a minimum of ten years of follow-up. *J Bone Joint Surg Am* 1999;81(1):74-82.

Zweymüller KA, Lintner FK, Semlitsch MF: Biologic fixation of a press-fit titanium hip joint endoprosthesis. *Clin Orthop Relat Res* 1988;(235):195-206.

Chapter 13
Parallel-Sided Femoral Stems

Christopher Grayson, MD
R. Michael Meneghini, MD

Indications

Total hip arthroplasty (THA) provides reliable pain relief in patients with end-stage degenerative joint disease of the hip. Options for femoral fixation in THA include cemented and noncemented femoral stems. Noncemented femoral implant designs include cylindric fully porous-coated, double-tapered, parallel-sided tapered, modular, and short femoral stems. Parallel-sided tapered stems (also known as blade-type stems or blade stems) are designed to gain initial press-fit fixation between the medial and lateral cortices of the femoral canal and are characterized by their thin anteroposterior dimension, relative to the much wider mediolateral dimension (**Figure 1**). The femur is prepared in a broach-only manner. Compared with other stem designs, these stems are generally considered bone sparing because they preserve a substantial amount of anterior and posterior femoral metaphyseal bone.

Indications for the use of parallel-sided tapered stems are the same as those for most noncemented primary THA procedures. The procedure is indicated in patients with substantial pain and radiographic evidence of degenerative joint disease in whom an appropriate course of nonsurgical treatment has been unsuccessful and who have adequate femoral bone stock to support the use of noncemented fixation in the proximal femur. The authors of this chapter use blade-type stems in all patients who do not have a substantial proximal femoral deformity that would preclude appropriate positioning of the stem with stable fixation. Because of the shorter length of some implant designs, these stems provide a good option for fixation in patients with malunion of a previous proximal femur fracture and avoid the need for osteotomy or the use of intraosseous hardware in the proximal femoral diaphysis (**Figure 2**).

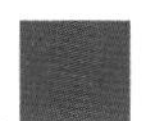

Contraindications

Blade-type stems have some relative contraindications. Some surgeons suggest that wide, capacious Dorr type C femoral anatomy is a relative contraindication to the use of noncemented femoral fixation and that these patients are best treated with cemented femoral fixation. In patients with very narrow Dorr type A femoral bone stock, the surgeon may have difficulty fully seating a broach-only stem if the canal isthmus is narrow as the result of robust thickness of the cortices. In these patients, the surgeon may be unable to obtain adequate press-fit fixation proximally, which will increase the risk of aseptic loosening resulting from the lack of bony integration. However, this anatomic variant may be overcome by opening the femoral isthmus in the metadiaphyseal region with flexible reamers or sharp broaches. Apart from these relative contraindications, adequate fixation can be attained with blade-type stems in most patients provided that the surgeon adheres to the principles that are essential for achieving axial and rotational stability of the implant against viable host bone.

Proximal femoral deformities may be a relative contraindication to the use of blade-type stems. These stems are tapered in the shape of a wedge and achieve fixation by interference fit within the tapered medial and lateral cortices of the proximal femoral metaphysis. Therefore, patients with altered femoral geometry, lack of appropriate contour, or substantial deformity of the proximal femur may not be good candidates for the use of this implant design and may require the use of a femoral stem that bypasses the altered anatomy and achieves stable fixation more distally. Patients with developmental dysplasia of the hip often have excessive femoral

Dr. Meneghini or an immediate family member has received royalties from, serves as a paid consultant to, and has received research or institutional support from Stryker, and serves as a board member, owner, officer, or committee member of The Knee Society. Neither Dr. Grayson nor any immediate family member has received anything of value from or has stock or stock options held in a commercial company or institution related directly or indirectly to the subject of this chapter.

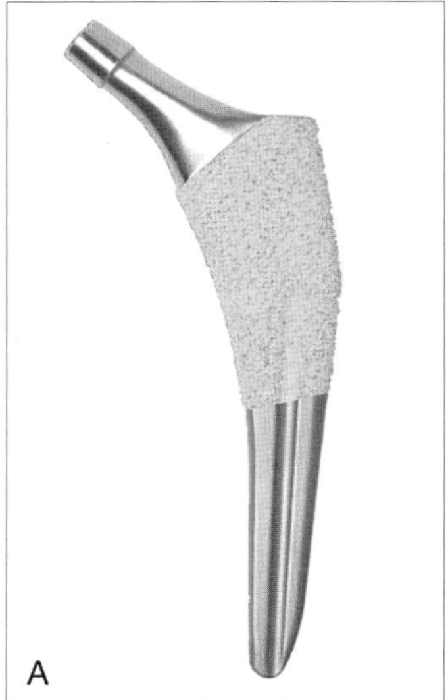

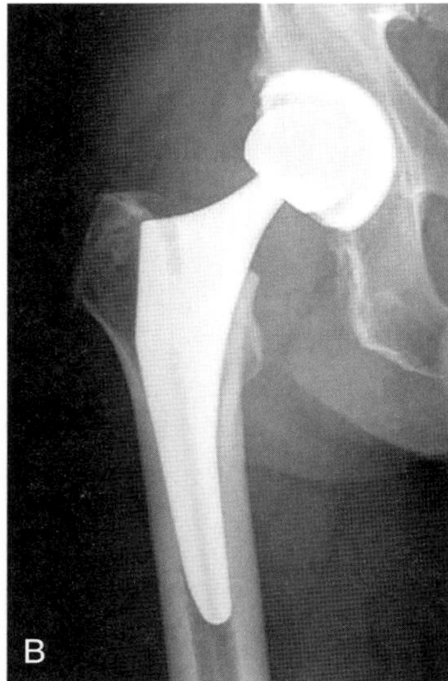

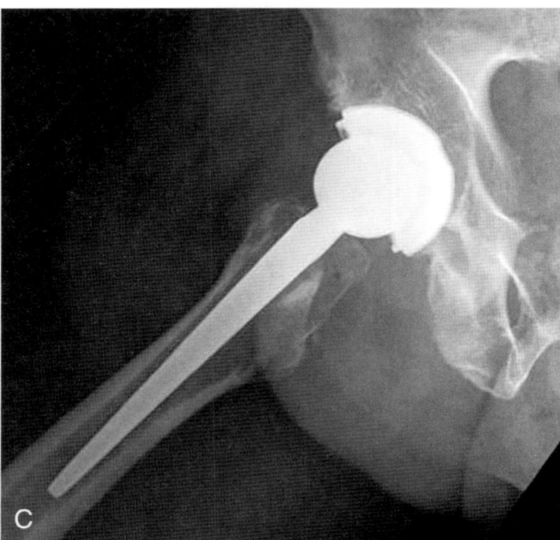

Figure 1 **A,** Photograph of a blade-type stem (Accolade II; Stryker) shows the characteristic roughened proximal surface to promote bony ingrowth and the smooth and tapered distal geometry of this stem type. Postoperative AP (**B**) and frog-lateral (**C**) radiographs of a right hip demonstrate a blade-type stem. **B,** On the AP view, the stem geometrically fills the proximal femoral canal. **C,** Frog-lateral view demonstrates the thin profile characteristic of a blade-type stem.

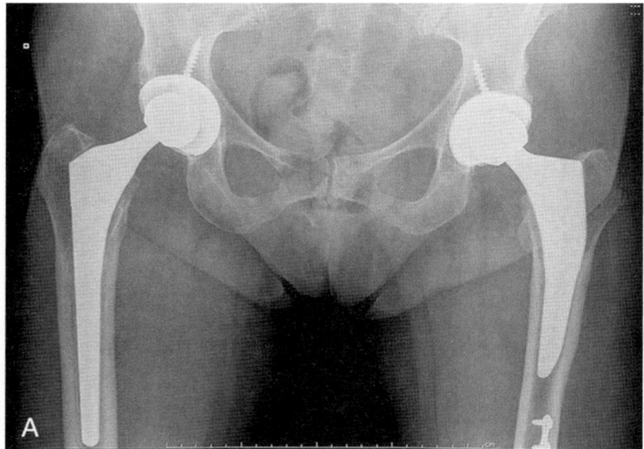

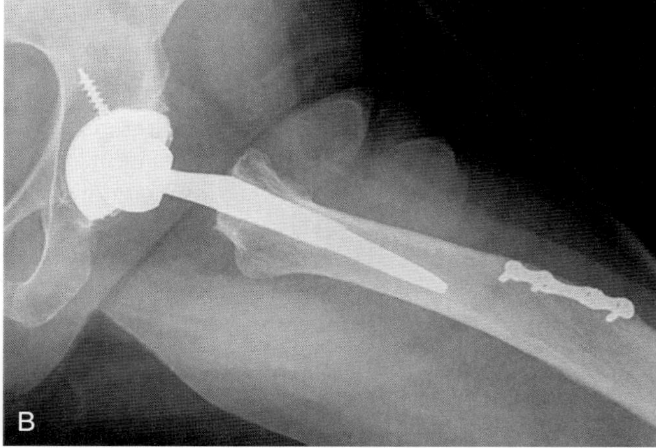

Figure 2 AP (**A**) and frog-lateral (**B**) radiographs demonstrate the use of a short blade-type stem to gain stable proximal fixation in the left hip with preexisting diaphyseal hardware. The AP pelvic radiograph demonstrates the benefit of the shorter stem in comparison with the longer fit-and-fill stem in the contralateral hip.

anteversion that cannot be corrected with a blade-type stem. Uncorrected excessive anteversion would increase the risk of instability. Blade-type stems should not be used in patients who require subtrochanteric osteotomy for high dislocation because of the inability to achieve fixation of the distal osteotomy fragment with a proximally fixed stem. Often, these patients are best treated with cylindric or modular stems that allow the surgeon to obtain distal fixation and independently set the stem anteversion. In patients with proximal femoral fractures that extend into the calcar or peritrochanteric region, a blade-type stem should not be used unless the surgeon can attain a stable reduction with cable fixation and the reduction reproduces the internal proximal femoral geometry sufficiently to allow mechanical stability of the stem.

Alternative Treatments

A variety of alternative noncemented femoral stem geometries is effective in primary THA. Fully porous-coated

Table 1 Results of Total Hip Arthroplasty With Parallel-Sided Femoral Stems

Authors (Year)	Number of Patients	Approach	Mean Patient Age in Years (Range)	Mean Follow-up in Years (Range)	Success Rate (%)[a]	Results
Teloken et al (2002)	42	Not specified	50.4 (25-72)	15 (14.5-16.9)	100	No revision for aseptic loosening of the femur 7 revisions were performed during acetabular revision 2% incidence of thigh pain
Parvizi et al (2004)	121	Direct lateral or Hardinge	60.8 (32-79)	11 (6-15)	100	No radiographic subsidence or loosening 1 femoral revision for osteolysis 3.6% incidence of thigh pain 99.1% survivorship
McLaughlin and Lee (2008)	138	Posterolateral	50 (20-75)	20 (18-22.6)	99	1 femoral revision for aseptic loosening 1 radiographically confirmed loose femur Survival rate of 87% at 22 yr
Casper et al (2011)	200	Anterolateral	68.5 (44-87)	7.6 (5-9)	99.5	1 revision for femoral aseptic loosening 2.6% overall failure rate

[a] Success is defined as the total number of femoral components not revised for aseptic loosening.

cylindric stems are reserved for patients with distorted proximal femoral anatomy, in which distal fixation into the diaphysis is required for successful fixation. Cylindric titanium tapered stems with fins (Wagner-type cone) can be used in patients with one of several anatomic variants, especially those with distorted proximal anatomy or neck anteversion abnormalities, such as in hip dysplasia. Another stem option for abnormal femoral neck version in patients with dysplasia is a modular sleeved stem that allows femoral implant version independent of the native neck through the modular proximal sleeve. Traditional fit-and-fill, or double-tapered, stems are proximal-fitting implants that require intact proximal femoral anatomy to gain appropriate fixation. A unique feature of fit-and-fill stems is a proximal anteroposterior dimension greater than that of blade type, or parallel-sided, stems. This dimensional feature necessitates both an awareness of the anteroposterior anatomy of the femur as seen on a lateral radiograph and an understanding that this dimension may be where the stem obtains its interference fit in some femora (unlike blade stems, which always gain fixation in the mediolateral dimension). Ultimately, the surgeon should be familiar with a variety of noncemented stem options and techniques to treat the variations observed in femoral anatomy among patients undergoing THA.

Results

Blade-type stems have been in use since the 1980s and have demonstrated excellent long-term survival (**Table 1**). In one study of 145 consecutive THAs in 138 patients treated with a blade-type stem, 65 hips in 58 patients were followed for an average of 20 years. The estimated survival rate was 87% at 22-year follow-up, with the end point defined as revision for any reason. Of the 13 revisions performed, only 1 was the result of aseptic loosening of the femur, which occurred in a patient with an unrecognized calcar fracture at the time of the initial procedure. Excellent clinical outcomes were reported, with a mean Harris hip score of 85.4 at latest follow-up.

In a retrospective review of 121 patients (129 hips) who underwent THA with a noncemented blade-type stem, only one femoral revision was reported, which was the result of proximal femoral osteolysis. No evidence of radiographic subsidence or loosening was found at mean 11-year follow-up. Similar results were demonstrated in a study of 42 patients (49 hips) with a mean 15-year follow-up after THA with a blade-type stem. No femoral revisions for aseptic loosening were reported. Two femoral implants had radiographic evidence of instability, and one was revised during revision for aseptic loosening of the acetabulum. Notably, no signs of loosening developed in any stem that was initially thought to have good bony ingrowth. Five stems had initial subsidence of greater than 3 mm, but three of those stems showed evidence of bony ingrowth at 2 years.

These studies demonstrate excellent clinical results with a blade-type stem and low rates of aseptic loosening at long-term follow-up. Some of these studies include femoral implants with nonmodular femoral head designs, which may limit the applicability to current designs. A more recent study with midterm follow-up of a modular stem design also showed a low revision rate for aseptic loosening and excellent overall survival of the femoral implants. In addition, a blade-type stem design may have clinical benefits related to outcomes. In two of the studies described previously, low rates of thigh pain were reported, with incidence of 3.6% and 2%. This incidence of thigh pain is substantially better than has been reported in studies using fully porous cylindric stems, in which the rate of thigh pain was as high as 16% to 27%. Blade-type stems also have a low incidence of subsidence. At the institution of the authors of this chapter, blade-type stems were found to have a lower mean subsidence compared with a standard fit-and-fill stem. The axial stability exemplified by the lack of subsidence is likely the result of the substantial metaphyseal fill and stability provided by the interference fit of the wedge-shaped stem into the proximal femoral geometry. Some surgeons have proposed that a more rapid and enhanced taper of the distal stem width is essential to optimize the proximal interference fit, particularly in patients with a narrow femoral isthmus.

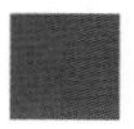

Technique

Setup/Exposure

- Blade-type stems can be implanted through any approach.
- The authors of this chapter prefer to use a posterolateral approach with the patient placed in the lateral decubitus position.
- Blade-type stems are also ideal for the direct anterior approach because of their shorter length and lateral proximal shoulder relief, which facilitate insertion in approaches with limited femoral visualization.
- Regardless of the approach used, the proximal femoral exposure should be as robust as feasible while minimizing soft-tissue trauma.
- Adequate exposure is attained, and the hip is dislocated posteriorly.
- The authors of this chapter use the lesser trochanter and the junction of the lateral femoral neck and greater trochanter as landmarks for the femoral neck osteotomy, the level of which is determined on the basis of preoperative templating to restore the hip biomechanics and ideal leg length.

Instruments/Equipment/ Implants Required

- The standard instrument sets provided by the manufacturer are the minimum required instruments for implantation of these stems.
- A box osteotome or similar device is helpful to remove cortical bone from the lateral femoral neck.
- A tapered canal finder is necessary to identify the optimal path of the broach during initial femoral preparation.
- In addition to the femoral broaches provided by the implant manufacturer, flexible reamers sometimes are required to open the distal diameter in patients with a narrow femoral isthmus to accommodate the distal implant width.

Procedure

FEMORAL PREPARATION

- Femoral preparation can be performed either before or after acetabular preparation.
- The authors of this chapter prefer to perform femoral preparation after successful placement of the acetabular implant and insertion of a trial acetabular liner.
- The proximal femur is exposed and elevated laterally with adequate retractors.
- Residual piriformis tendon and capsule are removed from the medial base of the greater trochanter to adequately expose the entire lateral femoral neck.
- A box osteotome is used to open the entry point in the posterolateral portion of the cut femoral neck. Care is taken to set appropriate anteversion with this step. Because most proximally coated femoral stems achieve an interference fit by maximizing the mediolateral dimension, the degree of anteversion closely approximates that of the native femoral neck. However, the surgeon may slightly increase the anteversion by biasing the entry point to a relatively posterior position on the lateral femoral neck.
- A canal finder is used to open the canal and demonstrate the appropriate path for broaching.
- Femoral broaches are inserted sequentially in increasing sizes. Care is taken to ensure that the first broach is inserted with the anteversion that is determined by the position of the posterolateral shoulder of the implant and the maximum medial neck dimension.
- Care is taken to hold the broaches with the appropriate anteversion and to insert and remove the broaches in a varus position to avoid fracture of the greater trochanter.
- With each sequential broach, care is taken to follow the same collinear path to prevent removal of bone in the anteroposterior direction, which can destabilize the final implant.

- After each broach has cleared the greater trochanter, lateral pressure is gently applied to prevent the broach from being seated in a varus position and to ensure clearing of the lateral femoral metaphyseal bone. Applying this gentle valgus force helps the surgeon avoid the tendency to undersize the stem, which can increase the risk of subsidence.
- While sequentially increasing the broach size, the surgeon must be attentive to the audible and tactile feedback. Maximal cortical contact is signaled by noticeable and discernible changes in the sound and feel of the broach. After this point is reached, the broach is worked in a repetitive in-and-out fashion to clear the teeth of the broach and allow the hoop stress of the femoral cortical bone to relax.
- The authors of this chapter have found that taking the time to ensure that the maximal mediolateral dimension is attained with the broach will maximize the axial and rotational stability of the implant and minimize the risk of postoperative subsidence. When the optimal size broach is reached, the stem should have no movement in the axial direction with repetitive impactions and should have minimal motion when a rotational torque is applied on the insertion handle.
- In patients with Dorr type A bone, the broaches may begin to get caught distally before appropriate proximal fit is achieved. In this scenario, flexible reamers are used to open the distal canal.
- Optimal broach size is characterized by axial and rotational stability of the implant, which is achieved by maximally filling the mediolateral dimension of the proximal femur at the level of the femoral neck cut to create proper biomechanics and leg length. However, in some patients, femoral geometry determines that the maximal mediolateral dimensional fill of the implant occur somewhat distal to the neck cut, most commonly just below or at the level of the lesser trochanter.
- After the final broach is seated, a calcar reamer is used if necessary, and attention is focused on trialing.
- The trial femoral head and neck are placed, and the trial implant is reduced.
- Leg lengths and stability are checked through the full range of motion. With the leg in full extension and external rotation, the femoral neck should be close to impingement on the posterior rim of the acetabulum. This position of the femoral neck indicates that the maximum combined anteversion has been attained.
- If intraprosthetic impingement occurs with maximal external rotation and hip extension, the acetabular implant may need repositioning.
- Stability is assessed with the hip in full flexion and with the hip in 90° of flexion with internal rotation.
- If instability is noted, care is taken to determine whether internal (intraprosthetic) or external (extra-articular) impingement occurs as the source of instability. The authors of this chapter have found that additional excision of anterior capsule or anterior osteophytes is often necessary to minimize extraprosthetic impingement and improve stability by allowing greater impingement-free range of motion with the hip in flexion, adduction, and internal rotation.

PROSTHESIS IMPLANTATION

- After adequate stability is attained with the trial implants, the broach and neck trial are removed.
- The femoral canal is cleared of debris with pulsatile lavage.
- Any obstructing soft tissue that may interfere with seating of the femoral implant is removed from the medial greater trochanter.
- The femoral prosthesis is inserted by hand into the path that was created by the broaches.
- A mallet is used to impact the stem into place. Care is taken to maintain consistent force with each impact of the mallet because the use of greater force as the implant nears its final position can result in calcar fracture.
- When the stem no longer advances on impact, it is considered to have reached the final position with maximal implant stability.
- The trunnion taper is thoroughly cleaned with pulsatile lavage and a dry laparotomy pad.
- The femoral head is impacted carefully on the trunnion.
- A bone hook is used to assist in reduction of the femur, taking care not to damage the femoral head during insertion.
- Stability is checked again.

Wound Closure

- Wound closure is performed in standard manner depending on the surgical approach used.
- If a posterior approach was used, meticulous repair of the short external rotators and posterior capsule is performed through drill holes in the posterior trochanter.
- The fascia lata, dermal layer, and skin are closed in a standard manner.

Postoperative Regimen

Postoperatively, patients are allowed to bear weight as tolerated and are encouraged to increase their physical activity as their symptoms allow. Postoperative radiographs are obtained in the recovery room for documentation of implant position and at the 4-week postoperative follow-up examination.

Avoiding Pitfalls and Complications

Because blade-type stems rely on initial proximal fixation to promote bony ingrowth, complications such as intraoperative fracture, aseptic loosening, and femoral implant subsidence are associated with this stem design and with other proximally porous-coated designs. The risk of these complications can be minimized with careful preoperative planning and meticulous surgical technique.

Some studies have reported that patients with Dorr type A bone are at risk of failure to achieve bony integration of the proximally coated femoral prosthesis. This finding is thought to be the result of the stem becoming fixed distally in the narrow femoral canal without achieving appropriate press-fit fixation proximally. Blade-type stems likely have a greater risk of this complication than other stem types because they are broach-only systems and their placement does not involve routine reaming of the femoral diaphysis. Some stem designs that have a greater distal stem width relative to the proximal stem width may have a greater risk of aseptic loosening and subsidence than other designs. For patients with Dorr type A bone, the authors of this chapter recommend having flexible reamers available for use in case they are needed to open the canal distally to achieve good proximal fill and fixation. However, when careful and aggressive broaching is performed, reaming often is not necessary.

Close attention must be paid to the calcar region during the process of broaching and during impaction of the final implant. Because of the need for tight proximal press-fit fixation of these stems, the risk of intraoperative fracture may be as high as 2%. A broach or implant that suddenly seats more deeply in the femur than during the previous mallet strike often indicates a fracture. If a fracture is identified, care must be taken to remove the broach or stem and identify the distal extent of the fracture. These fractures are most often incomplete, minimally displaced fractures isolated to the calcar region. A cable is passed around the proximal femur, and the stem is reintroduced into the canal.

Blade-type stems are also at risk of femoral subsidence because of their tapered, collarless design. In most patients, subsidence is minimal and the stem achieves bony ingrowth in a stable position. However, if subsidence is substantial, the stem may not achieve osseointegration or the hip may become unstable. To prevent subsidence, it is imperative to avoid or greatly minimize micromotion of the final broach during femoral preparation. The final broach should be tested with torque applied as described previously in this chapter. An appropriately sized stem that is fully seated in the femoral canal should have no motion. If care is taken to avoid motion when the final broach is seated, the patient is likely to have little or no subsidence of the stem.

Bibliography

Casper DS, Kim GK, Restrepo C, Parvizi J, Rothman RH: Primary total hip arthroplasty with an uncemented femoral component: Five- to nine-year results. *J Arthroplasty* 2011;26(6):838-841.

Cooper HJ, Jacob AP, Rodriguez JA: Distal fixation of proximally coated tapered stems may predispose to a failure of osteointegration. *J Arthroplasty* 2011;26(6 suppl):78-83.

Issa K, Pivec R, Wuestemann T, Tatevossian T, Nevelos J, Mont MA: Radiographic fit and fill analysis of a new second-generation proximally coated cementless stem compared to its predicate design. *J Arthroplasty* 2014;29(1):192-198.

Lettich T, Tierney MG, Parvizi J, Sharkey PF, Rothman RH: Primary total hip arthroplasty with an uncemented femoral component: Two- to seven-year results. *J Arthroplasty* 2007;22(7 suppl 3):43-46.

McLaughlin JR, Lee KR: Total hip arthroplasty with an uncemented tapered femoral component. *J Bone Joint Surg Am* 2008;90(6):1290-1296.

McLaughlin JR, Lee KR: Uncemented total hip arthroplasty using a tapered femoral component in obese patients: An 18-27 year follow-up study. *J Arthroplasty* 2014;29(7):1365-1368.

McLaughlin JR, Lee KR: Uncemented total hip arthroplasty with a tapered femoral component: A 22- to 26-year follow-up study. *Orthopedics* 2010;33(9):639.

Parvizi J, Keisu KS, Hozack WJ, Sharkey PF, Rothman RH: Primary total hip arthroplasty with an uncemented femoral component: A long-term study of the Taperloc stem. *J Arthroplasty* 2004;19(2):151-156.

Teloken MA, Bissett G, Hozack WJ, Sharkey PF, Rothman RH: Ten to fifteen-year follow-up after total hip arthroplasty with a tapered cobalt-chromium femoral component (Tri-lock) inserted without cement. *J Bone Joint Surg Am* 2002;84(12):2140-2144.

White CA, Carsen S, Rasuli K, Feibel RJ, Kim PR, Beaulé PE: High incidence of migration with poor initial fixation of the Accolade stem. *Clin Orthop Relat Res* 2012;470(2):410-417.

Chapter 14
Primary Total Hip Arthroplasty: Modular Stems

William P. Barrett, MD

Indications

Total hip arthroplasty (THA) implants with modular femoral head and neck designs were introduced in the early 1980s. A modular design offers several advantages, including the ability to adjust limb length and offset after the femoral implant is in place, use of a variety of head and stem materials, decreased stem inventory, simplified exposure in patients who require isolated acetabular revision, and the ability to adjust the femoral head size and femoral neck length to address instability. The disadvantages of modular implants include fretting and corrosion wear, generation of third-body wear debris, mechanical failure of the junction, dissociation of the femoral head, and decreased range of motion associated with use of skirted femoral heads. Fretting and corrosion wear depend on several factors, including load, number of loading cycles, contact stress distribution, and surface finish.

Several implant systems have modular stem-sleeve combinations. In these systems, a porous-coated metaphyseal sleeve is placed in the proximal femoral bone to maximize fit and fill. The cylindrical stem is placed through the proximal sleeve, and distal flutes on the stem engage the diaphyseal bone. The stem and sleeve are joined in a Morse taper junction, in which a truncated cone fits into a similarly shaped socket. The progressive wedge shape of the Morse taper results in mechanical interlock. Stability of the construct depends on bony ingrowth into the proximal porous sleeve, diaphyseal engagement of the stem flutes, and the stability of the Morse taper junction. The cylindrical stem is undersized proximally, allowing it to be inserted into the sleeve with any amount of version. Any sleeve can accommodate different stem lengths, offsets, and calcar lengths (**Figure 1**).

This chapter focuses on the S-ROM (DePuy Synthes) modular implant system because it is the most widely studied stem-sleeve implant for primary THA. The S-ROM system was introduced in the mid 1980s, and several midterm and long-term studies of this system are available. The principles discussed in this chapter apply to any modular stem-sleeve system, although specific techniques may need to be modified according to the recommendations of the manufacturer.

Modularity at the stem-sleeve junction can be particularly useful in patients in whom the femoral anatomy makes primary THA difficult. In these patients, modularity provides intraoperative flexibility because the hip biomechanics can be considered separately from implant position and fixation. Several reports document the usefulness and durability of these systems in performing challenging primary THA procedures. However, these systems carry the risk of modular failure, which can lead to malrotation, implant fracture, and corrosion or fretting with the potential for adverse reaction in the bone and soft tissue.

Modular noncemented stems can be used in any situation in which a noncemented stem is indicated. Often, selection is based on surgeon preference and experience. Typically, young, active patients with type A and B bone are good candidates for a noncemented stem. Modular stems allow the

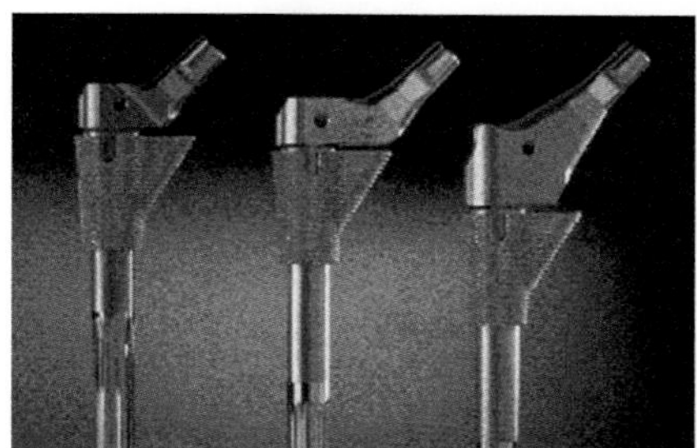

Figure 1 Photograph shows proximal modular implants. The fluted stem attaches to the metaphyseal sleeve via a Morse taper. Multiple sizes of sleeves are available for use with any stem. (Reproduced from Barrett WP: Primary total hip arthroplasty: Modular stems, in Lieberman JR, Berry DJ, eds: *Advanced Reconstruction: Hip.* Rosemont, IL, American Academy of Orthopaedic Surgeons, 2005, pp 85-90.)

Dr. Barrett or an immediate family member has received royalties from, is a member of a speakers' bureau or has made paid presentations on behalf of, serves as a paid consultant to, and has received research or institutional support from DePuy Synthes.

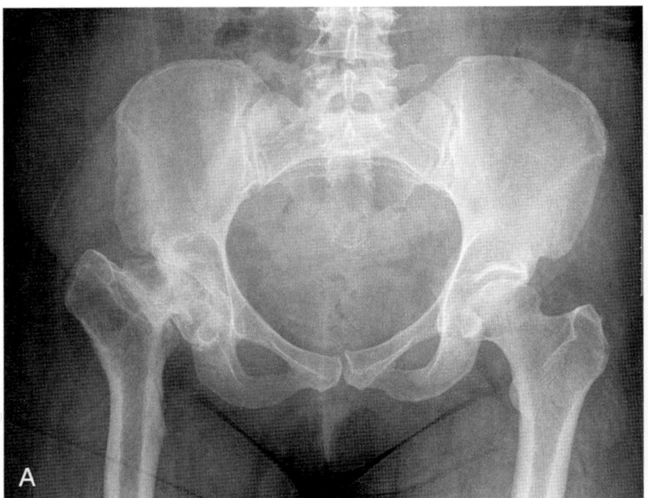

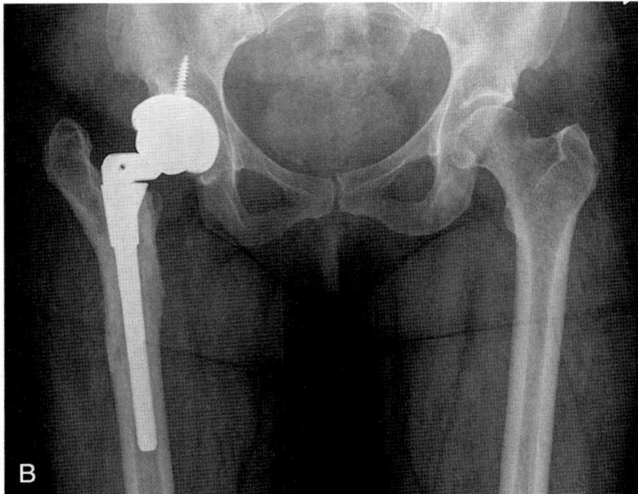

Figure 2 **A,** AP pelvic radiograph of a 46-year-old woman with developmental dysplasia of the hip demonstrates end-stage osteoarthritis of the right hip. **B,** AP pelvic radiograph of the same patient obtained 2 years postoperatively demonstrates noncemented arthroplasty of the right hip with the use of a modular stem.

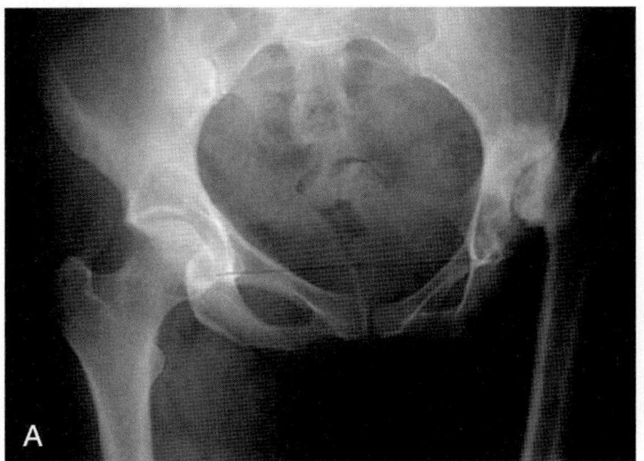

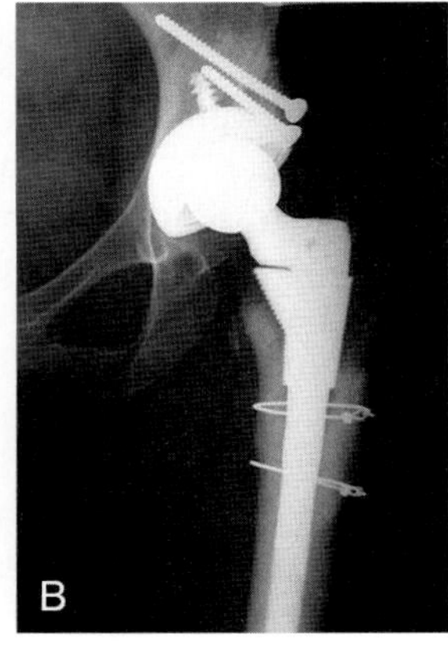

Figure 3 **A,** AP pelvic radiograph of a 42-year-old woman with developmental dysplasia of the left hip demonstrates symptomatic osteoarthritis. **B,** AP radiograph of the same patient obtained 5 years postoperatively demonstrates noncemented total hip arthroplasty with the use of a modular stem and a subtrochanteric shortening osteotomy. The proximal portion of the osteotomy demonstrates ingrowth into the metaphyseal sleeve. The distal portion is stabilized by the eight flutes on the modular stem. (Reproduced from Barrett WP: Primary total hip arthroplasty: Modular stems, in Lieberman JR, Berry DJ, eds: *Advanced Reconstruction: Hip.* Rosemont, IL, American Academy of Orthopaedic Surgeons, 2005, pp 85-90.)

surgeon to select the appropriate version to compensate for variation in the patient's anatomy, such as in patients with a history of a proximal femoral fracture or femoral osteotomy. A modular stem is indicated in patients with developmental dysplasia of the hip (DDH), juvenile rheumatoid arthritis, previous trauma surgery, or metabolic bone disease.

In patients with DDH, who typically have excessive anteversion of the femoral neck, altered anatomy of the femoral head and neck, and a proximal location of the femoral head, a modular implant is particularly helpful. The modular stem allows placement of the proximal metaphyseal sleeve in the best available bone. The stem can be placed in the diaphysis regardless of the metaphyseal anatomy, allowing correction of excessive anteversion (**Figure 2**). If a standard stem is implanted in the femur of a patient with DDH who has increased femoral anteversion, the result may be excessive anteversion of the femoral implant, which can lead to anterior instability. A modular stem allows placement of the stem in relative retroversion to compensate for the native femoral anteversion.

In patients with congenital hip dislocation, in whom anatomic placement of the acetabular implant is desired, a subtrochanteric shortening osteotomy can be performed to avoid excess stretch on soft-tissue and neurovascular structures (**Figure 3**). In these patients, the fluted distal stem allows independent fixation of the distal fragment of the osteotomy, and the proximal metaphyseal sleeve allows fixation to the portion above the osteotomy. Stability is provided by the modular junction, which has adequate strength to resist torsional load before the osteotomy heals.

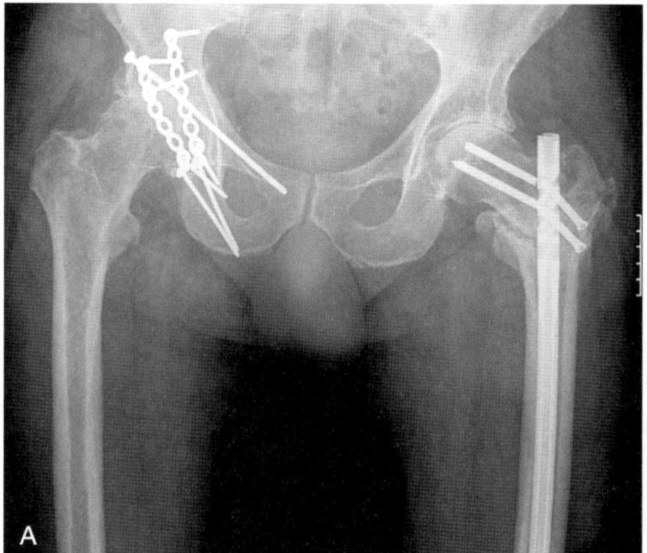

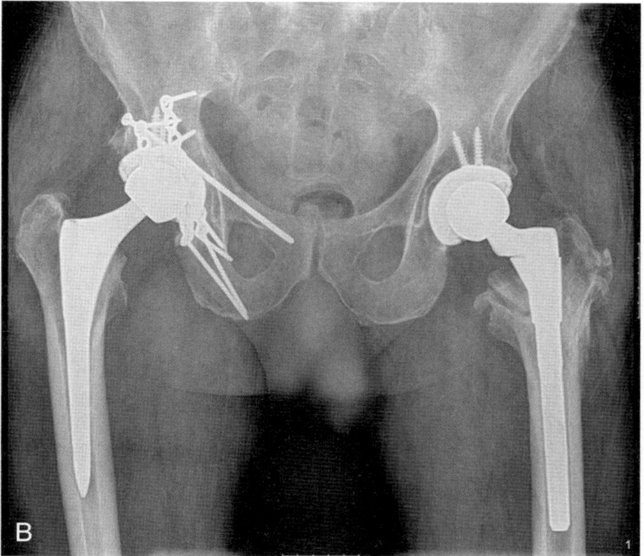

Figure 4 **A,** AP pelvic radiograph of a 52-year-old man who sustained polytrauma demonstrates a subtrochanteric nonunion of the left hip and posttraumatic osteoarthritis of the right hip after open reduction and internal fixation of a right acetabular fracture. **B,** AP pelvic radiograph of the same patient 1 year postoperatively demonstrates management of the nonunion of the left hip with hardware removal, bone grafting, and conversion to total hip arthroplasty with the use of a modular stem, which resulted in stable fixation of the stem and resolution of the nonunion.

In patients with juvenile rheumatoid arthritis, the proximal and distal femoral anatomy and overall bone quality are affected. A proximal modular system allows independent sizing of the distal and proximal femur, as well as correction of excess anteversion. In patients who have had previous trauma or surgery, the anatomy of the proximal femur often is distorted. The use of a modular implant allows the surgeon to bypass defects created by the presence of previously implanted hardware and address malrotation (**Figure 4**). The availability of varied stem lengths allows bypass of the lowest screw hole by at least two canal diameters. Proximal and distal fixation allows correction of angular or rotational malalignment with a corrective osteotomy. In patients with metabolic bone disease, bowing of the femur often precludes use of a monoblock stem. In these patients, the use of a modular stem facilitates corrective osteotomy, realignment, and rotational correction of the femur.

Contraindications

Contraindications to the use of modular noncemented stems are similar to those of any other noncemented stems in THA. A patulous femur that prevents the surgeon from obtaining either proximal or distal fixation precludes the use of a noncemented implant. When a modular stem is fixed both proximally and distally, the reported load to failure is similar to that of cemented stems inserted with third-generation cementing techniques. However, when the stem is fixed only proximally or only distally, the load to failure is only one-half of that obtained with both proximal and distal fixation.

Alternative Treatments

In most patients with excellent bone stock and typical endosteal anatomy, the monoblock stems currently available will achieve rigid fixation, which prevents micromotion and allows contact of the roughened femoral surface with endosteal bone. In these patients, the advantages of a modular system are not required, and the use of a monoblock stem reduces the risk of fretting, corrosion, and third-body wear that can lead to adverse local tissue reaction and osteolysis.

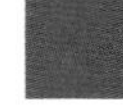

Results

Results of THA with the S-ROM prosthesis are summarized in **Table 1**. A 2001 study reported a 100% rate of ingrowth of metaphyseal sleeves and a 42% rate of proximal osteolysis at midterm follow-up. A 2008 study reported on the use of the S-ROM stem in anatomically difficult THAs; nine hips required a shortening femoral osteotomy. Long-term survivorship of the S-ROM stem was reported in 2011 (mean, 17 years). A 2013 study reported on the use of 9-mm-diameter S-ROM stems in 30 hips with very small femoral canals.

Table 1 Results of Primary Total Hip Arthroplasty With Modular Femoral Stems

Authors (Year)	Number of Hips	Procedure or Approach	Mean Patient Age in Years (Range)	Mean Follow-up in Years (Range)	Results
Tanzer et al (2001)	59	Posterolateral	56 (17-76)	8.5 (6-12.9)	Mean HHS, 88[a] 100% bone ingrowth 42% proximal osteolysis
Biant et al (2008)	55	NS	52.6 (23-81)	≥5[b]	Mean HHS was 83 at 5-yr follow-up and 85 at 10-yr follow-up 100% bone ingrowth 18% proximal osteolysis
Le et al (2011)	31	Posterolateral	52 (18-70)	17 (15-20)	Mean HHS, 83 100% bone ingrowth No femoral revisions 58% proximal osteolysis
Drexler et al (2013)	30	NS	42 (17-69)	19 (12-23)	Mean HHS, 83[a] 93% femoral survivorship 37% proximal osteolysis

HHS = Harris hip score, NA = not applicable, NS = not stated.
[a] Good to excellent results.
[b] 28 hips were followed for a mean of 10 years.

Techniques

Setup/Exposure

- A standard posterolateral, lateral, or anterior approach can be used, depending on surgeon preference.
- Care must be taken to protect the abductor muscles to avoid damage of reamers into the greater trochanter during lateralization.

Instruments/Equipment/Implants Required

- The S-ROM prosthesis is used in the procedure described here.
- If other implants are used, the specific techniques may need to be modified according to the recommendations of the manufacturer.

Procedure

FEMORAL PREPARATION

- A trial implant or a final implant with a trial liner is placed in the acetabulum.
- The femoral osteotomy for the S-ROM stem is made transverse to the longitudinal axis of the femur (**Figure 5**). A saw is used to make a definitive cut based on preoperative templating or a provisional cut that will be revised after the bone is prepared.
- The femur is prepared in a three-step reaming process that begins distally, continues proximally after the diaphysis is sized, and ends in the calcar area.
- Patients with type A bone often have a very narrow diaphyseal canal. In these patients, the diaphyseal canal is initially reamed with flexible reamers to avoid the step-off that can result from the use of a straight, rigid reamer.
- A bulb-tipped guide rod is inserted, and flexible reamers are used up to the minor diameter of the stem (the stem diameter minus the width of the flutes).
- Straight, rigid reamers (1 mm smaller than the final flexible reamer) are used to prepare the diaphysis to the minor diameter of the stem or 0.5 mm wider than the minor diameter of the stem, depending on bone quality. Care is taken to remain lateral as the reaming begins and avoid varus placement of the stem as the reaming progresses distally (**Figure 6**).
- Use of a bent Hohmann retractor over the tip of the greater trochanter protects the abductors and the gluteus medius during reaming.
- Reaming is progressed distally until the reference line on the reamer reaches the tip of the greater trochanter.
- Proximal reaming of the metaphysis is performed with cone reamers that are 5 mm larger than the distal stem size selected. The smallest cone reamer for a given size is attached to a pilot shaft that is the same size as the selected distal stem, and reaming is initiated (**Figure 7, A**).

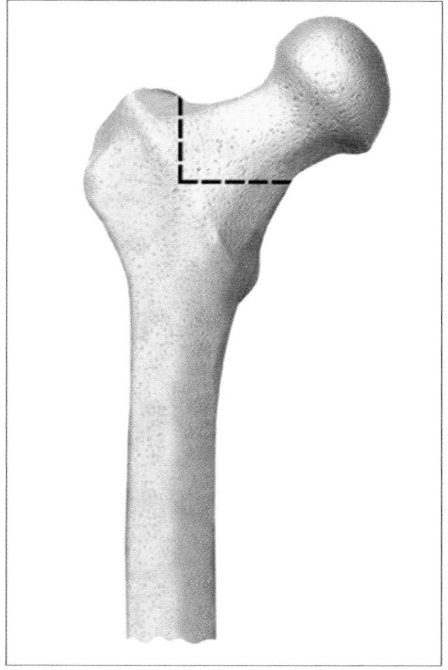

Figure 5 Illustration depicts the femoral neck osteotomy for a modular stem. The osteotomy (dashed lines) is made transverse to the longitudinal axis of the femur. (Reproduced from Barrett WP: Primary total hip arthroplasty: Modular stems, in Lieberman JR, Berry DJ, eds: *Advanced Reconstruction: Hip*. Rosemont, IL, American Academy of Orthopaedic Surgeons, 2005, pp 85-90.)

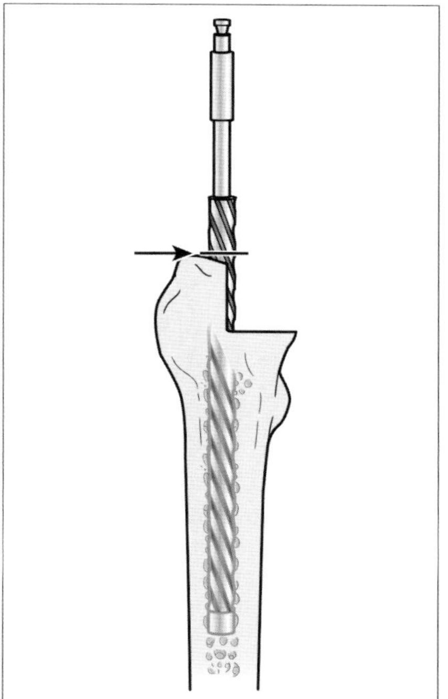

Figure 6 Illustration depicts distal reaming of the femoral diaphysis with a rigid reamer. Note the lateral starting point and avoidance of varus positioning. The arrow depicts the marking on the reamer indicating appropriate stem and neck length.

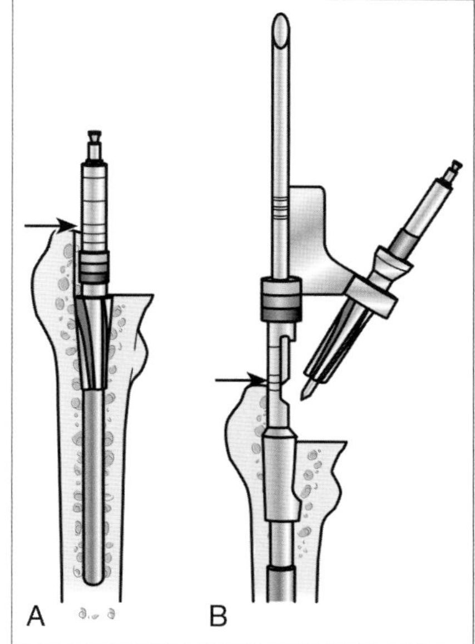

Figure 7 **A,** Illustration depicts proximal reaming of the femoral metaphysis with cone reamers. **B,** Illustration depicts the use of a milling reamer to prepare the calcar for the spout of the metaphyseal sleeve. The arrows indicate depth of reaming for desired neck length.

- Lateralization of the cone reamer into the medial side of the greater trochanter is important to avoid varus placement of the stem. This step requires retraction of the abductors with a rake or a bent Hohmann retractor.
- Progressively larger cone reamers are used until cortical contact is achieved. Anteriorly, cortical contact first occurs in the subtrochanteric region. Proximally, the cone reamer is advanced to a depth at which the reference line indicating the desired femoral neck length is level with the tip of the greater trochanter.
- The triangular portion of the proximal sleeve is prepared with the appropriate milling reamer until cortical contact is attained in the medial proximal femur. Because placement of the proximal sleeve does not determine stem anteversion, the triangular portion can be placed anywhere in the proximal femur to achieve fixation in the highest quality bone (**Figure 7, B**).

IMPLANTATION OF THE PROSTHESIS

- A trial proximal sleeve is placed on the sleeve introducer.
- The triangular portion of the sleeve is rotated to the appropriate position, and the sleeve is impacted into the metaphysis. Care is taken to avoid overzealous impaction because excessive impaction can cause the sleeve to act as a wedge, splitting the proximal femur.
- A trial stem with appropriate femoral neck length and offset is inserted with the desired anteversion (**Figure 8**).
- Trial reduction is performed.
- Stability is checked with the hip in flexion and internal rotation and in extension and external rotation. If stability is not adequate, the cup placement or stem version is adjusted (**Figure 9**).
- After adequate stability is achieved, the final implants are placed.
- The proximal sleeve is seated.
- The Morse taper junction is cleaned and dried to optimize the taper lock.
- The final stem is placed in the appropriate version and driven into the sleeve until the Morse taper is engaged. Appropriate engagement is confirmed audibly by a change in the pitch of impaction and visually by a gap of 1 to 3 mm between the sleeve and neck of the prosthesis.
- Because the stem has sharp flutes that engage the endosteal bone

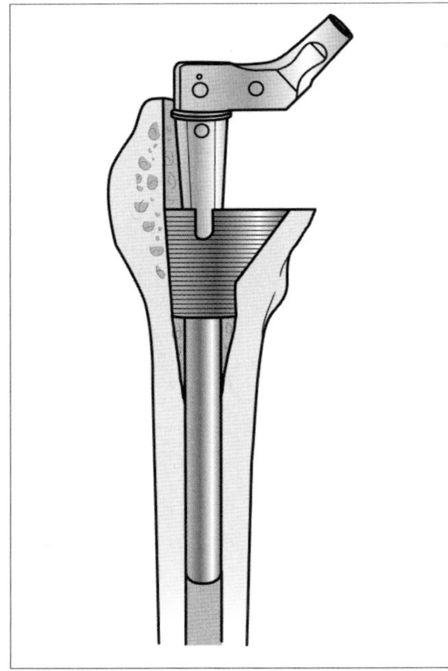

Figure 8 Illustration depicts insertion of a trial femoral stem into a trial metaphyseal sleeve. Stem version is independent of sleeve placement.

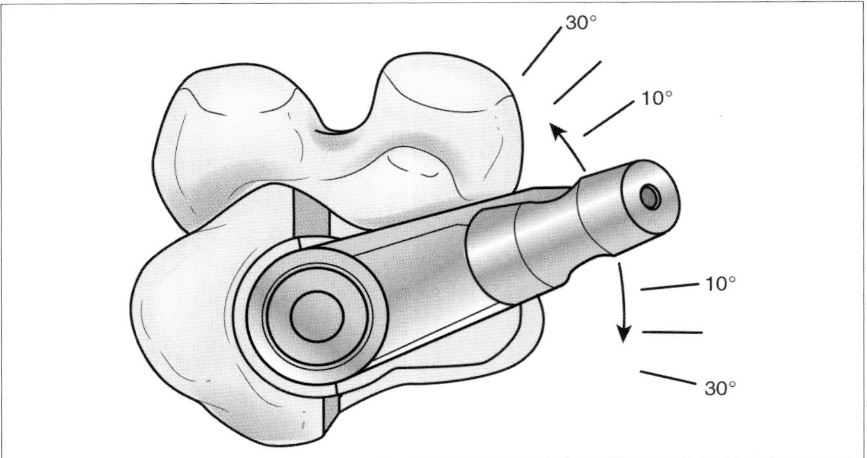

Figure 9 Illustration depicts adjustment of the femoral stem version. With trial implants in place, stem version can be adjusted to enhance stability or correct excess anteversion. The position of the trial implants is recorded and used to ensure proper orientation of the final implants.

early, version cannot be changed after the flutes have engaged the bone.

- The appropriate neck length and head size are chosen to restore limb length and offset.
- The femoral head and neck are placed in standard fashion, taking care to ensure that the modular junction is clean and appropriate impaction force is used.

Wound Closure

- If a posterior approach was used, the posterior capsule and short external rotators are reattached to the posterior trochanter or tendon of the gluteus medius with No. 5 nonabsorbable sutures.
- The quadratus femoris muscle is loosely tacked down to its stump with No. 1 bioabsorbable suture.
- The fascia lata is closed with No. 1 bioabsorbable suture.
- The subcutaneous tissue is closed with 2-0 bioabsorbable suture.
- The skin is closed with staples or subcuticular sutures.

Postoperative Regimen

Physical therapy is initiated the day of the procedure with the patient standing at the bedside and walking if tolerated. A home strengthening exercise program is prescribed before the patient leaves the hospital. If good fixation is obtained intraoperatively and no corrective osteotomy is required, then weight bearing as tolerated with a walker or crutches is allowed. When balance and strength allow, the patient may advance to using a cane as tolerated, typically at 2 to 3 weeks postoperatively. The patient uses a cane until abductor strength is adequate to walk without a substantial limp. If a corrective osteotomy is performed or if fixation is compromised because of bony deficiencies, protected weight bearing for at least 6 weeks postoperatively will be necessary. The duration of protected weight bearing is based on surgeon discretion. Hip precautions depend on the surgical approach used.

Avoiding Pitfalls and Complications

Varus placement of the stem is the most common technical error with the use of a modular stem system. Varus stem position can lead to undersizing of the stem and compromise fixation. This problem can be avoided by ensuring a lateral starting point for the reaming process and maintaining lateralization during distal and proximal reaming. If the stem position is in question, an intraoperative radiograph can be obtained with the trial implants in place. Overly aggressive reaming of the proximal bone with cone reamers can thin the anterior cortical bone, increasing the risk of fracture. Because of the triangular shape of the sleeve, forceful seating can cause the proximal sleeve to act as a wedge, splitting the proximal femur. Malrotation of the stem within the modular sleeve during seating can affect the stability of the hip construct. This problem can be avoided by assessing the proper stem version to achieve maximum stability of the hip construct with trial implants and replicating that amount of version when the final stem is impacted. Failure to engage the Morse taper of the sleeve can occur with inadequate over-reaming (that is, failure to over-ream the minor diameter of the stem by 0.5 mm) of the distal bone in type A femurs or when early three-point fixation of a long, bowed stem occurs, causing the stem to become stuck before fully seating. Failure to completely engage the Morse taper will severely affect rotational stability of the modular system. A small number of case reports have described failure of the stem-sleeve junction, leading to hip instability and/or pain.

Bibliography

Biant LC, Bruce WJ, Assini JB, Walker PM, Walsh WR: The anatomically difficult primary total hip replacement: Medium- to long-term results using a cementless modular stem. *J Bone Joint Surg Br* 2008;90(4):430-435.

Biant LC, Bruce WJ, Assini JB, Walker PM, Walsh WR: Primary total hip arthroplasty in severe developmental dysplasia of the hip: Ten-year results using a cementless modular stem. *J Arthroplasty* 2009;24(1):27-32.

Christie MJ, DeBoer DK, Trick LW, et al: Primary total hip arthroplasty with use of the modular S-ROM prosthesis: Four to seven-year clinical and radiographic results. *J Bone Joint Surg Am* 1999;81(12):1707-1716.

Drexler M, Dwyer T, Marmor M, et al: Nineteen year results of THA using modular 9 mm S-ROM femoral component in patients with small femoral canals. *J Arthroplasty* 2013;28(9):1667-1670.

Fabi DW, Goldstein WM, Gordon AC: Dislocation of an S-ROM total hip arthroplasty secondary to traumatic femoral stem dissociation from the metaphyseal sleeve. *J Arthroplasty* 2009;24(1):159.e19-159.e24.

Fraitzl CR, Moya LE, Castellani L, Wright TM, Buly RL: Corrosion at the stem-sleeve interface of a modular titanium alloy femoral component as a reason for impaired disengagement. *J Arthroplasty* 2011;26(1):113-119, 119.e1.

Imbuldeniya AM, Walter WK, Zicat BA, Walter WL: The S-ROM hydroxyapatite proximally-coated modular femoral stem in revision hip replacement: Results of 397 hips at a minimum ten-year follow-up. *Bone Joint J* 2014;96-B(6):730-736.

Kindsfater KA, Politi JR, Dennis DA, Sychterz Terefenko CJ: The incidence of femoral component version change in primary THA using the S-ROM femoral component. *Orthopedics* 2011;34(4):260.

Le D, Smith K, Tanzer D, Tanzer M: Modular femoral sleeve and stem implant provides long-term total hip survivorship. *Clin Orthop Relat Res* 2011;469(2):508-513.

Lim SJ, Moon YW, Eun SS, Park YS: Total hip arthroplasty using the S-ROM modular stem after joint-preserving procedures for osteonecrosis of the femoral head. *J Arthroplasty* 2008;23(4):495-501.

Patel A, Bliss J, Calfee RP, Froehlich J, Limbird R: Modular femoral stem-sleeve junction failure after primary total hip arthroplasty. *J Arthroplasty* 2009;24(7):1143.e1-1143.e5.

Pearce S, Jenabzadeh AR, Walter WL, Gillies RM: Spontaneous fracture of diaphyseal stem of S-ROM femoral prosthesis. *BMJ Case Rep* 2014.

Sporer SM, Obar RJ, Bernini PM: Primary total hip arthroplasty using a modular proximally coated prosthesis in patients older than 70: Two to eight year results. *J Arthroplasty* 2004;19(2):197-203.

Tamegai H, Otani T, Fujii H, Kawaguchi Y, Hayama T, Marumo K: A modified S-ROM stem in primary total hip arthroplasty for developmental dysplasia of the hip. *J Arthroplasty* 2013;28(10):1741-1745.

Tanzer M, Chan S, Brooks CE, Bobyn JD: Primary cementless total hip arthroplasty using a modular femoral component: A minimum 6-year follow-up. *J Arthroplasty* 2001;16(8 suppl 1):64-70.

Zhao ZS, Sun JY: Total hip arthroplasty using S-ROM prosthesis in elder patients with type C and B bone. *J Orthop* 2013;10(2):65-69.

Chapter 15
Primary Total Hip Arthroplasty With Short Stems

Adolph V. Lombardi, Jr, MD, FACS

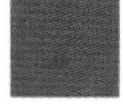

Indications

Total hip arthroplasty (THA) is a highly cost-effective and successful procedure. Most patients experience excellent clinical outcomes and long-term implant survivorship with well-designed prostheses. Although standard femoral stems have demonstrated successful results, innovations in femoral stem design have resulted from improved understanding of the biomechanics of native and artificial hips, advances in implant technology, and the increasing popularity of less invasive, tissue-sparing surgical techniques. Furthermore, the standard tapered stem design has several unresolved issues. Reasons to consider the use of short tapered stems in THA include conservation of existing bone stock, physiologic loading of the proximal femur, potential reduction of stress shielding, and the ability to address proximal-distal mismatch and other anatomic deformities.

Bone-conserving short stems can be categorized into four design styles (excluding resurfacing implants). Mayo-type stems are those influenced by the Mayo Conservative Hip (Zimmer) implant introduced in the early 1980s. This stem has a trapezoidal coronal shape that allows it to achieve multiple-point contact within the proximal femoral cavity while resisting varus-valgus stress by engaging the lateral femoral cortex. With the exception of the Mayo stem, which has long been marketed in the United States, short stems have been more widely used in Europe than in the United States until recently. Short curved femoral neck–sparing prostheses, such as the C.F.P. (Waldemar Link) collum femoris-preserving prosthesis, were developed for use in young (age 60 years or younger), active patients. The femoral neck–sparing design attains triplanar stability with an intact cortical cylindrical femoral neck that blocks varus-valgus and rotational movements. Another type of short stem is the short, bulky, non–femoral neck–sparing prosthesis, such as the Proxima (DePuy Synthes) prosthesis. This type of prosthesis engages the femur at the lateral trochanteric flare and transmits weight-bearing loads through the lateral femoral column. Short tapered stems, such as the Taperloc Microplasty and Taperloc Complete (Zimmer Biomet), use the proximal loading theory of tapered design to transmit loads to the proximal femur.

In the past decade, the author of this chapter has primarily used the Taperloc Microplasty stem, a collarless, mediolaterally tapered, wedge-shaped stem that allows self-seating for rotational stability. It is made of a titanium alloy (Ti-6Al-4V) with circumferential porous plasma-sprayed proximal coating. It uses broach-only femoral preparation, so no additional reaming is required after the femoral canal is opened. Femoral preparation is accomplished without the use of reamers by means of straightforward broaching of the canal. Stems are available in diameters ranging from 5 to 24 mm, with lengths ranging from 95 to 132 mm. Enhancements to this stem design in the Taperloc Complete stem, introduced in 2011, include reducing the caput-collum-diaphyseal femoral neck-shaft angle from 138° to 133° for improved offset, optimized neck taper and polished neck flats to increase range of motion, and reduced distal geometry to improve proximal canal fill and the gradual off-loading that is the goal of tapered geometry. Both generations of this stem design offer a high-offset option by means of a 7.8-mm medial shift of the taper trunnion.

Contraindications

As with standard-length tapered stems, short tapered stems can be extremely difficult to use in patients who have

Dr. Lombardi or an immediate family member has received royalties from Innomed, OrthoSensor, and Zimmer Biomet; serves as a paid consultant to OrthoSensor, Pacira Pharmaceuticals, and Zimmer Biomet; has received research or institutional support from Kinamed, Pacira Pharmaceuticals, and Zimmer Biomet; and serves as a board member, owner, officer, or committee member of The Hip Society, The Knee Society, Mount Carmel Education Center at New Albany, and Operation Walk USA.

Table 2 Results of Select Short Stem Designs in Total Hip Arthroplasty

Authors (Year)	Number of Patients (Hips)	Approach and Implant	Mean Patient Age in Years (Range)	Mean Follow-up in Years (Range)	Success Rate (%)[a]	Results
Gilbert et al (2009)	42 (49)	Anterolateral; Mayo Conservative Hip (Zimmer)	57.8 (44-77)	3.1 (2-5)	89.8	2 intraoperative fractures occurred 5 femoral stems in 4 patients required revision 18% of stems had ≥5° malalignment
Lombardi et al (2009)	591 (640)	Minimally invasive direct lateral or direct anterior; Taperloc Microplasty (Zimmer)	62.7 (27-91)	0.6 (0-3)	99.1	1 same-day stem revision because of perforation of the posterior femoral cortex 5 early stem revisions because of periprosthetic femoral fracture
Kendoff et al (2013)	149 (149)	Posterior; C.F.P. (Waldemar Link)	63.8 (33-83)	11.2 (9-15)	94.6	3 stems required revision (2 for aseptic loosening, 1 for infection) 5 additional stems were revised (indications for revision not specified) Mean HHS, 93
Kim et al (2013)	200 (226)	Posterolateral; Proxima (DePuy)	61.4 (31-91)	7.6 (6-9)	99.9	Younger patient group (mean age, 43.9 yr) had 1 intraoperative fracture and no stem revisions; mean HHS, 95 Older patient group (mean age, 78.9 yr) had 1 intraoperative fracture, and 1 stem revised for traumatic fracture at 5 days; mean HHS, 91
Hutt et al (2014)	69 (75)	Posterior; C.F.P.	52 (13-69)	9.3 (7-11)	100	1 periprosthetic lateral femoral wall fracture, which was managed nonsurgically No stems were revised Mean HHS, 91
Martins et al (2014)	44 (52)	Anterolateral; Mayo Conservative Hip (Zimmer)	48.5 (23-66)	6.1 (5-7.5)	92.3	1 deep infection, 1 sciatic nerve palsy, 2 incomplete metaphyseal fractures, and 4 stem failures resulting from aseptic loosening required revision Mean HHS, 94.5
Barreca et al (2015)	67 (74)	Anterolateral (82%), anterior (12%), or posterolateral (5%); Proxima	61 (31-82)	4 (3-8)	100	No revisions were performed 4 stems valgus, 4 stems varus 2 hips had infraction of greater trochanter 1 hip had subsidence and was stabilized 1 malpositioned stem that extended out of the posterior cortex was asymptomatic

HHS = Harris hip score.

[a] Success is defined as hips that were not revised owing to stem failure for any reason.

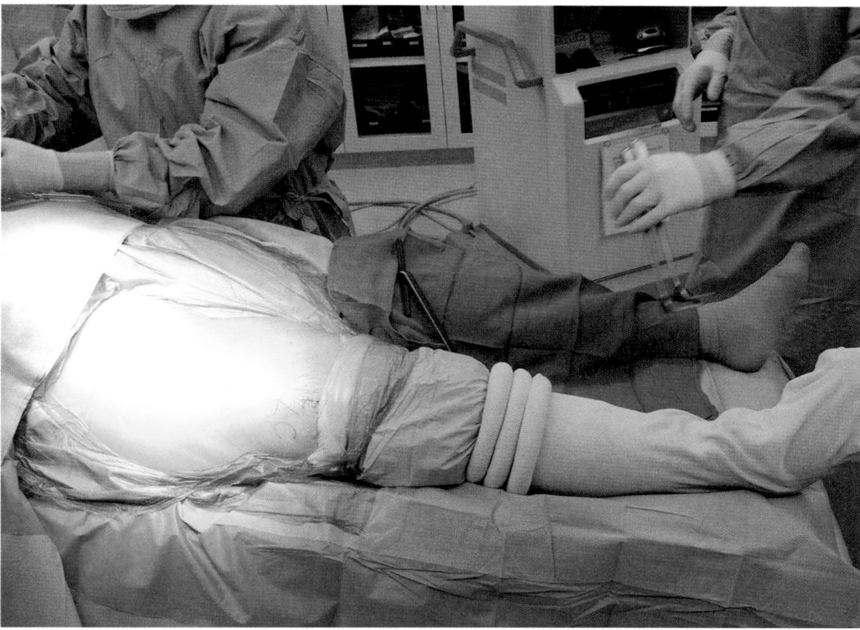

Figure 2 Intraoperative photograph shows patient positioning for the anterior supine intermuscular approach to the hip. The patient is supine on a standard radiolucent surgical table with the ischial tuberosities aligned at the break of the table.

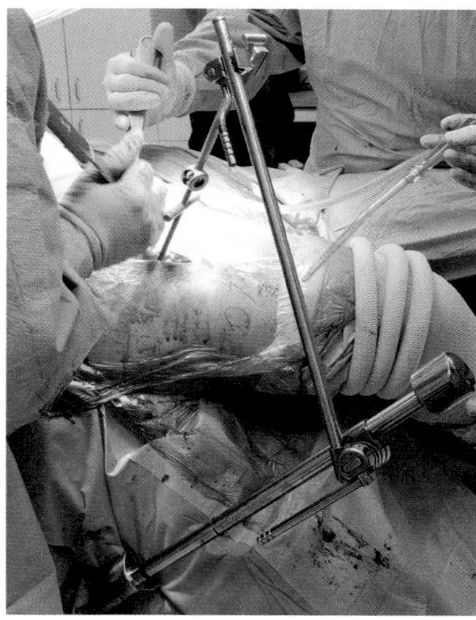

Figure 3 Intraoperative photograph shows the anterior supine intermuscular approach to the hip. To facilitate exposure of the femur, the foot of the bed has been dropped, the patient has been placed in the Trendelenburg position, and a table-mounted hook has been attached to the bed. The hook has been placed around the proximal femur just proximal to the gluteal sling.

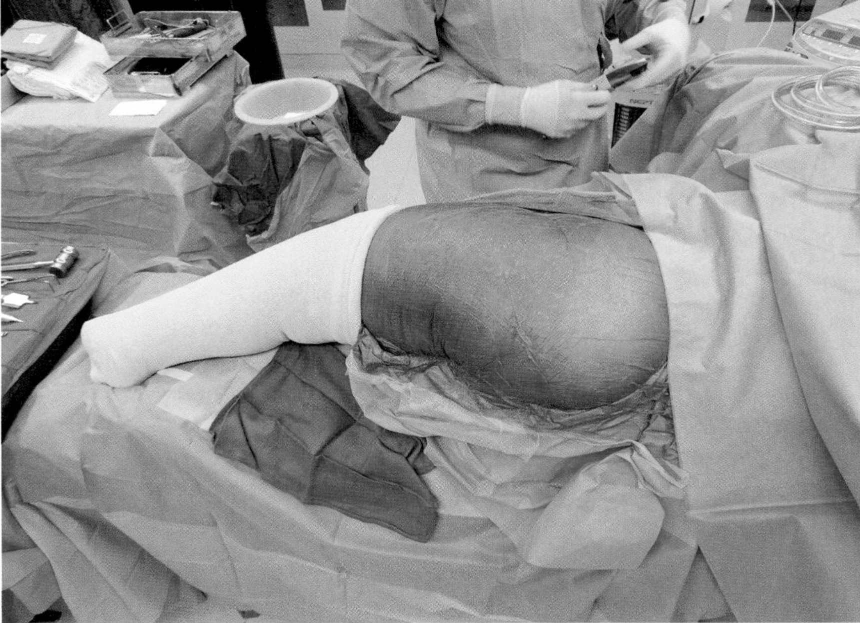

Figure 4 Intraoperative photograph shows patient positioning for the direct lateral approach to the hip. The patient is placed in the lateral decubitus position and secured with padded pegs.

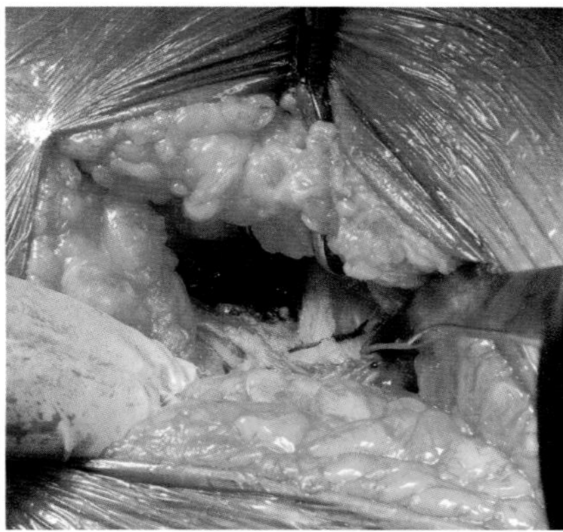

Figure 5 Intraoperative photograph shows the direct lateral approach. Dissection was begun at the level of the vastus ridge, and the vastus lateralis has been elevated in continuity with only the anterior third of the gluteus medius and minimus. The posterior two-thirds of the gluteus medius and minimus remain attached to the trochanter.

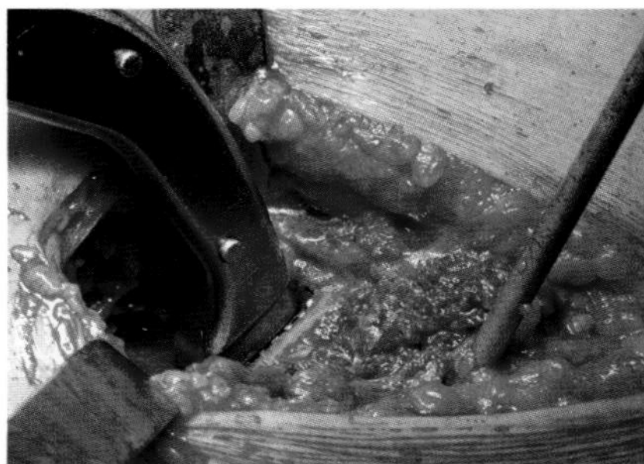

Figure 6 Intraoperative photograph shows broaching of the femoral canal.

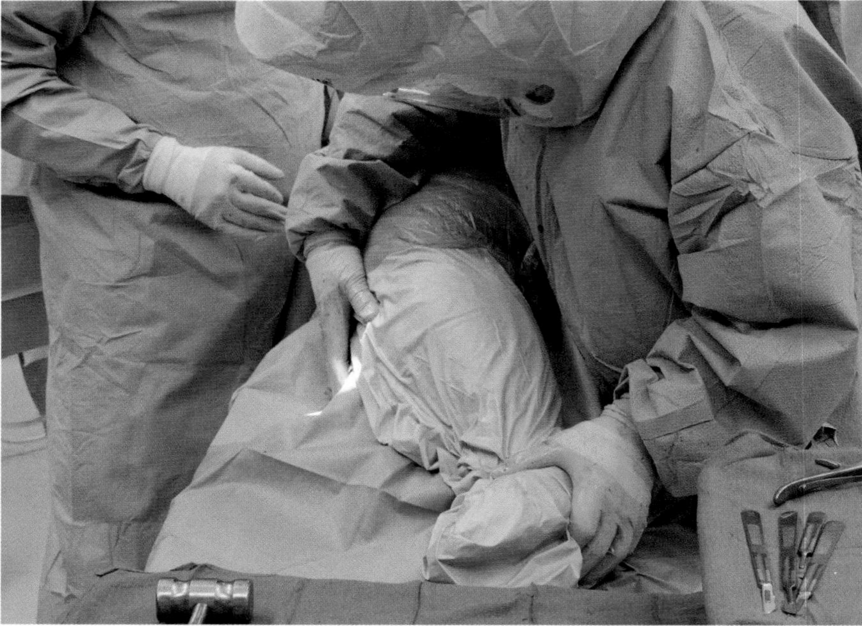

Figure 7 Intraoperative photograph shows positioning of the affected leg for assessment of limb length and stability in the direct lateral approach for total hip arthroplasty. The nonoperated leg, which lies beneath the surgical draping, is used as a reference, with the surgeon aligning the medial malleoli and palpating the patellar tendons for comparison with the preoperative estimate.

- A box chisel is used to facilitate adequate lateralization of the femoral implant and thereby avoid varus malalignment.
- An aggressive canal-finding rasp is used to open the femoral canal.
- Sequential broaching, starting with the smallest broach, is performed to enlarge the femoral canal until the medial and lateral cortices are engaged and the broach cannot be advanced deeper (**Figure 6**).
- Because the implant has a flat, tapered wedge shape, the anteversion tends to follow the patient's natural anteversion.
- During the process of sequential broaching, care is taken to work the broach laterally to prevent varus orientation.
- When the largest broach is in place, a calcar planer is inserted to finish the femoral neck cut.
- A femoral neck taper trunnion and trial femoral head based on the offset option selected via preoperative templating are placed for trial reduction using the shortest available femoral neck length.
- In the direct lateral approach, the surgeon can assess limb length and stability using the nonoperated leg as a reference by aligning the medial malleoli and palpating the patellar tendon for comparison with the preoperative estimate (**Figure 7**).
- In the anterior supine intermuscular approach, the surgeon can check the limb length while the patient is supine by palpating both malleoli and using fluoroscopic imaging (**Figure 8**).
- The noncemented short tapered stem is fully seated with a tight interference fit.
- Femoral head and neck trial units are selected and used to determine stability and equalize limb length. The author of this chapter uses a ceramic femoral head in most patients (**Figure 9**).
- After the femoral head-neck unit is inserted, the hip is reduced.
- The wound is copiously irrigated, and the intra-articular soft tissues are infiltrated with analgesic medication.

Wound Closure

- Meticulous wound closure is accomplished in layers.
- In the direct lateral approach, meticulous repair of the gluteus medius–vastus lateralis sleeve is extremely important. The gluteus minimus and attached capsule are repaired in continuity with nonabsorbable sutures, which are anchored into the tendinous portion of the gluteus medius and the tip of the greater trochanter.
- The continuity of the gluteus medius is reapproximated with nonabsorbable and absorbable sutures.
- The tensor fascia lata, subcutaneous tissue, and skin are approximated in layers.
- For skin closure, the author of this chapter prefers to use subcutaneous barbed sutures with cyanoacrylate tissue adhesive.
- In the anterior supine intermuscular approach, closure is simple. The fascia lata is repaired, and the subcutaneous tissue and skin are closed using the same sutures and adhesive used for the direct lateral approach.

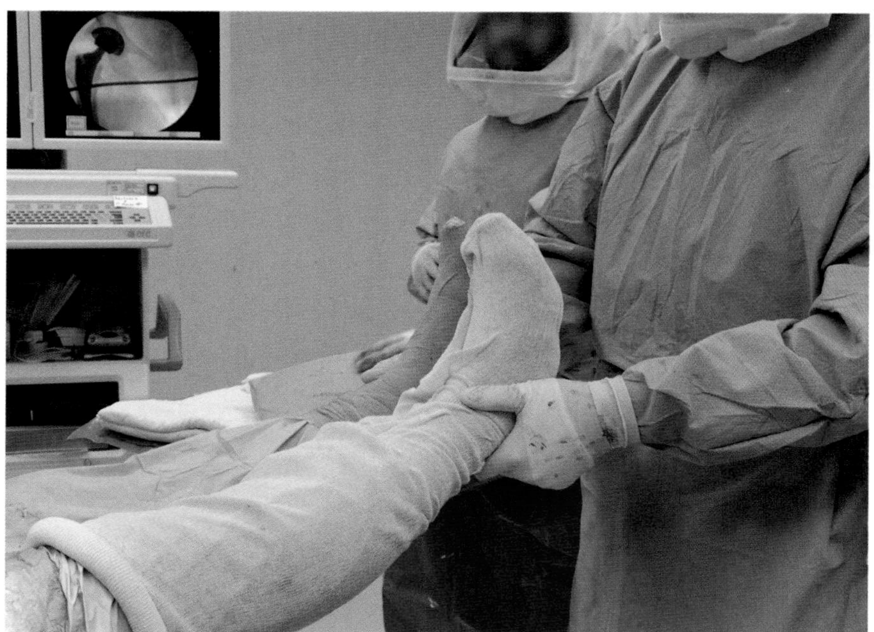

Figure 8 Intraoperative photograph shows assessment of limb length in the anterior supine intermuscular approach used in total hip arthroplasty. The surgeon palpates and compares the malleoli in the affected and nonoperated legs and uses fluoroscopic imaging.

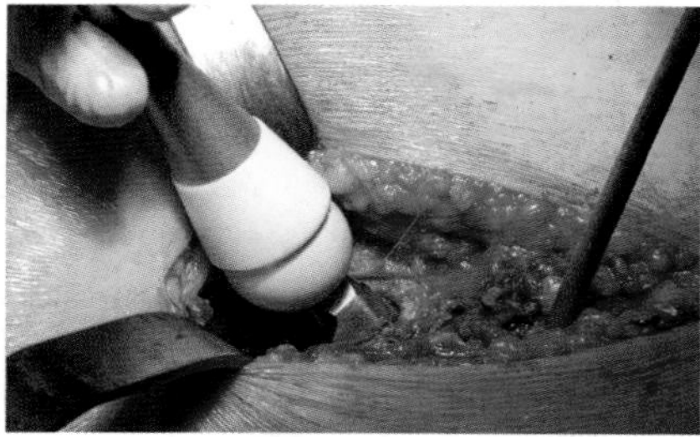

Figure 9 Intraoperative photograph shows insertion of the femoral implant. The short tapered stem is fully seated with a tight interference fit.

Postoperative Regimen

The patient is transferred to the gurney in the supine position. Abduction pillows are not used. The patient is taken to the postanesthesia care unit, and radiographs are obtained. At the institution of the author of this chapter, patients are placed on a multimodal pain management regime and mobilized within 2 hours of the surgical procedure. Patients are risk stratified for deep vein thrombosis prophylaxis. In most patients deemed to be low risk, aspirin (325 mg) is prescribed to be taken twice daily for 6 weeks postoperatively, and patients are discharged with instruction to use ambulatory calf compression pumps for 2 weeks postoperatively. In patients considered to be high risk, daily chemoprophylaxis is prescribed for 2 weeks postoperatively, followed by aspirin (325 mg) twice daily for an additional 4 weeks. In addition, these patients are discharged with instructions to use ambulatory calf compression pumps for the first 2 weeks postoperatively. All patients are instructed to use a walker or crutches initially and to advance to a cane at their discretion, and ultimately, to walk unassisted. Historical hip precautions are no longer used.

Avoiding Pitfalls and Complications

Preoperative templating is crucial in determining the level of femoral neck resection and the implant size. The author of this chapter typically uses a short tapered stem one or two sizes larger than the standard-length stem that would otherwise be used. The surgeon should use the largest-sized broach possible. Technical expertise must be exercised during broaching. Although studies have demonstrated that tapered designs are not susceptible to failure with varus placement, the surgeon can ensure adequate lateralization of the femoral implant to avoid varus malalignment by using a lateralizing rasp and driving the implant in valgus during insertion. This technique will prevent undersizing of the implant. If a fracture occurs during preparation of the femur, cerclage cables must be used for stabilization. In this scenario, the author of this chapter does not consistently change to the use of a standard-length stem. Because of the robust plasma-sprayed coating on the author's preferred implant, the selected implant may stop 1 to 2 mm above the desired final position of the implant. If the surgeon determines that limb lengths are equal and the hip is stable with the smallest femoral neck length, it may be helpful to place a stem one size smaller than the selected implant or to use a broach 1 mm larger than the desired implant size before final seating of the implant is attempted.

Acknowledgments

The author would like to thank his surgeon partners, Keith R. Berend, MD, and Michael J. Morris, MD, for their contribution of cases to the series reviewed, and Erin L. Ruh, MS, and Joanne B. Adams, BFA, CMI, for their assistance in preparation of this manuscript.

Bibliography

Banerjee S, Pivec R, Issa K, Harwin SF, Mont MA, Khanuja HS: Outcomes of short stems in total hip arthroplasty. *Orthopedics* 2013;36(9):700-707.

Barreca S, Ciriaco L, Ferlazzo M, Rosa MA: Mechanical and biological results of short-stem hip implants: Consideration on a series of 74 cases. *Musculoskelet Surg* 2015;99(1):55-59.

Barrington JW, Emerson RH Jr: The short and "shorter" of it: >1750 tapered titanium stems at 6- to 88-month follow-up. *J Arthroplasty* 2013;28(8 suppl):38-40.

Berend KR, Mallory TH, Lombardi AV Jr, Dodds KL, Adams JB: Tapered cementless femoral stem: Difficult to place in varus but performs well in those rare cases. *Orthopedics* 2007;30(4):295-297.

Chang RW, Pellisier JM, Hazen GB: A cost-effectiveness analysis of total hip arthroplasty for osteoarthritis of the hip. *JAMA* 1996;275(11):858-865.

Falez F, Casella F, Papalia M: Current concepts, classification, and results in short stem hip arthroplasty. *Orthopedics* 2015;38(3 suppl):S6-S13.

Frye BM, Berend KR, Lombardi AV Jr, Morris MJ, Adams JB: Do sex and BMI predict or does stem design prevent muscle damage in anterior supine minimally invasive THA? *Clin Orthop Relat Res* 2015;473(2):632-638.

Gilbert RE, Salehi-Bird S, Gallacher PD, Shaylor P: The Mayo Conservative Hip: Experience from a district general hospital. *Hip Int* 2009;19(3):211-214.

Hutt J, Harb Z, Gill I, Kashif F, Miller J, Dodd M: Ten year results of the collum femoris preserving total hip replacement: A prospective cohort study of seventy five patients. *Int Orthop* 2014;38(5):917-922.

Kendoff DO, Citak M, Egidy CC, O'Loughlin PF, Gehrke T: Eleven-year results of the anatomic coated CFP stem in primary total hip arthroplasty. *J Arthroplasty* 2013;28(6):1047-1051.

Khalily C, Lester DK: Results of a tapered cementless femoral stem implanted in varus. *J Arthroplasty* 2002;17(4):463-466.

Khanuja HS, Banerjee S, Jain D, Pivec R, Mont MA: Short bone-conserving stems in cementless hip arthroplasty. *J Bone Joint Surg Am* 2014;96(20):1742-1752.

Kim YH, Choi Y, Kim JS: Comparison of bone mineral density changes around short, metaphyseal-fitting, and conventional cementless anatomical femoral components. *J Arthroplasty* 2011;26(6):931-940.e1.

Kim YH, Oh JH: A comparison of a conventional versus a short, anatomical metaphyseal-fitting cementless femoral stem in the treatment of patients with a fracture of the femoral neck. *J Bone Joint Surg Br* 2012;94(6):774-781.

Kim YH, Park JW, Kim JS: Behaviour of the ultra-short anatomic cementless femoral stem in young and elderly patients. *Int Orthop* 2013;37(12):2323-2330.

Lombardi AV Jr, Berend KR, Adams JB: A short stem solution: Through small portals. *Orthopedics* 2009;32(9):1-4.

Martins LG, Garcia FL, Picado CH: Aseptic loosening rate of the Mayo femoral stem with medium-term follow up. *J Arthroplasty* 2014;29(11):2122-2126.

McCalden RW, Korczak A, Somerville L, Yuan X, Naudie DD: A randomised trial comparing a short and a standard-length metaphyseal engaging cementless femoral stem using radiostereometric analysis. *Bone Joint J* 2015;97-B(5):595-602.

McElroy MJ, Johnson AJ, Mont MA, Bonutti PM: Short and standard stem prostheses are both viable options for minimally invasive total hip arthroplasty. *Bull NYU Hosp Jt Dis* 2011;69(suppl 1):S68-S76.

Molli RG, Lombardi AV Jr, Berend KR, Adams JB, Sneller MA: A short tapered stem reduces intraoperative complications in primary total hip arthroplasty. *Clin Orthop Relat Res* 2012;470(2):450-461.

Morrey BF, Adams RA, Kessler M: A conservative femoral replacement for total hip arthroplasty: A prospective study. *J Bone Joint Surg Br* 2000;82(7):952-958.

Pipino F: CFP prosthetic stem in mini-invasive total hip arthroplasty. *J Orthop Traumatol* 2004;5(3):165-171.

Rometsch E, Bos PK, Koes BW: Survival of short hip stems with a “modern”, trochanter-sparing design: A systematic literature review. *Hip Int* 2012;22(4):344-354.

Tahim AS, Stokes OM, Vedi V: The effect of femoral stem length on duration of hospital stay. *Hip Int* 2012;22(1):56-61.

van Oldenrijk J, Molleman J, Klaver M, Poolman RW, Haverkamp D: Revision rate after short-stem total hip arthroplasty: A systematic review of 49 studies. *Acta Orthop* 2014;85(3):250-258.

Chapter 16
Hip Resurfacing Arthroplasty

Paul E. Beaulé, MD, FRCSC
Alex Pagé, MD, FRCSC

Indications

Hip resurfacing arthroplasty replaces only the diseased portions of the hip joint, whether the femoral head alone or the femoral head and the acetabular surface, using nonmodular components in which the femoral implant matches the inner diameter of the acetabular implant. The optimal patient for hip resurfacing arthroplasty is a young (typically younger than 60 years), active man with osteoarthritis and a history of hip pain. Hip resurfacing in women remains highly controversial. The senior author (P.E.B.) considers women 40 to 50 years of age with degenerative arthritis and a femoral implant size larger than 48 mm to have results that are as good as those of men. Studies of the National Joint Registry for England and Wales and the Australian Orthopaedic Association National Joint Replacement Registry support this opinion. Women younger than 55 years without hip dysplasia represent a small percentage of candidates for hip resurfacing arthroplasty. Patients should be counseled that frequent impact activity can increase the risk of femoral failure. In one study, impact activity was associated with up to a fourfold increase in the revision rate at a mean follow-up of 10 years.

Physical examination should include assessment of the patient's neurovascular status, limb-length discrepancy, muscle strength (specifically of the abductors), and range of motion. At the institution of the authors of this chapter, the standard radiographic evaluation of patients with hip pathology consists of an AP pelvic radiograph, a cross-table lateral radiograph, and/or a Dunn radiograph (**Figure 1**). Most patients who undergo hip resurfacing have insufficient femoral head-neck offset and an underlying cam deformity that contributed to the development of arthritis. Digital templating is necessary to ensure that a femoral implant of sufficient size is chosen. A femoral implant that is too small can result in femoral notching and undersizing of the acetabular implant. The final implant size is chosen intraoperatively with the use of femoral head size gauges typically used in open surgical procedures for the correction of cam deformities of the hip (**Figure 2**). In addition to sizing, preoperative planning can help ensure relative valgus positioning of the femoral implant of 5° to 10° to minimize tensile stresses. Preoperative planning also can reveal a lack of concavity at the anterior femoral head-neck junction. If anterior offset is not corrected, patients can experience persistent pain secondary to impingement and a decreased range of motion.

The choice of the surgical approach is critical to ensure proper implant position and to preserve or minimize damage to key functional structures. When performing hip resurfacing, the surgeon must preserve the blood supply to the femoral head (especially the deep branch of the medial circumflex artery and the inferior gluteal neurovascular bundle). Although the posterior approach has been associated with femoral neck fracture, it remains the most commonly used approach. With the Steffen modification of the technique, described later in this chapter, the risk of fracture of the femoral neck is less than 1%. The senior author of this chapter (P.E.B.) has used the Ganz trochanteric flip osteotomy approach and continues to use it on select patients undergoing joint-preserving surgery of the hip in whom intraoperative conversion to joint arthroplasty may be necessary. However, this technique is associated with a risk of nonunion because of the trochanteric osteotomy.

Dr. Beaulé or an immediate family member has received royalties from Corin USA, Medacta USA, and MicroPort; is a member of a speakers' bureau or has made paid presentations on behalf of Medacta USA, MicroPort, and Smith & Nephew; serves as a paid consultant to Corin USA, DePuy Synthes, Medacta USA, Smith & Nephew, and Zimmer Biomet; and has received research or institutional support from Corin USA, DePuy Synthes, and MicroPort. Neither Dr. Pagé nor any immediate family member has received anything of value from or has stock or stock options held in a commercial company or institution related directly or indirectly to the subject of this chapter.

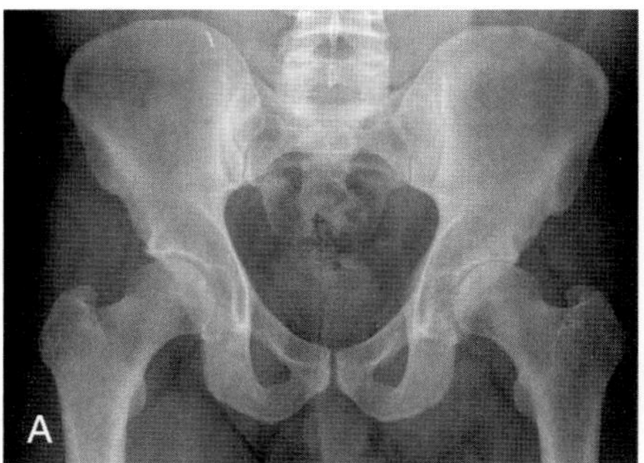

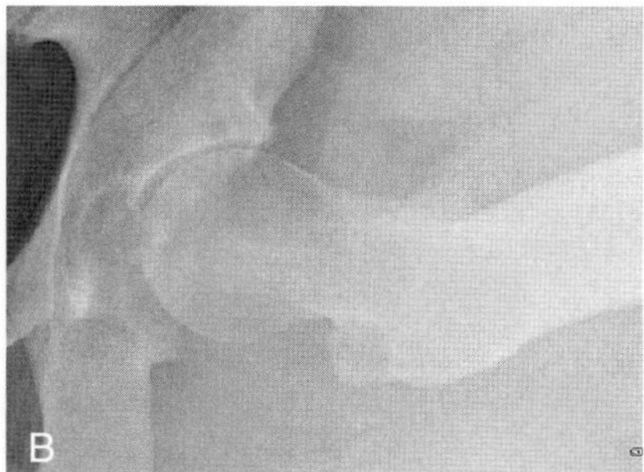

Figure 1 AP pelvic radiograph (**A**) and Dunn radiograph of a left hip (**B**) demonstrate advanced arthritis of the left hip in a 43-year-old man.

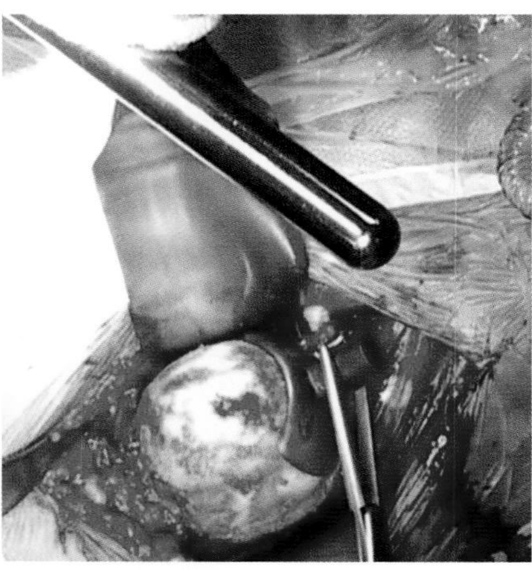

Figure 2 Intraoperative photograph of a hip shows the use of a spherometer to determine femoral head size prior to hip resurfacing.

Contraindications

Hip resurfacing is contraindicated in patients with severe cystic or atrophic changes in the femoral head or neck, which are associated with a high risk of femoral failure. Patients with renal failure or proven hypersensitivity to metal also are not suitable candidates. Hip dysplasia is a relative contraindication because associated torsional deformities of the femur and acetabulum make optimal implant position challenging to obtain, and because these patients often require small implant sizes, which increase the risk of early failure. The use of a metal-on metal interface should be avoided in women of childbearing age. Patients with smaller bone structures would likely benefit from total hip arthroplasty (THA) instead of hip resurfacing. In many studies, femoral implant size smaller than 48 mm has been correlated with poor outcomes.

Alternative Treatments

Most candidates for hip resurfacing have the option of THA or hip resurfacing. THA provides additional choices of cup, stem, and interface not available with hip resurfacing. Resurfacing is a bone-conserving approach and in some patients allows more accurate biomechanical reconstruction than THA would.

Results

Currently, two metal-on-metal hip resurfacing systems are commonly used worldwide: Birmingham Hip Resurfacing (BHR; Smith & Nephew), which uses hybrid fixation, and the Conserve Plus (MicroPort), which has hybrid and noncemented fixation options. The four most relevant studies are summarized in **Table 1**.

In a 2014 study of hip resurfacing, high rates of implant survivorship at 15 years were reported for both men and women, although the rate was somewhat lower for women. Osteonecrosis of the femoral head and dysplasia were risk factors for failure. Patients with osteoarthritis had the best results, with 99.4% survivorship at 15 years compared with patients diagnosed with dysplasia and osteonecrosis. In a study of 100 hip resurfacings, the 10-year Kaplan-Meier survivorship rate was 88.5%. No failures occurred in the 28 hips with femoral implants larger than 46 mm and good femoral bone quality (cyst size less than 1 cm). The results of this latter study are consistent with data from the Australian Orthopaedic Association National Joint Replacement Registry.

The authors of a 2012 study reported the influence of acetabular implant positioning on implant survival with revision as the end point at 5-year follow-up in patients treated with the Conserve Plus (mean age, 48.6 years). At a mean 8.9-year follow-up, 12 hips required conversion to THA, with loosening of the acetabular implant in 5 hips, femoral neck fracture in 2 hips, femoral loosening in 2 hips, and adverse tissue reaction in 3 hips. Implants with a contact patch–to–rim distance of less than 10 mm were at increased risk of revision. The incidence of adverse tissue reaction was 1%.

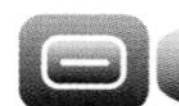

Video 16.1 Surgical Technique: Hip Resurfacing Postero-Lateral Approach. Antonio Moroni, MD; Giovanni Micera, MD; Maria Teresa Miscione, MD; Riccardo Orsini, MD (22 min)

Techniques

Setup/Exposure

MODIFIED POSTERIOR APPROACH

- This approach preserves a substantial portion of the blood supply to the femoral head.
- A standard incision for the extended posterior approach is made.
- The fascia lata and gluteus maximus are split in line with their fibers.

Table 1 Results of the Largest Clinical Series of Metal-on-Metal Hip Resurfacing

Author(s) (Year)	Number Treated	Implant Type	Mean Patient Age in Years (Range)	Mean Follow-up in Years (Range)	Results
Amstutz et al (2010)	89 patients (100 hips)	Conserve Plus (Wright Medical Technology)[a]	49.1 (15-71)	11.7 (10.8-12.9)	10-yr Kaplan-Meier survivorship rate of 88.5% 11 hips were converted to total hip arthroplasty because of femoral implant loosening, femoral neck fracture, recurrent subluxation, or late infection
Amstutz et al (2012)	178 patients (200 hips)	Conserve Plus	48.6 (15-78)	8.9 (2.1-11.5)	10-yr implant survivorship rate of 94.3% (95% CI: 89.2-97) Cup positioning affected outcomes, with contact patch–to–rim distance of <10 mm associated with implant failure
Canadian Arthroplasty Society (2013)	2,450 patients (2,773 hips)	Conserve Plus, Durom (Zimmer), Birmingham Hip Resurfacing (Smith & Nephew), ASR (DePuy)	50.5 (18-82)	3.4 (2.0-10.1)	5-yr implant survivorship rate of 97.4% in men and 93.6% in women Overall implant survivorship rate of 96.4% (95% CI: 96.1-96.9) The Durom and ASR implants were recalled and are no longer available
Daniel et al (2014)	886 patients (1,000 hips)	Birmingham Hip Resurfacing	53 (15-84)	13.7 (12.3-15.3)	15-yr implant survivorship rate of 98.0% in men (95% CI: 97.4-98.6) and 91.5% in women (95% CI: 89.8-93.2) Overall implant survivorship rate of 95.8% (95% CI: 95.1-96.5)
Mehra et al (2015)	120 hips	Birmingham Hip Resurfacing	50 (28-63)	10.8 (10-14)	10-yr implant survivorship rate of 96.1 (95% CI: 91.5-99.8)

CI = confidence interval.
[a] Currently, this device is manufactured by MicroPort.

- The gluteus maximus tendon is partially divided where it inserts into the linea aspera.
- The deep branch of the medial femoral circumflex artery is visualized and is divided with the use of electrocautery.
- The quadratus femoris is divided at a point 5 to 8 mm from its insertion.
- The piriformis muscle is detached at its insertion on the femur.
- The remaining short external rotator muscles are divided 5 to 8 mm from their insertion.
- A cuff of soft tissue or muscle is preserved on the femur.
- The capsule is incised approximately 10 mm from the posterior wall of the acetabulum with a scalpel, taking care to cut against the femoral head and not in the soft tissues around the femoral neck.
- The hip is dislocated.
- A circumferential incision is made carefully in the capsule. The capsule itself is preserved.
- The soft tissues around the femoral neck are preserved.
- Care is taken throughout the procedure to minimize dissection around the femoral neck to avoid damage to the branches of the circumflex vessels.

ANTERIOR APPROACH

- The senior author of this chapter (P.E.B.) uses the anterior (Hueter) approach with the patient positioned supine on an orthopaedic surgical positioning table because this method provides full preservation of both the musculature and the structures that supply blood to the femoral head.
- An incision is made 1 to 2 cm posterolateral and 2 cm distal to the anterior superior iliac spine. The incision runs obliquely and follows the orientation of the tensor fascia lata (TFL).
- An incision is made in the fascia

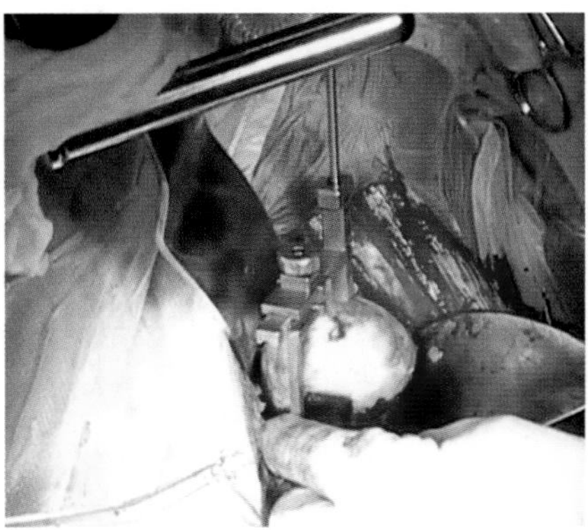

Figure 3 Intraoperative photograph of a hip shows placement of a guidewire with the use of a spin-around gauge for the appropriate-size femoral implant. The entry point is placed in the midaxis of the femoral neck to ensure proper implant version and to avoid notching of the femoral neck. The correct starting point is usually one fingerbreadth (approximately 2 cm) above the fovea.

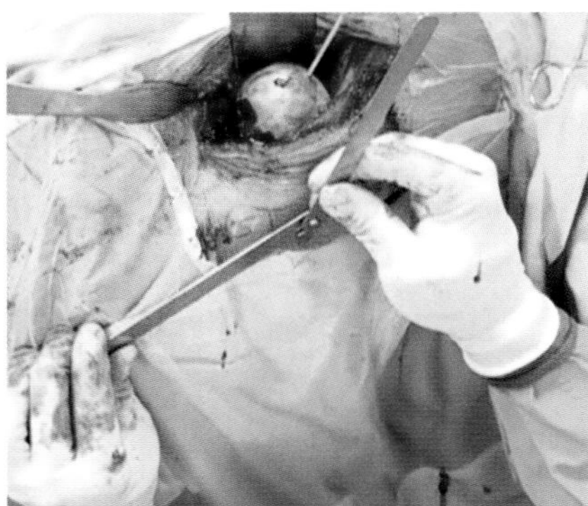

Figure 4 Intraoperative photograph of a hip shows the use of a goniometer to confirm valgus positioning of the femoral implant.

over the TFL in line with the fibers of the muscle.

- The fibers of the TFL are gently teased off the fascial sleeve with sharp dissection.
- The interval between the TFL and rectus femoris muscles is developed, exposing the aponeurosis of the rectus femoris.
- A large cobra retractor is placed behind the lateral part of the iliac wing to retract the TFL laterally.
- The fascia over the rectus femoris is incised.
- The ascending branches of the lateral circumflex vessels are meticulously identified and ligated.
- The reflected head of the rectus femoris is released to expose the hip capsule and facilitate visualization of the anterior acetabular rim.
- A lateral capsulectomy is performed to expose the femoral head and neck.
- With the use of a large metal skid placed intra-articularly, the hip is dislocated with pure external rotation and no traction. The femoral head is levered out of the acetabulum with the metal skid.
- Careful distal release of the fascia of the rectus femoris is performed. This release permits medial retraction of the rectus femoris and inferomedial capsular release to facilitate external rotation of the leg and optimize exposure of the femoral head-neck junction.
- For femoral preparation, the affected leg is placed in extension with the foot externally rotated approximately 160°. Occasionally in men of large body size, the origin of the TFL at the anterior superior iliac spine is partially released (1 to 2 cm) to avoid damaging the muscle.
- For acetabular preparation, the affected leg is placed in slight flexion and the foot is placed at rest in external rotation.

Procedure

PREPARATION OF THE FEMORAL HEAD

- After the capsular releases have been performed, the femoral head is exposed with the use of an elevator or long, curved retractors.
- The femoral head size is determined with the use of femoral head size gauges in correlation with preoperative templating.
- A guidewire is passed into the femoral head. If the posterior approach is used, commercial jigs are available for use in this step. If the anterior approach is used, limited exposure of the femoral head prevents the use of a jig, and the Kirschner wire is placed freehand with the use of landmarks for reference (**Figure 3**).
- The Kirschner wire can be inserted in approximately 5° to 10° of valgus relative to the native femoral neck-shaft angle, resulting in a final angle of approximately 140°. This measurement is checked with the use of a goniometer (**Figure 4**).
- A spin-around guide corresponding with the planned femoral head size is used to check for any impinging osteophytes at the inferomedial femoral neck and to check for clearance at the anterior and inferior femoral neck.
- Care is taken to avoid unnecessary débridement of osteophytes or bone that would expose cancellous bone in the femoral neck, which could result in the development of a stress riser or femoral neck fracture.
- The femoral head typically is prepared with the use of cylindric and chamfer reamers. However, implant manufacturers may specify different techniques for preparation of the femoral head.
- If the surgeon is unsure of the acetabular sizing, the femoral head may be reamed initially to one size larger than planned and finalized after the acetabulum is prepared.
- After the femoral head is prepared to the final size, a trial implant is placed and checked for notching, osteophytes, and seating position.

PREPARATION OF THE ACETABULUM AND PLACEMENT OF THE ACETABULAR IMPLANT

- In the posterior approach, a superolateral pocket is created by elevating the capsule off the superolateral acetabular surface. This step facilitates placement of the reamed femoral head during preparation of the acetabulum. The subsequent steps are similar to performing a THA.

- A long, curved Hohmann retractor is placed over the anteromedial lip of the acetabulum at approximately the 3- to 4-o'clock position in the right hip or the 8- to 9-o'clock position in the left hip (**Figure 5**).
- A second Hohmann retractor is placed under the posterior wall at the 9-o'clock position in the right hip or the 3-o'clock position in the left hip.
- Reaming begins in reverse mode to ensure adequate bony contact, after which forward reaming is performed.
- The targeted extent of reaming is initially three sizes smaller than the planned size of the acetabulum based on the size of the femoral implant.
- The reamers allow the surgeon to approximate the anteversion and inclination of the host socket.
- A curet is used between reamings to remove soft tissue and determine the depth of reaming.
- Line-to-line reaming is typically performed to provide press-fit fixation of 0.75 mm. However, the depth of reaming can vary according to manufacturer guidelines. Because patients often have sclerotic bone, reaming often is performed to one size larger than the implant size to ensure proper seating of the implant.
- After the bony bed is prepared, the acetabulum is cleaned with pulsatile lavage.
- The final implant is impacted into place.
- Implant anteversion and inclination are assessed with the use of a guide specific to the surgical approach.
- The authors of this chapter strongly recommend obtaining an intraoperative radiograph to ensure correct orientation and seating of the acetabular implant.
- All four quadrants of the acetabular cup are stressed manually with a punch to ensure initial stability of the implant.

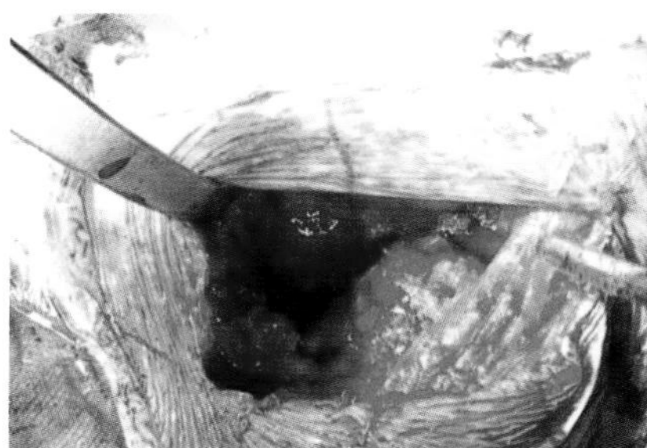

Figure 5 Intraoperative photograph of a left hip shows the acetabulum with the femoral neck posteriorly and a curved Hohmann retractor anteriorly.

PLACEMENT OF THE FEMORAL IMPLANT

- The femoral head is thoroughly irrigated, all debris is removed, and the bony bed is dried.
- Any sclerotic areas are prepared by making drill holes with a 2.5-mm drill bit.
- A noncemented or cemented femoral implant can be used. A recent study demonstrated equivalent results of noncemented, porous-coated femoral implants and cemented femoral implants at short-term follow-up. The authors of this chapter have recently begun using noncemented femoral implants with satisfactory anecdotal outcomes.
- If a noncemented femoral implant is chosen, it is impacted into place (**Figure 6**).
- If a cemented femoral implant is chosen, the cement is applied when it has a doughlike consistency. If the cement is applied before it has hardened to a doughlike consistency, overpenetration of the cement can cause thermal necrosis.
- The partially cement-filled femoral implant is impacted. Excessive cement is removed. The hip is reduced quickly to allow dissipation of the heat generated by the curing of the cement.

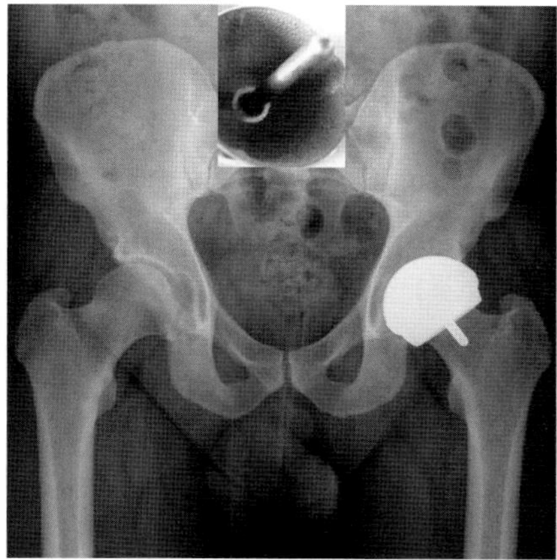

Figure 6 Postoperative AP pelvic radiograph demonstrates hip resurfacing with a noncemented femoral implant. Inset, photograph of a noncemented femoral implant.

Wound Closure

- After the final implants have been placed, an intraoperative radiograph is obtained to evaluate implant position.
- Closure is performed in standard fashion according to the approach used.

Postoperative Regimen

The patient is mobilized on postoperative day 1 and receives prophylaxis for deep vein thrombosis. A physical therapist evaluates the patient to determine if the patient can be discharged safely. If the anterior approach was used, the patient is restricted to partial (50%) weight bearing with the use of crutches or a walker for approximately 4 weeks postoperatively. If the posterior approach was used, the patient is allowed to bear weight as tolerated. Athletic activity or aggressive physical activity is delayed until 12 weeks postoperatively to allow some bony remodeling of the femoral neck.

Avoiding Pitfalls and Complications

Certain intraoperative complications can be avoided if the blood supply to the femoral head is maintained during femoral preparation. Care must be taken to preserve the retinacular vessels to prevent osteonecrosis of the femoral head, especially when the posterior approach is used. Overly aggressive barrel reaming must be avoided to prevent notching of the femoral neck, which can result in the development of a stress riser and result in femoral neck fracture. Because the size of the femoral head corresponds with fixed sizes of the acetabular cup, careful evaluation is required to avoid inappropriate sizing of the cup. Oversizing of the cup can lead to the loss of bony coverage anteriorly and result in recurrent psoas tendinitis, whereas undersizing of the cup can lead to poor press-fit fixation and result in loosening of the cup.

Before the anterior approach is used, the surgeon is strongly advised to observe expert use of the approach and to undergo specialized training. Among patients who undergo hip resurfacing through the anterior approach, more than two-thirds report hypoesthesia in the distribution of the lateral femoral cutaneous nerve. Most of these patients regain sensitivity in the region within 4 to 6 months postoperatively.

Adverse local tissue reactions remain a concern with hip resurfacing. However, this complication can be detected early with ultrasonographic imaging, and the overall incidence remains low.

Bibliography

Amstutz HC, Le Duff MJ, Campbell PA, Gruen TA, Wisk LE: Clinical and radiographic results of metal-on-metal hip resurfacing with a minimum ten-year follow-up. *J Bone Joint Surg Am* 2010;92(16):2663-2671.

Amstutz HC, Le Duff MJ, Johnson AJ: Socket position determines hip resurfacing 10-year survivorship. *Clin Orthop Relat Res* 2012;470(11):3127-3133.

Australian Orthopaedic Association National Joint Replacement Registry: *Annual Report.* Adelaide, Australia, Australian Orthopaedic Association, 2013. Available at https://aoanjrr.sahmri.com/documents/10180/127202/Annual%20Report%202013?version=1.2&t=1385685288617. Accessed July 28, 2016.

Beaulé PE, Campbell P, Lu Z, et al: Vascularity of the arthritic femoral head and hip resurfacing. *J Bone Joint Surg Am* 2006;88(suppl 4):85-96.

Beaulé PE, Campbell P, Shim P: Femoral head blood flow during hip resurfacing. *Clin Orthop Relat Res* 2007;456:148-152.

Beaulé PE, Harvey N, Zaragoza E, Le Duff MJ, Dorey FJ: The femoral head/neck offset and hip resurfacing. *J Bone Joint Surg Br* 2007;89(1):9-15.

Benoit B, Gofton W, Beaulé PE: Hueter anterior approach for hip resurfacing: Assessment of the learning curve. *Orthop Clin North Am* 2009;40(3):357-363.

Canadian Arthroplasty Society: The Canadian Arthroplasty Society's experience with hip resurfacing arthroplasty: An analysis of 2773 hips. *Bone Joint J* 2013;95-B(8):1045-1051.

Canadian Hip Resurfacing Study Group: A survey on the prevalence of pseudotumors with metal-on-metal hip resurfacing in Canadian academic centers. *J Bone Joint Surg Am* 2011;93(suppl 2):118-121.

Daniel J, Pradhan C, Ziaee H, Pynsent PB, McMinn DJ: Results of Birmingham hip resurfacing at 12 to 15 years: A single-surgeon series. *Bone Joint J* 2014;96-B(10):1298-1306.

de Steiger RN, Hang JR, Miller LN, Graves SE, Davidson DC: Five-year results of the ASR XL Acetabular System and the ASR Hip Resurfacing System: An analysis from the Australian Orthopaedic Association National Joint Replacement Registry. *J Bone Joint Surg Am* 2011;93(24):2287-2293.

Ganz R, Gill TJ, Gautier E, Ganz K, Krügel N, Berlemann U: Surgical dislocation of the adult hip: A technique with full access to the femoral head and acetabulum without the risk of avascular necrosis. *J Bone Joint Surg Br* 2001;83(8):1119-1124.

Girard J, Lavigne M, Vendittoli PA, Roy AG: Biomechanical reconstruction of the hip: A randomised study comparing total hip resurfacing and total hip arthroplasty. *J Bone Joint Surg Br* 2006;88(6):721-726.

Goulding K, Beaulé PE, Kim PR, Fazekas A: Incidence of lateral femoral cutaneous nerve neuropraxia after anterior approach hip arthroplasty. *Clin Orthop Relat Res* 2010;468(9):2397-2404.

Le Duff MJ, Amstutz HC: The relationship of sporting activity and implant survivorship after hip resurfacing. *J Bone Joint Surg Am* 2012;94(10):911-918.

Matharu GS, McBryde CW, Pynsent WB, Pynsent PB, Treacy RB: The outcome of the Birmingham Hip Resurfacing in patients aged < 50 years up to 14 years post-operatively. *Bone Joint J* 2013;95-B(9):1172-1177.

Mehra A, Berryman F, Matharu GS, Pynsent PB, Isbister ES: Birmingham Hip Resurfacing: A single surgeon series reported at a minimum of 10 years follow-up. *J Arthroplasty* 2015;30(7):1160-1166.

Sedrakyan A, Romero L, Graves S, et al: Survivorship of hip and knee implants in pediatric and young adult populations: Analysis of registry and published data. *J Bone Joint Surg Am* 2014;96(suppl 1):73-78.

Smith AJ, Dieppe P, Howard PW, Blom AW; National Joint Registry for England and Wales: Failure rates of metal-on-metal hip resurfacings: Analysis of data from the National Joint Registry for England and Wales. *Lancet* 2012;380(9855):1759-1766.

Steffen RT, De Smet KA, Murray DW, Gill HS: A modified posterior approach preserves femoral head oxgenation during hip resurfacing. *J Arthroplasty* 2011;26(3):404-408.

Zylberberg AD, Nishiwaki T, Kim PR, Beaulé PE: Clinical results of the Conserve Plus metal on metal hip resurfacing: An independent series. *J Arthroplasty* 2015;30(1):68-73.

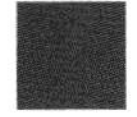

Video Reference

Moroni A, Micera G, Miscione MT, Orsini R: Video. *Surgical Technique: Hip Resurfacing Postero-Lateral Approach.* Bologna, Italy, 2016.

Chapter 17
Bearing Surfaces

Joshua J. Jacobs, MD
Rishi Balkissoon, MD, MPH
Brett R. Levine, MD, MS

Introduction

Although total hip arthroplasty (THA) is highly successful in most patients, the increasing use of the procedure in patients younger than 60 years with high activity demands and increased life expectancy has raised concerns related to bearing surfaces. A higher prevalence of periprosthetic osteolysis and aseptic loosening has been observed in these patients. These concerns have prompted the search for bearing surfaces with favorable wear properties that minimize wear rates and decrease adverse local tissue reactions to particulate debris. The current success rates of THA are largely the result of improvements in bony integration surfaces, sterilization processes, and articular surface properties that have resulted in increased implant longevity. However, these advancements in implant design have brought new challenges. To address articular wear, a wide variety of bearing surfaces has been used with varied success. Surface materials include polytetrafluoroethylene, ultra-high–molecular-weight polyethylene (UHMWPE, including variations such as carbon fiber–reinforced and extended chain recrystallized), ceramics, titanium alloys (including nitrided and ion-implanted versions), cobalt-chromium (CoCr) alloys, oxygen diffusion–hardened zirconium alloy, and highly cross-linked polyethylene (XLPE).

Research over the past two decades has resulted in better understanding of the mechanisms of bearing surface wear, joint lubrication, osteolysis, and local tissue reactions to particulate and ionic debris. In joint arthroplasty, bearing surface wear occurs at the articular surface, which may be affected by adjacent and remote modular junctions. The variables that affect articular wear include implant design factors (materials, geometry, manufacture), environmental factors (patient-related factors such as bone structure and quality, weight, and activity level), and combined factors (implant position, surgical technique, third-body interactions). Design requirements for successful joint arthroplasty articulation include minimization of contact stresses, optimization of the contact area, optimization of constraint, maintenance of an acceptable range of motion, and preferably fluid film lubrication. Even with the best-conceived implant designs, wear performance often is compromised by factors such as impingement, third-body damage (cement, bone, and metal particles), and the breakdown of lubricating surfaces. Precision is essential in manufacturing because mismatches in congruency of articular couples can result in early wear, and poor locking mechanisms and roughened surfaces can cause backside wear (**Figure 1**). The goal is to minimize the generation of wear debris, which will decrease adverse local tissue reactions, including osteolysis, necrosis, and pseudotumors.

Terminology

An understanding of the terminology associated with tribology is fundamental in the discussion of bearing surfaces and wear properties in joint arthroplasty. The process resulting in loss of material as a consequence of two surfaces rubbing against one another is known as wear. Types of wear relevant to THA include adhesion, abrasion,

Dr. Jacobs or an immediate family member has stock or stock options held in Implant Protection; has received research or institutional support from Medtronic, NuVasive, and Zimmer Biomet; and serves as a board member, owner, officer, or committee member of The Hip Society. Dr. Levine or an immediate family member serves as a paid consultant to Link Orthopaedics, McGraw-Hill, OrthoView, and Zimmer Biomet; has received research or institutional support from Zimmer Biomet; and serves as a board member, owner, officer, or committee member of the American Association of Hip and Knee Surgeons and Council of Orthropaedic Residency Directors. Neither Dr. Balkissoon nor any immediate family member has received anything of value from or has stock or stock options held in a commercial company or institution related directly or indirectly to the subject of this chapter.

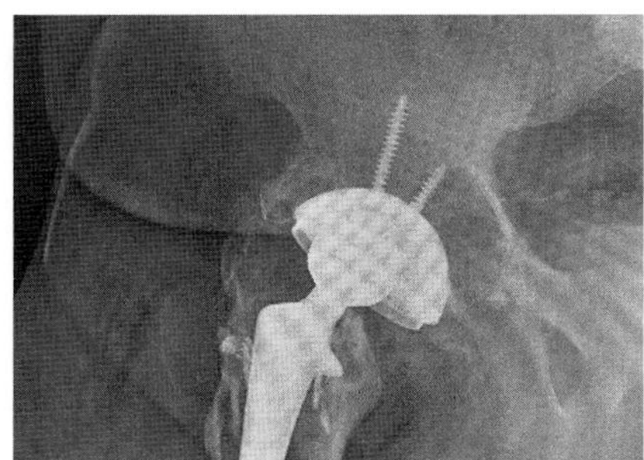

Figure 1 AP radiograph of a right hip demonstrates massive retroacetabular osteolysis. The acetabular cup used in this patient has been found to have a weak locking mechanism that results in substantial backside wear and is often associated with osteolysis.

third-body wear, fatigue, and tribocorrosion. Adhesion occurs when material is transferred from the weaker surface to the stronger surface in the bearing couple during loading. Abrasion occurs when asperities in the material of the stronger surface cut the surface of the weaker material. Fatigue wear occurs when local strains result in subsurface stresses that cause delamination after repetitive cycling. Third-body involvement occurs when trapped particulate debris results in increased local stress concentrations, which also contribute to fatigue-type wear. Tribocorrosion is the synergistic combination of mechanical and electrochemical processes that occur on a metal surface in contact with other surfaces.

Because of the favorable lubrication properties of articular cartilage, a native human hip joint has a low coefficient of friction, ranging from 0.002 to 0.04. The goal of joint arthroplasty is to re-create the process of elastohydrodynamic lubrication. In this process, the surfaces of the loaded joint experience elastic strain with a constant film separating the surfaces at all times, such that the lubricant properties of the film determine the coefficient of friction. This lubrication minimizes direct contact of the bearing surfaces and thereby minimizes wear. Historically, THA articulations have exhibited boundary lubrication, whereby the loading forces at the hip joint create an environment in which the synovial fluid does not fully separate the bearing surfaces. Accelerated wear resulting from suboptimal lubrication may affect long-term outcomes and the generation of adverse local tissue reactions.

Material properties of the bearing largely determine the wear properties of a particular articulation. The surface roughness of a material refers to the average deviation measured from the center line along the surface; a low value is ideal for an articular bearing. Scratching and wear increase the surface roughness of a material. The modulus of elasticity of a material measures its resistance to elastic deformation when a force is applied to it. The hardness of a material is a numeric value indicating the ability of the material to resist plastic deformation. Scratch resistance is directly related to the hardness of a material. Among joint arthroplasty materials, ceramics have greater scratch resistance than CoCr, which has greater scratch resistance than titanium. Yield strength refers to the level of stress a material experiences before it undergoes plastic deformation. Wettability is the ability to maintain contact between a liquid and a surface as a result of the molecular interactions between the liquid and the surface, determined by a balance of adhesive and cohesive forces. An ideal bearing surface would be wettable and have high scratch resistance, hardness, and yield strength.

Particle-Induced Osteolysis

A brief introduction to the pathogenesis of wear-induced periprosthetic osteolysis provides a framework for understanding the rationale of the so-called alternative bearing surfaces. The process of wear generates primarily polyethylene particles that vary in shape from spheroids to fibrils and range in size from 0.1 μm to several millimeters. Local macrophages respond to particles that can be phagocytosed, whereas giant cells form around larger particles. Local cellular activity incites a cascade of events that can ultimately result in local osteolysis (**Figure 2**). Tissue histology surrounding failed implants as a result of particulate-induced osteolysis demonstrates a chronic granulomatous inflammatory response characterized by macrophages, fibroblasts, foreign-body giant cells, and lymphocytes in a connective tissue matrix. Chemical mediators that have been isolated from tissue surrounding aseptic, failed arthroplasty implants notably include tumor necrosis factor α (TNF-α) and interleukin 1 (IL-1), which stimulate osteoclast differentiation and maturation via a marked increase in expression of receptor-activated nuclear factor–κB ligand (RANKL) and its receptor (receptor-activated nuclear factor–κB [RANK]), and matrix metalloproteinases, which are responsible for bone matrix degradation. Activation of the RANK-RANKL pathway promotes osteoclastogenesis, resulting in local overactivity of osteoclasts; particulate debris also can downregulate osteoblastic activity. Together, these processes can result in periprosthetic osteolysis. Clinically, wear-induced osteolysis is usually silent; however, in advanced stages it can result in pain, implant instability, major local bone loss, and catastrophic failure of implants requiring revision arthroplasty. Thus, minimizing wear in THA is of utmost importance to enhance implant longevity.

Bearing Surfaces

Polyethylene

CONVENTIONAL UHMWPE

Conventional UHMWPE, the first successful bearing surface with favorable wear properties, previously dominated the joint arthroplasty market and was widely used in THA. Polyethylene is a repeating chain of ethylene monomer molecules. Ultra-high–molecular-weight refers to the molecular weight, chain length, and arrangement of polymer chains. The condensed polymers have crystalline lamellae interspersed with amorphous regions. The crystalline lamellae are connected to one another by tie molecules that provide additional strength and means for load transfer. Conventional UHMWPE has been used extensively in THA, and numerous long-term follow-up studies have reported good results in wear, osteolysis, and subsequent aseptic loosening (**Figure 3**). Recent studies evaluating the long-term performance of UHMWPE in THA demonstrate survival rates of up to 89% at 10 years and 60% at 15 years postoperatively. In THA, research has focused on improving the material properties of UHMWPE because most wear debris originates from the polyethylene component.

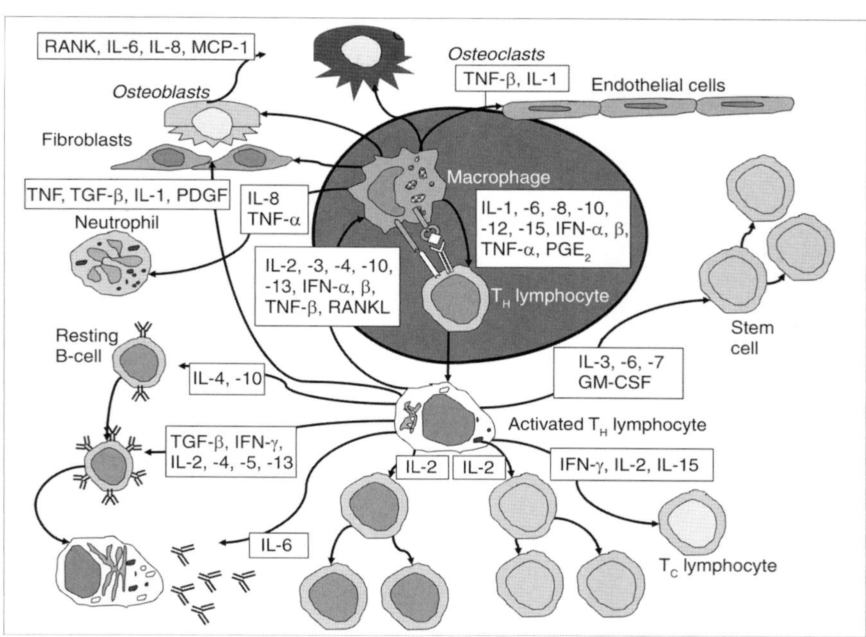

Figure 2 Diagram depicts the complex interrelationship of wear products and the cells of the innate and adaptive immune systems. GM-CSF = granulocyte monocyte–colony-stimulating factor, IFN = interferon, IL = interleukin, MCP = monocyte chemoattractant protein, PDGF = platelet-derived growth factor, PGE_2 = prostaglandin E_2, RANKL = receptor-activated nuclear factor–κB ligand, T_C = cytotoxic T lymphocyte, TGF = transforming growth factor, T_H = T helper lymphocyte, TNF = tumor necrosis factor. (Reproduced from Jacobs JJ, Campbell PA, Konttinen YT; Implant Wear Symposium 2007 Biologic Work Group: How has the biologic reaction to wear particles changed with newer bearing surfaces? *J Am Acad Orthop Surg* 2008;16[suppl 1]:S49-S55.)

Linear wear rates of conventional UHMWPE have been reported to be 0.18 mm per year for the first 5 years postoperatively and 0.1 mm per year thereafter. Wear rates vary depending on patient age, activity level, adjacent joint degenerative changes, sterilization techniques, implant positioning, and implant design. Minimizing contact stresses in articular couples will minimize material wear. Researchers have found that maximal contact stress is lowered when the modulus of elasticity of UHMWPE is decreased, thickness is increased, and the articular surfaces have greater conformity. Despite the high inherent conformity of THA surfaces and typical clearance of approximately 0.1 mm, the implants generate approximately 100 million microscopic UHMWPE wear particles daily—a heavy burden of foreign debris on the local tissues. Using elasticity theory and finite element models, researchers have demonstrated that if perfect conformity at the articular couple is achieved, the contact stresses are independent of the modulus of elasticity of UHMWPE. With a fixed head size and larger inner diameter of the acetabular component, stresses are independent of UHMWPE thickness. However, with a fixed acetabular shell diameter and larger femoral head size, the contact stresses are reduced because the load is distributed over a greater area. This finding is particularly relevant because of the current emphasis on using larger-diameter femoral heads to improve stability in THA.

Femoral head size is an important consideration in the calculation of volumetric wear,

$$v = \pi r^2 w$$

where w = linear wear rate and r = radius of femoral head. Despite improved surface area contact and therefore better load distribution, larger femoral heads result in a substantial increase in volumetric wear. Three-dimensional finite element modeling has demonstrated that volumetric wear in THA increases 4% to 6% with each millimeter increase in femoral head size, in linear proportion to the diameter of the femoral head. Although dislocation rates are reportedly lower with larger-diameter femoral heads, clinicians must consider the long-term effects of wear, particulate debris generation, and osteolysis and the need for future revision surgery when choosing a femoral head size. Additionally, increasing femoral head size necessitates a decrease in thickness of the polyethylene liner for the same cup size. The minimum allowable thickness of the liner depends on factors such as wear resistance, locking mechanism

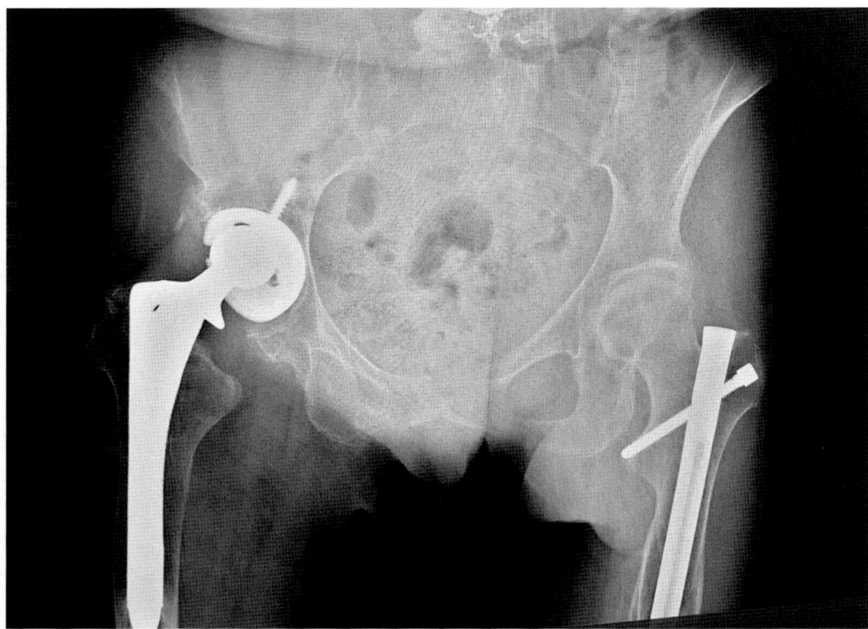

Figure 3 AP pelvic radiograph demonstrates substantial eccentric polyethylene wear of the arthroplasty implant in the right hip with migration and loss of fixation of the acetabular component at 18-year follow-up.

design, implant orientation (vertical cups demonstrate greater edge loading, wear, and contact forces), head diameter, and stiffness of the acetabular implant.

Implant manufacture can substantially affect wear. Several studies have demonstrated lower linear wear rates of liners manufactured with direct compression molding compared with those machined from extruded bar stock. The sterilization and packaging of UHMWPE also affect wear characteristics and survivorship. Early implants were irradiated with 2.5 to 4 Mrad (25 to 40 kGy) in a standard room-air environment. The gamma radiation sterilized the implants while creating intrasubstance free radicals from cleavage of the covalent bonds in the UHMWPE. The free radicals undergo oxidation in air, which results in truncation of the large polymer chains and a reduction in fracture strength. Oxidation occurs 0.5 to 2 mm below the implant surface (resulting in so-called white bands) and is responsible for fatigue cracks and delamination. Irradiation is now performed in inert environments to avoid the deleterious effects of oxidation. Alternatively, diffused ethylene oxide gas can be used for sterilization, but the process requires more than 40 hours to complete. A third technique, gas-plasma surface sterilization, takes between 1.2 and 4 hours and functions by oxidizing biologic matter. Studies have shown increased wear rates of UHMWPE sterilized with gamma radiation in air compared with UHMWPE sterilized with a gas-plasma technique (0.19 and 0.097 mm/yr, respectively).

Despite wear rates that may limit the long-term success of conventional UHMWPE in THA, a recent meta-analysis demonstrated similar clinical and radiographic outcomes of these implants compared with modern metal-on-metal implants. Patients with metal-on-metal implants were 3.37 times more likely than patients with UHMWPE implants to experience a complication. Similarly, in a randomized clinical trial comparing conventional UHMWPE with XLPE at 10-year follow-up, researchers found a lower wear rate in the XLPE group compared with the UHMWPE group (0.005 and 0.056 mm/yr, respectively) but no differences in cup migration, radiolucencies, or functional scores at latest follow-up. Despite adequate midterm and long-term results, conventional UHMWPE is limited by the concerns of premature polyethylene wear and periprosthetic osteolysis.

XLPE

As noted previously, the use of ionizing radiation to sterilize UHMWPE produces highly reactive free radicals. These free radicals combine with oxygen in the environment, resulting in chain scission and degradation of the mechanical and wear performance of the UHMWPE. However, when ionizing radiation is introduced in an oxygen-free environment, the free radicals are more likely to combine with free radicals on adjacent polymer chains, forming XLPE, which has a cross-linked molecular structure that has proved to be more resistant to wear. The results of many hip simulation studies indicate an inverse correlation between the dose of radiation and the rate of polyethylene wear. However, the reduction in wear is accompanied by decreased fatigue strength and fracture toughness of the polyethylene. The dose of radiation must be optimized to leverage the beneficial effects of cross-linking (reduction of wear) without substantially compromising other mechanical properties. Compared with the dose of gamma radiation used for sterilization of conventional UHMWPE, radiation doses of 5 to 10 Mrad (50 to 100 kGy) have shown improved wear properties in XLPE. No further improvements were noted with doses greater than 10 Mrad (100 kGy). Similarly, mechanical properties improved with doses of 5 to 7.5 Mrad (50 to 75 kGy) and decreased with higher doses of radiation. This improved wear performance has resulted in the widespread use of XLPE since its approval by the US FDA for use in THA in 1997. Advantages of XLPE include reduced articular wear rates, potential decreases in backside wear, and greater resistance to surface pitting and delamination.

Thermal treatment of UHMWPE affects the mechanical properties of the material. Thermal treatments such as remelting (heating above the melting-point temperature) or annealing (heating to just below the melting point) enhance cross-linking and reduce the presence of free radicals. Remelting better eliminates free radicals but results in a reduction in the mechanical and fatigue properties of the material, whereas annealing better maintains the mechanical properties at the cost of an increase in residual free radicals and subsequently increased oxidation in vivo. Changes in material properties may result in greater crack propagation and catastrophic failure, particularly in areas with thinner XLPE (**Figure 4**). Laboratory studies have shown a reduction in wear rates for femoral heads ranging in diameter from 22 to 46 mm with the use of XLPE compared with conventional polyethylene. Additional studies have confirmed reduced wear with XLPE compared with conventional UHMWPE and no difference in wear rates with 28- and 32-mm femoral heads. These findings have led to the adoption of larger-diameter femoral heads (36 mm or larger) in primary THA and the use of thinner polyethylene liners to reduce the rates of dislocation and limb-length discrepancy.

Further laboratory studies testing XLPE liners in adverse conditions, such as in the presence of third-body particles or with roughened femoral heads, have demonstrated favorable results in wear compared with conventional UHMWPE. Such testing also emphasizes the need for intraoperative protection of the femoral head and the importance of minimizing the potential for third-body wear. Another concern is related to implant positioning and the increased stress on the focal areas of XLPE liners. Vertical placement or malpositioning of acetabular implants can result in implant impingement, which can lead to fracture of thinner XLPE liners (**Figure 4**).

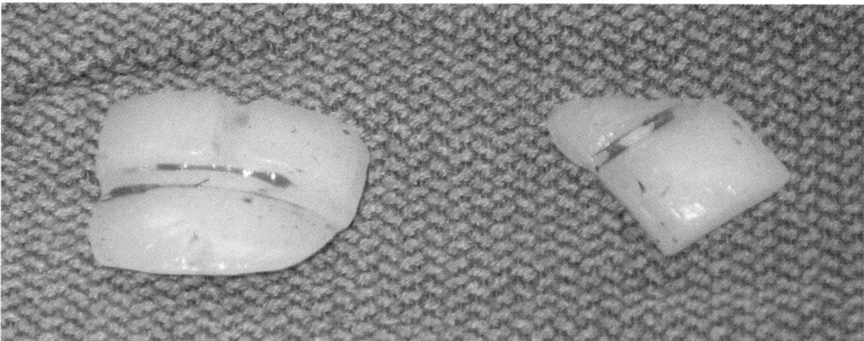

Figure 4 Clinical photograph shows a fractured highly cross-linked polyethylene liner that was used in a vertically placed acetabular cup. The fracture occurred at the locking ring cutout, which is the thinnest portion of the liner.

Currently available XLPE THA liners and dual-mobility femoral heads are fabricated by means of proprietary methods by each manufacturer. Clinical studies have shown equivalent functional and pain scores and significantly lower rates of polyethylene wear at mid-term follow-up. A recent prospective, double-blind, randomized controlled trial using radiostereometric analysis found significantly less linear wear at 10 years postoperatively in patients with XLPE liners than in patients with UHMWPE liners (0.003 mm/yr and 0.030 mm/yr, respectively; $P < 0.001$). The corresponding volumetric wear was significantly lower in the XLPE group (14 mm^3 and 98 mm^3, respectively), and no differences in Oxford Hip Score were found between groups. A review comparing linear wear rates of XLPE and conventional UHMWPE demonstrated a weighted average of 0.042 mm/yr for XLPE in 28 studies and a weighted average of 0.137 mm/yr for conventional UHMWPE in 18 studies. In addition, the authors of the study found an 87% reduction in risk of osteolysis with XLPE. A similar review highlighted overall wear reduction rates of 40% to 85% with the use of XLPE compared with conventional UHMWPE. Continued follow-up will be necessary to ensure that the trend toward the use of larger-diameter femoral heads with XLPE does not increase the rate of adverse long-term outcomes.

Manufacturing techniques such as sequential irradiation and annealing or doping with vitamin E may reduce wear without adversely affecting mechanical properties. Implants using some of these methods to enhance the performance of XLPE are commercially available. Ongoing research will determine whether these techniques ultimately reduce wear while maintaining favorable mechanical properties.

Ceramic

Ceramics are inorganic, chemically inert materials noted for their resistance, strength, biocompatibility, wettability, and high resistance to wear and corrosion. Compared with metal-on-polymer bearing surfaces, ceramics are an appealing option in THA because of their superior lubrication, smoother surfaces, and low susceptibility to third-body wear resulting from increased hardness. Ceramics are stiffer than the metal alloys currently used in THA and are therefore better able to maintain congruence, which allows for distribution of forces over a larger area and ultimately results in decreased wear. Furthermore, a surface protein monolayer develops in vivo and improves lubrication of the joint. Aluminum oxide (Al_2O_3) and zirconium oxide (ZrO_2) have been used in THA. Early ceramic designs demonstrated poor survivorship with failure rates of 16% to 25% at 10-year follow-up, which were attributed to high rates of aseptic loosening, and ceramic fracture, which occurred in up to 5% of patients. Modern improvements in material design have focused on reducing the grain size and inclusions while improving taper tolerances, yielding more successful ceramic-on-ceramic bearings. Numerous studies report favorable outcomes in THA for current ceramic-on-ceramic bearing options with 10-year survival rates of up to 98%; however, audible squeaking of implants is a concern. Linear wear rates of modern ceramic-on-ceramic couples are approximately 5 µm/yr, several orders of magnitude less than those of metal-on-polyethylene bearings.

ALUMINA-ON-ALUMINA

The favorable material properties of alumina support the trend toward the use of large-diameter femoral heads in THA to enhance stability because they have shown no clinically relevant increase in wear, a higher resistance to fracture, and a low potential for metal ion release. Furthermore, the use of alumina bearing surfaces results in less separation of the femoral head and the liner because of the wettability of the alumina surface. Long-term studies evaluating alumina ceramic-on-ceramic bearings in THA have shown favorable survival rates. The authors of one study reported a 20-year survival rate of 85.6% for 33 alumina noncemented acetabular cups with revision for any reason as the end point. The authors of a more recent series of 104 THAs with an alumina-on-alumina articulation documented a 98.9% survival rate at 15.9 years postoperatively, with good clinical results and no measurable wear or periprosthetic osteolysis and no implant fracture. However, 14 THAs in the study were lost to follow-up. Assuming revision for any cause of all 14 THAs lost to follow-up, the authors note an 85.5% survival rate at 15.9 years postoperatively.

Key limitations of ceramic-on-ceramic bearings in THA are well documented and have diminished their acceptance. Concerns include limited implant options and reports of implant fracture, chipping on insertion, and squeaking. Restoration of the normal anatomy and hip biomechanics is critically important in THA; however, intraoperative fine-tuning is limited by the restricted options available with ceramic-on-ceramic bearing surfaces, such as limited neck lengths and the lack of elevated rim liners.

Peripheral chipping of ceramic liners may occur intraoperatively as a result of forceful impaction of a liner that is not fully seated. This phenomenon has been observed in 1.2% of patients. Encasing the ceramic liner within a titanium sleeve substantially reduces the concern of insertional chipping and fracture but increases the risk of impingement. The risk of postoperative implant fracture is approximately 1 in 2,000 to 3,000 for femoral heads and 1 in 6,000 to 8,000 for acetabular liners. One manufacturer noted the following trends in fracture risk on the basis of information from nearly 2 million distributed implants: 83% of fractures occur within 36 months of implantation, femoral heads are more likely to fracture than acetabular liners are, 28-mm femoral heads have greater rates of fracture than 32-mm and 36-mm femoral heads have, and femoral heads have greater rates of fracture when used with very short or very long femoral necks. Revision surgery after implant fracture requires thorough synovectomy and complete debris removal to avoid substantial future third-body wear. Typically, in patients undergoing revision, a new ceramic femoral head should be paired with a metal sleeve to avoid mating a ceramic femoral head with a damaged trunnion taper and either a new ceramic liner or a polyethylene liner.

A common concern with alumina-on-alumina bearings is squeaking, reported in 0.45% to 7% of patients. The squeaking phenomenon has been linked to edge loading and stripe wear resulting from microseparation of the femoral head and the liner. This scenario is typically associated with acetabular malpositioning, failure to restore hip biomechanics, and impingement. However, multiple factors have been cited as the cause of squeaking in THAs with ceramic-on-ceramic bearings. Laboratory simulation of roughened articular surfaces and dry articulations causing microseparation as well as retrieval studies have confirmed that squeaking occurs in the presence of stripe wear and edge loading.

ZIRCONIA-ALUMINA COMPOSITE

The addition of zirconia to alumina ceramic bearings affords better resistance to crack propagation and improved ability to dissipate energy. The latest zirconia-alumina ceramic bearings are composed of 82% alumina, 17% ZrO_2, 0.3% chromium oxide, and 0.6% strontium oxide. This composite offers improved fracture toughness, burst strength, and four-point bend strength and maintains the same surface hardness as its alumina predecessors. Implant fracture rates with the use of zirconia-alumina bearings have been reported to decline from 0.086% to 0.025% for acetabular liners and from 0.18% to 0.0013% for femoral heads, compared with prior alumina-only ceramic bearings.

Ceramic-on-Polyethylene

Both alumina and zirconia femoral heads have an extensive history of use with polyethylene liners in THA. Historically, alumina femoral heads had a better track record because of reports of fracture of zirconia heads related to a manufacturing process and because a phase transformation of zirconia can occur over time, leading to accelerated wear. Current studies of ceramic-on-polyethylene bearings have revealed mixed results compared with those of metal-on-polyethylene bearings. However, ceramic femoral heads remain a preferred option in patients younger than 60 years because of the favorable biomaterial properties of these femoral heads. The risk of fracture of ceramic femoral heads paired with polyethylene liners has been found to be lower than that of ceramic femoral heads paired with ceramic liners, and ceramics are generally more resistant to third-body wear than CoCr. The wear of ceramic-on-polyethylene bearings is substantially less than that of metal-on-polyethylene bearings. A recent comparison of early wear rates between ceramic-on-ceramic bearings and ceramic-on-polyethylene bearings in patients undergoing THA revealed a linear wear rate of 30.5 µm/yr with no radiographic sign of wear in 44.9% of patients in the ceramic-on-ceramic group compared with a linear wear rate of 218.2 µm/yr and no radiographic sign of wear in 6% of patients in the ceramic-on-polyethylene group. However, squeaking was a problem in 3.1% of patients in the ceramic-on-ceramic group, whereas no patients in the ceramic-on-polyethylene group experienced implant-related noise. Ceramic-on-polyethylene bearings have seen a recent surge in usage because of the increasing awareness of mechanically assisted crevice corrosion occurring with modular CoCr alloy femoral heads.

Metal-on-Metal (CoCr)

Originally used in the early 1960s, metal-on-metal bearings fell out of favor because of high rates of implant loosening and concerns regarding biologic reaction to the alloy constituents. Interest in metal-on-metal articulations was renewed in the late 1980s because of concerns regarding polyethylene wear debris from metal-on-polyethylene articulations, particularly because hip simulator studies demonstrated substantially improved articular surface wear rates of metal-on-metal bearings. Commercially available metal-on-metal bearing surfaces use a CoCr alloy combined with molybdenum, which enhances the CoCr alloy by decreasing grain size and increasing strength. CoCr alloys are among the strongest, hardest, and most fatigue resistant of the metals used for arthroplasty implants. CoCr alloys also are more corrosion resistant than stainless steel. Carbon is sometimes added in smaller amounts in the form of carbide, which strengthens the metal and improves wear resistance.

Favorable material properties of metal bearings, like those of ceramics, include strength and rigidity that afford the ability to use large-diameter femoral heads with thinner liners than can be used with metal-on-polyethylene bearings. Large-diameter femoral heads enhance stability and reduce dislocation rates. Large metal femoral heads are also more likely to develop an optimal mode of lubrication, which will minimize articular wear. Smaller femoral head sizes may result in suboptimal lubrication and a greater likelihood of adhesive and abrasive wear.

Modern metal-on-metal implant designs have demonstrated wear rates and particulate debris generation that are drastically lower than those of metal-on-polymer articulations in THA. The use of metal-on-metal bearing surfaces also has resulted in the reemergence of hip resurfacing arthroplasty, which offers the potential advantage of femoral bone preservation. A potential complication related to the use of large metal femoral heads is higher frictional torque and corrosion at the femoral head-neck junction (**Figure 5**). This finding may explain the trunnion-related problems (mechanically assisted crevice corrosion and locally related adverse tissue reactions) seen more frequently with metal-on-metal bearings in THA than in resurfacing procedures. The process of wear in metal-on-metal THA has two distinct phases. The initial period, called the run-in phase, consists of relatively elevated initial wear for up to 2×10^6 cycles. The run-in phase is followed by a steady-state phase, during which wear stabilizes at a much lower rate, reported to range from 1 to 5 µm/yr for typical metal-on-metal articulations. The wear of metal-on-metal bearings in THA is 2% of the wear seen under similar conditions with metal-on-polyethylene implants using conventional UHMWPE. Also contributing to lower wear rates is the ability of metal-on-metal bearings to self-polish surface asperities, which improves the initial surface finish to a highly polished surface with decreased friction.

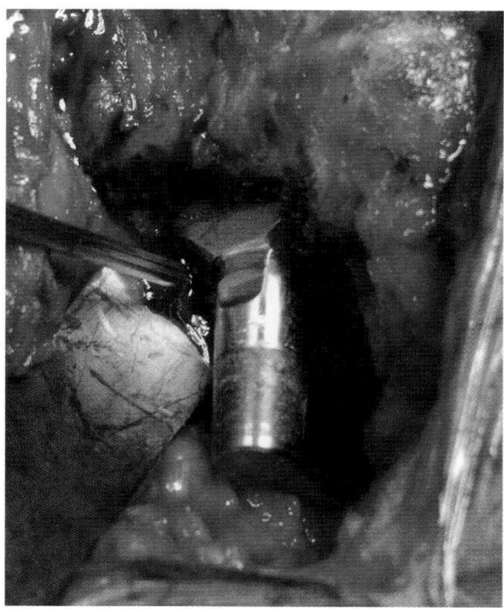

Figure 5 Intraoperative photograph shows corrosion of the femoral neck in a failed metal-on-metal total hip arthroplasty implant. Increased frictional torque and mechanically assisted crevice corrosion are thought to be responsible for this trunnion damage.

The favorable attributes of metal-on-metal bearings in THA are supported by numerous studies demonstrating excellent implant durability at midterm follow-up. However, concerns with the

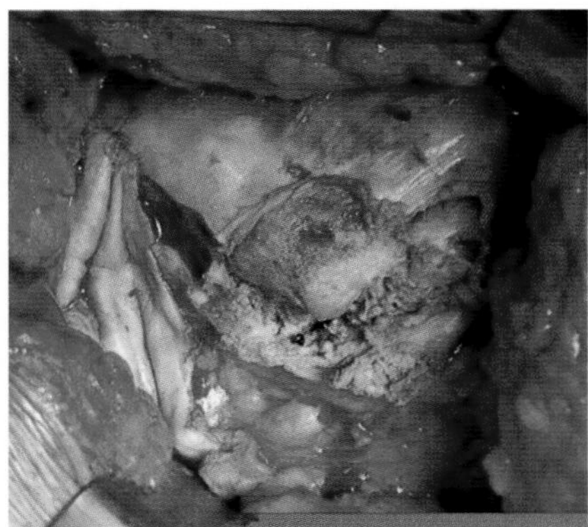

Figure 6 Intraoperative photograph shows a pseudotumor in a patient undergoing revision total hip arthroplasty after failure of a metal-on-metal implant.

use of metal-on-metal bearings have become apparent. Recently, multiple metal-on-metal implant designs have demonstrated high rates of catastrophic failure in THA. THA designs using monoblock CoCr acetabular implants have demonstrated poor implant fixation, possible deformation on insertion, and unacceptably high rates of early failure. These findings have led to the recall of multiple metal-on-metal THA and hip resurfacing arthroplasty devices. Also, accelerated wear and corrosion can occur with modern metal-on-metal THA designs under conditions such as implant malposition.

Patients undergoing conventional metal-on-polyethylene THA have been found to have elevated serum metal ion levels, not from passive dissolution, but from taper corrosion of modular implants. With metal-on-metal THA, these levels are further increased by metal debris generated at the articular surface. In patients with a well-functioning metal-on-metal THA implant, serum metal levels tend to increase in the first 6 months postoperatively, peak at 4 to 5 years postoperatively, and then decrease to a steady-state level that is elevated from the norm. Healthy control subjects have been shown to have a mean serum cobalt level of 0.24 µg/L and a mean serum chromium level of 0.28 µg/L. Safe serum metal ion levels for cobalt and chromium have been difficult to define. Serum cobalt levels after metal-on-metal joint arthroplasty typically range from 1 to 2 µg/L, elevated compared with that of healthy control subjects.

Metal particles from metal-on-metal bearings are smaller than debris generated from metal-on-polyethylene bearings. As a result, the total number of particles released from metal-on-metal articular couples is greater than 100 times the amount released from conventional bearings. Locally, the pattern of inflammation seen in periarticular tissues surrounding metal-on-metal implants is distinctly different from that seen in tissues surrounding metal-on-polyethylene bearings and is characterized by perivascular lymphocytic infiltration, the clinical relevance of which remains unclear. Local reactions to CoCr particles have been described as metallosis, aseptic lymphocyte-dominated vasculitis-associated lesions, adverse reaction to metal debris, adverse local tissue reactions, and pseudotumors (**Figure 6**). Direct or indirect DNA damage as well as genomic instability may occur in the presence of metal wear debris via a chemical effect of CoCr particles. However, no direct correlation has been established between elevated serum cobalt and chromium levels and the risk of development of malignant tumors. Additionally, changes in lymphocyte counts have been noted in patients with elevated serum cobalt and chromium levels. Serum metal levels are associated with transplacental transfer and are present in the milk of breast-feeding mothers but have not been linked to teratogenic effects. Further epidemiologic studies are needed to better clarify the clinical relevance of these concerns.

Local tissue reactions range from small fluid collections to massive destructive lesions. Pseudotumors have been observed in up to 42% of patients who are asymptomatic after metal-on-metal THA and can result in compression of local neurovascular bundles, hip abductor dysfunction, and/or a large potential dead space after excision. Management of these difficult masses can be challenging, depending on the extent of bone and soft-tissue destruction. Recently, recommendations for the surveillance and management of metal-on-metal THA have been proposed by the American Association of Hip and Knee Surgeons, the American Academy of Orthopaedic Surgeons, and The Hip Society on the basis of a consensus of expert practitioners. The risk stratification and management recommendations are based on patient factors, patient symptoms, clinical examination, implant type, radiographs, infection workup, serum metal ion testing, and cross-sectional imaging. Although revision rates vary, widespread warnings and recalls have led to a dramatic decrease in the use of metal-on-metal implants. At the peak of their use in 2007, nearly one-third of primary THA procedures in the United States used metal-on-metal implants, whereas their use decreased to 10% of THA procedures in 2010 and to 1% in 2012. Because of the substantial concerns with the use of metal-on-metal bearings and the known and unknown consequences of metal debris, the indications for the use of metal-on-metal bearings are limited. For hip resurfacing arthroplasty, the only bearing couple commercially available in the United States is metal-on-metal, and its use may be indicated in patients with characteristics matching those of patient populations in whom results of the procedure have been satisfactory, such as men younger than 60 years with osteoarthritis.

Summary

The new bearing surfaces in THA implants have demonstrated improved wear performance compared with that of conventional metal-on-polyethylene articulations. However, each of the newer low-wear bearing couples has potential drawbacks, including diminished fracture toughness (XLPE and ceramic-on-ceramic bearing surfaces) and elevated systemic metal levels (metal-on-metal bearing surfaces). These concerns, together with the lack of long-term clinical evidence definitively demonstrating improved function or survival, have tempered the enthusiasm for widespread use of these couples, with the exception of XLPE, which almost universally demonstrates favorable wear rates and low rates of osteolysis. Determination of the ultimate safety and efficacy of the newer bearing couples will require long-term studies, including survivorship and outcome data from national implant registries and adequately powered, high-quality clinical trials.

Bibliography

Amanatullah DF, Landa J, Strauss EJ, Garino JP, Kim SH, Di Cesare PE: Comparison of surgical outcomes and implant wear between ceramic-ceramic and ceramic-polyethylene articulations in total hip arthroplasty. *J Arthroplasty* 2011;26(6 suppl):72-77.

American Academy of Orthopaedic Surgeons: *Current Concerns With Metal-on-Metal Hip Arthroplasty.* Rosemont, IL, American Academy of Orthopaedic Surgeons, 2012. Available at: http://www.aaos.org/about/papers/advistmt/1035.asp. Accessed August 1, 2016.

Aqil A, Sidiqui M: A critical appraisal of the evidence regarding the choice of common bearing couples available for total hip arthroplasty. *J Pak Med Assoc* 2012;62(8):829-834.

Bartel DL, Bicknell VL, Wright TM: The effect of conformity, thickness, and material on stresses in ultra-high molecular weight components for total joint replacement. *J Bone Joint Surg Am* 1986;68(7):1041-1051.

Bernstein M, Desy NM, Petit A, Zukor DJ, Huk OL, Antoniou J: Long-term follow-up and metal ion trend of patients with metal-on-metal total hip arthroplasty. *Int Orthop* 2012;36(9):1807-1812.

Blumenfeld TJ, McKellop HA, Schmalzried TP, Billi F: Fracture of a cross-linked polyethylene liner: A multifactorial issue. *J Arthroplasty* 2011;26(4):666.e5-666.e8.

Bosker BH, Ettema HB, Boomsma MF, Kollen BJ, Maas M, Verheyen CC: High incidence of pseudotumour formation after large-diameter metal-on-metal total hip replacement: A prospective cohort study. *J Bone Joint Surg Br* 2012;94(6):755-761.

Bozic KJ, Browne J, Dangles CJ, et al: Modern metal-on-metal hip implants. *J Am Acad Orthop Surg* 2012;20(6):402-406.

Brown TD, Bartel DL; Implant Wear Symposium 2007 Engineering Work Group: What design factors influence wear behavior at the bearing surfaces in total joint replacements? *J Am Acad Orthop Surg* 2008;16(suppl 1):S101-S106.

Cai P, Hu Y, Xie J: Large-diameter Delta ceramic-on-ceramic versus common-sized ceramic-on-polyethylene bearings in THA. *Orthopedics* 2012;35(9):e1307-e1313.

Callaghan JJ, Forest EE, Sporer SM, Goetz DD, Johnston RC: Total hip arthroplasty in the young adult. *Clin Orthop Relat Res* 1997;344:257-262.

Calvert GT, Devane PA, Fielden J, Adams K, Horne JG: A double-blind, prospective, randomized controlled trial comparing highly cross-linked and conventional polyethylene in primary total hip arthroplasty. *J Arthroplasty* 2009;24(4):505-510.

Campbell DG, Field JR, Callary SA: Second-generation highly cross-linked X3™ polyethylene wear: A preliminary radiostereometric analysis study. *Clin Orthop Relat Res* 2010;468(10):2704-2709.

Charnley J, Halley DK: Rate of wear in total hip replacement. *Clin Orthop Relat Res* 1975;112:170-179.

Chevillotte C, Pibarot V, Carret JP, Bejui-Hugues J, Guyen O: Hip squeaking: A 10-year follow-up study. *J Arthroplasty* 2012;27(6):1008-1013.

Corten K, MacDonald SJ: Hip resurfacing data from national joint registries: What do they tell us? What do they not tell us? *Clin Orthop Relat Res* 2010;468(2):351-357.

D'Antonio JA, Capello WN, Manley MT, Naughton M, Sutton K: A titanium-encased alumina ceramic bearing for total hip arthroplasty: 3- to 5-year results. *Clin Orthop Relat Res* 2005;441:151-158.

D'Antonio JA, Sutton K: Ceramic materials as bearing surfaces for total hip arthroplasty. *J Am Acad Orthop Surg* 2009;17(2):63-68.

deSouza RM, Wallace D, Costa ML, Krikler SJ: Transplacental passage of metal ions in women with hip resurfacing: No teratogenic effects observed. *Hip Int* 2012;22(1):96-99.

Dumbleton JH, Manley MT: Metal-on-metal total hip replacement: What does the literature say? *J Arthroplasty* 2005;20(2):174-188.

Garino J, Rahaman MN, Bal BS: The reliability of modern alumina bearings in total hip arthroplasty. *Semin Arthroplasty* 2006;17(3-4):113-119.

Geerdink CH, Grimm B, Vencken W, Heyligers IC, Tonino AJ: Cross-linked compared with historical polyethylene in THA: An 8-year clinical study. *Clin Orthop Relat Res* 2009;467(4):979-984.

Glyn-Jones S, Thomas GE, Garfjeld-Roberts P, et al: Highly crosslinked polyethylene in total hip arthroplasty decreases long-term wear: A double-blind randomized trial. *Clin Orthop Relat Res* 2015;473(2):432-438.

Haddad FS, Thakrar RR, Hart AJ, et al: Metal-on-metal bearings: The evidence so far. *J Bone Joint Surg Br* 2011;93(5):572-579.

Hamadouche M, Boutin P, Daussange J, Bolander ME, Sedel L: Alumina-on-alumina total hip arthroplasty: A minimum 18.5-year follow-up study. *J Bone Joint Surg Am* 2002;84(1):69-77.

Hannouche D, Hamadouche M, Nizard R, Bizot P, Meunier A, Sedel L: Ceramics in total hip replacement. *Clin Orthop Relat Res* 2005;430:62-71.

Hermida JC, Bergula A, Chen P, Colwell CW Jr, D'Lima DD: Comparison of the wear rates of twenty-eight and thirty-two-millimeter femoral heads on cross-linked polyethylene acetabular cups in a wear simulator. *J Bone Joint Surg Am* 2003;85(12):2325-2331.

Holt G, Murnaghan C, Reilly J, Meek RM: The biology of aseptic osteolysis. *Clin Orthop Relat Res* 2007;460:240-252.

Hopper RH Jr, Young AM, Orishimo KF, Engh CA Jr: Effect of terminal sterilization with gas plasma or gamma radiation on wear of polyethylene liners. *J Bone Joint Surg Am* 2003;85(3):464-468.

Jacobs JJ, Skipor AK, Patterson LM, et al: Metal release in patients who have had a primary total hip arthroplasty: A prospective, controlled, longitudinal study. *J Bone Joint Surg Am* 1998;80(10):1447-1458.

Jasty MJ, Floyd WE III, Schiller AL, Goldring SR, Harris WH: Localized osteolysis in stable, non-septic total hip replacement. *J Bone Joint Surg Am* 1986;68(6):912-919.

Jazrawi LM, Kummer FJ, DiCesare PE: Alternative bearing surfaces for total joint arthroplasty. *J Am Acad Orthop Surg* 1998;6(4):198-203.

Johanson PE, Digas G, Herberts P, Thanner J, Kärrholm J: Highly crosslinked polyethylene does not reduce aseptic loosening in cemented THA 10-year findings of a randomized study. *Clin Orthop Relat Res* 2012;470(11):3083-3093.

Kang BJ, Ha YC, Ham DW, Hwang SC, Lee YK, Koo KH: Third-generation alumina-on-alumina total hip arthroplasty: 14 to 16-year follow-up study. *J Arthroplasty* 2015;30(3):411-415.

Kurtz SM, Gawel HA, Patel JD: History and systematic review of wear and osteolysis outcomes for first-generation highly crosslinked polyethylene. *Clin Orthop Relat Res* 2011;469(8):2262-2277.

Kwon YM, Lombardi AV, Jacobs JJ, Fehring TK, Lewis CG, Cabanela ME: Risk stratification algorithm for management of patients with metal-on-metal hip arthroplasty: Consensus statement of the American Association of Hip and Knee Surgeons, the American Academy of Orthopaedic Surgeons, and the Hip Society. *J Bone Joint Surg Am* 2014;96(1):e4.

Lachiewicz PF, Geyer MR: The use of highly cross-linked polyethylene in total knee arthroplasty. *J Am Acad Orthop Surg* 2011;19(3):143-151.

Lehil MS, Bozic KJ: Trends in total hip arthroplasty implant utilization in the United States. *J Arthroplasty* 2014;29(10):1915-1918.

Levine BR, Singh K, Jacobs JJ: Bearing surface materials for hip and knee replacement, in Cannada LK, ed: *Orthopaedic Knowledge Update 11*. Rosemont, IL, American Academy of Orthopaedic Surgeons, 2014, pp 61-75.

Malviya A, Ramaskandhan JR, Bowman R, et al: What advantage is there to be gained using large modular metal-on-metal bearings in routine primary hip replacement? A preliminary report of a prospective randomised controlled trial. *J Bone Joint Surg Br* 2011;93(12):1602-1609.

Malviya A, Ramaskandhan J, Holland JP, Lingard EA: Metal-on-metal total hip arthroplasty. *J Bone Joint Surg Am* 2010;92(7):1675-1683.

Massin P, Lopes R, Masson B, Mainard D; French Hip & Knee Society (SFHG): Does Biolox Delta ceramic reduce the rate of component fractures in total hip replacement? *Orthop Traumatol Surg Res* 2014;100(6 suppl):S317-S321.

Maxian TA, Brown TD, Pedersen DR, Callaghan JJ: A sliding-distance-coupled finite element formulation for polyethylene wear in total hip arthroplasty. *J Biomech* 1996;29(5):687-692.

McAuley JP, Szuszczewicz ES, Young A, Engh CA Sr: Total hip arthroplasty in patients 50 years and younger. *Clin Orthop Relat Res* 2004;418:119-125.

Meding JB, Keating EM, Davis KE: Acetabular UHMWPE survival and wear changes with different manufacturing techniques. *Clin Orthop Relat Res* 2011;469(2):405-411.

Meyer H, Mueller T, Goldau G, Chamaon K, Ruetschi M, Lohmann CH: Corrosion at the cone/taper interface leads to failure of large-diameter metal-on-metal total hip arthroplasties. *Clin Orthop Relat Res* 2012;470(11):3101-3108.

Milošev I, Kovač S, Trebše R, Levašič V, Pišot V: Comparison of ten-year survivorship of hip prostheses with use of conventional polyethylene, metal-on-metal, or ceramic-on-ceramic bearings. *J Bone Joint Surg Am* 2012;94(19):1756-1763.

Muratoglu OK, Kurtz SM: Alternative bearing surfaces in hip replacement, in Sinha RK, ed: *Hip Replacement: Current Trends and Controversies.* New York, NY, Marcel Dekker, 2002, pp 1-46.

Mutimer J, Devane PA, Adams K, Horne JG: Highly crosslinked polyethylene reduces wear in total hip arthroplasty at 5 years. *Clin Orthop Relat Res* 2010;468(12):3228-3233.

Nikolaou VS, Petit A, Debiparshad K, Huk OL, Zukor DJ, Antoniou J: Metal-on-metal total hip arthroplasty: Five- to 11-year follow-up. *Bull NYU Hosp Jt Dis* 2011;69(suppl 1):S77-S83.

Parfitt DJ, Wood SN, Chick CM, Lewis P, Rashid MH, Evans AR: Common femoral vein thrombosis caused by a metal-on-metal hip arthroplasty-related pseudotumor. *J Arthroplasty* 2012;27(8):1581.e9-1581.e11.

Rieker CB, Schön R, Köttig P: Development and validation of a second-generation metal-on-metal bearing: Laboratory studies and analysis of retrievals. *J Arthroplasty* 2004;19(8 suppl 3):5-11.

Silva M, Heisel C, McKellop H, Schmalzried TP: Bearing surfaces, in Callaghan JJ, Rosenberg AG, Rubash HE, eds: *The Adult Hip*, ed 2. Philadelphia, PA, Lippincott Williams & Wilkins, 2007, vol 1, pp 247-266.

Small SR, Berend ME, Howard LA, Tunc D, Buckley CA, Ritter MA: Acetabular cup stiffness and implant orientation change acetabular loading patterns. *J Arthroplasty* 2013;28(2):359-367.

Voleti PB, Baldwin KD, Lee GC: Metal-on-metal vs conventional total hip arthroplasty: A systematic review and meta-analysis of randomized controlled trials. *J Arthroplasty* 2012;27(10):1844-1849.

Walter A: On the material and the tribology of alumina-alumina couplings for hip joint prostheses. *Clin Orthop Relat Res* 1992;282:31-46.

Walter WL, O'Toole GC, Walter WK, Ellis A, Zicat BA: Squeaking in ceramic-on-ceramic hips: The importance of acetabular component orientation. *J Arthroplasty* 2007;22(4):496-503.

Williams DH, Greidanus NV, Masri BA, Duncan CP, Garbuz DS: Prevalence of pseudotumor in asymptomatic patients after metal-on-metal hip arthroplasty. *J Bone Joint Surg Am* 2011;93(23):2164-2171.

Ziaee H, Daniel J, Datta AK, Blunt S, McMinn DJ: Transplacental transfer of cobalt and chromium in patients with metal-on-metal hip arthroplasty: A controlled study. *J Bone Joint Surg Br* 2007;89(3):301-305.

Chapter 18
Optimizing Stability and Limb Length

C. Anderson Engh, Jr, MD

Introduction

Instability and limb-length discrepancy are common complications after total hip arthroplasty (THA). Hip dislocation has been reported to be the most common cause of revision surgery after THA. The 6-month postoperative dislocation rate is 2%. Not all patients who experience dislocations will require revision surgery. Dislocation is a multifactorial problem influenced by patient factors, surgical technique, and implant design. The surgical approach is among the most important factors influencing postoperative dislocation. Historically, the posterior approach has had the highest dislocation rate. However, the advent of posterior capsular repair has substantially reduced the rate of dislocation after THA performed via the posterior approach. The use of implants with large-diameter femoral heads in combination with cross-linked polyethylene has decreased the occurrence of dislocations. Historically, large-diameter femoral heads were associated with increased polyethylene wear and osteolysis, resulting in late failure. In the 1990s, the preferred femoral head size was 28 mm. Cross-linked polyethylene appears to be sufficiently wear resistant that 32- and 36-mm femoral heads can be used without the increased risk of osteolysis that is historically associated with large femoral heads.

Limb-length discrepancy is a common cause of patient dissatisfaction after THA, leading to malpractice claims. A change in limb length less than 1 cm is generally tolerated by a patient. However, if the limb is lengthened 1 cm or more, patients are more likely to complain and complications such as nerve injury, limp, and back pain are more frequent. Unlike dislocation, which is multifactorial and partially related to patient behavior, the change in limb length is related to the surgical procedure and, therefore, often is perceived as surgeon error. Occasionally, surgeons must compromise limb length to obtain stability of the hip joint. Sometimes the hip must be lengthened to obtain enough soft-tissue tension to avoid dislocation.

Postoperative limb-length difference and instability are interrelated complications. To minimize these complications, a successful THA requires a complete preoperative evaluation, including a thorough history, a physical examination, and radiographic studies; patient counseling; preoperative planning; and appropriate surgical technique.

Evaluation

Although most of the information related to stability and limb length is derived from the physical and radiographic evaluation, patient-related factors should be reviewed for every THA candidate. Patient factors that increase the risk of dislocation include alcohol or drug abuse and neurologic disorders. Patients with dementia, Parkinson disease, a previous stroke, or cerebral palsy may be unable to comply with postoperative instructions and have an increased risk for dislocation. Patients should be asked if they are aware of a limb-length difference and if they have spine or knee disease. Scoliosis, prior spine surgery, and spine stiffness can cause coronal or sagittal tilt of the pelvis, which may influence limb length and hip stability. As surgeons better understand the influence of sagittal pelvic tilt on hip stability, cup position parameters likely will change to match pelvic tilt.

Key components of the physical examination include gait observation, assessment of the hip range of motion (ROM; especially contractures), limb-length assessment, and a brief

Dr. Engh or an immediate family member has received royalties from, serves as a paid consultant to, and has stock or stock options held in DePuy Synthes; has received research or institutional support from DePuy Synthes and Smith & Nephew; and serves as a board member, owner, officer, or committee member of the American Academy of Orthopaedic Surgeons, the American Association of Hip and Knee Surgeons, and The Hip Society.

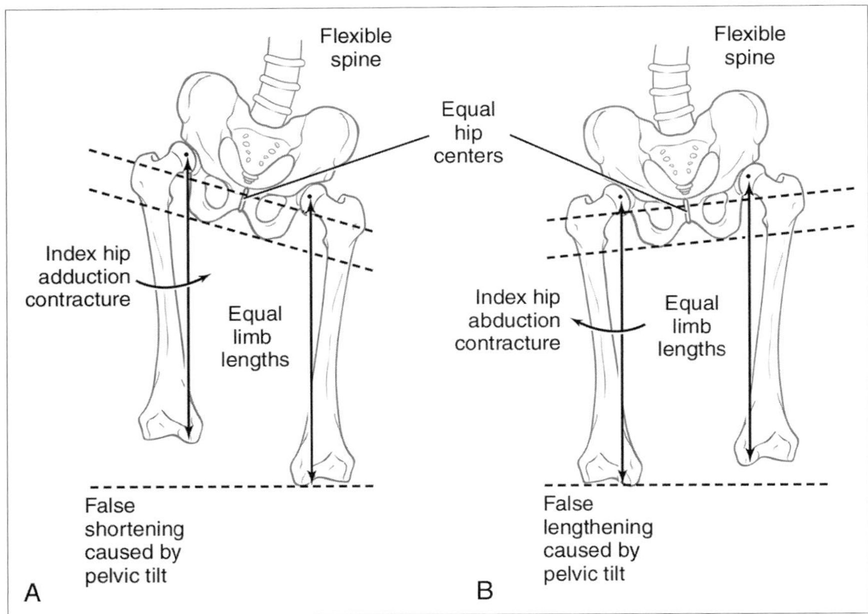

Figure 1 **A,** Illustration shows a hip adduction contracture, which causes a patient to perceive the involved leg as shortened. **B,** Illustration shows a hip abduction contracture, which causes a patient to perceive the involved leg as lengthened. If a patient has a flexible spine, these false limb-length differences should not be corrected with implants. After surgery, the contracture will resolve, the spine will adjust, and limb lengths will be equal. (Reproduced from Engh CA Sr: Optimizing stability and limb length, in Lieberman JR, Berry DJ, eds: *Advanced Reconstruction: Hip*. Rosemont, IL, American Academy of Orthopaedic Surgeons, 2005, pp 105-112.)

examination of the spine. Analysis of a patient's gait should include more than just an observation for an antalgic or Trendelenburg gait. Characteristics of a patient's gait can direct the examiner to focus on limb length or spinal aspects of the examination. An unsteady or widely based gait may indicate an underlying neurologic issue. Walking with one hip or iliac crest higher than the other may indicate scoliosis or a hip adduction or abduction contracture. The presence of a forward-flexed gait or the simple inability to stand up straight is almost always an indication of a hip flexion contracture that may cause a patient to perceive the involved leg as shorter than the uninvolved leg. Assessment of hip ROM and the presence or absence of pain with motion are basic aspects of the examination to document the medical necessity for surgery.

The surgeon must assess a patient for hip contractures, which can result in false or functional limb-length differences. A Thomas test should be performed to assess for hip flexion contracture, which can confound preoperative limb-length determination if not identified. Identification of an abduction or adduction contracture is equally important (**Figure 1**). A patient who cannot spread his or her legs or who experiences increased pain if the involved leg is abducted may have an adduction contracture that may cause the patient to perceive the involved leg as shorter. A patient who has difficulty bringing the legs together or who experiences pain with passive adduction likely has an abduction contracture. This patient may perceive the involved leg as longer. These scenarios are examples of a false or functional limb-length discrepancy that should not be corrected during surgery.

Examination of limb length is an absolute requirement to provide medicolegal documentation. The author of this chapter always tells patients when he is examining limb length preoperatively in the hope that the patient will remember that the limb length was assessed. Historically, limb length has been evaluated with the patient supine by measuring the distance from the anterior superior iliac spine to the medial malleolus. The author of this chapter prefers to measure limb length with the patient standing (**Figure 2**). The patient is asked if he or she perceives a length difference as blocks of different thickness are placed under the involved and uninvolved legs. If the patient perceives the legs as level, the anterior superior iliac spines can be palpated to confirm that the pelvis is level with the floor. In patients with a small length difference or no difference, the author of this chapter moves a 5-mm wedge from side to side and asks if the patient notices the difference more on one side (the longer side) than the other side. Some patients have equal limb lengths but can easily tolerate a 5-mm block placed under one leg. Knowing that a patient can tolerate a small amount of lengthening allows more flexibility intraoperatively. The standing limb-length measurement actively involves the patient in the preoperative examination, setting the stage for a discussion of potential limb-length difference. The standing or supine measurement of limb length is always reconciled with other aspects of the physical examination and radiographic measurement of hip length. To determine if a limb-length difference is a true (structural) or false limb-length discrepancy, the surgeon must consider the limb-length examination in combination with hip contractures, pelvic obliquity, and the radiographic hip length difference. A true limb-length discrepancy can be corrected intraoperatively by

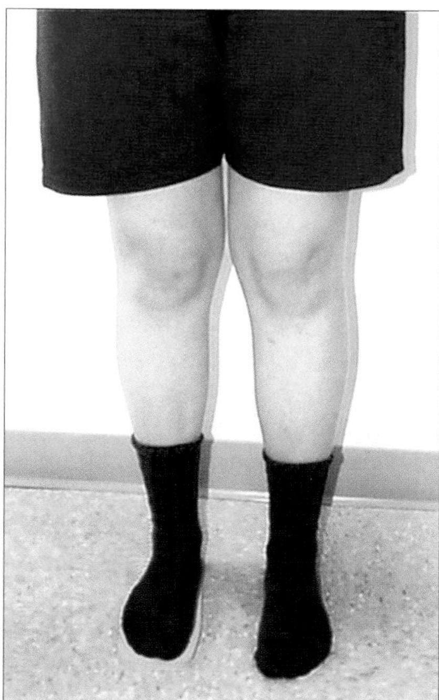

Figure 2 Clinical photograph shows measurement of limb lengths with the patient standing, using a block of the correct thickness placed under the right leg to achieve patient perception of equal leg length and a level pelvis. After the patient feels that the pelvis is level, the thickness and side of the block are recorded. The surgeon must reconcile this measurement with the involved hip side, the radiographic hip length, and patient contractures to determine a planned surgical length correction.

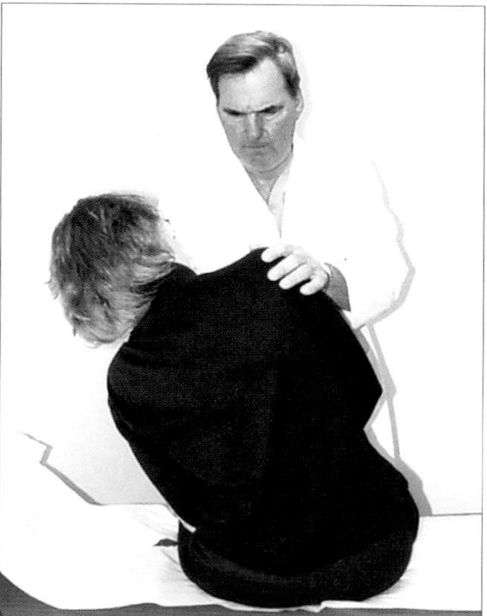

Figure 3 Clinical photograph shows examination of spinal motion with the patient seated (seated side-bending examination). This position eliminates the influence of hip contractures, allowing the surgeon to better determine if a preoperative limb-length discrepancy is the result of fixed lumbar scoliosis.

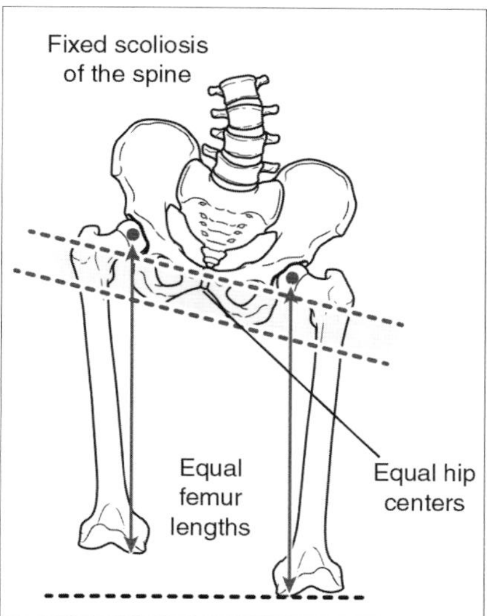

Figure 4 Illustration shows noncorrectable false limb-length difference. The patient has equal femur length and a pelvic tilt resulting from fixed scoliosis. Although the right side can be lengthened slightly with total hip arthroplasty to decrease the discrepancy, shortening the left side would cause hip instability.

lengthening the involved hip, whereas a false limb-length difference typically should not be corrected.

Examination of the spine is important in the assessment of limb-length discrepancy and hip joint stability. If pelvic obliquity is noted either during examination of the patient's gait or on the radiographic evaluation, a seated side-bending examination is recommended to determine the flexibility of the lumbar spine (**Figure 3**). Pelvic obliquity with a flexible lumbar spine is commonly the result of a hip adduction or abduction contracture. After the THA procedure and resolution of the contracture, the limb-length difference should resolve. However, patients with a limb-length difference caused by a fixed pelvic obliquity must be counseled that their limp and limb-length difference is a combination of hip arthritis and a fixed pelvic obliquity and may persist postoperatively (**Figure 4**). Although the arthritis is corrected, the fixed pelvic obliquity, which is usually the result of lumbar disease, will continue to contribute to the limb-length difference. Pelvic tilt, as observed on lumbar examination in the sagittal plane, contributes to hip joint instability. In a patient who has a stiff lumbar spine or decreased lumbar lordosis, the pelvis does not tilt or roll back when the patient moves from standing to sitting. In these patients, a slightly vertical and more anteverted acetabular cup position may be less likely to dislocate. The author of this chapter attempts to obtain 45° rather than 40° of inclination, and 40° rather than 35° of combined anteversion.

An AP pelvic radiograph is the primary image used for preoperative planning. This radiograph consists of a low pelvic view centered on the pubic symphysis. A patient is asked to internally rotate the legs 15° if possible. If the femurs are internally rotated 10° to 15°, the radiographic projection of the femur will be in the same anatomic plane as the template, which facilitates templating of the femoral metaphyseal size and femoral offset (**Figure 5**). If the femur is properly rotated, the anterior and posterior aspects of the greater trochanter are superimposed, and the posteriorly located lesser trochanter has a reduced profile (**Figure 6**). If the patient is unable to internally rotate the arthritic hip, the contralateral, nonarthritic hip is templated and the plan is reproduced on the arthritic side. An AP pelvic radiograph is used to compare right and left hip length. The hip-length difference is determined with either the interischial line, which intersects both

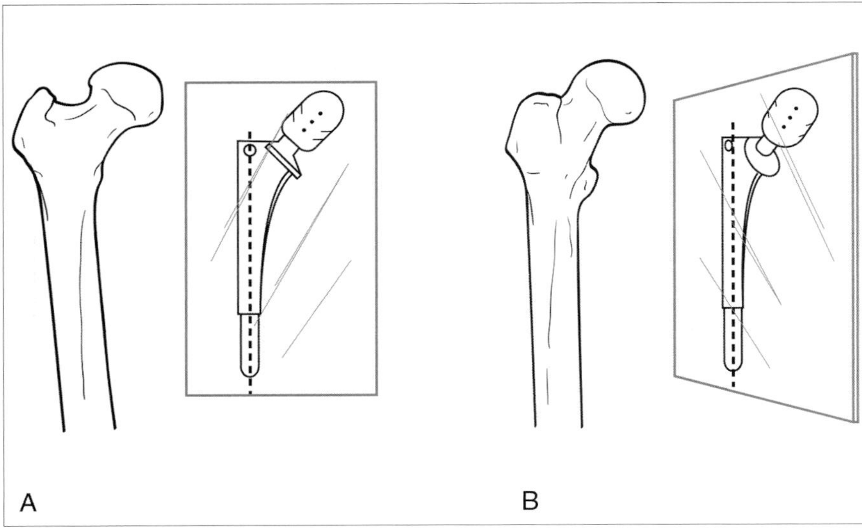

Figure 5 Illustrations of a femur show correct (**A**) and incorrect (**B**) femoral rotation of 10° to 15° for templating femoral metaphyseal size and offset. **A,** The rotation of the femur for radiographic imaging matches the template rotation. **B,** The external rotation of the femur does not match the plane of the template. Femoral metaphyseal size and offset cannot be templated based on this view. (Reproduced from Engh CA Sr: Optimizing stability and limb length, in Lieberman JR, Berry DJ, eds: *Advanced Reconstruction: Hip*. Rosemont, IL, American Academy of Orthopaedic Surgeons, 2005, pp 105-112.)

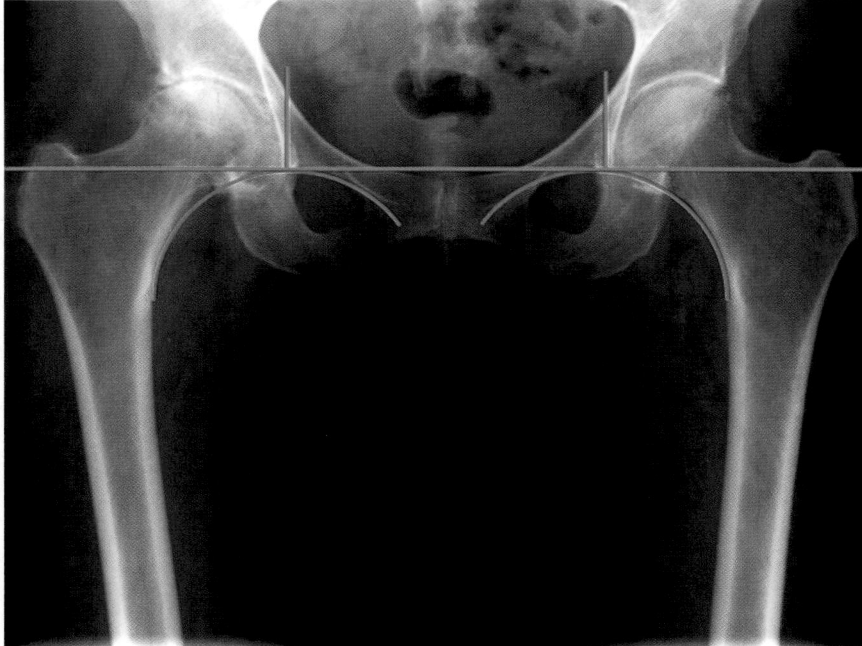

Figure 6 AP pelvic radiograph demonstrates proper rotation of the femurs. The intersection of the interteardrop line (blue line) with the greater trochanters indicates that the right hip length is slightly shorter than the left hip length. The Shenton line (curved red lines) is a helpful measure of proper hip offset. (Reproduced from Engh CA Sr: Optimizing stability and limb length, in Lieberman JR, Berry DJ, eds: *Advanced Reconstruction: Hip*. Rosemont, IL, American Academy of Orthopaedic Surgeons, 2005, pp 105-112.)

lesser trochanters, or the interteardrop line, which intersects both greater trochanters. If the radiographic hip length matches the limb-length difference observed on physical examination, the arthritic shortening represents a true limb-length discrepancy that can be corrected surgically (**Figure 7**). In patients with an obvious difference between the radiographic hip length and the physical limb-length, some portion of the difference likely represents a false limb-length discrepancy that should not be corrected (**Figure 8**). This scenario usually occurs secondary to a hip adduction or abduction contracture.

Pelvic tilt on an AP pelvic radiograph is often the first clue that a false limb-length discrepancy exists. The tilt occurs because the stiff hip does not allow the femur to rest perpendicular to the pelvis when the patient is positioned for the radiograph with the legs parallel. Increasingly, surgeons also are concerned with the sagittal orientation of the pelvis on an AP pelvic radiograph. For example, a patient with a stiff lumbar spine and without normal lordosis may have an AP pelvic radiograph that appears similar to an outlet view, with obturator foramina that appear tall. In addition, the pubic symphysis will be closer to or superimposed on the sacrum rather than lying below it. In this scenario, if the acetabular implant is placed vertical or with excessive anteversion, a patient may have an increased risk for anterior dislocation.

Patient Counseling

The risk of instability and postoperative limb-length difference should be specifically discussed as part of the process of obtaining informed consent. With a systematic approach to THA that includes planning and intraoperative measurements, 97% of hips should have a postoperative limb-length discrepancy of less than 1 cm. The author of this chapter typically tells patients that the chances are 80% that they will perceive the legs to be equal postoperatively and 20% that they will notice a difference. The author also informs patients that only one-half of patients who notice a difference, or 10% overall, will require a small lift in one shoe. Additionally, the author of this chapter mentions that in the first 3 to 4 months postoperatively, the surgical hip may be perceived as longer because the hip is stiff and the patient's gait has not normalized. This scenario is considered a transient functional limb-length discrepancy. The author provides additional counseling for patients with less common anatomic or developmental causes of arthritis that make it difficult to obtain equal limb length. These patients include those with coxa vara and coxa breva, both of whom have an increased risk for lengthening of the hip. The author also discusses limb length with obese patients because exposure and palpation of the intraoperative landmarks required to obtain equal limb length can be difficult in these patients. Additionally, patients are informed that hip stability and limb lengths are interrelated and that, in rare instances, the surgeon may need to lengthen the leg to attain a stable joint.

Patients should be counseled that postoperative dislocation can occur and that few patients require additional surgical treatment. Dislocation rates range from 0.5% to 3%. Patients in whom the posterior approach is used have the highest rate of dislocation; however, the rate has decreased with posterior capsular repair and the use of 32- or 36-mm femoral heads. Specific counseling about the risk of dislocation is necessary for patients who are elderly, have neurologic disorders, have a history of substance abuse, have had prior surgical treatment, or have hip dysplasia. The risk of dislocation also should be discussed with patients with hyperflexibility and tall or large male patients with high native hip offset.

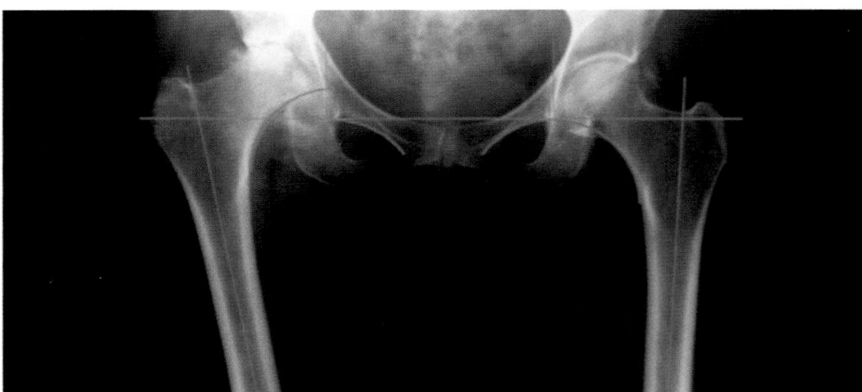

Figure 7 AP pelvic radiograph demonstrates shortening of the right hip that is similar to the shortening measured with the use of blocks with a patient standing. The lumbar spine is flexible. This scenario represents true limb-length discrepancy resulting from acetabular and femoral bone loss that should be corrected with total hip arthroplasty. The vertical blue lines define the femoral axis, which make it easier for the surgeon to recognize a probable adduction contracture of the hip. The horizontal blue line is the interteardrop line. The curved red lines represent the Shenton line. The disruption of the Shenton line in the patient's right hip is caused by both right-side hip shortening and the adduction contracture. (Reproduced from Engh CA Sr: Optimizing stability and limb length, in Lieberman JR, Berry DJ, eds: *Advanced Reconstruction: Hip*. Rosemont, IL, American Academy of Orthopaedic Surgeons, 2005, pp 105-112.)

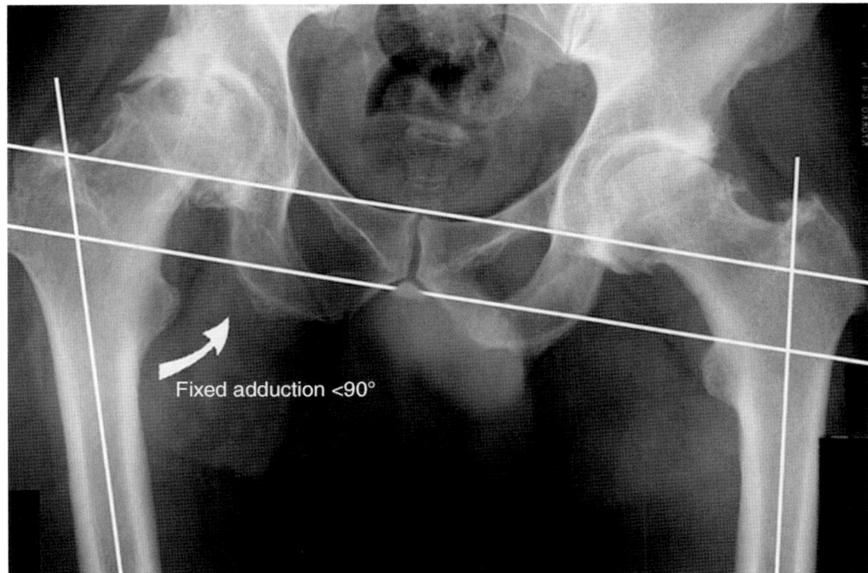

Figure 8 AP pelvic radiograph of a patient who has a short right leg as measured with blocks, a right hip adduction contracture, and a flexible lumbar spine. The white interteardrop line and a line parallel to the obturator foramen indicate that the right hip joint may be longer than the left. The shortening of the right leg is false and should not be corrected. The vertical white lines represent the femoral axis, which make it easier to recognize the adducted position of the right femur relative to the interteardrop line. The white arrow highlights the decreased angle between the femoral axis and the interteardrop line, which is caused by the adduction contracture. (Reproduced from Engh CA Sr: Optimizing stability and limb length, in Lieberman JR, Berry DJ, eds: *Advanced Reconstruction: Hip*. Rosemont, IL, American Academy of Orthopaedic Surgeons, 2005, pp 105-112.)

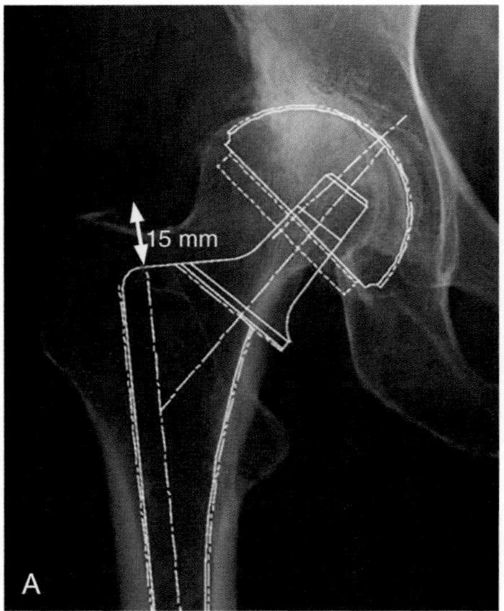

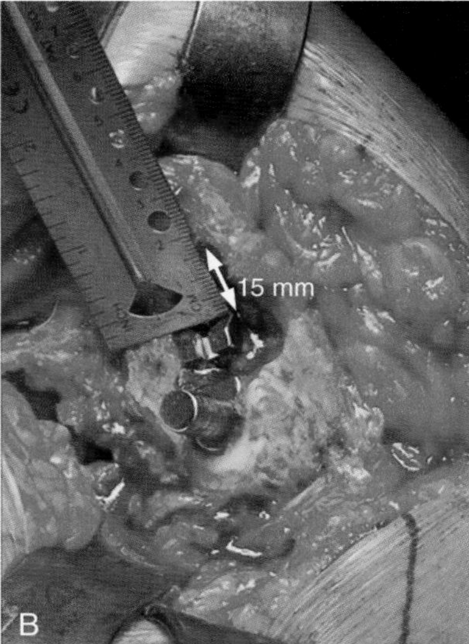

Figure 9 **A,** AP radiograph of a right hip demonstrates the seating level of the femoral template. The femoral template is 15 mm distal to the proximal aspect of the femur. The red circles indicate the centers of the femoral head and acetabular implant. In this patient, the femoral offset may be increased because the femoral center is medial to the acetabular center. **B,** Intraoperative photograph of a hip shows re-creation of the templated distance from the tip of the greater trochanter to the lateral aspect of the femoral broach.

Preoperative Templating

Preoperative templating improves implant positioning and limits postoperative limb-length discrepancies. With the implant templates superimposed on an AP pelvic radiograph, the surgeon can reference intraoperative bony landmarks such as the greater or lesser trochanters and the superior lateral edge of the acetabulum to execute the templated plan. Intraoperative hip navigation systems provide the ultimate form of templating; however, navigation technology can be cumbersome and expensive and does not improve patient outcomes. Therefore, it has not been widely adopted by surgeons. The discussion of templating in this chapter focuses on issues related to limb length and stability.

The surgeon uses the planned hip length correction, which takes into account the true length discrepancy identified during the patient examination, to determine the height of the femoral implant in the femoral canal. This requires reconciliation of the limb length observed on physical examination and the radiographic hip length difference. After the acetabular template is positioned in the center of the acetabulum, the femoral template is lowered along the femoral axis until the femoral head overlies the acetabular center to obtain equal limb length or is above the acetabular center to lengthen the hip. With the femoral position templated, the author of this chapter measures the distance from the lateral aspect of the femoral template to the proximal aspect of the greater trochanter (**Figure 9**). This distance is re-created intraoperatively when the femoral broach is seated.

Hip joint stability is affected by templating. If a patient's femur has proper internal rotation on an AP pelvic radiograph, templating allows the surgeon to determine whether a standard or high-offset stem should be used. If a standard offset template shows that the center of the femoral head is positioned lateral to the center of the acetabular template, then hip offset will be reduced with a resultant decrease in soft-tissue tension and an increased risk for hip instability. If this scenario occurs, a high-offset femoral template will better restore hip anatomy. Occasionally, a patient is unable to internally rotate the involved leg for the radiograph, making it impossible to determine whether a standard or high-offset stem should be selected. For such patients, the surgeon can place the template at the proper depth to adjust limb length and intraoperatively test standard and high-offset trial implants for tension and stability. However, the author of this chapter prefers to template the correctly rotated contralateral hip to determine the femoral offset required before acetabular preparation (**Figure 10**). In some patients (typically tall men), a high-offset stem does not fully re-create femoral offset. If this scenario is identified preoperatively, the author of this chapter places the acetabular implant slightly more lateral than the standard position and may consider an offset acetabular insert to accommodate the need for increased offset.

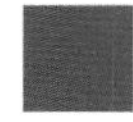

Surgical Techniques

Achieving a stable hip joint with equal limb length requires surgical execution of the plan that was developed preoperatively. The hip joint shuck test and assessment of quadriceps tightness as measures of length and stability are not sufficient. Intraoperative assessment tools include anatomic landmarks for the acetabulum and the femur, measurement of limb length, determination of offset combined with ROM using trial implants, and the increasingly frequent use of intraoperative radiographs. The author of this chapter always performs an examination with trial acetabular and femoral implants in place so that adjustments can be made to either component.

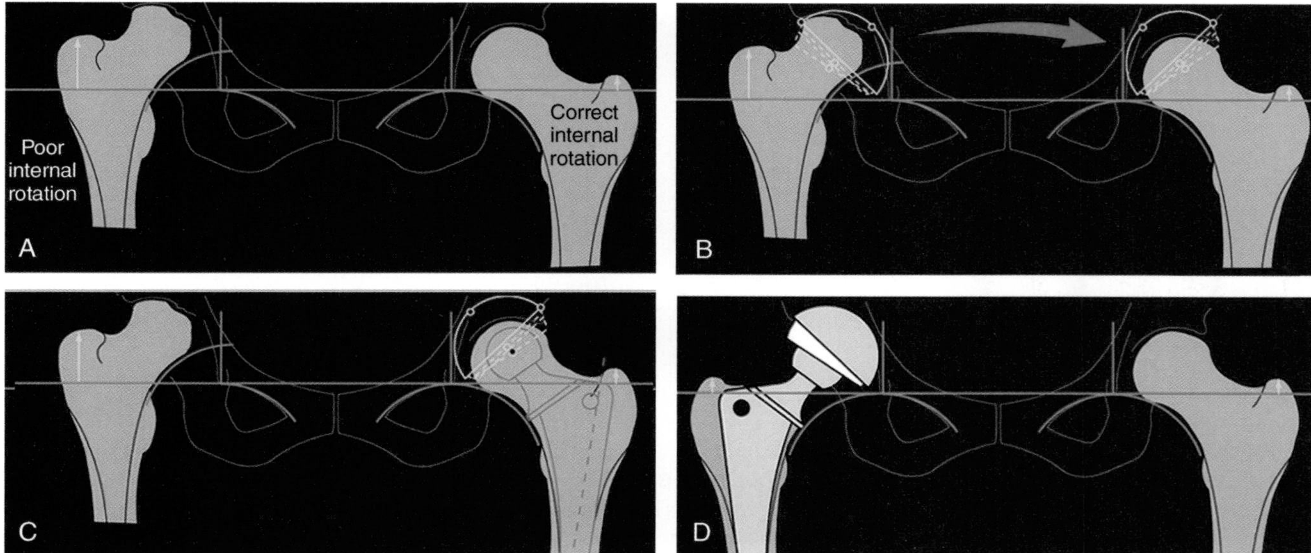

Figure 10 Sequential illustrations show templating of a patient's contralateral hip. **A,** The right hip has poor internal rotation as a result of acetabular and femoral bone loss. The patient has a true limb-length discrepancy. **B,** The position of the acetabular cup is determined on the right (involved) hip and is transferred to the left (contralateral) hip, at which the center of the acetabular cup is marked. The center of the acetabular cup is higher in the left hip because of the acetabular bone loss in the right hip. **C,** The seating level and head position of the femoral implant are templated in the left hip in relation to the marked center of the elevated acetabular cup. **D,** The templated positions are re-created intraoperatively in the involved hip. (Reproduced from Engh CA Sr: Optimizing stability and limb length, in Lieberman JR, Berry DJ, eds: *Advanced Reconstruction: Hip*. Rosemont, IL, American Academy of Orthopaedic Surgeons, 2005, pp 105-112.)

A reliable, easy-to-use intraoperative femoral landmark is the distance from the tip of the greater trochanter to the lateral aspect of the femoral trial implant, which is determined during templating (**Figure 9**). A similar distance from the lesser trochanter to the medial aspect of the stem is often used; however, the round or sloping aspect of the lesser trochanter can make this measurement less reproducible. The best intraoperative landmark for acetabular inclination is the anterosuperior edge of the acetabulum. In general, the acetabular implant will be slightly uncovered superiorly and posteriorly. The proximal edge of the acetabular implant should match the superior lateral aspect of the labrum, and the inferior edge of the acetabular implant should be in contact with the transverse acetabular ligament. Placing the acetabular shell parallel to and touching the transverse acetabular ligament is an easy way to obtain proper inclination and anteversion in many patients. If the transverse acetabular ligament is not visible, the surgeon can ensure that the anteroinferior aspect of the acetabular implant is just inside the anteroinferior acetabular wall.

To augment the intraoperative landmarks for the femoral and acetabular implants, the hip is examined with trial implants in place. At the start of the procedure, before hip dislocation, the lengths of the surgical and nonsurgical legs are compared. Advocates of the supine position for THA (without the use of a specialized surgical table) advocate the ease of obtaining this measurement via palpation of the anterior superior iliac spines and malleoli. If the lateral decubitus position is used, the relative lengths of the femurs are recorded (**Figure 11**). In addition, with the patient in the lateral decubitus position, the author of this chapter places a pin in the ilium and bends the pin to touch the greater trochanter, providing a reference for the measurement of limb length and offset.

After the trial implants are placed and limb length and offset changes are documented, hip stability is checked. This check of hip stability is performed in all approaches for THA, with the exception of the direct anterior approach with the use of a specialized surgical table. ROM is documented for both anterior and posterior stability. For posterior stability, the hip should not dislocate if placed in 20° of adduction, 45° of flexion, and 50° of internal rotation. For anterior stability, the hip should not dislocate if extended 15°, adducted 10°, and externally rotated 25°. Depending on the surgical approach used, the intact anterior or posterior capsule may limit testing of hip joint stability. For example, surgeons cannot always test anterior hip stability in THA performed via the posterior approach because the intact anterior hip capsule prevents extension and external rotation. This scenario creates the possibility for excessive acetabular anteversion. For this reason,

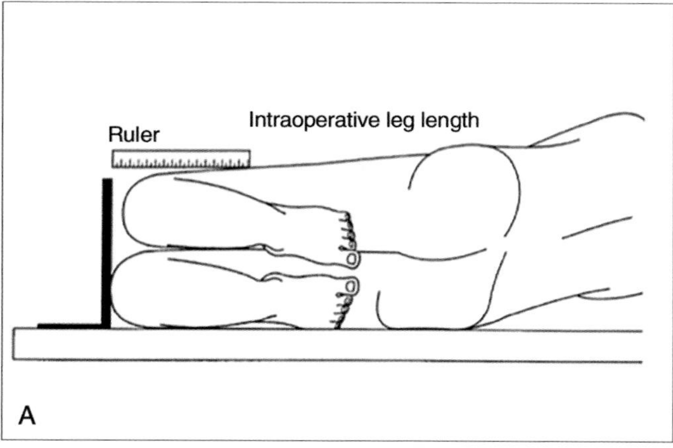

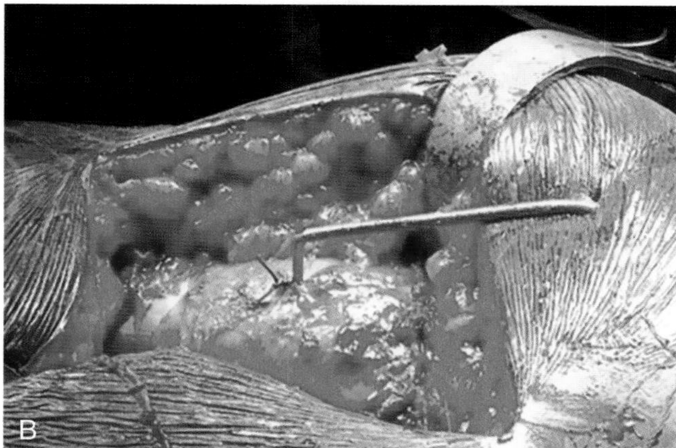

Figure 11 **A,** Illustration of a lower extremity shows intraoperative comparison of limb lengths with the patient in the lateral decubitus position. The relative position of the femurs is recorded. **B,** Intraoperative photograph of a hip shows measurement of limb length and offset. Before the hip is dislocated, a pin in the ileum is bent to touch the left greater trochanter, providing a reference for the measurement of length and offset. These measurements are re-created with trial implants.

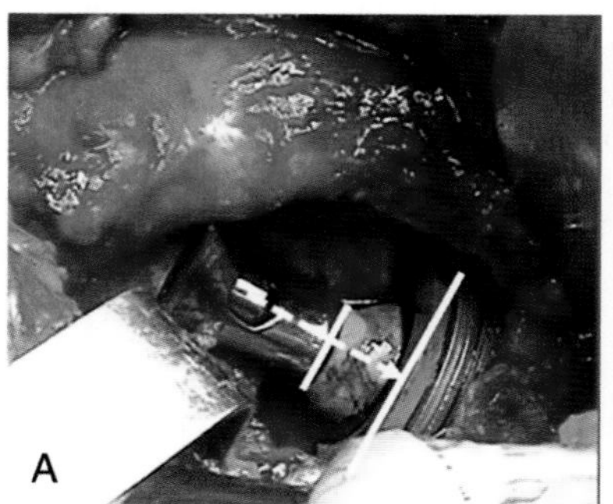

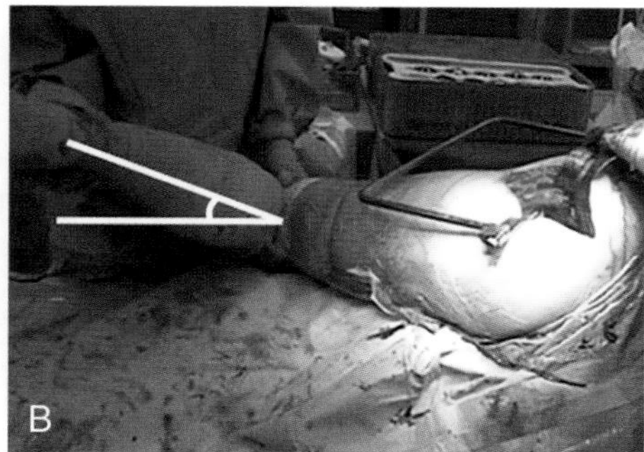

Figure 12 Intraoperative photographs of a hip show assessment of the combined anteversion of the acetabular and femoral implants. **A,** The hip has been rotated until the femoral neck is perpendicular to the face of the trial acetabular implant (dashed arrow). **B,** In that position, the angle created by the tibia and a line parallel to the floor (white line segments) is the combined anteversion. It is important to note that it is presumed the pelvis is firmly positioned and the frontal pelvic plane is vertical.

surgeons should assess the combined anteversion of the acetabular and femoral implants (**Figure 12**). The recommended combined anteversion is 25° to 50° and is measured by internally rotating the femur until the trial femoral neck is perpendicular to the face of the acetabular implant. Proper combined anteversion can decrease dislocation and edge loading of the bearing surface. This test is more helpful for THA performed via the posterior approach than for THA performed via anterior approaches because the greater trochanter usually obscures visibility of the trial neck in THA performed via anterior approaches. The author of this chapter recommends trial reduction with a 28-mm femoral head. If the hip is stable with a 28-mm–diameter femoral head, it will be stable with a larger-diameter femoral head. Additionally, the smaller trial head size makes visualization of impingement of the prosthetic components on each other or impingement of the femoral implant on the pelvis easier. Multiple trial reductions may be necessary to optimize hip joint stability, and reduction of a 28-mm trial implant is easier than reduction of a 36-mm trial implant.

Intraoperative radiography is perhaps the best way to verify implant positioning to achieve the desired limb length and stability. If the patient is in the supine position, fluoroscopy is commonly used because it does not add much time to the procedure. Fluoroscopy is more difficult to use if the patient is in the lateral decubitus position. With lateral decubitus positioning, a portable radiography machine is used. Some surgeons find that the time required for the radiograph to be obtained and processed is prohibitive. Furthermore, acetabular inclination, anteversion, and limb length are only estimated. The time required for radiography has decreased with the advent of digital radiographs that can be projected onto screens in the operating room without delay. Radiographic systems with software that measures rather than estimates limb length and implant position have recently become available and are the preferred technique of the author of this chapter for determining acetabular inclination and leg length.

Avoiding Pitfalls and Complications

Attaining a stable hip joint and equal leg length is a process that must begin preoperatively. The patient must be involved during the physical examination and counseled about the risks of instability and leg length inequality during the office visit. The surgeon should obtain a thorough history and provide a running description of findings during the physical examination to facilitate the discussion of limb length and instability as part of the informed consent process. The availability of digital radiography in the examination room allows a surgeon to show patients their hip length and, with some systems, the process of templating. Patients should be informed that in rare instances the leg must be lengthened to attain hip joint stability. Surgeons should note the presence of specific disease processes that may influence hip joint stability, such as dementia and Parkinson disease. Childhood hip disease and spine disease may influence the discussion of limb length and stability. The surgical procedure should be planned and executed using as many measurements and tools as necessary to ensure a stable hip joint and the best possible limb length. The author of this chapter recommends the use of intraoperative radiographs in all primary hip replacements to confirm proper leg length and acetabular implant positioning.

Bibliography

Archbold HA, Mockford B, Molloy D, McConway J, Ogonda L, Beverland D: The transverse acetabular ligament: An aid to orientation of the acetabular component during primary total hip replacement. A preliminary study of 1000 cases investigating postoperative stability. *J Bone Joint Surg Br* 2006;88(7):883-886.

Berry DJ, von Knoch M, Schleck CD, Harmsen WS: Effect of femoral head diameter and operative approach on risk of dislocation after primary total hip arthroplasty. *J Bone Joint Surg Am* 2005;87(11):2456-2463.

Bozic KJ, Kurtz SM, Lau E, Ong K, Vail TP, Berry DJ: The epidemiology of revision total hip arthroplasty in the United States. *J Bone Joint Surg Am* 2009;91(1):128-133.

Clark CR, Huddleston HD, Schoch EP III, Thomas BJ: Leg-length discrepancy after total hip arthroplasty. *J Am Acad Orthop Surg* 2006;14(1):38-45.

Ezzet KA, McCauley JC: Use of intraoperative x-rays to optimize component position and leg length during total hip arthroplasty. *J Arthroplasty* 2014;29(3):580-585.

Goel A, Lau EC, Ong KL, Berry DJ, Malkani AL: Dislocation rates following primary total hip arthroplasty have plateaued in the Medicare population. *J Arthroplasty* 2015;30(5):743-746.

Kanawade V, Dorr LD, Wan Z: Predictability of acetabular component angular change with postural shift from standing to sitting position. *J Bone Joint Surg Am* 2014;96(12):978-986.

Lazennec JY, Brusson A, Rousseau MA: Lumbar-pelvic-femoral balance on sitting and standing lateral radiographs. *Orthop Traumatol Surg Res* 2013;99(1 suppl):S87-S103.

Legaye J: Influence of the sagittal balance of the spine on the anterior pelvic plane and on the acetabular orientation. *Int Orthop* 2009;33(6):1695-1700.

Lucas DH, Scott RD: The Ranawat sign. *J Orthop Tech* 1994;2(2):1-3.

McGee HM, Scott JH: A simple method of obtaining equal leg length in total hip arthroplasty. *Clin Orthop Relat Res* 1985;(194):269-270.

Ng VY, Kean JR, Glassman AH: Limb-length discrepancy after hip arthroplasty. *J Bone Joint Surg Am* 2013;95(15):1426-1436.

O'Brien S, Kernohan G, Fitzpatrick C, Hill J, Beverland D: Perception of imposed leg length inequality in normal subjects. *Hip Int* 2010;20(4):505-511.

Ranawat CS, Rodriguez JA: Functional leg-length inequality following total hip arthroplasty. *J Arthroplasty* 1997;12(4):359-364.

Upadhyay A, York S, Macaulay W, McGrory B, Robbennolt J, Bal BS: Medical malpractice in hip and knee arthroplasty. *J Arthroplasty* 2007;22(6 suppl 2):2-7.

Woolson ST, Hartford JM, Sawyer A: Results of a method of leg-length equalization for patients undergoing primary total hip replacement. *J Arthroplasty* 1999;14(2):159-164.

SECTION 2

Complex Total Hip Arthroplasty

Jay R. Lieberman, MD

Chapter 19
Total Hip Arthroplasty: Developmental Dysplasia of the Hip

Daniel J. Berry, MD
Miguel E. Cabanela, MD

Indications

The indications for total hip arthroplasty (THA) in patients with developmental dysplasia of the hip (DDH) and subluxation without dislocation are the same as those in patients with any other form of hip disease. Clinical symptoms must be sufficient to warrant surgical intervention, and radiologic changes must be of sufficient magnitude to make alternative solutions impossible. Pain is usually the most important factor in surgical decision making. Limb-length inequality is a concern in some patients but should not be the principal reason for THA.

Degenerative disease secondary to hip dysplasia occurs at an early age. Most patients who require THA undergo the procedure when they are younger than 50 years. In these patients, THA often requires special techniques and is associated with a higher failure rate than in patients with degenerative joint disease. The higher failure rate is likely related to the altered anatomy of patients with this condition.

Several methods of classifying the bony anatomic abnormalities of patients with DDH have been proposed. Most classification systems focus on the amount of femoral subluxation or dislocation relative to the normal anatomic hip center. The authors of this chapter prefer the Hartofilakidis classification, which defines three types of DDH in adults on the basis of the relationship between the femoral head and the acetabulum (**Table 1**). In patients with dysplasia, the femoral head is in contact with the true (anatomic) acetabulum, also known as the paleoacetabulum. In patients with low dislocation, the femoral head is partially in contact with the true acetabulum and partially in contact with the false acetabulum (neoacetabulum) formed by the femoral head in its abnormal position on the lateral pelvic wall. This type of deformity is the most severe. In patients with high dislocation, the femoral head and the true acetabulum have no contact, and the femoral head has migrated superiorly and posteriorly. In patients with this deformity, the true acetabulum often is reasonably well preserved but is underdeveloped and osteoporotic. The Crowe classification of DDH is based on the amount of proximal migration of the femoral head calculated on an AP pelvic radiograph (**Table 1**). In Crowe type I DDH, the femoral head is subluxated 50%; this type is equivalent to Hartofilakidis type I DDH. In Crowe types II and III DDH, the femoral head is subluxated between 50% and 75% and between 75% and 100%, respectively; both types are equivalent to the low subluxation of Hartofilakidis type II DDH. In Crowe type IV DDH, the subluxation is greater than 100%, which is equivalent to the high dislocation of Hartofilakidis type III DDH.

Changes in the bony anatomy are associated with changes in the soft tissues. The more severe the bony abnormality, the more severe the changes in the soft tissues will be. All patients will have hypertrophy of the psoas tendon and some capsular thickening. Shortening of the hamstring, adductor, and rectus femoris tendons is common. The abductors are oriented transversely because of the upward position of the femoral head and the proximal femur but are less foreshortened than might be expected. The femoral and sciatic nerves may be shortened and therefore vulnerable to intraoperative injury.

Contraindications

Radiologic joint deformity alone is not a sufficient indication for THA in patients with adequate cartilage space remaining. In these patients, nonsurgical or alternative conservative surgical treatment should be considered.

Dr. Berry or an immediate family member has received royalties from, serves as a paid consultant to, and has received research or institutional support from DePuy Synthes; and serves as a board member, owner, officer, or committee member of the American Joint Replacement Registry, the Hip Society, and the Mayo Clinic. Dr. Cabanela or an immediate family member serves as a board member, owner, officer, or committee member of the Mid-America Orthopaedic Association.

Table 1 The Degree of Severity of Developmental Dysplasia of the Hip According to the Crowe and Hartofilakidis Classifications

Hartofilakidis Classification	Crowe Type	Percentage of Vertical Diameter of Femoral Head
Dysplasia	Type I	<50%
Low dislocation	Type II	50%-75%
	Type III	75%-100%
High dislocation	Type IV	>100%

Adapted from MacDonald SJ, Parvizi J, Ghanem E, Mears DC: Total hip arthroplasty in unusual medical and surgically challenging condition, in Glassman AH, Lachiewicz PF, Tanzer M, eds: *Orthopaedic Knowledge Update: Hip and Knee Reconstruction 4*. Rosemont, IL, American Academy of Orthopaedic Surgeons, 2011, pp 233-261.

Alternative Treatments

Alternative joint-sparing procedures should be considered in patients who experience pain with activity but not at rest and who have adequately preserved joint space and reasonable range of motion. Redirection pelvic (acetabular) osteotomies are indicated in patients with DDH that principally affects the acetabulum and is characterized by lack of coverage of the femoral head, subluxation, lateralization of the hip joint center, and well-preserved cartilage. Conversely, in patients with coxa valga luxans (that is, excess proximal femoral valgus but adequate articular cartilage), a varus femoral osteotomy (sometimes combined with medial derotation in patients with excess femoral anteversion) is the procedure of choice. These alternative treatments are not appropriate for patients with advanced joint destruction. THA should be reserved for patients in whom alternative joint-preserving procedures are not feasible.

Results

Longer-term results are available for cemented acetabular implants than for noncemented acetabular implants. Relatively high failure rates of 12% to 52% have been reported at 10 to 20 years postoperatively. The high failure rates may be the result of the young age of the patients and the quality of the bone available for cement fixation. The use of femoral head autografts to improve coverage of the cemented implant has not improved implant longevity, but several studies have noted that it improves the bone stock for future revision.

Noncemented acetabular implants have fared well in studies with up to 20-year follow-up. **Table 2** summarizes select published results of acetabular reconstruction with noncemented implants with and without femoral head autograft augmentation. Rates of loosening and mechanical failure (revision for loosening plus revision for other causes) are moderate. Notably, the most common cause of failure of noncemented acetabular implants is wear and osteolysis, whereas the most common cause of failure of cemented acetabular implants is loosening. The advent of alternative bearing materials, such as highly cross-linked polyethylene, allows the use of thinner inserts and has reduced the rates of wear and resulting osteolysis.

Few studies have reported on the technique of cotyloplasty (medialization of the acetabular reconstruction by cracking the medial wall), and its use has been limited. The reported results are excellent, with satisfactory long-term follow-up at more than 20 years postoperatively. However, this technique results in decreased bone stock, which can complicate revision.

Mild elevation of the hip center has provided acceptable results at 12-year follow-up. Concerns associated with this technique include altered hip mechanics, which increases the risk of dislocation, and rapidly diminishing bone stock as the center of rotation is moved upward.

Results of cemented femoral reconstruction in patients with dysplasia have been better than those of acetabular reconstruction. Failure rates of 2% to 20% have been reported for cemented femoral reconstruction with up to 20-year follow-up. Modern noncemented stem designs, including tapered, modular, and conic stems, have demonstrated very good results with more than 10-year follow-up.

Techniques

Setup/Exposure

- In patients with mild to moderate DDH, a standard anterolateral approach or a posterolateral approach can be used depending on surgeon preference.
- Occasionally, patients who have a very stiff hip or patients who have undergone previous surgical procedures, such as a varus-producing osteotomy, may require a transtrochanteric approach.
- When a transtrochanteric approach is necessary, the surgeon must ensure that enough bone remains laterally on the femur after implantation of the prosthesis to allow reattachment of the trochanter onto a bony base. A flat osteotomy of the trochanter usually is preferred to a more complex geometric osteotomy because flat osteotomy facilitates anterior translation of a posteriorly displaced trochanter.
- In patients with mild to moderate dysplasia, subtrochanteric

Table 2 Results of Noncemented Acetabular Reconstruction in Patients With Developmental Dysplasia of the Hip

Authors (Year)	Number of Hips	Implant Type	Mean Patient Age in Years (Range)	Mean Follow-up in Years (Range)	Results
Silber and Engh (1990)	19	Noncemented with acetabular augmentation	45 (NR)	3 (2-6.3)	5% required revision for loosening 26% had mechanical failure
Morsi et al (1996)	17	Noncemented with acetabular augmentation	50.3 (36-65)	6.6 (5.1-9.8)	No revision for loosening No mechanical failure
Anderson and Harris (1999)	20	Noncemented	52 (25-87)	6.9 (5.3-8.5)	No revision for loosening No mechanical failure
Spangehl et al (2001)	44	Noncemented with acetabular augmentation	39 (12-67)	7.5 (5-12.3)	4.5% required revision for loosening 9% had mechanical failure
Karachalios et al (2013)	61	Noncemented with cotyloplasty	46.7 (23-68)	24.3 (20-32)	45.9% required revision for loosening 47.4% had mechanical failure
Abdel et al (2014)	35	Noncemented with acetabular augmentation	43 (12-60)	21.3 (13.1-26)	2.9% required revision for loosening 34% had mechanical failure
Nawabi et al (2014)	24	Noncemented with high hip center	49 (28-77)	12 (10-21)	No revision for loosening No mechanical failure

NR = not reported.

shortening femoral osteotomies are not necessary.

Instruments/Equipment/ Implants Required

- Standard instruments are used.

Procedure: Acetabular Reconstruction

- Most surgeons in North America prefer noncemented acetabular fixation over cemented acetabular fixation for patients of all ages, but particularly for younger patients with DDH.
- In most patients, the acetabular implant should be placed as close to the anatomic hip center as possible.
- However, in patients with moderate DDH, the center of rotation can be placed slightly proximally. Some authors have suggested that a proximal and medial location is better than a proximal and lateral position.

BONE PREPARATION

- If the acetabular bone stock is insufficient (that is, if anterolateral coverage of the implant is deficient), several alternatives are available, including augmentation with bone grafting, reconstruction with a high hip center, and medialization of the acetabular cup (**Figure 1**).
- If the construct is stable, mild deficiency of the anterolateral support of the acetabular cup is acceptable (**Figure 2**).
- If superior coverage of the implant is severely deficient, three options are available.
- The first option, medialization of the acetabulum beyond the Köhler line, produces a mild, deliberate perforation of the medial pelvic wall. Cotyloplasty or reaming of the medial wall can be performed and the implant translated slightly medially to a deliberate protrusio position. This approach is relatively simple and provides good coverage of the acetabular cup on host bone. However, it sacrifices bone stock, which can make revision surgery difficult. It also increases the risk of weakening of the acetabulum, which can result in failure by means of early protrusion of the acetabular cup into the pelvis.
- The second option involves placement of a small, noncemented acetabular implant in a high hip center location. In this position, the acetabular implant is completely covered by host bone, which facilitates bony integration and avoids the need for grafting. Disadvantages of this approach include decreased polyethylene thickness associated with the small acetabular implant, difficult equalization of limb lengths, altered hip mechanics, and hip instability related to femoropelvic impingement in flexion or extension.

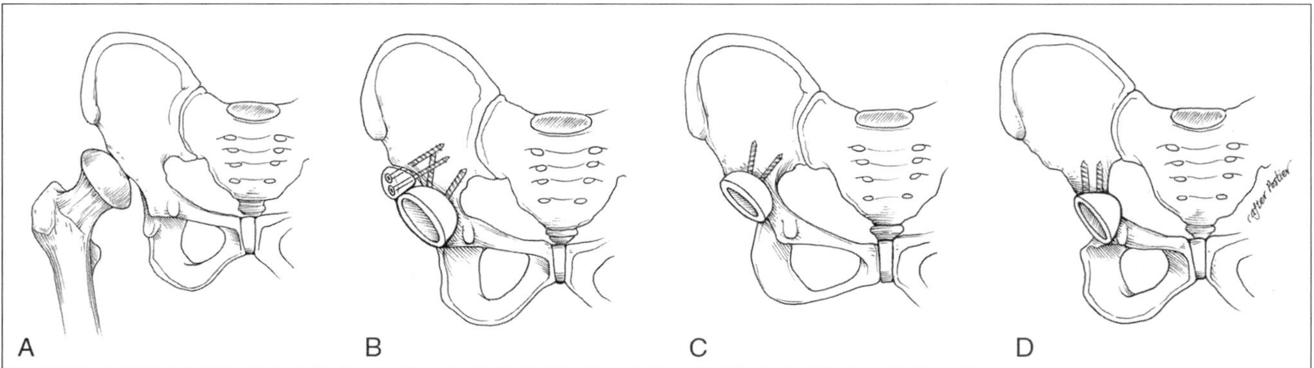

Figure 1 Illustrations depict a Crowe type II and III dysplastic acetabulum (**A**) and three methods of reconstruction of these types: augmentation with bone grafting (**B**), reconstruction with a high hip center (**C**), and medialization of the acetabular cup (**D**). (Reproduced from Sanchez-Sotelo J, Berry DJ, Trousdale RT, Cabanela ME: Surgical treatment of developmental dysplasia of the hip in adults: II. Arthroplasty options. *J Am Acad Orthop Surg* 2002;10[5]:334-344.)

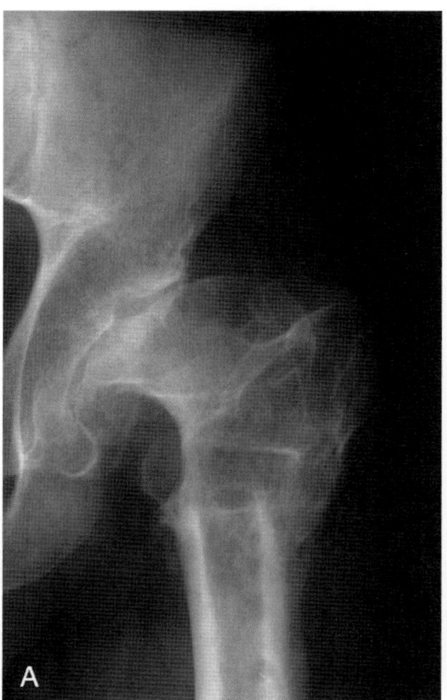

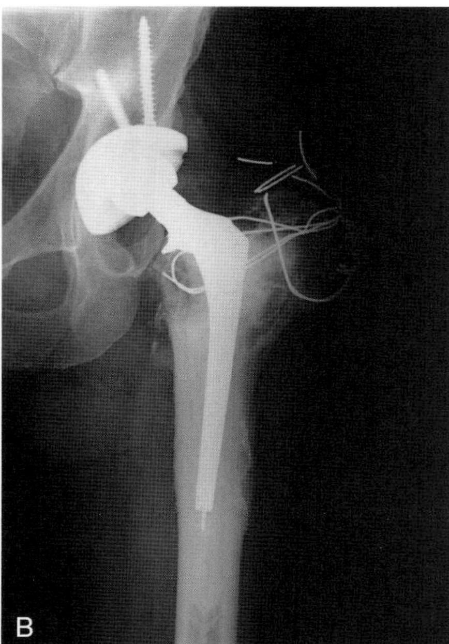

Figure 2 **A,** AP radiograph demonstrates the left hip of a 42-year-old man 15 years after he underwent a varus femoral osteotomy. Note the poor coverage of the deformed femoral head. **B,** AP radiograph demonstrates the left hip of the same patient after total hip arthroplasty. Medialization to the Köhler line without perforation of the medial wall provided satisfactory coverage of the noncemented acetabular implant. The femoral deformity was corrected with a cemented implant in a slight valgus position. A trochanteric osteotomy was used for the approach and was fixed with Vitallium wires. (Reproduced from Cabanela ME: Total hip arthroplasty: Degenerative dysplasia of the hip, in Lieberman JR, Berry DJ, eds: *Advanced Reconstruction: Hip*. Rosemont, IL, American Academy of Orthopaedic Surgeons, 2005, pp 115-120.)

- The third option is augmentation of superior coverage with bone graft. The graft usually is obtained from the patient's femoral head and is fixed to the lateral pelvic wall with cancellous screws (**Figure 3**). This technique restores the center of rotation and the hip mechanics. In addition, bone stock is increased, which can be valuable in patients requiring acetabular revision. Graft healing is predictable, and resorption is minimal at long-term follow-up.

GRAFT PLACEMENT

- The acetabulum is reamed with the goal of preserving the anterior wall. Reaming should extend into the ischium and the posterior column because bone is typically thicker in patients with DDH than in most patients requiring THA.
- Reamer coverage is assessed to determine if augmentation with bone graft is necessary.
- If bone grafting is necessary, the femoral head is divided along the weight-bearing trabeculae and fashioned so that it can be grafted onto the prepared lateral pelvic wall. This step typically augments superior and anterior coverage, where the most common deficiencies are located.
- The femoral head is temporarily fixed to the pelvic wall with two 3.2-mm drill bits or two small Steinmann pins, with care taken to leave enough grafted bone overhanging

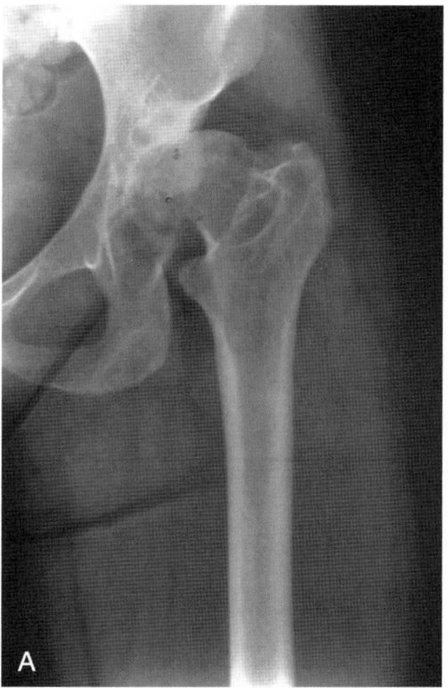

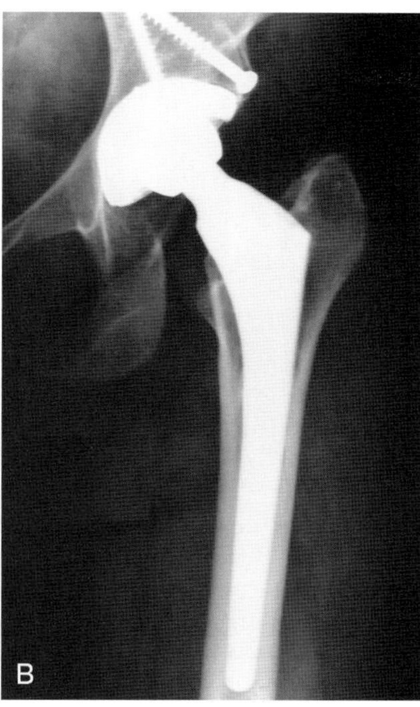

Figure 3 **A,** AP radiograph demonstrates the left hip of a 27-year-old woman with osteoarthritis secondary to developmental dysplasia of the hip. The dysplasia is classified as Hartofilakidis and Crowe type II. **B,** AP radiograph demonstrates the left hip of the same patient 2 years postoperatively. A femoral head autograft was used for acetabular coverage. A standard press-fit metaphyseal-filling femoral implant was used because of the minimal deformity of the patient's femoral anatomy. (Reproduced from Cabanela ME: Total hip arthroplasty: Degenerative dysplasia of the hip, in Lieberman JR, Berry DJ, eds: *Advanced Reconstruction: Hip*. Rosemont, IL, American Academy of Orthopaedic Surgeons, 2005, pp 115-120.)

inferiorly for later reaming. The pins, and later the screws, are directed in a medial and superior direction toward the sacroiliac joint to provide mechanical stability.

- One of the pins or drills is changed to a 6.5-mm cancellous screw. The smooth portion of the screw traverses the bone graft and the threaded portion engages the pelvis. If possible, the screw is placed with no threads present in the grafted bone.
- After the first screw is in place, additional reaming is performed to complete the preparation of the acetabulum. Typically, a congruous junction of the bone graft and the native acetabulum is obtained.
- The acetabular implant is placed.
- Press-fit fixation is augmented with two or three screws.
- A second 6.5-mm cancellous screw is placed through the graft.
- Placement of the graft overhanging the acetabular implant provides no advantage because it will not be mechanically stressed and will likely resorb.

Procedure: Femoral Reconstruction

BONE PREPARATION

- The femoral anatomy often is distorted with excessive anteversion, coxa valga, and a small medullary canal, which may have a peculiar shape (typically narrow with a mediolateral diameter smaller than the anteroposterior diameter). The greater trochanter may be located posteriorly.
- The degree of anteversion must be carefully assessed. Increased acetabular anteversion can result in excessive anteversion of the implants, which can lead to anterior instability of the reconstructed hip. In addition, anteversion of the femoral implant can result in an internal rotation contracture of the hip.

PROSTHESIS IMPLANTATION

- Either cemented or noncemented implants can be used in patients with DDH who have dysplasia or low dislocation (Hartofilakidis type I or II).
- Cemented implants allow the surgeon to address femoral deformities, especially increased anteversion.
- Many implant systems have cemented stems specially designed for patients with DDH. To accommodate the distorted femoral anatomy, these implants typically are smaller and straighter than standard implants, and have minimal metaphyseal flare.
- Alternatively, downsizing the implant allows the surgeon to place the implant in less anteversion than that of the native femur.
- A noncemented implant can be used. However, proximally (metaphyseally) fitted implants may not allow correction of the anteversion. In patients with severe femoral anteversion in extreme situations, these implants may require a simultaneous femoral derotation osteotomy to correct the abnormal femoral anteversion.
- In some patients, the use of a distally fixed, extensively coated implant allows correction of the abnormal anteversion by bypassing the proximal femur and obtaining fixation in the diaphysis.
- With some modular implants, the proximal and distal femur can be

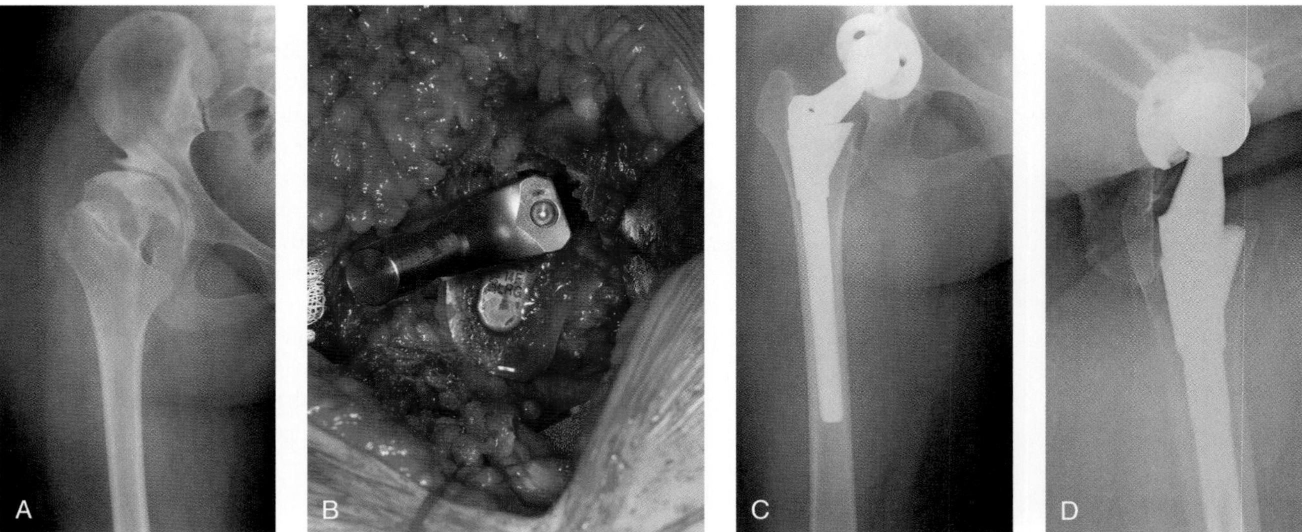

Figure 4 **A,** AP radiograph demonstrates the right hip of a 34-year-old woman with substantial anteversion of the proximal femur. **B,** Intraoperative photograph of the proximal femur shows the modular femoral implant and the marked mismatch between the femoral anteversion and the anteversion of the prosthesis. The modular sleeve is oriented to the anatomy of the patient, and the prosthesis is derotated to re-create normal femoral anteversion. AP (**C**) and lateral (**D**) postoperative radiographs of the same patient demonstrate the modular prosthesis and the mismatch between the bony anatomy and the prosthetic anteversion. (Reproduced from Cabanela ME: Total hip arthroplasty: Degenerative dysplasia of the hip, in Lieberman JR, Berry DJ, eds: *Advanced Reconstruction: Hip*. Rosemont, IL, American Academy of Orthopaedic Surgeons, 2005, pp 115-120.)

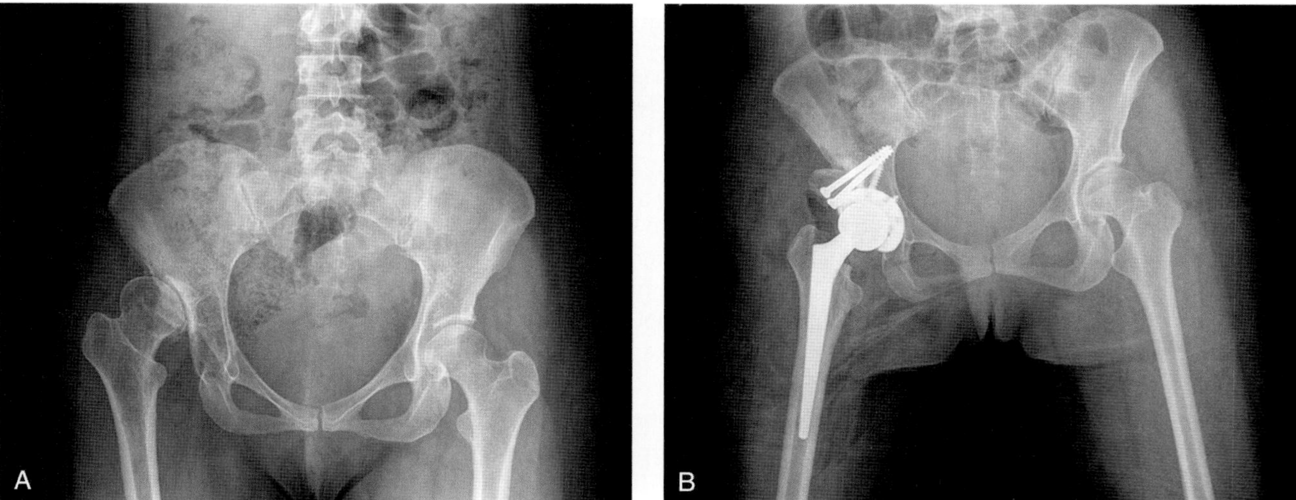

Figure 5 **A,** AP pelvic radiograph demonstrates a highly symptomatic low dislocation in a 36-year-old woman. **B,** Postoperative AP pelvic radiograph demonstrates the same patient after total hip arthroplasty with a Wagner-type conic stem. To manage the excessive femoral anteversion, the stem was rotated in a posterior direction at the time of insertion.

fitted separately, which allows simultaneous accommodation and correction of the femoral deformity. Modular implants allow the anteversion of the femoral implant to be adjusted independent of the patient's anatomy and can be useful in this scenario (**Figure 4**).

- Another useful implant type is the conic Wagner style stem, which can be inserted regardless of the femoral version (**Figure 5**).

Wound Closure

- Routine layered wound closure is performed.
- Use of drains is optional and depends on the amount of intraoperative bleeding.

Avoiding Pitfalls and Complications

As noted previously, most patients who undergo THA for the management of DDH are younger than 50 years. Therefore, a well-performed reconstruction is critically important to ensure long-lasting satisfactory results. As deformity of the acetabular and femoral anatomy increases, the technical difficulty of the reconstruction also increases.

Following the abnormal anatomy of the acetabulum too closely, such as with excessive anteversion of the acetabular implant, can result in anterior instability. A substantial amount of acetabular deformity can be present despite a relatively normal-looking AP radiograph. The surgeon must be aware of this possibility and plan the procedure accordingly. Following the outline of the anterior and posterior acetabular walls on the AP pelvic radiograph typically provides a sufficient indication of the amount of anteversion present. If any doubt remains, a preoperative false-profile radiograph will yield the best estimate of the extent of acetabular anteversion.

Femoral anteversion may be difficult to assess. Even if the AP radiograph appears normal, substantial femoral antetorsion can be present. Attempting to fit a proximally coated noncemented stem in a deformed proximal femur can result in proximal femoral fracture. Use of a cemented stem or a modular or conic stem, as discussed previously, can help avoid this complication.

Nerve injury is a risk in these patients. Avoidance of excessive lengthening may reduce this risk. Optimization of hip biomechanics and implant stability improves the potential to restore normal gait postoperatively and reduces the substantial long-term risk of implant loosening in these young patients.

Bibliography

Abdel MP, Stryker LS, Trousdale RT, Berry DJ, Cabanela ME: Uncemented acetabular components with femoral head autograft for acetabular reconstruction in developmental dysplasia of the hip: A concise follow-up report at a mean of twenty years. *J Bone Joint Surg Am* 2014;96(22):1878-1882.

Abolghasemian M, Drexler M, Abdelbary H, et al: Revision of the acetabular component in dysplastic hips previously reconstructed with a shelf autograft: Study of the outcome with special assessment of bone-stock changes. *Bone Joint J* 2013;95-B(6):777-781.

Anderson MJ, Harris WH: Total hip arthroplasty with insertion of the acetabular component without cement in hips with total congenital dislocation or marked congenital dysplasia. *J Bone Joint Surg Am* 1999;81(3):347-354.

Crowe JF, Mani VJ, Ranawat CS: Total hip replacement in congenital dislocation and dysplasia of the hip. *J Bone Joint Surg Am* 1979;61(1):15-23.

Dorr LD, Tawakkol S, Moorthy M, Long W, Wan Z: Medial protrusio technique for placement of a porous-coated, hemispherical acetabular component without cement in a total hip arthroplasty in patients who have acetabular dysplasia. *J Bone Joint Surg Am* 1999;81(1):83-92.

Dunn HK, Hess WE: Total hip reconstruction in chronically dislocated hips. *J Bone Joint Surg Am* 1976;58(6):838-845.

Hartofilakidis G, Stamos K, Karachalios T, Ioannidis TT, Zacharakis N: Congenital hip disease in adults: Classification of acetabular deficiencies and operative treatment with acetabuloplasty combined with total hip arthroplasty. *J Bone Joint Surg Am* 1996;78(5):683-692.

Karachalios T, Roidis N, Lampropoulou-Adamidou K, Hartofilakidis G: Acetabular reconstruction in patients with low and high dislocation: 20- to 32-year survival of an impaction grafting technique (named cotyloplasty). *Bone Joint J* 2013;95-B(7):887-892.

Morsi E, Garbuz D, Gross AE: Total hip arthroplasty with shelf grafts using uncemented cups: A long-term follow-up study. *J Arthroplasty* 1996;11(1):81-85.

Nawabi DH, Meftah M, Nam D, Ranawat AS, Ranawat CS: Durable fixation achieved with medialized, high hip center cementless THAs for Crowe II and III dysplasia. *Clin Orthop Relat Res* 2014;472(2):630-636.

Numair J, Joshi AB, Murphy JC, Porter ML, Hardinge K: Total hip arthroplasty for congenital dysplasia or dislocation of the hip: Survivorship analysis and long-term results. *J Bone Joint Surg Am* 1997;79(9):1352-1360.

Pak P, de Steiger R: Cone femoral prosthesis for osteoarthritis of the hip with femoral dysplasia. *J Orthop Surg (Hong Kong)* 2008;16(2):206-210.

Silber DA, Engh CA: Cementless total hip arthroplasty with femoral head bone grafting for hip dysplasia. *J Arthroplasty* 1990;5(3):231-240.

Sochart DH, Porter ML: The long-term results of Charnley low-friction arthroplasty in young patients who have congenital dislocation, degenerative osteoarthrosis, or rheumatoid arthritis. *J Bone Joint Surg Am* 1997;79(11):1599-1617.

Spangehl MJ, Berry DJ, Trousdale RT, Cabanela ME: Uncemented acetabular components with bulk femoral head autograft for acetabular reconstruction in developmental dysplasia of the hip: Results at five to twelve years. *J Bone Joint Surg Am* 2001;83(10):1484-1489.

Ström H, Mallmin H, Milbrink J, Petrén-Mallmin M, Nivbrant B, Kolstad K: The cone hip stem: A prospective study of 13 patients followed for 5 years with RSA. *Acta Orthop Scand* 2003;74(5):525-530.

Chapter 20

Total Hip Arthroplasty in Patients With High Hip Dislocation

James L. Howard, MD, MSc, FRCSC

Indications

In patients with untreated or unsuccessfully treated high-riding developmental dysplasia of the hip (DDH), symptomatic secondary arthritis frequently develops. Total hip arthroplasty (THA) may be considered in adult patients with high-riding (or high) hip dysplasia who have progressive pain and dysfunction secondary to degenerative changes at the hip. Nonsurgical management including activity modification, analgesics, NSAIDs, and walking aids should be attempted before surgical intervention is considered. Patients with high-riding hip dysplasia may become symptomatic later in life (age range, 40 to 59 years), whereas patients with lower-grade dysplasia may become symptomatic earlier (age range, 20 to 39 years). Patients are frequently women of childbearing age with active lifestyles. Some may have undergone previous surgical procedures such as femoral or acetabular osteotomies. Often the dysplastic high hip occurs bilaterally; therefore, staged bilateral reconstruction may be necessary. Because of the young age of patients undergoing this type of THA, counseling regarding the likelihood of future revision is recommended.

The anatomy of severely dysplastic hips increases the complexity of THA. Reconstruction of a high-riding dysplastic hip with THA is one of the most technically demanding procedures an arthroplasty surgeon can perform. Two radiographic classifications of hip dysplasia are commonly used. The Hartofilakidis classification has three categories: dysplasia, low dislocation, and high dislocation. In high dislocations, articulation of the femoral head with the lateral pelvis creates a false acetabulum proximal to the true acetabulum. The Crowe system further classifies high dislocations as Crowe type III or IV on the basis of proximal migration relative to the radiographic teardrop. In patients with Crowe type III dislocation, the femoral head has eroded a portion of the superolateral true acetabulum. Structural grafts may be required to improve implant coverage in these patients. In patients with Crowe type IV dislocation, this bone remains intact and provides more host bone for implant coverage.

Typically, the true acetabulum is hypoplastic, the femur has a small canal diameter and often has abnormal anteversion, and the soft tissues surrounding the hip joint are contracted because of the chronic dislocation. The surgical technique includes reconstruction of an anatomic hip center to maximize durability and a subtrochanteric femoral shortening osteotomy to avoid overlengthening of the leg, which can result in neurologic compromise (**Figure 1**). Proximal femoral anteversion can be corrected with the use of a subtrochanteric osteotomy to place the greater trochanter and abductors in an anatomic lateral position and restore the abductor lever arm. The technique preserves metaphyseal fixation and avoids the need for trochanteric osteotomy and advancement techniques.

Contraindications

A history of infection at the surgical site is a potential contraindication to THA for the management of high-riding hip dysplasia. In patients with a history of infection at the surgical site, the possibility of low-grade chronic infection should be investigated before the procedure is performed. If infection is identified at the surgical site, it must be treated appropriately and cleared before arthroplasty is performed. Any remote sites of infection that are currently active should be treated before the procedure is performed.

Appropriate evaluation and counseling is necessary when arthroplasty is considered in patients with high-riding hip dysplasia. Some patients with a high-riding dysplastic hip have minimal

Dr. Howard or an immediate family member is a member of a speakers' bureau or has made paid presentations on behalf of, serves as a paid consultant to, and has received research or institutional support from DePuy Synthes; and has received nonincome support (such as equipment or services), commercially derived honoraria, or other non–research-related funding (such as paid travel) from DePuy Synthes, MicroPort, Smith & Nephew, Stryker, and Zimmer Biomet.

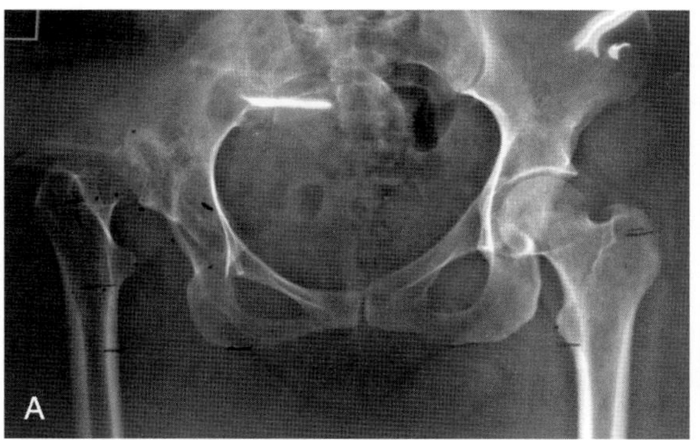

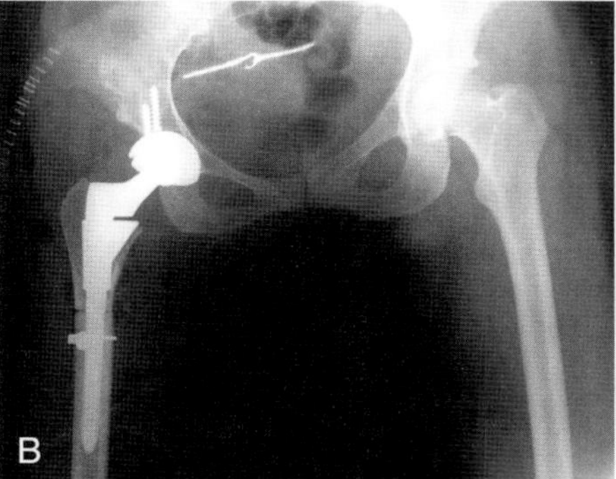

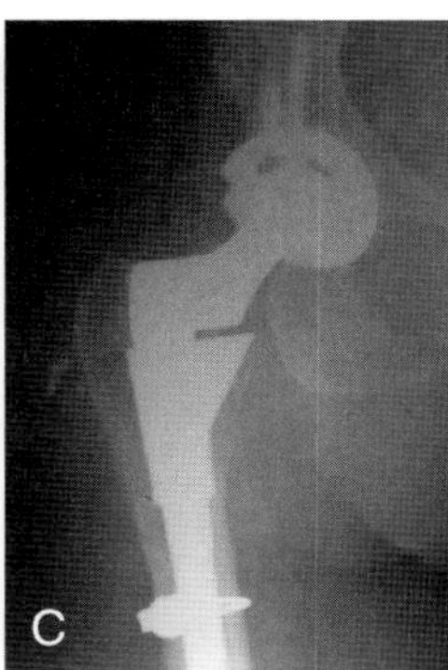

Figure 1 **A,** Preoperative AP pelvic radiograph demonstrates unilateral Crowe type IV developmental dysplasia of the right hip in a 32-year-old woman. **B,** AP pelvic radiograph obtained after transverse subtrochanteric osteotomy demonstrates reconstruction of the affected hip with total hip arthroplasty at the true (anatomic) hip center. **C,** AP hip radiograph obtained 1 year postoperatively demonstrates complete union at the osteotomy site.

pain but are concerned about their limb-length discrepancy and/or gait pattern. Nonsurgical measures such as shoe modification, physical therapy, and gait aids should be considered in these patients. Surgical treatment should be delayed until symptoms consistent with degenerative changes develop in the dysplastic hip. The technique described in this chapter is not indicated if conventional THA can be performed by placing the acetabular implant at the desired location and placing the femoral implant in a location that preserves the proximal femoral anatomy and avoids excessive limb lengthening.

Alternative Treatments

Early screening and prevention programs are critical in avoiding high-riding DDH and subsequent degenerative problems requiring complex reconstruction. If DDH is identified early, most children can be successfully treated to restore the hip to its anatomic center, maintain congruity of the joint, and maximize femoral head coverage.

If DDH is not identified and managed early, high-riding hip dysplasia can develop in adulthood. Few alternative procedures are available to manage this challenging condition. Periacetabular and femoral osteotomies that have been successful in patients with low-grade dysplasia are contraindicated in patients with high-riding hip dysplasia. Similarly, although Chiari osteotomies have been described for the management of low-riding hip dysplasia with less than 2 cm of proximal migration, the procedure is inappropriate in patients with high-riding hip dysplasia. Hip fusion is a potential alternative procedure. However, the challenge of obtaining successful fusion combined with the functional limitations imposed on the patient generally make this option less desirable. Girdlestone resection arthroplasty with soft-tissue releases can be considered in low-demand, nonambulatory patients with conditions such as cerebral palsy. In these patients who have symptomatic degenerative changes resulting from high-riding hip dysplasia, substantial pain relief and improved personal hygiene can be achieved with a resection arthroplasty.

Reconstruction of the hip using a high hip center has been described as an alternative to the technique presented in this chapter. The use of a high hip center decreases the need for femoral shortening osteotomy. However, concerns associated with this technique include limited bone available for screw fixation, abnormal biomechanics resulting in early loosening, and impingement in flexion (anterior superior iliac spine) or extension (ischial tuberosity). Because of these concerns, many surgeons prefer to perform reconstruction at the true hip center.

Results

Patients with high-riding hip dysplasia managed with THA generally experience substantial pain relief postoperatively. Improved clinical outcome scores are generally noted in most series. Patients with substantial stiffness preoperatively may have residual stiffness. Complication rates of THA in patients with high-riding hip dysplasia are higher than those in patients with lower-grade dysplastic hips. **Table 1** summarizes the results of some previous investigations of THA in patients with high-riding hip dysplasia.

Techniques

Preoperative Templating

- To calculate the existing limb-length discrepancy, a horizontal line is drawn connecting the radiographic teardrops on the preoperative AP pelvic radiograph. Distances are measured from this reference line to similar fixed points on each

Table 1 Results of Total Hip Arthroplasty in Patients With High Hip Dislocation

Authors (Year)	Number of Hips	Approach	Implant Type	Mean Patient Age in Years (Range)	Mean Follow-up in Years (Range)	Results
Stans et al (1998)	70	Transtrochanteric (63), anterolateral (5), posterior (2)	Cemented acetabulum and femur (several designs)	50 (21-75)	16.6 (5-23)	All Crowe type III dysplasia No shortening osteotomies Trochanteric union rate, 87% Aseptic loosening developed in 53% of acetabular cups and 40% of femoral stems Acetabular failure was higher when outside true acetabulum 1 sciatic nerve injury and 1 sciatic/femoral nerve injury 2 dislocations
Anderson and Harris (1999)	20	Posterior (3), trochanteric osteotomy (17)	Noncemented acetabulum (Harris-Galante) Noncemented and cemented femur	52 (25-87)	6.9 (5.3-8.5)	Hartofilakidis low and high type hips No shortening osteotomies Mean HHS, 90 Trochanteric union rate, 88% 1 femoral/sciatic nerve palsy 1 dislocation No acetabular failures 1 femoral implant loosening
Masonis et al (2003)	21	Lateral (13), posterior (8)	Noncemented acetabulum (several designs) Noncemented and cemented femur (several designs)	48 (21-69)	5.8 (2-11.2)	Crowe type III and IV hips All had subtrochanteric osteotomy Femoral osteotomy union rate, 91% 33% underwent acetabular grafting Mean HHS, 74 3 dislocations 5 hips required revision surgery No neurologic compromise
Krych et al (2010)	28	Posterior (26), anterolateral (2)	Noncemented acetabulum (several designs) Noncemented (S-ROM; DePuy) and extensively porous-coated femoral designs	48 (30-72)	4.8 (2-13.4)	Crowe type IV hips All had subtrochanteric osteotomy Osteotomy union rate, 93% Mean HHS, 89 4 dislocations 6 hips required revision surgery No neurologic compromise
Sofu et al (2015)	73	Posterior	Noncemented acetabulum (Trident; Stryker) Noncemented femur (Omnifit; Stryker)	47 (31-69)	5.1 (3-7.6)	Crowe type III and IV hips All had subtrochanteric osteotomy Femoral osteotomy union rate, 94.5% Mean HHS, 84 6 femoral implants required revision No neurologic compromise

HHS = Harris hip score.

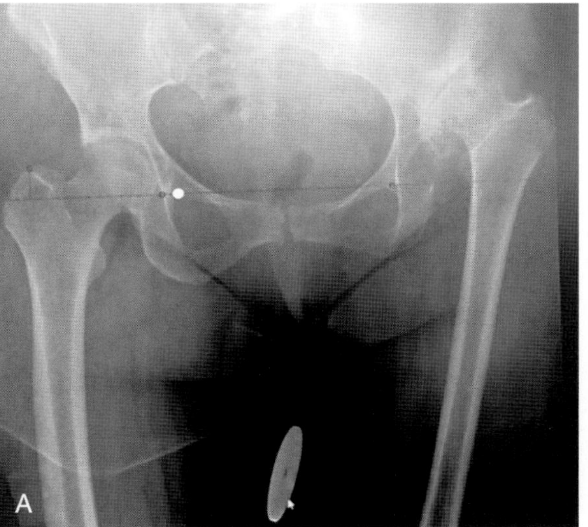

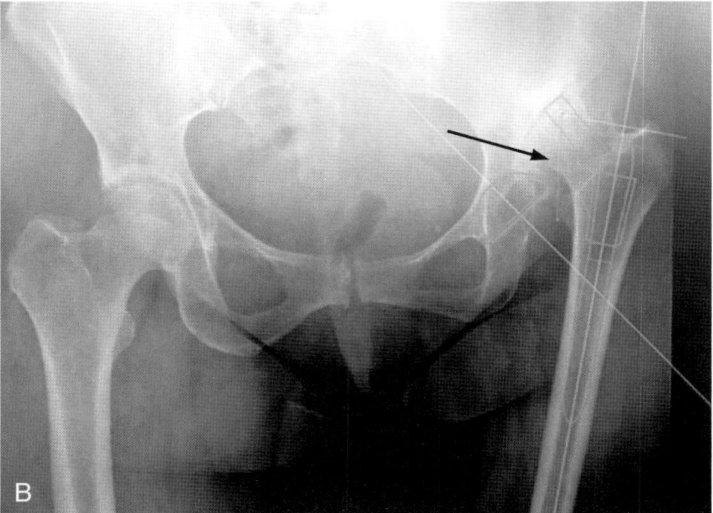

Figure 2 AP pelvic radiographs demonstrate calculation of the preoperative limb-length discrepancy in a patient with high hip dysplasia. **A,** A horizontal line is drawn connecting the radiographic teardrops of the hips. Distances are measured from this reference line to similar fixed points on each femur to determine the limb-length discrepancy. **B,** The vertical distance between the center of rotation of the templated acetabular implant and the femoral implant represents the length that will be gained as a result of the procedure. Subtrochanteric osteotomy should be considered in all patients with an anticipated gain of more than 2 to 2.5 cm.

femur to determine the limb-length discrepancy (**Figure 2, A**).

- An appropriately sized acetabular implant template is positioned at the true acetabulum. The amount of medialization required and the amount of the implant left uncovered are noted.
- An appropriately sized proximal sleeve and stem template are selected for the femur.
- A vertical line is drawn from the center of rotation of the femoral implant template to the center of rotation of the acetabular implant template and is measured (**Figure 2, B**). This distance represents the length that can be gained without a shortening osteotomy.
- Partial or complete sciatic or femoral nerve palsies have been reported in patients with DDH who have undergone THA, especially when the limb is lengthened more than 4 cm or 6% of the limb length. Therefore, shortening osteotomy should be considered in all patients in whom lengthening of more than 2 to 2.5 cm is anticipated.

Setup/Exposure

- The patient is placed in the lateral decubitus position with the affected hip facing up and the long axis of the body parallel to the surgical table.
- Pelvic support devices are applied to keep the pelvis stable in that position for the duration of the procedure.
- The location of the surgical incision for a posterior approach to the hip is marked. To do so, the patient's hip is flexed, and a line is drawn along the long axis of the femur. The incision curves posteriorly near the tip of the trochanter when the leg is brought back to a slightly flexed position.
- The skin and subcutaneous tissue are incised.
- The fascia is opened in line with the incision.
- The fibers of the gluteus maximus are divided proximally.
- The bursa is elevated off the short external rotators.
- Any obvious vessels are cauterized.
- The gluteus medius and gluteus minimus muscles are retracted anteriorly. These muscles often are underdeveloped and have a horizontal or reverse oblique vector of pull.
- The sciatic nerve is palpated posteriorly in the soft tissues. To avoid devascularization, dissection of the nerve is not recommended. The baseline tension in the nerve before dislocation is noted to allow comparison with the tension after the reconstruction is complete.
- The piriformis is identified. The capsule is opened proximally in an oblique manner, and the opening is continued distally to the greater trochanter. Capsular hypertrophy is often present, and there is an hourglass constriction between the femoral head and the true acetabulum.
- The piriformis and the short external rotators are released off the femur in a single soft-tissue sleeve. These muscles may be severely dysplastic.
- Progressive internal rotation of the femur facilitates the dissection.
- It is often helpful to place tag sutures in the soft-tissue sleeve consisting

of the piriformis, the capsule, and the short external rotators.
- The hip is dislocated from the false acetabulum with internal rotation.

Instruments/Equipment/ Implants Required

ACETABULAR IMPLANT

- Noncemented acetabular fixation is generally preferred. The use of modular, noncemented porous-coated acetabular implants with multiple screw holes increases the options for fixation in poor-quality bone.
- Extra-small acetabular implants are often required (38 to 46 mm).
- Smaller femoral heads (22 and 28 mm) are often required to maintain adequate polyethylene thickness.

FEMORAL IMPLANT

- Noncemented femoral fixation is generally preferred. The technique described in this chapter is based on a modular system that provides proximal metaphyseal support, distal fluted fixation, and anteversion adjustment (for example, S-ROM [DePuy Synthes] or Emperion [Smith & Nephew]).
- Alternatively, noncemented extensively porous-coated implants with a narrow proximal flare can be used.
- Cemented femoral fixation has been described. However, the use of cement in combination with an osteotomy increases the risk of nonunion.

Procedure

INITIAL FEMORAL PREPARATION

- A femoral neck osteotomy is performed at a level that is determined by using the preoperative template.
- Several anatomic differences in patients with DDH must be accounted for. These patients typically have a small femoral head, coxa valga, excessive anteversion, and a posterior trochanter. The metaphyseal flare is often decreased and narrows to a tight isthmus. The femoral canal is narrow, with a smaller mediolateral than AP diameter.
- A box osteotome is used to open the femoral canal.
- Intramedullary canal reaming is completed with blunt-tipped reamers until cortical fit is achieved. The diameter of the final reamer determines the diaphyseal stem size (**Figure 3, A**).
- Proximal femoral reaming is completed with a cone reamer and a milling reamer to prepare the femur for the proximal femoral sleeve (**Figure 3, B**).
- A trial proximal sleeve is placed. Often, the sleeve must be placed in excessive anteversion to match the native anatomy (**Figure 4, A**).
- A transverse subtrochanteric femoral osteotomy is performed 1 to 2 cm below the distal aspect of the sleeve (**Figure 3, B**).

ACETABULAR PREPARATION

- The proximal femoral segment is mobilized anteriorly.
- Careful dissection is completed to release the capsule anteriorly. Release of the psoas tendon off the lesser trochanter may be required.
- The true hip center is identified by following the remnant of the ligamentum teres to the fovea. Alternatively, the surgeon can pass a finger inferiorly through the hourglass constriction in the capsule to localize the true acetabulum.
- The true acetabulum is small and can be difficult to identify. An intraoperative radiograph can be obtained to confirm the location of the true acetabulum.
- Retractors are placed anteriorly and inferiorly to expose the true acetabulum (**Figure 4, B**). In patients with high-riding hip dysplasia, the deep femoral artery becomes proximally displaced and is at risk of injury at the inferior margin of the acetabulum. Dissection in this area must be performed with great care.
- The capsule is elevated posteriorly. Headed pins can be placed in the posterior column to facilitate retraction.
- The fat pad is resected to identify the medial wall of the acetabulum.
- To estimate the amount of bone available for medialization, a 2.5-mm hole can be drilled through the medial wall. A depth gauge is then used to measure the thickness of the medial wall before reaming.
- Sequential acetabular reaming is completed. Small-diameter reamers (38 to 46 mm) are often required. The bone is often osteopenic, and care must be taken not to overream the acetabulum.
- The host acetabulum is often anteverted, with relative deficiency of the anterior wall and anterior column. To achieve adequate coverage of the implant, preferential posterior reaming may be required.
- Options to improve implant coverage and stability in Crowe type III hips with deficient superolateral coverage are a controlled medial protrusio technique or the use of a femoral head autograft superolaterally.
- A hemispheric, porous-coated acetabular implant is impacted into position, with care taken to ensure appropriate anteversion and closure of the socket.
- Supplementary screw fixation of the acetabulum is recommended to augment the press-fit fixation.
- A trial acetabular liner (often 22 or 28 mm) is placed in the socket.

FINAL FEMORAL PREPARATION

- A trial femoral head and neck are placed on the trial femoral sleeve. The proximal segment is reduced into the acetabulum.

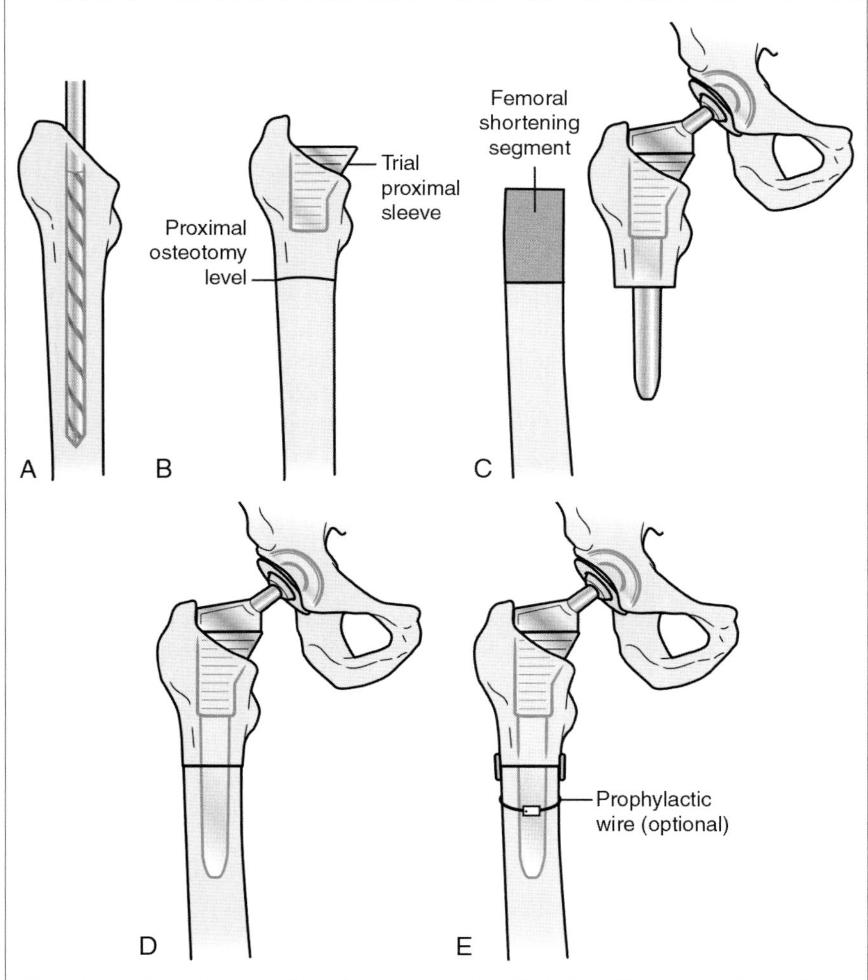

Figure 3 Illustrations depict femoral reconstruction to manage high hip dysplasia. **A,** The intramedullary canal is reamed with blunt-tipped reamers until cortical contact is achieved. **B,** Proximal femoral reaming is completed with a cone reamer and a milling reamer to prepare the femur for the proximal femoral sleeve. After a trial proximal sleeve is placed, a transverse subtrochanteric femoral osteotomy is performed 1 to 2 cm below the distal aspect of the sleeve. **C,** A trial stem is inserted through the sleeve. After the proximal segment is reduced into the acetabulum, the overlap between the proximal and distal segments represents the required amount of shortening. **D,** The trial construct is reduced after the distal segment has been shortened and a trial stem has been placed across the osteotomy. **E,** The final implants have been placed with careful attention to the final anteversion of the femoral implant and the final position of the proximal fragment. A prophylactic wire can be placed around the distal segment before the final femoral implant is placed. Autogenous bone graft is placed around the osteotomy site.

- Gentle traction is applied to the leg, and the amount of overlap between the proximal and distal segments is evaluated (**Figures 3, C** and **4, C**). This overlap represents the amount of bone that should be removed with the shortening osteotomy. Generally, slightly less bone is removed initially because additional bone can be removed later in the procedure if required.
- The trial femoral implant is dislocated from the acetabulum.
- A second transverse osteotomy is performed in the distal segment on the basis of the overlap measurement, with care taken to remain parallel to the plane of the first osteotomy.
- Diaphyseal reaming is completed to prepare the distal segment of the femur in which the femoral stem will engage.
- The final reamer size is defined by the implant size chosen for the proximal sleeve. Because the femur is shortened, a portion of the anterior bow of the femur is removed. Therefore, in some patients, slight underreaming of 0.5 to 1.0 mm can help ensure engagement of the stem in the distal segment.
- A definitive trial implant is assembled and inserted through the proximal segment and into the distal femur.
- The trial implant is reduced into the acetabulum (**Figure 3, D**).
- With the trial construct reduced, limb lengths are compared by palpating the knees and the bottom of the feet. Despite the shortening procedure, the leg is usually lengthened. The lengthening is compared with the lengthening that was planned on the basis of preoperative templating.
- The sciatic nerve is palpated posteriorly to assess the amount of tension in comparison with the amount of tension that was present before reconstruction.
- Hip stability and abductor tension are evaluated.
- The osteotomy site is assessed to evaluate the amount of contact between the proximal and distal segments. Small corrections to the osteotomy planes are made as needed to maximize contact between the segments.
- The hip is dislocated, and the trial implants are removed.

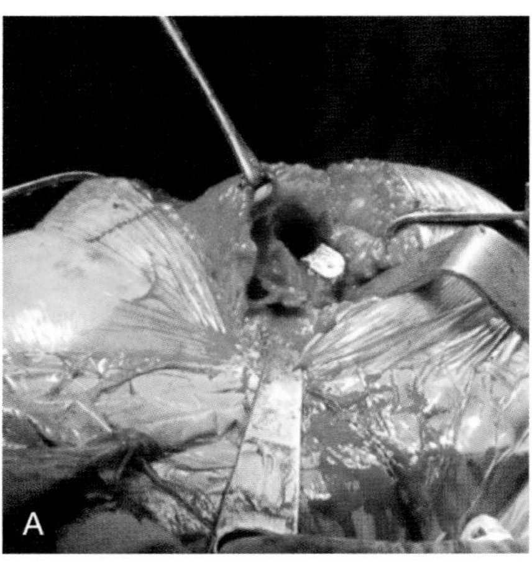

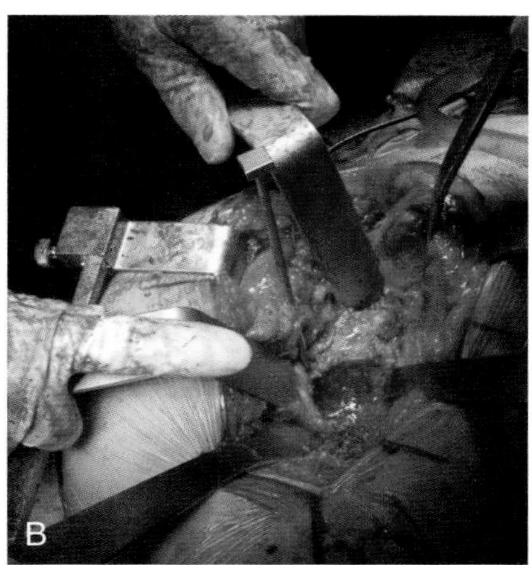

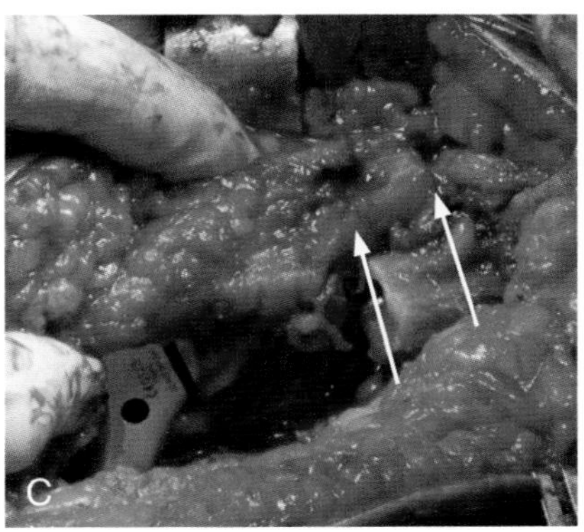

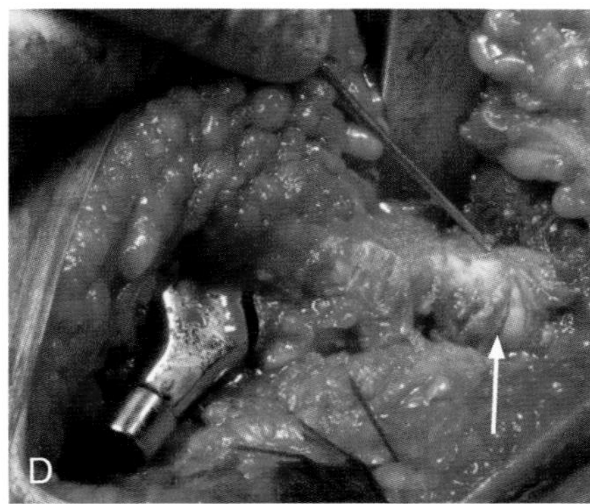

Figure 4 Intraoperative photographs of different hips show steps in femoral reconstruction to manage high hip dysplasia. **A,** A trial proximal femoral sleeve is placed in the femur. The sleeve is placed in excessive anteversion to match the anatomy of the proximal femur. **B,** Retractors are placed for acetabular exposure after reaming has been completed. **C,** The proximal femoral segment is reduced into the acetabulum. The amount of overlap between the proximal and distal femoral segments indicates the amount of distal resection required (arrows). **D,** The definitive proximal sleeve and stem are placed. The proximal segment has been derotated to an appropriate amount of anteversion. The osteotomy site is well approximated (arrow).

FINAL IMPLANT INSERTION

- The definitive acetabular liner is placed into the acetabular cup.
- The definitive metaphyseal sleeve is impacted into the proximal segment.
- The femur is positioned for insertion of the final femoral stem. The lower leg and foot are positioned vertically to serve as an easy reference for anteversion.
- A clamp is placed on the proximal segment to provide rotational control. The proximal segment is derotated to an appropriate amount of anteversion.
- The definitive stem is inserted through the proximal sleeve and into the distal segment in appropriate anteversion. After the stem begins to gain fixation in the distal segment, no further changes of version will be possible. A prophylactic wire can be placed on the distal segment before definitive impaction of the stem (**Figure 3, E**).
- The stem is impacted into the distal segment until the osteotomy closes (**Figure 4, D**).
- Additional fixation of the osteotomy site typically is not required. If additional fixation is necessary, the resected segment of femur can be divided and secured to the femur with wires as an onlay strut autograft. If the segment of resected bone is small, a cortical strut allograft or a short locking plate with unicortical screws can be used to augment the osteotomy fixation.
- Cancellous graft from the acetabular and femoral reamers is placed at the osteotomy site (**Figure 3, E**).
- The definitive head is placed on the trunnion, and the hip is relocated into position.
- Final limb length and stability as well as soft-tissue and sciatic nerve tension are assessed.

Wound Closure

- The piriformis, short external rotators, and capsule are reapproximated with nonabsorbable suture by means of either drill holes in the trochanter or side-to-side soft-tissue repair.
- The fascia and subcutaneous tissues are closed with running absorbable sutures.
- The skin is closed with staples.

Postoperative Regimen

Patients are mobilized immediately postoperatively with physical therapy. Prophylactic antibiotics are administered for 24 hours postoperatively. Patients are maintained on deep vein thrombosis prophylaxis per the American College of Chest Physicians guidelines. Patients with residual limb-length discrepancy may require assessment for shoe lifts or modifications. Staples are removed 14 days postoperatively. Patients should continue toe-touch weight bearing for a minimum of 6 weeks. Patients are seen for radiographic follow-up at 6 weeks, and weight bearing is advanced on the basis of healing visualized at the osteotomy site.

Avoiding Pitfalls and Complications

During acetabular preparation, the surgeon must remain aware of the deficiency of the anterior column and anterior wall in these patients compared with that of other patients. Preferential posterior reaming may be required to maximize implant coverage. Care must be taken to avoid overreaming the anterior and medial walls, and the superolateral rim of the host acetabulum. The bone at the true acetabulum is usually soft, and the use of reamers in a reverse mode may be helpful. This method will help preserve bone stock by expanding the acetabulum and compacting rather than removing bone.

Intraoperative femur fractures can occur in both the proximal and distal segment. Preparation for the metaphyseal sleeve can weaken the proximal segment because of the size of the sleeve required to match the diaphyseal fixation distally. If bone quality is poor, prophylactic wiring of the proximal segment before definitive placement of the proximal sleeve should be considered. Fractures can occur in the distal femoral segment during femoral preparation and placement of the femoral implant. Some surgeons routinely place a cerclage cable prophylactically just distal to the distal osteotomy site before femoral preparation and implant impaction.

Nonunion of a transverse subtrochanteric osteotomy occurs infrequently. Nonunion may be the result of inadequate fixation in the diaphysis or poor bone contact at the osteotomy site. Reliable fixation in the distal femur can usually be obtained with a diaphyseal locking press-fit stem (with either extensive porous coating or sharp antirotation flutes). Adjunctive techniques such as cortical onlay autograft or allograft segments, or the use of locking plates, can be used intraoperatively to augment stability as needed. Additionally, the surgeon should focus specific attention to the amount of bone-to-bone contact at the subtrochanteric osteotomy site. Apposition at the osteotomy site should be checked with the trial implant in place and with the proximal and distal fragments in the anticipated final rotational position. If necessary, the bone ends of the osteotomy should be trimmed before definitive placement of the implant. Treatment of nonunion includes revision of the stem to a longer or larger-diameter stem to achieve stability, cancellous bone grafting at the osteotomy site, and augmentation of fixation with cortical allograft struts or compression plating.

Dislocation rates of 5% to 11% have been reported after THA in patients with severe dysplasia. Factors related to the soft tissue, bone, and implant all contribute to the instability in these patients. Trial reductions are important to confirm implant position, soft-tissue tension, osteotomy position, and stability before definitive implant placement. Final rotational alignment of the implants and bone fragments is essential to obtain optimal stability and an optimal arc of motion of the hip. In particular, the surgeon must verify the rotational position of the final stem early in the impaction process because changes to the version will not be possible after the stem begins to engage the diaphysis.

Sciatic and femoral nerve palsies (both partial and complete) have been reported as a complication of THA in patients with high-riding DDH. These complications are more frequent in patients with limb lengthening of more than 4 cm. The sciatic nerve is dysplastic with abnormal vascularity and may be tethered as a result of previous surgical treatment. In patients with high hip dysplasia, the femoral nerve exits from the pelvis more superolaterally than in most patients, and the use of anterior retractors may place this nerve at risk. Care must be taken when passing cerclage wires around the femur to avoid damage to the sciatic nerve and when placing anterior retractors to avoid damage to the femoral nerve. The use of the wake-up test, somatosensory-evoked potentials, and electromyographic monitoring in the operating room remains controversial. Patients with complete palsy may warrant a return to the operating room to undergo assessment for compression hematoma or, if the surgeon thinks that the nerve is under substantial residual tension, to undergo further shortening.

Bibliography

Anderson MJ, Harris WH: Total hip arthroplasty with insertion of the acetabular component without cement in hips with total congenital dislocation or marked congenital dysplasia. *J Bone Joint Surg Am* 1999;81(3):347-354.

Crowe JF, Mani VJ, Ranawat CS: Total hip replacement in congenital dislocation and dysplasia of the hip. *J Bone Joint Surg Am* 1979;61(1):15-23.

Hartofilakidis G, Stamos K, Karachalios T, Ioannidis TT, Zacharakis N: Congenital hip disease in adults: Classification of acetabular deficiencies and operative treatment with acetabuloplasty combined with total hip arthroplasty. *J Bone Joint Surg Am* 1996;78(5):683-692.

Kearon C, Akl EA, Comerota AJ, et al; American College of Chest Physicians: Antithrombotic therapy for VTE disease: Antithrombotic Therapy and Prevention of Thrombosis, 9th ed: American College of Chest Physicians Evidence-Based Clinical Practice Guidelines. *Chest* 2012;141(2 suppl):e419S-e494S.

Krych AJ, Howard JL, Trousdale RT, Cabanela ME, Berry DJ: Total hip arthroplasty with shortening subtrochanteric osteotomy in Crowe type-IV developmental dysplasia. *J Bone Joint Surg Am* 2009;91(9):2213-2221.

Krych AJ, Howard JL, Trousdale RT, Cabanela ME, Berry DJ: Total hip arthroplasty with shortening subtrochanteric osteotomy in Crowe type-IV developmental dysplasia: Surgical technique. *J Bone Joint Surg Am* 2010;92(suppl 1 pt 2):176-187.

Masonis JL, Patel JV, Miu A, et al: Subtrochanteric shortening and derotational osteotomy in primary total hip arthroplasty for patients with severe hip dysplasia: 5-year follow-up. *J Arthroplasty* 2003;18(3 suppl 1):68-73.

Sanchez-Sotelo J, Berry DJ, Trousdale RT, Cabanela ME: Surgical treatment of developmental dysplasia of the hip in adults: II. Arthroplasty options. *J Am Acad Orthop Surg* 2002;10(5):334-344.

Sofu H, Kockara N, Gursu S, Issin A, Oner A, Sahin V: Transverse subtrochanteric shortening osteotomy during cementless total hip arthroplasty in Crowe type-III or IV developmental dysplasia. *J Arthroplasty* 2015;30(6):1019-1023.

Stans AA, Pagnano MW, Shaughnessy WJ, Hanssen AD: Results of total hip arthroplasty for Crowe type III developmental hip dysplasia. *Clin Orthop Relat Res* 1998;(348):149-157.

Chapter 21
Protrusio Acetabuli

Michael H. Huo, MD
Timothy S. Brown, MD
Matthew Landrum, MD

Indications

Protrusio acetabuli is the medial migration of the acetabular floor into the true pelvis that was first described in a pathologic specimen in 1824. The overall prevalence of the condition is difficult to estimate, but it is much more common in females than males. Causes of secondary protrusio acetabuli include Marfan syndrome, Ehlers-Danlos syndrome, osteogenesis imperfecta, neurofibromatosis, rheumatoid arthritis, and ankylosing spondylitis (**Table 1**).

Radiographic definitions of and parameters in protrusio acetabuli are varied, but consistently reported characteristics include a center-edge angle greater than 40°, an acetabular floor medial to the ilioischial line by 3 mm in males and 6 mm in females, a femoral head positioned at or medial to the ilioischial line, and a negative acetabular roof angle (**Figure 1**). Coxa profunda is a condition that lies on the spectrum between a normal hip and protrusio acetabuli. It describes the finding of the acetabular floor medial to the ilioischial line with the femoral head lateral to the ilioischial line.

The normal joint reaction force across the hip during the stance phase of gait acts in a direction in line with the direction of protrusio progression. In 1965, primary protrusio was hypothesized to be related to an incomplete or delayed closure of the triradiate cartilage, resulting in an inability for the medial acetabulum to resist the normal joint reaction forces. Iatrogenic causes of protrusio can result from total hip arthroplasty (THA) and hemiarthroplasty (**Figure 2**).

Patients with protrusio acetabuli typically have activity-related groin pain and loss of motion. As the condition progresses, stiffness and contractures about the hip predominate, and often pain is reported as a secondary concern. Flexion contracture can result in excessive lordosis of the lumbar spine and mechanical back pain. Difficulty with hip abduction causes substantial functional impairment and, in women with protrusio acetabuli, often is diagnosed at their yearly gynecologic visit.

Because of the strong association

Table 1 Causes of Secondary Protrusio Acetabuli

Iatrogenic
Postoperative
Neoplastic
Neurofibromatosis
Metastatic disease
Infectious
Gram positive
Gram negative
Mycobacterial
Genetic
Marfan syndrome
Ehlers-Danlos syndrome
Sickle cell disease
Traumatic
Acetabular fractures
Metabolic
Osteogenesis imperfecta
Paget disease
Osteomalacia
Hyperparathyroidism
Inflammatory
Rheumatoid arthritis
Juvenile idiopathic arthritis
Ankylosing spondylitis
Psoriatic arthritis

Adapted from Huo MH: Total hip arthroplasty: Protrusio acetabulum, in Lieberman JR, Berry DJ, eds: *Advanced Reconstruction: Hip*. American Academy of Orthopaedic Surgeons, Rosemont, IL, 2005, pp 131-136.

Dr. Huo or an immediate family member is a member of a speakers' bureau or has made paid presentations on behalf of Johnson & Johnson; serves as a paid consultant to Zimmer Biomet and DePuy Synthes; has received research or institutional support from Zimmer Biomet; and serves as a board member, owner, officer, or committee member of the American Academy of Orthopaedic Surgeons. Dr. Landrum or an immediate family member has stock or stock options held in Abbott. Neither Dr. Brown nor any immediate family member has received anything of value from or has stock or stock options held in a commercial company or institution related directly or indirectly to the subject of this chapter.

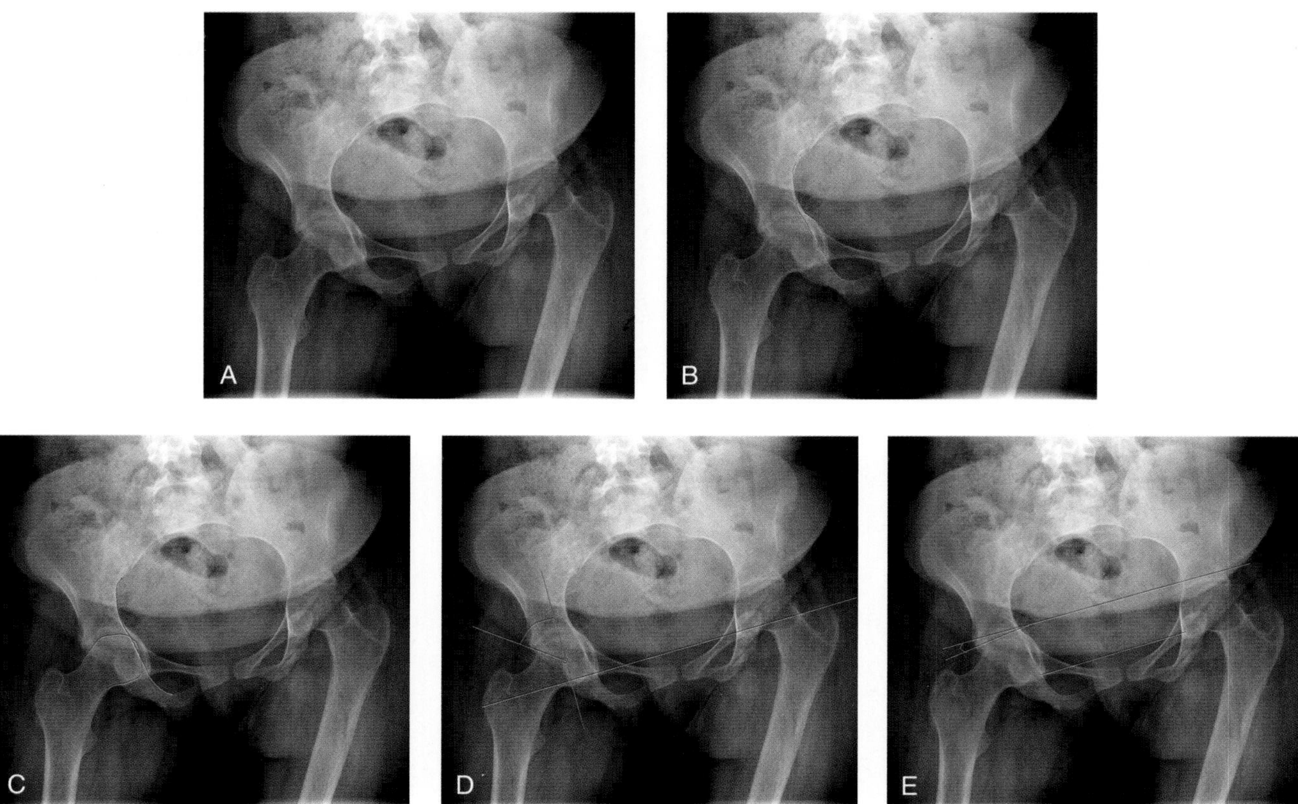

Figure 1 **A,** AP pelvic radiograph from a patient with protrusio acetabuli. **B** through **E,** The same AP pelvic radiograph with red markings indicating parameters in protrusio acetabuli. **B,** Medialization of the acetabular floor greater than 6 mm past the ilioischial line. **C,** Medialization of the femoral head past the ilioischial line. **D,** The lateral center-edge angle (angle of Wiberg). **E,** The negative acetabular roof angle.

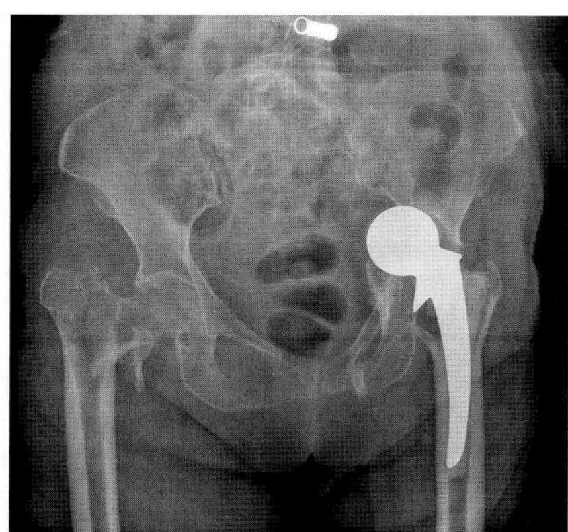

Figure 2 AP pelvic radiograph demonstrates iatrogenic protrusio acetabuli in a left hip after cemented hemiarthroplasty. The patient had little motion in the affected hip, which was asymptomatic. The protrusio acetabuli was detected radiographically when the patient was evaluated for fracture on the contralateral side.

between secondary protrusio acetabuli and several metabolic, genetic, and rheumatologic conditions, a complete history and physical examination always should be performed in patients with protrusio acetabuli. Physical examination of the patient with protrusio acetabuli shows an antalgic or Trendelenburg gait secondary to the shortened lever arm of the abductors. Examination of the lumbar spine frequently shows hyperlordosis and a fixed flexion contracture across the affected hip. Hip range of motion (ROM) is notably decreased in abduction and external rotation. Further workup consisting of laboratory studies or referral to a specialist can be decided on an individual basis, depending on abnormal findings in the examination or history.

THA is an effective surgical option and has become the standard treatment for symptomatic protrusio acetabuli, especially in patients older than 40 years (**Figure 3**). The preoperative planning is similar to that for other diagnoses managed with THA. Specific considerations for patients with protrusio acetabuli include flexion and adduction contractures, loss of motion at the hip, limb-length discrepancy, and whether the protrusio is unilateral or bilateral. Loss of motion combined with flexion and adduction contractures often results in difficult surgical exposure. Adequate soft-tissue releases and bone resection are necessary to ensure safe dislocation of the femoral head. Specific considerations include the size of the acetabular cup (optimal

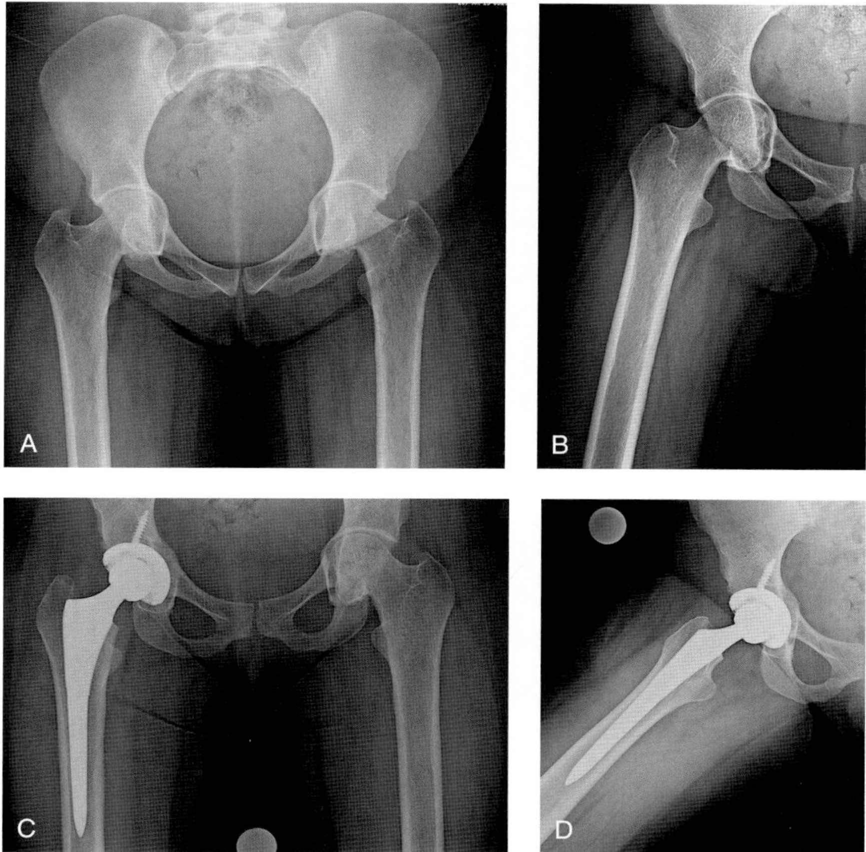

Figure 3 Preoperative AP pelvic (**A**) and lateral hip (**B**) radiographs demonstrate protrusio acetabuli of the right hip. AP pelvic (**C**) and lateral hip (**D**) radiographs obtained after the patient underwent total hip arthroplasty.

size is necessary for contact at the periphery of the acetabulum); location of the hip center (it should be lateralized to achieve rim fit of the cup); and femoral offset, paying close attention to the femoral offset and the overall joint lateralization.

Contraindications

Contraindications for THA in patients with protrusio acetabuli are similar to those for other diseases. Active infection is an absolute contraindication. Relative contraindications include neuropathic conditions, substantial myopathy, deficient or paralytic hip abductor mechanism, advanced medical comorbidities that are not correctable, morbid obesity, and a psychosocial profile that is risky for patient compliance.

Alternative Treatments

Nonsurgical management of pain and immobility resulting from protrusio acetabuli starts with activity modification, use of anti-inflammatory medications, and physical therapy. Stretching and strengthening the muscles that cross the hip joint can relieve symptoms in patients with mild protrusio acetabuli.

Options for surgical management of protrusio acetabuli depend on patient age and clinical severity. For symptomatic skeletally mature patients younger than 40 years, valgus intertrochanteric osteotomy is an option. Early recognition of the disease has led to other joint-preserving options for young patients, including surgical hip dislocation, acetabuloplasty, relative femoral neck lengthening, femoral osteotomy, arthroscopy with osteochondroplasty, and reverse periacetabular osteotomy.

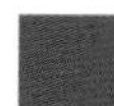

Results

High rates of clinical success have been reported after THA to manage protrusio acetabuli (**Table 2**). An early study of 253 cemented Charnley low-friction arthroplasties with a minimum follow-up of 5 years reported no difference in outcomes between THA done for protrusio acetabuli and THAs performed for other diagnoses. Another early study reported midterm results (mean, 4.3 years) of cemented THAs performed in patients who had both rheumatoid arthritis and protrusio acetabuli, with data demonstrating that restoration of the anatomic hip center was imperative for long-term survival.

Technique for noncemented cup fixation changed rapidly in the 1980s and 1990s. Early reports of this type of fixation in patients with protrusio acetabuli showed good clinical outcomes and low rates of radiographic loosening. A study published in 2007 reported no cup loosening at a mean follow-up of 4.2 years. A retrospective study published in 2008 reported no loosening in 29 THAs in which a dual-geometry noncemented cup was used (mean follow-up, 4 years). In 2011, a retrospective study of 135 THAs in 127 patients reported good overall clinical outcomes in 80% to 85% of THAs and signs of radiographic loosening in 7.4% of THAs at a mean follow-up of 12.7 years.

In a study published in 2014, long-term results were reported for 53 patients (65 hips) with protrusio acetabuli who underwent THA with a noncemented acetabular implant. Autograft was

Table 2 Implant Survivorship in Primary Total Hip Arthroplasty for Protrusio Acetabuli

Author(s) (Year)	Number of Hips	Mean Patient Age in Years (Range)	Mean Follow-up in Years (Range)	Success Rate (%)[a]	Results
Heywood (1980)	9	58 (37-71)	1.3 (0.3-2)	100	No complications
Mullaji and Marawar (2007)	30	46 (NA)	4.2 (2-10)	90	Postoperative hematoma developed in 1 hip, which required incision and drainage 1 hip required secondary suturing because of skin necrosis All acetabular implants were considered stable with no instance of graft resorption
Krushell et al (2008)	29	66 (40-82)	4 (2-9.2)	93	Peroneal nerve palsy developed in 1 hip Recurrent dislocation developed in 1 hip 1 hip underwent late revision surgery for polyethylene wear and secondary osteolysis
Dutka et al (2011)	135	55.2 (30-72)	12.7 (NA)	80-85	Loosening developed in 6 hips Complications other than aseptic loosening developed in 25 hips
Baghdadi et al (2015)	65	66 (NA)	15.4 (10-24)	70	6 hips underwent cup revision: 3 for aseptic loosening of the acetabular component, 2 for polyethylene wear, and 1 for recurrent instability 85.4% survival rate for the acetabular implant

NA = not available.
[a] Success is defined as survival from revision for any reason.

used in 58 hips. At a mean follow-up of 15 years, the survival rate from revision for any cause was 85.4% for the acetabular implant.

Technique

Setup/Exposure

- Surgical exposure can be difficult because of hip contractures and medialization of the hip center. In a patient with a prominent adduction contracture, the authors of this chapter perform percutaneous adductor tenotomy while the patient is supine, before shifting the patient to the lateral position.
- The authors of this chapter favor an anterolateral approach in patients with protrusio acetabuli because we believe the in situ neck cut is easier with this approach.
- The prominent greater trochanter, reduced ROM, and bony impingement against the femoral neck make ROM for visualization of the entire gluteus medius difficult.
- Dislocation of the femoral head must be done carefully to reduce the risk for femoral fracture. In most patients with protrusio, an in situ femoral neck osteotomy is the safest technique for dislocation.
- Visualization of the lesser trochanter often is challenging in the setting of hip flexion contracture in these patients, and care is taken to clearly define the landmark for making the definitive neck cut.
- In patients in whom the protrusio acetabuli is so severe that access to the femoral neck is impossible, a trochanteric osteotomy is recommended, after which an in situ neck cut can be performed.

Instruments/Equipment/Implants Required

- The authors of this chapter do not use any special equipment when managing protrusio acetabuli.
- Standard hip instrumentation is used for both the femur and the acetabulum. Retractors are used in the technique.

Procedure

ACETABULAR PREPARATION

- Acetabular exposure and preparation are critical to achieve optimal peripheral rim fit and lateralize the hip center of rotation without weakening the acetabulum by overreaming it medially or peripherally.
- While using a bone hook to maintain posterior traction on the femur, an intracapsular Hohmann retractor is placed posteriorly into the ischium, anterior to the femur,

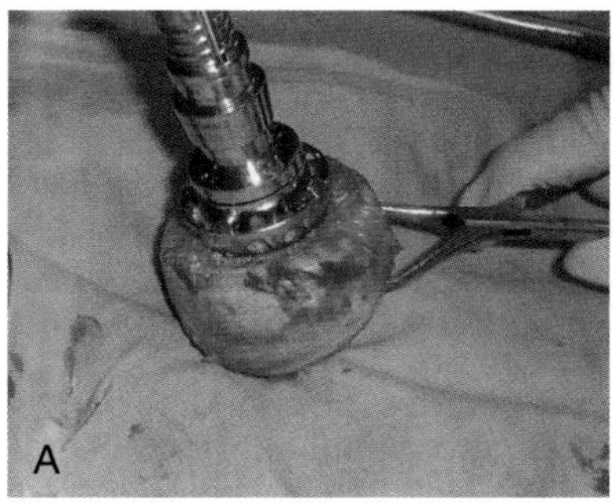

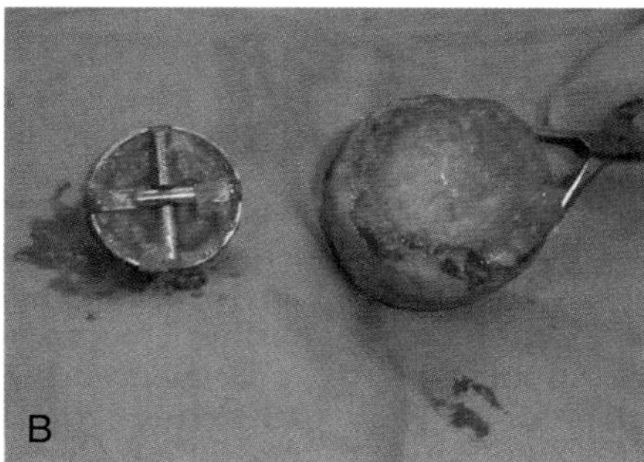

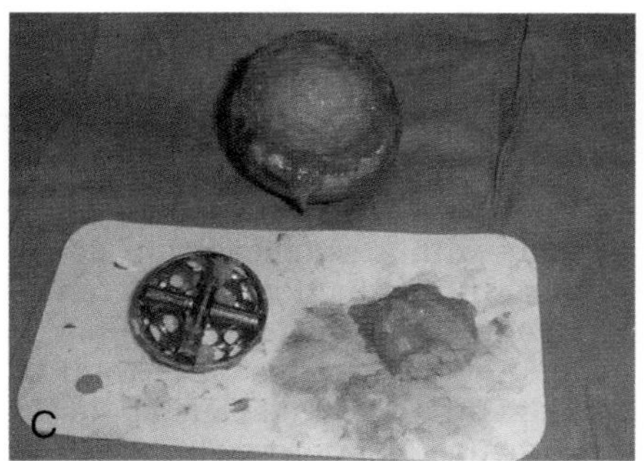

Figure 4 Photographs show preparation of the resected femoral head for morcellized autograft on a back table. **A,** The femoral head is stabilized with a penetrating towel clip, and the smallest reamer in the set is used to begin obtaining autograft. **B,** The appearance of the acetabular reamer (left) filled with graft and the femoral head (right) after bone removal. **C,** The autograft is shown after removal from the reamer. (Reproduced with permission from Padgett D: Protrusio acetabuli, in Berry DJ, Lieberman JR, eds: *Surgery of the Hip.* St. Louis, MO, Elsevier Saunders, 2013, pp 996-1004.)

to maintain femoral retraction for access to the acetabulum.

- Another intracapsular Hohmann retractor is placed anteriorly into the pubis to retract the gluteus medius anteriorly.
- An inferior retractor is placed under the transverse acetabular ligament to displace the inferior capsule.
- If necessary, yet another Hohmann retractor is placed superiorly into the ilium for 360° exposure of the acetabulum.
- In many patients, the acetabulum is deep and has a thin medial wall. The authors of this chapter recommend minimal medialization with the initial reamers, because often the goal is to lateralize the hip center in these patients.
- Acetabular reaming is done with care to minimize removal of subchondral bone.
- Reaming is done to the templated size and solid peripheral fit is ensured. If the fixation is questionable, two or three screws may be placed.

ACETABULAR BONE GRAFTING AND POSITIONING

- Acetabular bone grafting is recommended. Typically, autograft is obtained from the resected femoral head.
- The femoral head is morcellized with sequential acetabular reamers (**Figure 4**).
- Impaction and reverse reaming of the graft in the acetabulum is recommended to fill the defect.
- The cup is positioned in approximately 40° of abduction and 15° of anteversion similar to all total hip replacements, with care taken to lateralize the hip center.
- Adjunct screw fixation is advisable.

FEMORAL PREPARATION AND RECONSTRUCTION

- Femoral preparation is done in the same manner as for other routine primary THAs.
- Implant positioning is important to avoid impingement at one or a combination of the implant-implant, implant-bone, bone-bone, or implant–soft-tissue interfaces.
- Particular attention is paid to potential areas of impingement, and hip ROM is checked during trial reduction.

Wound Closure

- Wound closure can be difficult because lateralization of the hip center and the greater trochanter can put excessive tension on the lateral soft tissues, including the skin.
- The gluteus medius and deep approach are closed with two interrupted nonabsorbable sutures through the anterior greater trochanter.
- The fascia is closed with two interrupted nonabsorbable sutures followed by a running barbed No. 1 polydioxanone suture.
- The subcutaneous dermis is closed with interrupted 2-0 monofilament absorbable suture, and the skin is closed with a running 3-0 monofilament absorbable suture.

Postoperative Regimen

Rehabilitation protocols are similar to those for routine THAs. Stretching contracted soft tissues is critical to restore the proper hip joint biomechanics and gait kinematics, and it should continue for several months postoperatively. Iliotibial band stretching is important to decrease pain that may arise from lateralization of the hip center. No restrictions are placed on weight bearing postoperatively.

Avoiding Pitfalls and Complications

Surgical exposure and hip dislocation often are challenging in patients with protrusio acetabuli. The surgeon must take particular care to avoid complications that can result from forceful dislocation attempts. Lateralization of the hip center and restoration of offset are critical, and preoperative templating helps ensure restoration of hip biomechanics. Penetration of the thin medial wall during acetabular preparation must be avoided. Autologous bone graft from the femoral head should be placed behind the cup and noncemented fixation should rely on the peripheral rim fit. Proper seating of the femoral stem is important to avoid contributing to excessive lengthening of the leg. Overlengthening can potentially result in sciatic neuropathy. Implant positioning also is important to avoid impingement at any interface.

Bibliography

Alexander C: The aetiology of primary protrusio acetabuli. *Br J Radiol* 1965;38:567-580.

Baghdadi YM, Larson AN, Sierra RJ: Long-term results of the uncemented acetabular component in a primary total hip arthroplasty performed for protrusio acetabuli: A fifteen year median follow-up. *Int Orthop* 2015;39(5):839-845.

Dutka J, Sosin P, Skowronek P, Skowronek M: Total hip arthroplasty with bone grafts for protrusio acetabuli. *Ortop Traumatol Rehabil* 2011;13(5):469-477.

Egan KJ, Kummer FJ, Frankel VH: Biomechanics of total hip arthroplasty. *Semin Arthroplasty* 1993;4(4):288-301.

Gates HS III, Poletti SC, Callaghan JJ, McCollum DE: Radiographic measurements in protrusio acetabuli. *J Arthroplasty* 1989;4(4):347-351.

Heywood AW: Arthroplasty with a solid bone graft for protrusio acetabuli. *J Bone Joint Surg Br* 1980;62(3):332-336.

Hooper JC, Jones EW: Primary protrusion of the acetabulum. *J Bone Joint Surg Br* 1971;53(1):23-29.

Krushell RJ, Fingeroth RJ, Gelling B: Primary total hip arthroplasty using a dual-geometry cup to treat protrusio acetabuli. *J Arthroplasty* 2008;23(8):1128-1131.

Leunig M, Nho SJ, Turchetto L, Ganz R: Protrusio acetabuli: New insights and experience with joint preservation. *Clin Orthop Relat Res* 2009;467(9):2241-2250.

McBride MT, Muldoon MP, Santore RF, Trousdale RT, Wenger DR: Protrusio acetabuli: Diagnosis and treatment. *J Am Acad Orthop Surg* 2001;9(2):79-88.

Mullaji AB, Marawar SV: Primary total hip arthroplasty in protrusio acetabuli using impacted morsellized bone grafting and cementless cups: A medium-term radiographic review. *J Arthroplasty* 2007;22(8):1143-1149.

Mullaji AB, Shetty GM: Acetabular protrusio: Surgical technique of dealing with a problem in depth. *Bone Joint J* 2013;95-B(11 suppl A):37-40.

Pomeranz MM: Intrapelvic protrusion of the acetabulum (Otto pelvis): 1932. *Clin Orthop Relat Res* 2007;465:6-15.

Ranawat CS, Dorr LD, Inglis AE: Total hip arthroplasty in protrusio acetabuli of rheumatoid arthritis. *J Bone Joint Surg Am* 1980;62(7):1059-1065.

Sotelo-Garza A, Charnley J: The results of Charnley arthroplasty of hip performed for protrusio acetabuli. *Clin Orthop Relat Res* 1978;(132):12-18.

Chapter 22
Total Hip Arthroplasty in Patients With Paget Disease

Sharon Walton, MD
Richard Iorio, MD
Ajit Deshmukh, MD

Indications

Paget disease of bone is a metabolic disorder characterized by an increase in bone turnover. Although the etiology is unknown, the disorder was originally suggested to be the result of an inflammatory process. It has been hypothesized that the disease is caused by a viral infection (paramyxovirus) acquired years before the patient becomes symptomatic. Hereditary factors also play a role, with the genes *SQSTM1* and *RANK* and specific regions of chromosomes 5 and 6 identified as associated with the disease. A pathologic increase in the number and cellular activity of osteoclasts and osteoblasts causes a disorganized bone structure, resulting in trabecular hypertrophy, osteosclerosis, and cystic degeneration.

Paget disease can be monostotic or polyostotic. Many cases of Paget disease remain undetected because the patient has only mild involvement of bone and no symptoms. When symptoms occur, they can be similar to those of arthritis or other conditions. The disease can cause bone pain, deformity, fractures, neoplastic degeneration, and degenerative joint disease. The disorder is most common in Europe and North America, with an incidence of 2% to 4% in patients older than 40 years. Among symptomatic patients, greater than 50% report joint dysfunction at the time of diagnosis. Degenerative hip disease develops in up to 50% of patients with Paget disease. Several mechanisms have been proposed through which Paget disease may result in arthritis. First, uniform enlargement of the subchondral bone may cause compromise of the joint space. Second, asymmetric enlargement of the subchondral bone causes cartilage fracture and necrosis. Lastly, altered joint biodynamics resulting from the bowed nature of pagetoid bone may alter pressure contact points within the joint. Pseudofractures occur in 10% of patients with Paget disease. These pseudofractures are commonly found in the femoral neck and are usually transverse in nature.

It is important to discern the etiology of hip pain in patients with Paget disease. Active Paget disease can be characterized by high metabolic bone turnover, stress fractures, lumbar spinal compression with neurologic sequelae, and possibly sarcomatous degeneration, which can cause pain about the hip. Localized enlargement of the proximal femur or acetabulum with accompanying sclerosis is indicative of Paget disease of the hip. If the origin of pain is unclear, intra-articular injection of local anesthesia under fluoroscopy can help locate the origin of pain.

Total hip arthroplasty (THA) can be used with predictable success in the surgical management of painful degeneration of the hip secondary to Paget disease. Certain characteristics must be considered when THA is performed in patients with Paget disease of the hip. On the femoral side, the patient may have coxa vara, diaphyseal bowing, fractures of the neck or shaft, and/or a sclerotic medullary canal. Characteristics that may be present on the acetabular side include enlargement of the pelvis, cavitary cystic degeneration, acetabular protrusion, and hypovascularity (**Figure 1**). Hypervascularity can cause excessive bleeding; thus, preoperative medical management of active Paget disease may minimize active bleeding and facilitate intraoperative evaluation of the bone-implant interface.

Contraindications

Patients with Paget disease can have variable phases of bone resorption

Dr. Iorio or an immediate family member has received research or institutional support from OrthoSensor and Pacira Pharmaceuticals, and serves as a board member, owner, officer, or committee member of the American Association of Hip and Knee Surgeons and The Hip Society. Neither of the following authors nor any immediate family member has received anything of value from or has stock or stock options held in a commercial company or institution related directly or indirectly to the subject of this chapter: Dr. Walton and Dr. Deshmukh.

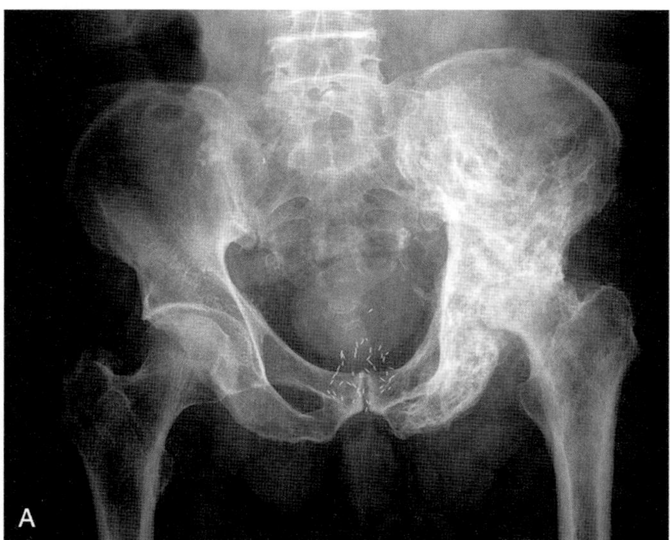

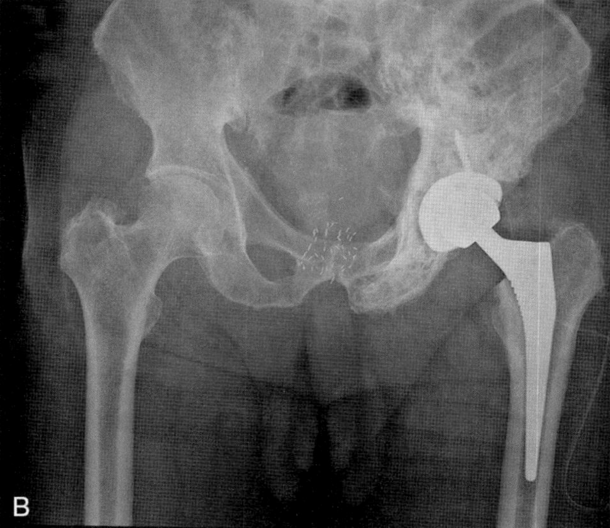

Figure 1 **A,** AP pelvic radiograph demonstrates Paget disease of the hip with degenerative joint disease and mostly acetabular involvement. **B,** AP pelvic radiograph obtained 1 year after noncemented total hip arthroplasty using a coated hemiarthroplasty stem for the management of Paget disease.

resulting from hyperactive osteoclasts and new bone formation resulting from an osteoblast proliferation. The active lytic phase of bone resorption is associated with vascular proliferation, and this phase of hypervascularity may be associated with bone pain. The presence of serum alkaline phosphatase is a marker for bone formation, whereas the presence of urinary hydroxyproline is a marker for resorption. A bone scan also can demonstrate the extent of pagetoid lytic activity. THA performed on pagetoid bone during the hypervascular phase may be associated with increased intraoperative blood loss, increased postoperative bone-related pain, and an increased risk for osteolysis. Thus, preoperative medical management of active Paget disease may decrease the risk of complications. Sarcomatous degeneration of pagetoid bone is seen in less than 1% of patients. If bone changes become rapidly destructive and increasingly painful, or if cortical erosions are present with an accompanying soft-tissue mass, the presence of sarcomatous degeneration must be considered.

Alternative Treatments

Medical management of Paget disease includes the use of calcitonin, plicamycin, gallium nitrate, and diphosphonates. Patients with bone pain secondary to Paget disease who do not respond to anti-inflammatory or pain medications are candidates for antiresorptive therapy. Bone deformity, risk of fracture, and preparation for surgical treatment are indications for pharmaceutical therapy. Decreased bone turnover, indicated by a decrease in biochemical markers, alters the disease progression. If bone turnover is decreased and pain and deformity are prevented, the need for surgical intervention may be avoided. After THA is performed, management of pagetoid bone in the resorptive phase may decrease vascularity of the affected bone and decrease the incidence of bone-related pain and postoperative bone resorption.

Severe varus deformity of the proximal femur and bowing of the femoral shaft are commonly seen in patients with Paget disease of the hip. These deformities can result in malalignment with subsequent abnormal stress on the hip joint, stress fracture, impingement, and limited range of motion. When pagetoid involvement of the femur results in malalignment, and articular cartilage in the hip joint shows no sign of degeneration, corrective osteotomy may be an alternative to THA. Metaphyseal osteotomies heal faster than diaphyseal osteotomies in patients with Paget disease. Nonsurgical management of degenerative arthritis associated with Paget disease is the same as that of idiopathic osteoarthritis and may include NSAIDs, activity modification, and the use of gait aids.

Results

In patients with degeneration resulting from Paget disease, THA with cemented or noncemented implants is generally associated with good outcomes (**Table 1**). However, failure rates with cemented implants are higher than those seen in patients with osteoarthritis who undergo primary THA.

Table 1 Results of Total Hip Arthroplasty (THA) in Patients With Paget Disease

Authors (Year)	Number of Patients (Hips)	Procedure or Approach	Mean Patient Age in Years (Range)	Mean Follow-up in Years (Range)	Success Rate (%)[a]	Results
Hozack et al (1999)	5	Posterolateral noncemented acetabular implant (3 primary, 2 revision)	68.3 (NR)	5.8 (4.8-8.8)	100	No patients had clinical symptoms referable to the acetabular component HHS not reported
Wegrzyn et al (2010)	32 (39)	Posterolateral noncemented hydroxyapatite fully coated THA (37 primary, 2 revision)	74.2 (55-89)	6.6 (2-16)	99	Mean HHS improved from 54 to 89
Imbuldeniya et al (2014)	27 (33)	Posterolateral noncemented primary THA	72.1 (NR)	12.3 (10-17)	100	14 hips in 14 patients were available for follow-up Mean HHS improved from 56 to 83

HHS = Harris hip score, NR = not reported.

[a] Success is defined as no revision surgery at the time of follow-up and is based on number of hips.

Hypervascularity, bone resorption, and bone deformity can affect the endurance of the THA. Bone deformity and the unpredictability of bone ingrowth make routine use of noncemented femoral implants controversial. Reported revision rates at intermediate-term follow-up are lower for noncemented implants than for cemented implants. In a long-term follow-up study of 33 noncemented THA procedures in 27 patients with Paget disease, mean Harris hip scores improved from 56 preoperatively to 83 postoperatively. Three revisions were required (one for aseptic loosening and two for periprosthetic fractures). Radiographic examination demonstrated ingrowth of all surviving implants. These findings suggest good long-term outcomes of noncemented THA in patients with Paget disease.

A retrospective study of 39 noncemented hydroxyapatite fully coated THA implants in patients with Paget disease of the hip at mean follow-up of 6.6 years demonstrated significant improvement in functional scores and excellent clinical outcome, measured with the Harris hip score, in 84% of patients. In a review of five patients with Paget disease localized to the acetabulum in which all patients underwent THA with noncemented acetabular implants, all acetabular implants were well fixed radiographically with no migration or loosening at an average of 5.8 years postoperatively.

Techniques

Setup/Exposure

- Approaches that can be used include the anterior, lateral, and posterolateral approaches to the hip. The authors of this chapter prefer the posterolateral approach.
- In patients with Paget disease of the hip without femoral deformity, the THA procedure is similar to any routine arthroplasty.
- Coxa vara, or bowing of the femur, may make entrance to the canal more difficult than it would be in other patients. In the pagetoid hip, osteotomy of the greater trochanter can be performed to facilitate dislocation of the hip and access to the femoral canal.
- Advancement of the greater trochanter improves the biomechanics of the pagetic hip with coxa vara. The incidence of nonunion of trochanteric osteotomy after THA has been reported to be 13% in patients with Paget disease compared with 6% in patients without Paget disease.
- Acetabular protrusion can be encountered in the pagetoid hip and, when combined with coxa vara, can make dislocation difficult.
- Before dislocation is attempted, care must be taken to remove osteophytic bone around the acetabulum.
- If the combination of acetabular protrusion and coxa vara is severe, in situ femoral neck osteotomy is performed before dislocation and/or trochanteric osteotomy to facilitate dislocation and avoid fracture.

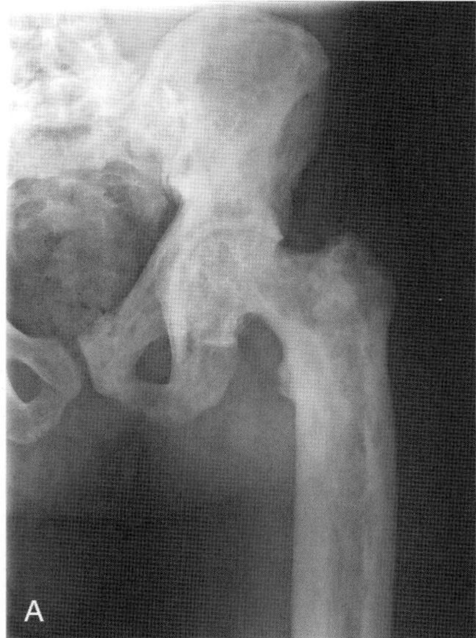

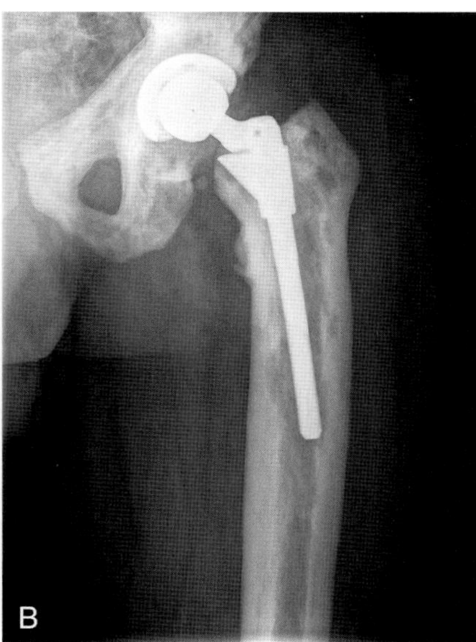

Figure 2 **A,** AP radiograph of the left hip obtained from a patient with Paget disease. The patient has coxa vara, diaphyseal bowing, and a sclerotic medullary canal. **B,** AP radiograph obtained immediately after noncemented total hip arthroplasty. The femur was reconstructed with a modular femoral stem with a metaphyseal sleeve. Reaming of the femoral canal was extremely difficult. In this patient, the use of a high-speed burr was insufficient to remove the sclerotic island of bone on the medial aspect of the greater trochanter. Because removal of all the sclerotic bone could result in fracture of the greater trochanter, varus positioning of the stem was accepted.

Instruments/Equipment/ Implants Required

- Fluoroscopy or standard radiography should be available if needed to help localize anatomic structures.
- Primary and revision arthroplasty implants including modular stems should be available.
- Cerclage wires and trochanteric osteotomy plates should be readily available for use if femoral osteotomy is performed.

Procedure

- In patients with Paget disease, the acetabulum often is enlarged and may be medialized. To avoid causing added protrusion, reaming is performed to expand the periphery without deepening the socket.
- Cystic changes also can be encountered in patients with pagetoid bone. If present, the bone is curetted to remove fibrous tissue and grafted with host bone reamings.
- Preparation of the femoral canal depends on eradication of fibrous pagetoid tissue and the ability to shape the sclerotic, enlarged femoral canal. Safe penetration of sclerotic bone with broaches may not be possible.
- Intraoperative fluoroscopic evaluation may help with proper placement of the trial femoral implant.
- The use of high-speed burrs or rotatory reamers may be necessary to avoid varus placement of the stem, resulting from the presence of sclerotic bone in the canal (**Figure 2**).
- The use of a modular stem has the advantage that no broaching is needed (**Figures 3** and **4**).
- As noted, bowing of the femur may necessitate osteotomy to allow implantation of the femoral stem. Proximal femoral osteotomy for the management of coxa vara and multiple diaphyseal osteotomies for the management of femoral bowing have been reported with both cemented and noncemented techniques.
- Femoral healing after diaphyseal osteotomies can be protracted. However, attempts to avoid osteotomy by using a customized curved cemented femoral stem to match the femoral geometry in patients with Paget disease have been unsuccessful because of subsequent periprosthetic fracture.
- If cement is used for femoral fixation in association with an osteotomy, care must be taken to prevent cement intrusion into the osteotomy sites, which will impair healing. Strut grafting may be a valuable adjunct to osteotomy.
- The authors of this chapter prefer noncemented fixation of femoral implants. If osteotomy is required to accommodate the prosthesis, a metaphyseal osteotomy spanned by a modular implant and supported with adjunctive fixation and strut grafting is advisable.
- If multiple diaphyseal osteotomies are necessary, long-stemmed femoral fixation may provide a more stable construct.
- An attempt should be made to bypass all pseudofractures with the femoral prosthesis. Alternatively, pseudofractures may be supported by strut grafts and/or adjunctive fixation. Struts can be invaded by pagetoid bone as they revascularize and may be best supported with the use of an intramedullary femoral stem. In the acetabulum, the inability to produce a dry acetabular bone interface may preclude the successful implantation of a cemented cup. Long-term results of noncemented acetabular implants have not been reported in patients with Paget disease; however, intermediate-term results appear promising.

- Underreaming can increase the risk of fracture of sclerotic acetabular pagetoid bone.
- The authors of this chapter prefer noncemented fixation of the acetabulum with supplemental screw fixation when hemispheric contact can be maintained (**Figure 3, B**).

Wound Closure

- Wound closure is performed in a routine manner.

Postoperative Regimen

After osteotomy in conjunction with THA, protected weight bearing is recommended until evidence of radiographic union is present, usually 3 to 6 months postoperatively. Increased pain or increased bone resorption resulting from active Paget disease can be prevented with calcitonin or diphosphonates to prevent stress fractures or periprosthetic resorption. Heterotopic ossification can occur after THA in patients with Paget disease. Prophylaxis with either NSAIDs or perioperative irradiation is recommended.

Avoiding Pitfalls and Complications

Excessive blood loss is common with preparation of pagetoid bone. Therefore, meticulous technique with closure is required to minimize blood loss and prevent hematoma. Blood salvage techniques may be helpful when hypervascular bone is encountered. Excessive intraoperative bleeding can be minimized by treating patients with active disease and hypervascularity with a preoperative medical regimen. Varus positioning of the femoral implant, which leads to early failure, can be avoided by checking the position of trial implants with intraoperative radiography. If trochanteric osteotomy or power reaming of sclerotic Paget bone is not sufficient to provide a femoral shape that correctly positions the implant, femoral osteotomy may be necessary to properly position the stem. Because osteotomy of the femoral diaphysis is susceptible to nonunion, care must be taken to attain adequate bone-to-bone contact and to prevent cement intrusion into

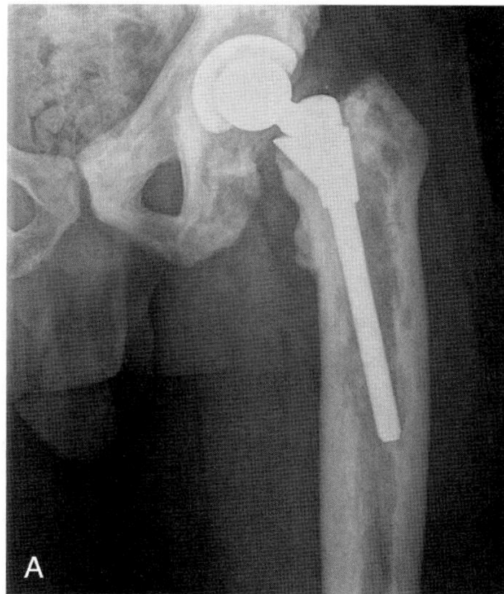

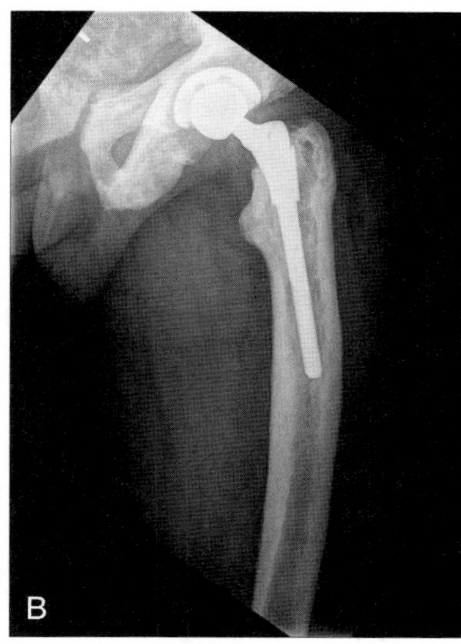

Figure 3 Postoperative AP (**A**) and lateral (**B**) radiographs obtained from the same patient in Figure 2 demonstrate the left hip 1 year after total hip arthroplasty with a modular stem. Note the disappearance of the dark zone that was seen in the immediate postoperative radiograph (Figure 2, B), which indicates bony integration of the medial aspect of the sleeve.

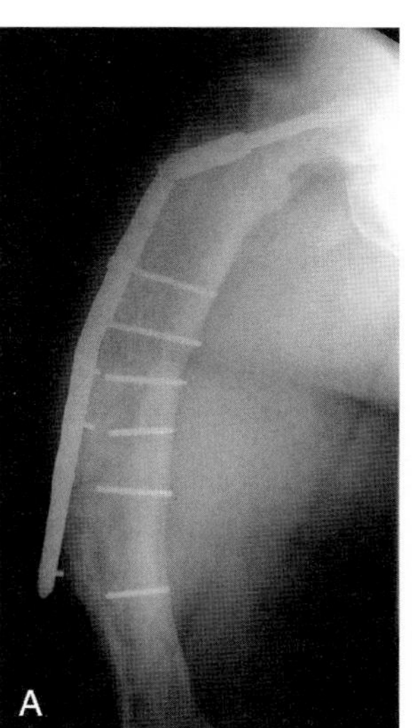

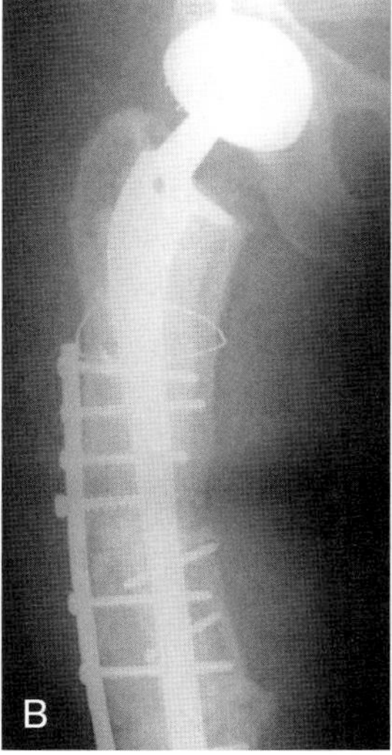

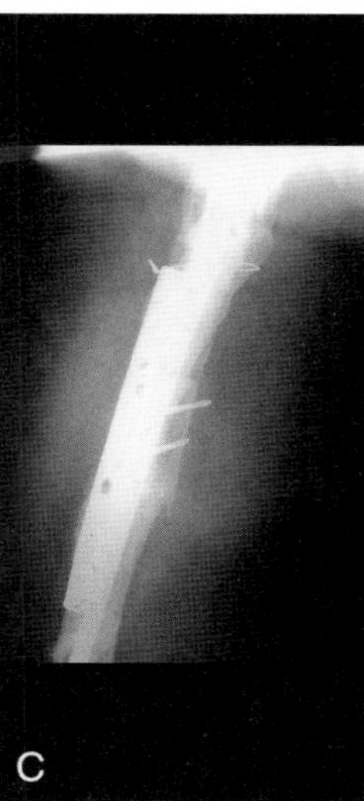

Figure 4 **A,** AP radiograph of a right hip demonstrates Paget disease with degenerative joint disease several years after the patient underwent a femoral osteotomy. Femoral bowing and varus deformity are evident. AP (**B**) and lateral (**C**) radiographs obtained 6 months after cemented total hip arthroplasty with a modular stem. (Reproduced from Iorio R, Healy WL: Total hip arthroplasty: Paget's disease, in Lieberman JR, Berry DJ: *Advanced Reconstruction: Hip*. Rosemont, IL, American Academy of Orthopaedic Surgeons, 2005, pp 137-141.)

the osteotomy site. Strut grafts must be augmented with either intramedullary or plate fixation to ensure long-term femoral reinforcement.

Symptomatic heterotopic ossification may cause substantially decreased functional hip scores in patients with Paget disease compared with unaffected control subjects. Therefore, heterotopic ossification prophylaxis in the form of NSAIDs or irradiation is strongly recommended.

Bibliography

Alexakis PG, Brown BA, Hohl WM: Porous hip replacement in Paget's disease: An 8-2/3-year followup. *Clin Orthop Relat Res* 1998;(350):138-142.

Altman RD: Musculoskeletal manifestations of Paget's disease of bone. *Arthritis Rheum* 1980;23(10):1121-1127.

Hozack WJ, Rushton SA, Carey C, Sakalkale D, Rothman RH: Uncemented total hip arthroplasty in Paget's disease of the hip: A report of 5 cases with 5-year follow-up. *J Arthroplasty* 1999;14(7):872-876.

Imbuldeniya AM, Tai SM, Aboelmagd T, Walter WL, Walter WK, Zicat BA: Cementless hip arthroplasty in Paget's disease at long-term follow-up (average of 12.3 years). *J Arthroplasty* 2014;29(5):1063-1066.

Kirsh G, Kligman M, Roffman M: Hydroxyapatite-coated total hip replacement in Paget's disease: 20 patients followed for 4-8 years. *Acta Orthop Scand* 2001;72(2):127-132.

Ludkowski P, Wilson-MacDonald J: Total arthroplasty in Paget's disease of the hip: A clinical review and review of the literature. *Clin Orthop Relat Res* 1990;(255):160-167.

Lusty PJ, Walter WL, Walter WK, Zicat B: Cementless hip arthroplasty in Paget's disease at medium-term follow-up (average of 6.7 years). *J Arthroplasty* 2007;22(5):692-696.

McDonald DJ, Sim FH: Total hip arthroplasty in Paget's disease: A follow-up note. *J Bone Joint Surg Am* 1987;69(5):766-772.

Merkow RL, Pellicci PM, Hely DP, Salvati EA: Total hip replacement for Paget's disease of the hip. *J Bone Joint Surg Am* 1984;66(5):752-758.

Mills BG, Singer FR, Weiner LP, Holst PA: Immunohistological demonstration of respiratory syncytial virus antigens in Paget disease of bone. *Proc Natl Acad Sci U S A* 1981;78(2):1209-1213.

Namba RS, Brick GW, Murray WR: Revision total hip arthroplasty with correctional femoral osteotomy in Paget's disease. *J Arthroplasty* 1997;12(5):591-595.

Parvizi J, Frankle MA, Tiegs RD, Sim FH: Corrective osteotomy for deformity in Paget disease. *J Bone Joint Surg Am* 2003;85(4):697-702.

Parvizi J, Schall DM, Lewallen DG, Sim FH: Outcome of uncemented hip arthroplasty components in patients with Paget's disease. *Clin Orthop Relat Res* 2002;(403):127-134.

Ralston SH, Langston AL, Reid IR: Pathogenesis and management of Paget's disease of bone. *Lancet* 2008;372(9633):155-163.

Wegrzyn J, Pibarot V, Chapurlat R, Carret JP, Béjui-Hugues J, Guyen O: Cementless total hip arthroplasty in Paget's disease of bone: A retrospective review. *Int Orthop* 2010;34(8):1103-1109.

Chapter 23
Total Hip Arthroplasty After Acetabular Fracture

Adam A. Sassoon, MD, MS
George J. Haidukewych, MD

Indications

Total hip arthroplasty (THA) is sometimes necessary in the management of acetabular fractures. After an acetabular fracture, THA typically is performed at one of four junctures: acutely, as part of initial management (usually in conjunction with columnar plating); in a delayed manner, after an initial period of nonsurgical management; semiacutely, after failure of fixation; or much later, after the development of posttraumatic arthritis.

In patients with acute acetabular fracture, THA should be considered if open reduction and internal fixation (ORIF) cannot accomplish the goals of anatomic restoration of the acetabular articular surface, congruent and stable location of the femoral head within the acetabulum, and restoration of limb offset, length, and alignment of the involved extremity. Anatomic reduction of the articular surface can be particularly difficult to achieve in patients with certain fracture patterns, including central dislocation of the hip through the quadrilateral plate (**Figure 1**), fractures with extensive articular comminution, and fractures with impaction of the weight-bearing portion of the articular surface, indicated radiographically by the so-called gull sign. The ability to restore the articular surface to within 2 mm is critical in preventing posttraumatic arthritis; therefore, THA should be considered when this restoration cannot be reliably achieved. Associated injuries on the femoral side of the hip joint may also be a reason to perform THA acutely. Patients with articular impaction or fractures of the femoral head, especially cephalad to the fovea, and fractures of the femoral neck may benefit from THA rather than combined ORIF procedures. Preexisting arthritis, dysplasia, or inflammatory arthritides are also reasons to consider acute THA. In addition, acetabular fractures in the geriatric population have a high mortality rate and a high rate of conversion to THA, thereby warranting consideration of acute THA as a primary treatment modality in elderly patients.

Delayed THA in patients with acetabular fracture occurs after a trial of nonsurgical management has failed or after a period of benign neglect in which the fracture heals primarily in a nonanatomic fashion. In this clinical scenario, indications for THA are the development of a symptomatic malunion, or compromised function because of impingement, which often results from medialization of the femoral head. In these patients, the potential of the acetabular fracture to result in a secondary femoral neck fracture over time is a concern.

Semiacute THA after failure of fixation is indicated in patients in whom articular reduction has been lost, especially in patients with one of the aforementioned fracture types that have a poor prognosis with ORIF. Failure of fixation is sometimes accompanied by instability of the hip, especially in patients with a fracture pattern that involves the posterior wall of the acetabulum (**Figure 2**). Involvement of the posterior wall can result in either posterior subluxation or frank dislocation of the femoral head. If this scenario occurs in conjunction with preservation of fixation of an associated column fracture, the surgeon may prefer to delay the conversion to THA to allow healing of the column fracture.

Finally, and most commonly, THA is performed remotely after acetabular fracture fixation to manage posttraumatic arthritis. Remote THA is indicated in patients with a painful hip joint that compromises the patient's ability to perform

Dr. Haidukewych or an immediate family member has received royalties from DePuy Synthes; serves as a paid consultant to DePuy Synthes and Zimmer Biomet; has stock or stock options held in the Institute for Better Bone Health and OrthoPediatrics; has received nonincome support (such as equipment or services), commercially derived honoraria, or other non–research-related funding (such as paid travel) from DePuy Synthes; and serves as a board member, owner, officer, or committee member of the American Academy of Orthopaedic Surgeons. Neither Dr. Sassoon nor any immediate family member has received anything of value from or has stock or stock options held in a commercial company or institution related directly or indirectly to the subject of this chapter.

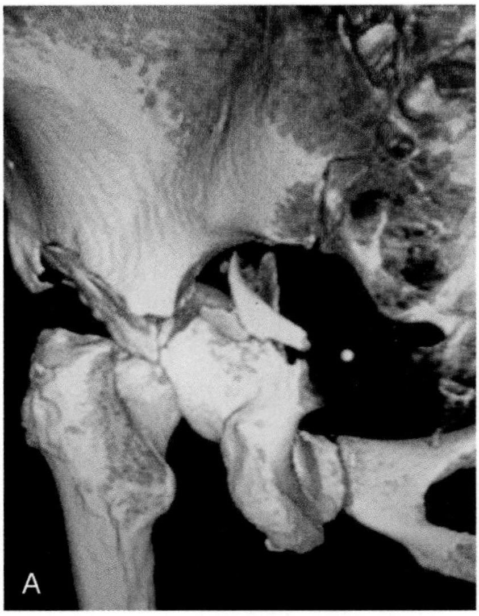

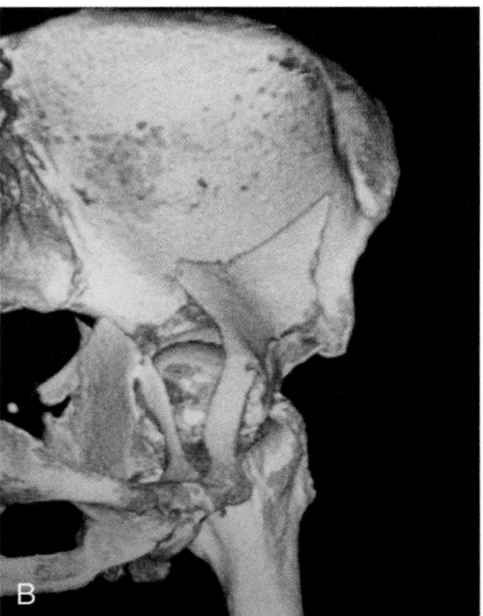

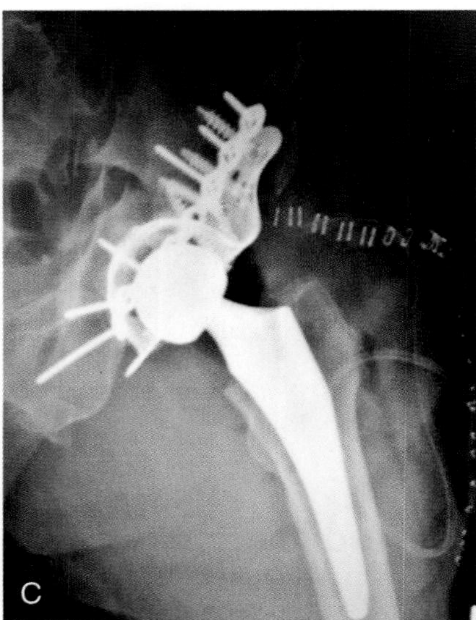

Figure 1 **A** and **B,** Three-dimensional CT reconstructions of a left hip demonstrate a central fracture-dislocation of the hip through the quadrilateral plate and associated both-column fracture of the acetabulum. **C,** AP hip radiograph obtained after acute total hip arthroplasty with the use of an anti-protrusio cage. This was performed as a salvage procedure because the patient had both a central defect of the medial wall and an acetabular rim that could not be reconstructed to obtain a chamfer fit of a standard acetabular implant.

activities of daily living and pursue a reasonable quality of life, in conjunction with the hallmark radiographic findings of arthritis: joint-space narrowing, subchondral sclerosis, subchondral cysts, and osteophyte formation.

Contraindications

The contraindications to THA in patients with acetabular fracture are similar to those for elective THA performed for the management of osteoarthritis. Active infection, either remotely or at the site of previously placed hardware, must be ruled out before arthroplasty is performed. When delayed or remote THA is performed, serum inflammatory markers should be measured, and hip aspiration should be performed if these values are elevated. Additionally, if the patient has low functional demand, such as in patients with concomitant spinal cord injuries or patients with chronic disability, the risks incurred as a result of THA may not outweigh the potential benefits. Other relative contraindications are tobacco use and drug or alcohol abuse, which can reduce the likelihood of successful THA.

Alternative Treatments

Alternative treatment options include ORIF in patients with acute acetabular fractures, revision ORIF in patients with failed fixation, and comprehensive nonsurgical management (physical therapy, weight loss, activity modification, and occasional intra-articular corticosteroid injections) in patients with posttraumatic arthritis.

Results

The results of THA after acetabular fracture are generally favorable in achieving improvement of pain and function but are inferior to the results of elective THA in patients with arthritis. The results must be interpreted carefully because the timing of the THA procedure relative to when the fracture was sustained is a distinguishing factor and has implications for the technical aspects of the procedure. Therefore, reported results should be considered given whether the THA procedure was performed in patients with acute fracture or remotely after the development of posttraumatic arthritis (**Table 1**).

In a study of acute THA using noncemented acetabular implants in 57 patients with acetabular fracture, 79% of patients achieved an excellent or good outcome at a mean follow-up of 8 years. No revisions were performed for mechanical loosening; however, one acetabular cup required revision for multiple dislocations. In a study of combined ORIF and THA for displaced acetabular fractures in 22 elderly patients with a mean 29-month follow-up, 5 patients required revision for osteolysis and/or instability. A recent study of the functional results of acute THA in 33 patients with acetabular fractures at 1- to 14-year follow-up demonstrated good to excellent functional outcomes using the Oxford Hip Score in 93% of patients. In this series, functional outcomes did not correlate with initial fracture pattern or age at the time of fracture.

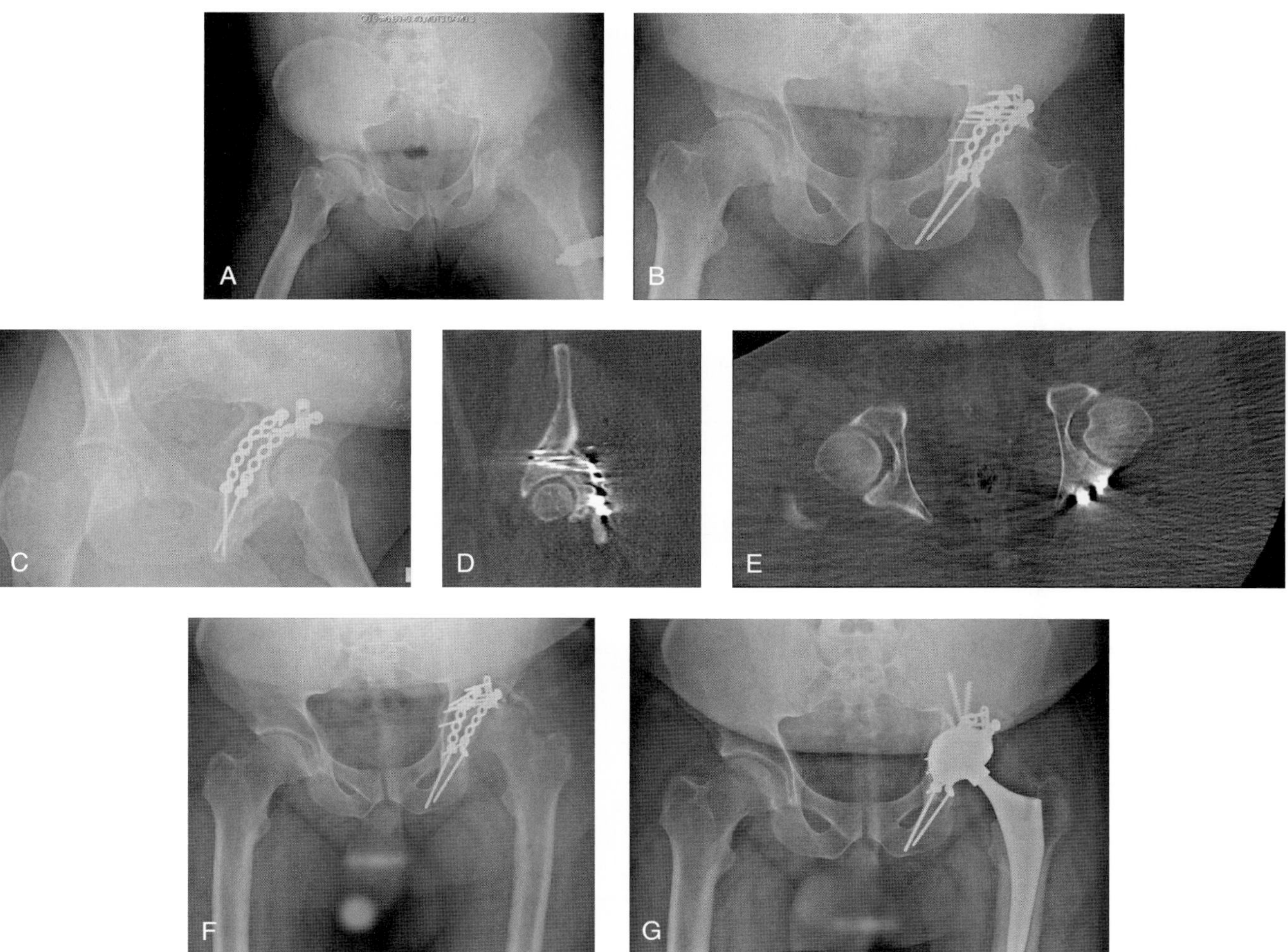

Figure 2 **A,** AP pelvic radiograph demonstrates a combined posterior column and posterior wall fracture of the acetabulum. AP pelvic radiograph (**B**) and iliac oblique pelvic radiograph (**C**) demonstrate subsequent fixation with dual posterior column plates and a spring plate. Sagittal (**D**) and axial (**E**) postoperative CT scans demonstrate excellent reduction. However, the fixation of the posterior wall fracture failed, resulting in dislocation of the hip, demonstrated on an AP pelvic radiograph (**F**). After a period of non–weight bearing to allow the column fracture to heal, the patient underwent total hip arthroplasty with retention of most of the previously placed hardware, demonstrated on an AP pelvic radiograph (**G**). Because of the patient's prolonged dislocation, a dual-mobility prosthesis was used to enhance stability.

More literature is available regarding the results of THA performed remotely in patients with posttraumatic arthritis resulting from acetabular fracture than for THA performed acutely in patients with acetabular fracture. The results of these studies vary depending on the type of fixation used for the acetabular implant, with noncemented implants generally showing better results than cemented implants. In a study of 55 hips with degenerative arthritis secondary to acetabular fracture, the acetabular implants, which were predominantly cemented, required revision in 14% at mean 7.3-year follow-up. Radiographic and symptomatic acetabular loosening was noted in 53% and 28% of patients, respectively. The authors of a recent study from the same institution reported long-term results of THA in patients with coxarthrosis related to acetabular fracture. Femoral or acetabular revision was required in 19 of 25 patients at a mean 20-year follow-up. Of these revisions, 18 were performed for mechanical loosening or osteolysis.

Noncemented acetabular implants have shown favorable results in patients undergoing delayed THA for posttraumatic arthritis. In a study of 32 patients undergoing delayed THA, 5-year implant survivorship was 97% with aseptic loosening as the end point; however, overall implant survivorship was only 79%. A more recent study of porous metal acetabular implants demonstrated

Table 1 Results of Total Hip Arthroplasty (THA) in Patients With Acetabular Fractures

Authors (Year)	Number of Patients	Procedure and Timing	Mean Patient Age in Years (Range)	Mean Follow-up (Range)	Success Rate (%)[a]	Results
Romness and Lewallen (1990)	53 (55 hips)	Delayed THA in patients with post-traumatic arthritis	56.2 (19-91)	7.3 yr (7 d to 16.6 yr)	73	73% of hips had no symptomatic loosening
Mears and Velyvis (2002)	57	Acute THA with or without ORIF	69 (26-89)	8.1 yr (2-12 yr)	98	98% without mechanical loosening Mean HHS at final follow-up, 89
Ranawat et al (2009)	32	Delayed THA in patients with post-traumatic arthritis	52 (20-87)	4.7 yr (2.0-9.7 yr)	79	97% without mechanical loosening Mean HHS, 82
Herscovici et al (2010)	22	ORIF and acute THA	75.3 (60-95)	29.4 mo (13-67 mo)	77	77% without mechanical loosening Mean HHS, 74
Lin et al (2015)	33	ORIF and acute THA	66 (47-92)	5.6 yr (1-14.3 yr)	94	94% without mechanical loosening
von Roth et al (2015)	25	Delayed THA in patients with post-traumatic arthritis	52 (19-80)	20 yr (3-42 yr)	57	71% without mechanical loosening Mean HHS at final follow-up was 80
Yuan et al (2015)	30	Delayed THA in patients with post-traumatic arthritis	45 (23-75)	5 yr (2-11 yr)	88	100% without mechanical loosening Median HHS at final follow-up was 82

HHS = Harris hip score, ORIF = open reduction and internal fixation.

[a] Success is defined as implant survivorship without revision.

improved results, with overall 5-year implant survivorship of 88% and no mechanical loosening at a mean 5-year follow-up.

Techniques

Setup/Exposure

- The fracture pattern and/or fracture healing and the extent of columnar involvement must be understood before the procedure begins. Pelvic CT with three-dimensional reconstruction is extremely helpful.
- A posterior approach is used in patients with a posterior or both-column fracture pattern, whereas an anterolateral approach is used in patients with a fracture pattern predominantly involving the anterior column.
- The patient is placed in a lateral decubitus position on either a pegboard positioner or a beanbag.
- The affected leg is kept in a position of hip extension and knee flexion to relieve tension on the sciatic nerve during the procedure. Careful attention must be given to the nerve tension throughout the procedure.

Instruments/Equipment/Implants Required

- Intraoperative cell salvage is used routinely because the potential for blood loss is high.
- The surgeon should be prepared for columnar plating. A range of options including anti-protrusio cup-cage constructs should be available. Pelvic reconstruction plates, plate benders, long screws, and pelvic reduction clamps are required for successful columnar plating.
- In delayed THA procedures, a broken screw removal set can be helpful. Additionally, a metal-cutting burr is helpful to contour screw tips that may impede seating of the acetabular implant.
- The authors of this chapter prefer noncemented acetabular fixation and recommend the use of a porous metal implant with multiple screw options.
- Acetabular augmentation and bone

graft are important in the management of associated defects.
- Femoral fixation is determined by the quality of the femoral bone stock and any associated fractures. In patients with Dorr type C (stovepipe-shaped) femoral bone, cemented fixation may be required.

Procedure

ACUTE THA IN PATIENTS WITH ACETABULAR FRACTURE

- After exposure and plating of the affected column, reaming is performed.
- If the medial wall of the acetabulum has been compromised, such as in a central dislocation through the quadrilateral plate, reaming of a chamfer around the acetabular rim will be necessary. If rim fit cannot be achieved, press-fit fixation may be unattainable.
- A trial implant is used to check the stability of the acetabular cup. The acetabular implant should withstand an axial load without migrating posterolaterally or medially into the pelvis. In the rare patients in whom this requirement is not met, an anti-protrusio cage should be used to prevent cup migration and promote ingrowth.
- Liberal bone grafting is performed with the use of acetabular bone obtained during reaming, femoral head autograft, or allograft bone.
- The final acetabular cup is inserted. Because the acetabular cup serves as a hemispheric plate for the acetabular fracture, multiple screws are placed through the cup to improve stability.

DELAYED THA IN PATIENTS WITH POSTTRAUMATIC ARTHRITIS

- Delayed THA varies in technical difficulty depending on the existing anatomy and hardware.
- In patients with successful column healing, the conversion to THA can be straightforward. Usually, previously placed hardware can be left in place. If the articular surface has settled to the level of indwelling screws, a high-speed burr can be used to remove the screws to prevent interference with preparation and seating of the acetabular cup.
- In patients with acetabular nonunion, THA is technically demanding. In these patients, revision fixation may be required to support the acetabular implant.
- An anti-protrusio cage (**Figure 1**) or triflange implants may be required depending on the remaining bone stock.
- Triflange constructs are particularly useful when nonunion or malunion has resulted in the migration of the femoral head through the medial wall in patients with a defect of the acetabular rim.
- Another relative indication for a custom triflange construct is if a constrained liner is required in patients with moderate bone loss.

Wound Closure

- Layered, watertight closure is paramount. Often, a running barbed suture is used for reinforcement of interrupted suture in fascial closure.
- Incisional, negative-pressure wound therapy devices are used liberally for the first 4 to 6 days postoperatively to enhance healing.

Postoperative Regimen

Postoperatively, the patient is placed in a hip abduction pillow, which is left in place until the patient can be fitted for a hip abduction brace. The brace is set with a 60° flexion limit and is used for 6 weeks postoperatively. Antibiotics are administered intravenously for 24 hours after acute THA or until negative intraoperative cultures are obtained after delayed THA. Pharmacologic deep vein thrombosis prophylaxis is administered for 6 weeks postoperatively in all patients. Patients are restricted to flat-foot weight bearing of 20 lb (9.1 kg) on the surgical extremity for 6 to 12 weeks to protect the implants during ingrowth, fracture healing, and bone graft consolidation.

Avoiding Pitfalls and Complications

A thorough understanding of the acetabular fracture pattern is necessary. The surgeon should obtain advanced imaging to assist in preoperative planning. A variety of implants, augmentation methods, and fixation options should be available. The surgeon must be mindful of tension on the sciatic nerve throughout the procedure. A noncemented porous metal acetabular implant with multiple screws should be used whenever possible. Postoperatively, limited weight bearing and the use of a hip abduction brace can help promote implant ingrowth and prevent dislocation.

Bibliography

Anglen JO, Burd TA, Hendricks KJ, Harrison P: The "Gull Sign": A harbinger of failure for internal fixation of geriatric acetabular fractures. *J Orthop Trauma* 2003;17(9):625-634.

Giannoudis PV, Grotz MR, Papakostidis C, Dinopoulos H: Operative treatment of displaced fractures of the acetabulum: A meta-analysis. *J Bone Joint Surg Br* 2005;87(1):2-9.

Herscovici D Jr, Lindvall E, Bolhofner B, Scaduto JM: The combined hip procedure: Open reduction internal fixation combined with total hip arthroplasty for the management of acetabular fractures in the elderly. *J Orthop Trauma* 2010;24(5):291-296.

Lin C, Caron J, Schmidt AH, Torchia M, Templeman D: Functional outcomes after total hip arthroplasty for the acute management of acetabular fractures: 1- to 14-year follow-up. *J Orthop Trauma* 2015;29(3):151-159.

Matta JM: The goal of acetabular fracture surgery. *J Orthop Trauma* 1996;10(8):586.

Mears DC, Velyvis JH: Acute total hip arthroplasty for selected displaced acetabular fractures: Two to twelve-year results. *J Bone Joint Surg Am* 2002;84(1):1-9.

O'Toole RV, Hui E, Chandra A, Nascone JW: How often does open reduction and internal fixation of geriatric acetabular fractures lead to hip arthroplasty? *J Orthop Trauma* 2014;28(3):148-153.

Ranawat A, Zelken J, Helfet D, Buly R: Total hip arthroplasty for posttraumatic arthritis after acetabular fracture. *J Arthroplasty* 2009;24(5):759-767.

Romness DW, Lewallen DG: Total hip arthroplasty after fracture of the acetabulum: Long-term results. *J Bone Joint Surg Br* 1990;72(5):761-764.

Schnaser E, Scarcella NR, Vallier HA: Acetabular fractures converted to total hip arthroplasties in the elderly: How does function compare to primary total hip arthroplasty? *J Orthop Trauma* 2014;28(12):694-699.

von Roth P, Abdel MP, Harmsen WS, Berry DJ: Total hip arthroplasty after operatively treated acetabular fracture: A concise follow-up, at a mean of twenty years, of a previous report. *J Bone Joint Surg Am* 2015;97(4):288-291.

Yuan BJ, Lewallen DG, Hanssen AD: Porous metal acetabular components have a low rate of mechanical failure in THA after operatively treated acetabular fracture. *Clin Orthop Relat Res* 2015;473(2):536-542.

Chapter 24
Total Hip Arthroplasty After Hip Fusion

Mark J. Spangehl, MD
Matthew C. Niesen, MD

Indications

Despite increased patient expectations and improved results of total hip arthroplasty (THA), arthrodesis of the hip remains a viable option for young adults with unilateral hip disease. Arthrodesis provides patients with long-term pain relief and allows adequate function in patients who are not yet candidates for THA. However, the long-term disability resulting from hip fusion may necessitate conversion of hip arthrodesis to THA.

The long-term sequelae of hip fusion include increased low back, ipsilateral knee, and contralateral hip pain secondary to degenerative joint disease resulting from the increased stress placed on the joints juxtaposed to the fused hip. In addition, patients with a fused hip have higher energy expenditure during gait compared with patients without a fused hip and, over time, may desire conversion to a more mobile hip.

The most common indication for conversion of hip arthrodesis to THA is disabling back pain. Additional indications include increasing knee pain or contralateral hip pain secondary to degenerative joint disease, a malpositioned arthrodesis resulting in functional disability, or painful pseudarthrosis. Whether conversion of a fused hip should be performed before ipsilateral knee arthroplasty remains controversial. Poor range of motion (ROM) has been documented after knee arthroplasty in patients with ipsilateral hip arthrodesis, and some studies advocate conversion of the hip fusion to THA before knee arthroplasty is performed. Even patients without the previously mentioned indications may seek conversion of hip arthrodesis to THA because of increased dissatisfaction with the inconvenience of activities of daily living and the increased energy expenditure required during gait as a result of hip arthrodesis.

Conversion of hip arthrodesis to THA is technically demanding. Important considerations include adequate exposure with maintenance or restoration of abductor function, removal of hardware if present, and careful identification of bony landmarks to ensure proper implant positioning. Surgeons should be familiar with the technique that was used for hip arthrodesis because it may influence the exposure and need for bone removal, particularly in patients with an extra-articular arthrodesis.

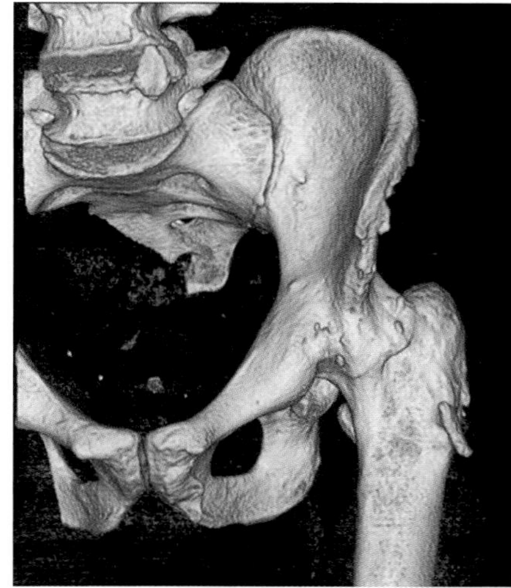

Figure 1 Three-dimensional CT reconstruction of a left hip demonstrates arthrodesis. Awareness of the bony landmarks, particularly inferiorly and posteroinferiorly, will help the surgeon localize them intraoperatively.

Preoperative CT helps identify extra-articular bone bridges, bony landmarks around the fused hip, and the status of the abductor muscles. Three-dimensional CT reconstruction is widely available and clearly demonstrates the bony anatomy and landmarks (**Figure 1**). In addition, CT-based surgical navigation can be used to help identify landmarks as well as determine the level of the femoral neck osteotomy and the location of the acetabulum.

Dr. Spangehl or an immediate family member has received research or institutional support from DePuy Synthes, Stryker, and Teleflex Vidacare. Neither Dr. Niesen nor any immediate family member has received anything of value from or has stock or stock options held in a commercial company or institution related directly or indirectly to the subject of this chapter.

Contraindications

Absolute contraindications for conversion of hip arthrodesis to THA are similar to those of primary or revision THA. Active or suspected infection and poor medical health are contraindications. Relative contraindications include young age in a patient with a hip that is fused in an acceptable position (20° of flexion, 5° of external rotation, neutral abduction/adduction), particularly if the patient will return to heavy labor; severely distorted anatomy that would preclude restoration of near-normal hip biomechanics or would result in a high risk of failure; and poor or absent abductor musculature.

Some studies have recommended the use of electromyography to assess preoperative gluteal muscle function; however, other studies have demonstrated that the use of electromyography is of limited value and does not correlate well with postoperative abductor muscle function. Postoperative abductor muscle function can be predicted via preoperative palpation of the abductor musculature during contraction and, more importantly, via intraoperative assessment of the muscles. The intraoperative assessment has been reported to correlate well with return of postoperative abductor muscle function. Even patients who have severely atrophied muscle can recover acceptable abductor muscle function if the muscle otherwise appears intact and healthy (bleeding and red in appearance and without fatty degeneration).

Patients who expect complete or near complete relief of symptoms in the surrounding joints or a normally functioning hip must be counseled with regard to the expected outcome of conversion. Typically, the outcomes of patients who undergo conversion of hip arthrodesis to THA are not comparable with those of patients who undergo primary THA. Although a patient can expect great improvement in symptoms in the surrounding joints, particularly low back pain, complete relief of symptoms is unlikely.

Alternative Treatments

Alternatives to conversion of hip arthrodesis to THA involve management of the symptomatic joint or joints around the fused hip. Typically, conversion is undertaken after nonsurgical management of symptomatic joints fails. Failed nonsurgical management of low back pain is the most common reason for conversion. Surgical management of mechanical low back pain should not be considered until after conversion of hip arthrodesis to THA because surgical management of mechanical low back pain before conversion is unlikely to be successful as a result of the ongoing stress that the hip arthrodesis places on the lumbar spine. In addition, spine fusion would result in increased disability because of the loss of compensatory motion in the low back, which is necessary in patients with fused hips. Pain relief in the ipsilateral knee or the contralateral hip is less predictable compared with improvement in low back pain after conversion. Surgical management of the ipsilateral knee or the contralateral hip, either before or after conversion of the fused hip, may be required depending on the pathology and the severity of symptoms in those joints.

Results

Conversion of hip fusion to THA usually is performed to relieve pain in the surrounding joints as well as to improve function and gait efficiency. Therefore, results of conversion of hip fusion to THA can be separated into relief of symptoms in the surrounding joints, hip function and pain, survival of the THA, and overall patient satisfaction.

Pain Relief in the Surrounding Joints

Low back pain is the most common complaint after long-standing hip fusion. Most patients demonstrate substantial improvement in lower back symptoms after conversion of hip fusion to THA. However, patients need to be counseled that as many as one-third of patients may have no improvement in their lower back symptoms because of advanced degenerative changes. Pain relief in other surrounding joints is less predictable and depends mostly on the primary pathology of the affected joint. Patients with degenerative changes may eventually require surgical treatment in those joints. In one study, ipsilateral knee pain improved in only 33% of patients. The authors of a different study reported somewhat more favorable results, with decreased knee pain in 10 of 15 patients who had knee pain before conversion. Five patients in this study required total knee arthroplasty after conversion. Similarly, relief of contralateral hip pain depends on the extent of degenerative changes in the hip.

Function and Pain of the Converted Hip

In general, patients are satisfied with the function of the converted hip and typically accept somewhat inferior results compared with those of routine primary THA to obtain increased hip mobility and relief of symptoms in the surrounding joints. Because of the wide variability and case mix of patients with converted hips, reported functional results vary widely. The authors of one recent study reported that the results of conversion of hip fusion to THA were similar to the results of primary THA based on a wide variety of outcome scores. However, the authors of a different recent study compared the results of conversion of hip fusion to THA with the results of primary THA and the results of first-time revision THA and reported that the results of conversion of hip fusion to

THA were inferior compared with those of first-time revision THA.

Despite good patient satisfaction, patients who undergo conversion of hip fusion to THA have less satisfactory muscle strength, a greater need for walking aids, and less satisfactory ROM compared with patients who undergo primary THA. Abductor muscle strength may continue to improve for years postoperatively, and some studies have reported improvement in abductor muscle strength as many as 3 years after conversion. Despite this improvement, many patients require walking aids and continue to limp after conversion. In several studies, 46% to 62% of patients required a walking aid postoperatively. Other studies have shown that 12% of patients (5 of 41) and 74% of patients (34 of 46) required greater walking aid support postoperatively than they did preoperatively. Reduced ROM, compared with that typically reported after routine primary THA, is commonly present after conversion of hip fusion to THA, with mean flexion arcs ranging from 76° to 88°. Limb-length discrepancy usually is improved after conversion of hip fusion to THA. In general, the side of the fusion is the shorter limb, and conversion lessens the limb-length discrepancy. The ability to equalize the leg lengths depends on the preoperative limb-length discrepancy, the amount of bony deficiency (however, contemporary implants usually can compensate for deficiency), the amount of scarring, and the ability to release soft tissues without excessively lengthening the limb and putting the femoral or sciatic nerves at risk. The authors of several studies have reported improvement in limb-length inequality, with a mean lengthening of the limb of approximately 2.5 cm reported without complications. The amount of pain in a converted hip is generally small; however, pain is somewhat more common after conversion of hip fusion to THA than after routine primary THA. In a study of 208 conversions, 79% of patients were pain free or had minimal pain. In a study of 45 conversions, 96% of patients had no postoperative pain in the converted hip.

Survival of the Converted THA

Survival of a converted THA varies depending on the study. The authors of a large study of 208 conversions reported 96% and 90% implant survival at 10 years and 15 years postoperatively, respectively, with revision for any reason as the end point. A study of 45 consecutive conversions reported a 10-year implant survival rate of 91%. Other studies have been less encouraging. In a study of 60 hips that underwent conversion of hip fusion to THA, the authors reported mechanical failure in 11 hips at a 9- to 15-year follow-up. The authors of a different study reported a 15% failure rate at a similar length of follow-up (7 of 46 hips). The authors of the latter study attributed most of the failures to the use of inferior prostheses. Better implant survival rates noted in more recent studies may be the result of the use of improved implants, which provide more reliable fixation in patients with compromised bone quality or bone deformities.

Overall Patient Satisfaction

Despite outcomes that are less predictable compared with those of primary THA as well as the common occurrence of a limp and the need for a walking aid in many patients postoperatively, overall satisfaction in patients who undergo conversion of hip fusion to THA is high. In general, patients are satisfied with the mobility of the converted hip; the improved symptoms in other joints, particularly back pain; and the improved function. Reported patient satisfaction rates after conversion of hip fusion to THA range from approximately 72% to 93%.

Risk factors for poorer clinical outcome include male sex, older patient age at the time of fusion, longer duration of fusion, age younger than 50 years at the time of conversion, multiple surgeries, fusion to manage sepsis, and surgical arthrodesis. In general, better outcomes are reported in patients who are older at the time of conversion, patients in whom a spontaneous fusion occurred, and patients in whom the abductors were in relatively good condition (**Table 1**).

Complications

Complications after conversion of hip arthrodesis to THA are similar to complications after primary THA that is performed to manage degenerative joint disease. However, the incidence of complications after conversion of hip arthrodesis to THA is generally greater compared with that observed after routine THA. The incidence of infection after conversion of hip arthrodesis to THA is generally higher compared with that observed after routine primary THA, and reported rates of infection vary from 1.4% to 13%. Nerve palsy is more commonly observed after conversion of hip arthrodesis to THA compared with after routine primary THA. The authors of a large study reported a 7% incidence of nerve palsy, with an almost equal number of femoral and sciatic nerve palsies reported. Rates of trochanteric nonunion as high as 14% have been reported; however, the authors of most studies report an incidence of trochanteric nonunion of approximately 5%.

The rate of dislocation observed after conversion of hip fusion to THA does not appear to be substantially greater than that observed after primary THA, which may be related to the fact that the mean ROM in patients who undergo conversion of hip fusion to THA is less than that in patients who undergo primary THA. However, patients with very deficient or absent abductors may have an increased risk for dislocation. In one large study of 208 conversions, four of five dislocations occurred in patients who were younger than 15 years at the

Table 1 Results of Total Hip Arthroplasty (THA) After Hip Fusion

Authors (Year)	Number of Hips	Procedure or Approach	Mean Patient Age in Years (Range)[a]	Mean Follow-up in Years (Range)	Results
Strathy and Fitzgerald (1988)	80	NR	50 (21-70)	10.4 (9-15)	Age <50 yr at time of conversion was associated with a higher failure rate Effect of age at fusion on outcome NR Duration of fusion had no effect on outcome 20 spontaneous and 60 surgical fusions; surgical fusion was associated with a higher failure rate (1 failure in a spontaneously fused hip versus 20 failures in surgically fused hips) 9 deep infections 30 hips had poor results
Kilgus et al (1990)	41	Transtrochanteric	53 (24-75)	7 (2-16.5)	Age <50 yr at time of conversion was associated with a higher failure rate Effects of age at fusion and duration of fusion on outcome NR 13 spontaneous and 28 surgical fusions; surgical fusion was associated with a higher failure rate 4 deep infections 5 mechanical failures Decreased Trendelenburg sign in patients whose abductor moment arm was restored 74% required a walking aid postoperatively
Reikerås et al (1995)	46	Lateral or posterior	58 (33-75)	8 (5-13)	Younger age at fusion was associated with greater patient satisfaction Effects of age at conversion and fusion type on outcome NR Mean duration of fusion, 17 yr (range, 7-28 yr); shorter duration of fusion was associated with greater patient satisfaction 76% good or excellent results 85% satisfied 74% used a walking aid postoperatively 15.2% required revision
Hamadouche et al (2001)	45	Transtrochanteric	55.8 (28-80)	8.5 (5-21)	Age at fusion and age at conversion had no effect on outcome Mean duration of fusion, 36 yr (range, 3-65 yr); trend of higher functional scores with shorter duration of fusion 20 spontaneous and 25 surgical fusions; fusion type had no effect on outcome 91% 10-yr implant survival Walking ability was associated with quality of gluteal muscle intraoperatively Walking improved for 2 to 3 yr postoperatively 50% used a cane postoperatively
Joshi et al (2002)	208	Transtrochanteric	51 (20-80)	9.2 (2-26)	Age at fusion ≤15 yr associated with a poorer outcome, possibly related to underdeveloped abductors; age >15 yr associated with better functional scores (mean age at fusion, 21.3; range, 2-56) Effects of age at conversion and duration of fusion on outcome NR 48 spontaneous and 160 surgical fusions; spontaneous fusion was associated with slightly better functional results 96% 10-yr and 90% 15-yr implant survival 5 dislocations (4 in patients with fusion at age <15 yr) 15 nerve palsies 79% had minimal pain or were pain free 83% had good or excellent function

NR = not reported.

[a] Age at conversion.

Table 1 Results of Total Hip Arthroplasty (THA) After Hip Fusion (*continued*)

Authors (Year)	Number of Hips	Procedure or Approach	Mean Patient Age in Years (Range)[a]	Mean Follow-up in Years (Range)	Results
Peterson et al (2009)	30	Transtrochanteric (15), direct lateral (10), posterior (5)	52.5 (27-70)	10.4 (2-20.5)	Mean age at fusion, 19.9 yr (range, 2-42 yr); effect on outcome NR Age <50 yr at conversion associated with a higher failure rate but better function Mean duration of fusion, 32.6 yr (range, 1-42 yr); duration of fusion <30 yr was associated with higher failure rate but better function 5 spontaneous and 25 surgical fusions; surgical fusion associated with higher failure rate 86% 5-yr and 75% 10-yr implant survival 10 unsuccessful (3 for pain, 7 for failure) 2 dislocations
Fernandez-Fairen et al (2011)	48	Anterolateral (21), transtrochanteric (15), posterolateral (12)	52 (31-68)	17 (10-29)	Mean age at fusion, 26 yr (range, 17-41 yr); effect on outcome NR Effect of age at conversion on outcome NR Mean duration of fusion, 26 yr (range, 3-47 yr); effect on outcome NR 18 spontaneous and 30 surgical fusions; effect of fusion type on outcome NR Conversion cohort was compared with 50 primary THAs, with similar results between the two cohorts for numerous outcome scores 11 converted hips and 12 hips with primary THA required revision (23% and 25%, respectively)
Richards and Duncan (2011)	17	Transtrochanteric or direct lateral	49 (25-74)	9 (2-21)	Mean age at fusion, 29 yr (range, 7-46 yr) Effects of age at conversion, duration of fusion, and fusion type on outcome NR Conversion cohort was compared with primary THA and first-time revision THA cohorts; conversion cohort had the poorest outcome scores 74% 10-yr implant survival 54% had complications
Aderinto et al (2012)	18	Trochanteric slide osteotomy	53 (21-77)	5 (2-15)	Age at fusion and age at conversion had no effect on outcome Mean duration of fusion, 33 yr (range, 11-60 yr); duration of fusion had no effect on outcome 4 spontaneous and 14 surgical fusions; no effect of fusion type on outcome 2 (11%) had peroneal nerve injury 2 (11%) required revision 7 (39%) had heterotopic bone with 1 complete fusion
Villanueva et al (2013)	21	Posterolateral	58.5 (21-77)	8 (3-14)	Mean age at fusion, 18.8 yr (range, 12-37 yr); age at fusion had no effect on outcome Age at conversion and duration of fusion had no effect on outcome Spontaneous fusion had better flexion than surgical fusion but no difference in clinical scores 8 (38%) had perioperative complications

NR = not reported.

[a] Age at conversion.

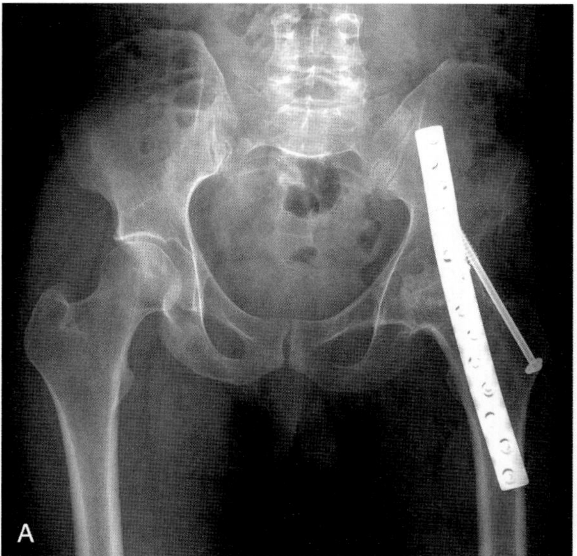

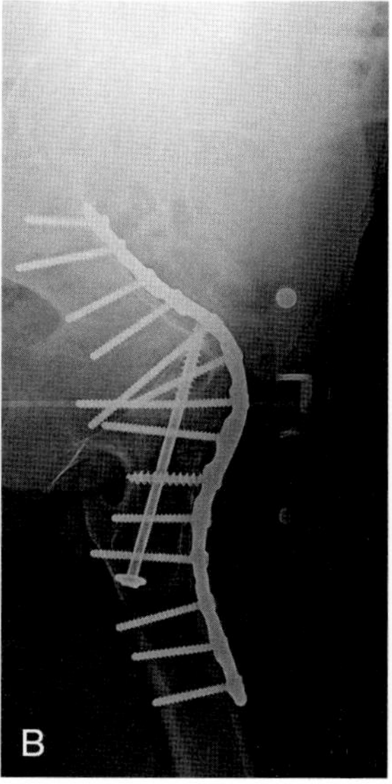

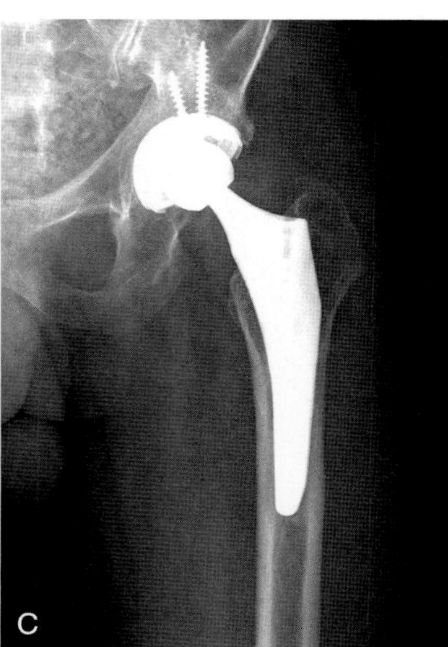

Figure 2 Preoperative AP pelvic radiograph (**A**) and lateral radiograph of the left hip (**B**) demonstrate hip arthrodesis that was performed via an anterior approach, with the plate placed over the anterior femur and the hip joint extending proximally onto the inner aspect of the iliac wing. **C,** AP radiograph of the left hip obtained 1 year after conversion to total hip arthroplasty via the direct anterior approach. The normal proximal femoral anatomy allowed the use of a conventional wedge-shaped tapered stem.

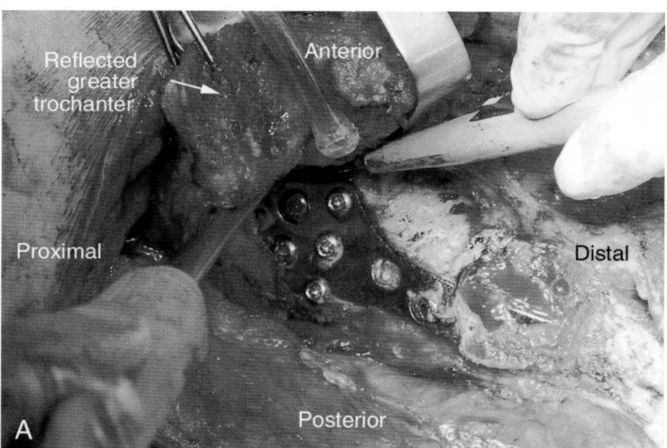

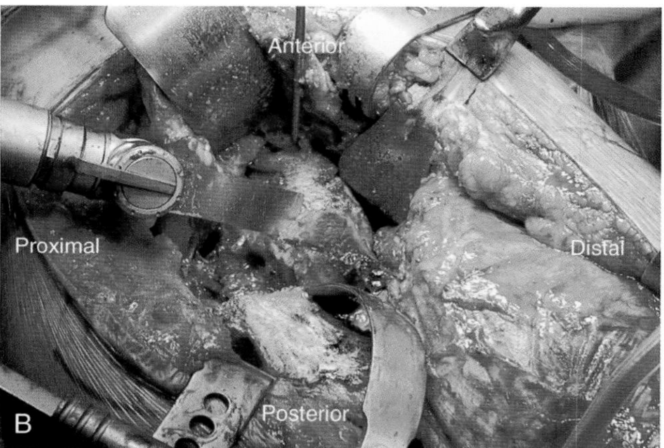

Figure 3 **A,** Intraoperative photograph of a hip shows a classic trochanteric osteotomy, which is used to facilitate hardware removal. The plate was located beneath the trochanter. **B,** Intraoperative photograph of the same hip shows a femoral neck osteotomy. Retractors are placed anteriorly and posteriorly, and the osteotomy is performed just proximal to the superior aspect of the trochanteric osteotomy. (Courtesy of Clive Duncan, MD, MSc, FRCSC, Vancouver, British Columbia, Canada.)

time of hip fusion. The authors of the study concluded that the underdeveloped abductors increased the patients' risk for dislocation.

A large study reported heterotopic ossification in 13% of patients who underwent conversion of hip fusion to THA. No prophylactic measures against heterotopic ossification were used in any of the patients. Only 3 of 28 hips had Brooker class III heterotopic ossification, and the remainder of the hips had less heterotopic ossification. Furthermore, heterotopic ossification did not result in functional limitation in any of the patients. A more recent study of 18 patients who underwent conversion of hip fusion to THA reported a 37% incidence of heterotopic ossification, including one instance of complete ankylosis. No prophylactic measures against heterotopic ossification were used in any of the patients.

Techniques

Setup/Exposure

- Conversion of hip fusion to THA usually is performed with the

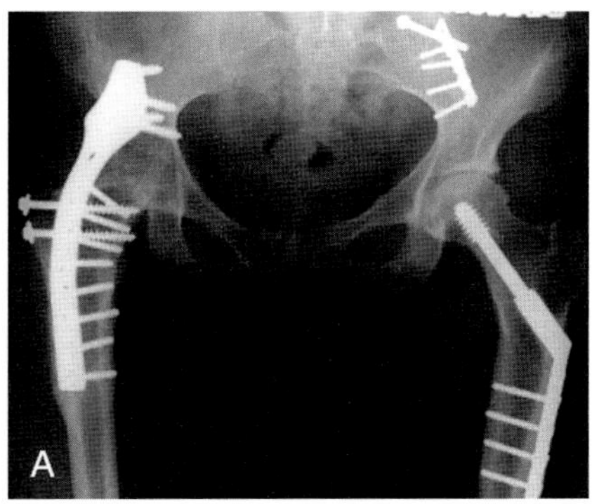

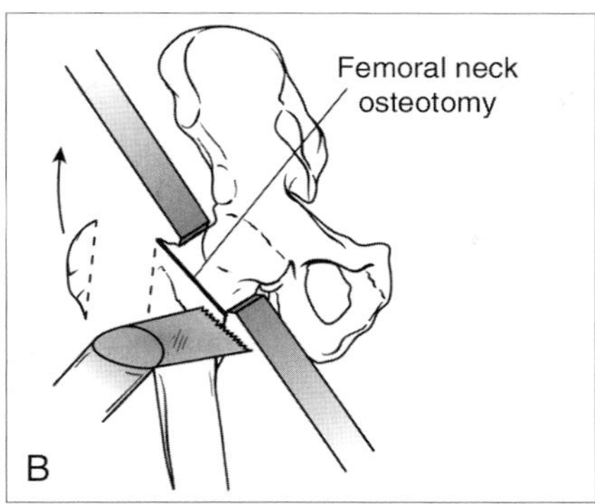

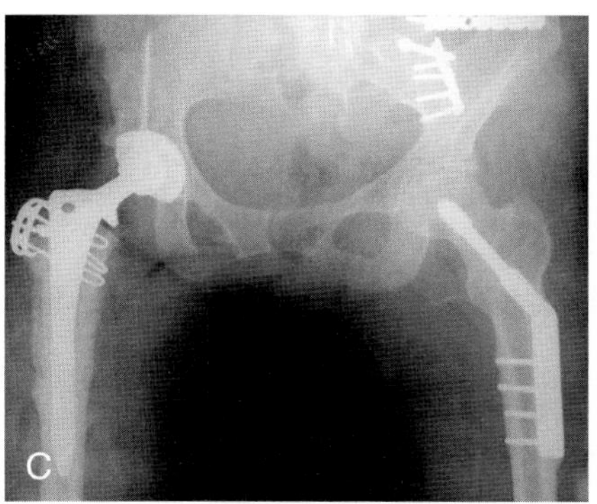

Figure 4 **A,** AP pelvic radiograph demonstrates fusion of the right hip with the use of a cobra plate. The greater trochanter was reattached over the lateral aspect of the plate. **B,** Illustration of a hip shows a femoral neck osteotomy. The fusion mass is exposed with the use of retractors that are placed superiorly and inferiorly, after which the superior and inferior aspects of the femoral neck are identified and the femoral neck osteotomy is performed. Landmarks for the femoral neck osteotomy include the trochanteric osteotomy site (proximal aspect), the lesser trochanter, and the screw holes from removed hardware. **C,** Postoperative AP pelvic radiograph demonstrates the use of an extensively porous-coated implant to address metaphyseal distortion and bypass the removed plate. (Courtesy of Clive Duncan, MD, MSc, FRCSC, Vancouver, British Columbia, Canada.)

patient placed in the lateral decubitus position.

- The supine position may be used if a direct anterior approach is preferred, especially if removal of anterior hardware is required (**Figure 2**).
- The skin incision is dictated by the previous incisions and the need for hardware removal. If a spontaneous arthrodesis occurred and no incision is present, then a posterolateral incision typically is used because it allows the use of more extensile exposures as necessary.
- Any hardware overlying the trochanter and proximal femur is removed. If a previous trochanteric osteotomy was performed at the time of fusion and hardware is beneath the trochanter, then a classic trochanteric osteotomy is required (**Figure 3**). Otherwise, a posterior approach can be used.
- If exposure is difficult, a trochanteric slide osteotomy with the use of anterior retraction generally allows adequate exposure and avoids further violation of the abductors.
- A short extended osteotomy may be performed to facilitate closure and healing of the osteotomy. However, a more formal or longer extended osteotomy may be required if deformity in the proximal femur requires correction.
- Soft tissues are cleared from the arthrodesis and the proximal femur to allow identification of the femoral neck.
- If a bony bridge exists between the femur and the ischium, the bridge is osteotomized before the femoral neck osteotomy is performed. Care is taken to protect the sciatic nerve in this region.
- A femoral neck osteotomy is performed somewhat more proximal than the anticipated final osteotomy. Further release of soft tissues around the proximal femur will improve exposure (**Figure 4**).
- Based on preoperative templating and identification of bony landmarks (either the greater or lesser trochanter), the definitive femoral neck osteotomy is performed, which provides the surgeon additional room to prepare the acetabulum.

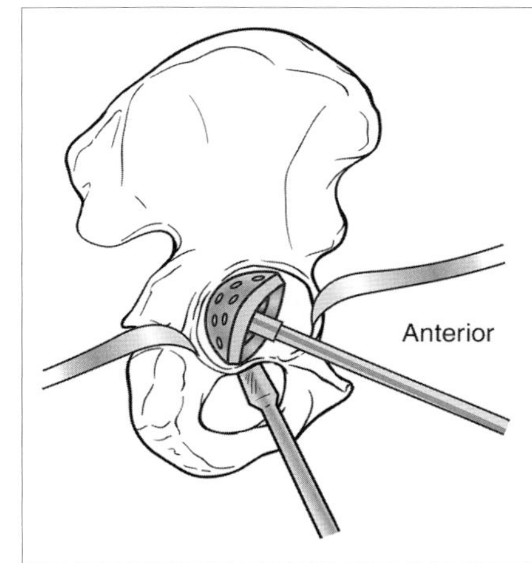

Figure 5 Illustration shows identification of the inferior aspect of the acetabulum to ensure proper orientation before reaming. A blunt retractor may be placed beneath the teardrop. The anterior and posterior aspects of the acetabulum also are identified for orientation in the coronal plane. (Reproduced from Spangehl MJ: Total hip arthroplasty after hip fusion, in Lieberman JR, Berry DJ: *Advanced Reconstruction: Hip*. Rosemont, IL, American Academy of Orthopaedic Surgeons, 2005, pp 151-157.)

Instruments/Equipment/ Implants Required

- The equipment typically required for the implants must be available.
- Metal-cutting burrs, broken-screw extractors, and fluoroscopy may be required to remove hardware or identify bony landmarks.

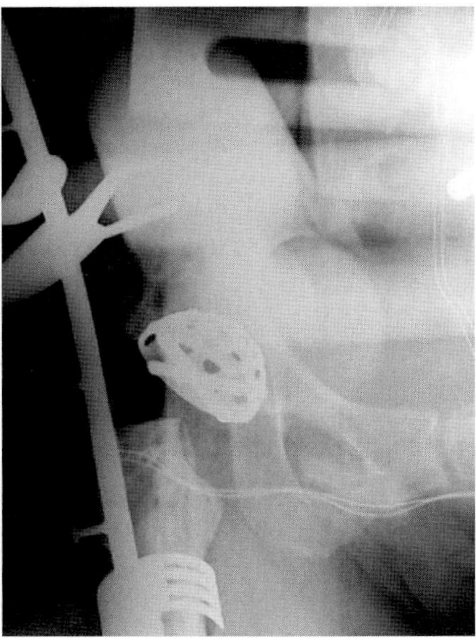

Figure 6 Intraoperative AP radiograph of the right hip of the patient shown in Figure 3 demonstrates proper positioning of the reamer. (Courtesy of Clive Duncan, MD, MSc, FRCSC, Vancouver, British Columbia, Canada.)

- As already mentioned, CT-based surgical navigation may be helpful.

Procedure

BONE PREPARATION

- Bone preparation begins on the acetabular side.
- Identification of the inferior aspect of the acetabulum is critical but may be difficult because of the bone overlying the floor of the acetabulum. The inferior aspect of the acetabulum can be located via identification of the superior aspect of the obturator foramen and placement of a hooked retractor around the most inferior portion of the acetabulum (the so-called teardrop).
- Before reaming begins, the anterior and posterior walls of the acetabulum must be identified for proper placement of the reamer. A blunt retractor that is carefully placed over the anterior wall often helps maintain exposure and identify the anterior wall for proper orientation (**Figure 5**).
- The acetabulum is carefully deepened and widened with the use of reamers. Often, especially in patients in whom a spontaneous fusion occurred, soft tissues (the transverse acetabular ligament or remnants of the ligamentum teres) are recognized in the floor of the acetabulum as the acetabulum is deepened.
- Careful attention to the thickness of the anterior and posterior walls is necessary during preparation of the socket. An intraoperative radiograph or fluoroscopy may aid in early preparation of the socket to ensure proper positioning of the reamer in the superoinferior plane (**Figure 6**).
- In patients with severely distorted anatomy, the placement of a Kirschner wire as a marker before

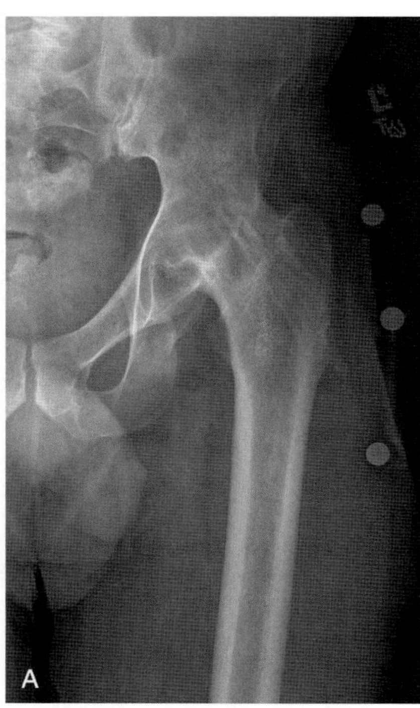

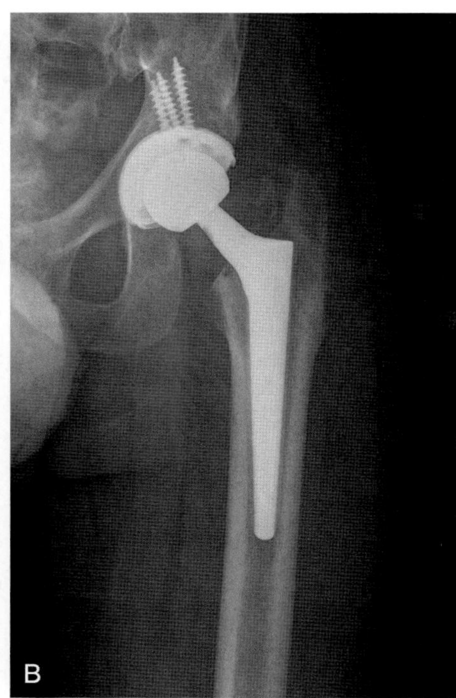

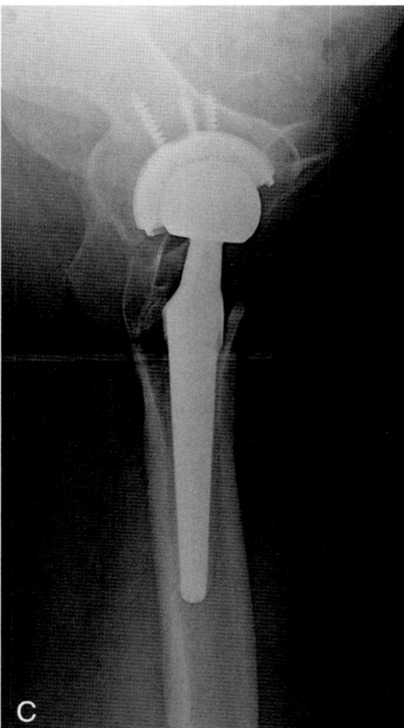

Figure 7 **A,** Preoperative AP radiograph of a left hip demonstrates a somewhat distorted proximal diaphysis as a result of prior surgical treatment and hardware, which was previously removed. Postoperative AP (**B**) and lateral (**C**) radiographs of the left hip demonstrate fixation with a fluted, tapered stem that engages in the proximal diaphysis, which bypasses the distorted proximal bone.

a radiographic image is obtained will assist in orientation.

- After the acetabulum is prepared, a trial socket is inserted.
- Femoral preparation is performed according to the type of femoral implant that will be used.

IMPLANTATION OF THE PROSTHESIS

- Prosthesis selection depends on a patient's bone quality, the presence of any cortical defects or stress risers that are related to hardware removal, the amount of deformity in the proximal femur, and any steps that were taken to address the deformity. A patient's age and activity level as well as a surgeon's preferred implant fixation method also are factors that should be considered in the selection of the prosthesis.
- Similar to primary or revision THA, noncemented fixation can be used on the acetabular side.
- On the femoral side, implant choice and fixation vary. In general, a noncemented implant is preferred because most patients who undergo conversion are relatively young and/or have sufficient bone quality to support stable fixation of a noncemented implant.
- Patients with distortion of the proximal metaphysis as a result of deformity or prior hardware require metadiaphyseal or diaphyseal implant fixation (**Figure 7**).
- Distal fixation also is necessary if an extended trochanteric osteotomy was required for exposure because of deformity.
- If a long plate was removed from the proximal femur, the presence of multiple stress risers and the likelihood of stress-shielded bone under the plate make distal fixation a good option.
- A larger femoral head and liner (36 mm or larger), a dual-mobility bearing, or a constrained acetabular liner may be considered in patients in whom the abductors are absent or if a patient has a high risk for postoperative instability.
- Before final implant placement, a trial reduction is performed to determine the appropriate femoral neck length to achieve the desired soft-tissue tension and limb length.
- The sciatic nerve is palpated to ensure that it is mobile with the hip slightly flexed and the knee extended. If excess tension on the sciatic nerve is noted, the femoral neck length or femoral implant position may need to be adjusted. The risk of stretching the sciatic nerve likely depends on the amount of shortening and the age of the patient at the time of arthrodesis.
- Although the limb in which the conversion is performed is shorter than the contralateral limb in most patients, excessive lengthening (2 cm or more) should be avoided because it increases the risk of injury to the sciatic and femoral nerves and can increase the difficulty of trochanteric reattachment if an osteotomy was required.

Wound Closure

- Before the wound is closed, the hip is taken through a ROM into the positions of risk for dislocation and is carefully inspected for bony impingement.
- Immediately after conversion, the hip will lack the usual ROM of a primary THA. Motion usually improves with time but typically not to the extent observed in patients who undergo primary THA. Because this increase in motion can result in bony impingement, potential areas of bony impingement should be removed at the time of conversion even if direct bony impingement is not observed.
- The trochanteric osteotomy is closed with the use of wires or cables.
- The use of a claw or grip device should be avoided if a short extended osteotomy was performed.
- If the trochanter is absent, then the abductors, if present and not overly shortened, are sutured to the proximal femur.
- Alternatively, the tensor fascia lata can be sutured to the trochanter or the proximal femur.
- An adductor tenotomy or release of the psoas tendon may be required in patients with limited hip abduction and patients with a persistent flexion deformity in whom shortening of the limb is not desired or would leave the hip unstable.

Postoperative Regimen

Weight bearing after conversion of hip fusion to THA depends on the type of implants used; the surgeon's preference with regard to weight bearing after THA; and, if a trochanteric osteotomy was performed, the adequacy of fixation of the trochanteric fragment. Partial weight bearing may be allowed in patients with good trochanteric fixation; however, if the quality of fixation is in doubt, weight bearing should be delayed until 6 to 8 weeks postoperatively. Active abduction is delayed until 8 weeks postoperatively to allow adequate trochanteric or abductor healing.

Most patients who undergo conversion of hip arthrodesis to THA will have remaining stiffness and lack the usual motion observed after primary THA. Therefore, the risk for early dislocation may be decreased. However, patients with severely deficient or absent abductors may have an increased risk for dislocation; in these patients, a hip abduction orthosis may be used for 6 to 12 weeks postoperatively to restrict flexion and adduction.

Routine antibiotics and thromboembolic prophylaxis should be administered. Prophylaxis against heterotopic ossification is not routinely required. However, prophylactic perioperative radiation therapy or anti-inflammatory drugs should be used in patients in whom a spontaneous arthrodesis occurred and patients at risk for heterotopic ossification.

Avoiding Pitfalls and Complications

The use of a trochanteric slide osteotomy with maintenance of the vastus lateralis attachment or the use of a short extended trochanteric osteotomy that allows for wire or cable fixation of the proximal lateral cortex and maintains the soft-tissue attachments may help reduce the risk for trochanteric nonunion.

Bibliography

Aderinto J, Lulu OB, Backstein DJ, Safir O, Gross AE: Functional results and complications following conversion of hip fusion to total hip replacement. *J Bone Joint Surg Br* 2012;94(suppl 11-A):36-41.

Akiyama H, Kawanabe K, Ito T, Goto K, Nangaku M, Nakamura T: Computed tomography-based navigation to determine the femoral neck osteotomy and location of the acetabular socket of an arthrodesed hip. *J Arthroplasty* 2009;24(8):1292.e1-1292.e4.

Brewster RC, Coventry MB, Johnson EW Jr: Conversion of the arthrodesed hip to a total hip arthroplasty. *J Bone Joint Surg Am* 1975;57(1):27-30.

Fernandez-Fairen M, Murcia-Mazón A, Torres A, Querales V, Murcia A Jr: Is total hip arthroplasty after hip arthrodesis as good as primary arthroplasty? *Clin Orthop Relat Res* 2011;469(7):1971-1983.

Garvin KL, Pellicci PM, Windsor RE, Conrad EU, Insall JN, Salvati EA: Contralateral total hip arthroplasty or ipsilateral total knee arthroplasty in patients who have a long-standing fusion of the hip. *J Bone Joint Surg Am* 1989;71(9):1355-1362.

Gore DR, Murray MP, Sepic SB, Gardner GM: Walking patterns of men with unilateral surgical hip fusion. *J Bone Joint Surg Am* 1975;57(6):759-765.

Hamadouche M, Kerboull L, Meunier A, Courpied JP, Kerboull M: Total hip arthroplasty for the treatment of ankylosed hips: A five to twenty-one-year follow-up study. *J Bone Joint Surg Am* 2001;83(7):992-998.

Jain S, Giannoudis PV: Arthrodesis of the hip and conversion to total hip arthroplasty: A systematic review. *J Arthroplasty* 2013;28(9):1596-1602.

Joshi AB, Markovic L, Hardinge K, Murphy JC: Conversion of a fused hip to total hip arthroplasty. *J Bone Joint Surg Am* 2002;84(8):1335-1341.

Kilgus DJ, Amstutz HC, Wolgin MA, Dorey FJ: Joint replacement for ankylosed hips. *J Bone Joint Surg Am* 1990;72(1):45-54.

Peterson ED, Nemanich JP, Altenburg A, Cabanela ME: Hip arthroplasty after previous arthrodesis. *Clin Orthop Relat Res* 2009;467(11):2880-2885.

Reikerås O, Bjerkreim I, Gundersson R: Total hip arthroplasty for arthrodesed hips: 5- to 13-year results. *J Arthroplasty* 1995;10(4):529-531.

Richards CJ, Duncan CP: Conversion of hip arthrodesis to total hip arthroplasty: Survivorship and clinical outcome. *J Arthroplasty* 2011;26(3):409-413.

Rittmeister M, Starker M, Zichner L: Hip and knee replacement after longstanding hip arthrodesis. *Clin Orthop Relat Res* 2000;371:136-145.

Sirikonda SP, Beardmore SP, Hodgkinson JP: Role of hip arthrodesis in current practice: Long term results following conversion to total hip arthroplasty. *Hip Int* 2008;18(4):263-271.

Strathy GM, Fitzgerald RH Jr: Total hip arthroplasty in the ankylosed hip: A ten-year follow-up. *J Bone Joint Surg Am* 1988;70(7):963-966.

Villanueva M, Sobrón FB, Parra J, Rojo JM, Chana F, Vaquero J: Conversion of arthrodesis to total hip arthroplasty: Clinical outcome, complications, and prognostic factors of 21 consecutive cases. *HSS J* 2013;9(2):138-144.

Waters RL, Barnes G, Husserl T, Silver L, Liss R: Comparable energy expenditure after arthrodesis of the hip and ankle. *J Bone Joint Surg Am* 1988;70(7):1032-1037.

Whitehouse MR, Duncan CP: Conversion of hip fusion to total hip replacement: Technique and results. *Bone Joint J* 2013;95(suppl 11-A):114-119.

Chapter 25

Total Hip Arthroplasty in Patients With Femoral Deformity

Joshua L. Carter, MD
Bryan D. Springer, MD

Indications

Deformity of the proximal femur creates unique challenges in total hip arthroplasty (THA). Factors that must be considered include anatomic and exposure issues, implant fit and fixation challenges, and stability concerns. The pertinent challenges to THA in patients with femoral deformity and a strategy to appropriately manage these challenges must be identified preoperatively to ensure a successful outcome.

Indications for THA in patients with proximal femoral deformity include end-stage osteoarthritis with pain and loss of function that cannot be managed nonsurgically. The Berry classification of proximal femoral deformity describes proximal femoral deformity based on location, geometry, and etiology (**Table 1**). These factors are interrelated, with the etiology of femoral deformity generally determining both the geometry and location of femoral deformity. Femoral deformity may be the result of neoplastic causes.

Preoperative planning for THA is important and includes a thorough preoperative medical evaluation, physical examination, and appropriate imaging studies. In patients with femoral deformity in particular, preparation for THA requires thorough preoperative templating based on appropriate radiographs. Surgeons may choose to use specialized implants, which require time to obtain and process. Some patients may require custom implants. The choice of THA technique and implant is largely determined by the exact location of the femoral deformity.

Femoral neck deformities include increased varus (coxa vara), valgus (coxa valga), and a shortened femoral neck (coxa breva). A varus femoral neck deformity is defined as a femoral neck-shaft angle less than 120° (**Figure 1**) and may result from congenital pathologies (skeletal dysplasia) or acquired pathologies (posttraumatic pathology, osteomyelitis, rickets, fibrous dysplasia, slipped capital femoral epiphysis, osteogenesis imperfecta, Paget disease; **Figure 2**). The primary goal in the treatment of patients with a coxa vara deformity is to recognize and restore femoral offset. The failure to maintain femoral offset may result in hip instability (secondary to laxity in the soft tissues) and/or increased leg length (required to achieve stability).

Table 1 Berry Classification of Proximal Femoral Deformity

Site of deformity
Greater trochanter
Femoral neck
Metaphysis
Diaphysis
Geometry of deformity
Torsional
Angular
Translational
Size abnormality
Etiology of deformity
Developmental (dysplasia)
Metabolic (Paget disease)
Previous osteotomy
Previous fracture

Adapted with permission from Berry DJ: Total hip arthroplasty in patients with proximal femoral deformity. *Clin Orthop Relat Res* 1999;(369):262-272.

A coxa valga deformity is defined as a femoral neck-shaft angle greater than 135° (**Figure 3**). The primary causes of acquired coxa valga are developmental dysplasia of the hip and neurologic disorders, such as cerebral palsy and spinal muscular atrophy. The goals in the treatment of patients with a coxa valga deformity include attaining hip stability and ensuring femoral stem fixation.

Dr. Springer or an immediate family member is a member of a speakers' bureau or has made paid presentations on behalf of CeramTec and DePuy Synthes; serves as a paid consultant to ConvaTec, Polaris Medical, and Stryker; has received nonincome support (such as equipment or services), commercially derived honoraria, or other non–research-related funding (such as paid travel) from Joint Purification Systems; and serves as a board member, owner, officer, or committee member of the American Joint Replacement Registry. Neither Dr. Carter nor any immediate family member has received anything of value from or has stock or stock options held in a commercial company or institution related directly or indirectly to the subject of this chapter.

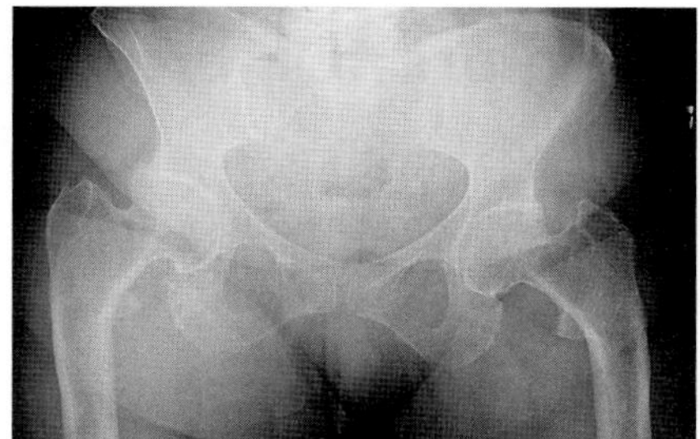

Figure 1 AP pelvic radiograph demonstrates a substantial coxa vara deformity of both proximal femurs.

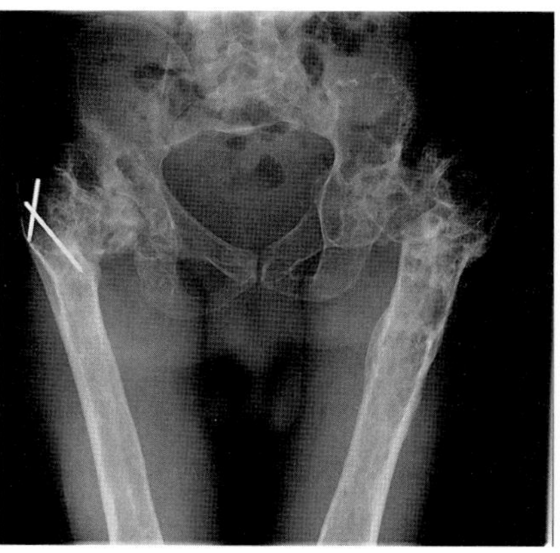

Figure 2 AP pelvic radiograph from a patient with bilateral fibrous hip dysplasia demonstrates substantial shepherd's crook deformity of the proximal femur.

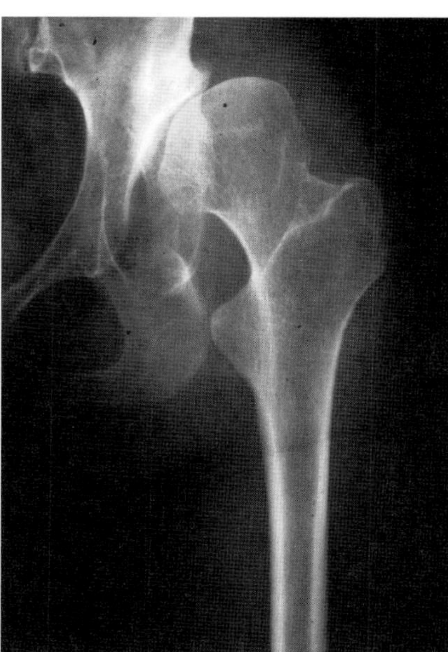

Figure 3 AP radiograph of a left hip demonstrates an increased femoral neck-shaft angle, which is associated with coxa valga deformity.

Appropriate assessment of the rotation and anteversion of the coxa valga deformity is necessary.

A coxa breva deformity indicates a short femoral neck, which is common in patients with Legg-Calvé-Perthes disease (**Figure 4**). The primary surgical considerations for patients who have a coxa breva deformity involve navigating a difficult exposure. Exposure techniques for patients with a stiff and short femoral neck are discussed later in this chapter.

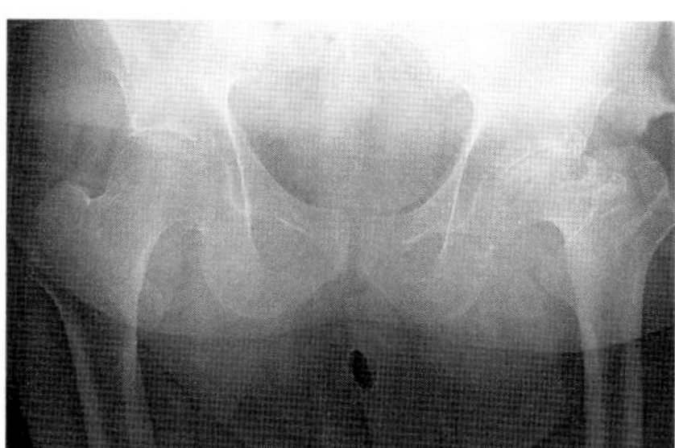

Figure 4 AP pelvic radiograph demonstrates a coxa breva deformity, which resulted from prior Legg-Calvé-Perthes disease of the left hip.

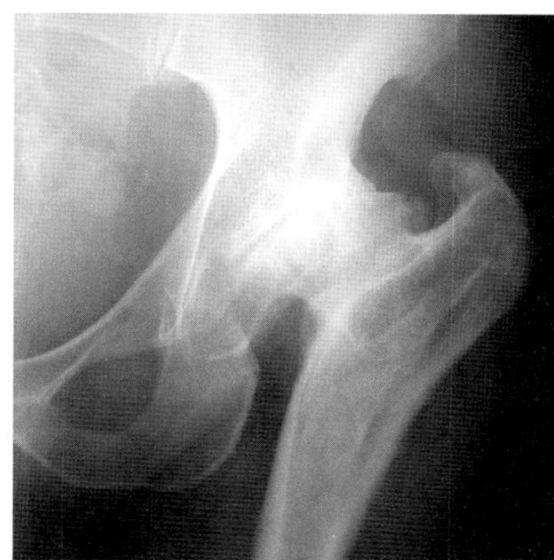

Figure 5 AP radiograph of a left hip demonstrates a greater trochanter overhanging the femoral canal, which makes canalization of the femoral diaphysis with the use of a straight stem difficult.

Deformity of the greater trochanter generally results in a high-riding or overhanging trochanter (**Figure 5**). Deformity of the greater trochanter may result from idiopathic, posttraumatic, or postoperative causes or may be associated with a varus proximal femur. Management of an overhanging trochanter involves safely accessing the femoral canal with the use of reamers and broaches and avoiding varus malpositioning of the femoral implant. A high-riding or anteriorly positioned trochanter may result in anterior impingement that causes hip instability; debulking of the bone with the use of a high-speed burr or rongeur may be required to decrease the impingement.

Deformity of the proximal femoral metadiaphysis creates complex challenges in THA. Deformity of the proximal femoral metadiaphysis may result from metabolic, neoplastic, posttraumatic, or infectious causes but most commonly is the result of prior intertrochanteric hip fractures or osteotomies. The Dorr classification is used to describe the shape of the proximal femur. Diaphyseal deformity may result from femoral expansion and metadiaphyseal mismatch ranging from Dorr type A (champagne flute) to type C (stovepipe) femurs, prior trauma, prior osteotomies, dysplasia, or substantial femoral bowing. Modular implants that allow for intraoperative control of femoral anteversion, such as the S-ROM Modular Hip System (DePuy Synthes) (**Figure 6**), are excellent tools for managing complex deformity in the metadiaphysis. Custom implants also may be beneficial in these patients. Similarly, deformity in the proximal femoral metadiaphysis may be managed by positioning implants proximal to the deformity with the use of a short stem or via hip resurfacing or by reorienting the deformity with an osteotomy.

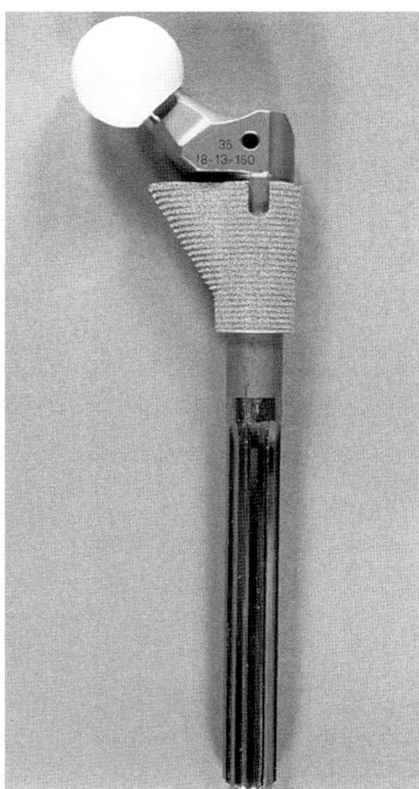

Figure 6 Photograph shows an example of a modular femoral stem (S-ROM Modular Hip System; DePuy Synthes). (Reproduced with permission from Christine MJ, DeBoer DK, Trick LW, et al: Primary total hip arthroplasty with the use of the modular S-ROM prosthesis: Four to seven-year clinical and radiographic results. *J Bone Joint Surg Am* 1999;81[12]:1707-1716.)

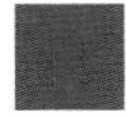

Contraindications

Patients with femoral deformity have the same contraindications for THA as patients with normal anatomy; however, many patients with femoral deformity are younger than the typical arthroplasty candidate and, therefore, may place higher demands on the implant. A careful preoperative discussion with the patient of the goals and expectations of THA is necessary. Patients without end-stage arthritis and patients with radiographic features of arthritis or deformity without clinical correlation of pain or loss of function may not be appropriate candidates for THA. Known active infection, uncontrolled diabetes mellitus, severe cardiac or pulmonary disease, undiagnosed neoplasm, or other substantial medical problems may increase a patient's perioperative risk for complications and are potential contraindications to elective THA. Appropriate patient selection and surgical skills are critical to ensure the long-term success of THA in patients with femoral deformity.

Alternative Treatments

Nonsurgical treatment options for the management of osteoarthritis in patients with deformity of the proximal femur are the same as those in patients with normal anatomy. Patients with deformity of the proximal femur may benefit from control of arthritic symptoms via weight loss, NSAIDs, acetaminophen, physical therapy, and joint injections.

Results

Few well-designed comparative studies of THA in patients with femoral deformity have been published. Although some studies have been published on THA in patients with hip dysplasia (which is not the focus of this chapter), most of the literature involves small series or case reports of patients with unique deformities. In a study published in 1989, the mean Harris Hip score improved from 41 to 94 in three primary dysplastic hips managed with femoral osteotomy and noncemented implants. In a 1996 study reporting on 20 primary dysplastic hips that were managed in the same manner, time to healing was 30 weeks for most osteotomies. Several studies on primary THA in patients with femoral deformity resulting from prior osteotomy are available in the literature (**Table 2**). These studies have reported that the results of THA in patients who underwent a varus-producing osteotomy of the proximal femur are inferior, especially in patients with more than 10 mm of femoral shaft medialization. In patients who underwent a prior valgus osteotomy, however, THA is generally successful and results in outcomes similar to those of THA in patients without deformity. Furthermore, several studies have reported that THA with cemented stems in patients who underwent a prior osteotomy results in higher failure rates compared with patients treated with noncemented stems. Moreover, THA with noncemented stems in patients who underwent a prior valgus intertrochanteric osteotomy for hip dysplasia has resulted in reasonably good outcomes. The authors of one study reported a 4% failure rate in 48 hips at 16 years postoperatively, and another study reported no failures at a mean follow-up of 7 years after THA in patients who underwent a prior valgus intertrochanteric osteotomy to manage hip dysplasia.

The results of THA with modular noncemented stems were reported in a study of 125 hips, most without deformity. At a mean follow-up of 5.3 years postoperatively, 98% of patients had stable bone ingrowth, and only 7% of patients had osteolysis proximal to the sleeve of the implant.

Techniques

Setup/Exposure

- Typically, a posterior approach to the hip is used. For this approach, the patient is positioned with his or her pelvis secured in the lateral decubitus position on a standard surgical table. Other approaches to the hip may be used depending on the surgical plan and surgeon preference.
- The patient is prepared and draped in a manner that creates a large

Table 2 Results of Primary Total Hip Arthroplasty (THA) in Patients With Femoral Deformity Resulting From Prior Osteotomy

Authors (Year)	Number of Hips	Procedure	Mean Patient Age in Years (Range)	Mean Follow-up in Years (Range)	Success Rate (%)[a]	Results
Ferguson et al (1994)	305 (290 patients)	Conversion to THA with cemented components after intertrochanteric osteotomy	61.4 (NR)	10.1 (all >5)	81.9	Good to excellent results in 79% of hips Total probability of failure was 20.6% at 10 yr
Boos et al (1997)	74 (matched with 74 control hips)	Conversion to THA with cemented Müller femoral component after intertrochanteric osteotomy	Study group: 57.4 (34-79) Control group: 61.6 (33-82)	Study group: 6.9 (4.8-9.7) Control group: 7.3 (4.7-12.2)	10 yr: 82	Mean HHS in the study group improved from 42.9 to 87.7 Mean HHS in the control group improved from 40.7 to 90.1 Study group had longer surgical times and more trochanteric osteotomies compared with control group Control group had a trend toward better implant survivorship compared with the study group
Shinar and Harris (1998)	22	Conversion to THA with cemented femoral and acetabular components after subtrochanteric or intertrochanteric osteotomy	53 (17-73)	15.5 (11.5-19.2)	Femoral implants: 89.5 Acetabular implants: 73.7	Mean postoperative HHS was 80.4 No femoral revisions Acetabular loosening rate was 47.4% at 15.5 yr
Iwase et al (1999)	30	Conversion to THA after valgus osteotomy (12 cemented femoral components, 18 noncemented femoral components)	57 (43-76)	7 (2-18)	83	Mean HHS improved from 54 to 86 3 noncemented stems failed 2 cemented acetabular cups failed
Suzuki et al (2007)	30 (27 patients)	Conversion to THA with noncemented femoral and acetabular components after valgus osteotomy	57 (37-70)	7 (5-20)	96.7	Mean HHS improved from 43 to 93 100% survivorship of femoral stems 1 acetabular revision for aseptic loosening
Parsch et al (2008)	48 (45 patients)	Conversion to THA with noncemented tapered femoral stem and noncemented or cemented acetabular implant after intertrochanteric osteotomy	50 (26-67)	16 (10-20)	Femoral stems: 90 Acetabular cups: 52	Median HHS was 76 at final follow-up Stem survivorship was 91% at 15- and 20-yr follow-up

HHS = Harris hip score, NR = not reported.

[a] Success is defined as THAs not requiring revision at latest follow up.

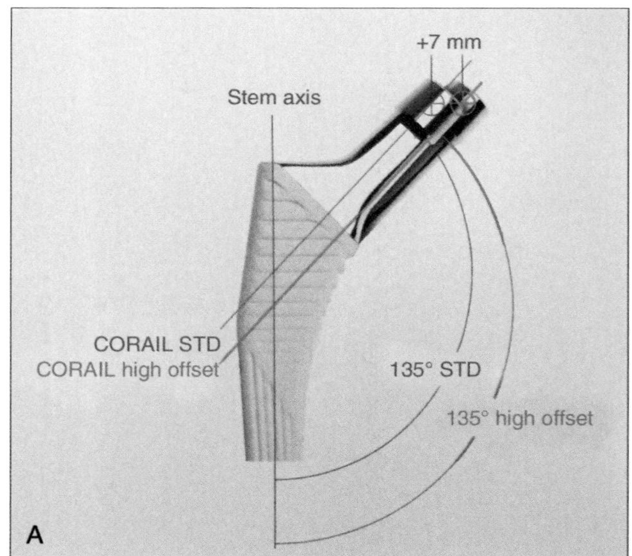

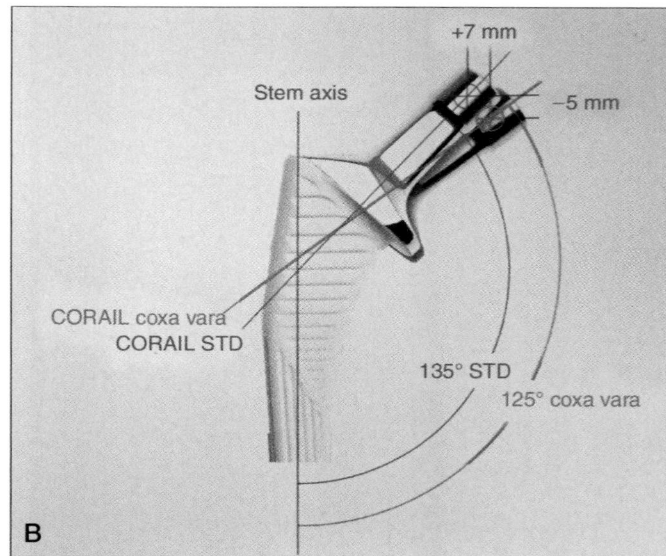

Figure 7 Photographs show an example of a femoral stem (CORAIL Hip System; DePuy Synthes) with three different offset options. **A,** Offset options for a standard stem (STD) compared with a high-offset stem. **B,** Offset options for a standard stem (STD) compared with a coxa vara stem.

surgical field. The surgical field should include the knee if the surgeon believes that a femoral osteotomy may be necessary.

- To achieve adequate femoral exposure in a patient with a stiff hip, several techniques may be useful, including removal of osteophytes, tendinous release of contracted muscles (piriformis, conjoined tendon, iliopsoas tendon, adductor tendons), release and later repair of the gluteus maximus insertion, wide capsulotomy, and in situ femoral neck osteotomy.
- Techniques used to achieve adequate acetabular exposure include a wide capsulotomy, release of the reflected head of the rectus femoris off the anterosuperior aspect of the acetabulum, a radial release in the inferior capsule, and the use of specialized acetabular retractors.

Instruments/Equipment/ Implants Required

- The S-ROM Modular Hip System offers intraoperative control of version and optimizes bony fixation. A modular implant is particularly helpful in the management of most metaphyseal deformities.
- Patients with a varus femoral neck deformity may require low femoral neck osteotomies and a femoral stem with high-offset or varus options (**Figure 7**).
- Severe metadiaphyseal deformities that cannot be managed with a standard distal stem can be managed with short, so-called microplasty femoral stems or femoral resurfacing implants.

Procedure

- If the use of a short proximal femoral stem or a femoral resurfacing arthroplasty is necessary because the patient has a more distal deformity, the surgical procedure remains the same as that with other implants. However, the surgeon must remain aware of the potential for an abnormal femoral neck and canal.
- If a modular stem is used and an osteotomy will be performed, proximal femoral preparation should be complete before the osteotomy is performed to allow for control of the proximal fragment. Proximal femoral preparation for a modular stem includes distal reaming and preparation of the proximal sleeve.
- The osteotomy site is identified based on bony landmarks that are observed on preoperative imaging.
- Rotational alignment is noted with the use of a Bovie electrocautery mark or by scoring the femur with a saw.
- After adequate exposure of the femur has been attained via elevation of the vastus lateralis and the periosteum, the osteotomy is performed with the use of an oscillating saw, drill holes, and an osteotome, or with a Gigli saw.
- The distal fragment is prepared with the use of straight reamers until solid cortical contact is attained. Overreaming the canal will result in loss of rotational control of the distal fragment. Underreaming the

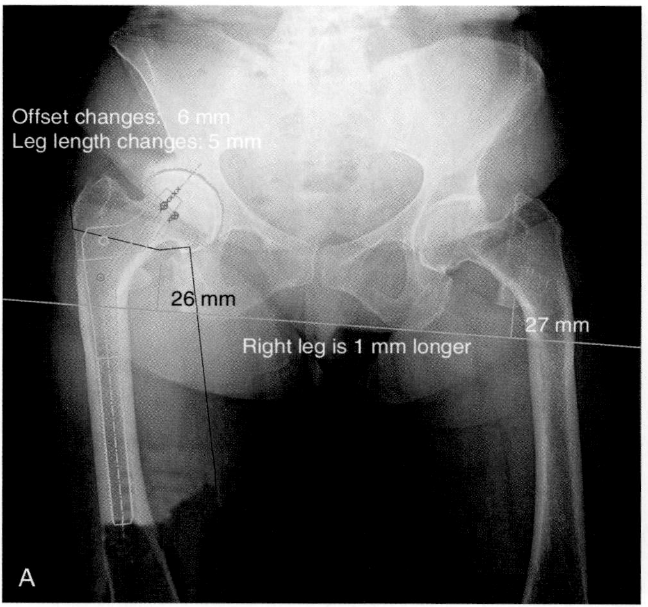

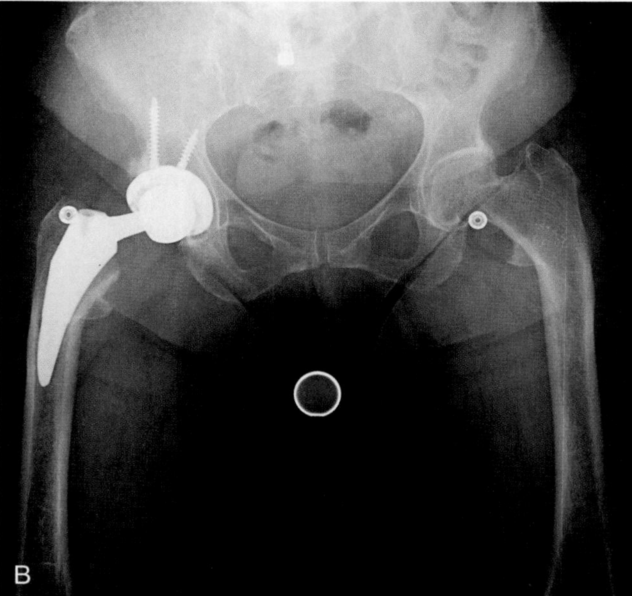

Figure 8 AP pelvic radiographs from a patient with diaphyseal deformity in whom femoral hemiresurfacing failed. **A,** Templated preoperative radiograph demonstrates the surgical plan for femoral osteotomy. **B,** Postoperative radiograph demonstrates a modular femoral stem and a diaphyseal osteotomy with cerclage wires.

canal will increase the risk for femoral shaft fracture.

- In patients who have poor bone quality, the use of prophylactic cerclage wires or cables in either the metaphyseal or diaphyseal segments may help avoid iatrogenic fracture.
- The stem is inserted through the proximal sleeve, across the osteotomy site, and into the distal shaft (**Figure 8**).

Wound Closure

- After thorough irrigation, anatomic repair of the posterior capsule and the external rotators is attempted.
- If the gluteus maximus tendon was divided, it is repaired anatomically.
- If possible, the vastus lateralis fascia and the iliotibial tract are reapproximated about the osteotomy site with the use of interrupted or running barbed absorbable suture.
- The wound is irrigated and closed in layers.

Postoperative Regimen

The postoperative regimen after THA in patients with femoral deformity is similar to that of patients who undergo routine primary THA. Weight bearing is determined based on a patient's bone quality and the quality of implant fixation obtained intraoperatively, particularly if an osteotomy was performed. Routine postoperative radiographs are obtained at 4 to 6 weeks postoperatively, at which time any weight-bearing restrictions are lifted.

Avoiding Pitfalls and Complications

Because of the importance of preoperative planning and templating, adequate radiographs are paramount in patients with femoral deformity who undergo THA. Radiographic imaging must be obtained with appropriate and symmetric patient positioning, recognition of magnification error, and correct placement of a standardized marker.

In a patient with femoral deformity, a femoral osteotomy may be required to gain access to the femoral canal for the placement of a straight stem. If possible, modular, custom-designed, or short femoral stems should be used to avoid the morbidity of femoral osteotomy, which includes limited weight bearing, increased blood loss, increased surgical time, altered biomechanics, and possible nonunion.

Awareness of trochanteric overhang is critical to avoid varus malpositioning of the implant, trochanteric fracture, and femoral canal perforation. Thorough exposure of the site of femoral osteotomy is necessary to avoid neurovascular injury or accidental damage to the perforator vessels. In a patient who has poor bone quality, the use of prophylactic cerclage cables or wires may help avoid propagation of a fracture.

Intraoperative orthogonal radiographs can be obtained to confirm stem size, avoid cortical perforation, and prevent varus malpositioning of the implant. Despite normal-appearing AP radiographs, lateral radiographs may reveal compromise of the anterior femoral cortex as a result of femoral bowing.

Bibliography

Aarabi M, Rauch F, Hamdy RC, Fassier F: Coxa vara in osteogenesis imperfecta. *Orthopaedic Proceedings* 2008;90(suppl I):81.

Berry DJ: Total hip arthroplasty in patients with proximal femoral deformity. *Clin Orthop Relat Res* 1999;369:262-272.

Boos N, Krushell R, Ganz R, Müller ME: Total hip arthroplasty after previous proximal femoral osteotomy. *J Bone Joint Surg Br* 1997;79(2):247-253.

Christie MJ, DeBoer DK, Trick LW, et al: Primary total hip arthroplasty with use of the modular S-ROM prosthesis: Four to seven-year clinical and radiographic results. *J Bone Joint Surg Am* 1999;81(12):1707-1716.

Della Valle AG, Padgett DE, Salvati EA: Preoperative planning for primary total hip arthroplasty. *J Am Acad Orthop Surg* 2005;13(7):455-462.

Dorr LD, Faugere MC, Mackel AM, Gruen TA, Bognar B, Malluche HH: Structural and cellular assessment of bone quality of proximal femur. *Bone* 1993;14(3):231-242.

Ferguson GM, Cabanela ME, Ilstrup DM: Total hip arthroplasty after failed intertrochanteric osteotomy. *J Bone Joint Surg Br* 1994;76(2):252-257.

Holtgrewe JL, Hungerford DS: Primary and revision total hip replacement without cement and with associated femoral osteotomy. *J Bone Joint Surg Am* 1989;71(10):1487-1495.

Iwase T, Hasegawa Y, Iwasada S, Kitamura S, Iwata H: Total hip arthroplasty after failed intertrochanteric valgus osteotomy for advanced osteoarthrosis. *Clin Orthop Relat Res* 1999;(364):175-181.

Mattingly DA: The S-ROM modular stem for femoral deformities. *Orthopedics* 2005;28(9 suppl):s1059-s1062.

Mehlhoff MA, Sledge CB: Comparison of cemented and cementless hip and knee replacements. *Arthritis Rheum* 1990;33(2):293-297.

Mont MA, Ragland PS, Etienne G, Seyler TM, Schmalzried TP: Hip resurfacing arthroplasty. *J Am Acad Orthop Surg* 2006;14(8):454-463.

Papagelopoulos PJ, Trousdale RT, Lewallen DG: Total hip arthroplasty with femoral osteotomy for proximal femoral deformity. *Clin Orthop Relat Res* 1996;(332):151-162.

Parsch D, Jung AW, Thomsen M, Ewerbeck V, Aldinger PR: Good survival of uncemented tapered stems for failed intertrochanteric osteotomy: A mean 16 year follow-up study in 45 patients. *Arch Orthop Trauma Surg* 2008;128(10):1081-1085.

Shinar AA, Harris WH: Cemented total hip arthroplasty following previous femoral osteotomy: An average 16-year follow-up study. *J Arthroplasty* 1998;13(3):243-253.

Søballe K, Boll KL, Kofod S, Severinsen B, Kristensen SS: Total hip replacement after medial-displacement osteotomy of the proximal part of the femur. *J Bone Joint Surg Am* 1989;71(5):692-697.

Suzuki K, Kawachi S, Matsubara M, Morita S, Jinno T, Shinomiya K: Cementless total hip replacement after previous intertrochanteric valgus osteotomy for advanced osteoarthritis. *J Bone Joint Surg Br* 2007;89(9):1155-1157.

Weinstein JN, Kuo KN, Millar EA: Congenital coxa vara: A retrospective review. *J Pediatr Orthop* 1984;4(1):70-77.

Chapter 26
Total Hip Arthroplasty in Patients With Failed Hip Fracture Fixation

Daniel A. Oakes, MD
Michael D. Stefl, MD

Indications

In the past decade, primary total hip arthroplasty (THA) has been increasingly used in the management of displaced subcapital femoral head fractures, femoral neck fractures, and some high intertrochanteric fractures. This approach has been validated in several studies and may be based in part on the high risk of complications, specifically higher dislocation rates, seen in previous studies of the conversion of failed fracture fixation to THA. The conversion of failed hip fracture fixation to THA remains a challenging endeavor (**Table 1**).

Presentation of failed hip fracture fixation can vary. Patients with united fractures can have posttraumatic degenerative disease with or without osteonecrosis. The fracture may have resulted in nonunion or malunion. The hardware may be loose or well-fixed and may consist of a plate-and-screw construct or an intramedullary device. Most patients have clear abnormality of the hip mechanics (hip center of rotation, femoral offset, leg length, and/or position or integrity of the greater trochanter). The goal of conversion to THA is to provide a pain-free hip with restoration of hip mechanics to as near normal as possible. When possible, records of the prior implant or reports of the previous surgical procedure are consulted to help plan for the extraction of the existing hardware.

Contraindications

Although the clinical outcomes and survivorship of THA have continued to improve, the surgeon should always strive to preserve or salvage a viable hip joint whenever possible, particularly in young patients (45 years or younger). In patients with a well-preserved joint space and a viable femoral head devoid of osteonecrosis, a joint-preserving salvage osteotomy should be performed if possible.

If the native femoral head is deemed unsalvageable, the most important contraindication to conversion of failed fracture fixation to THA is the presence of active infection. The workup for infection is identical to that performed in patients in whom infected THA is suspected. If an infection is identified, the conversion procedure should be done in a two-stage manner with either a temporary resection arthroplasty or placement of an antibiotic spacer (either articulating or nonarticulating).

Because conversion procedures are associated with increased surgical times and blood loss, comprehensive medical optimization is a critical part of the preoperative workup.

Alternative Treatments

Revision Open Reduction and Internal Fixation

Revision open reduction and internal fixation should be considered in patients 45 years or younger who have a viable femoral head, preserved articular joint space, and reasonable bone stock. Revision fixation is not repeat fixation. The revision fixation may require corrective intertrochanteric osteotomy to convert shear forces that may have contributed to the failure of the initial construct into compressive forces. Successful revision fixation typically requires restoration of normal hip mechanics, which must be considered as part of the preoperative planning process.

Revision fixation will usually require a fixed-angle device such as a blade plate, dynamic hip screw, dynamic compression screw, or intramedullary device. Bone grafting may be required.

Dr. Oakes or an immediate family member serves as a paid consultant to Zimmer Biomet and serves as a board member, owner, officer, or committee member of the American Association of Hip and Knee Surgeons. Neither Dr. Stefl nor any immediate family member has received anything of value from or has stock or stock options held in a commercial company or institution related directly or indirectly to the subject of this chapter.

Table 1 Results of Surgical Management of Failed Hip Fracture Fixation

Authors (Year)	Number of Patients	Procedure	Mean Patient Age in Years (Range)	Mean Follow-up in Years (Range)	Success Rate (%)	Results
Gebhard et al (1992)	166	Hemiarthroplasty (122) or THA (44)	Hemiarthroplasty group: 76.2 (NR) THA group: 75.2 (NR)	Hemiarthroplasty group: 4.8 (NR) THA group: 4.5 (NR)	THA: 97.8[a] Cemented hemiarthroplasty: 92.1[a] Noncemented hemiarthroplasty: 87[a]	Dislocation rates were 2.3% for THA and 4.9% for hemiarthroplasty
Haidukewych and Berry (2003)	60	Failed fixation of intertrochanteric fractures converted with bipolar or unipolar hemiarthroplasty	58 (21-86)	2.3 (0.3-10)	10-yr survivorship: 87.5	5 revisions 1 dislocation
Mabry et al (2004)	84	Proximal femoral (hip) fractures converted to Charnley THA	68 (36-92)	1.0 (0.2-2.4)	10-yr survivorship: 93 20-yr survivorship: 76	9 dislocations
Winemaker et al (2006)	36	Failed fixation of femoral neck or intertrochanteric fractures converted to THA	71 (SD, 12.5)	NR	94.4[a]	5 fractures, 1 infection, and no dislocations 1 yr postoperatively
Watson et al (2008)	37	THA to manage displaced femoral neck fractures	80 (50-98)	NR	83.9[b]	5 dislocations 1 nonfatal myocardial infarction
Hopley et al (2010)	1,890	THA or hemiarthroplasty to manage displaced intracapsular hip fractures	NR	NR	NR	Lower revision rate after THA compared with hemiarthroplasty
Rutz et al (2010)	53	THA to manage acute fracture of the proximal femur	Men: 75.1 (61-90) Women: 78.2 (61-91)	4.6 (NR)	98.1[a]	3 dislocations 1 revision for hematoma 1 revision for aseptic loosening of the femoral stem
Carroll et al (2011)	972	THA or hemiarthroplasty to manage primary intracapsular hip fractures	NR	NR	NR	Meta-analysis demonstrated a significant increase in the risk of dislocation ($P = 0.01$) but a significant reduction in the risk of revision ($P = 0.0003$) in patients treated with THA compared with patients treated with hemiarthroplasty

NR = not reported, SD = standard deviation, THA = total hip arthroplasty.

[a] Success rate based on the percentage of patients in whom revision was not performed.

[b] Success rate based on the percentage of patients who did not have complications.

Table 1 Results of Surgical Management of Failed Hip Fracture Fixation (*continued*)

Authors (Year)	Number of Patients	Procedure	Mean Patient Age in Years (Range)	Mean Follow-up in Years (Range)	Success Rate (%)	Results
Burgers et al (2012)	986	Hemiarthroplasty or THA to manage displaced femoral neck fractures in healthy elderly patients	NR	NR	THA: 96[a] Hemiarthroplasty: 93[a]	Pooled data showed a trend toward a lower incidence of revision surgery in patients who underwent THA compared with patients who underwent hemiarthroplasty
Yu et al (2012)	1,320	THA or hemiarthroplasty to manage displaced femoral neck fractures	NR	NR	THA: 95.4[a] Hemiarthroplasty: 91.4[a]	Higher rate of dislocation in patients who underwent THA compared with patients who underwent hemiarthroplasty (7.6% and 3.5%, respectively)
Zi-Sheng et al (2012)	1,208	Hemiarthroplasty or primary THA to manage displaced femoral neck fractures in elderly patients	NR (69-81)	NR (1-13)	NR	Dislocation rate of 4.5% in the hemiarthroplasty group and 17.2% in the THA group
Archibeck et al (2013)	102	Failed fixation of femoral neck fractures (63) or failed fixation of intertrochanteric fractures (39) converted to THA	70 (30-96)	3.2 (2-18)	93.2[a]	10 complications, 4 fractures, 5 dislocations, and 7 revisions at 2-yr follow-up 33 hips required a revision-type femoral stem
DeHaan et al (2013)	46	Failed fixation of femoral neck fractures with cannulated screws (18), failed fixation of intertrochanteric fractures (16), or failed fixation of intertrochanteric fractures with intramedullary hip screws (12) converted to THA	64 (22-91)	0.7 (NR)	87[a]	4 intraoperative fractures 2 dislocations 6 revisions
Pui et al (2013)	91	Failed fixation of intertrochanteric fractures with sliding hip screws (60) or with intramedullary hip screws (31) converted to THA	Sliding hip screw group: 64.8 (23-86) Intramedullary hip screw group: 65.1 (24-90)	Sliding hip screw group: 3.1 (NR) Intramedullary hip screw group: 2.9 (NR)	Sliding hip screw group: 88.3[b] Intramedullary hip screw group: 58.1[b]	8 complications in the sliding hip screw group 15 complications in the intramedullary hip screw group

NR = not reported, SD = standard deviation, THA = total hip arthroplasty.

[a] Success rate based on the percentage of patients in whom revision was not performed.

[b] Success rate based on the percentage of patients who did not have complications.

Vascularized transfer of the quadratus femoris and vascularized fibular grafts have been described in the management of nonunion of the femoral neck.

Although these surgical procedures can salvage a viable femoral head, they require a prolonged recovery period and carry the risk of osteonecrosis.

Hemiarthroplasty

Historically, hip fractures not amenable to fracture fixation were managed with hemiarthroplasty. An emerging body of evidence has shown that these patients may be better treated with THA.

A patient in whom hip fracture fixation has failed will often have nonunion of the femoral neck or osteonecrosis. In these patients, the articular joint space may appear well preserved. However, the articular surface is unlikely to have been loaded normally and is unlikely to have normal cartilage function.

Long-term results of hemiarthroplasty in young or active patients demonstrate a high incidence of groin pain and a high rate of future conversion to THA. Although hemiarthroplasty may have a lower rate of dislocation than THA has, the increased use of larger-diameter femoral heads seems to have narrowed the difference in dislocation rates between hemiarthroplasty and THA. In addition, most hemiarthroplasty devices use non–cross-linked polyethylene in the device, whereas most THA implants have a highly cross-linked bearing surface.

Although the use of hemiarthroplasty in the conversion of failed hip fracture fixation has decreased, hemiarthroplasty may still be used to treat medically infirm patients, patients with extraordinarily low demands, or patients who cannot reasonably be expected to follow basic precautions against dislocation.

Resection Arthroplasty (Girdlestone)

Girdlestone resection arthroplasty is usually the treatment of last resort because it typically has a poor functional outcome. It may be the best treatment option for patients with recalcitrant infection. In medically infirm patients, it may be the most expedient procedure. The surgeon should evaluate all other treatment options before performing resection arthroplasty.

Results

Most studies demonstrate higher complication rates for conversion of failed proximal femoral fixation to THA than for routine primary arthroplasty (**Table 1**). This finding is consistent for cemented and noncemented reconstruction techniques. The conversion procedure is least complicated when revising failed femoral neck fractures that were previously managed with cannulated screw fixation, because this procedure is most similar to routine primary arthroplasty. Conversion of failed intertrochanteric fractures managed with sliding hip screws or intramedullary hip screws is a more complicated procedure that often requires the use of revision femoral implants. Several studies have indicated that conversion of failed intramedullary hip screw fixation to THA may be the most difficult conversion procedure. Common complications include intraoperative fractures and dislocations.

Techniques

Setup/Exposure

- Conversion of a failed hip fracture to THA is most commonly performed with the patient placed in the lateral decubitus position.
- The patient is held in position with any of a variety of positioning devices.
- The most common surgical approaches used in the conversion of failed hip fracture fixation to THA are the posterolateral approach and the anterolateral approach.
- The posterolateral approach offers the most extensile options.
- The anterolateral approach preserves the posterior structures and can potentially reduce the rate of postoperative dislocation; however, this strategy is best used by surgeons for whom this approach is their standard hip arthroplasty approach.
- Although the supine anterior approach has gained popularity for routine primary THA procedures, it is not recommended for a conversion procedure because it lacks the extensile options of the posterolateral and anterolateral approaches.
- When possible, old incisions are used for improved cosmesis.
- The surgical incision will be longer than the standard primary THA incision because the most distal part of the incision must extend past the most distal hardware.
- For the management of failed femoral neck fractures and posttraumatic osteonecrosis, the authors of this chapter prefer a posterolateral approach, which is their standard hip arthroplasty approach. As in primary THA procedures, the posterior sleeve should be released, tagged, and repaired to reduce the risk of postoperative dislocation with this approach. The approach follows the standard primary arthroplasty dissection down to the hip capsule. The hip is dislocated with the hardware in place.
- Dislocating the hip with the hardware in place is important because hip dislocation may be slightly more difficult than it would be in a primary THA procedure. Removing the hardware before the dislocation maneuver is performed can result in a fracture through bone defects created by the previously placed hardware.
- After the hip is dislocated and the

hip capsule is released off the femoral neck, the hip is relocated and the retained hardware is located. This step usually will require elevating the vastus lateralis from the lateral femur at the vastus ridge.

- All hardware must be identified before removal begins.
- If the failed fixation is a series of cannulated screws, the screws are removed with the appropriate screwdriver. If the most distal screw is below the level of the lesser trochanter and the patient's bone is osteoporotic, a prophylactic cerclage wire or cable may be used. If the hip is stiff, release of the gluteus maximus insertion into the femur can facilitate mobilization of the femur.
- If the failed fixation is a sliding hip screw and plate, the plate is removed first and the hip screw second. The surgeon should consider placing a prophylactic cerclage wire or cable over each screw hole or at least over the most distal screw hole. The authors of this chapter prefer to place the crimps of the cerclage cable overlying the screw holes so that the cable will also act as a plug against cement extrusion if a cemented device is used.
- In some patients, partial removal of hardware proximally is a reasonable option but will require cutting the plate with a high-speed burr.
- If the failed fixation is an intramedullary nail, fluoroscopy can help locate the tip of the nail if it is not easily identified. This method can help avoid additional damage to the trochanter and abductors. Fluoroscopy can assist with placement of a guidewire into the tip of the nail for localization of the nail and placement of the appropriate insertion or extraction device.
- In patients with failed intertrochanteric fractures managed with either plate or intramedullary nail fixation, flexibility regarding the best approach to the hip joint is necessary. In these patients, it is important to assess the integrity of the trochanter and the abductors during the approach. In a patient with trochanteric nonunion, it is often advantageous to mobilize this fragment as if it were a conventional trochanteric osteotomy.
- In a patient with trochanteric malunion, a conventional trochanteric osteotomy should be considered because it will enhance the exposure and allow more anatomic repositioning of the trochanter after the final THA prosthesis has been implanted.
- When mobilizing the trochanter, the surgeon has three options. The vastus slide involves preserving the attachment of the vastus lateralis to the trochanter and facilitates anterior or posterior mobilization of the trochanter. If the vastus is detached, the exposure will allow either posterior release of the short external rotators or preservation of the rotators with release of the anterior third of the abductors. Either of these maneuvers will allow superior reflection of the trochanter and dissection in the plane beneath the musculature and above the capsule. The senior author of this chapter (D.A.O.) prefers to dissect this plane with electrocautery (**Figure 1**).
- After the hip has been dislocated and the hardware has been removed, the femoral neck osteotomy

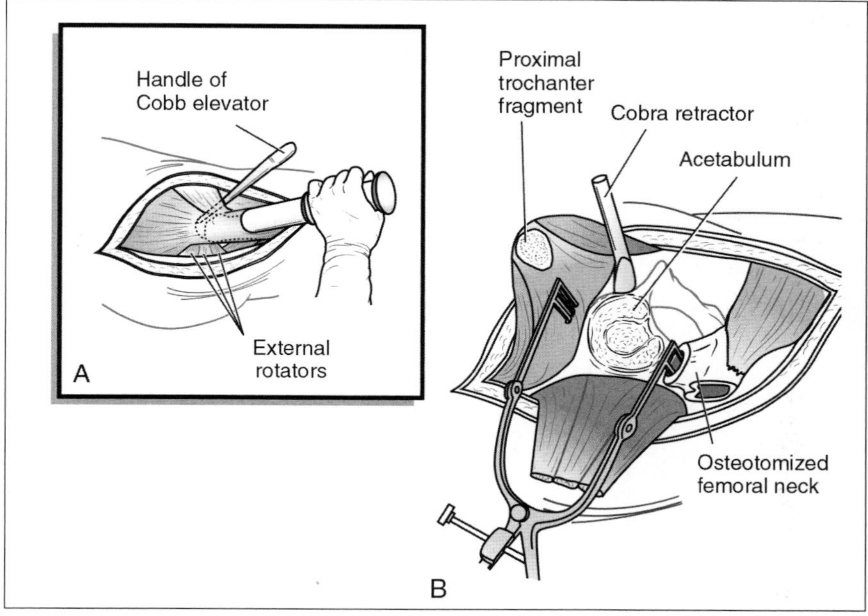

Figure 1 Illustrations depict the conventional trochanteric osteotomy technique for surgical exposure in total hip arthroplasty after failed hip fracture fixation. **A,** A Cobb elevator is placed deep to the entire gluteus musculature and superficial to the hip capsule to orient the direction of a dome-shaped osteotome. The vastus lateralis is elevated distally before the trochanteric cut is made at the level of its attachment. **B,** A self-retaining retractor is placed between the femur and the gluteus muscle. Ideally, a Charnley (or modified Charnley) self-retaining retractor should be used. The gluteus retraction can be aided by fastening a wet laparotomy sponge proximal and distal to the muscle (under the self-retaining retractor). (Reproduced from Kelley SS: Total hip arthroplasty after failed hip fracture fixation, in Lieberman JR, Berry DJ, eds: *Advanced Reconstruction: Hip.* Rosemont, IL, American Academy of Orthopaedic Surgeons, 2005, pp 167-174.)

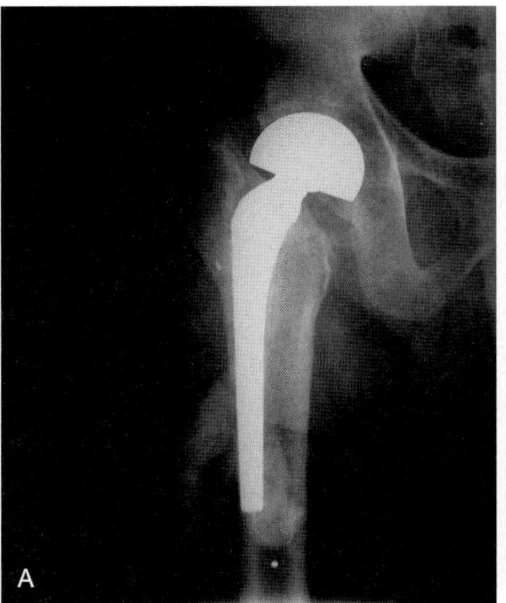

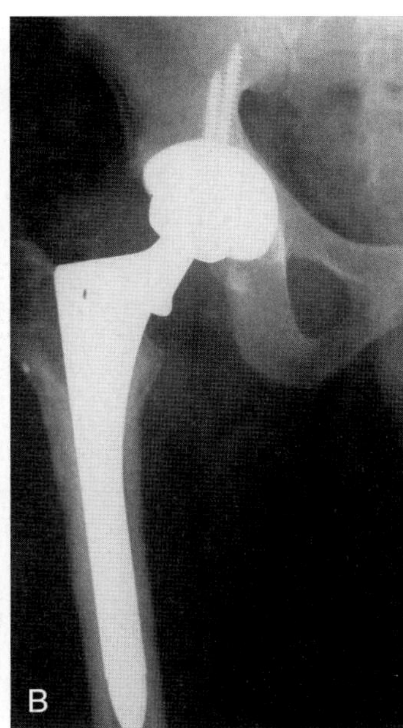

Figure 2 AP radiographs of a right hip demonstrate a pitfall of converting prior hip fracture fixation to arthroplasty. The patient was originally treated with a dynamic hip screw, which subsequently failed. He underwent conversion to cemented hemiarthroplasty (**A**). The surgeon incorrectly identified the intramedullary canal and instead cemented the stem in an extramedullary position. This misplacement required conversion to total hip arthroplasty with a fully porous-coated stem (**B**).

is performed. The most reliable landmark is the lesser trochanter. The level of the osteotomy is based on preoperative templating. It may be helpful to use the contralateral hip as a reference.

Instruments/Equipment/Implants Required

- Some devices have specific extraction instrumentation that can facilitate hardware removal.
- If the implant record is not available, an array of instruments, including a universal extraction system, a slap hammer with vise grip, and a metal-cutting burr system, should be available for use in the extraction of hardware.

Procedure

ACETABULAR RECONSTRUCTION

- The acetabular reconstruction is performed in a standard manner.
- In most hips, adequate exposure can be achieved with a posterior paddle retractor, an anterior C-shaped or snake retractor placed on the anterior column, and a superior retractor or self-retaining retractor. Alternatively, pins may be used. A consistent exposure can be obtained with the help of a single skilled assistant.
- The labrum is removed with a long-handled knife or electrocautery.
- The pulvinar is removed with electrocautery.
- Circumferential exposure of the acetabular rim is necessary.
- The transverse acetabular ligament should be preserved if possible because it is a useful landmark for determining proper cup position.
- The acetabulum is reamed and prepared for a noncemented or cemented acetabular implant. In North America, noncemented fixation is more common than cemented fixation.
- Because the acetabular bone is often osteoporotic from disuse, care must be taken while reaming.
- The authors of this chapter favor the placement of at least two acetabular screws through the cup.

FEMORAL RECONSTRUCTION

- The femoral reconstruction begins with assessment of the femur, which includes determining the extent of bone loss resulting from the failed fixation and removal of the hardware, whether a primary implant can be used, whether proximal or diaphyseal fixation will be used, whether a standard-length implant can be used or a longer revision implant will be needed, and whether a calcar replacement implant will be necessary. Ideally, these questions will have been answered in the preoperative planning process. The purpose of the intraoperative assessment is to confirm that the appropriate equipment is present in the operating room.
- The first step is to reestablish and define the femoral canal. The failed implant may have created lateral pathways out of the canal or sclerotic margins that can prevent in-line preparation of the canal (**Figure 2**). A high-speed burr and a canal-finding awl are helpful in this process. Radiography or fluoroscopy can also be helpful for localization.
- After the canal is opened, a flexible guide rod is placed in the canal, and flexible reamers are used to ensure in-line preparation of the canal.
- In the conversion of failed open reduction and internal fixation of a fracture of the femoral head or neck, femoral preparation is routine. Almost any cemented or noncemented femoral stem design can be used (**Figure 3**). If a femoral screw track is present laterally

below the lesser trochanter, a prophylactic cerclage cable or wire can be placed at the level of the screw hole to reduce the risk of fracture during broaching or stem insertion.

- In the conversion of a failed intramedullary device or lateral plate, the surgeon should use a stem that can achieve bypass fixation below the most distal cortical defect if possible (**Figure 4**). Bypassing the defect by two cortical diameters is an effective strategy. To achieve distal fixation, it is often necessary to use a revision-type stem with either a fully porous-coated or a splined tapered design. Placement of a prophylactic cerclage wire at or just distal to the most distal cortical defect is recommended.
- If the prior hardware is well overgrown with bone and/or is long, selective hardware removal can be performed. A high-speed burr with a metal-cutting tip is essential for this approach. Care is taken to limit the spread of metal debris in the wound. After selective hardware removal, a standard or short noncemented or cemented stem can be used (**Figure 5**).
- Calcar replacement devices are often helpful for managing proximal medial defects in patients with failed fixation of intertrochanteric fractures. The use of a calcar replacement proximal stem body is less crucial when distal noncemented fixation is used than when cemented fixation is used.
- The authors of this chapter prefer to reconstruct the femur with noncemented fixation. The technique for cemented fixation is more demanding because it is difficult to achieve cement pressurization and prevent cement extrusion. A technique for making custom molds with a surgical glove and bone cement to reduce the risk of cement extrusion

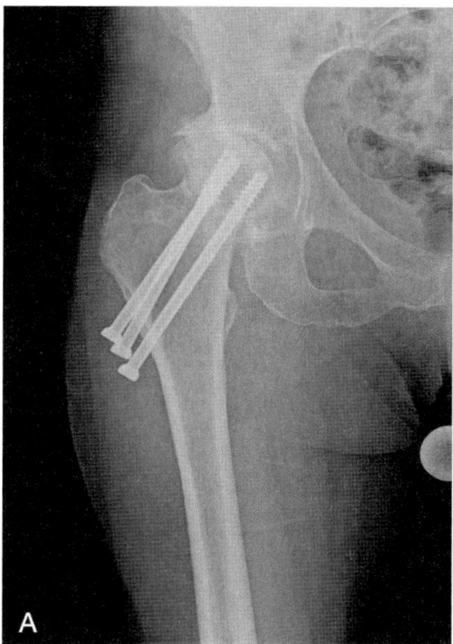

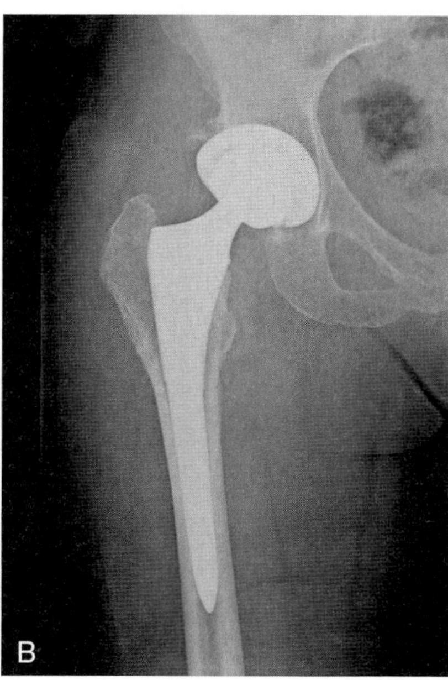

Figure 3 AP radiographs of a right hip demonstrate conversion of failed open reduction and internal fixation of a fracture of the femoral neck (**A**) to total hip arthroplasty (**B**). Because the removal of hardware did not result in a substantial bone defect, the conversion could be performed with a noncemented primary total hip arthroplasty implant.

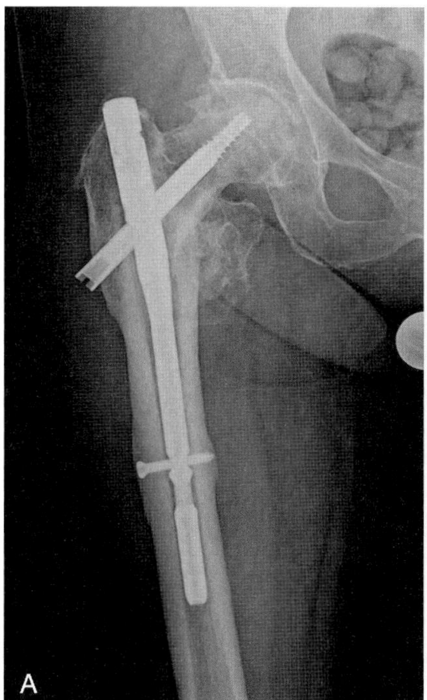

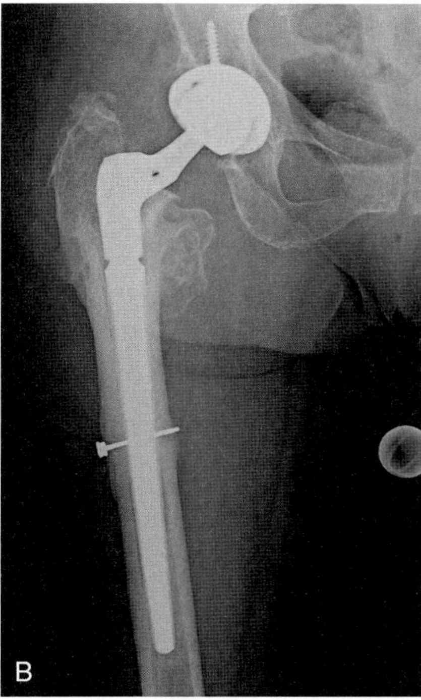

Figure 4 AP radiographs of a right hip demonstrate conversion of intramedullary hip screw fixation (**A**) to total hip arthroplasty (**B**) in a patient with osteonecrosis of the femoral head after fracture fixation. **B,** A noncemented splined tapered modular revision stem was used to restore the hip center, femoral length, and femoral offset. A prophylactic cerclage wire was placed over the screw hole at the site of the distal interlock. The stem bypasses the screw hole by two cortical diameters.

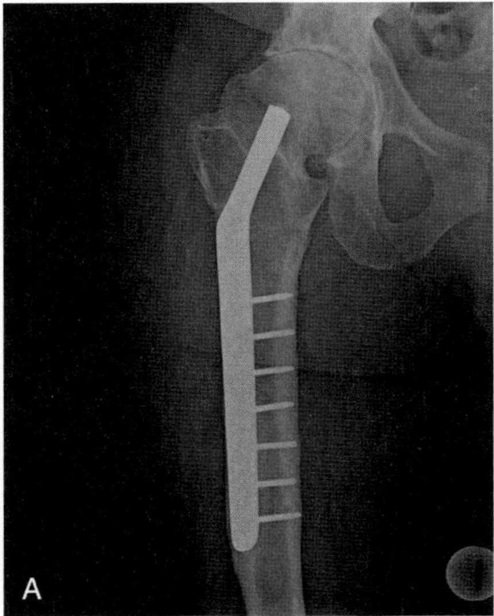

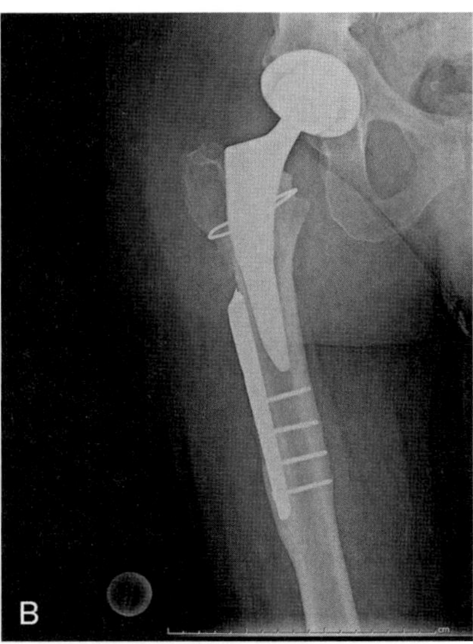

Figure 5 AP radiographs of a right hip demonstrate conversion of prior blade plate fixation (**A**) to total hip arthroplasty (**B**). **A,** The plate was in place for more than 20 years, and posttraumatic degenerative joint disease developed. Because the plate was encased in bone and was long, removal of the plate would have required substantial bone destruction and the use of a long revision-type stem. **B,** By cutting the plate and performing selective hardware removal, the surgeon was able to use a shorter, primary noncemented stem. A prophylactic cerclage wire was placed over the lateral cortical defect from the blade of the plate.

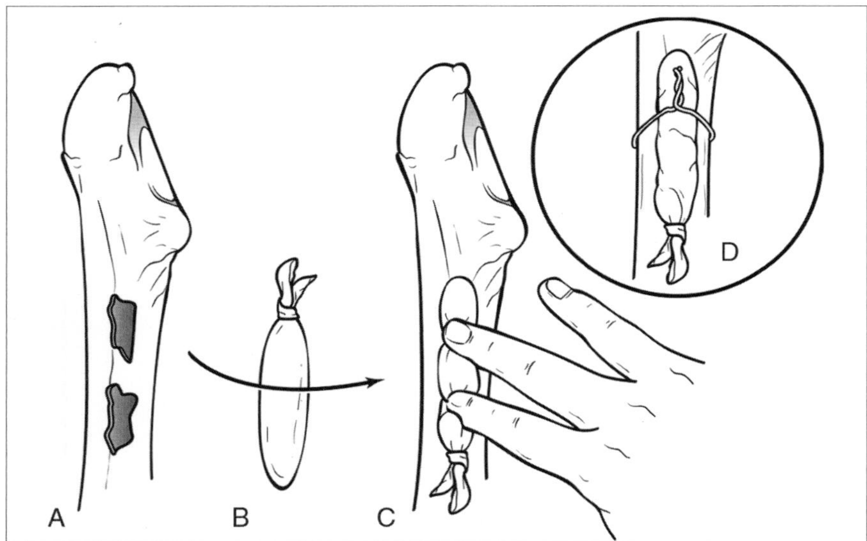

Figure 6 Illustrations depict a cement plugging technique. **A,** The appearance of the femoral bone defects. **B,** The cement plug is created by injecting polymethyl methacrylate cement into the finger of a surgical glove, which is then tied off as a balloon would be. **C,** The doughlike, latex-encased polymethyl methacrylate cement is pressed firmly into the defects and held until it polymerizes, leaving a custom mold of the bone defects. **D,** The mold can be wired in place temporarily with a single cerclage wire or held in place by the surgeon during the next steps of the procedure. (Reproduced from Kelley SS: Total hip arthroplasty after failed hip fracture fixation, in Lieberman JR, Berry DJ, eds: *Advanced Reconstruction: Hip*. Rosemont, IL, American Academy of Orthopaedic Surgeons, 2005, pp 167-174.)

from prior screw holes has been described (**Figure 6**).

Wound Closure

- After final implantation of the prosthesis, the wound is thoroughly irrigated with pulsatile lavage containing an antibiotic.
- Remaining bone defects from the prior hardware can be grafted with bone reamings from the acetabulum or the resected femoral head.
- Trochanteric osteotomies can be reconstructed with a classic cerclage wire technique, a trochanteric claw with cables, or a claw plate with cables. All are excellent options. The greater the proximal medial bone loss, the better it is to use longer fixation with a claw plate with cables.
- The use of drains is controversial. The authors of this chapter favor the use of a deep drain because the creation of the surgical field for this procedure requires extensive dissection, which may result in bleeding in the early postoperative period.

Postoperative Regimen

Weight bearing is determined based on subjective assessment of the quality of the bone and the presence or absence of trochanteric fixation. Patients who have undergone conversion of failed fixation of femoral head and neck fractures are typically allowed to progress weight bearing as tolerated without restrictions in a manner identical to that of patients who have undergone routine primary THA. Patients with subjectively determined osteoporosis and trochanteric fixation are placed on toe-touch weight bearing for 4 to 6 weeks. A hip abduction brace is used in any patient with abductor damage or trochanteric fixation.

Avoiding Pitfalls and Complications

The first step in avoiding complications in this patient population is to acknowledge the difficulty of these procedures. Prior surgical procedures have been performed and failed. These patients are less mobile than the typical THA patient and are more likely to be infirm. It is critical to achieve adequate medical optimization of the patient for the planned surgical procedure.

Preoperative planning, intraoperative organization, intraoperative patience, and adherence to a thoughtful surgical plan are necessary for success. If the complex THA procedure is not commonly performed by the surgeon and the team, a preoperative conference among the team members or a written surgical plan posted in the operating room may be helpful.

The surgical procedure must restore the hip center, leg length, and offset. Because these patients are prone to instability, the use of a larger-diameter femoral head and the restoration of hip mechanics often help achieve a successful outcome.

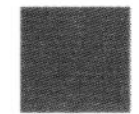

Bibliography

Archibeck MJ, Carothers JT, Tripuraneni KR, White RE Jr: Total hip arthroplasty after failed internal fixation of proximal femoral fractures. *J Arthroplasty* 2013;28(1):168-171.

Burgers PT, Van Geene AR, Van den Bekerom MP, et al: Total hip arthroplasty versus hemiarthroplasty for displaced femoral neck fractures in the healthy elderly: A meta-analysis and systematic review of randomized trials. *Int Orthop* 2012;36(8):1549-1560.

Carroll C, Stevenson M, Scope A, Evans P, Buckley S: Hemiarthroplasty and total hip arthroplasty for treating primary intracapsular fracture of the hip: A systematic review and cost-effectiveness analysis. *Health Technol Assess* 2011;15(36):1-74.

DeHaan AM, Groat T, Priddy M, et al: Salvage hip arthroplasty after failed fixation of proximal femur fractures. *J Arthroplasty* 2013;28(5):855-859.

Gebhard JS, Amstutz HC, Zinar DM, Dorey FJ: A comparison of total hip arthroplasty and hemiarthroplasty for treatment of acute fracture of the femoral neck. *Clin Orthop Relat Res* 1992;(282):123-131.

Haidukewych GJ, Berry DJ: Hip arthroplasty for salvage of failed treatment of intertrochanteric hip fractures. *J Bone Joint Surg Am* 2003;85(5):899-904.

Hopley C, Stengel D, Ekkernkamp A, Wich M: Primary total hip arthroplasty versus hemiarthroplasty for displaced intracapsular hip fractures in older patients: Systematic review. *BMJ* 2010;340:c2332.

Mabry TM, Prpa B, Haidukewych GJ, Harmsen WS, Berry DJ: Long-term results of total hip arthroplasty for femoral neck fracture nonunion. *J Bone Joint Surg Am* 2004;86(10):2263-2267.

Pui CM, Bostrom MP, Westrich GH, et al: Increased complication rate following conversion total hip arthroplasty after cephalomedullary fixation for intertrochanteric hip fractures: A multi-center study. *J Arthroplasty* 2013;28(8 suppl):45-47.

Rutz E, Leumann A, Rutz D, Schäfer D, Valderrabano V: Total hip arthroplasty for fractures of the proximal femur in older patients. *Hip Int* 2010;20(2):215-220.

Slater RR, Morrison J, Kelley SS: Custom-made molds that prevent cement extrusion through bone defects. *Clin Orthop Relat Res* 1995;(317):126-130.

Watson D, Bostrom M, Salvati E, Walcott-Sapp S, Westrich G: Primary total hip arthroplasty for displaced femoral neck fracture. *Orthopedics* 2008;31(10):31.

Winemaker M, Gamble P, Petruccelli D, Kaspar S, de Beer J: Short-term outcomes of total hip arthroplasty after complications of open reduction internal fixation for hip fracture. *J Arthroplasty* 2006;21(5):682-688.

Yu L, Wang Y, Chen J: Total hip arthroplasty versus hemiarthroplasty for displaced femoral neck fractures: Meta-analysis of randomized trials. *Clin Orthop Relat Res* 2012;470(8):2235-2243.

Zi-Sheng A, You-Shui G, Zhi-Zhen J, Ting Y, Chang-Qing Z: Hemiarthroplasty vs primary total hip arthroplasty for displaced fractures of the femoral neck in the elderly: A meta-analysis. *J Arthroplasty* 2012;27(4):583-590.

Chapter 27

Total Hip Arthroplasty for Management of Osteonecrosis of the Femoral Head

Bernard N. Stulberg, MD

Indications

Osteonecrosis of the femoral head with accompanying femoral head collapse can result from a variety of etiologies. The resulting structural compromise can be a source of substantial pain and functional limitation for the patient. Etiologies that lead to collapse in young patients (younger than 50 years) include ongoing disease states and their treatment, such as systemic lupus erythematosus, hemophilia, and sickle cell disease, which have low likelihood of stabilization or reversibility, as well as potentially modifiable factors such as alcohol abuse or episodic steroid treatment. Osteonecrosis and collapse of the femoral head in young patients is frequently mediated through venous or bone marrow abnormalities. In these patients, total hip arthroplasty (THA) is appropriate in patients either with femoral head collapse or with late precollapse disease with substantial involvement of the femoral head (greater than 30%; University of Pennsylvania [that is, Steinberg] stage IIC), for whom joint-preserving treatment options will be less predictable. In older patients (50 years or older), osteonecrosis is more commonly mediated by arterial abnormalities. In this patient population, THA is the treatment of choice, even in patients with University of Pennsylvania stage IIC disease (precollapse but with quantitatively defined head involvement), when nonsurgical interventions have been unsuccessful in alleviating pain or improving function.

The most common classification systems used to characterize and quantify the location and extent of osteonecrosis of the femoral head are Ficat and Arlet, University of Pennsylvania, and ARCO (Association Research Circulation Osseous), all of which are helpful in both educating the patient and determining treatment options. Proper staging requires the use of plain radiographs and MRI. All three systems classify precollapse of the subchondral plate as stage II. Stage II disease should be confirmed by CT because variability in MRI acquisition and reading can hinder accurate determination of collapse. In addition, the author of this chapter is of the opinion that after collapse of the subchondral plate has been confirmed (Ficat and Arlet stage III, University of Pennsylvania stage IV, ARCO stage IV), THA is indicated because no predictable alternative approach is available to stabilize or reverse even minimal compromise of the subchondral plate.

In patients with documented collapse or partial collapse of the femoral head, the decision to perform THA is based on the surgeon's judgment that the articular surface has been damaged to the extent that adequate repair to provide long-term function of the hip is not possible. In patients with late-stage osteonecrosis, the need for THA is clear. In patients with Ficat and Arlet late stage II and early stage III osteonecrosis, the decision to perform THA can be controversial. Thorough discussion of the concerns in a shared decision-making process is particularly important when arthroplasty is being considered in patients younger than 50 years (**Table 1**).

Contraindications

The only absolute contraindication to THA in a patient with osteonecrosis is the presence of active infection in or about the hip. Relative contraindications occur when the patient's physical or mental state, or local conditions around the hip joint, would increase the risk of failure of the arthroplasty. In patients aged 50 years and older, relative contraindications include health status that would make the patient an unsuitable candidate for a major surgical

Dr. Stulberg or an immediate family member has received royalties from and serves as a paid consultant to Exactech, is a member of a speakers' bureau or has made paid presentations on behalf of Medtronic and Pacira Pharmaceuticals, and has received research or institutional support from Corin USA.

Table 1 Results of Total Hip Arthroplasty (THA) in Patients With Osteonecrosis

Authors (Year)	Number of Patients (Hips)	Procedure or Approach	Mean Patient Age in Years (Range)	Mean Follow-up in Years (Range)	Success Rate (%)[a]	Results
Seyler et al (2006)	Group 1: 146 (158) Group 2: 50 (52)	Group 1: THA with alumina-on-alumina bearings in patients with osteonecrosis or osteoarthritis Group 2: THA with cobalt-chromium bearings on UHMWPE in patients with osteonecrosis or osteoarthritis	Group 1: 45.2 (21-67) with osteonecrosis, 46.5 (30-67) with osteoarthritis Group 2: 44 (24-75) with osteonecrosis, 44.8 (28-74) with osteoarthritis	Last, 7	Group 1: 95.5 in patients with osteonecrosis, 89.4 in patients with osteoarthritis Group 2: 92.3 in patients with osteonecrosis, 92.9 in patients with osteoarthritis	Comparable 7-yr survivorship results in patients with osteoarthritis and those with osteonecrosis, and for the two bearing surface types
Baek and Kim (2008)	60 (71)	THA with alumina-on-alumina bearings	39.1 (18-49)	7.1 (6-9)	100	Mean Harris hip score, 97 at last follow-up 20% of hips had squeaking
Millar et al (2010)	48 (48)	THA with alumina-on-alumina ceramic bearings in patients with osteonecrosis (24) or osteoarthritis (24)	Osteonecrosis group: 46 (33-54) Osteoarthritis group: 50 (40-58)	Osteonecrosis group: 2.8 (2.1-4.2) Osteoarthritis group: 2.9 (2.2-4.3)	100 in both groups	Harris hip score and Oxford Hip Score at 6 mo postoperatively were good to excellent in 85% of patients with osteonecrosis and 90% of patients with osteoarthritis; no significant difference at 24 mo postoperatively
Johannson et al (2011)	2,593 (3,277)	Systematic review of THA for management of osteonecrosis before 1990 vs after 1990	44 (16-86)	8 (0.7-28)	83 before 1990 97 after 1990	Results after 1990 are equal to those in publicly reported THA registries, including all causes resulting in THA
Kim et al (2011)	71 (73)	THA with alumina ceramic on cross-linked UHMWPE	45.5 (20-50)	8.5 (7-9)	100	Mean ± SD linear UHMWPE penetration, 0.05 ± 0.02 mm/yr
Byun et al (2012)	41 (56)	THA with alumina-on-alumina bearings	25.6 (16-29)	7.7 (6.0-8.5)	100	39 patients returned to their preoperative occupation No loosening or osteolysis
Solarino et al (2012)	61 (68)	THA with alumina-on-alumina bearings for osteonecrosis	50 (29-72)	13 (11-15)	100	No revisions for wear 1 revision for infection 1 revision for excessive cup abduction No loosening

UHMWPE = ultra-high–molecular-weight polyethylene.

[a] Success is defined as no mechanical failure resulting from wear, loosening, or instability.

Table 1 Results of Total Hip Arthroplasty (THA) in Patients With Osteonecrosis (*continued*)

Authors (Year)	Number of Patients (Hips)	Procedure or Approach	Mean Patient Age in Years (Range)	Mean Follow-up in Years (Range)	Success Rate (%)[a]	Results
Issa, Naziri, et al (2013)	34 (44) in HIV-positive group, 70 (78) in non-HIV group	THA for management of osteonecrosis in patients with or without HIV diagnosis	HIV-positive group: 48 (34-80) Non-HIV group: 43 (18-71)	7 (4-11)	5 yr: 100 in HIV-positive group vs 98 in non-HIV group 10 yr: 95 in HIV-positive group vs 96.5 in non-HIV group	Late infection is a potential concern in HIV-positive patients Otherwise equivalent results
Kim et al (2013)	50 (60)	THA with alumina ceramic on highly cross-linked UHMWPE	28 (21-29)	10.8 (10-12)	100	Mean ± SD linear UHMWPE wear rate, 0.031 ± 0.004 mm/yr
Min et al (2013)	162 hips	THA with alumina ceramic on highly cross-linked UHMWPE for management of osteonecrosis	51.5 (20-74)	7.2 (5.0-10.6)	100	Mean linear UHMWPE wear rate, 0.038 mm/yr
Kim et al (2015)	430 patients	Systematic review of hemiresurfacing arthroplasty from 1950 to 2014 (14 published articles)	37 (12-72)	5.8 (1-28)	74	21% revision rate

UHMWPE = ultra-high–molecular-weight polyethylene.

[a] Success is defined as no mechanical failure resulting from wear, loosening, or instability.

procedure, active sources of infection elsewhere in the body, morbid obesity that has not been treated (even if attempts are unsuccessful), poorly controlled diabetes mellitus, or other medical conditions known to be associated with poorer short-term outcomes. In young patients, relative contraindications are present when the medical risks are substantial, such as in patients with systemic disease who are on immunomodulation medications and in patients with hemophilia, in whom controlling the underlying disease may be difficult. In extremely young patients (younger than 25 years), nonarthroplasty approaches may be sufficient to alleviate pain and allow deferral of definitive THA until later in the patient's life. In these patients, decision making is challenging, and patients (and family members when appropriate) should be fully informed of the short- and long-term risks of arthroplasty.

Alternative Treatments

Nonarthroplasty options for management of early-stage osteonecrosis are not discussed in this chapter. The arthroplasty surgeon must fully understand the importance of these options in young patients (younger than 40 years) who have precollapse osteonecrosis with a stabilized etiology. In young patients who have severe pain with limited involvement of the femoral head, the surgeon may attempt to perform THA to manage the pain even if the structural integrity of the femoral head is intact and the articular surface is normal. Nonarthroplasty approaches are available to manage these large lesions. However, care must be taken to ensure that the treatment will not compromise any subsequent arthroplasty procedure, which can subject the patient to multiple arthroplasty procedures and their many inherent risks. Nonarthroplasty options that preserve the external geometry of the proximal femur will not compromise future noncemented THA procedures, and these limited approaches can provide patients decades of pain relief if timed and performed properly.

On the basis of more than 30 years of experience with multiple treatment options in patients with osteonecrosis of the femoral head, the author of this chapter has concluded that attempts to alter the biologic and/or mechanical environment of the upper femur (not discussed in this chapter) can be successful in certain patients. The challenge has

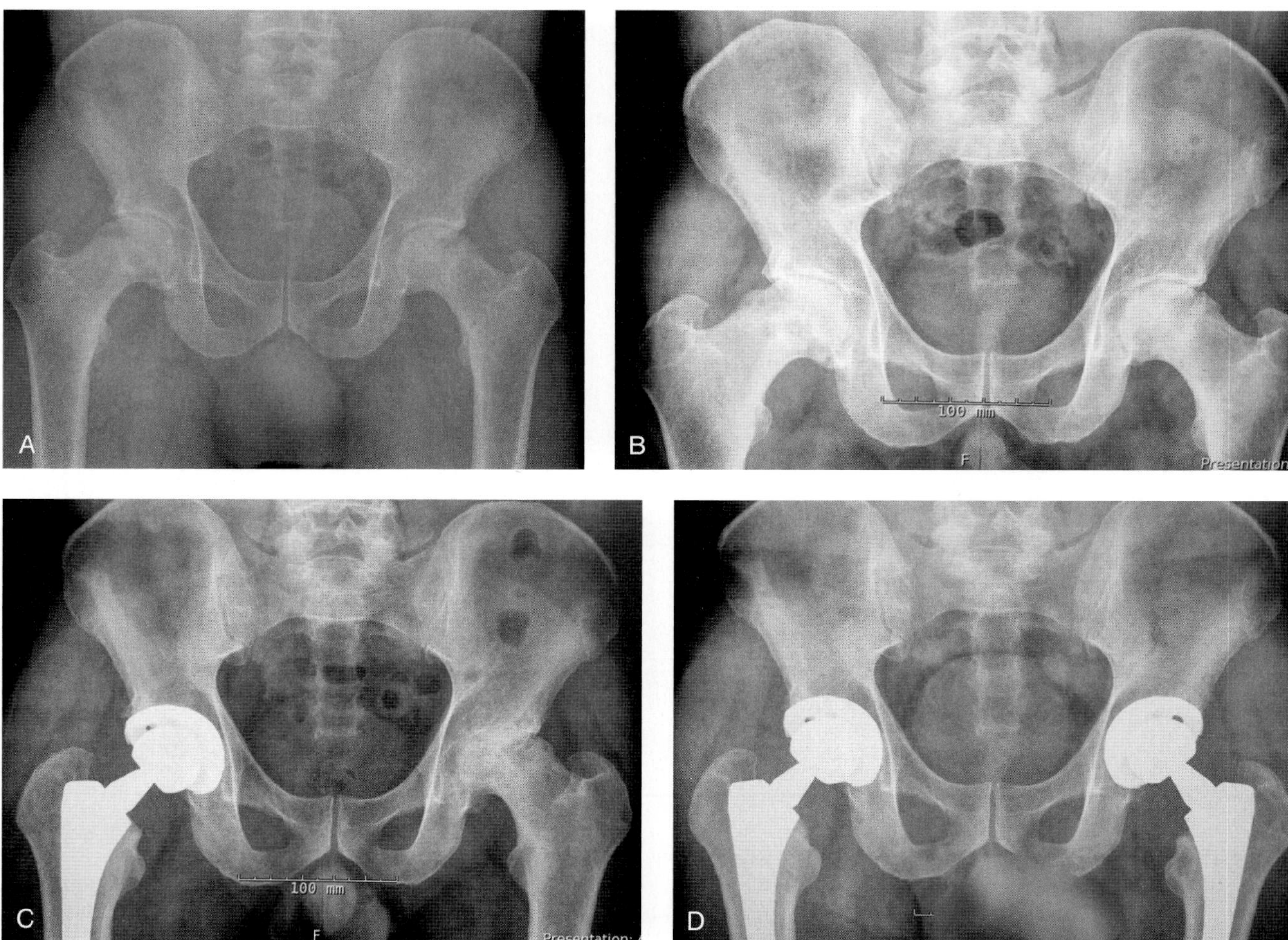

Figure 1 **A,** AP pelvic radiograph demonstrates bilateral University of Pennsylvania stage IV osteonecrosis, with greater than 30% involvement of the femoral head, in a 42-year-old man with a history of psoriatic arthritis and alcohol abuse. The patient was treated nonsurgically until his pain increased. **B,** AP pelvic radiograph obtained 4 months later demonstrates bilateral stage V osteonecrosis. Because the patient's symptoms had become severe and radiographs demonstrated advanced collapse of both femoral heads, staged bilateral noncemented total hip arthroplasty (THA) was performed. **C,** AP pelvic radiograph obtained 1 month after the radiograph in panel **B** demonstrates THA of the right hip, with continued progression of osteonecrosis in the left hip. **D,** AP pelvic radiograph obtained 4 months after the radiograph in panel **C** demonstrates THA of the left hip. The THA procedures were performed with dual modular neck hydroxyapatite-coated femoral stems and noncemented acetabular implants with ceramic femoral heads and highly cross-linked ultra-high–molecular-weight polyethylene bearing surfaces. The femoral implants subsequently were the subject of a product recall. The patient underwent revision of the femoral implants 5 years after implantation.

been to make these approaches predictable in any given patient. Careful staging (which has required advances in diagnostic capability) and aggregation of patient populations to obtain consistency of application and assessment (such as has been done in studies of the Japanese Arthroplasty Register) will help define the appropriate conditions to ensure the predictable use of such approaches. Currently, the author of this chapter prefers nonarthroplasty options in patients with stage I and some stage II lesions (those that are smaller in volume and involve less surface area) and sees only a very limited role of hemiarthroplasty. In patients with extensive involvement of the femoral head, THA represents the most predictable means of obtaining pain-free function for 15 to 20 years postoperatively. In patients with collapse of the femoral head, THA provides long-term pain relief and durable fixation. Some surgeons perform hip resurfacing in these patients, but the metal debris generated over time is a concern. In patients younger than 50 years, this option is unlikely to be a definitive solution but can be part of a lifelong strategy of management (**Figures 1** and **2**).

Results

Over the past decade, the results of contemporary approaches to THA in patients younger than 50 years have become clearer over a broad range of diagnoses and implantation approaches. The results are similar in patients with osteonecrosis and in patients of comparable status with diagnoses other than osteonecrosis. However, certain disease states associated with osteonecrosis may be associated with greater perioperative morbidity. Young patients with osteonecrosis, good bone quality, and high activity levels have results equal to those of patients with osteoarthritis and similar characteristics. Patients with inflammatory arthritis (that is, systemic lupus erythematosus or rheumatoid arthritis) and osteonecrosis may have poor bone quality; however, long-term implant fixation usually occurs (**Table 1**). The decision to use noncemented or cemented fixation depends on the quality of the patient's femoral bone stock. Many surgeons choose noncemented fixation because of younger patient age.

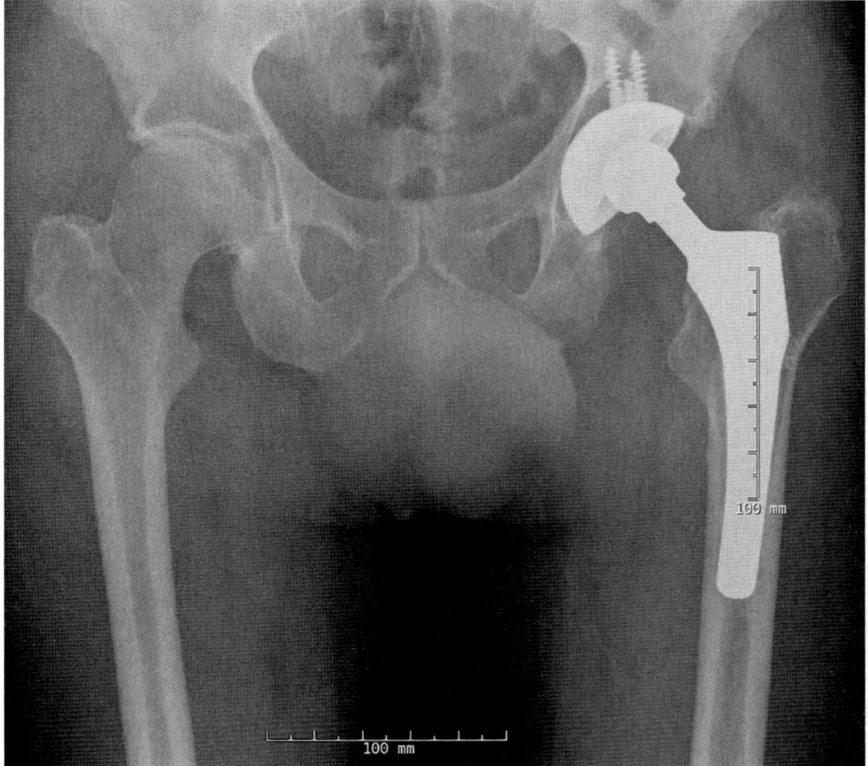

Figure 2 AP pelvic radiograph demonstrates long-term follow-up of a patient who was diagnosed initially at age 25 years with idiopathic osteonecrosis, late Ficat and Arlet stage II, when pain persisted after lumbar diskectomy. The patient was initially treated with a nonvascularized fibular graft, which failed at 4 years postoperatively. He therefore underwent primary left total hip arthroplasty (THA) with a first-generation noncemented cobalt-chromium implant in late 1984. Careful debulking of the fibular graft at the lateral flare was performed with a burr. The patient underwent acetabular revision 15 years after the primary procedure. The AP pelvic radiograph shown here, obtained 30 years after primary THA, demonstrates no evidence of osteolysis. At age 60 years, the patient reported no hip symptoms. The remnant of a fibular graft is seen laterally, with evidence of excellent fixation of the acetabular and femoral implants and no evidence of polyethylene wear.

Techniques

Setup/Exposure

- In patients with osteonecrosis, THA can be performed successfully through any of the established surgical approaches.
- The author of this chapter prefers to use a posterolateral approach because it allows safe and straightforward exposure of the acetabulum with minimal muscle disruption. A posterolateral approach also offers excellent direct visualization of the upper femur, where the greatest variation of geometry is likely to occur and in which prior treatment can alter the patient's natural environment. Even straightforward treatments such as core decompression with or without bone grafting can alter the lateral endosteal cortex. Such alteration, if not treated, can result in varus positioning of a femoral stem and fracture of the medial/calcar metaphysis during insertion of the broaches or the final implant. This concern is particularly important with proximally filling devices and tapered stems. Additionally, if a fracture occurs, it can be easily managed from a posterolateral approach.
- For the posterolateral approach, the patient is positioned in the lateral decubitus position, and a gently posteriorly curving incision is made over the greater trochanter.
- Retractors are positioned about the femoral neck to isolate it and allow measurement of the resection level and subsequent resection of the femoral neck.
- The surgeon must be aware of any prior procedures in which bone grafting or hardware has been

used. In general, these prior procedures present minimal additional difficulty.
- Prior femoral osteotomy will distort the geometry of the femoral neck. In these patients, proper resection of the femoral neck through the osteotomized upper femur requires thoughtful preoperative planning.

Instruments/Equipment/ Implants Required

- The basic instrumentation required for THA in this patient population is the same as that used for THA through a posterolateral approach in all patients.
- Several additional instruments will be helpful if the patient has undergone prior surgical treatment.
- If the upper femur has been distorted by means of upper femoral osteotomy, the use of a proximally modular femoral implant can help stabilize the implant within the femur with the allowance for independent adjustment of limb length, version, and offset proximally. Because upper femoral osteotomy is no longer frequently performed in the United States, this scenario is not typical.
- The use of a high-speed burr is helpful in patients in whom prior decompression, fibular grafting, or similar mechanical augmentation has been used to stabilize the collapsed or collapsing segments. These patients will have lateral endosteal hypertrophy, which, if not trimmed back to the normal anatomic lateral flare, will affect proper positioning of a proximally coated femoral stem and can result in potential varus positioning and fracture.
- Standard acetabular implants are used in these patients. Hemispheric implants will accommodate most anatomic abnormalities that may be encountered.

Procedure

- After resection of the femoral head and neck is completed, a key elevator is placed on the anterior femoral neck (with the hip held in 90° of internal rotation), and the anterior capsule is separated from the femoral neck bluntly.
- An angled retractor is used anteriorly to retract the femur superiorly and anteriorly to allow exposure of the anterior aspect of the acetabulum.
- A flanged retractor is used posteriorly (intracapsularly).
- A long, pointed retractor is used inferior to the transverse ligament.
- The placement of these retractors usually provides complete visualization of the acetabulum to allow preparation and implantation.
- The use of additional superior retraction (a single large Steinmann pin) or additional release of the reflected head of the rectus femoris superiorly or release of the capsule, gluteus maximus tendon insertion, and/or iliopsoas tendon inferiorly can aid in improving exposure but is rarely necessary in these patients.

ACETABULAR PREPARATION

- For much of the procedure, acetabular preparation is routine. However, the surgeon must take into consideration several unique features of this disease state.
- First, the patient may have minimal cartilage damage on the acetabulum, which allows the surgeon to take a minimalist approach to preparation, consisting of thorough curetting of the cartilage off the subchondral bone and slightly less aggressive reaming into the subchondral bone superomedially, which will allow for a combination of subchondral and cancellous bone.
- Second, the patient may have substantial inflammatory changes, resulting in a hyperemic and hypertrophic pulvinar. Before manipulating the pulvinar, the surgeon should cauterize it, use a long rigid curet to release its upper attachment, sweep it down to the transverse ligament, and transect it using electrocautery.
- Hyperemia and inflammatory synovitis can result in substantial osteopenia of the acetabular bone stock (particularly in patients with inflammatory arthritic or steroid-related osteonecrosis). In this scenario, curettage of the cartilage surface followed by careful reaming, with care taken to avoid overreaming, is important to avoid inadvertent compromise of the posterior or medial walls of the acetabulum.
- In most patients, a hemispheric titanium acetabular shell and a highly cross-linked, neutral ultra-high–molecular-weight polyethylene liner are used. The femoral head size is chosen such that the ultra-high–molecular-weight polyethylene is at least 6 mm thick and has an inner diameter of up to 36 mm.

FEMORAL PREPARATION

- In most patients, the author of this chapter uses a broach-only technique, usually with a tapered stem.
- Any trimming that is required because of prior surgical alteration of the metaphyseal/diaphyseal flare of the proximal femur is done with the use of a burr or a milling device. To ensure stability of the implant, these patients may require a stem that bypasses that area.
- Proximally filling implants or modular implants that require the surgeon to ream the bony bed during preparation of the femoral canal can be used.
- In some patients, the proximal-distal dimensions of the femur are not suitable to be used with a

standard hip stem (although this scenario has become much less common with the advent of current implant designs). In these patients, modular or customized devices are occasionally necessary.

- An intraoperative plain radiograph is obtained if potential varus positioning of the broach is a concern.
- To achieve optimal positioning of the acetabular and femoral implants, the surgeon should aim for combined anteversion of 35° to 45°.
- Implants with titanium fixation surfaces and a ceramic femoral head are typically used in patients younger than 65 years.

Wound Closure

- Careful attention to development of the capsular and muscular intervals as part of the exposure makes secure closure of the capsule a straightforward proposition.
- After the implants are positioned properly and the implant size, positioning, and offset and limb-length restoration have been confirmed by means of intraoperative radiography, hemostasis is rechecked.
- Local analgesic infiltration is used for pain control.
- The capsule is closed by tagging the superior and inferior capsule and external rotators, then bringing the four doubled strands of the nonabsorbable braided suture through drill holes in the posterior greater trochanter (two superiorly, two inferiorly).
- The capsular and muscular layers are tied separately to the back of the greater trochanter, with the affected limb held in flexion, abduction, and external rotation.
- The interval is oversewn with No. 1 absorbable braided sutures.
- The remainder of the wound closure is routine, with local analgesic infiltration in the fascia and subcutaneous tissue, and a subcuticular closure.

Postoperative Regimen

With the use of current technologies and approaches, the author of this chapter allows patients to return to full weight-bearing activity as soon as they can comfortably do so. Patients begin with full weight bearing as tolerated with crutches the day of the procedure and are allowed to progress to the use of a single crutch or cane as preferred. Strengthening is allowed as soon as tolerated, and walking is encouraged. The author of this chapter does not restrict positioning postoperatively. Higher-impact activities are avoided for 3 months postoperatively. Low and moderate activities are allowed as tolerated.

Avoiding Pitfalls and Complications

Successful THA in patients with osteonecrosis requires adequate exposure and attention to the many details that make arthroplasty successful in any patient. In muscular men with osteonecrosis (often ethanol induced), acetabular exposure can sometimes be challenging. Implant malposition or eccentric reaming can occur if the femur is not freed sufficiently to allow clearance of the handles of the acetabular reamers. The previously noted releases and their extensions can be helpful.

In patients with inflammatory arthritis, in whom the acetabular bone can be of poor quality, removal of the cartilage from the subchondral bone before reaming can minimize the risk of overreaming and perforation or damage to the medial or posterior walls of the acetabulum. In these patients, underreaming or reverse reaming to size may be necessary to ensure a secure fit and stability of the acetabular shell.

Awareness of endosteal buildup after a prior (and perhaps seemingly minimal) surgical intervention is important. The rasp must be centered in the femoral canal to avoid varus positioning and potential fracture during implantation. Standard broaches usually cannot remove this buildup, and the use of curved rasps or high-speed burrs can be helpful. If a lateral perforation occurs, it must be carefully bypassed with the stem, and cancellous bone grafting can be performed. If a femoral crack occurs, cerclage wires can be placed as needed.

In preoperative assessment, the effects of prior surgical intervention on the patient's femoral geometry usually are clear. However, because alterations will be three-dimensional, both AP and lateral radiographs should be carefully evaluated to assess the potential fit of standard implants. Modular implants can usually address these alterations.

Occasionally, diaphyseal/metaphyseal mismatch may be a concern. Because osteonecrosis affects a variety of patients and because bone geometry and integrity ranges from severely osteopenic to substantially osteosclerotic, the surgeon must carefully examine the upper femoral geometry to ensure an appropriate choice of implant. No single implant style or fixation method is appropriate in all patients with osteonecrosis. The surgeon may need to assess the wide range of implant designs available to select an appropriate and predictable choice for the patient.

In general, osteonecrosis in elderly patients can result from several potential etiologic influences, and arteriolar disease and venous and marrow alterations play a role in its development. THA is the treatment of choice in these patients. However, bone compromise is more likely in elderly patients than in other patients, and the surgeon must be attentive to the previously discussed concerns related to the shape and integrity of the bone.

Bibliography

Baek SH, Kim SY: Cementless total hip arthroplasty with alumina bearings in patients younger than fifty with femoral head osteonecrosis. *J Bone Joint Surg Am* 2008;90(6):1314-1320.

Byun JW, Yoon TR, Park KS, Seon JK: Third-generation ceramic-on-ceramic total hip arthroplasty in patients younger than 30 years with osteonecrosis of femoral head. *J Arthroplasty* 2012;27(7):1337-1343.

Ficat RP, Arlet J: Ischemia and necrosis of bone, in Hungerford DS, ed: *Ischemia and Necroses of Bone*. Baltimore, MD, Williams & Wilkins, 1980.

Issa K, Naziri Q, Rasquinha V, Maheshwari AV, Delanois RE, Mont MA: Outcomes of cementless primary THA for osteonecrosis in HIV-infected patients. *J Bone Joint Surg Am* 2013;95(20):1845-1850.

Issa K, Pivec R, Kapadia BH, Banerjee S, Mont MA: Osteonecrosis of the femoral head: The total hip replacement solution. *Bone Joint J* 2013;95-B(11 suppl A):46-50.

Johannson HR, Zywiel MG, Marker DR, Jones LC, McGrath MS, Mont MA: Osteonecrosis is not a predictor of poor outcomes in primary total hip arthroplasty: A systematic literature review. *Int Orthop* 2011;35(4):465-473.

Johnson AJ, Mont MA, Tsao AK, Jones LC: Treatment of femoral head osteonecrosis in the United States: 16-year analysis of the Nationwide Inpatient Sample. *Clin Orthop Relat Res* 2014;472(2):617-623.

Kim SJ, Kang DG, Park SB, Kim JH: Is hemiresurfacing arthroplasty for osteonecrosis of the hip a viable solution? *J Arthroplasty* 2015;30(6):987-992.

Kim YH, Choi Y, Kim JS: Cementless total hip arthroplasty with alumina-on-highly cross-linked polyethylene bearing in young patients with femoral head osteonecrosis. *J Arthroplasty* 2011;26(2):218-223.

Kim YH, Park JW, Patel C, Kim DY: Polyethylene wear and osteolysis after cementless total hip arthroplasty with alumina-on-highly cross-linked polyethylene bearings in patients younger than thirty years of age. *J Bone Joint Surg Am* 2013;95(12):1088-1093.

Millar NL, Halai M, McKenna R, McGraw IW, Millar LL, Hadidi M: Uncemented ceramic-on-ceramic THA in adults with osteonecrosis of the femoral head. *Orthopedics* 2010;33(11):795.

Min BW, Lee KJ, Song KS, Bae KC, Cho CH: Highly cross-linked polyethylene in total hip arthroplasty for osteonecrosis of the femoral head: A minimum 5-year follow-up study. *J Arthroplasty* 2013;28(3):526-530.

Seyler TM, Bonutti PM, Shen J, Naughton M, Kester M: Use of an alumina-on-alumina bearing system in total hip arthroplasty for osteonecrosis of the hip. *J Bone Joint Surg Am* 2006;88(suppl 3):116-125.

Solarino G, Piazzolla A, Notarnicola A, et al: Long-term results of 32-mm alumina-on-alumina THA for avascular necrosis of the femoral head. *J Orthop Traumatol* 2012;13(1):21-27.

Steinberg ME, Hayken GD, Steinberg DR: A quantitative system for staging avascular necrosis. *J Bone Joint Surg Br* 1995;77(1):34-41.

Chapter 28

Management of Metastases and Neoplasms in the Hip

Mary I. O'Connor, MD
Courtney E. Sherman, MD
Cody L. Martin, MD

Indications

Tumor destruction of bone can be the result of a primary benign or malignant bone tumor or can occur secondary to metastatic bone disease. Although metastatic bone disease is far more common, primary bone tumors may be encountered in any orthopaedic practice. Suspicion of neoplasm should be elevated if the patient has progressive pain that is unrelieved by rest and is most pronounced at night. Because up to 50% loss of trabecular bone can occur before lesions are visualized on plain radiographs, a neoplasm diagnosis should be high on the list of differential diagnoses for the patient who has a radiograph that appears to be negative for neoplasm but does not respond to therapies that have been deemed appropriate for the working diagnosis. Tumors that cause a permeative pattern of bone destruction, such as lymphoma and Ewing sarcoma, often are very difficult to identify on plain radiographs. In the patient with continued symptoms (particularly if the symptoms are progressive), repeat plain radiographs are recommended, and bone scintigraphy or MRI can be helpful.

Osteoarthritis, metastatic bone disease, and chondrosarcoma all commonly affect elderly patients. A history of prior malignancy (particularly a primary malignancy that tends to metastasize to bone, such as lung, breast, prostate, kidney, or thyroid cancer) should alert the surgeon to the possibility of metastatic bone disease. The predilection of chondrosarcoma for the periacetabular region should be noted and patterns of referred pain considered.

Establishing the Diagnosis

After a bone tumor has been identified, a thorough diagnostic and staging evaluation is necessary before a needle or an open biopsy. Patients in whom a primary bone sarcoma is suspected should be referred to an orthopaedic oncologist before biopsy. The hazards of biopsy by nonspecialists are well documented. In patients with known metastatic bone disease, tissue to confirm the diagnosis may be obtained at the time of surgical treatment of impending or actual fracture. Guidelines are less defined in patients with a primary carcinoma without known metastases or in patients with a remote history of malignancy. In patients with malignancy or a history of malignancy and who have multiple bone lesions, a working diagnosis of metastatic bone disease is reasonable, and tissue can be obtained for histologic confirmation via needle biopsy or at the time of surgical intervention. However, if such patients have a solitary bone lesion, a primary bone sarcoma remains possible, particularly if the history of malignancy is remote. If the orthopaedic surgeon is not knowledgeable regarding the principles of needle or bone biopsy, the patient should be referred to an orthopaedic oncologist.

Primary Bone Tumors

Benign bone tumors develop around the hip and often require excision or curettage and bone grafting. Primary bone sarcomas are managed with wide en bloc resection followed by complex reconstruction. These procedures should be performed by a surgeon who understands the principles of tumor surgery. Most patients are appropriately referred to an orthopaedic oncologist. However, orthopaedic surgeons who treat patients with hip disease will see and need to manage metastatic bone disease about the hip. Therefore, the management of metastatic bone disease in the pelvis and proximal femur is the focus of this chapter.

Metastatic Bone Disease

Indications for surgical management of metastatic bone disease about the

Dr. O'Connor or an immediate family member serves as a paid consultant to or is an employee of Zimmer Biomet; and serves as an unpaid consultant to and has stock or stock options held in Accelalox. Neither of the following authors nor any immediate family member has received anything of value from or has stock or stock options held in a commercial company or institution related directly or indirectly to the subject of this chapter: Dr. Sherman and Dr. Martin.

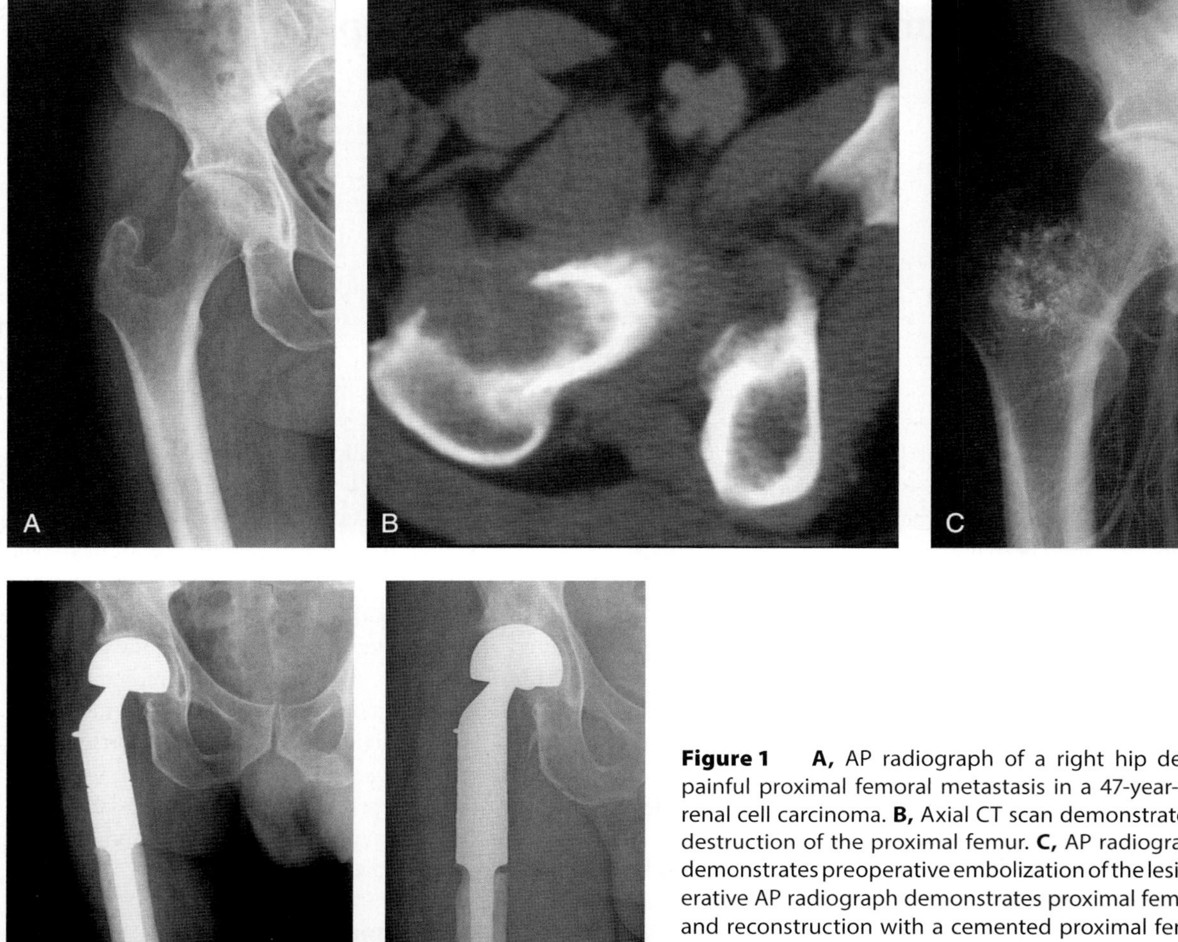

Figure 1 **A,** AP radiograph of a right hip demonstrates a painful proximal femoral metastasis in a 47-year-old man with renal cell carcinoma. **B,** Axial CT scan demonstrates the cortical destruction of the proximal femur. **C,** AP radiograph of the hip demonstrates preoperative embolization of the lesion. **D,** Postoperative AP radiograph demonstrates proximal femoral resection and reconstruction with a cemented proximal femoral implant with a bipolar femoral head. **E,** AP radiograph obtained 13 years postoperatively demonstrates mild stress shielding proximally and a well-fixed implant. Degenerative acetabular changes are noted. Prolonged survival can be seen in patients with renal cell carcinoma who undergo resection of a solitary metastasis. (Copyright the Mayo Foundation for Education and Research, Rochester, MN.)

hip include mechanical instability because of pathologic fracture; impending pathologic fracture; and symptomatic lesions that have not responded to nonsurgical and minimally invasive treatments, such as chemotherapy, diphosphonate agents, external radiation therapy, hormone therapy, immunotherapy, thermal therapy, ethanol therapy, radiofrequency ablation, cryoablation, and acetabuloplasty. The goals of surgical management are to relieve pain, restore maximal function in the shortest possible time, prevent pathologic fracture, and avoid treatment-related complications. The patient's life expectancy is a factor in the consideration of surgical treatment. Although no rigid guidelines have been established for the minimum life expectancy to justify surgical intervention, patients with acetabular metastases should have an expected survival of 3 to 6 months to undergo surgical treatment, and patients with disease of the proximal femur should have an expected survival of 2 to 3 months. Select patients with a shorter expected survival but acute fracture may still be candidates for surgical treatment because of pain management and nursing care issues. Very rarely, select patients with a solitary metastasis from thyroid carcinoma or renal cell carcinoma (**Figure 1**) may be candidates for wide en bloc resection in an attempt to cure and should be referred to an orthopaedic oncologist. A multidisciplinary approach to the treatment of these patients, particularly with input from medical oncology and radiation oncology specialists, is appropriate.

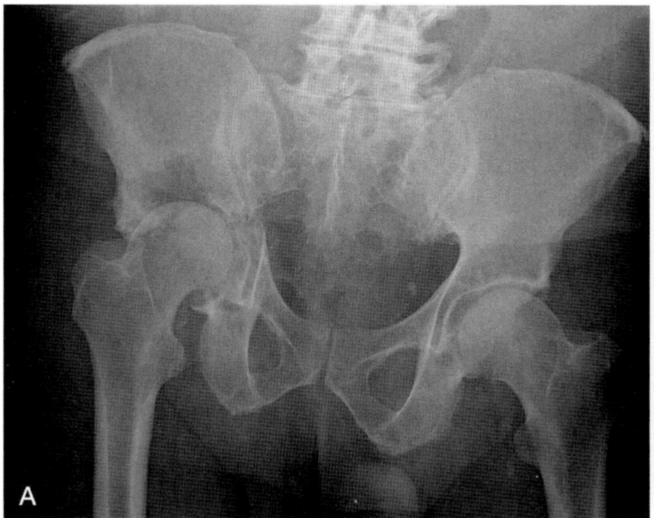

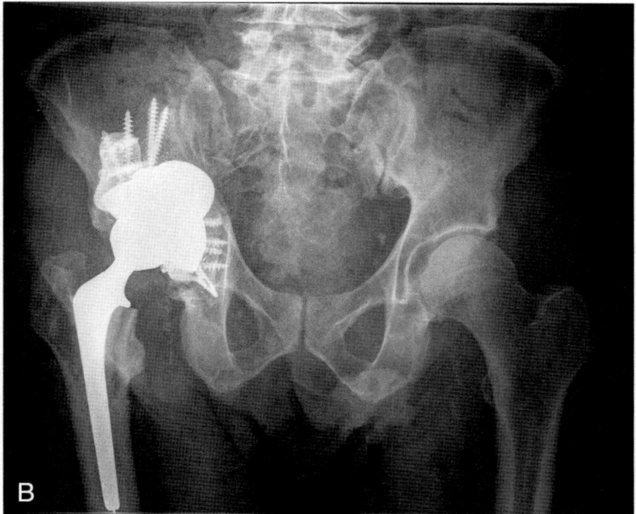

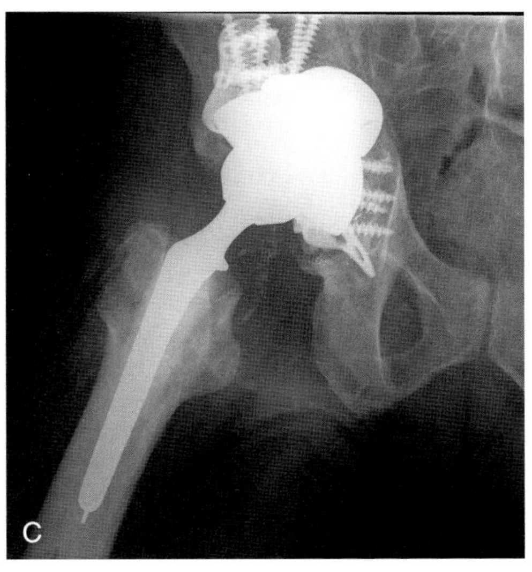

Figure 2 **A,** Preoperative AP pelvic radiograph demonstrates metastatic renal cell carcinoma and pathologic acetabular fracture in a 69-year-old man. Postoperative AP pelvic (**B**) and oblique hip (**C**) radiographs demonstrate reconstruction with a trabecular metal acetabular implant with trabecular metal augmentation, multiple screws, and an anti-protrusio cage. (Copyright the Mayo Foundation for Education and Research, Rochester, MN.)

PERIACETABULAR METASTASES

Although metastases can occur in other areas of the pelvis, periacetabular lesions are often painful and limit weight bearing. Destruction of the superior dome, medial wall, posterior column, or a combination thereof may result in collapse of the articular surface, protrusio acetabuli, or acute fracture. The extent of bone destruction that should be present to justify prophylactic intervention has not been established. CT and MRI are recommended in patients being considered for surgical intervention. The use of MRI allows optimal assessment of soft-tissue extension of the tumor and other areas of metastasis within the pelvis and sacrum. CT is helpful in defining the degree of cortical bone compromise.

The indications for specific surgical techniques about the acetabulum are determined by the extent of bone destruction. The principles of reconstruction are to transfer weight-bearing stress away from the diseased bone to the remaining intact pelvis; avoid bone grafting and procedures that require bony healing, which could be impaired by postoperative radiation therapy and require postoperative functional restrictions; and minimize the risk of postoperative complications.

Typically, acetabular reconstruction of metastatic destruction involves thorough curettage of the tumor and diseased bone and reconstruction of the bone defect with implants and polymethyl methacrylate cement. Implants such as an anti-protrusio cage, Steinmann pins, or screws are used to transfer stress from the defect into intact (generally superior) bone. Cement is then used to fill the remaining defect and incorporate the implants (**Figure 2**). Small lesions may require only polymethyl methacrylate and an anti-protrusio cage. To minimize the risk of postoperative dislocation, the use of a constrained liner should

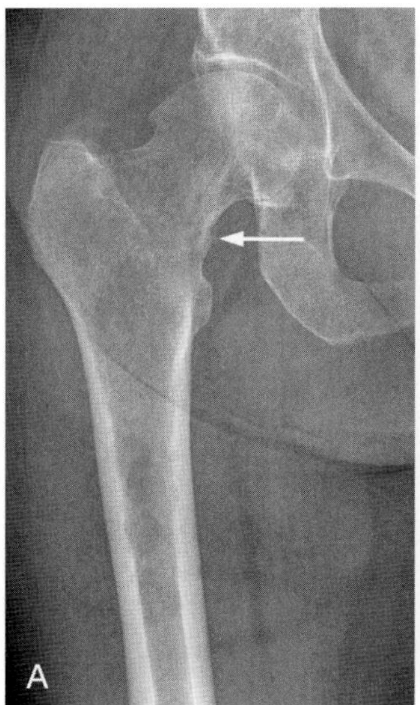

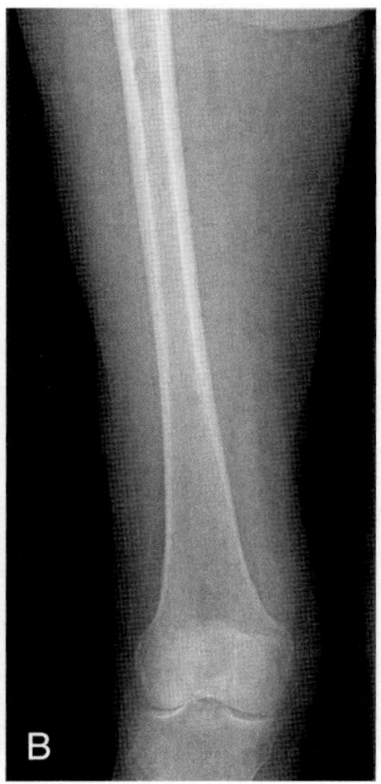

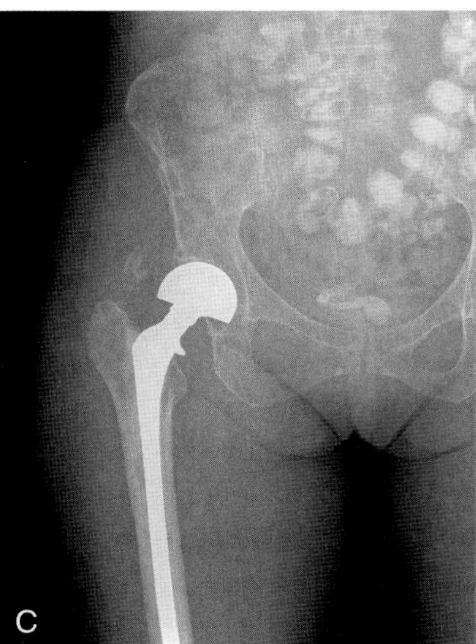

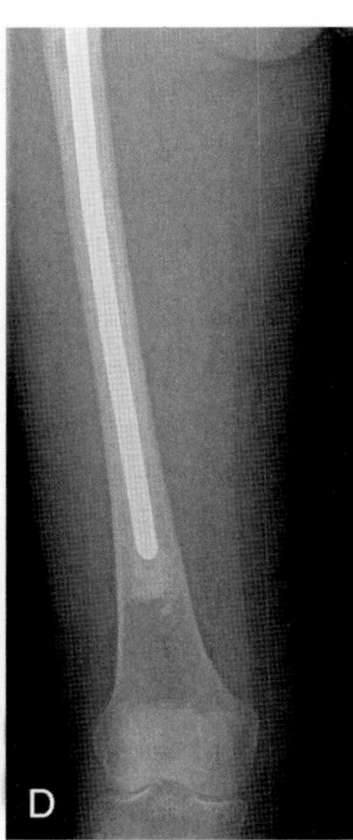

Figure 3 **A,** AP radiograph of a right hip demonstrates lytic breast cancer metastasis with pathologic fracture of the femoral neck (arrow) in a 64-year-old woman. **B,** AP radiograph of the mid and distal femur demonstrates the distal extent of the metastases. Postoperative AP hip (**C**) and AP femoral (**D**) radiographs demonstrate the use of long-stemmed, cemented bipolar hemiarthroplasty to protect the visualized metastatic lesions of the femur. (Copyright the Mayo Foundation for Education and Research, Rochester, MN.)

be considered. In patients who are not candidates for acetabular reconstruction, a Girdlestone procedure may be considered for palliation; however, the procedure will result in limb shortening, and pain relief is variable. If the patient has sufficient bone in the ilium but destruction of the acetabular columns, a saddle prosthesis may be used for reconstruction. Results of reconstruction with a saddle prosthesis have been mixed, and currently, few surgeons use this device. Porous tantalum implants have been used successfully in patients with metastatic disease to reconstruct acetabuli with severe bone loss and pelvic discontinuity.

METASTASES IN THE PROXIMAL FEMUR

Substantial metastatic destruction of the femoral neck or intertrochanteric region places the patient at great risk of pathologic fracture; therefore, prophylactic intervention should be considered in these patients. The extent of bone destruction needed for prophylactic intervention is not well defined for these patients. Historically, the criteria for impending fracture included cortical destruction greater than 50% or a lesion larger than 2.5 cm. The Mirels scoring system can be used to assess the need for prophylactic fixation on the basis of the location, type, and size of the lesion and the amount of pain associated with the lesion. Compromise of the medial cortex (including avulsion of the lesser trochanter) usually results in fracture because the lateral cortex cannot withstand the compression loads. Destruction of both the medial and lateral cortex warrants consideration of surgical management. CT is particularly helpful in determining the need for prophylactic intervention.

The surgical technique is determined by the extent of bone destruction and the location of the lesion. Compromise of the femoral head or neck is best managed with hip arthroplasty because internal fixation is not likely to achieve rigid fixation, and progression of the tumor may result in fracture or hardware failure. A bipolar or unipolar articulation may be used in patients without substantial metastatic acetabular involvement and with satisfactory acetabular cartilage (**Figures 1** and **3**). Acetabular micrometastases are not uncommon and often can be controlled with radiation therapy and other nonsurgical measures. If metastatic involvement of the acetabulum is a concern, a cemented acetabular implant can be placed. If preoperative MRI demonstrates no evidence of metastatic acetabular involvement, a noncemented acetabular implant may be used. The noncemented acetabular implant should be shielded during postoperative radiation therapy.

The femoral implant should be cemented. Indications for standard, calcar-replacement, long-stemmed, and proximal femoral implants depend on the location and extent of bone destruction (**Figure 1**). The entire femur should be imaged preoperatively; plain radiographs and advanced imaging such as MRI or bone scintigraphy can be used. In patients with compromise of the calcar, a calcar-replacement stem is indicated. If metastatic foci are present elsewhere in the femur, a long-stemmed femoral implant should be used. In patients with longer life expectancy, such as patients with breast carcinoma metastases, a long-stemmed femoral implant

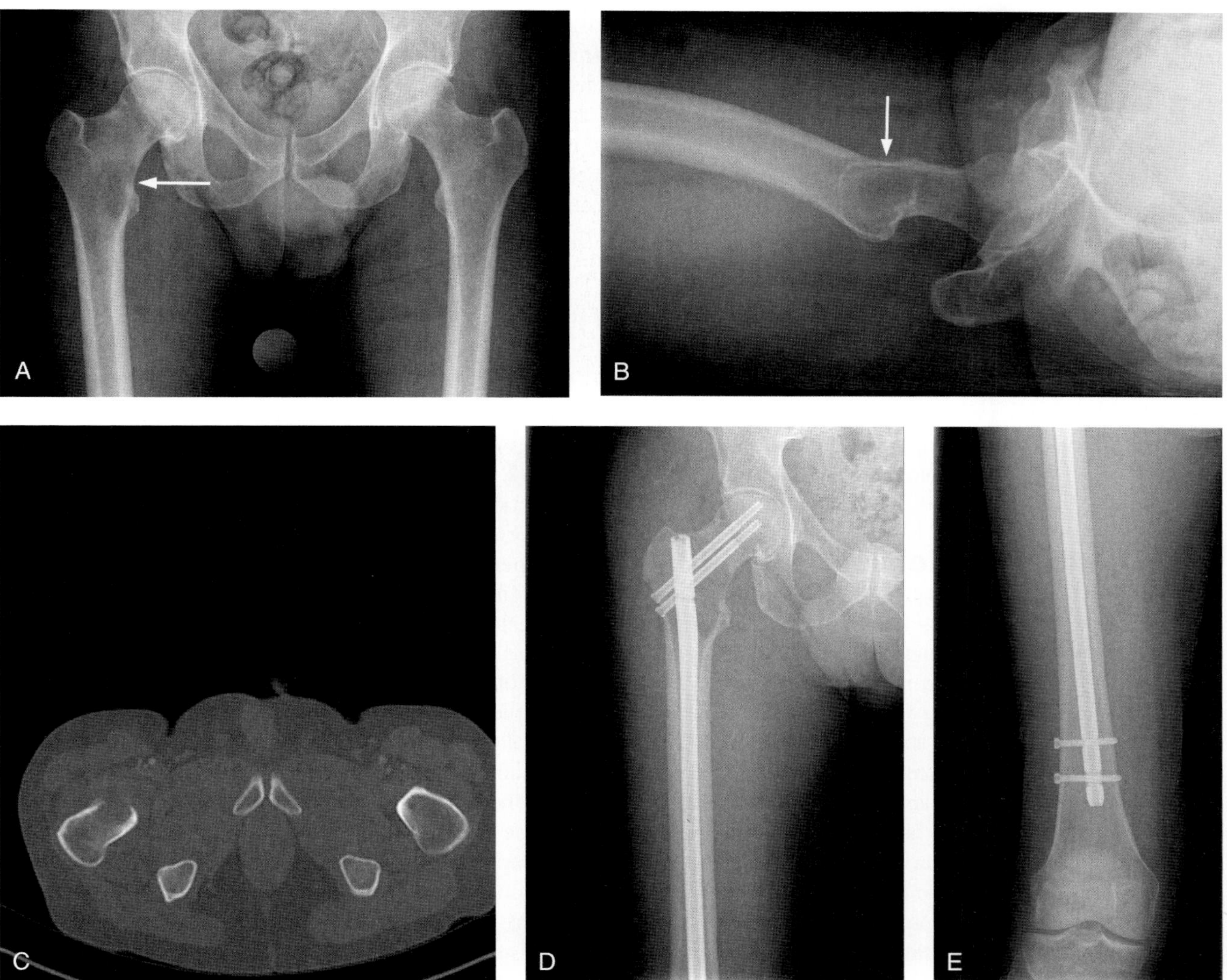

Figure 4 Preoperative AP pelvic (**A**) and lateral hip (**B**) radiographs demonstrate impending pathologic fracture of the right intertrochanteric proximal femur (arrow) in a 58-year-old man with metastatic lung carcinoma. **C,** Axial CT scan demonstrates the cortical destruction. Postoperative AP hip (**D**) and AP femoral (**E**) radiographs demonstrate stabilization with an intramedullary nail device with proximal screw fixation into the femoral head. Because the hardware fixation had good, stable purchase and adequately spanned the lesion, cement was not used. In addition, because of the cortical bone destruction, the cement would not have been contained. The patient underwent postoperative radiation therapy. (Copyright the Mayo Foundation for Education and Research, Rochester, MN.)

should be considered because it will prophylactically address most of the femur in the event that future metastatic sites develop (**Figure 3**). Because the use of cemented long-stemmed femoral implants is associated with an increased risk of embolization of marrow contents and cardiopulmonary events, a hole can be drilled into the distal femur to help vent medullary contents during cementation of the implant. Aggressive medullary lavage, intraoperative canal suctioning, and slow, controlled insertion of long-stemmed prosthesis can help minimize cement-related emboli. Communication with the anesthesiologist is important. In patients with known cardiopulmonary compromise and a limited life expectancy, the authors of this chapter use a standard or midlength femoral implant, if adequate for the extent of bone destruction, to minimize the risk of an intraoperative cardiopulmonary event.

Metastatic involvement of the intertrochanteric region can be addressed with a calcar-replacement femoral stem, as noted previously. In patients with lesions but minimal compromise of the adjacent cortical bone, the authors of this chapter typically use an intramedullary nail device with fixation into the femoral head (**Figure 4**), potentially with adjuvant methyl methacrylate inserted into the intertrochanteric region via a proximal lateral screw hole. Use of methyl methacrylate to fill metastatic defects and augment internal fixation is an off-label, non–FDA-approved use of bone cement. Adjunctive polymethyl methacrylate cement use for pathologic fracture fixation and improvement of pullout strength has been well documented. For patients with extensive destruction of the entire proximal femur, a proximal femoral prosthesis, combined with a bipolar or constrained liner to minimize the risk of postoperative dislocation, is the implant of choice.

Contraindications

Sclerotic metastases pose less risk for fracture than other types of metastases do and typically are managed nonsurgically. Surgical treatment is not appropriate for patients with a short life expectancy or medical compromise that would likely prevent the patient from surviving the procedure. Other contraindications to surgical intervention are the presence of metastatic disease elsewhere in the body that would continue to limit functional restoration, such as spinal metastases with epidural cord compression, and extensive bone destruction in the pelvis, which would prevent a mechanically sound reconstruction. In general, nonsurgical treatment is appropriate if the goals of surgical treatment (pain relief, pain maintenance, or restoration of function) cannot be realistically achieved.

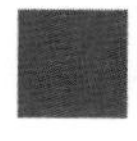

Alternative Treatments

Alternatives to surgical management of metastatic disease of the hip include the nonsurgical measures mentioned previously and embolization therapy. Because many pelvic metastases are vascular (particularly renal cell carcinoma, myeloma, and thyroid carcinoma), embolization often is performed before surgical intervention. Embolization also may be a specific nonsurgical treatment of patients with vascular metastases because it can improve pain and slow disease progression. Serial embolization may be performed.

Results

Published series of patients with periacetabular metastases show improvement in pain in most patients with surgical intervention (**Table 1**). Functional status is generally maintained or, in some patients, improves postoperatively. However, patient survival is limited in all series, making true assessment of the efficacy of the procedure difficult to determine. Most series note median postoperative survival of less than 12 months. The presence of visceral metastases results in early death, which in one study occurred at a median of 3 months postoperatively. The morbidity associated with these complex procedures is substantial, and most series include a perioperative death.

In patients with metastases in the proximal femur, surgical intervention typically results in improved pain and maintenance or restoration of ambulation. In general, more favorable results are achieved in the management of an impending pathologic fracture than in the management of an existing fracture. In addition, fewer treatment failures have been associated with endoprosthetic reconstruction compared with intramedullary nailing or open reduction and internal fixation for the management of pathologic proximal femur fractures. However, some studies contradict these results. Assessment of the results of surgical treatment in this region is limited by patient mortality. In a series of surgical treatment of patients with metastatic disease of the femur, patient survival rates at 1 and 2 years postoperatively were 35% and 19%, respectively, in patients with impending fractures, compared with 25% and 10%, respectively, in patients with completed fractures. In a different study, the patient survival rate at 1 year after surgical treatment with a proximal femoral implant was 53.3% in patients with metastatic disease and 82.3% in patients with a primary bone tumor. Results of prosthetic management of pathologic or impending fractures of the hip have been favorable, with ambulation restored or maintained in most patients and a low incidence of complications (**Table 2**).

Techniques

Discussion of all surgical techniques used in the management of metastatic disease in the hip region is beyond the scope of this chapter. The modified Harrington technique of acetabular reconstruction and the use of a proximal femoral implant in patients with extensive metastases in the proximal femur are presented. The technique for the use of calcar-replacement femoral stems is not discussed.

Acetabular Reconstruction

SETUP/EXPOSURE

- Preoperative embolization is performed in any patient in whom a vascular metastasis is suspected.
- The surgical approach should allow sufficient exposure for thorough access to the lesion and placement of an anti-protrusio cage.
- A trochanteric osteotomy may be needed. If the osteotomy is performed, it should be shielded during postoperative radiation therapy.

INSTRUMENTS/EQUIPMENT/ IMPLANTS REQUIRED

- Cancellous screws (and/or threaded Steinmann pins), polymethyl methacrylate, and an anti-protrusio cage are used for reconstruction of the defect.

PROCEDURE

- The hip is dislocated, and a femoral neck osteotomy is performed.
- Thorough curettage of the gross tumor and involved bone is performed. The tumor is removed as completely as possible to minimize the risk of subsequent local disease progression, which would result in fixation failure.
- Reconstruction of the defect is determined by the extent of the bone loss and can include cancellous screws, threaded Steinmann pins, polymethyl methacrylate, and an anti-protrusio cage. The goal of the reconstruction is to transfer weight-bearing stress to the intact proximal bone.
- Screws or pins are driven from within the defect proximally toward the sacroiliac joint for fixation into the strong intact posterior iliac bone.
- In patients with compromise of the acetabular columns, screws or pins are placed in an antegrade fashion from the iliac wing distally into the superior pubic ramus for reconstruction of the anterior column and into the ischium for reconstruction of the posterior column. A triangulation guide can be used for antegrade screw or pin placement.
- A portion of the anti-protrusio cage should rest on intact host bone; at a minimum, the flanges should contact intact bone. The cage is precontoured.
- Screws are drilled and measured for both the iliac and ischial flanges of the anti-protrusio cage.
- These screws and the anti-protrusio cage are removed.
- If necessary, mesh can be placed medially before insertion of the cement and anti-protrusio cage to prevent extrusion of the cement.
- Because an anti-protrusio cage typically is seated against the pelvis in a vertical fashion, cementation of the polyethylene acetabular liner within the cage requires particular attention. If a liner designed for cementation is not available, the back surface of a press-fit liner can be roughened to provide better cement fixation.
- Cement is placed in the defect, incorporating any previously placed screws or pins, and the anti-protrusio cage is placed.
- The two initial flange screws are quickly replaced to provide initial fixation to the anti-protrusio cage.
- Additional screws are quickly inserted through the anti-protrusio cage and through the doughlike cement into intact bone. Dome screws are placed first. Flange screws are subsequently placed because they are typically inserted into host bone.
- The liner is cemented into the anti-protrusio cage. Because an anti-protrusio cage typically is seated against the pelvis in a vertical manner, cementation of the polyethylene acetabular liner within the cage requires particular attention. If a liner designed for cementation is not available, the back surface of a press-fit liner can be roughened to provide better cement fixation.
- The surgical technique for the femoral component is not described in this section.
- A trial reduction is performed with particular attention to joint stability. The authors of this chapter typically use a larger diameter femoral head to promote stability. A constrained liner is used if necessary for stability.

WOUND CLOSURE

- Wound irrigation and closure are performed in the standard manner.

Proximal Femoral Replacement Implant

SETUP/EXPOSURE

- A standard approach to the hip with distal extension typically is sufficient to access the midshaft to proximal femur.
- The abductor tendons are preserved.
- If possible, a portion of the greater trochanter is retained with the tendons.

INSTRUMENTS/EQUIPMENT/ IMPLANTS REQUIRED

- Reconstruction of the extensive metastatic destruction of the proximal femur is best achieved with the use of a proximal femoral implant. This device allows immediate weight bearing and rehabilitation.
- An allograft-prosthetic composite should not be used in patients with metastatic disease because postoperative radiation therapy will negatively affect healing at the allograft–host bone junction.
- In patients with intact acetabular cartilage and no substantial metastatic compromise of the acetabulum, a bipolar articulation of the proximal femoral implant is recommended to enhance stability.
- If acetabular reconstruction is performed, the use of a constrained liner should be considered.
- A modular implant system is used to provide intraoperative flexibility.

PROCEDURE

- Before the hip is dislocated, the rotational position of the femur is marked for use as an aid during cementation of the implant.
- The hip is dislocated.
- The diseased portion of the proximal femur is resected en bloc.
- If possible, the length of the resected segment is measured to aid in selection of proper length of the implant.
- The canal is reamed sufficiently to allow a 2-mm cement mantle.

Table 1 Results of Surgical Treatment of Patients With Periacetabular Metastases

Author(s) (Year)	No. of Patients	Procedure or Approach	Adjunctive Treatment	Mean Patient Age in Years (Range)	Survival	Results
Harrington (1981)	58[a]	Conventional THA (11) THA with isolated anti-protrusio cage (19) Cemented and pin-reinforced THA with anti-protrusio cage (28) 3 patients underwent internal hemipelvectomy	All patients received local radiation therapy	58 (40-82)	Mean patient, 19 mo	Good or excellent pain relief was attained in 37 patients 6 mo postoperatively and in 24 patients 2 yr postoperatively 45 patients were ambulatory 6 mo postoperatively, and 26 patients were ambulatory 2 yr postoperatively 5 patients had loosening secondary to tumor recurrence 2 patients died
Kunisada and Choong (2000)	37 (40 hips)	Cemented THA with modified Harrington reconstruction and pelvic reconstruction	None	61 (35-86)	1 patient died during surgery Median survival of remaining patients, 8 mo	Hip pain, analgesic use, ambulation, and mobility improved in all patients 3 patients experienced complications, including 1 intraoperative death
Marco et al (2000)	55	Hemipelvic endoprosthesis (1) Cemented THA with anti-protrusio cage (3) Cemented THA with modified Harrington reconstruction with anti-protrusio cage and long retrograde screws (15) Cemented THA with modified Harrington reconstruction with anti-protrusio cage and antegrade pins or screws (36)	12 patients underwent selective embolization 54 patients underwent chemotherapy or radiation therapy either preoperatively or postoperatively	62 (43-82)	Median patient, 9 mo	45 patients were available at 3-mo follow-up 34 patients experienced pain relief 14 patients experienced disease progression 14 patients experienced early complications 1 perioperative death occurred 30 of 32 patients who were ambulatory preoperatively retained the ability to walk 9 of 13 patients who were nonambulatory preoperatively regained the ability to walk 33 patients were available at 6-mo follow-up 25 patients experienced pain relief 19 patients maintained the ability to walk and function in the community 21 patients had more than 12 mo of follow-up 14 patients experienced pain relief 12 patients maintained the ability to walk and function in the community
Nilsson et al (2000)	32	Cemented THA with Harrington reconstruction with pins	13 patients underwent preoperative radiation therapy	62 (29-82)	Median patient, 11 mo	13 patients lived ≥1 yr postoperatively, of whom 10 were pain free at rest and when weight bearing, 6 walked with support, 7 walked without support, and 11 lived outside of a healthcare facility at 1 yr postoperatively 7 patients had complications

MSTS = Musculoskeletal Tumor Society, THA = total hip arthroplasty.
[a] Patients also had pathologic fracture.
[b] Patients also had Harrington type III deficiency.

Table 1 Results of Surgical Treatment of Patients With Periacetabular Metastases (*continued*)

Author(s) (Year)	No. of Patients	Procedure or Approach	Adjunctive Treatment	Mean Patient Age in Years (Range)	Survival	Results
Tillman et al (2008)	19	Cemented THA with modified Harrington reconstruction	5 patients with metastasis of renal carcinoma underwent preoperative embolization Most patients received preoperative radiation (total not reported)	66 (48-83)	Mean patient, 16 mo	All patients were able to ambulate indoors independently postoperatively 1 patient required revision Need for analgesics was less postoperatively At 6-mo follow-up, 4 patients required opiate pain medication because of progression of malignancy No patients had dislocation, deep infection, or injury to major vessels or nerves or the bladder
Clayer (2010)	29	Cemented THA with anti-protrusio cage	15 patients received radiation before surgery 13 patients received radiation after surgery No radiation treatment at surgical site within 6 wk of surgery 1 patient did not receive radiation 11 patients received preoperative chemotherapy	67 (30-82)	Median patient, 12 mo	5 patients experienced dislocations 1 patient experienced loss of fixation Deep infection developed in 3 patients Postoperatively, 10 patients became indoor ambulators, 17 became community ambulators, 2 remained chairbound, and 1 remained bedbound
Ho et al (2010)	37[b]	Cemented THA with modified Harrington reconstruction and periacetabular screws	31 patients received chemotherapy, radiation therapy, or both preoperatively	63 (35-83)	24 mo: 59% implant, 55% patient 60 mo: 49% implant, 39% patient	Mean MSTS score improved from 14 to 20 Significant improvement was achieved in pain ($P < 0.0001$), mobility ($P < 0.0385$), and function ($P < 0.0186$) 12 patients experienced complications
Kiatisevi et al (2015)	22	Cemented THA with multiple screws and anti-protrusio cage (19, with long screws in 4 patients and no Steinmann pins) Cemented THA with multiple screws without anti-protrusio cage (3)	All patients underwent preoperative embolization and postoperative radiation therapy	54 (33-71)	Median patient, 11 mo	Eastern Cooperative Oncology Group score improved from 3.1 to 1.7 Visual analog scale score improved from 8.4 to 2.2 Mean MSTS score, 70 2 patients had complications 20 patients were ambulatory

MSTS = Musculoskeletal Tumor Society, THA = total hip arthroplasty.
[a] Patients also had pathologic fracture.
[b] Patients also had Harrington type III deficiency.

Table 2 Results of Surgical Treatment of Patients With Metastases in the Proximal Femur

Authors (Year)	Number of Patients	Procedure or Approach	Adjunctive Treatment	Patient Age in Years (Range)	Survival	Results
Lane et al (1980)	163[a] (167 femora)	Endoprosthetic replacement	81 patients received chemotherapy and 46 received radiotherapy prior to surgery	Women: mean, 52.6 (NA) Men: mean, 60.7 (NA)	Median patient, 5.6 mo	All patients experienced pain relief 72% of patients who were ambulatory preoperatively were able to walk independently or with assistance postoperatively 46% of the patients who were nonambulatory preoperatively were ambulatory postoperatively Deep infection developed in 1.2% of patients No dislocations, loosening, or device failure
Wedin and Bauer (2005)	142 (146 femora)	Endoprostheses (hemiarthroplasty, bipolar prosthesis, total hip arthroplasty, tumor prosthesis, or reconstruction prosthesis; 109) Osteosynthetic devices (reconstruction nails, locked IM nails, or hip screws; 37)	NR	Median, 69 (33-91)	Median survival of patients not requiring revision surgery, 5 mo Median survival of patients requiring revision surgery, 15 mo	15 of the 146 procedures failed necessitating revision surgery 16.2% failure rate of osteosynthetic devices compared with 8.3% failure rate of endoprostheses 2-yr risk of revision surgery was 0.35 for osteosynthesis and 0.18 for endoprostheses
Chandrasekar et al (2009)	65 (metastatic disease) 25 (primary bone tumors) 10 (other malignant conditions)	Modular proximal femoral implant	Chemotherapy was administered as appropriate 11 patients received radiotherapy	Mean, 56.3 (16-84)	Median patient, 21 mo	Patient survival rates: 63.6% at 1 yr and 23.1% at 5 yr Patients with a primary bone tumor had significantly higher 1-yr survival compared with those with metastatic disease (82.3% and 53.3%, respectively; $P = 0.003$) Six patients (7%) required revision surgery Estimated 5-yr implant survival rate with revision as the end point was 90.7%

IM = intramedullary, MSTS = Musculoskeletal Tumor Society, NA = not available, NR = not reported, ORIF = open reduction and internal fixation.
[a] Patients had hip fractures or impending fractures.
[b] Patients had femoral fractures.
[c] There is a discrepancy in the source article, with 146 reported in the abstract but a summed total in text of 144.
[d] Patients had proximal femur fractures or impending fractures.

Table 2 Results of Surgical Treatment of Patients With Metastases in the Proximal Femur (*continued*)

Authors (Year)	Number of Patients	Procedure or Approach	Adjunctive Treatment	Patient Age in Years (Range)	Survival	Results
Sarahrudi et al (2009)	142[b] (146 femora[c])	IM nailing (94 femora) Sliding hip screws (15 femora) Other extramedullary fixation (dynamic condylar screw or conventional plate; 7 femora) Arthroplasty for metastatic femur fracture (23 femora) Nonsurgical (5 femora)	Additional cementation was performed in 11 patients with extramedullary implants and 4 IM implants	Median, 72 (36-89)	Mean patient, 3.7 mo	Patient survival rates: 17% at 1 yr and 6% at 2 yr Complication rates: 3.2% after IM nailing, 20% after sliding hip screw fixation, and 8.6% after arthroplasty Implant failures occurred an average of 9.5 mo postoperatively Differences in pre- and postoperative mobility were not statistically different
Harvey et al (2012)	158 (159 femora)	IM nailing (46) Endoprosthetic reconstruction (113)	IM nailing: All received 30-Gy radiation therapy 3 wk postoperatively Both groups: Patients received chemotherapy if indicated by their disease	Mean, 60 (17-91)	Patient survival rates: 51% at 1 yr, 29% at 2 yr, and 11% at 5 yr	Endoprosthetic reconstruction: 18% complication rate, no mechanical failures, and 100% 5-yr endoprosthesis survival rate. Mean MSTS, 21 of 30 IM nailing: 26% complication rate, 11% mechanical failure rate, and 85% 5-yr nail survival rate. Mean MSTS, 24 of 30
Steensma et al (2012)	298[d]	IM nailing (82) Endoprosthetic reconstruction (197) ORIF (19)	IM nailing: radiation therapy in 41% Endoprosthetic reconstruction: radiation therapy in 28% ORIF: radiation therapy in 26%	IM nailing: median, 61.8 Endoprosthetic reconstruction: median, 62.4 ORIF: median, 55.7	NR	The 3.1% failure rate of endoprosthetic reconstruction was significantly lower than that of the other treatment methods (6.0% for IM nailing and 42.1% for ORIF) Revisions requiring implant exchange: 0.5% for endoprosthetic, 6.0% for IM nailing, and 42.1% for ORIF ($P < 0.01$)

IM = intramedullary, MSTS = Musculoskeletal Tumor Society, NA = not available, NR = not reported, ORIF = open reduction and internal fixation.
[a] Patients had hip fractures or impending fractures.
[b] Patients had femoral fractures.
[c] There is a discrepancy in the source article, with 146 reported in the abstract but a summed total in text of 144.
[d] Patients had proximal femur fractures or impending fractures.

The implant should be seated on solid cortical bone with no gross evidence of disease.
- An intramedullary stem of length 135 to 200 mm with an anterior bow is used unless the level of the resection is distal to the middle of the diaphysis.
- A trial reduction is performed to assess limb length and hip stability. Although patients are counseled preoperatively that limb lengthening will occur, care is taken to avoid excessive lengthening.
- In patients with a more proximal resection level, a cement restrictor is used.
- In patients with more distal resections, the use of a cement restrictor may not be functional or necessary.
- The implant is cemented in approximately 15° to 20° of anteversion.
- The bipolar articulation is impacted onto the femoral implant and the final reduction is performed.
- Soft-tissue reconstruction is performed to optimize postoperative function. The acetabular capsule, iliopsoas tendon, and short external rotators are closed in a purse-string manner around the neck of the implant.
- The abductor tendon (or the greater trochanter) is secured to the trochanteric portion of the implant with nonabsorbable suture. Implants with trabecular metal pads in the greater trochanteric region may facilitate healing of the abductor soft tissues to the implant.
- The vastus lateralis is reapproximated to the trochanteric portion of the implant. The implant should be completely enclosed by the deep soft tissues, which should be sutured at a physiologic length. Postoperatively, scarring of the deep soft tissues can result in surprisingly good function after sufficient healing and rehabilitation.

WOUND CLOSURE

- The wound is irrigated and closed in the standard manner.

Postoperative Regimen

Patients are promptly mobilized postoperatively. If a constrained liner was used in acetabular reconstruction, bracing is not necessary. Rehabilitation should emphasize ambulation. Hip range of motion and abduction exercises should be delayed until several months after the procedure, depending on the extent of the bone resection and reconstruction and soft-tissue reconstruction. Because survival typically is not long enough for patients to develop hip strength, a Trendelenburg gait is common, and patients are advised that they will require an assistive device for ambulation.

Avoiding Pitfalls and Complications

Appreciation of the extent of metastatic bone disease is critical to surgical planning. Access to good preoperative imaging studies will allow the surgeon to anticipate additional bone compromise beyond that which is visible in the images (similar to the appreciation of debris-induced osteolysis). Thorough gross tumor removal is necessary. Weak, compromised, and diseased bone should be removed. Particularly in patients with diseases that do not typically respond to adjuvant therapies, these techniques will minimize the risk of local tumor progression, which would compromise fixation and ultimately result in failure of the reconstruction. A variety of implants and internal fixation devices should be available intraoperatively in the event that additional bone removal is necessary or a fracture occurs.

Instability of the hip, particularly after complex acetabular reconstruction, can be minimized with appropriate positioning of the acetabular implant, avoidance of impingement at the femoral neck, and the use of large-diameter femoral heads and constrained acetabular liners. The authors of this chapter recommend use of a constrained liner in patients who have metastatic bone disease, limited life expectancy, and a higher risk of hip instability.

Good surgical planning and technique can reduce the risk of some complications. Extensive intraoperative blood loss can occur during surgical procedures in the pelvic region. Preoperative angiography with embolization is essential in patients with vascular metastases. Even with embolization, substantial bleeding may occur. Rapid removal of the tumor is critical because bleeding will usually subside markedly after the tumor is removed. If bleeding remains problematic after tumor removal, a layer of bone cement may be placed to cauterize the bleeding bone. The anesthesia team must be prepared for the potential for substantial intraoperative blood loss and sudden cardiopulmonary events. Fat embolization, particularly during preparation and cementation of a long-stemmed femoral implant, can result in intraoperative cardiac arrest. Techniques that can help to minimize the risk of embolism include slow reaming of the femoral canal with narrow, fluted reamers; frequent suction of the medullary contents out of the canal; avoidance of the use of a cement restrictor; distal venting of the medullary contents; and controlled insertion of the implant.

Bibliography

Chandrasekar CR, Grimer RJ, Carter SR, Tillman RM, Abudu A, Buckley L: Modular endoprosthetic replacement for tumours of the proximal femur. *J Bone Joint Surg Br* 2009;91(1):108-112.

Clayer M: The survivorship of protrusio cages for metastatic disease involving the acetabulum. *Clin Orthop Relat Res* 2010;468(11):2980-2984.

Harrington KD: The management of acetabular insufficiency secondary to metastatic malignant disease. *J Bone Joint Surg Am* 1981;63(4):653-664.

Harvey N, Ahlmann ER, Allison DC, Wang L, Menendez LR: Endoprostheses last longer than intramedullary devices in proximal femur metastases. *Clin Orthop Relat Res* 2012;470(3):684-691.

Ho L, Ahlmann ER, Menendez LR: Modified Harrington reconstruction for advanced periacetabular metastatic disease. *J Surg Oncol* 2010;101(2):170-174.

Kiatisevi P, Sukunthanak B, Pakpianpairoj C, Liupolvanish P: Functional outcome and complications following reconstruction for Harrington class II and III periacetabular metastasis. *World J Surg Oncol* 2015;13:(4).

Kunisada T, Choong PF: Major reconstruction for periacetabular metastasis: Early complications and outcome following surgical treatment in 40 hips. *Acta Orthop Scand* 2000;71(6):585-590.

Lane JM, Sculco TP, Zolan S: Treatment of pathological fractures of the hip by endoprosthetic replacement. *J Bone Joint Surg Am* 1980;62(6):954-959.

Marco RA, Sheth DS, Boland PJ, Wunder JS, Siegel JA, Healey JH: Functional and oncological outcome of acetabular reconstruction for the treatment of metastatic disease. *J Bone Joint Surg Am* 2000;82(5):642-651.

Nilsson J, Gustafson P, Fornander P, Ornstein E: The Harrington reconstruction for advanced periacetabular metastatic destruction: Good outcome in 32 patients. *Acta Orthop Scand* 2000;71(6):591-596.

Sarahrudi K, Greitbauer M, Platzer P, Hausmann JT, Heinz T, Vécsei V: Surgical treatment of metastatic fractures of the femur: A retrospective analysis of 142 patients. *J Trauma* 2009;66(4):1158-1163.

Steensma M, Boland PJ, Morris CD, Athanasian E, Healey JH: Endoprosthetic treatment is more durable for pathologic proximal femur fractures. *Clin Orthop Relat Res* 2012;470(3):920-926.

Tillman RM, Myers GJ, Abudu AT, Carter SR, Grimer RJ: The three-pin modified 'Harrington' procedure for advanced metastatic destruction of the acetabulum. *J Bone Joint Surg Br* 2008;90(1):84-87.

Ward WG, Holsenbeck S, Dorey FJ, Spang J, Howe D: Metastatic disease of the femur: Surgical treatment. *Clin Orthop Relat Res* 2003;(suppl 415):S230-S244.

Wedin R, Bauer HC: Surgical treatment of skeletal metastatic lesions of the proximal femur: Endoprosthesis or reconstruction nail? *J Bone Joint Surg Br* 2005;87(12):1653-1657.

Chapter 29

Total Hip Arthroplasty in Patients With Inflammatory Arthritis and Other Conditions Affecting Bone Quality

Michael E. Berend, MD

Indications

Inflammatory arthropathies often affect the hip joint and lead to symptomatic degenerative changes that result in the need for total hip arthroplasty (THA). The condition is frequently bilateral. In patients with inflammatory arthritis of the hip, reconstruction with THA is challenging with regard to surgical exposure, hip dislocation, acetabular preparation and bone grafting, and restoration of leg length and offset.

Inflammatory arthropathies have many etiologies. A common diagnosis is rheumatoid arthritis. The disease is characterized by abnormal immune response in a host with a genetic predisposition. It leads to chronic and progressive synovial inflammation and subsequent destruction of joint surfaces and surrounding tissues. Management of rheumatoid arthritis centers on modification of the immune mediator pathways. The mechanism of joint destruction occurs at a cellular level, resulting in damage to the articular cartilage, ligaments, and bone. In a series of 8,102 THAs performed at the institution of the author of this chapter, 74% were performed to manage osteoarthritis and 6% were performed to manage inflammatory arthritic conditions of the hip, with rheumatoid arthritis representing approximately 3%. Other authors have reported that rheumatoid arthritis represents 3% of diagnoses leading to THA. The radiographic appearance of inflammatory arthritis of the hip often demonstrates loss of joint space without osteophyte formation. The indication for THA is deterioration of quality of life, function, and ambulatory status to an extent that nonsurgical treatments are no longer effective.

Inflammatory arthritis of the hip may be associated with the specific anatomic pathoanatomy called acetabular protrusion, or protrusio acetabuli, in which the femoral head has migrated medial to the medial wall or floor of the acetabulum (**Figure 1**). Acetabular protrusion, also known as arthrokatadysis and Otto disease, is commonly seen in patients with lupus, ankylosing spondylitis, and rheumatoid arthritis (**Figure 1**). It occurs bilaterally more often than unilaterally. Inflammatory arthritis with associated acetabular protrusion presents unique surgical challenges during primary THA.

Evaluation of the patient with inflammatory arthritis includes a thorough history and physical examination. The history and physical examination should focus on the manifestations of underlying systemic inflammatory disease, which often affects the spine and other joints. These manifestations often result in fixed flexion deformity of the hip and limited mobility of the spine. Emerging evidence suggests that fixed spinal deformity may influence postoperative functional status, limb length, and risk of dislocation after THA. Gait and limb lengths should be carefully assessed with the patient both standing and supine to ensure proper correction of functional limb length during THA. Upper extremity range of motion (ROM), strength, and functional capacity are important considerations for postoperative rehabilitation after THA. Special modifications such as the use of a walker often are necessary, and patient education preoperatively is helpful to avoid postoperative limitations on rehabilitation. Such limitations may exist due to other joint involvement (such as the shoulders and elbows) that may limit use of a postoperative assistive device.

ROM of the hip should be carefully quantified. Hip flexion contractures and limited motion about the hip are more commonly seen in patients with bilateral inflammatory disease than in patients with osteoarthritis or monoarticular inflammatory arthropathies.

Dr. Berend or an immediate family member has received royalties from and serves as a paid consultant to Zimmer Biomet; has stock or stock options held in OrthAlign; has received research or institutional support from Johnson & Johnson, Stryker, and Zimmer Biomet; and serves as a board member, owner, officer, or committee member of the American Association of Hip and Knee Surgeons, the Joint Replacement Surgeons of Indiana Research Foundation, and the Piedmont Orthopedic Society.

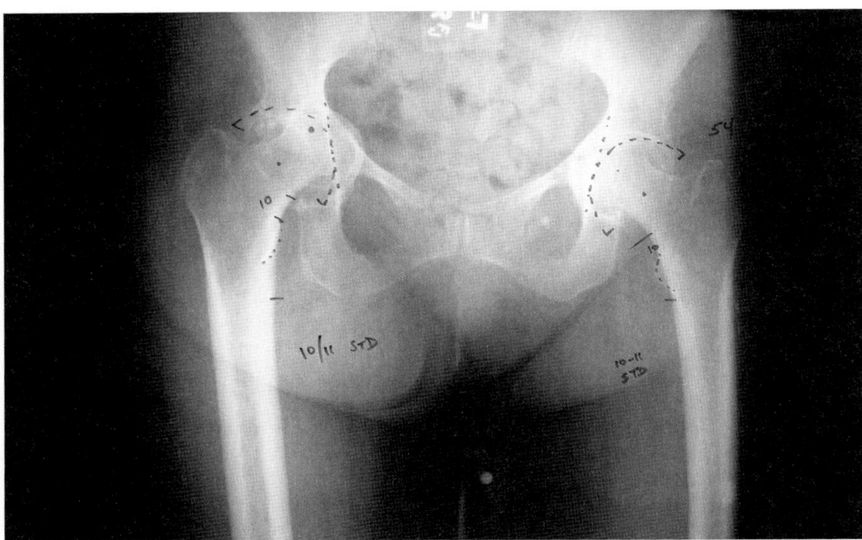

Figure 1 AP pelvic radiograph demonstrates bilateral acetabular protrusion in a patient with rheumatoid arthritis. Both femoral heads are medial to the ilioischial line. Inflammatory arthritis of the hip has resulted in loss of joint space without osteophyte formation. Preoperative templating is done in preparation for placing a noncemented acetabular implant into the anatomic position. The dashed hemispheres represent the planned acetabular cup placement. The marks on the femoral neck represent the planned femoral neck osteotomy level and the implant sizing for the system used. Preoperative tempting aids in formulating a surgical plan to correct the underlying deformity.

Adduction contractures with limited passive and active abduction are common and must be noted and managed intraoperatively. Supine and standing evaluation is helpful to complete the dynamic assessment of the severity and interaction of the deformities associated with acetabular protrusion. When THA is performed in a patient with severe adduction contracture, adductor tenotomy may be required to improve abduction postoperatively.

Hip reconstruction in a patient with inflammatory arthritis requires a detailed and stepwise radiographic examination. AP radiographs are evaluated to assess the position of the acetabulum, limb-length inequality, femoral offset, and femoral bone stock. The qualitative signs of osteopenia are assessed because osteopenia may influence implant fixation and surgical risks. Additionally, the endosteal geometry may be affected. Potential mismatch of metaphyseal and diaphyseal geometry can influence the femoral implant selection.

The routine femoral and acetabular landmarks of the hip and pelvis are identified. The ilioischial or Köhler line should be outlined. This line begins in the sciatic notch and proceeds distally along the posterior column and onto the medial border of the ischium. Acetabular protrusion is present if the medial aspect of the femoral head is at or medial to the Köhler line. In severe cases, the trochanteric region of the femur is adjacent to the pelvis (**Figure 1**). Radiographic limb-length discrepancy is measured, as is femoral offset relative to the contralateral hip. Often little offset is present, which brings the sciatic nerve closer to the surgical exposure of the acetabulum and makes the surgical exposure more challenging. Fixed pelvic obliquity should be noted. The center of rotation of the femoral head is also identified.

Contraindications

The contraindications to THA in patients with inflammatory arthritis are active infection, poor overall medical status, open skin ulcerations, and insufficient bone stock to support a functional THA on the femoral or acetabular side of the reconstruction. Factors to consider when determining whether to perform THA in patients with inflammatory arthropathy of the hip include the duration of disease, involvement of other joints, immunosuppressive medications, prior surgical treatment, motor strength, and functional capacity. In younger patients (younger than 30 years) with symmetric joint space of the hip, rheumatologic evaluation may be warranted if an inflammatory condition is ruled out. Disease-modifying agents used to treat inflammatory conditions place these patients at increased risk of infection and must be stopped before THA is performed.

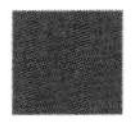

Alternative Treatments

In general, nonsurgical medical management should be exhausted before surgical intervention is attempted. The goals of nonsurgical treatment are twofold. The first goal is control of joint pain and swelling, and the second goal is limiting joint damage and delaying hip arthroplasty. NSAIDs inhibit inflammation cascades and reduce symptoms from synovitis but do not modify the disease itself. Alternatively, disease-modifying antirheumatic drugs such as the tumor necrosis factor-α antagonists are effective in many patients.

Results

The functional improvement resulting from THA performed for the management of inflammatory arthritis typically

Table 1 Results of Total Hip Arthroplasty (THA) in Patients With Inflammatory Arthritis

Authors (Year)	Number Studied	Procedure or Approach	Mean Patient Age in Years (Range)	Mean Follow-up in Years (Range)	Results
McCollum et al (1980)	25 patients (32 hips)	THA with acetabular augmentation with femoral head autograft	Women: 50 Man: 57	NA (2-8)	Demonstrated viability of femoral head autograft in restoring acetabular bone stock All grafts appeared united within 3 mo, and the protrusion did not progress
Johnsson et al (1984)	25 patients (26 hips)	THA with cancellous bone grafting	56 (29-76)	2 (1-4)	Demonstrated value of cancellous bone grafting in restoring acetabular bone stock during THA In 25 hips, the bone grafts demonstrated radiographic healing and no further protrusion occurred
Berend et al (2006)	2,551 hips (2,191 patients)	Cemented or noncemented THA	Cemented: 70.4 Noncemented: 54.1	6.8 (2-16.2)	Elevated risk of periprosthetic fracture in patients with rheumatoid arthritis compared with patients with osteoarthritis (5.5% and 2.1%, respectively)
Eskelinen et al (2006)	1,893 patients (2,557 hips)	THA to manage rheumatoid arthritis	<55	9.7 (0-24)	Finnish Arthroplasty Register report Proximally circumferentially porous-coated, noncemented stems had a 15-yr survival rate of 89% with aseptic loosening as the end point Risk of stem revision resulting from aseptic loosening was higher with cemented stems than with proximally porous-coated noncemented stems (relative risk, 2.4) Cox regression analysis showed that the risk of cup revision with any cup revision as the end point was higher for all noncemented cup designs than for all-polyethylene cemented cups
Rud-Sørensen et al (2010)	1,661 hips in patients with rheumatoid arthritis and 64,858 hips in patients with osteoarthritis	THA to manage rheumatoid arthritis or osteoarthritis	NA	<14	Danish Hip Arthroplasty Registry report Overall survival of primary THA in patients with rheumatoid arthritis was similar to that of patients with osteoarthritis Stem survival appeared to be better in patients with rheumatoid arthritis, whereas survival of the entire THA was not significantly different between the two groups Among patients with rheumatoid arthritis, risk of revision appeared to be greater in men than women

NA = not available.

is excellent; however, the perioperative risks may be different from those in patients with other diagnoses (**Table 1**). The risk of early infection has been reported to be 1.3 times higher in patients who undergo THA for inflammatory arthritis than in patients who undergo THA for osteoarthritis. Long-term THA implant survivorship is comparable for rheumatoid arthritis and osteoarthritis. The authors of meta-analyses examining revision rates, hip dislocation, infection, 90-day mortality, and venous thromboembolic events found that patients with rheumatoid arthritis are at increased risk of dislocation after THA compared with patients with osteoarthritis (adjusted odds ratio 2.16 [95%

confidence interval, 1.52–3.07]). These authors identified some evidence supporting an increased risk of infection in patients with rheumatoid arthritis compared with patients with osteoarthritis. No evidence suggested any differences in the rates of revision at later time points, 90-day mortality, or rates of venous thromboembolic events after THA in patients with rheumatoid arthritis and patients with osteoarthritis. The same authors reported similar results in a claims analysis, suggesting increased risk of dislocation and infection.

Clinical outcomes of cemented and noncemented femoral and acetabular implants in patients with rheumatoid arthritis have been published. The risk of revision after primary THA is multifactorial and may be related to the combined effects of young age and the diagnosis of rheumatoid arthritis. Larger femoral head sizes (32 mm or larger) may help reduce dislocation risk, but this effect has not been well studied.

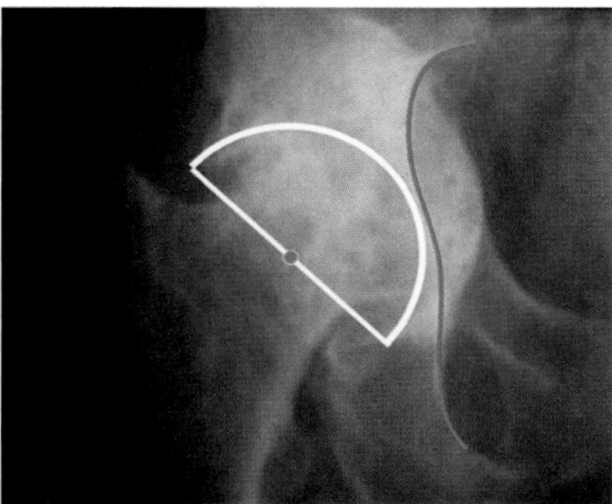
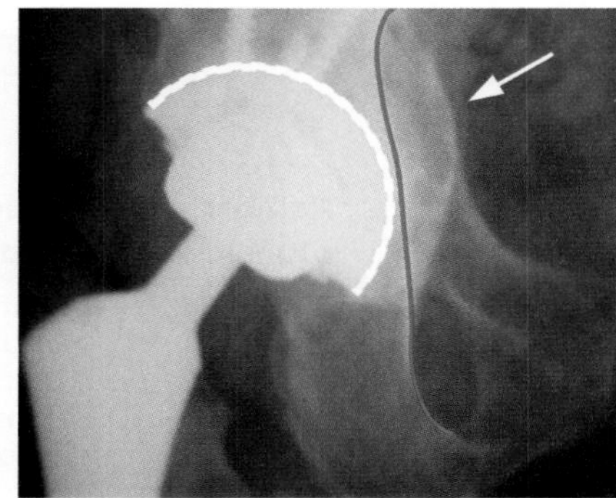

Figure 2 **A,** Preoperative AP radiograph demonstrates acetabular protrusion in the right hip of a patient with degenerative hip arthritis. The femoral head is medial to the ilioischial (Köhler) line. Preoperative templating demonstrates planned placement of a noncemented acetabular implant into the anatomic position with medial bone graft. **B,** Postoperative AP radiograph of the same hip demonstrates total hip arthroplasty with noncemented implants and medial bone graft (arrow). The implant is positioned lateral to the ilioischial line.

Techniques

Setup/Exposure

- The surgical approach to the hip should be carefully chosen on the basis of surgeon preference, surgeon experience, and the degree of deformity.
- Dislocation of the hip for primary THA is often challenging in patients with substantial synovitis and acetabular protrusion. Hip ROM is often markedly limited in these patients. The sciatic nerve is much closer to the femur and to the surgical exposure, especially if a posterior approach is used.
- Satisfactory capsular release must be performed around the acetabular rim and proximal femur to enhance hip ROM and the opportunity for safe dislocation.
- Patients with inflammatory arthritis often have osteopenia or osteoporosis secondary to the disease, disuse, and/or the pharmacologic agents that are prescribed. The hip should be dislocated using appropriate visualization and careful application of traction forces to avoid fracture of the femur or acetabulum.
- If dislocation is difficult, an in situ femoral neck osteotomy may be performed. Before an in situ femoral neck osteotomy is done, retractors are inserted to protect the surrounding tissues. A napkin-ring osteotomy is performed with parallel neck cuts and removal of a central portion of the femoral neck. The femoral head is then removed with a threaded Steinmann pin, a corkscrew, or acetabular reamers.
- In patients with severe ankylosis or severe acetabular protrusion, a trochanteric osteotomy may help increase exposure.

Instruments/Equipment/ Implants Required

- Noncemented acetabular implants have proven durable compared with cemented acetabular implants in midterm to long-term follow-up studies of hips with acetabular protrusion.
- Acetabular and femoral implant sizing can be estimated with digital or acetate templates.
- Acetabular implants with various screw configurations should be available.
- Femoral implants with variable offset and endosteal geometries are used, depending on the patient's anatomic variation.
- The author of this chapter uses noncemented stems with variable metaphyseal geometries and femoral offsets to more closely match the patient's bony and soft-tissue anatomy after correction of the deformity.

Procedure

- In patients with inflammatory arthritis with or without acetabular protrusion, the goal of surgical reconstruction is to place the functional hip center of the THA near its anatomic position. This method will move the center of rotation of the acetabulum laterally and distally.
- One way to quantify this goal of acetabular reconstruction is to

place the medial portion of the cup adjacent to the Köhler line (**Figure 2**).
- Numerous treatment options aimed at restoring bone stock, including solid and morcellized cancellous bone grafting, have been used over the past three decades.
- Offset and leg length will be increased proportionally to the deformity correction after the femoral reconstruction is completed. Trial reductions often demonstrate decreased ROM compared with that of patients with dysplasia, who have greater preoperative ROM.

ACETABULAR PREPARATION

- With the goal of repositioning the hip center of rotation as close as possible to the anatomic location, the acetabular implant is often placed more laterally than the native acetabulum, with fixation obtained on the acetabular rim.
- Medial acetabular reaming is performed carefully because the medial wall is thin. Areas of degenerative medial cartilage and soft tissue are gently removed with reamers and curets to expose healthy bleeding bone for bone graft incorporation and cup fixation with biologic ingrowth/ongrowth.
- The acetabular rim is prepared with reamers that are slightly (1 to 2 mm) larger than the diameter of the depth of the acetabular cavity. During preparation of the acetabular rim, the reamers are held in the position that will be used for the final reamer to ensure placement of the final cup in the appropriate anatomic position.
- The final reamer is often 1 mm smaller than the size of the acetabular implant that will be placed, depending on the design of the cup.
- Trial implants are inserted to confirm the positioning.
- An intraoperative radiograph is obtained for further confirmation if necessary.

BONE GRAFTING

- Medial central bone grafting is often necessary in patients with acetabular protrusion.
- Patients with acetabular profusion who are undergoing primary THA have ample bone available in the resected femoral head. This bone can be morcellized with acetabular reamers or a bone mill.
- The author of this chapter has found that bone grafts that are loaded by the acetabular implant remodel nicely and reconstitute the deficient acetabulum. Grafts that are not loaded tend to resorb over time. Medial grafts have proved viable in biopsy studies.
- Depending on the severity of the protrusion, morcellized bone graft can be inserted after initial acetabular preparation and medial to the acetabular implant.
- The graft is placed into the depth of the acetabular cavity.
- A 2- to 4-mm hemispheric reamer is used in reverse to adequately disperse and impact the graft into the depth of the acetabulum.
- Satisfactory host bone should be exposed on the native acetabular rim to allow direct fixation of the noncemented acetabular implant to the pelvis.

PLACEMENT OF ACETABULAR IMPLANT

- The cup is impacted into the prepared socket, obtaining fixation on the rim.
- The use of cups with adjuvant fixation such as fins or pegs may aid in obtaining initial press-fit stability.
- Supplemental screw fixation should be used for additional initial cup support in patients who have undergone substantial bone grafting.
- The appropriate acetabular liner for the desired femoral head size is inserted.

FEMORAL PREPARATION AND IMPLANT PLACEMENT

- The femur is prepared in the standard manner for the desired femoral implant.
- Care is taken to assess leg length and femoral offset as the reconstruction is trialed and the final femoral neck length is selected.
- Femoral preparation depends on the choice of stem geometry and cemented or noncemented fixation. Templating should include assessment of bone density and cortical thickness.
- The author of this chapter often places a cerclage wire around the femoral metaphysis before trial implant broaching and insertion of the final noncemented stem. In the chapter author's experience, patients with diagnoses other than osteoarthritis are at increased risk of intraoperative fracture. Prophylactic cerclage wiring may help prevent fracture propagation and subsequent stem loosening.

Wound Closure

- Wound closure is performed in the standard manner for THA procedures.

Postoperative Regimen

In patients who undergo THA for the management of inflammatory arthritis, postoperative weight bearing generally begins with a walker or crutches, and advances to the use of a cane as tolerated. The author of this chapter no longer uses hip precautions in any patients. When the restoration of the hip center has resulted in increased offset and leg length, care is taken to monitor the status of the motor function in the lower extremity and keep the knee bent and the hip extended to reduce tension on the sciatic nerve. This position maintains better blood supply to the nerve, which may have been lengthened when the hip was reconstructed. Follow-up radiographs are obtained at 3 months postoperatively, 1 year postoperatively, and every 2 years thereafter.

Avoiding Pitfalls and Complications

Hip reconstruction with THA in patients with inflammatory arthropathy with or without associated acetabular protrusion is challenging. Common complications include periprosthetic fracture related to decreased bone density, increased risk of infection resulting from immune suppression, and increased risk of damage to the sciatic nerve because of acetabular protrusion. The likelihood of implant loosening may be increased in these patients because of poor bone density and intraoperative difficulties. In a study performed at the chapter author's institution, rates of periprosthetic fracture after THA were 2.1% in patients with osteoarthritis and 5.5% in patients with rheumatoid arthritis. The author of this chapter often places a prophylactic cerclage wire to help prevent intraoperative fracture and possible postoperative femoral fracture and implant subsidence.

Bibliography

Berend ME: Acetabular protrusio: A problem in depth. *Orthopedics* 2008;31(9):895-896.

Berend ME: Indications for primary total hip arthroplasty, in Hozack WJ, Parvizi J, Bender B, eds: *Surgical Treatment of Hip Arthritis: Reconstruction, Replacement, and Revision.* Philadelphia, PA, Saunders Elsevier, 2010, pp 87-92.

Berend ME, Smith A, Meding JB, Ritter MA, Lynch T, Davis K: Long-term outcome and risk factors of proximal femoral fracture in uncemented and cemented total hip arthroplasty in 2551 hips. *J Arthroplasty* 2006;21(6 suppl 2):53-59.

Eskelinen A, Paavolainen P, Helenius I, Pulkkinen P, Remes V: Total hip arthroplasty for rheumatoid arthritis in younger patients: 2,557 replacements in the Finnish Arthroplasty Register followed for 0-24 years. *Acta Orthop* 2006;77(6):853-865.

Johnsson R, Ekelund L, Zygmunt S, Lidgren L: Total hip replacement with spongious bone graft for acetabular protrusion in patients with rheumatoid arthritis. *Acta Orthop Scand* 1984;55(5):510-513.

McCollum DE, Nunley JA, Harrelson JM: Bone-grafting in total hip replacement for acetabular protrusion. *J Bone Joint Surg Am* 1980;62(7):1065-1073.

Ravi B, Croxford R, Hollands S, et al: Increased risk of complications following total joint arthroplasty in patients with rheumatoid arthritis. *Arthritis Rheumatol* 2014;66(2):254-263.

Ravi B, Escott B, Shah PS, et al: A systematic review and meta-analysis comparing complications following total joint arthroplasty for rheumatoid arthritis versus for osteoarthritis. *Arthritis Rheum* 2012;64(12):3839-3849.

Rosenberg WW, Schreurs BW, de Waal Malefijt MC, Veth RP, Slooff TJ: Impacted morsellized bone grafting and cemented primary total hip arthroplasty for acetabular protrusion in patients with rheumatoid arthritis: An 8- to 18-year follow-up study of 36 hips. *Acta Orthop Scand* 2000;71(2):143-146.

Rud-Sørensen C, Pedersen AB, Johnsen SP, Riis AH, Overgaard S: Survival of primary total hip arthroplasty in rheumatoid arthritis patients. *Acta Orthop* 2010;81(1):60-65.

Schrama JC, Fenstad AM, Dale H, et al: Increased risk of revision for infection in rheumatoid arthritis patients with total hip replacements. *Acta Orthop* 2015;86(4):469-476.

Van De Velde S, Fillman R, Yandow S: The aetiology of protrusio acetabuli: Literature review from 1824 to 2006. *Acta Orthop Belg* 2006;72(5):524-529.

Chapter 30
Total Hip Arthroplasty in Obese Patients

Michael Bolognesi, MD
Alexander R. Vap, MD

Indications

Total hip arthroplasty (THA) has provided good quality and consistent results in patients with degenerative hip disease. The number of THA procedures performed annually in the United States is projected to increase to nearly 572,000 by 2030. The increasing proportion of obese patients seeking THA has contributed to this increase in demand. The United States has seen a marked increase in the prevalence of Americans who are considered obese. The mean national body mass index (BMI), calculated as a person's weight in kilograms divided by height in meters squared, has increased to more than 30 in the United States (**Figure 1**). A 24% increase in the mean national BMI occurred over the 3-year period from 2001 to 2004. Age-adjusted prevalence of obesity has been reported to be 33% for men and 36% for women.

Biomechanical studies have shown that patients with excessive BMI place greater stress on articular cartilage. In addition, obese patients are thought to have higher levels of proteins that accelerate the process of joint inflammation and destruction. The authors of one study reported a peak relative risk of THA 8.5 times higher in patients with BMI 40 or more compared with patients with BMI less than or equal to 25. The exact relationship between obesity and degenerative joints is not fully understood. Accurately defining obesity is part of the challenge. BMI greater than or equal to 30 has been the most common measurement used to classify a patient as obese.

The World Health Organization classification of obesity has three main categories (**Table 1**). Although this system provides a framework for categorizing patients, it does not identify key body habitus characteristics that can influence the technical aspects of hip arthroplasty, and it does not distinguish between healthy patients who happen to have a high BMI and those who have both a high BMI and associated medical comorbidities. Usually, obesity is not an isolated condition. Patients who are obese have an increased rate of associated chronic diseases, including diabetes mellitus, hyperlipidemia, hypertension, and coronary artery disease, all of which increase the baseline surgical risk.

Specific indications for THA in obese patients are the same as those in nonobese patients. Key indications for surgical management include intra-articular hip pain, radiographic evidence of joint degradation (**Figure 2**), functional limitation, and unsuccessful nonsurgical management. Underlying etiologies of joint degeneration are similar to those found in nonobese patients (**Table 2**). One study showed that obese patients who undergo THA are, on average, 13 years younger than nonobese patients who undergo THA. Other studies have supported the finding of the younger age of obese patients who undergo arthroplasty. The surgeon must keep this finding about the likelihood of future revision surgery in mind when counseling patients before the index procedure.

Contraindications

No definitive study has identified a BMI value as a specific contraindication to

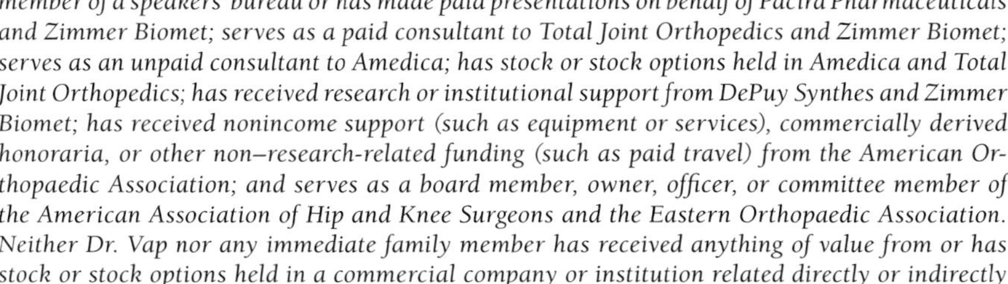

Dr. Bolognesi or an immediate family member has received royalties from Zimmer Biomet; is a member of a speakers' bureau or has made paid presentations on behalf of Pacira Pharmaceuticals and Zimmer Biomet; serves as a paid consultant to Total Joint Orthopedics and Zimmer Biomet; serves as an unpaid consultant to Amedica; has stock or stock options held in Amedica and Total Joint Orthopedics; has received research or institutional support from DePuy Synthes and Zimmer Biomet; has received nonincome support (such as equipment or services), commercially derived honoraria, or other non–research-related funding (such as paid travel) from the American Orthopaedic Association; and serves as a board member, owner, officer, or committee member of the American Association of Hip and Knee Surgeons and the Eastern Orthopaedic Association. Neither Dr. Vap nor any immediate family member has received anything of value from or has stock or stock options held in a commercial company or institution related directly or indirectly to the subject of this chapter.

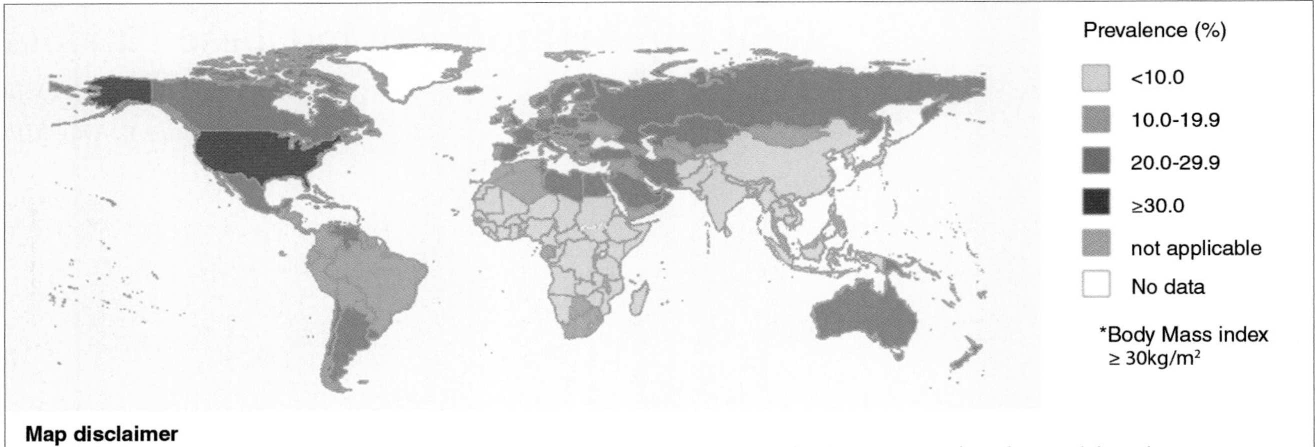

Map disclaimer
The boundaries and names shown and the designations used on this map do not imply the expression of any opinion whatsoever on the part of the World Health Organization concerning the legal status of any country, territory, city or area or of its authorities, or concerning the delimitation of its frontiers or boundaries. Dotted and dashed lines on maps represent border lines for which there may not yet be full agreement. The borders of the map provided reflect the current political geographic status as of the date of publication (2015). However, the technical health information is based on data accurate with respect to the year indicated (2014). The disconnect in this arrangement should be noted but no implications regarding political or terminological status should be drawn from this arrangement as it is purely a function of technical and graphical limitations.

Figure 1 Prevalence of obesity*, ages 18+, 2014 (age standardized estimate). Both sexes: 2014. (Reproduced with permission from World Health Organization: Prevalence of Obesity*, Ages 18+, 2014 [Age Standardized Estimate]: Both Sexes. Geneva, Switzerland, World Health Organization, 2015. http://gamapserver.who.int/gho/interactive_charts/ncd/risk_factors/obesity/atlas.html.)

Table 1 World Health Organization Classification of Obesity

Classification	Body Mass Index[a]	Risk of Comorbidities
Underweight	<18.50	Low (but risk of other clinical problems increased)
Normal range	18.50-24.99	Average
Overweight	≥25.00	—
Preobese	25.00-29.99	Increased
Obese class I	30.00-34.99	Moderate
Obese class II	35.00-39.99	Severe
Obese class III	≥40.00	Very severe

[a] Body mass index is calculated as the weight in kilograms divided by height in meters squared.

Adapted with permission from World Health Organization: *Obesity: Preventing and Managing the Global Epidemic. Report of a WHO Consultation*. Geneva, Switzerland (WHO Technical Report Series 894), 1999.

THA. Although reported complication rates have been mixed, the general trend in the literature has shown an increased risk of perioperative complications, including infection and revision rates, in patients with BMI greater than 35. Therefore, an American Association of Hip and Knee Surgeons workgroup recommended that patients with BMI greater than 40 be counseled regarding weight loss before surgical management.

Alternative Treatments

NSAIDs are the first line of symptomatic treatment of degenerative joint disease in any patient, irrespective of weight. Physical therapy, improved conditioning, and weight loss can help decrease the biomechanical stress on joints. If surgical intervention is ultimately performed, improved preoperative conditioning could have a positive effect on postoperative recovery and rehabilitation. Intra-articular corticosteroid injection has been shown to provide symptomatic relief. It also provides diagnostic information to support or confirm the physical examination and radiographic findings of a degenerative hip as the source of a patient's symptoms. However, the clinical benefit of injections has been shown to decrease over time and no prospective randomized controlled study has shown significant efficacy of injections. Bariatric surgery has been performed to lower a patient's BMI before THA. However, bariatric surgery has not been shown to be associated with improvement in postoperative complications or revision rates. In a study evaluating the effect of nonsurgical weight loss on outcomes,

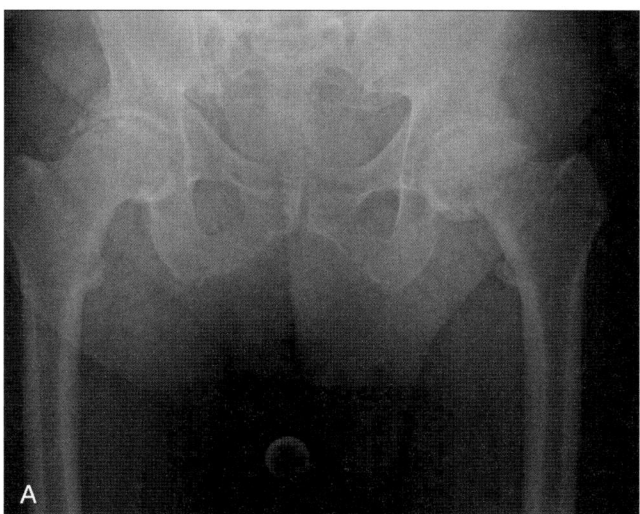

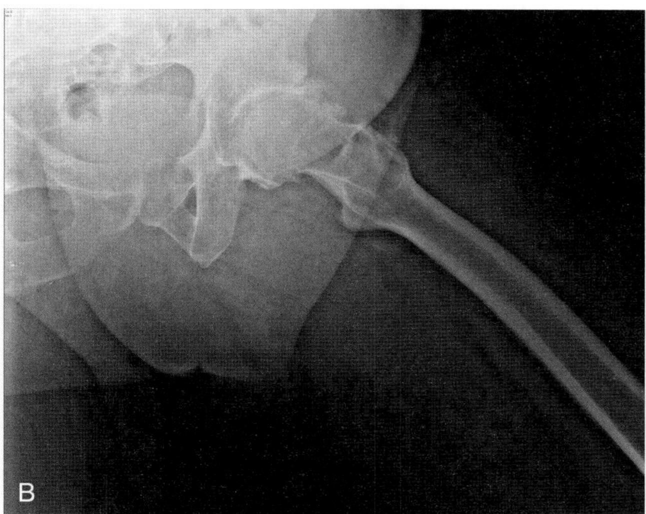

Figure 2 **A,** Low AP pelvic radiograph demonstrates substantial joint space loss with osteophyte formation in a left hip. A radiographic marker ball has been placed for use in digital templating. **B,** Lateral radiograph of the left hip demonstrates substantial joint space narrowing with posterior and anterior osteophytes.

no significant improvement in surgical site infection or readmission rates was found in obese patients who underwent THA or total knee arthroplasty after preoperative weight change (gain or loss).

Results

Results of THA in obese patients are summarized in **Table 3**. Early studies that examined outcomes of obese patients (BMI greater than 30) who underwent THA (cemented and noncemented) did not show significant differences in survivorship, complication rates, or functional and clinical outcome. Patients with BMI 30 or more who underwent THA experienced symptomatic improvement and satisfaction comparable with that of patients with BMI less than 30 in terms of outcome measures such as Harris hip score (HHS), Oxford Hip Score, Medical Outcomes Study 12-Item Short Form, pain scores, and patient satisfaction. Postoperative pain and function scores in obese patients are often substantially lower than those of nonobese patients; however, the mean changes within the groups from preoperative to postoperative status often are equivalent.

Table 2 Etiologies and Options for Management of Femoral and Acetabular Degenerative Disease

Etiology	Treatment Options
Osteoarthritis	NSAIDs, corticosteroids, physical therapy, arthroplasty
Rheumatoid arthritis	NSAIDs, disease-modifying antirheumatic drugs, arthroplasty
Osteonecrosis	Core decompression, vascularized graft, arthroplasty
Posttraumatic arthritis	NSAIDs, corticosteroids, physical therapy, arthroplasty
Slipped capital femoral epiphysis	Osteotomy, arthroplasty
Legg-Calvé-Perthes disease	Pelvic acetabular osteotomy, arthroplasty

A recent case-control study found that obese patients (BMI 30 or more) were significantly younger at the time of surgery. However, no difference was found in HHS improvement, patient satisfaction, orientation or radiologic loosening of the prosthesis, or incidence of postoperative complications. A recent large review of the New Zealand Joint Registry showed a significant difference in the age of patients undergoing THA, with younger age at time of surgery in patients with higher BMI. The study also showed surgical times for morbidly obese patients were up to 17.54 minutes longer, significantly higher 2-year revision rates in obese and morbidly obese patients, and significantly worse Oxford Hip Scores in obese and morbidly obese patients compared with nonobese patients. Data suggest that the degree of obesity can influence outcomes. In a study of 42 primary THA procedures in so-called super-obese patients (BMI 50 or more), the super-obese patients had a substantially increased risk of complication (hazard ratio 5.6; 95% confidence interval [CI], 2.8-11.0)

Table 3 Results of Total Hip Arthroplasty (THA) in Obese Patients

Authors (Year)	Number of Patients (Hips)	Procedure or Approach	Mean Body Mass Index[a]	Mean Patient Age in Years (Range)	Mean Follow-up (Range)	Results
Andrew et al (2008)[b]	BMI <30: 1,069 hips BMI 30-40: 330 hips BMI ≥40: 18 hips	Cemented primary THA Anterolateral or posterior approach	BMI <30: 25.1 BMI 30-40: 33.2 BMI ≥40: 44.8	BMI <30: 69.1 (21.3-94.9) BMI 30-40: 65.5 (33.4-86.9) BMI ≥40: 60.6 (28.5-78.0)	5 yr (NR)	No significant difference in dislocation rate, deep infection rate, calculated blood loss, DVT, pulmonary embolism, revision rate, implant position, LOS, or mean change of OHS between groups Patients with BMI ≥40 longer surgical time ($P = 0.005$)
Jackson et al (2009)[b]	BMI <30: 1,301 (1,612) BMI ≥30: 358 (414)	Noncemented primary THA Posterior approach	BMI <30: 25.0 BMI ≥30: 33.8	BMI <30: 68 (34-93) BMI ≥30: 63 (24-89)	6.3 yr (0-11.71 yr)	Complication rates NR No significant difference in survivorship rate between nonobese and obese patients at 11-yr follow-up (95.2% and 96.7%, respectively) The mean HHS was significantly higher in the nonobese group than in the obese group (93.2 and 89.9, respectively; $P < 0.001$) No significant difference in patient satisfaction between groups
Chee et al (2010)[c]	BMI <30 (control group): 53 BMI >40 alone or >35 and 1 medical comorbidity (study group): 53 (55)	Cemented primary THA Anterolateral approach	Control group: 25.5 Study group: 37.9	Control group: 63.7 (45-83) Study group: 63.6 (45-83)	5 yr (NR)	The complication rate was significantly higher in the study group than in the control group (22% and 5%, respectively; $P = 0.012$) HHS and SF-36 scores improved significantly in all groups ($P < 0.001$, for all) No significant difference in the mean improvement in HHS between study and control groups
Davis et al (2011)[c]	BMI <25: 455 BMI 25-29.9: 641 BMI 30-34.9: 373 BMI ≥35: 148	Cemented THA Anterolateral approach	NR	69 (34-96)	5 yr (NR)	Approximately 70% of patients were evaluated at mean 5-yr follow-up No significant increase in revision rate or deep infection rate Superficial infection rate was 3.37 times higher in patients with BMI >35 Dislocation rate increased by 113% per 10 units of BMI Surgical time increased by 3.16 minutes per 10 units of BMI Change in HHS decreased by 0.302 points per 1 unit of BMI but showed overall mean improvement
McCalden et al (2011)[c]	BMI <25: 647 BMI 25.0-29.9: 1,212 BMI 30.0-39.9: 1,225 BMI >40.0: 206	Cemented or noncemented primary THA Direct lateral approach	NR	BMI <25: 71.0 (23.77-95.74) BMI 25.0-29.9: 68.5 (23.33-94.46) BMI 30.0-39.9: 66.1 (23.1-90.1) BMI >40.0: 59.7[d] (26.51-82.36)	8.4 yr (2.0-20.3)	Revision rate highest for patients with BMI >40, but no significant difference between groups Patients with BMI >40 had lowest survivorship at 1, 2, 5, and 15 yr postoperatively Patients with BMI >40 had significantly higher rate of failure because of sepsis ($P = 0.045$) All groups had significant improvement in WOMAC, HHS, and SF-12 scores ($P < 0.001$, for all) Significant improvement in mean change of WOMAC ($P < 0.001$) and HHS ($P < 0.001$) in patients with BMI >40.0

BMI = body mass index, DVT = deep vein thrombosis, HHS = Harris hip score, LOS = length of stay, NR = not reported, OHS = Oxford Hip Score, SF-12 = Medical Outcomes Study 12-Item Short Form, SF-36 = Medical Outcomes Study 36-Item Short Form, WOMAC = Western Ontario and McMaster Universities Osteoarthritis Index.

[a] Body mass index is calculated as the weight in kilograms divided by height in meters squared.
[b] Level III evidence.
[c] Level II evidence.
[d] Significant difference.
[e] Level IV evidence.

Table 3 Results of Total Hip Arthroplasty (THA) in Obese Patients (*continued*)

Authors (Year)	Number of Patients (Hips)	Procedure or Approach	Mean Body Mass Index[a]	Mean Patient Age in Years (Range)	Mean Follow-up (Range)	Results
Michalka et al (2012)[c]	BMI <30: 113 BMI 30-34.99: 57 BMI ≥35: 21	Cemented or noncemented primary THA Approach NR	NR	BMI <30: 67.7 BMI 30-34.99: 67.6 BMI ≥35: 65.4	6 wk (NR)	Mean improvement was equivalent between groups for OHS, SF-12, pain score, and patient satisfaction No significant difference between groups in complication rate, LOS, calculated blood loss, or surgical time
Rajgopal et al (2013)[b]	BMI 18.5-24.9: 39 (39) BMI 30-39.90: 39 (39) BMI ≥50: 30 (39)	Noncemented primary THA Lateral or posterior approach	NR	BMI 18.5-24.9: 53.1 (29-72) BMI 30-39.90: 52.6 (30-72) BMI ≥50: 53.0 (31-72)	4.2 yr (2.0-11.7 yr)	Compared with obese and normal weight patients, super-obese patients had significantly higher major ($P = 0.01$) and minor ($P = 0.02$) mean complication rates, LOS ($P = 0.01$), and requirement for rehabilitation after leaving the hospital ($P < 0.001$) No significant differences between groups in changes of HHS or WOMAC
Arsoy et al (2014)[b]	Study group: 40 (42) Control group: 84	Noncemented primary THA Posterior or anterior approach	Study group: 53.2 Control group: 26.0	Study group: 56.4 (19-77) Control group: 56.7 (27-77)	5.2 yr (3.0-12.2 yr)	Study group had significantly increased risk of complications (hazard ratio 5.6; 95% CI, 2.8-11.0) 52% complication rate 12% required additional procedures Mean HHS improved from 35.0 to 74.8 in the study group ($P < 0.01$) and from 55.0 to 89.6 in the control group ($P < 0.01$)
McLaughlin and Lee (2014)[b]	105 (119)	Noncemented primary THA Posterolateral approach	34	NR	23 yr (18-27 yr)	47 patients (55 hips) were evaluated at 18-yr follow-up 91% implant survivorship and 99% survivorship with aseptic loosening as end point at 27 yr postoperatively At 23 yr postoperatively, HHS range was 56-87 2% complication rate No dislocation No wound issues
Murgatroyd et al (2014)[e]	BMI ≤18.5: 131 BMI 18.5-24.9: 1,136 BMI 25-29.99: 2,126 BMI 30-39.90: 1,745 BMI 40-49.99: 219	Noncemented or hybrid primary THA Approach NR	NR	BMI ≤18.5: 70.72 BMI 18.5-24.9: 69.28 BMI 25-29.99: 67.14 BMI 30-39.90: 64.43 BMI 40-49.99: 59.95	2.0 yr (NR)	2-yr revision rate significantly higher for obese (2.0%) and morbidly obese (2.3%) than for other groups ($P = 0.027$) OHS significantly lower in obese (39.5) and morbidly obese (36.7) groups than in other groups ($P < 0.001$)
Tai et al (2014)[b]	Study group: 82 Control group: 162	Noncemented primary THA Posterior approach	Study group: 34.2 Control group: 24.8	Study group: 58.8 Control group: 60.4	10.9 yr (NR)	Mean HHS improved from 52.4 to 88.9 in the study group ($P < 0.001$) and from 58.7 to 94.1 in the control group ($P < 0.001$) No significant increase in complications in the study group

BMI = body mass index, DVT = deep vein thrombosis, HHS = Harris hip score, LOS = length of stay, NR = not reported, OHS = Oxford Hip Score, SF-12 = Medical Outcomes Study 12-Item Short Form, SF-36 = Medical Outcomes Study 36-Item Short Form, WOMAC = Western Ontario and McMaster Universities Osteoarthritis Index.

[a] Body mass index is calculated as the weight in kilograms divided by height in meters squared.

[b] Level III evidence.

[c] Level II evidence.

[d] Significant difference.

[e] Level IV evidence.

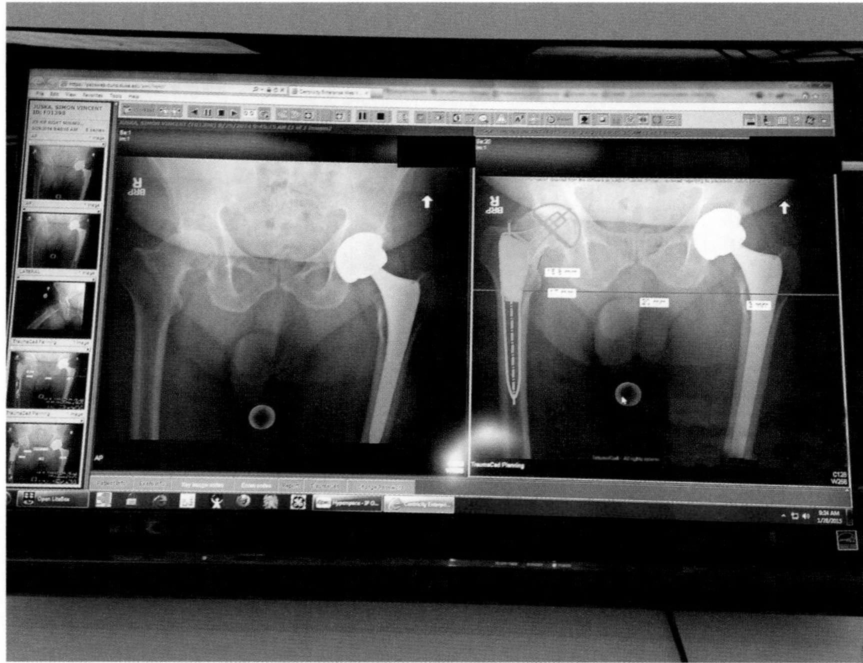

Figure 3 Photograph shows a preoperative low AP pelvic radiograph that demonstrates joint space narrowing with subchondral sclerosis of the right hip and previous total hip arthroplasty in the left hip (left image) and a low AP pelvic radiograph of the same patient with digital arthroplasty templating (right image), displayed in the operating room.

Table 4 Surgical Approaches for Total Hip Arthroplasty in Obese Patients

Approach	Patient Positioning	Positioning Devices	Assistive Devices
Anterior	Supine	Specialized surgical table for anterior approach	Abdominal binder/corset Retractable adhesive tape
Anterolateral	Lateral decubitus	None	None
Direct lateral	Lateral decubitus	Hip positioner	Foam padding
Posterior	Lateral decubitus	Hip positioner	Foam padding

when compared with a matched control group, despite significant improvement in mean HHS from 35 to 74.8. Additionally, the average length of hospital stay was significantly longer in the obese group than in the control group (6.4 and 4.3 days, respectively). Similar results for patients with BMI greater than 40 also have been reported in earlier studies that examined outcomes in morbidly obese patients.

Techniques

Setup/Exposure

- Preoperative planning and templating is highly recommended for THA in obese patients to ensure the availability of appropriate implant sizes and provide insight into potential intraoperative complications.
- Preoperative low AP pelvic and lateral radiographs and a preoperative low AP pelvicradiograph with overlying implant templating should be displayed in the operating room (**Figure 3**). The radiographs provide intraoperative reference for pelvic and femoral anatomy and implant positioning and sizing.
- Any of the approaches listed in **Table 4** can be used in obese patients. The choice of surgical approach is based on the surgeon's preference. However, preoperative evaluation of a patient's body habitus and fat distribution may influence the selection of the approach.
- Patient positioning and the use of positioning devices depend on surgeon preference and the surgical approach (**Table 4**).
- Pelvic stability is paramount in obese patients. Lack of pelvic stability can affect acetabular cup positioning and the ability to reduce trial and final implants (**Figure 4**).
- Prepping and draping of an extensive surgical field is important in obese patients to provide an adequate sterile area for an extensile surgical approach. A large surgical field also provides flexibility to alter the surgical plan if an intraoperative complication occurs (**Figure 5**).
- The authors of this chapter recommend that an extensile approach be used in obese patients even if a small-incision technique is the surgeon's standard practice in nonobese patients.

Instruments/Equipment/Implants Required

- The choice of surgical table depends on the surgical approach.
- The use of inflatable sliding devices can expedite preoperative and postoperative patient positioning.
- Large retractors and self-retaining retractors with deep blades should be available for use (**Figure 6**).

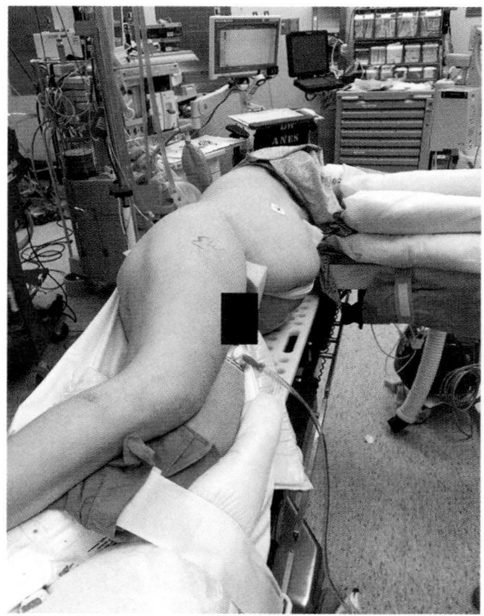

Figure 4 Intraoperative photograph shows a patient in the lateral decubitus position. Pelvic stability is critical, and pressure areas are well padded to prevent pressure sores.

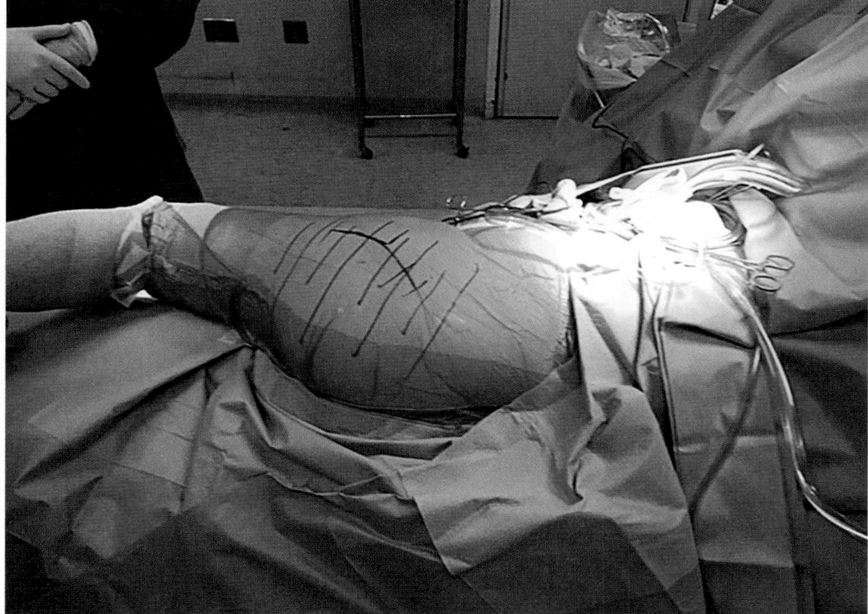

Figure 5 Intraoperative photograph shows an extensive surgical field, which allows use of an extensile approach if necessary.

- Intraoperative radiography (low AP pelvic view) can provide real-time information to verify implant positioning and sizing (**Figure 7**).
- Implants of appropriate size must be available. Standard implants can be used according to surgeon preference.
- Standard surgical tables are adequate for most patients.
- The presence of an extra surgical assistant in the operating room is helpful.

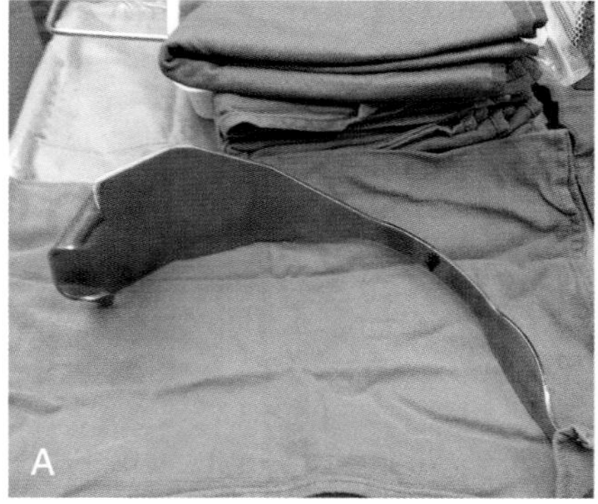

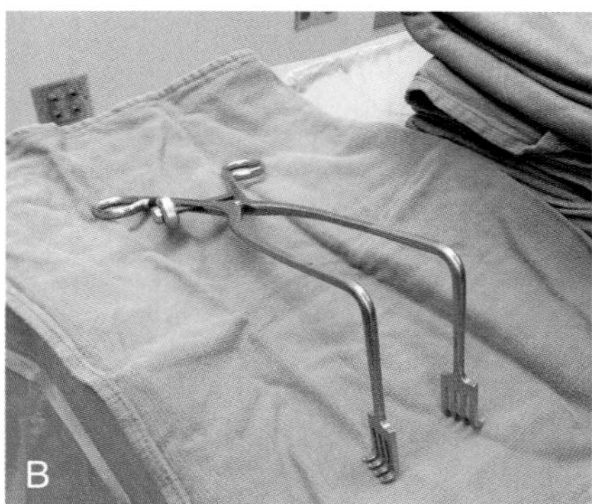

Figure 6 Photographs show a large-belly cobra retractor (**A**) and a large self-retaining retractor (**B**).

Procedure

ACETABULAR PREPARATION

- Appropriate acetabular exposure is critical to ensure appropriate positioning of the cup in 35° to 45° of abduction and 10° to 20° of anteversion.
- Retractors are placed superiorly, anteriorly, and inferiorly to enable adequate visualization.
- Labral tissues are removed to prevent soft-tissue interposition during placement of the acetabular cup.
- The cotyloid fossa must be adequately visualized. If preoperative radiographs demonstrate osteophyte concealment of the medial wall and teardrop, the osteophytes are resected with an osteotome or curet before reaming.
- Acetabular preparation begins with medialization. Reaming begins with the use of a reamer 4 to 5 mm smaller than the templated cup size or intraoperative femoral head size measurement.
- Medialization is carried nearly to the floor of the cotyloid fossa. The center of rotation for the acetabulum should be placed in 35° to 45° of abduction and 10° to 20° of anteversion. In obese patients, appropriate positioning of reamers is paramount during this step. Surgical dissection is extended if needed to prevent poor cup positioning.
- After the center of rotation has been established, the reamer size is incrementally increased

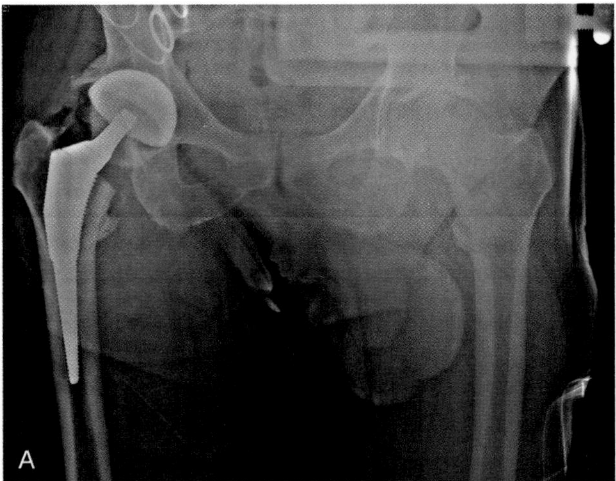

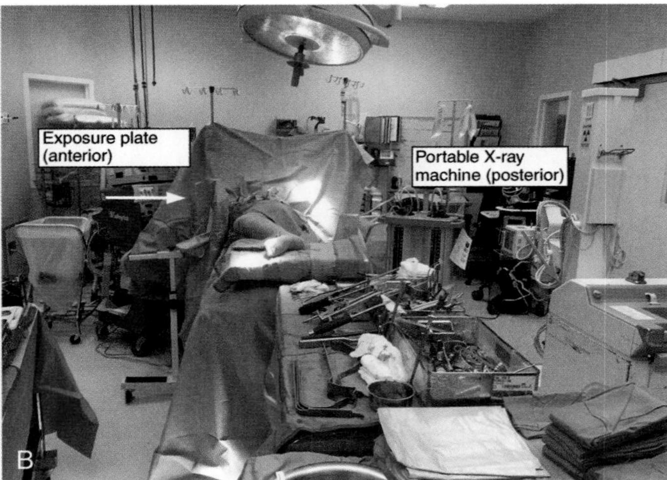

Figure 7 **A,** Intraoperative AP pelvic radiograph demonstrates the position and sizing of implants. A low AP pelvic radiograph allows visualization of both femurs (for limb-length evaluation) and the pelvis. **B,** Intraoperative photograph shows the use of a portable radiographic machine positioned near the posterior aspect of the patient's hip (red arrow). The radiographic exposure plate is placed anteriorly (white arrow). A sterile drape is used to prevent contamination of the surgical field. The green towel that has been placed on the patient provides a reference point for the radiography technician to ensure correct plate alignment superoinferiorly.

until circumferential reaming shows subchondral bleeding from the acetabulum.

- The final implant size should be 1 to 2 mm greater than the size of the last reamer.

FEMORAL PREPARATION

- Femoral preparation in obese patients is similar to that in nonobese patients.
- Adequate exposure is paramount to ensure protection of surrounding soft tissues and allow optimal sizing and positioning of the femoral implant.
- Femoral preparation depends on the surgeon's preference of proximal or diaphyseal fixation of the femoral prosthesis.
- A femoral canal finder is placed to help prevent cortical breach resulting from the use of reamers and/or broaches.
- Lateralization throughout the femoral preparation process helps avoid subsequent varus positioning of the implant.
- If possible, femoral broaches are placed in approximately 10° to 15° of anteversion to ensure appropriate version of the final implant.

IMPLANT TRIALING

- The hip is reduced and assessed for stability, leg length, range of motion, and anterior or posterior impingement.
- If necessary, adjustments can be made to change from a standard to a high-offset femoral neck and/or exchange the implant for different femoral head and neck sizes.
- Intraoperative radiography can be used to evaluate acetabular and femoral implant sizing and positioning.

Wound Closure

- The wound is thoroughly irrigated.
- If there is substantial fluid extravasation from the tissues at the end of the procedure, a drain should be placed.
- The deep fascial layer is closed completely and tightly with nonabsorbable suture in a figure-of-8 fashion or a barbed monofilament suture.
- The large subcutaneous tissue and the dead space are closed with a running or interrupted absorbable or monofilament suture to facilitate approximation of the skin.
- The subcutaneous tissue is closed with an absorbable or monofilament suture.
- The skin edges are carefully everted at the time of wound closure.
- Skin may be closed with subcuticular stitches or staples, per the surgeon's preference.

Postoperative Regimen

Because obese patients are at higher risk of dislocation than nonobese patients, strict hip precautions are instituted postoperatively. The use of a hip abduction pillow is recommended for 24 hours postoperatively or until physical therapy begins. A comprehensive physical therapy team that is experienced in working with THA patients is paramount. In the early postoperative rehabilitation period, additional physical therapists and/or precautions are necessary when physical therapists work with obese patients because of the physical demands on the therapists themselves.

Because the concern for implant subsidence has not been supported in the literature, patients are allowed to bear weight as tolerated. However, if the surgeon prefers, weight bearing can be restricted for 6 weeks postoperatively. A comprehensive fall precaution plan should be in place, and all nursing and support staff should be aware of the plan to help prevent in-hospital falls.

Because of the high incidence of comorbidities in obese patients, postoperative medical management is critical. Tight blood glucose control is important in patients with diabetes. Primary medical management by in-hospital internal medicine specialists is recommended.

Deep vein thrombosis (DVT) prophylaxis is critical. At the institution of the authors of this chapter, patients typically are placed on aspirin at 325 mg bid, which is continued for 35 days postoperatively. A sequential compression device is used while the patient is in the hospital. Additional prophylaxis is necessary in sedentary patients. Patients with a history of DVT or pulmonary embolism are placed on prophylactic weight-based dosing of enoxaparin at discharge.

Avoiding Pitfalls and Complications

Meticulous wound closure is crucial to limit wound-healing complications. If the patient's nutritional status is identified preoperatively as a concern, a preoperative evaluation is useful to facilitate postoperative wound healing.

Two studies have shown increased infection rates in patients considered to be morbidly obese. In one study, the risk of wound infection after THA was 1.6% in nonobese patients and 3.5% in obese patients. If infection is suspected in the early postoperative period, the authors of this chapter recommend aggressive management with early irrigation and débridement and liner exchange.

Obese patients have a high rate of obstructive sleep apnea, which has been shown to increase the complication rate in patients undergoing total joint arthroplasty. It is recommended that all obese patients undergo a complete evaluation and workup for obstructive sleep apnea prior to THA. Patients who use assistive breathing devices at home are instructed to bring their device to use during their hospital stay. A respiratory therapist should be consulted postoperatively to ensure proper evaluation and management of the patient's needs.

Obese patients are at increased risk of dislocation, and the risk is higher in women than men. This risk has been shown to increase as BMI increases. To reduce the risk of dislocation, the patient is placed on a hip abduction pillow postoperatively. Before early mobilization, the patient is evaluated and treated by physical and occupational therapists who have extensive experience with hip arthroplasty patients and take the necessary precautions to prevent dislocation. To reduce the risk of periprosthetic fracture, the authors of this chapter recommend a comprehensive fall prevention program on all postoperative care floors of the hospital.

One study showed a trend toward combined insufficient anteversion and overabduction of the acetabular cup in patients with BMI greater than 35. Preoperative templating, consistent patient positioning, and intraoperative radiography can help ensure correct implant positioning.

Obesity is one of the two most common risk factors associated with venous thromboembolism. In one study, obesity increased the risk of DVT and pulmonary embolism from 2.2% to 3.3%. As discussed previously, the use of anticoagulants and a sequential compression device is essential. If the patient is sedentary, an anticoagulant that is more potent than aspirin should be used.

Bibliography

Andrew JG, Palan J, Kurup HV, Gibson P, Murray DW, Beard DJ: Obesity in total hip replacement. *J Bone Joint Surg Br* 2008;90(4):424-429.

Arsoy D, Woodcock JA, Lewallen DG, Trousdale RT: Outcomes and complications following total hip arthroplasty in the super-obese patient, BMI >50. *J Arthroplasty* 2014;29(10):1899-1905.

Bourne R, Mukhi S, Zhu N, Keresteci M, Marin M: Role of obesity on the risk for total hip or knee arthroplasty. *Clin Orthop Relat Res* 2007;465:185-188.

Changulani M, Kalairajah Y, Peel T, Field RE: The relationship between obesity and the age at which hip and knee replacement is undertaken. *J Bone Joint Surg Br* 2008;90(3):360-363.

Chee YH, Teoh KH, Sabnis BM, Ballantyne JA, Brenkel IJ: Total hip replacement in morbidly obese patients with osteoarthritis: Results of a prospectively matched study. *J Bone Joint Surg Br* 2010;92(8):1066-1071.

Davis AM, Wood AM, Keenan AC, Brenkel IJ, Ballantyne JA: Does body mass index affect clinical outcome post-operatively and at five years after primary unilateral total hip replacement performed for osteoarthritis? A multivariate analysis of prospective data. *J Bone Joint Surg Br* 2011;93(9):1178-1182.

Elson LC, Barr CJ, Chandran SE, Hansen VJ, Malchau H, Kwon YM: Are morbidly obese patients undergoing total hip arthroplasty at an increased risk for component malpositioning? *J Arthroplasty* 2013;28(8 suppl):41-44.

Inacio MC, Paxton EW, Fisher D, Li RA, Barber TC, Singh JA: Bariatric surgery prior to total joint arthroplasty may not provide dramatic improvements in post-arthroplasty surgical outcomes. *J Arthroplasty* 2014;29(7):1359-1364.

Jackson MP, Sexton SA, Yeung E, Walter WL, Walter WK, Zicat BA: The effect of obesity on the mid-term survival and clinical outcome of cementless total hip replacement. *J Bone Joint Surg Br* 2009;91(10):1296-1300.

McCalden RW, Charron KD, MacDonald SJ, Bourne RB, Naudie DD: Does morbid obesity affect the outcome of total hip replacement? An analysis of 3290 THRs. *J Bone Joint Surg Br* 2011;93(3):321-325.

McLaughlin JR, Lee KR: Uncemented total hip arthroplasty using a tapered femoral component in obese patients: An 18-27 year follow-up study. *J Arthroplasty* 2014;29(7):1365-1368.

Michalka PK, Khan RJ, Scaddan MC, Haebich S, Chirodian N, Wimhurst JA: The influence of obesity on early outcomes in primary hip arthroplasty. *J Arthroplasty* 2012;27(3):391-396.

Moran M, Walmsley P, Gray A, Brenkel IJ: Does body mass index affect the early outcome of primary total hip arthroplasty? *J Arthroplasty* 2005;20(7):866-869.

Murgatroyd SE, Frampton CM, Wright MS: The effect of body mass index on outcome in total hip arthroplasty: Early analysis from the New Zealand Joint Registry. *J Arthroplasty* 2014;29(10):1884-1888.

Parvizi J, Trousdale RT, Sarr MG: Total joint arthroplasty in patients surgically treated for morbid obesity. *J Arthroplasty* 2000;15(8):1003-1008.

Rajgopal R, Martin R, Howard JL, Somerville L, MacDonald SJ, Bourne R: Outcomes and complications of total hip replacement in super-obese patients. *Bone Joint J* 2013;95-B(6):758-763.

Severson EP, Singh JA, Browne JA, Trousdale RT, Sarr MG, Lewallen DG: Total knee arthroplasty in morbidly obese patients treated with bariatric surgery: A comparative study. *J Arthroplasty* 2012;27(9):1696-1700.

Tai SM, Imbuldeniya AM, Munir S, Walter WL, Walter WK, Zicat BA: The effect of obesity on the clinical, functional and radiological outcome of cementless total hip replacement: A case-matched study with a minimum 10-year follow-up. *J Arthroplasty* 2014;29(9):1758-1762.

Wallace G, Judge A, Prieto-Alhambra D, de Vries F, Arden NK, Cooper C: The effect of body mass index on the risk of post-operative complications during the 6 months following total hip replacement or total knee replacement surgery. *Osteoarthritis Cartilage* 2014;22(7):918-927.

Workgroup of the American Association of Hip and Knee Surgeons Evidence Based Committee: Obesity and total joint arthroplasty: A literature based review. *J Arthroplasty* 2013;28(5):714-721.

Chapter 31
Total Hip Arthroplasty in Patients With Sickle Cell Hemoglobinopathy

Gregory G. Polkowski, MD, MSc
Adam C. Brekke, MD

Indications

Osteonecrosis of the femoral head is a common musculoskeletal manifestation of sickle cell hemoglobinopathy. Advanced osteonecrosis causes substantial pain, reduced activity levels, and limited functional capability, and patients with sickle cell disease are affected at an especially young age (average range, 20 to 29 years). Total hip arthroplasty (THA) in patients with sickle cell disease presents challenges different from those encountered in typical patients with osteoarthritis. These challenges historically have resulted in complications or suboptimal outcomes of THA in many patients with sickle cell disease. With advances in preoperative, intraoperative, and postoperative management, THA has become increasingly effective in the management of femoral head osteonecrosis in patients with sickle cell disease.

Pathophysiology

The underlying pathophysiology of sickle cell disease and the consequent associated syndromes create an environment that predisposes patients to femoral head osteonecrosis and other musculoskeletal conditions. An understanding of the pathophysiology is essential for effective treatment. Sickle cell hemoglobinopathies can result in anemia, recurrent painful crises, and chronic end-organ dysfunction. Anemia results from intravascular hemolysis of the rigid, sickle-shaped red blood cells and the decreased hematopoietic potential resulting from splenic infarction. Painful crises result from the sickling of red blood cells in an environment of low oxygen tension and increased stress. Chronic end-organ failure can result from multiple ischemic episodes.

Musculoskeletal manifestations of sickle cell hemoglobinopathy include pyogenic infection, bone marrow hyperplasia, and osteonecrosis. Pyogenic infections occur secondary to splenic autoinfarction, which increases susceptibility to polysaccharide-encapsulated pathogens such as *Streptococcus pneumoniae*, *Salmonella*, and *Klebsiella*. Bacteremia can result in subsequent hematogenous bacterial seeding in bones and joints. This disease-specific susceptibility can present challenges in joint arthroplasty. Bone marrow hyperplasia results from splenic autoinfarction and the secondary increase in bone erythropoiesis. Characteristic widening of the medullary canal and thinning of the trabeculae and cortices are especially prominent in metaphyseal long bone such as the proximal femur.

A common manifestation of sickle cell disease is osteonecrosis, which results from vascular thrombosis and infarction. Hypoxia induces the sickling of red blood cells, which, in combination with the extravascular compression of the intraosseous blood supply caused by medullary hyperplasia, leads to microvascular occlusion, ischemia, and bone infarction. Repeated episodes of this occlusion result in focal and patchy areas of sclerosis. Medullary hyperplasia and osteonecrosis can occur concurrently, resulting in medullary widening and an obliterated metadiaphyseal canal. These disease processes pose challenges in intramedullary reaming and prosthesis fitting, insertion, and fixation during THA.

The incidence of femoral head osteonecrosis related to sickle cell disease ranges from 3% to 50%, with high rates seen not only in patients who are homozygous for the sickle cell gene but also in patients who are heterozygous for the sickle cell gene and in those with sickle β-thalassemia. The clinical severity depends on the rate and extent of polymerization of hemoglobin S molecules and the disturbance in erythrocyte architecture.

Dr. Polkowski or an immediate family member serves as a board member, owner, officer, or committee member of the American Association of Hip and Knee Surgeons. Neither Dr. Brekke nor any immediate family member has received anything of value from or has stock or stock options held in a commercial company or institution related directly or indirectly to the subject of this chapter.

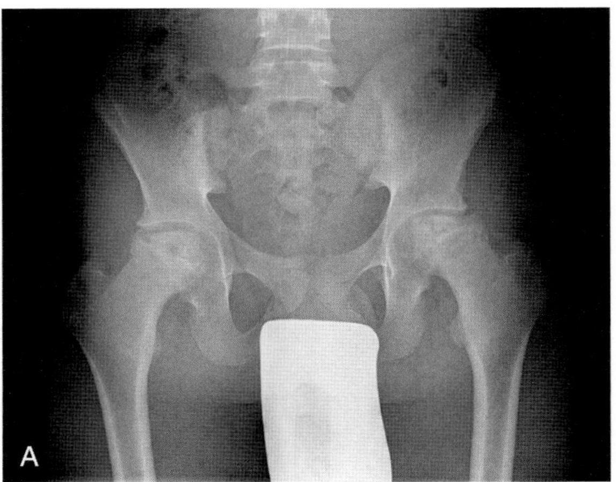

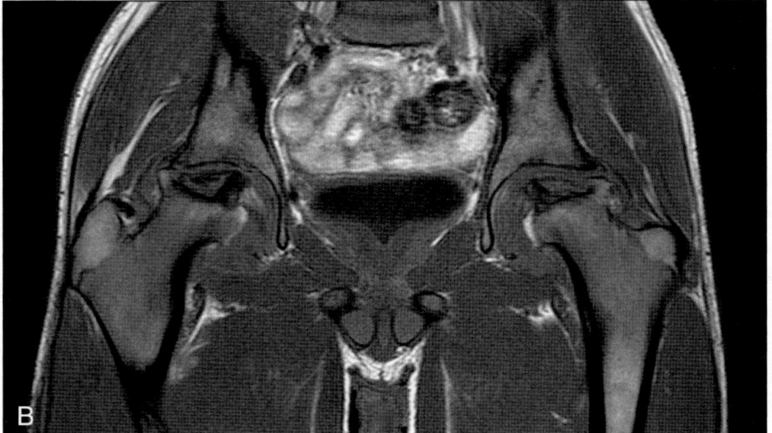

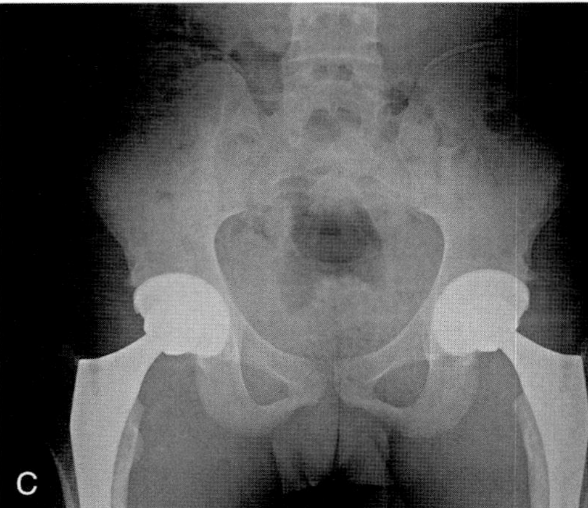

Figure 1 **A,** AP pelvic radiograph demonstrates advanced osteonecrosis with bilateral femoral head collapse, resulting in bilateral hip pain in a 13-year-old boy with sickle cell disease. **B,** Coronal T1-weighted MRI demonstrates a region of osteonecrosis limited to the femoral head. No areas of bone infarction are present in the remainder of the proximal femurs. **C,** Postoperative AP pelvic radiograph demonstrates the same patient after staged bilateral total hip arthroplasty performed over a 1-year period.

Clinical Presentation and Management

Patients with sickle cell disease who have femoral head osteonecrosis report characteristic symptoms similar to those reported by patients with osteonecrosis resulting from other etiologies. These symptoms can include groin pain, difficulty of ambulation, and painful and limited hip range of motion. Nonsurgical treatment consists of pain management, usually with NSAIDs and/or opiates, and the use of assistive devices for ambulation. After hip osteonecrosis becomes symptomatic in patients with sickle cell disease, the likelihood of progression to femoral head collapse is high. At the time of presentation, more than 40% of the femoral head is likely already affected. Without surgical intervention, the underlying bony infarctions persist and the degenerative changes advance, resulting in worsening symptoms and marked disability. Therefore, the primary indication for surgical treatment is intractable, persistent, and disabling hip pain refractory to nonsurgical treatment in a patient with a severely damaged hip joint. Because the root pathophysiology is systemic, hip involvement is often bilateral. Even if symptoms are unilateral, patients often have early radiographic evidence of bilateral involvement (**Figure 1**).

Contraindications

Surgical intervention is contraindicated in patients with sickle cell disease who are not medically fit for surgical treatment.

Alternative Treatments

Alternative surgical treatments include core decompression, femoral osteotomy, arthrodesis, hemiarthroplasty, and resection arthroplasty. The utility of core decompression has been questioned. One study showed no clinical improvement after core decompression and physical therapy versus physical therapy alone, with no significant differences in occurrences of major complications or episodes of acute chest syndrome. The author of a different study postulated that although core decompression can alleviate elevated intraosseous pressures resulting from marrow hyperplasia, it does not address the vaso-occlusion and the often diffuse femoral head involvement or reduce the strong probability of future infarctions. Arthrodesis is an undesirable option because of the frequency of bilateral hip involvement. Hemiarthroplasty often results in poor outcomes because of the soft acetabular bone stock in patients with chronic marrow hyperplasia. Femoral osteotomy can relieve only focal areas of osteonecrosis, whereas most patients with sickle cell disease have more diffuse involvement and can expect chronic progression. These options are not recommended except in unusual circumstances. Resection arthroplasty is best reserved as a salvage procedure for use after failure of THA. It is rarely indicated as a primary treatment both because of the likelihood of bilateral involvement and because the potential benefits are less than those of THA.

Results

Most published studies of THA in patients with sickle cell disease are level IV case series. Historically, the results of THA for the management of femoral head osteonecrosis in patients with sickle cell disease were fraught with intraoperative complications, medical complications, and infections, and demonstrated poor survivorship compared with that of conventional THA. The nature of the disease inherently predisposes patients to complications. After adjustment to account for confounders, the odds ratio for all complications after THA is 2.52 in patients with sickle cell disease compared with patients without sickle cell disease. Advances in medical management and surgical technique have improved results. Recent studies have shown good to excellent outcomes, with greatly improved survivorship, and have demonstrated that contemporary THA is an effective, beneficial therapy in patients with sickle cell disease (**Table 1**).

The debate regarding cemented versus noncemented implants has not been conclusively resolved in the literature. Advocates of cemented fixation argue that it avoids the risks associated with noncemented fixation, such as canal perforation during preparation and poor biologic ingrowth in bone that is compromised by osteonecrosis. A study of cemented implants published in 2008, with an extensive reported patient database and a comprehensive perioperative management protocol, demonstrated improvement from the results of earlier studies in which cemented implants were used. However, most surgeons in the United States use noncemented implants, citing substantially lower rates of loosening and failure and a decreased infection rate. No randomized controlled trials comparing the two fixation methods have been performed.

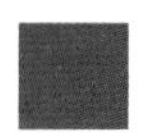

Techniques

Setup/Exposure

- Antibiotics consisting of a first-generation cephalosporin and vancomycin are initiated before induction of anesthesia. The use of prophylactic vancomycin in addition to a cephalosporin is a practice used at the chapter authors' institution at the recommendation of hospital epidemiologists because of the high institutional prevalence of methicillin-resistant staphylococcal species.
- Neuraxial anesthesia should be used instead of general anesthesia when possible because the temporary sympathectomy provided by the use of neuraxial anesthesia can reduce the likelihood of a sickle cell crisis.
- The patient is positioned in accordance with the surgical approach that will be used.
- The choice of surgical exposure and approach depends on the preference and experience of the surgeon. For most patients, the surgeon's preferred approach for THA should be used.
- However, in patients with extensive femoral sclerosis that extends into the metaphyseal region of the femur (**Figure 2**), the surgeon should use an approach that facilitates access to the proximal femur in case it is necessary to perform reaming of the femoral canal for femoral preparation.
- The authors of this chapter prefer a posterior approach because of the versatility of this approach and the relative ease with which adjuvant stem preparation techniques, such as high-speed burr disruption of sclerotic bone in alignment with the proximal femur, can be incorporated into the procedure.
- The patient is prepped and draped in the standard manner.
- Initial exposure is obtained in the standard manner.

Instruments/Equipment/Implants Required

- The choice of instrumentation should be consistent with the usual practice of the surgeon.
- Because of the high incidence of sclerotic bone in the proximal femur, the authors of this chapter recommend the use of a radiolucent table for all THA procedures in patients with sickle cell disease so that fluoroscopy can be used to assist with alignment and implant preparation.

Table 1 Results of Total Hip Arthroplasty in Patients With Sickle Cell Hemoglobinopathy[a]

Authors (Year)	Number of Patients (Hips)	Implant Type	Mean Patient Age in Years (Range)	Mean Follow-up in Years (Range)	Success Rate (%)[b]	Results
Clarke et al (1989)	15 (27)	13 cemented, 14 noncemented	33 (19-56)	>2	41	23% loosening rate 59% revision rate
Acurio and Friedman (1992)	25 (25)	17 cemented, 18 noncemented	30 (16-45)	8.6 (2-18)	60 overall (cemented, 41; noncemented, 78)	49% complication rate 20% infection rate 94% of cemented implants were loose or required revision 39% of noncemented implants were loose or required revision
Moran et al (1993)	12 (15)	13 cemented, 2 noncemented	37 (17-58)	4.8 (2.2-10.4)	62	Mean HHS, 88 13% intraoperative complication rate 30% aseptic loosening rate 8% infection rate All revisions were of cemented implants
Sanjay and Moreau (1996)	21 (26)	Noncemented	27 (15-47)	4.6 (2.1-7)	92	Mean HHS, 88 65% complication rate 19.2% intraoperative complication rate
Hickman and Lachiewicz (1997)	10 (15)	13 noncemented, 2 cemented	40 (21-50)	6 (2-12)	66	75% early postoperative complication rate (≤2 yr) 3 noncemented and 2 cemented implants required revision
Al-Mousawi et al (2002)	28 (35)	Cemented	27.5 (19-42)	9.5 (5-15)	80	Mean HHS, 86 (range, 68-97)
Ilyas and Moreau (2002)	18 (36)	Noncemented	28 (17-39)	5.7 (2-10)	97.3	25% complication rate 2.7% intraoperative complication rate 5.5% medical complication rate 5.5% infection rate Revisions were aseptic
Hernigou et al (2008)	244 (312)	Cemented	32 (18-51)	13 (5-25)	83.5	28% medical complication rate 13% intraoperative complication rate 7.7% postoperative complication rate 9.9% late postoperative complication rate (time postoperatively was not defined) 3% of revisions were septic
Issa et al (2013)	32 (42)	Noncemented	37 (18-58)	7.5 (5-11)	88.1	Mean HHS, 87 (range, 78-100) Mean Medical Outcomes Study 36-Item Short Form scores: physical, 43 (range, 34-55); mental, 59 (range, 53-64) No intraoperative complications 4.7% of revisions were septic

HHS = Harris hip score.

[a] Level of evidence is IV for all studies.

[b] Success is defined as procedures not requiring revision.

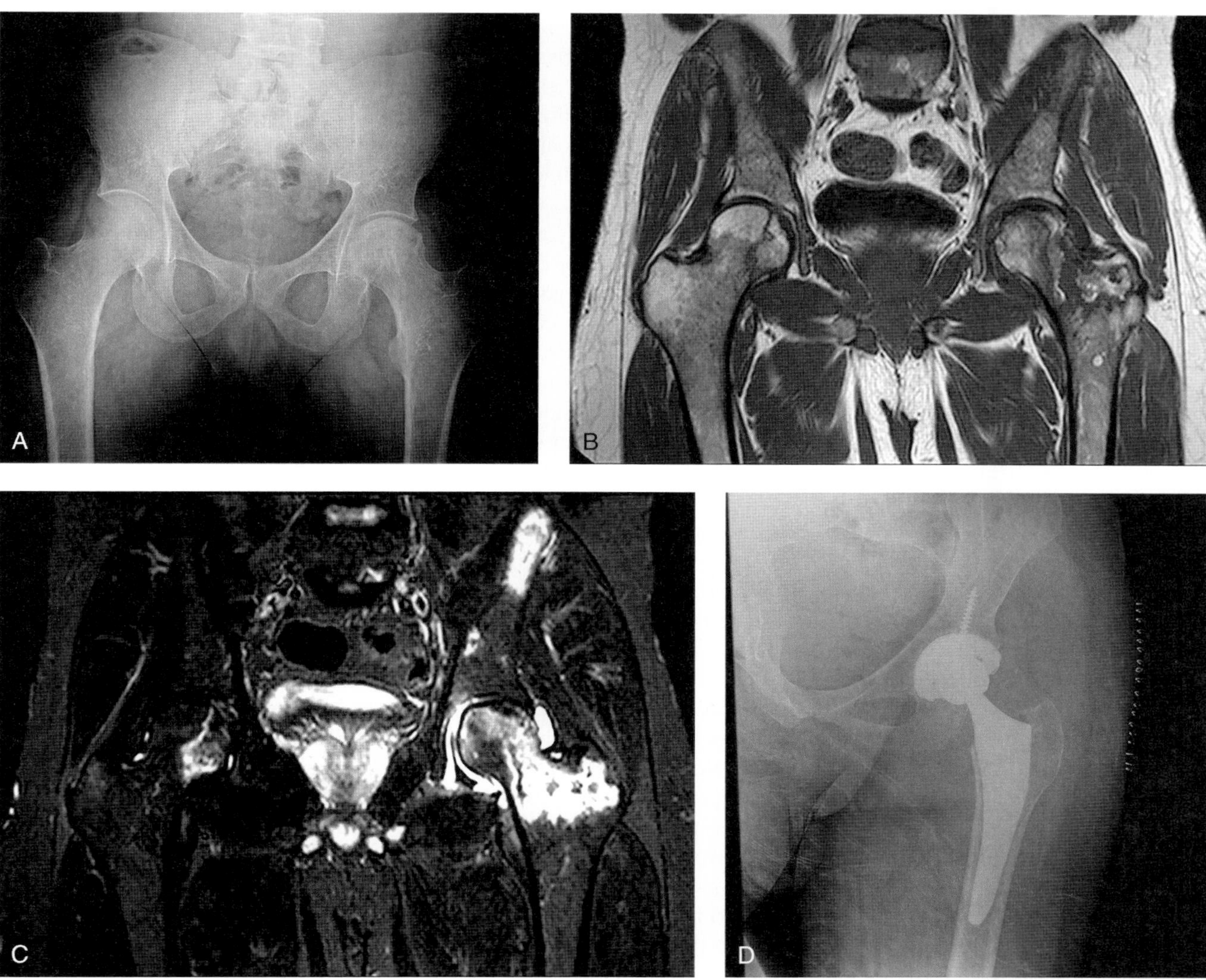

Figure 2 **A,** AP pelvic radiograph demonstrates symptomatic left hip osteonecrosis with femoral head collapse in a 32-year-old man with sickle cell disease. Coronal T1-weighted (**B**) and short tau inversion recovery (**C**) MRI demonstrate the extension of osteonecrosis from the femoral head into the femoral neck and the upper portion of the intertrochanteric region. Because of this condition, the use of a high-speed burr was required for assistance in femoral preparation. **D,** Postoperative AP radiograph demonstrates the same patient after total hip arthroplasty of the left hip. Because the affected bone was limited to the most proximal extent of the intertrochanteric region and healthy bone was present distally, a standard proximally coated, tapered stem was used.

- In addition to routine THA equipment, a high-speed burr, drill bits of varied sizes, and extra reamers should be available to assist with femoral preparation through frequently sclerotic metaphyseal femoral bone.
- Because of the improvements in noncemented femoral fixation, the authors of this chapter prefer to use noncemented implants for THA in patients with sickle cell disease. Proximally coated tapered stems can be used if observation of the bone quality after femoral preparation reveals viable bleeding bone, which is necessary to ensure adequate stem ingrowth. In patients with severe proximal femoral necrosis, fully coated stems may be necessary.
- Most patients with sickle cell disease who require THA are younger than the average patient requiring THA for the management of osteoarthritis. Although many bearing surface options are available for use in young patients, the authors of this chapter prefer the use of zirconia-alumina ceramic on highly cross-linked polyethylene.
- Adjuvant screw fixation of the acetabular implant is recommended if

the acetabular preparation reveals areas of sclerotic, necrotic bone.

Procedure

- Acetabular exposure and reaming are performed with careful inspection of acetabular bone.
- Adjuvant screw fixation of the acetabular implant is recommended in patients with acetabular osteonecrosis.
- Femoral preparation is begun in standard manner.
- In patients in whom the diseased femoral bone is isolated to the femoral head, routine femoral stem preparation can be accomplished.
- In patients with sclerotic islands of necrotic metaphyseal bone, care is taken to avoid perforation of the femoral cortex. Intraoperative fluoroscopy can be helpful in reestablishing the femoral canal. Broaching in sclerotic femoral bone can result in intraoperative fracture. If sclerotic bone is encountered, removal with a high-speed burr can facilitate femoral preparation.
- Intraoperative fluoroscopy or plain radiography can be helpful to confirm appropriate positioning of the canal finder and/or broach.
- If extensive necrotic metaphyseal bone is encountered, a fully coated, diaphyseally engaging femoral stem is used.

Wound Closure

- The wound is closed in layers in standard manner.
- Use of a deep surgical drain depends on surgeon preference.

Postoperative Regimen

The typical postoperative regimen after THA is followed in terms of activity and rehabilitation goals. An exercise program is performed independently or under the supervision of a physical therapist until the patient's gait normalizes. The choice of deep vein thrombosis prophylaxis is made on an individual basis. In patients with a history of deep vein thrombosis or pulmonary embolism, aggressive chemical prophylaxis in the form of warfarin or low-molecular-weight heparin should be considered. In patients who will undergo a rapid rehabilitation protocol with early ambulation and who do not have a history of thrombosis, the use of aspirin and mechanical prophylaxis can be considered. Routine postoperative hematology consultations are necessary to assist in managing the disease and preventing sickle cell crises. Hematologic management typically includes liberal red blood cell transfusion thresholds and aggressive pulmonary hygiene to maintain adequate oxygen delivery and blood oxygenation and to prevent sickle cell crises and acute chest syndrome. Postoperative pain management can be challenging because many patients with sickle cell disease are narcotic dependent preoperatively because of frequent pain crises related to the disease. Involvement of the hematologist in postoperative care can be beneficial in determining narcotic requirements because the hematologist typically is familiar with the patient's narcotic consumption requirements.

Avoiding Pitfalls and Complications

Preoperative Strategies

With careful attention to preoperative planning, THA can be accomplished successfully in patients with sickle cell disease. Preoperative planning aims to address the multisystem nature of sickle cell hemoglobinopathy and often requires a multidisciplinary approach. The authors of this chapter routinely request evaluation by the hematologist and anesthesiologist before the patient is cleared for surgical treatment. The patient's cardiac status and fluid balance should be assessed because congestive heart failure and cardiomegaly can develop secondary to chronic anemia. Preoperative resuscitation may be necessary and adequate oxygenation should be ensured to avoid acidosis, which can propagate a sickle cell crisis. Preoperative red blood cell transfusion or plasmapheresis is commonly performed to reduce the concentration of hemoglobin S. Transfusion thresholds of hemoglobin level greater than 11 g/dL or hematocrit level greater than 30% and a goal hemoglobin S concentration of less than 30% have been described. Reducing the concentration of hemoglobin S and increasing the normal hemoglobin level will increase oxygen carrying capacity and reduce the likelihood of a sickle cell crisis. Blood products should be tested to determine ABO, Rh, and Kell phenotypes and should be screened for antibodies to avoid alloimmunization and transfusion reactions. As noted, neuraxial anesthesia should be used instead of general anesthesia when possible because neuraxial anesthesia can help prevent red blood cell sickling and subsequent crises via temporary sympathectomy.

Preoperative screening for infection is advisable. Chronic stasis ulcers of the lower extremities are commonly seen in patients with sickle cell disease and can be a source of hematogenous spread of infection. Infected ulcers should be treated before the surgical procedure is performed. Gallbladder infections are a major source of secondary bone infection. A protocol including cholecystectomy has been described for patients who have evidence of gallstones preoperatively.

Intraoperative Strategies

Several strategies can help address characteristics of the diseased hip that can result in intraoperative complications. Bone marrow hyperplasia can drastically undermine the bone quality of the acetabulum and the femur, increasing the risk of fracture during implantation of the prosthesis. Patchy sclerosis or necrosis of the acetabulum may be present and require eccentric reaming. If protrusio acetabuli is present, hip dislocation is more difficult, and osteotomy of the femoral head or neck may be necessary to facilitate dislocation. Protrusio acetabuli also limits the medial extent of acetabular reaming, and the surgical plan may need to include medial bone grafting or the use of a structural acetabular support. Smaller femoral implants may be necessary if marrow hyperplasia and cortical thinning exist at the proximal femoral metaphysis.

Femoral reaming and implant placement can be particularly challenging in patients with sickle cell disease because patchy sclerosis occasionally results in false canals or completely obliterated canals. In these patients, care must be taken to avoid femoral fracture or perforation during reaming, broaching, and implant insertion. Introduction of a drill bit under fluoroscopy can be a valuable aid before a guidewire can be inserted. If canal perforation is suspected, radiographic confirmation of proper guidewire placement is essential before reaming is performed. A novel technique in which direct visualization is achieved by means of a femoral cortical window has been described. Long-term results of this strategy in hip arthroplasty for patients with sickle cell disease have not been published.

The use of prophylactic antibiotics should begin intraoperatively. Because the bone marrow of patients with sickle cell disease may harbor latent bacteria such as *Staphylococcus* and *Salmonella* species, some authors have described an aggressive protocol to combat infection. The authors of one study routinely obtain bone cultures and histologic analyses intraoperatively to rule out osteomyelitis before implantation of the prosthesis. Antibiotics are continued postoperatively until the culture data are available, at which point they are either discontinued or adjusted on the basis of culture sensitivities. Other surgeons described a similar practice in which smears, aspirates, cultures to determine the presence of aerobes and anaerobes, and histologic sections were obtained intraoperatively before antibiotic administration. If cemented fixation is used, impregnation of the cement with antibiotics reduces the risk of infection.

Intraoperative blood loss is a greater concern in patients with sickle cell disease than in other patients because of their vulnerability to anemia and hypoxia. Moreover, technical demands specific to the disease, such as hip dislocation in the presence of osteophytes or protrusion and difficult femoral canal and acetabular preparation, have the potential to increase surgical time and blood loss. Communication with the anesthesia team is critical because volume resuscitation and transfusion can reduce cardiopulmonary and central nervous system complications.

Postoperative Strategies

Strategies to mitigate postoperative risks are similar to the preoperative strategies and focus on reducing the risk of sickle cell crises and infections. Vigilant monitoring for sickle cell–related complications is warranted, especially perioperatively. Vaso-occlusive pain crises and acute chest syndromes occur in 17% of patients with sickle cell disease who undergo THA, and increased wound drainage and hematoma are reported in 14% to 18%. Indications for postoperative red blood cell transfusion are generally postoperative hemorrhage, hemoglobin level less than 10 g/dL, or symptoms of anemia (such as tachycardia, syncope, and angina). Transfusion also should be considered if symptoms of acute hypoxia or acute chest syndrome arise. Involvement of a hematology consultant, preferably one who is familiar with the patient, is essential. Some surgeons administer prophylactic antibiotics in the form of a first-generation cephalosporin for 24 to 72 hours or until cultures obtained intraoperatively are found to be negative.

Bibliography

Acurio MT, Friedman RJ: Hip arthroplasty in patients with sickle-cell haemoglobinopathy. *J Bone Joint Surg Br* 1992;74(3):367-371.

Al-Mousawi F, Malki A, Al-Aradi A, Al-Bagali M, Al-Sadadi A, Booz MM: Total hip replacement in sickle cell disease. *Int Orthop* 2002;26(3):157-161.

Chung SM, Alavi A, Russell MO: Management of osteonecrosis in sickle-cell anemia and its genetic variants. *Clin Orthop Relat Res* 1978;(130):158-174.

Clarke HJ, Jinnah RH, Brooker AF, Michaelson JD: Total replacement of the hip for avascular necrosis in sickle cell disease. *J Bone Joint Surg Br* 1989;71(3):465-470.

Hernigou P, Bachir D, Galacteros F: The natural history of symptomatic osteonecrosis in adults with sickle-cell disease. *J Bone Joint Surg Am* 2003;85(3):500-504.

Hernigou P, Habibi A, Bachir D, Galacteros F: The natural history of asymptomatic osteonecrosis of the femoral head in adults with sickle cell disease. *J Bone Joint Surg Am* 2006;88(12):2565-2572.

Hernigou P, Zilber S, Filippini P, Mathieu G, Poignard A, Galacteros F: Total THA in adult osteonecrosis related to sickle cell disease. *Clin Orthop Relat Res* 2008;466(2):300-308.

Hickman JM, Lachiewicz PF: Results and complications of total hip arthroplasties in patients with sickle-cell hemoglobinopathies: Role of cementless components. *J Arthroplasty* 1997;12(4):420-425.

Hug KT, Gupta AK, Wellman SS, Bolognesi MP, Attarian DE: Creation of a femoral cortical window to facilitate total hip arthroplasty in patients with sickle cell hemoglobinopathies. *J Arthroplasty* 2013;28(2):323-325.

Ilyas I, Moreau P: Simultaneous bilateral total hip arthroplasty in sickle cell disease. *J Arthroplasty* 2002;17(4):441-445.

Issa K, Naziri Q, Maheshwari AV, Rasquinha VJ, Delanois RE, Mont MA: Excellent results and minimal complications of total hip arthroplasty in sickle cell hemoglobinopathy at mid-term follow-up using cementless prosthetic components. *J Arthroplasty* 2013;28(9):1693-1698.

Jeong GK, Ruchelsman DE, Jazrawi LM, Jaffe WL: Total hip arthroplasty in sickle cell hemoglobinopathies. *J Am Acad Orthop Surg* 2005;13(3):208-217.

Mont MA, Zywiel MG, Marker DR, McGrath MS, Delanois RE: The natural history of untreated asymptomatic osteonecrosis of the femoral head: A systematic literature review. *J Bone Joint Surg Am* 2010;92(12):2165-2170.

Moran MC: Osteonecrosis of the hip in sickle cell hemoglobinopathy. *Am J Orthop (Belle Mead NJ)* 1995;24(1):18-24.

Moran MC, Huo MH, Garvin KL, Pellicci PM, Salvati EA: Total hip arthroplasty in sickle cell hemoglobinopathy. *Clin Orthop Relat Res* 1993;(294):140-148.

Neumayr LD, Aguilar C, Earles AN, et al; National Osteonecrosis Trial in Sickle Cell Anemia Study Group: Physical therapy alone compared with core decompression and physical therapy for femoral head osteonecrosis in sickle cell disease: Results of a multicenter study at a mean of three years after treatment. *J Bone Joint Surg Am* 2006;88(12):2573-2582.

Ould Amar K, Rouvillain JL, Loko G: Perioperative transfusion management in patients with sickle cell anaemia undergoing a total hip arthroplasty: Is there a role of red-cell exchange transfusion? A retrospective study in the CHU of Fort-de-France Martinique. *Transfus Clin Biol* 2013;20(1):30-34.

Perfetti DC, Boylan MR, Naziri Q, Khanuja HS, Urban WP: Does sickle cell disease increase risk of adverse outcomes following total hip and knee arthroplasty? A nationwide database study. *J Arthroplasty* 2015;30(4):547-551.

Sanjay BK, Moreau PG: Bipolar hip replacement in sickle cell disease. *Int Orthop* 1996;20(4):222-226.

Chapter 32
Total Hip Arthroplasty in Patients With Neurologic Conditions

Andrew I. Spitzer, MD

Indications

Neuromuscular disorders often result in degenerative disease of the hip. These conditions are either congenital or acquired and are classified according to their effect on muscle tone. Disorders characterized by increased muscle tone, muscle contractures, or movement abnormalities include cerebral palsy, Parkinson disease, and stroke. Disorders involving decreased muscle tone include polio, Down syndrome, myelomeningocele, and spinal cord injury. Neurologic disorders that do not alter muscle tone include dementia, confusion, and psychoses. Each disease process presents unique but often similar challenges during surgical hip reconstruction.

As many as 10% of patients undergoing total hip arthroplasty (THA) are reported to have neuromuscular disorders. Historically, surgeons have been reluctant to treat these patients surgically because of perceived risks of dislocation, aseptic loosening, heterotopic ossification, and perioperative complications, as well as poor rehabilitation potential and uncertain functional outcomes. However, because medical advances have dramatically improved survival after stroke and in patients with Parkinson disease, and because patients with other neuromuscular disorders are living longer and have higher expectations, increasingly arthroplasty surgeons have begun to encounter the challenges of reconstruction in these patients. Although the literature is still relatively sparse, multiple recent publications have elucidated the role of THA in patients with neuromuscular disease and have demonstrated reliable and durable pain relief and generally improved functional outcomes. In addition, many of these studies have addressed technologic innovations and have clarified the nature and risks of complications and methodologies for the prevention of complications in this complex patient population.

Hip degeneration can occur in patients with neuromuscular disorders either as a result of the underlying disease process or independently but concurrent with the disease process. In patients with cerebral palsy, profound muscle imbalance and spasticity present since childhood cause the stronger hip flexors, adductors, and internal rotators to overpower the extensors, abductors, and external rotators. This imbalance results in progressive subluxation of the hip, increased concentrated forces on the hip joint, degeneration of the acetabular and femoral head cartilage, soft-tissue contractures, and bony abnormalities such as acetabular dysplasia, coxa valga, persistent fetal femoral anteversion, shortened femoral neck, and decreased femoral offset. In 70% to 79% of these patients, disabling pain results in decreased ambulation and interferes with sitting tolerance, perineal hygiene, transfers, and nursing care. In contrast, patients who have had polio or who experience postpolio syndrome may have similarly unbalanced muscular forces, but the general flaccidity of the muscles reduces forces across the hip, reducing the likelihood of degeneration.

The indications for THA in patients with neurologic disease are similar to those in most patients with osteoarthritis. However, to optimize surgical outcome, the surgeon needs to consider the unique manifestations of a patient's neurologic disorder and the patient's specific medical conditions. The classic indications for THA include radiographically confirmed degenerative disease of the hip joint accompanied by pain unresponsive to nonsurgical management and substantial activity and functional limitations. Physical examination should confirm the hip as the source of pain. Additional indications include progressive pain in a degenerated dysplastic, subluxated, or dislocated hip; subcapital hip fracture (**Figure 1**), with or without underlying arthritis; failed fixation of hip fractures with nonunion, malunion, or osteonecrosis; and painful

Dr. Spitzer or an immediate family member is a member of a speakers' bureau or has made paid presentations on behalf of Sanofi-Aventis; serves as a paid consultant to DePuy Synthes and Sanofi-Aventis; and has received research or institutional support from DePuy Synthes.

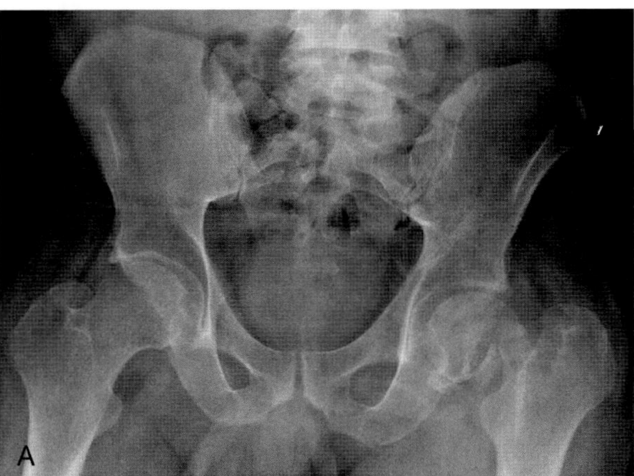

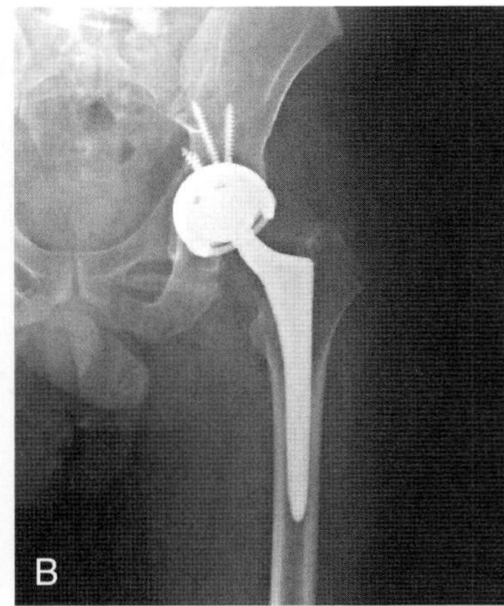

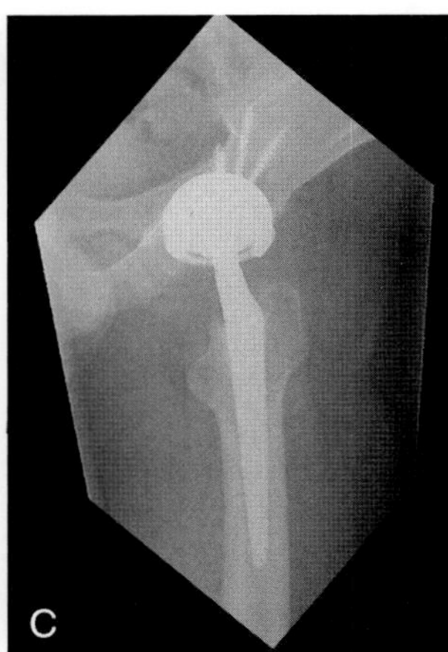

Figure 1 **A,** Preoperative AP pelvic radiograph demonstrates nonunion of a nonsurgically managed, comminuted, displaced, subcapital left hip fracture that was sustained as a result of a twisting injury during transfer in a patient with incomplete spinal cord injury and C6-C7 paraplegia resulting from a rollover vehicular accident with ejection 3 years earlier. Postoperative AP (**B**) and lateral (**C**) radiographs of the left hip after noncemented, constrained total hip arthroplasty was performed via an anterior approach. (Courtesy of Daniel Chris Allison, MD, Los Angeles, CA.)

arthritis that prevents comfortable positioning of the patient for perineal care or prevents functional activities such as sitting, standing, and ambulating. Ideally, patients should possess some active motor control of the limb and have functional abductors. Cognitive capacity to participate in rehabilitation and adhere to precautions to prevent dislocation is preferable.

A frank discussion between the surgeon and the patient and/or caregivers about realistic expectations is critical. The risk of postoperative complications, such as dislocation in patients with severe muscle imbalance, spasticity, or cognitive impairment, or decubitus ulceration in patients with altered sensation or difficulty with independent mobilization, must be weighed against the benefits of THA. Alternative surgical options may need to be considered depending on an individual patient's needs, activity level, and expectations. Despite the pain relief and improved function that THA provides these patients, the pain and disability resulting from the arthritic hip must be severe enough to outweigh the increased risk of complications of the procedure.

Contraindications

Absolute contraindications to THA in any patient include active or chronic infection in the hip joint, as well as active or chronic distant infection, such as skin breakdown and decubitus ulcers. In addition, Charcot neuropathic arthropathy, although rare in the hip, can occur as a result of syphilitic tabes dorsalis; diabetes mellitus; syringomyelia; peripheral neuritis resulting from alcoholism, diabetes mellitus, or vitamin deficiency; peripheral nerve injury; congenital absence of pain; myelodysplasia; and repeated intra-articular steroid injections. Charcot arthropathy is typically considered a contraindication to THA because the few reported results of THA in these patients have been uniformly poor.

Relative contraindications specific to patients with neurologic disease must be individually assessed with consideration of potential complications, activity level, age, and medical risk. Substantial abductor weakness resulting from polio, myelomeningocele, stroke, or multiple sclerosis increases the risk of dislocation and may require the use of constrained implants, which increase the risk of loosening or irreducible dislocation. Alternative treatments may be preferable in these patients. Patients who are cognitively impaired and patients who are noncompliant because of either unwillingness or inability to comply with restrictions may have a high risk for dislocation, particularly if they have preexisting substantial muscle imbalance, spasticity, paresis, or paralysis. Patients with minimal activity demands, those who are bedridden or nonambulatory, and those who have positioning requirements that place the hip at risk for dislocation may be best treated with an alternative strategy. Young age, although historically considered a risk factor for early failure, is of less concern in this patient population because the patients' relatively low activity levels should foster longevity of the prosthesis. Medical risk should be carefully considered, particularly in elderly patients who have sustained a stroke or have a progressive neurologic disorder, such as Parkinson disease or multiple sclerosis. The patient's underlying medical or neurologic condition should be optimized, and perioperative management should be designed to prevent cardiac, pulmonary, gastrointestinal, urinary, thromboembolic, and other general complications. Patients who have a high risk for medical complications should participate actively in the surgical decision-making process.

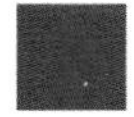

Alternative Treatments

Nonsurgical management should always be optimized before surgical treatment is considered. Judicious use of NSAIDs, analgesic agents, intra-articular steroid injections, and/or viscosupplementation; weight loss; activity modifications; and the use of ambulatory assistive devices and physical therapy to maintain motion, mobility, and strength may delay the need for surgical intervention. If nonsurgical management is unsuccessful, surgical intervention is indicated. In most ambulatory patients, THA will provide the most reliable and successful outcomes. However, in patients with neuromuscular conditions who have more profound impairment, alternative surgical strategies to address the arthritic hip include osteotomy, resection with or without interposition arthroplasty, and arthrodesis. These procedures, similar to THA, are designed to relieve pain and restore function, improving the patient's ability to stand, walk, or sit comfortably. Arthrodesis is relatively contraindicated in patients with arthritis and congenital neuromuscular disease because patients with increased muscle tone and spasticity frequently have bilateral hip disease and deformity along with spinal deformity and disease. Although arthrodesis remains an option for patients with unilateral hip arthritis, THA will provide a more functional result and greater satisfaction in these patients. Resection arthroplasty is reserved for patients who are bedridden or those who, at most, can be transferred to a sitting posture to permit comfortable positioning and facilitate hygiene and perineal care. Girdlestone resection arthroplasty has uniformly poor results. Proximal femoral resection below the level of the lesser trochanter with interposition of the vastus muscles, the hip capsule, the abductors, and the psoas muscles provides more reliable pain relief. Subtrochanteric valgus femoral osteotomy with femoral head resection also may be useful in nonambulatory patients. Complications include heterotopic ossification, the risk of which can be effectively reduced with a single dose of radiation or the use of oral NSAIDs for 3 to 6 weeks, and recurrent pain.

Results

The results of THA in patients with neuromuscular conditions are favorable (**Table 1**). Well-performed THA in properly selected patients with neuromuscular disease can result in successful long-term outcomes. Pain relief is reliably and durably achieved in most patients, with greater than 10-year follow-up. Caregivers also are routinely satisfied because the procedure facilitates perineal hygiene, transfers, and overall nursing care. Function routinely improves as a result of THA, and most patients are able to return to preoperative functional levels. However, in patients with Parkinson disease, function deteriorates over time because of the inexorable progression of the disease. In addition, patients with Parkinson disease, especially those with hip fracture, experience a perioperative complication rate as high as 36% and a 6-month mortality of approximately 6% because of medical complications, such as urinary tract infections, pneumonia, and decubitus ulcers resulting from immobility.

Vigilant attention to patient selection, surgical technique, implant choice and placement, and soft-tissue balance are all critical factors in optimizing outcomes and reducing complications. The use of larger femoral head articulations, dual-mobility implants, constrained articulations, and possibly hip resurfacing have substantially reduced the risk of dislocation even in patients with spasticity resulting from upper motor neuron disorder, who are at highest risk for dislocation, without increasing the rate of implant loosening or adverse local tissue reaction. Similar results have been achieved with cemented femoral stems implanted with modern cementing techniques and noncemented femoral stems.

Specific patient populations pose characteristic challenges. Spasticity, especially with muscle imbalance, increases the risk of dislocation. Although concerns of dislocation in patients with a prior stroke or with Parkinson disease have been prominent, the data suggest that these patients do not have an increased risk for dislocation, perhaps because of decreased mobility and activity levels. Nevertheless, patients with a prior stroke in particular have an increased risk for heterotopic ossification. Outcomes of THA in patients with flaccid paralysis, such as that resulting from polio, spinal cord injury, and myelomeningocele, are not well studied, but the risk of complications in these patients is thought to be extremely high.

Technique

Preoperative Planning

- A careful history and thorough physical examination are necessary to identify muscle imbalance, spasticity, contractures, paresis, or paralysis and to assess the patient's functional status and rehabilitative potential. A frank discussion of realistic expectations with the patient, family, and caregivers is necessary.
- If the source of the pain or the anticipated result of the procedure is in question, a diagnostic intra-articular local anesthetic injection can help predict the extent of pain

Table 1 Results of Total Hip Arthroplasty (THA) in Patients With Neuromuscular Disorders

Authors (Year)	Number of Hips (Patients)	Procedure or Approach	Mean Patient Age in Years (Range)	Mean Follow-up in Years (Range)	Success Rate (%)[a]	Results
Weber et al (2002)	107 (98)	56 anterolateral, 36 transtrochanteric, 12 posterior, and 3 direct lateral approaches in patients with Parkinson disease for 58 primary THAs, 19 failed endoprostheses, 10 instances of aseptic loosening, 18 femoral neck fractures, and 2 other diagnoses Tenotomy was performed in 8 hips 94 acetabuli and 103 femurs were cemented	72 (57-87)	7 (2-21)	97	6 hips had instability or dislocation (none in primary THA) 3 hips had aseptic loosening (1 femur, 1 acetabulum, 1 both femur and acetabulum) 5 other revisions (1 trochanteric nonunion, 1 instability, 1 wire removal, 1 periprosthetic fracture, 1 deep infection) 6% mortality at 6 mo 2 patients used braces postoperatively 93% survivorship rate at 5 yr postoperatively 93% had good to excellent pain relief 36% overall complication rate (26% of primary THAs, 47% of THAs for other indications) Functional outcome deteriorated over time as disease progressed
Hernigou et al (2010)	164 (144) with constrained implant and 132 (120) with nonconstrained implant	Posterolateral approach in patients with neurologic or cognitive impairment Tenotomy was performed in 28 hips managed with constrained implants and 25 hips managed with nonconstrained implants	Constrained implant group: 67 (24-98) Nonconstrained implant group: 70 (21-92)	Constrained implant group: 7 (5-10) Nonconstrained implant group: 12 (10-15)	5 yr: 95-100 7 yr: 91-97	Retrospective comparison of cohorts 3 hips with constrained implants and 33 hips with nonconstrained implants had instability or dislocation No postoperative immobilization or bracing Study authors concluded that a constrained liner provides durable protection against dislocation without increasing loosening at midterm follow-up
Raphael et al (2010)	59 (56)	Transtrochanteric posterolateral approach in patients with cerebral palsy Tenotomy was performed in 28 hips	30.7 (14-61)	9.7 (2-28)	85	8 hips had instability or dislocation Pain improved in all patients and was eliminated in 81% of patients Durable pain relief and improved function Postoperative immobilization with spica cast for 46 hips, abduction brace for 10 hips, and knee immobilizer for 2 hips; 1 hip was not immobilized

[a] Success is defined as implant survivorship free of pain and aseptic loosening.

Table 1 Results of Total Hip Arthroplasty (THA) in Patients With Neuromuscular Disorders (*continued*)

Authors (Year)	Number of Hips (Patients)	Procedure or Approach	Mean Patient Age in Years (Range)	Mean Follow-up in Years (Range)	Success Rate (%)[a]	Results
Schroeder et al (2010)	18 (16)	Supine transgluteal lateral Bauer approach in patients with ambulatory cerebral palsy Tenotomy was performed in 6 hips	42 (32-58)	10 (2-18)	78	2 hips had instability or dislocation Substantial reduction in pain and improvement in function over the long term 7 patients used spica cast or abduction brace for 6 wk postoperatively
Prosser et al (2012)	20 (19)	Posterior approach in patients with cerebral palsy No tenotomy Hip resurfacing with varus subtrochanteric osteotomy and derotation and shortening	37 (13-57)	8 (2.7-11.6)	75	2 hips had instability or dislocation 16 of the 18 patients who were contacted reported pain relief, thought that the surgery was worthwhile, and reported improved perineal care 35% of hips had substantial surgical complications No heterotopic ossification 10 patients used broomstick casts for 6 wk postoperatively
Sanders et al (2013)	10 (8)	Posterolateral approach in patients with cerebral palsy Tenotomy was performed in 1 hip Dual-mobility cup to prevent dislocation	54 (43-61)	3.3 (1.8-4.7)	100	No instability or dislocation 90% had pain reduction and improved function
Tudor et al (2013)	11 (9)	Total hip resurfacing through the posterolateral approach in patients with cerebral palsy, spinal cord injury, polio, head injury, hereditary spastic paraparesis, or extrapyramidal disorder Tenotomy was performed in 7 hips	33.1 (13-49)	5.3 (3.4-7.4)	91	1 hip had instability or dislocation 10 hips had good clinical results and improved pain and function, and caregivers reported good to excellent satisfaction 1 hip had recurrent dislocation and loose cup managed with resection arthroplasty 2 patients used broomstick casts, and 7 patients used abduction braces postoperatively

[a] Success is defined as implant survivorship free of pain and aseptic loosening.

Table 1 Results of Total Hip Arthroplasty (THA) in Patients With Neuromuscular Disorders (*continued*)

Authors (Year)	Number of Hips (Patients)	Procedure or Approach	Mean Patient Age in Years (Range)	Mean Follow-up in Years (Range)	Success Rate (%)[a]	Results
Alosh et al (2014)	30 (27)	Posterior approach in patients with spasticity (upper motor neuron disease) Adductor tenotomy was performed in 11 hips Iliopsoas tenotomy was performed in 6 hips Preoperative pharmacologic blockade (phenol or botulinum toxin) was used in 14 patients to control post-operative spasticity and improve compliance with hip precautions	48.6 (29.1-75)	2.7 (2.1-12.1)	100	No instability or dislocation All patients used postoperative muscle relaxation, abduction pillow, and knee immobilizer Abduction brace used for 6 wk in patients with cognitive impairment All patients went to postoperative rehabilitation facility Significant improvement in pain, function, and range of motion ($P < 0.01$) Mobility improved in nearly all patients 1 patient required resection arthroplasty for deep infection No instability or dislocation Study authors concluded that risk of instability can be minimized with careful patient selection, implant positioning, and management of soft-tissue contractures
Park et al (2014)	19 (19)	Modified minimally invasive two-incision approach in patients with dementia, Parkinson disease, or stroke Large femoral head with metal-on-metal articulation for management of displaced femoral neck fracture (mean femoral head diameter, 44 mm; all >38 mm) Tenotomy was performed in 4 hips	72.6 (62-81)	1.4 (1.0-1.3)	100	No instability or dislocation No metal hypersensitivity or osteolysis Abduction pillow used postoperatively
Mohammed et al (2015)	44 (41)	20 primary THAs and 24 revision THAs via a modified lateral posterior approach in patients with central nervous system conditions (Parkinson disease, stroke, dementia), dislocation of prior THA, severe fixed hip deformity, or peripheral neuropathy	70.8 (56-84)	1.8 (0.5-5.3)	100	No dislocations or revisions occurred

[a] Success is defined as implant survivorship free of pain and aseptic loosening.

relief expected as a result of surgical intervention.
- Preoperative pharmacologic blockade with CT-guided injections of phenol or botulinum toxin A into the hip flexor and adductor muscles may relieve spasticity for as long as 8 weeks and may be repeated postoperatively to facilitate safe positioning, maintain hip precautions, and reduce the risk of dislocation. However, the literature provides limited data and no consensus regarding dosing and location.
- Complete radiographic evaluation is essential to identify acetabular dysplasia or deficiency, hip subluxation or dislocation, abnormal femoral rotation or version, and osteopenia. Cross-sectional CT and/or MRI may be required to fully elucidate these abnormalities and detect injury patterns not evident on plain radiographs. Radiographic templating is used to determine a formal surgical plan and the best choice of implants to achieve a sound structural, biomechanical, and functional hip reconstruction.
- A thorough and formal preoperative medical evaluation is necessary.
- To minimize the risk of perioperative complications resulting from underlying medical and neurologic conditions in patients with Parkinson disease and those who have sustained a stroke, neurologic clearance should be obtained before surgical intervention is performed.

Setup/Exposure

- To reduce the risk of complications and dislocation, a surgical approach with which the surgeon is facile, familiar, and experienced should be chosen.
- Both anterior and posterior approaches can be successfully used, but the chosen approach must be extensile to permit flexibility and facilitate management of the complex bony and soft-tissue anatomy characteristic of this patient population. For this reason, the direct anterior approach is not recommended.
- The posterior approach, which can be used in a limited transgluteal fashion to minimize tissue trauma or can be extended to provide wide exposure to address bony deficiencies, soft-tissue contractures, and intraoperative complications, is the mainstay of these procedures, especially in patients in whom THA is complex. However, anterolateral and direct lateral approaches may facilitate extensive anterior releases of severe contractures in patients whose primary posture is sitting.
- Combination anterior and posterior (two-incision) approaches have been used to exploit the benefits of both approaches while minimizing tissue dissection.
- The surgeon must focus special attention on avoiding injury or excessive surgical trauma to the abductors, which are already compromised in patients with neuromuscular disorders. Injury or excessive trauma to the abductors can lead to residual weakness, a limp, or heterotopic ossification.
- To adequately expose the hip joint, tenotomies may be necessary as part of the primary approach. Release of the reflected head of the rectus femoris at its insertion on the anterosuperior acetabulum, the psoas tendon at its insertion on the lesser trochanter, and the anterosuperior capsule can facilitate mobilization of the femur and exposure of the acetabulum, help eliminate preoperative flexion contractures, and prevent flexion contractures from recurring postoperatively.

Instruments/Equipment/Implants Required

- The choice of implant should maximize the ability to achieve fixation, create a biomechanically sound hip reconstruction, and minimize the risk of dislocation, which is generally higher in this patient population than in other patients undergoing THA.
- Historically, acetabular reconstruction was accomplished with the use of cemented cups. However, recent data favor the use of noncemented cups. Ultraporous coatings and modular augments provide attractive options for achieving fixation and support in patients with acetabular deficiency.
- Adjunctive screw fixation is encouraged, especially if the use of a constrained implant is considered. Options such as bone grafts, cages, and oblong cups should be considered and available for use in the most complex patients.
- The largest possible femoral head size should be used to increase impingement-free motion and the jump distance of the femoral head and decrease the risk of postoperative dislocation.
- The use of hip resurfacing implants may facilitate the use of a larger femoral head in patients with relatively smaller anatomy; however, the use of a smaller femoral head in a metal-on-metal construct increases the risk of adverse local tissue reaction from metal debris and should be used with caution.
- Dual-mobility articulations also may play a substantial role in reducing dislocation rates, but longer-term follow-up is necessary before this technology is widely adopted.
- Constrained articulations have substantially reduced dislocation rates without increasing the risk of implant loosening, which is a theoretic concern with these implants.

Constrained implants have been particularly helpful in patients with cognitive impairment, decreased muscle tone, and lack of muscular limb control and in patients whose anatomy precludes the use of a larger femoral head articulation.

- Femoral fixation can successfully be achieved with both cemented and noncemented implants.
- Cemented stems may be preferred in patients with osteopenic bone, such as those with Parkinson disease and stroke. However, cemented stems require the use of meticulous contemporary cementing technique, including a broach-only technique, removal of loose cancellous debris, canal occlusion, pressurization of cement, and reduction of cement porosity.
- Noncemented modular femoral stems are favored in patients with better bone quality because they provide versatility in adjusting limb length, offset, and version independent of fixation within the bone, especially in patients with spasticity and a multitude of complex rotational, angular, and offset deformities. These stems also can eliminate the need for simultaneous femoral corrective osteotomies, which increase a patient's risk for hardware failure and nonunion.

Procedure

- Regardless of which approach is used, full exposure of the circumferential anatomy of the true acetabulum is necessary.
- The acetabulum is carefully and gently reamed, taking care to avoid overreaming of osteopenic bone, which is commonly present in these patients as a result of disuse.
- The size of the acetabular implant is determined by the size of the reamer that exposed punctate bleeding bone within the anterior and posterior walls. The surgeon should avoid attempting to reduce the extent of a superior deficiency by reaming to a larger hemisphere because doing so may dangerously thin the anterior and posterior walls of the acetabulum and substantially compromise the initial stability and long-term fixation of the acetabular implant.
- Bone graft, metal augments, or oblong cups are used to fill acetabular deficiencies. The surgeon should consider accepting a slightly higher hip center if offset, stability, and limb length can be restored with the femoral implant.
- In patients who spend most time sitting, regardless of the implant used, the acetabular implant is positioned in less than 45° of abduction, with additional anteversion to provide optimal posterior coverage and stability.
- After placement of the trial and final implants, soft-tissue balance, range of motion, and stability are meticulously assessed.
- Femoral modularity should be exploited to adjust limb length, offset, and version and to optimize stability.
- Releases of the psoas tendon from the lesser trochanter, the rectus femoris from the anterior acetabulum, and the anterior capsule from its acetabular and femoral insertions may be required to reduce a persistent flexion deformity and to prevent recurrence of the deformity, which can result in dislocation and loosening. Adduction contractures are addressed later in the procedure.

Wound Closure

- Secure repair of any bony or soft-tissue dissection that was performed for exposure is necessary to facilitate adequate healing and reduce the risk of postoperative dislocation.
- Especially if the posterior approach is used, careful reapproximation to bone of the posterior capsule and extensive soft-tissue repair of the posterior soft-tissue sleeve is necessary. Appropriate repair should reduce the risk of dislocation to less than 1%.
- The wound is closed in layers, taking care to ensure that the fascia is tightly sealed and any dead space is eliminated in the subcutaneous tissues.
- The skin closure technique is at the discretion of the surgeon. However, the use of staples may cause local irritation and lead to infection.
- Adhesive dressings are applied without tension to reduce the risk of shearing the skin and causing blisters.
- The patient is placed supine. If passive abduction to at least 30° is not easily obtainable, a percutaneous adductor tenotomy and release is performed (**Figure 2**).
- After sterile preparation and draping of the insertion of the adductors at the pubic tubercle, a tiny stab incision is made close to the pubis directly over the tight tendons with the tip of a No. 11 blade.
- The tip of the blade is rotated and angled to release the tight fibers until at least 45° of abduction is possible (**Figure 2, B**), maximizing the ability to keep the hip in the safe zone and avoid dislocation in the postoperative period and reducing the risk of recurrence of adduction contractures.
- Skin adhesives, such as topical skin adhesives or thin adhesive strips, are applied.
- The wound is covered with a small, sterile dressing.
- The use of sutures is discouraged to avoid the challenge of their removal in this area.

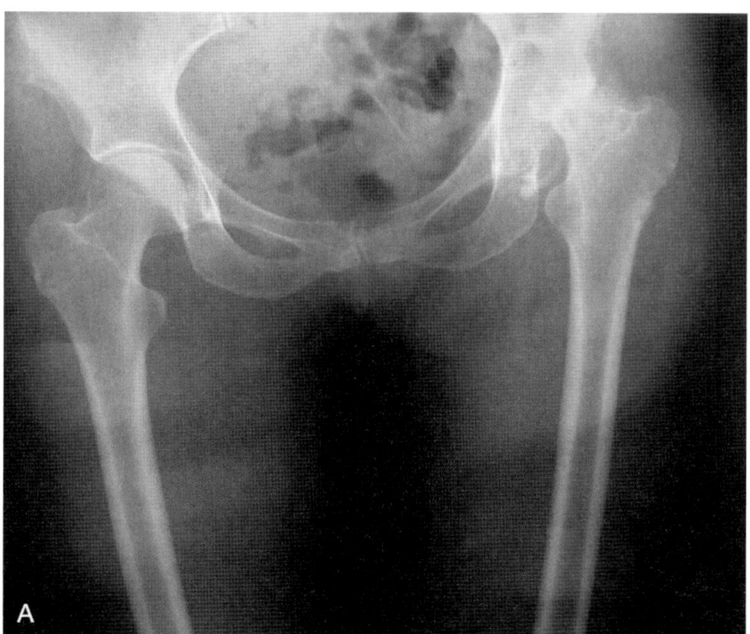

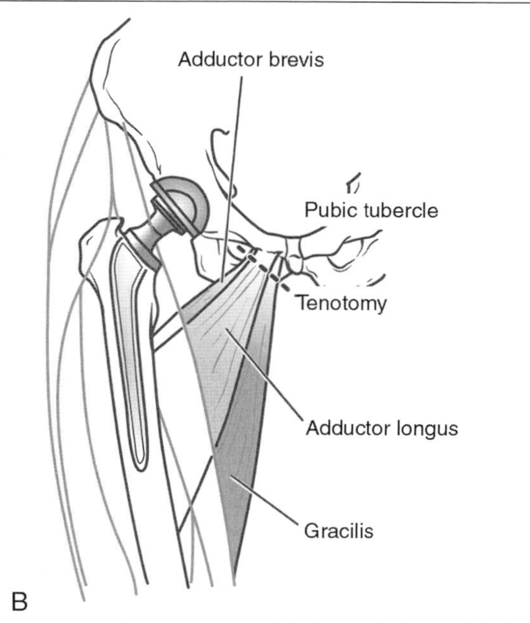

Figure 2 **A,** Preoperative AP pelvic radiograph demonstrates severe adduction contracture. **B,** Illustration of a hip shows the site of adductor tenotomy (dashed line) to manage such contracture. (Panel A reproduced from Spitzer A: Total hip arthroplasty in patients with neurologic conditions, in Lieberman JR, Berry DJ, eds: *Advanced Reconstruction: Hip*. Rosemont, IL, American Academy of Orthopaedic Surgeons, 2005, pp 211-219. Panel B reproduced with permission from Mayo Foundation for Medical Education and Research, Rochester, MN.)

Postoperative Regimen

The postoperative protocol in these patients is predicated, in part, on the nature of the underlying disease. Assuming no intraoperative complications occurred, postoperative precautions are directed at avoiding catastrophic complications, such as falling and dislocation. Disruption of bony or soft-tissue repair also is a concern, particularly in patients with spasticity and those who are noncompliant. Medical complications should be anticipated, with preventive measures taken to avoid them whenever possible. A multidisciplinary approach involving surgeons, medical and neurologic consultants, and the rehabilitation team helps to ensure a rapid, uncomplicated recovery. Postoperative analgesia and muscle relaxation and either preoperative or postoperative pharmacologic blockade of spastic muscles, described previously, can improve patient compliance with postoperative positioning and hip precautions to reduce the risk of postoperative hip dislocation.

Vigilance against infection is particularly important in this patient population, especially in patients with Parkinson disease, in whom a higher incidence of postoperative infections has been documented. Aggressive pulmonary toilet is important to avoid atelectasis and pneumonia. Depending on the extent of neurologic involvement, aspiration precautions also may be appropriate. The use of a urinary catheter for at least 1 day postoperatively may be advisable to minimize the likelihood of urinary retention; however, the catheter should be removed promptly to reduce the risk of subsequent urinary tract infections. Bowel management should be aggressive to avoid painful constipation or impaction and possible resulting bacteremia. Surgical drains should be removed promptly, preferably within 24 hours postoperatively. Perioperative antibiotics should be continued until all indwelling catheters are removed.

Prophylaxis against thromboembolic disease should be administered according to the surgeon's standard protocol, with additional consideration of any increased risk factors in the individual patient, such as anticipated prolonged immobilization, hypercoagulability risks, and family or personal history of a venous thromboembolic event. Choices of prophylaxis include mechanical devices, antiplatelet agents, low-molecular-weight heparins, vitamin K antagonists, direct thrombin inhibitors, and direct factor Xa inhibitors. The selection of these agents requires a balance between efficacy and the risk of bleeding.

The patient should be carefully and rapidly mobilized to minimize the risk of skin breakdown, pulmonary and urinary complications, and venous thromboembolic disease and to promote expeditious achievement of functional independence. The use of assistive devices for ambulation, which may be familiar to these patients and may be necessary because of the underlying disease even after the hip is rehabilitated, is mandatory to improve ambulatory stability and avoid falls, fractures, and dislocations. It may be necessary to modify these devices with troughs or other grasping mechanisms to accommodate upper extremity deformity, weakness, or spasticity. Full weight bearing is allowed immediately postoperatively unless protection of a bony or soft-tissue repair or reconstruction is necessary.

Cognitive impairment and unwillingness or inability to comply with postoperative hip precautions and positioning restrictions can lead to postoperative dislocation and compromise the final outcome of the surgical procedure. The decision to use an abduction hip brace with or without a knee immobilizer, or a spica cast, is made on an individual basis. Immobilization is strongly recommended and widely used if the patient has a substantial risk for postoperative dislocation or disruption of soft-tissue or bony repairs. Although inconvenient for the patient and caregivers, the use of such immobilization may substantially improve the long-term prognosis and eventual success of the reconstruction by helping to avoid these early complications.

Patients with a prior stroke have an increased risk for heterotopic ossification. Therefore, these patients benefit from a prophylactic regimen of either a single 700- to 800-cGy dose of perioperative external beam radiation in the period from 24 hours preoperatively to 72 hours postoperatively or the use of oral NSAIDs for 3 to 6 weeks postoperatively. Radiation is preferred in patients at risk for gastrointestinal complications from NSAIDs, but the implant surfaces must be properly shielded to avoid compromise of bony ingrowth.

Discharge of the patient to a familiar environment is ideal. However, many of these patients may benefit from inpatient rehabilitation before returning to their homes at the appropriate time. Caregivers should be thoroughly instructed regarding precautions and activity restrictions. Close follow-up should be arranged.

Avoiding Pitfalls and Complications

Efforts to avoid complications are critical in these patients, particularly because the underlying disease often increases their risk for complications. The key elements of success involve proper patient selection; meticulous attention to technical detail and execution, including implant choice and placement; and appropriate soft-tissue balancing and releases as described previously. A multidisciplinary, diligently managed postoperative regimen is necessary to avoid medical complications, falls, fractures, and dislocations and to optimize the rehabilitative outcome.

Bibliography

Alosh H, Kamath AF, Baldwin KD, Keenan M, Lee GC: Outcomes of total hip arthroplasty in spastic patients. *J Arthroplasty* 2014;29(8):1566-1570.

Cabanela ME, Weber M: Total hip arthroplasty in patients with neuromuscular disease. *Instr Course Lect* 2000;49:163-168.

DiCaprio MR, Huo MH, Zatorski LE, Keggi K: Incidence of heterotopic ossification following total hip arthroplasty in patients with prior stroke. *Orthopedics* 2004;27(1):41-43.

Eibach S, Krug H, Lobsien E, Hoffmann KT, Kupsch A: Preoperative treatment with Botulinum Toxin A before total hip arthroplasty in a patient with tetraspasticity: Case report and review of literature. *NeuroRehabilitation* 2011;28(2):81-83.

Hernigou P, Filippini P, Flouzat-Lachaniette CH, Batista SU, Poignard A: Constrained liner in neurologic or cognitively impaired patients undergoing primary THA. *Clin Orthop Relat Res* 2010;468(12):3255-3262.

Kraay MJ, Bigach SD: The neuromuscularly challenged patient: Total hip replacement is now an option. *Bone Joint J* 2014;96(11 suppl A):27-31.

Mathew PG, Sponer P, Kucera T, Grinac M, Knízek J: Total hip arthroplasty in patients with Parkinson's disease. *Acta Medica (Hradec Kralove)* 2013;56(3):110-116.

Meek RM, Allan DB, McPhillips G, Kerr L, Howie CR: Epidemiology of dislocation after total hip arthroplasty. *Clin Orthop Relat Res* 2006;447:9-18.

Mohammed R, Hayward K, Mulay S, Bindi F, Wallace M: Outcomes of dual-mobility acetabular cup for instability in primary and revision total hip arthroplasty. *J Orthop Traumatol* 2015;16(1):9-13.

Park KS, Seon JK, Lee KB, Yoon TR: Total hip arthroplasty using large-diameter metal-on-metal articulation in patients with neuromuscular weakness. *J Arthroplasty* 2014;29(4):797-801.

Prosser GH, Shears E, O'Hara JN: Hip resurfacing with femoral osteotomy for painful subluxed or dislocated hips in patients with cerebral palsy. *J Bone Joint Surg Br* 2012;94(4):483-487.

Queally JM, Abdulkarim A, Mulhall KJ: Total hip replacement in patients with neurological conditions. *J Bone Joint Surg Br* 2009;91(10):1267-1273.

Raphael BS, Dines JS, Akerman M, Root L: Long-term followup of total hip arthroplasty in patients with cerebral palsy. *Clin Orthop Relat Res* 2010;468(7):1845-1854.

Root L: Surgical treatment for hip pain in the adult cerebral palsy patient. *Dev Med Child Neurol* 2009;51(suppl 4):84-91.

Sanders RJ, Swierstra BA, Goosen JH: The use of a dual-mobility concept in total hip arthroplasty patients with spastic disorders: No dislocations in a series of ten cases at midterm follow-up. *Arch Orthop Trauma Surg* 2013;133(7):1011-1016.

Schroeder K, Hauck C, Wiedenhöfer B, Braatz F, Aldinger PR: Long-term results of hip arthroplasty in ambulatory patients with cerebral palsy. *Int Orthop* 2010;34(3):335-339.

Spitzer A: Total hip arthroplasty in patients with neurologic conditions, in Lieberman JR, Berry DJ, eds: *Advanced Reconstruction: Hip*. Rosemont, IL, American Academy of Orthopaedic Surgeons, 2005, pp 211-219.

Tudor F, Ariamanesh A, Potty A, Hashemi-Nejad A: Resurfacing hip arthroplasty in neuromuscular hip disorders: A retrospective case series. *J Orthop* 2013;10(3):105-110.

Weber M, Cabanela ME, Sim FH, Frassica FJ, Harmsen WS: Total hip replacement in patients with Parkinson's disease. *Int Orthop* 2002;26(2):66-68.

SECTION 3
Complications After Total Hip Arthroplasty
Daniel J. Berry, MD

Chapter 33
Management of Instability After Total Hip Arthroplasty

Paul F. Lachiewicz, MD
Cameron K. Ledford, MD

Indications

Instability is a frequent and disabling complication of primary and revision total hip arthroplasty (THA). A study of Medicare data demonstrated an overall dislocation rate of 3.9% after primary THA. The dislocation rate after revision THA has been reported to be approximately 9.8% but may be as high as 20% after isolated acetabular revision, acetabular liner exchange to manage wear, two-stage revision to manage infection, and revision of metal-on-metal THAs and resurfacing arthroplasties with large femoral heads. Recurrent hip instability was the most common indication for revision THA, accounting for 22.5% of such procedures in one study of 51,345 revisions. More than one-half of all dislocations occur within 3 months postoperatively, and more than 75% occur within 1 year postoperatively.

Factors associated with increased risk of dislocation can be categorized as patient related or procedure related. Patient-related factors include female sex, age greater than 75 years, neuromuscular disorders, cognitive disorders, substance abuse, and previous hip surgery. Higher rates of dislocation have been reported with the use of the posterior approach than with the use of the anterolateral or direct lateral approach. However, repair of the posterior capsule and short external rotator tendons decreases the rate of dislocation with the posterior approach to be closer to that of anteriorly based approaches (1% to 2%). The direct anterior approach has a dislocation rate of approximately 1%. Acetabular implant malposition may be the most important surgical factor related to instability. Increased cup abduction and excessive anteversion or retroversion of the acetabulum predispose patients to dislocation. The recommended safe acetabular cup abduction angle is 40° ± 10°, and the recommended anteversion is 20° ± 5°. An increased risk of cup malposition has been reported for procedures involving minimally invasive approaches, surgeons who perform the procedure infrequently, and obese patients. However, redislocation can occur even in patients in whom the acetabular cup is positioned correctly.

Restoration of the correct femoral offset to ensure appropriate soft-tissue tensioning is important for stability. If the soft tissues are lax or leg length is not restored, instability can occur even with appropriately placed implants. The role of the rotational position of the femoral implant is less well understood, likely because malposition is difficult to assess on plain radiographs. Femoral head diameter and acetabular liner profile can lead to impingement and dislocation. Impingement occurs when the prosthetic femoral neck or greater trochanter contacts a nonarticular surface at the extremes of the range of motion (ROM), levering the femoral head out of the socket. The use of a large-diameter femoral head (greater than 32 mm) without a skirted femoral neck will improve the femoral head-neck ratio and may result in reduced impingement and improved ROM. In a randomized controlled trial, the incidence of dislocation within 1 year after primary THA was significantly lower in patients with a 36-mm femoral head compared with that in patients with a 28-mm femoral head. Increased polyethylene volumetric wear is a concern associated with the use of large-diameter femoral heads (greater than 32 mm), even with highly cross-linked polyethylene. Polyethylene liners with a rim that is posteriorly elevated 10° have been reported to have reduced dislocation rates compared with those of neutral liners. However, routine

Dr. Lachiewicz or an immediate family member has received royalties from Innomed; is a member of a speakers' bureau or has made paid presentations on behalf of Mallinckrodt; serves as a paid consultant to Gerson Lehrman Group, Guidepoint Global Advisors, and Pacira Pharmaceuticals; has received research or institutional support from Zimmer Biomet; and serves as a board member, owner, officer, or committee member of The Hip Society and the Orthopaedic Surgery and Trauma Society. Neither Dr. Ledford nor any immediate family member has received anything of value from or has stock or stock options held in a commercial company or institution related directly or indirectly to the subject of this chapter.

use of liners with an elevated rim is not recommended because of the increased risk of impingement against the rim that can occur in extension and external rotation, which could lead to anterior dislocation or, in the longer term, increased polyethylene wear or implant loosening.

Approximately 16% to 33% of dislocations recur. The etiologies of recurrent instability have been categorized as follows: acetabular implant malposition, femoral implant malposition, abductor deficiency, impingement, late wear, and unknown etiology. Abductor deficiency and cup malposition are the most common etiologies. However, in many patients with recurrent dislocation, no specific cause can be determined.

The indications for acetabular implant revision in patients with recurrent dislocation are acetabular implant malposition (the lack of anteversion or the presence of any retroversion in patients with posterior dislocation, greater than 20° anteversion in patients with anterior dislocation, or abduction angle greater than 55°; **Figure 1**), implant loosening, and severe polyethylene wear. Indications for femoral implant revision are implant malposition or loosening. Less commonly, revision of the femoral implant may be required to establish adequate soft-tissue tension and stability. If soft-tissue and bony impingement is observed, the source of the impingement should be identified and removed after revision of any malpositioned implant.

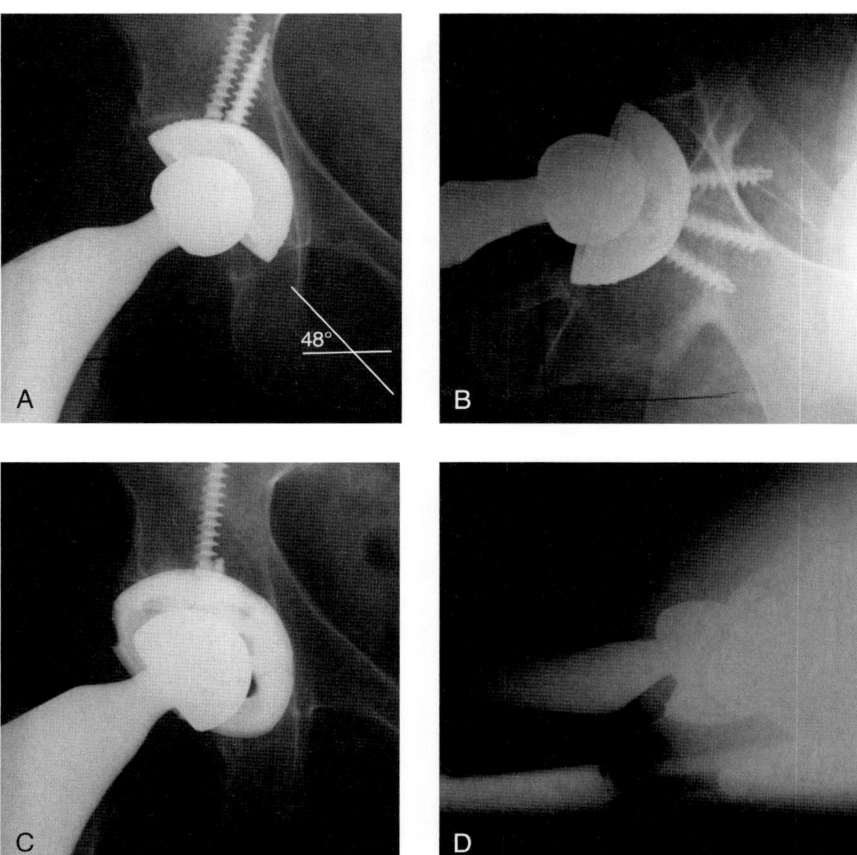

Figure 1 **A,** AP radiograph demonstrates the right hip of a 67-year-old woman with recurrent posterior dislocation after primary total hip arthroplasty. The acetabular abduction angle is 48°. **B,** Cross-table lateral radiograph demonstrates minimal anteversion. **C,** Postoperative AP radiograph demonstrates revision of the acetabular implant. The acetabular abduction angle is 38°. **D,** Postoperative cross-table lateral radiograph demonstrates approximately 20° anteversion. The femoral head size was increased from 28 mm to 32 mm.

Preoperative Evaluation

Careful clinical and radiographic evaluation is required before any surgical intervention to manage recurrent dislocation. A detailed patient history should include the mechanism of dislocation, any history of trauma, other previous episodes of instability, and symptoms of infection, such as pain, fever, or previous wound drainage. The time from the surgical procedure to dislocation may suggest the etiology; an early postoperative dislocation suggests implant malposition or impingement. Early dislocation also can result from patient behavior or activity. The index surgical note should be obtained because it may provide valuable details on the surgical approach, repair method, implant size, and any intraoperative complications.

Physical examination of both lower extremities should include evaluation of gait, ROM of the hip, side-lying abductor muscle strength, and limb lengths. The surgical incision and the patient's neurologic status also should be evaluated. The patient's serum erythrocyte sedimentation rate and C-reactive protein level should be measured to evaluate for possible infection. If results of these screening tests are abnormal and concomitant infection is suspected, hip joint aspiration should be performed to obtain a white blood cell count and cultures.

Standard radiographic evaluation should include AP pelvic, frog-lateral, and cross-table lateral views of the hip. The abduction angle and version angle of the acetabular implant should be measured if possible. Leg lengths and femoral implant offset should be measured. CT may provide a more accurate determination of acetabular implant version than plain radiographs and may be

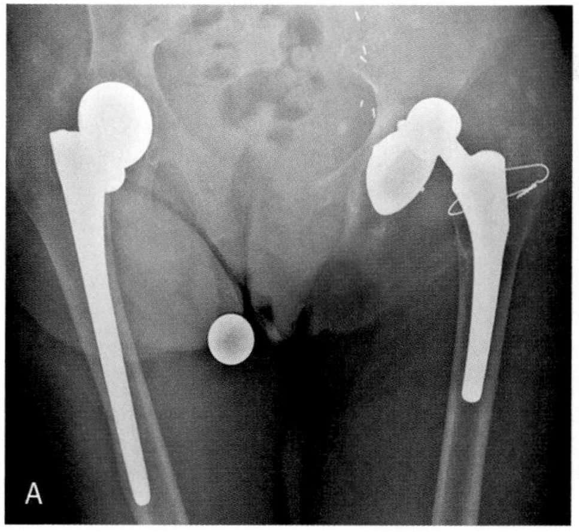

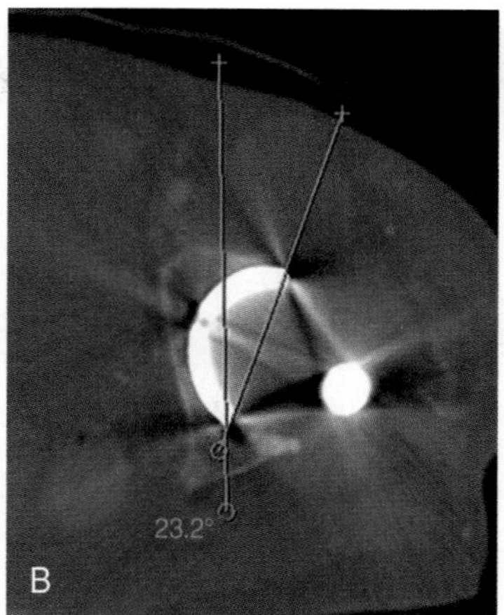

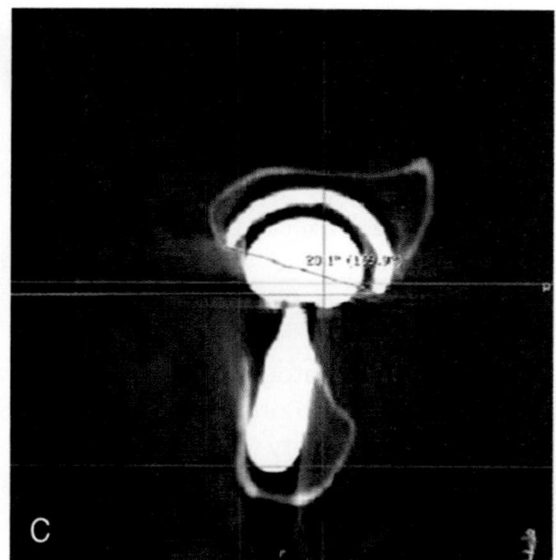

Figure 2 **A,** AP pelvic radiograph demonstrates recurrent posterior dislocation in a 52-year-old woman. **B,** Axial CT scan obtained before revision demonstrates excessive retroversion of the acetabular implant. **C,** CT scan from a different patient demonstrates appropriate acetabular cup anteversion of 20°. (Panel C reproduced with permission from Ghelman B, Kepler CK, Lyman S, Della Valle AG: CT outperforms radiography for determination of acetabular cup version after THA. *Clin Orthop Relat Res* 2009;467[9]:2362-2370.)

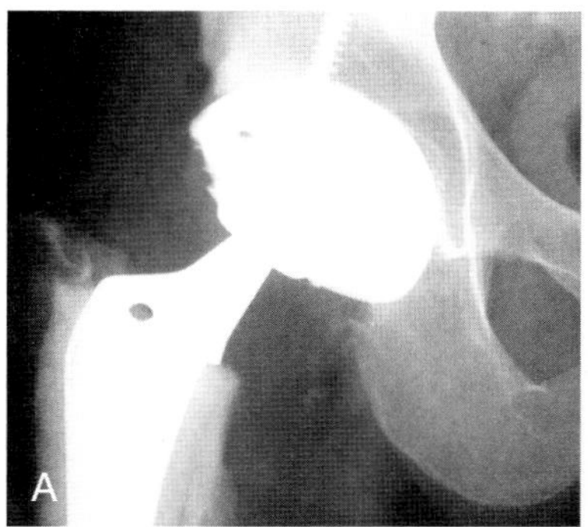

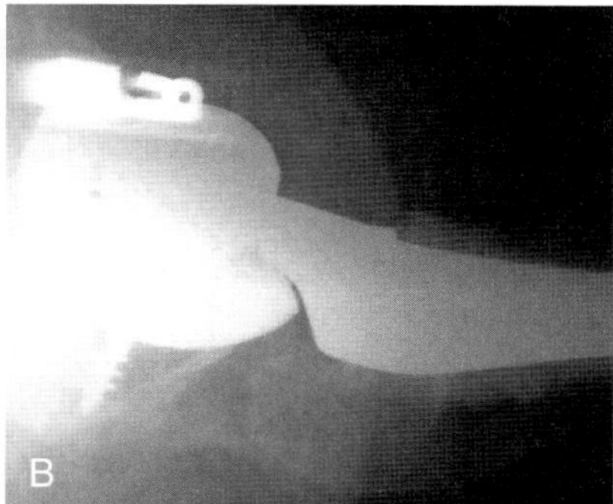

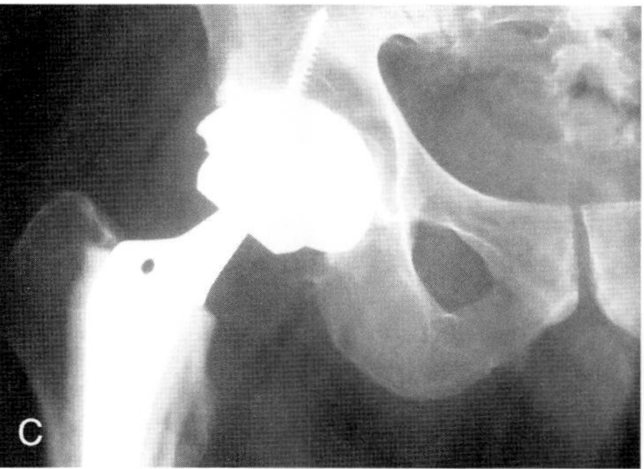

Figure 3 Radiographs of a 76-year-old man who has recurrent posterior dislocation 6 years after undergoing primary total hip arthroplasty through a posterior approach. **A,** AP view of the right hip demonstrates acceptable implant abduction. **B,** Cross-table lateral view demonstrates adequate anteversion. **C,** Postoperative AP view demonstrates modular implant revision with femoral head and acetabular liner exchange. The size of the femoral head was increased from 32 mm to 40 mm. The patient had no further dislocation at 3.5-year follow-up.

helpful for surgical planning (**Figure 2**). MRI, with metal artifact reduction sequences if necessary, can be helpful if abductor muscle avulsion or injury is suspected or if adverse local tissue reaction to metal debris (pseudotumor), which has been associated with late dislocation, is a concern.

Treatment Options

Modular exchange for the management of recurrent instability usually involves increasing the size of the femoral head and corresponding acetabular liner, sometimes involves using an acetabular liner with an elevated rim, and sometimes involves increasing the length and offset of the femoral neck. These methods also can be used in combination. The indications for modular exchange are not firmly established. However, the patient must have well-positioned and well-fixed implants with a relatively small femoral head (32 mm or smaller) and an intact abductor mechanism (**Figure 3**). The implants left in situ should have demonstrated favorable long-term results, and modular implants of various sizes must be available.

Constrained liners are generally indicated in patients with well-positioned implants and recurrent instability with no obvious cause (**Figure 4**). Other relative indications are recurrent dislocation resulting from insufficiency of the capsule or the abductor musculature; chronic nonunion of a greater trochanter osteotomy or fracture; cognitive disorder; neurologic motor disorder; late dislocation in the absence of implant loosening or malposition; failure of revision of a malpositioned implant; and failure of modular implant exchange.

Dual-mobility implants are a relatively new alternative to constrained implants in select patients with recurrent dislocation. The implant has a large polyethylene femoral head that

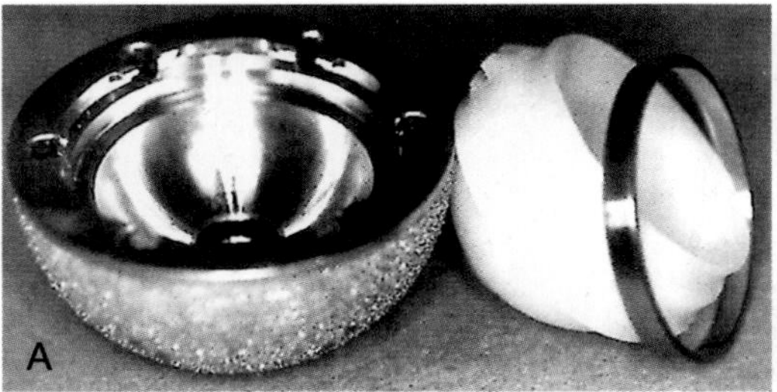
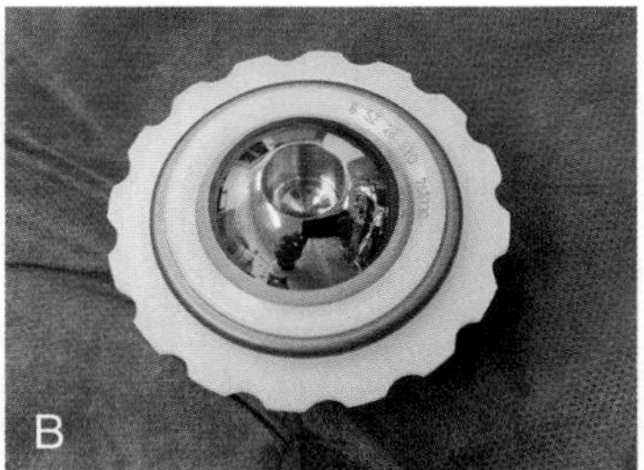
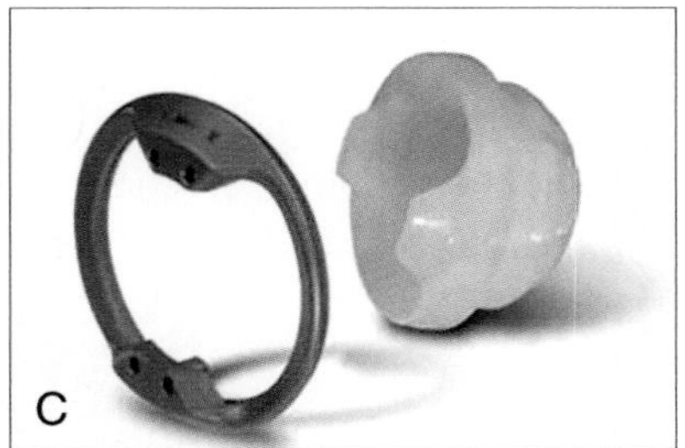

Figure 4 **A,** Photograph shows a constrained acetabular liner and a porous-coated acetabular implant. Extra polyethylene in the rim of the liner constrains the femoral head. Several companies manufacture these devices. Photographs show the Freedom (**B**; Zimmer Biomet) and Longevity (**C**; Zimmer Biomet) constrained liners. (Panel A reproduced with permission from Kaper BP, Bernini PM: Failure of a constrained acetabular prosthesis of total hip arthroplasty: A report of 4 cases. *J Bone Joint Surg* Am 1998:80[4]:561-565.)

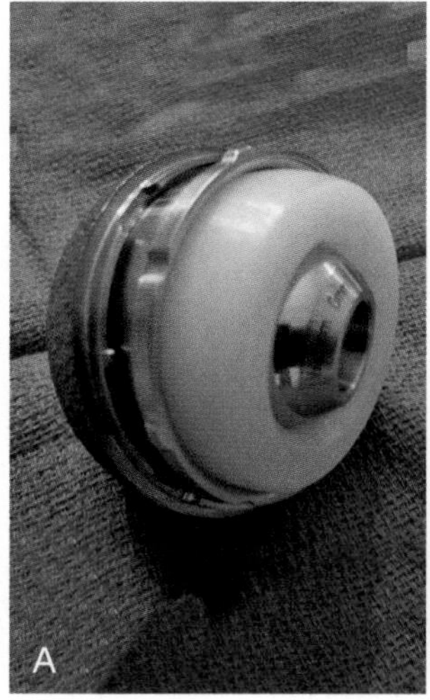
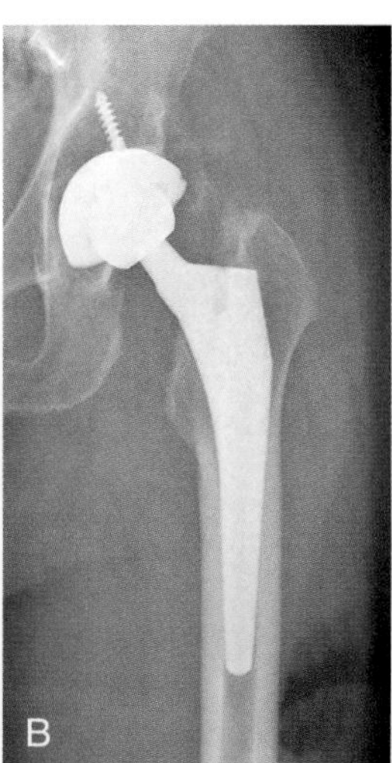
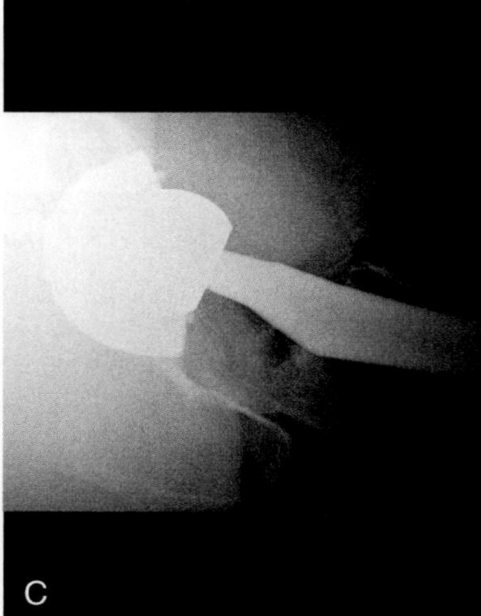
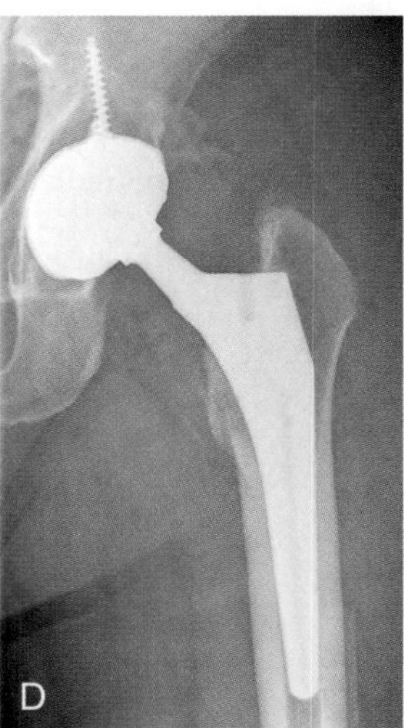
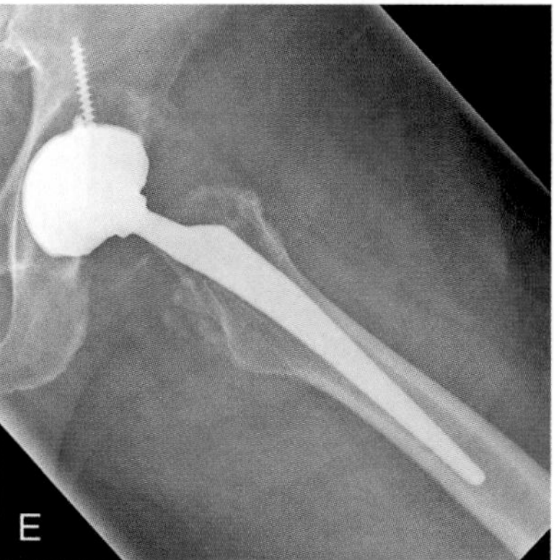

Figure 5 **A,** Photograph shows a dual-mobility implant. **B,** AP radiograph demonstrates the left hip of a 63-year-old man with recurrent dislocation that was unsuccessfully treated with the use of an abduction brace. **C,** Cross-table lateral radiograph demonstrates a minimally anteverted acetabular implant. Postoperative AP (**D**) and frog-lateral (**E**) radiographs demonstrate successful revision with a dual-mobility implant. (Panel A courtesy of Stryker Howmedica Osteonics, Rutherford, NJ.)

articulates with a polished acetabular component and an additional, smaller femoral head that snaps into the polyethylene ball (**Figure 5**). The biomechanical advantages of these implants have been theorized to include increased ROM and a larger jump distance before dislocation. A so-called third articulation is created when the femoral neck impinges or pushes against the large polyethylene ball at the extremes of motion. A similar—but not identical—construct involves a bipolar acetabular implant (usually with a 40-mm bipolar femoral head) articulating with a 40-mm highly cross-linked polyethylene liner. The primary indication for the use of dual-mobility implants is recurrent dislocation in patients who have an intact abductor mechanism. Dual-mobility implants also may be

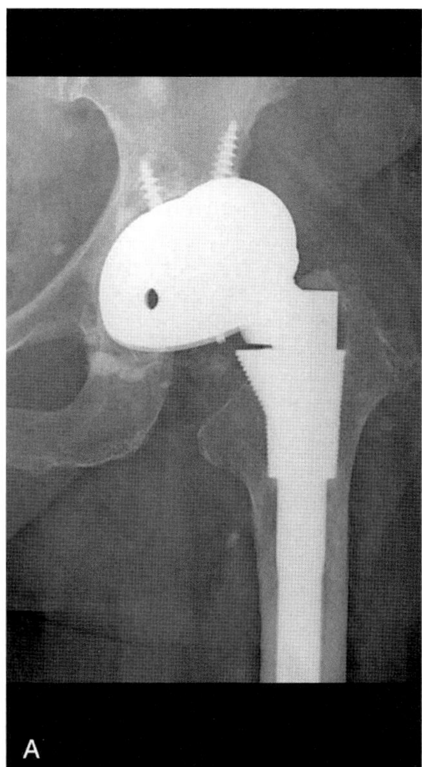

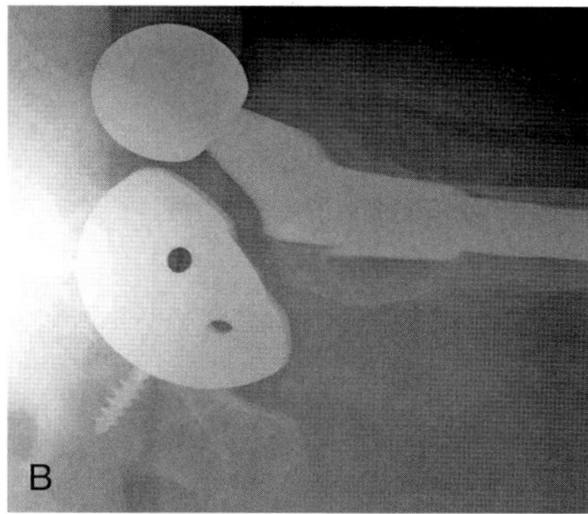

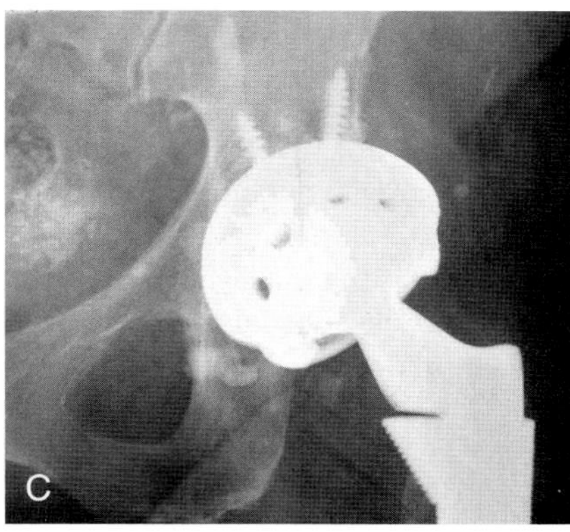

Figure 6 **A,** AP radiograph demonstrates the left hip of a 76-year-old woman who underwent jumbo acetabular revision for recurrent posterior dislocation and continued to experience recurrent anterior dislocation despite the use of a hip orthosis and a hip spica cast. **B,** Cross-table lateral radiograph demonstrates anterior dislocation. The patient underwent revision with the use of a constrained liner. **C,** AP radiograph obtained 10 years postoperatively demonstrates no further dislocation or complications.

indicated in patients with failed constrained implants, in patients undergoing modular exchange, and in patients requiring revision of malpositioned implants. Dual-mobility implants also have been used in revision procedures with a high risk of dislocation, such as revision of failed metal-on-metal resurfacing arthroplasty or THA, and second-stage reimplantation for the management of periprosthetic infection.

Contraindications

The contraindications for modular revision (liner or large femoral head exchange) include acetabular implant malposition, loosening of one or both implants, insufficient abductor musculature, chronic nonunion of the greater trochanter, history of cognitive or neurologic motor disorder, and inadequate intraoperative stability even with a large femoral head. The contraindication to the use of any constrained prosthesis is acetabular implant loosening or malposition. In such patients, revision of the acetabular implant is necessary. A constrained liner can be inserted into the revision acetabular implant to provide intraoperative stability if necessary. However, this constraint may result in lack of bony ingrowth and early loosening. In these patients, a large-diameter (36- or 40-mm) acetabular liner and femoral head can be used initially until bony ingrowth into the revision shell has occurred, with the understanding that a constrained liner may be needed later if recurrent dislocations occur (**Figure 6**). Alternatively, a malpositioned or loose acetabular implant could be managed initially with a new acetabular shell that can accommodate a dual-mobility implant. If the acetabular cup is well positioned and well fixed, a constrained liner can be cemented into the existing shell. Although the absence of a functioning abductor mechanism is considered a contraindication to the use of a dual-mobility implant, the senior author of this chapter (P.F.L.) has successfully used dual-mobility implants in such patients.

Dislocation associated with an acute avulsion of a greater trochanteric osteotomy or an acute fracture of the greater trochanter is managed with closed reduction and surgical repair or advancement. However, attempts to repair a chronic nonunion of the greater trochanter usually are unsuccessful. Therefore, dislocation in these patients is better managed with the use of a constrained liner or a dual-mobility implant.

Soft-tissue augmentation of the hip capsule with Achilles tendon allograft is no longer recommended for the management of recurrent dislocation.

Alternative Treatments

Early postoperative dislocation after primary or revision THA typically is managed with closed reduction either in the emergency department with the patient under intravenous sedation or in the operating room with the patient under general or regional anesthesia. Rarely, open reduction with the patient under general anesthesia may be required if closed reduction of the dislocation is not possible or if dislocation of a constrained liner has occurred. Plain radiographs or fluoroscopy should be used to confirm a concentric reduction, and the ROM of the reduced hip should be assessed

Table 1 Results of Modular Implant Exchange in Revision Total Hip Arthroplasty for the Management of Recurrent Dislocation

Authors (Year)	Number of Hips	Mean Patient Age in Years (Range)	Mean Follow-up in Years (Range)	Success Rate (%)[a]	Repeat Revision Surgery for Recurrent Instability
Toomey et al (2001)	13	59 (26-79)	5.8 (2.8-11.8)	77	1 hip (7.7%)
Earll et al (2002)	29	64 (22-90)	4.6 (2.0-10.2)	45	5 hips (17.2%)
Lachiewicz et al (2004)	17	60 (29-81)	4 (2-7)	82	2 hips (11.8%)
Biviji et al (2009)	48	69 (51-87)	4.7 (1.2-9.4)	67	13 hips (27.1%)

[a] Success is defined as the absence of repeat dislocation.

to determine a safe zone of motion in which subluxation does not occur. After reduction, many surgeons, including the senior author of this chapter (P.F.L.), place the patient in a hip orthosis or, rarely, in a hip spica cast for 6 weeks to limit ROM and encourage soft-tissue healing. The orthosis setting should be 0° to 70° for a posterior dislocation and −20° to 90° for an anterior dislocation. The senior author of this chapter (P.F.L.) sets the lateral hinge angle at neutral or 10° of adduction because orthosis settings with the thigh abducted will be poorly tolerated by the patient. However, immobilization has not been definitively proved to prevent recurrent dislocation. If extreme instability persists after reduction and the surgeon identifies an obvious cause of dislocation, the patient should be advised that early revision may be necessary.

In some patients, first-time dislocation may occur 5 years or later after THA. In one retrospective study, dislocation occurred 5 years or later after primary THA in 32% of dislocated hips. Risk factors included female sex, previous subluxation, substantial trauma, and the onset of cognitive or motor impairment. Radiographic evidence of polyethylene wear of greater than 2 mm, implant loosening, or initial malposition of the acetabular implant was associated with late first dislocation. The rate of recurrence after late dislocation is very high. Despite the poor success rate, closed reduction and the use of a hip orthosis for immobilization can be attempted for the management of first-time late dislocation in the absence of implant malposition or polyethylene wear.

Results

Historically, the results of surgical management of recurrent dislocation consisting of revision of one or both prosthetic components have been poor. However, improved results have become possible with the introduction of femoral heads larger than 32 mm with highly cross-linked polyethylene liners, modern constrained liners, and dual-mobility implants.

Only four studies of modular implant exchange for recurrent dislocation after primary THA have been published (**Table 1**). In two of these studies, with careful intraoperative assessment of ROM and possible impingement, 10 of 13 patients and 14 of 17 patients, at 5.8-year and 4-year follow-up, respectively, had no further dislocation. However, in the other two studies, 16 of 29 patients and 16 of 48 patients experienced further dislocation at nearly 5-year follow-up. The authors of this chapter are not aware of any study of modular implant exchange in which only femoral heads larger than 32 mm were used. This technique is relatively simple and should be considered for use in patients with recurrent dislocation and well-aligned prosthetic components. Patients should be carefully advised about the relative benefits and risks of this procedure. The use of a very large (36-mm, 38-mm, 40-mm, or larger) femoral head (either metal or ceramic alloy) and a highly cross-linked polyethylene liner may increase the success rate of modular implant exchange in patients with recurrent dislocation after primary THA. Modular implant exchange typically is not recommended for the management of recurrent dislocation after revision THA.

Numerous reports and literature reviews have examined a variety of constrained implant designs. Results are related to both the specific device and whether it was implanted to prevent dislocation after primary THA in high-risk patients or to manage recurrent dislocation after primary or revision THA. One type of constrained implant consists of a 28- or 32-mm (or larger) femoral head that snaps into a polyethylene liner, which is then sealed with a metal locking ring. The other type of constrained implant is tripolar. The results appear to be device specific. The rate of failure (recurrent dislocation) of constrained implants is less than 7% in most series (**Table 2**). However,

Table 2 Results of Constrained Implants in Revision Total Hip Arthroplasty for the Management of Recurrent Dislocation

Authors (Year)	Number of Hips	Mean Patient Age in Years (Range)	Mean Follow-up in Years (Range)	Success Rate (%)[a]	Repeat Revision Surgery for Mechanical Failure of Constrained Liner
Callaghan et al (2004)	31	72 (31-91)	3.9 (2-12.7)	100	2 hips (6.5%)
Goetz et al (2004)	56	71 (31-92)	10.2 (7-13.2)	98.3[b]	4 hips (7.1%)
Rady et al (2010)	15	57 (NA)	2.2 (NA)	93.3	NA
Munro et al (2013)	82	68 (14-94)	2.8 (2-4.1)	96.3	2 hips (2.4%)

NA = not available.

[a] Success is defined as the absence of repeat dislocation; if dislocation did occur, revision surgery was required because of the constrained implant.

[b] Report of one alleged dislocation but no confirmed clinical reports.

serious concerns regarding the use of constrained implants include the need for open reduction after dislocation, the limited impingement-free ROM, and the risk of loosening of the acetabular implant as a result of high interface forces.

Dislocation of a constrained implant can be very difficult to manage. Although successful closed reduction has been described in a few case reports, a surgical procedure usually is required to reduce the hip and revise a damaged locking ring, displaced liner, or acetabular cup (**Figure 7**). The range of hip motion usually is reduced with a constrained liner, and increased stress may be produced at the interface of the bone and the implant or polyethylene liner, resulting in increased wear and loosening of the acetabular or femoral implant. Some surgeons have reported breakage or dislodgement of the locking ring or dissociation of a tripolar constrained implant. Thus, constrained implants may be best reserved for use in elderly and debilitated patients, older patients with limited activity levels, patients with neurologic disorders, and patients with unreconstructable functional deficiency of the abductor musculature.

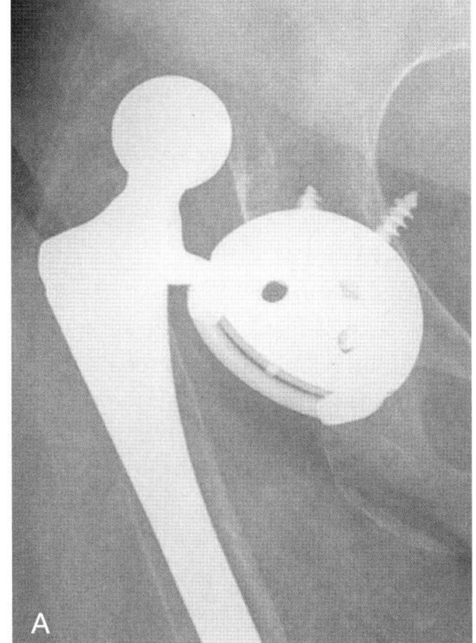

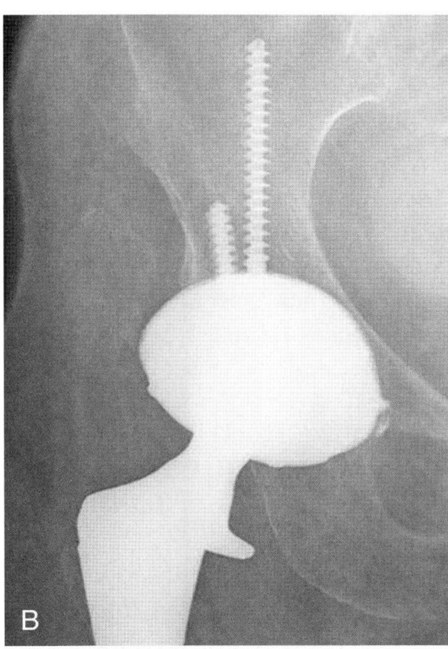

Figure 7 **A,** AP radiograph demonstrates dislocation of a constrained implant in an 82-year-old woman with deficiency of the greater trochanter. The femoral head pulled out of the liner without disruption of the locking ring. **B,** AP radiograph demonstrates acetabular revision to a dual-mobility implant. The patient remained without dislocation at 2.5-year follow-up.

The results of modern dual-mobility implants in patients with recurrent dislocation have been encouraging at short- to medium-term follow-up. Several studies have reported a success rate of approximately 98% in the prevention of further dislocation (**Table 3**). A report of the Swedish Hip Arthroplasty Register demonstrated a 2-year nondislocation rate of 99% and a 90% survival rate at 4 years postoperatively, with higher rates of failure in patients between ages 55 and 59 years and patients who underwent a prior revision THA. Dual-mobility devices can dislocate at the articulation of the large polyethylene ball and the metal shell (of which closed reduction often is possible) or at the articulation of the small metal head and the inner polyethylene ball (of which closed reduction is difficult or unlikely to succeed). A new, usually late, complication of dual-mobility implants, both in primary THA and in revision THA in patients with recurrent dislocation, is intraprosthetic dislocation resulting from wear or impingement of the femoral neck against the

Table 3 Results of Dual-Mobility Implants in Revision Total Hip Arthroplasty for the Management of Recurrent Dislocation

Authors (Year)	Number of Hips	Mean Patient Age in Years (Range)	Mean Follow-up in Years (Range)	Success Rate (%)[a]	Intraprosthetic Dislocation Rate
Guyen et al (2009)	54	65 (45-89)	4 (2.2-6.8)	98.2	2 hips (3.7%)
Hamadouche et al (2010)	47	71 (41-92)	4.3 (2.1-6.4)	98	1 hip (2.1%)
Leiber-Wackenheim et al (2011)	50	68 (47-88)	8 (6-11)	98.3	No intraprosthetic dislocation
Hailer et al (2012)	228	75 (NA)	2 (0-6)	98	Intraprosthetic dislocation rate not reported
Vasukutty et al (2012)	155	77 (42-89)	3.5 (1.5-5.7)	97.9	No intraprosthetic dislocation

NA = not available.

[a] Success is defined as the absence of repeat dislocation.

large polyethylene ball. Intraprosthetic dislocation must be managed with revision THA. Dual-mobility implants have been used to treat a variety of patients with recurrent dislocation but may be most suitable for use in younger, more active patients.

Techniques

Setup/Exposure

- Surgical treatment of a patient with recurrent dislocation can be performed through an anterolateral, posterior, direct anterior (in certain patients), or transtrochanteric (extended, slide, or standard) approach. The surgeon's experience and familiarity with the approach, the direction of dislocation, and the need for concomitant procedures influence the choice of approach.
- The senior author of this chapter (P.F.L.) uses the posterior approach, with repair of the posterior capsule and short external rotator tendons, in all procedures for the management of recurrent dislocation.
- Adequate soft-tissue exposure of the acetabular implant is necessary to completely visualize the circumference of the acetabulum.

Procedure

MODULAR REVISION

- The modular femoral head and acetabular liner are removed.
- Fixation of both components is checked with appropriate devices.
- A trial acetabular liner with the largest possible inner diameter is placed, with or without an elevated rim in the direction of the dislocation.
- A trial femoral head of the corresponding diameter and the same or longer femoral neck length is placed on the femoral implant.
- The hip is reduced.
- Generally, a skirted implant should not be used because it can result in impingement.
- The hip is manually moved through a full ROM to ensure stability in maximum flexion and both internal and external rotation.
- Any soft tissue or bone causing impingement should be excised.
- The final implants are placed.
- The hip is assessed for stability.
- If the hip remains unstable and the patient has a well-fixed acetabular shell, either a constrained liner or a dual-mobility prosthesis can be implanted if the device is compatible with the existing acetabular shell.
- If removal of a well-fixed, malpositioned acetabular implant is necessary, the safest method is to use a sharp, curved acetabular chisel system to minimize damage to the remaining acetabular bone structure.
- This same instrument can be used to remove a well-positioned acetabular implant that is incompatible with a modular exchange or a well-fixed acetabular shell in which a new dual-mobility or constrained acetabular implant cannot be securely placed.

CONSTRAINED IMPLANTS

- Several constrained acetabular liners are available that can be secured into a porous-coated acetabular implant. In several of these devices (for example, S-ROM [DePuy Synthes], Freedom [Zimmer Biomet], Longevity [Zimmer Biomet]), the rim contains extra polyethylene that serves to constrain the femoral head (**Figure 4**).
- A metal locking ring holds the polyethylene rim in place to provide

increased constraint. These rings are available in various sizes and designs.

- One constrained tripolar implant design consists of a polyethylene inner liner and a cobalt-chromium shell that articulates with another polyethylene liner within a porous acetabular shell. A 22-, 26-, or 28-mm femoral head can be used with the inner liner depending on the size of the shell. The locking ring is identical to the ring in a bipolar prosthesis.
- Any of these constrained liners can be cemented into a well-fixed and well-positioned metal acetabular shell.

DUAL-MOBILITY IMPLANTS

- Several dual-mobility implant designs have been used in primary THA. These devices consist of either a one-piece acetabular implant or a porous-coated titanium acetabular shell that has holes for screw fixation.
- Most surgeons in North America prefer to use modular acetabular implants for revision THA because these implants allow screw fixation of the acetabular cup, which is usually required in revision THA.
- A polished cobalt-chromium liner is impacted into the titanium shell.
- With the use of a clamp device, a 22- or 28-mm metal or ceramic femoral head is inserted into a large, highly cross-linked polyethylene ball that articulates with the cobalt-chromium acetabular liner.
- The use of the clamp device may require removal of an existing well-fixed acetabular implant or fixation with cement into an existing well-fixed and well-positioned acetabular shell.

Wound Closure

- If possible, the posterior capsule and available soft-tissue structures (external rotators) should be repaired to confer additional stability.
- The wound is closed in a standard, layered manner.

Postoperative Regimen

Weight bearing as tolerated with a walker or crutches is generally recommended for 4 to 6 weeks after revision THA for recurrent dislocation. The effect of patient precautions and use of an orthosis to limit ROM after revision to a constrained liner or dual-mobility implant has not been clearly demonstrated. The authors of this chapter usually recommend the use of a prefitted hip orthosis for 6 weeks postoperatively to prevent adduction greater than 10° and flexion greater than 70° and to allow soft-tissue healing.

Avoiding Pitfalls and Complications

A dislocated hip prosthesis requires prompt treatment. As noted, reduction can be performed in the emergency department with the patient under conscious sedation. However, forceful reduction maneuvers have been reported to result in dissociation of modular implants (dissociation of the femoral head from the trunnion or of the modular femoral neck from the stem) and disruption of acetabular or femoral fixation. If adequacy of conscious sedation is a concern or if the hip has been dislocated for more than 24 hours, the use of spinal or general anesthesia and intravenous muscle relaxation is strongly recommended. Reduction should be confirmed with the use of fluoroscopy or plain radiography because nonconcentric reductions can occur. After reduction, the hip should be moved through a gentle ROM to determine the range of safe motion and for prognostic reasons. If the hip subluxates with flexion less than 90°, early revision likely will be necessary. Although immobilization has not been demonstrated to reduce the risk of recurrent dislocation after a first-time early or late dislocation, the senior author of this chapter (P.F.L.) strongly recommends that the patient wear a well-fitted, padded hip orthosis to protect the soft tissues around the hip, facilitate healing, and avoid an early recurrence.

The risk of complications resulting from a modular implant exchange can be decreased by using the largest possible femoral head, carefully testing the ROM intraoperatively with trial implants, and removing any impinging bone or soft tissue. When constrained implants are used, the risk of complications can be decreased by ensuring correct positioning of the liner within the metal acetabular shell. Constrained implants should be avoided when fixation of the acetabular shell is a concern or when fixation is compromised by extensive pelvic osteolysis. Failure of a constrained implant usually requires open reduction and repeat revision, and patients should be advised preoperatively of this possible outcome. Complications resulting from the use of dual-mobility implants include painful psoas tendon impingement and the need for repeat revision because of late intraprosthetic dislocation.

Bibliography

Biviji AA, Ezzet KA, Pulido P, Colwell CW Jr: Modular femoral head and liner exchange for the unstable total hip arthroplasty. *J Arthroplasty* 2009;24(4):625-630.

Bozic KJ, Kurtz SM, Lau E, Ong K, Vail TP, Berry DJ: The epidemiology of revision total hip arthroplasty in the United States. *J Bone Joint Surg Am* 2009;91(1):128-133.

Callaghan JJ, Parvizi J, Novak CC, et al: A constrained liner cemented into a secure cementless acetabular shell. *J Bone Joint Surg Am* 2004;86(10):2206-2211.

Earll MD, Fehring TK, Griffin WL, Mason JB, McCoy T, Odum S: Success rate of modular component exchange for the treatment of an unstable total hip arthroplasty. *J Arthroplasty* 2002;17(7):864-869.

Goetz DD, Bremner BR, Callaghan JJ, Capello WN, Johnston RC: Salvage of a recurrently dislocating total hip prosthesis with use of a constrained acetabular component: A concise follow-up of a previous report. *J Bone Joint Surg Am* 2004;86(11):2419-2423.

Guyen O, Pibarot V, Vaz G, Chevillotte C, Béjui-Hugues J: Use of a dual mobility socket to manage total hip arthroplasty instability. *Clin Orthop Relat Res* 2009;467(2):465-472.

Hailer NP, Weiss RJ, Stark A, Kärrholm J: Dual-mobility cups for revision due to instability are associated with a low rate of re-revisions due to dislocation: 228 patients from the Swedish Hip Arthroplasty Register. *Acta Orthop* 2012;83(6):566-571.

Hamadouche M, Biau DJ, Huten D, Musset T, Gaucher F: The use of a cemented dual mobility socket to treat recurrent dislocation. *Clin Orthop Relat Res* 2010;468(12):3248-3254.

Howie DW, Holubowycz OT, Middleton R; Large Articulation Study Group: Large femoral heads decrease the incidence of dislocation after total hip arthroplasty: A randomized controlled trial. *J Bone Joint Surg Am* 2012;94(12):1095-1102.

Lachiewicz PF, Soileau E, Ellis J: Modular revision for recurrent dislocation of primary or revision total hip arthroplasty. *J Arthroplasty* 2004;19(4):424-429.

Leiber-Wackenheim F, Brunschweiler B, Ehlinger M, Gabrion A, Mertl P: Treatment of recurrent THR dislocation using of a cementless dual-mobility cup: A 59 cases series with a mean 8 years' follow-up. *Orthop Traumatol Surg Res* 2011;97(1):8-13.

Munro JT, Vioreanu MH, Masri BA, Duncan CP: Acetabular liner with focal constraint to prevent dislocation after THA. *Clin Orthop Relat Res* 2013;471(12):3883-3890.

Rady AE, Asal MK, Bassiony AA: The use of a constrained cementless acetabular component for instability in total hip replacement. *Hip Int* 2010;20(4):434-439.

Toomey SD, Hopper RH Jr, McAuley JP, Engh CA: Modular component exchange for treatment of recurrent dislocation of a total hip replacement in selected patients. *J Bone Joint Surg Am* 2001;83(10):1529-1533.

Vasukutty NL, Middleton RG, Matthews EC, Young PS, Uzoigwe CE, Minhas TH: The double-mobility acetabular component in revision total hip replacement: The United Kingdom experience. *J Bone Joint Surg Br* 2012;94(5):603-608.

Wera GD, Ting NT, Moric M, Paprosky WG, Sporer SM, Della Valle CJ: Classification and management of the unstable total hip arthroplasty. *J Arthroplasty* 2012;27(5):710-715.

Chapter 34
Periprosthetic Joint Infection: Diagnosis and Management

Mohammad Ali Enayatollahi, MD
Javad Parvizi, MD, FRCS

Introduction

Periprosthetic joint infection (PJI) is a substantial complication after total hip arthroplasty (THA). PJI is diagnosed in 15% of revision THAs in the United States and 13% in the United Kingdom. Complications resulting from PJI occur in approximately 0.88% to 2.22% of primary THAs and 4% to 6% of revision THAs.

PJI continues to occur despite the use of a clean-air operating room, perioperative antibiotics, and numerous other measures. Patients with PJI of the hip often require multiple surgical procedures, prolonged use of intravenous and oral antibiotics, and extended inpatient and outpatient rehabilitation. Clinical outcomes are worse in patients who undergo revision of an infected THA than in patients who undergo revision for aseptic failure. Recently, PJI has been found to increase patient mortality fivefold compared with that of patients with aseptic failure.

The economic burden associated with the treatment of PJI is substantial. In a database study based on the National Inpatient Sample, the average hospitalization charges for THA patients with infection were 1.76 times those of THA patients without infection. In an institutional database study, the direct medical costs associated with revision THA resulting from infection were 2.8 times those associated with revision THA for aseptic loosening and 4.8 times those associated with primary THA. Revision of an infected THA was associated with significantly longer length of stay in the hospital and more hospitalizations, surgical procedures, outpatient visits, outpatient costs, and complications compared with primary THA or revision for aseptic loosening. The authors of an institutional study from the United Kingdom reported that the mean total cost of septic revision THA was £21,937, whereas the mean total cost of aseptic revision THA was £11,897.

Definition of PJI

Numerous investigators have attempted to develop a unified definition of PJI. Three groups have presented guidelines and consensus-based evidence: the American Academy of Orthopaedic Surgeons (AAOS), a workgroup of the Musculoskeletal Infection Society (MSIS), and the International Consensus Meeting on Periprosthetic Joint Infection (ICM). The ICM adapted the MSIS definition of PJI and updated and revised the AAOS algorithmic approach to the diagnosis of PJI (**Figure 1**). The modified MSIS definition of an infected prosthetic joint is shown in **Table 1**. The presence of one of the criteria indicates infection. Although the modified MSIS diagnostic criteria have allowed the orthopaedic community to move toward a standard definition of PJI, some infections, especially those caused by indolent organisms such as *Propionibacterium acnes* or coagulase-negative *Staphylococcus aureus*, may exist without the presence of these signs of infection. Thus, clinicians must exercise judgment when evaluating patients in whom suspicion of PJI is high but these criteria do not provide a definitive diagnosis of infection.

The AAOS algorithm for the diagnosis of PJI categorizes patients as being at high or low risk of PJI on the basis of history, physical examination, radiographic

Dr. Parvizi or an immediate family member serves as a paid consultant to CeramTec, ConvaTec, Medtronic, Smith & Nephew, TissueGene, and Zimmer Biomet; has stock or stock options held in CD Diagnostics, Hip Innovation Technology, and PRN – Physician Recommended Nutriceuticals; has received research or institutional support from 3M, Cempra, CeramTec, DePuy Synthes, National Institutes of Health (National Institute of Arthritis and Musculoskeletal and Skin Diseases and National Institute of Child Health and Human Development), the Orthopaedic Research and Education Foundation, Smith & Nephew, StelKast, Stryker, and Zimmer Biomet; and serves as a board member, owner, officer, or committee member of the Eastern Orthopaedic Association and the M. E. Müller Foundation of North America. Neither Dr. Enayatollahi nor any immediate family member has received anything of value from or has stock or stock options held in a commercial company or institution related directly or indirectly to the subject of this chapter.

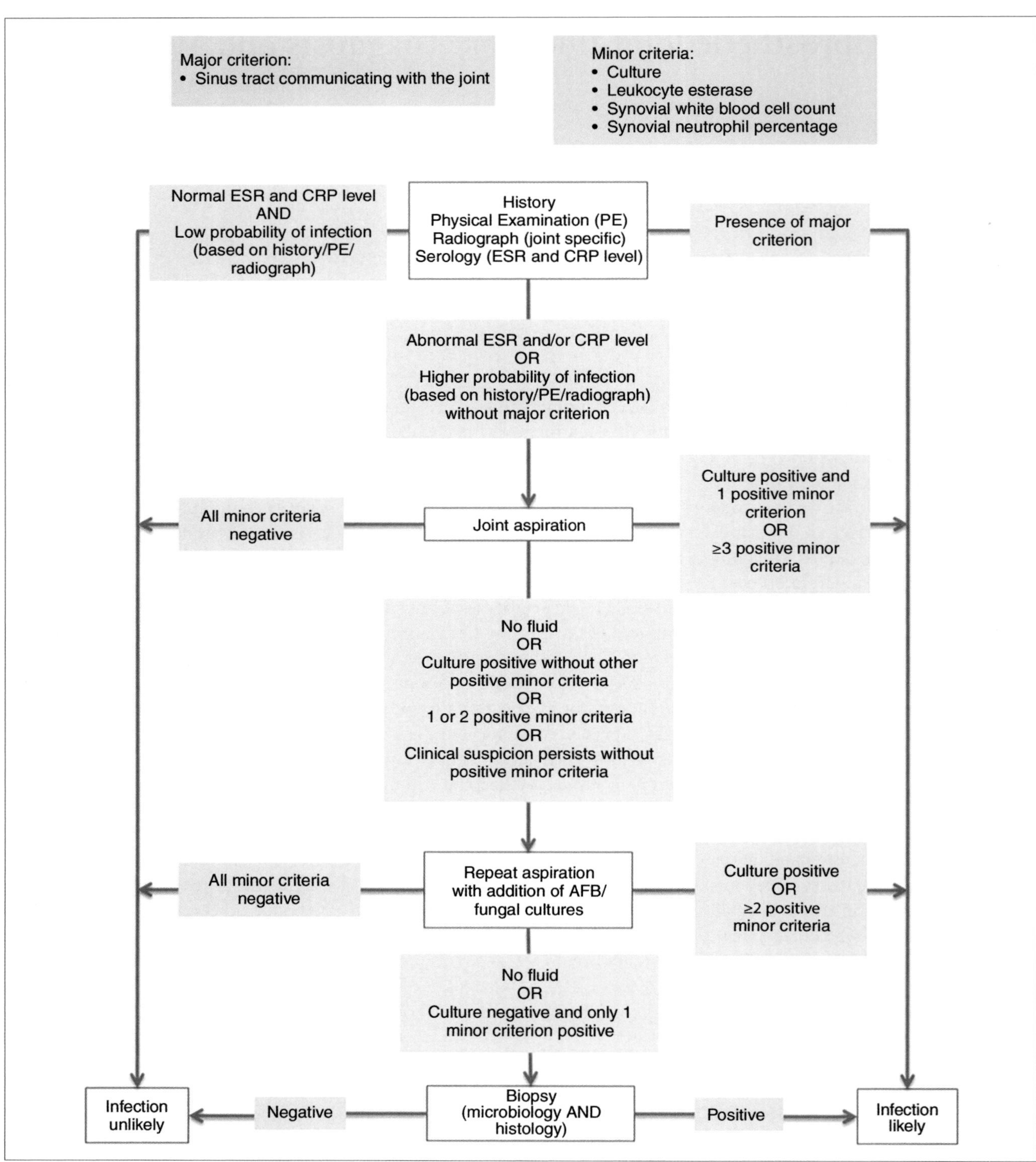

Figure 1 Algorithm demonstrates the approach to the diagnosis of periprosthetic joint infection recommended by the International Consensus Meeting on Periprosthetic Joint Infection. AFB = acid-fast bacillus, CRP = C-reactive protein, ESR = erythrocyte sedimentation rate. (Adapted with permission from Gehrke T, Parvizi J, eds: *Proceedings of the International Consensus Meeting on Periprosthetic Joint Infection.* Marentino, Italy, European Federation of National Associations of Orthopaedics and Traumatology [EFFORT], 2013. Available at: https://www.efort.org/wp-content/uploads/2013/10/Philadelphia_Consensus.pdf. Accessed April 27, 2016.)

Table 1 Criteria for an Infected Prosthetic Joint Based on the Modified Musculoskeletal Infection Society Definition[a]

Two positive cultures with a phenotypically identical organism
A sinus tract communicating with the prosthetic joint
Presence of three of the following five minor criteria:
Elevated serum C-reactive protein level and erythrocyte sedimentation rate
Elevated synovial fluid white blood cell count or a "++" result on leukocyte esterase test strip
Elevated synovial fluid polymorphonuclear neutrophil percentage
Positive histologic analysis of periprosthetic tissue
A single positive culture

[a] The presence of even one major criterion indicates infection.

imaging, and other tests. Despite the paucity of high-level data supporting risk stratification of patients, the identification of factors that can suggest a high probability of infection can assist the clinician in decision making and implementation of more extensive tests to diagnose PJI.

Diagnosis

Workup for PJI should be part of the evaluation of every patient with painful or failed THA. Differentiation of septic failure from aseptic failure is critical in the planning of revision THA. Because the treatment of a patient with an infected THA is markedly different from the treatment of a patient with aseptic failure, every effort must be made to accurately diagnose infection as the cause of failure. As noted, clinicians must rely on a combination of tests because no single test can consistently identify or rule out PJI in all patients. Diagnosis typically requires a combination of history and physical examination, serologic and synovial fluid tests, culture results, histology, and basic molecular techniques. **Figure 1** shows the assessment recommendations adapted from the AAOS algorithm for approaching a failed and/or painful joint arthroplasty.

History and Physical Examination

Findings in the history that should raise suspicion of PJI include a prolonged history of pain and/or stiffness in a prosthetic joint; history of prolonged wound drainage after index arthroplasty; recent history of bacteremia; multiple prior surgical procedures in the affected joint; history of PJI; comorbidities that can compromise the patient's innate immunity, such as diabetes mellitus, inflammatory arthropathy, or malnourishment; history of intravenous drug use; the presence of conditions that can affect the skin, such as ulcers, psoriasis, poor wound state, or chronic venous stasis; and history of prior surgical site infection.

Findings of the physical examination that are suggestive of PJI include swelling, warmth, redness, tenderness, and wound dehiscence or persistent wound discharge. The only physical examination finding that is pathognomonic for PJI is the presence of a sinus tract communicating with the prosthetic joint.

Serum Tests

Existing guidelines and recommendations endorse ESR and serum CRP level as the most appropriate screening tools for the diagnosis of PJI. Thus, these tests should be ordered for all patients in whom PJI is suspected and for all patients undergoing revision arthroplasty for any cause of failure. ESR and serum CRP level are sensitive but not specific biomarkers for the diagnosis of PJI. Both of these inflammatory markers are influenced by the presence of infection or inflammation in other organ systems, such as in patients with rheumatoid arthritis, neoplasm, coronary artery disease, polymyalgia rheumatica, or inflammatory bowel disease, or at a site other than the prosthetic joint. Thus, elevated ESR and CRP level are not always indicative of PJI. The combination of an elevated ESR and elevated serum CRP level has been found to be a better predictor of PJI than isolated elevation of either of these values. Negative results of ESR and serum CRP level are more accurate for ruling out infection than positive results of ESR and CRP level are for detecting infection. However, anecdotal evidence from the second author's (J.P.) institution suggests that the ESR and serum CRP level may be normal in up to 11% of patients with PJI. The CRP level is a better test than ESR for detecting PJI. Laboratories have different methods of measuring ESR and CRP. Furthermore, ESR may be influenced by patient age, sex, and medical comorbidities. The ESR and serum CRP level may be elevated for approximately 30 to 60 days postoperatively.

For the diagnosis of acute PJI (occurring less than 6 weeks postoperatively), the threshold for CRP level is greater than 100 mg/L, whereas ESR is not useful. For the diagnosis of chronic PJI, the ESR threshold is greater than 30 mm/h, and the CRP threshold is greater than 10 mg/L. Limited evidence suggests that the ESR and serum CRP thresholds remain applicable for diagnosing PJI in the presence of inflammatory diseases.

Synovial Fluid Tests

SYNOVIAL WBC COUNT AND PMN PERCENTAGE

Synovial white blood cell (WBC) count and polymorphonuclear neutrophil

(PMN) percentage are accurate predictors of PJI. However, different cutoff points for synovial WBC count and PMN percentage have been reported, resulting in inconsistent definitions of PJI according to laboratory results. Nonetheless, these thresholds are useful for diagnosis of PJI up to 6 weeks postoperatively despite elevated baseline levels because of surgery. The same thresholds for synovial WBC count and PMN percentage are used to predict PJI in patients with and without inflammatory disorders. Thresholds for the diagnosis of acute PJI (up to 6 weeks) are synovial WBC count greater than 10,000 cells/µL and synovial PMN percentage greater than 90. Thresholds for the diagnosis of chronic PJI (lasting 6 weeks or longer) are synovial WBC count greater than 3,000 cells/µL and synovial PMN percentage greater than 80.

To increase the accuracy of synovial WBC count and PMN percentage, two technical considerations should be kept in mind. First, if the synovial fluid is bloodstained, the WBC count should be adjusted for the presence of synovial red blood cell, serum red blood cell, and serum WBC counts according to the formula of Ghanem et al. Second, failed metal-on-metal bearings or corrosion of metal implants in THA may result in an elevated synovial WBC count and differential. Phagocytosed metal debris within monocytes may be read as neutrophils by some automated hematology instruments. In these instances, manual counts should be used for WBC analysis.

LEUKOCYTE ESTERASE TEST

Leukocyte esterase is a secretion of activated neutrophils in response to infections. A strip test for this enzyme is based on a chemical reaction with active leukocyte esterase that involves color change (**Figure 2**). The leukocyte esterase strip test has been used for the diagnosis of urinary tract infections since 1980. Applying synovial fluid to a simple urine strip test and reading the results for leukocyte esterase is a reliable test for PJI, with sensitivity between 81% and 93% and specificity between 87% and 100%. In addition, the leukocyte esterase concentration has shown a high correlation with ESR, CRP level, synovial WBC count, and synovial PMN percentage. The simple leukocyte esterase strip test thus appears to be fast, accurate, and inexpensive. A "++" result of the leukocyte esterase test is reflective of elevated synovial neutrophils and therefore is considered a minor criterion for the diagnosis of PJI.

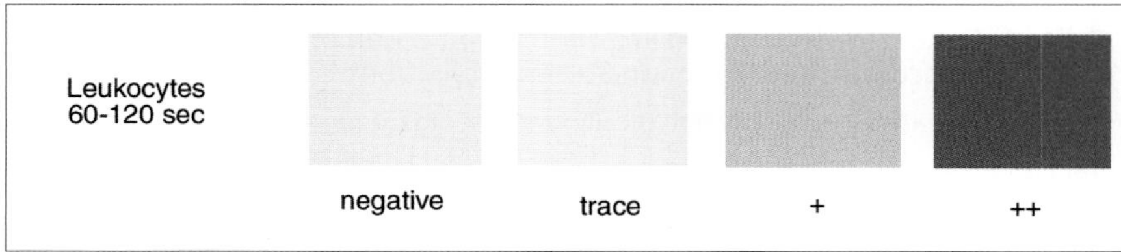

Figure 2 A colorimetric strip test measures the presence of leukocyte esterase, an enzyme secreted by activated neutrophils in response to infections. Any pink color is considered positive.

If the aspirated synovial fluid is contaminated with blood, which occurs in up to 33% of patients, a colorimetric strip test may be impractical. Centrifugation of the aspirate at 6,600 rpm for 2 to 3 minutes can help separate red blood cells from the synovial fluid and make the test feasible. Elevated synovial levels of protein and glucose and several antibiotics may interfere with the leukocyte esterase test.

Culture

In an attempt to identify the pathogens causing PJI, synovial fluid is processed for microbiologic culture. Routine cultures should be maintained for 5 days. In patients in whom culture-negative PJI or infection with low-virulence organisms is suspected, the culture should be maintained for at least 14 days. Extending cultures to 2 weeks will substantially increase sensitivity without increasing the risk of false-positive results. Investigation for unusual pathogens such as acid-fast bacillus and fungal infections should be reserved for patients at risk of these infections or in patients in whom typical pathogens have not been isolated but PJI is suspected on the basis of clinical findings. Even in presumed aseptic joints, routine acid-fast bacillus and fungal testing have not yielded clinically important results and are not cost effective.

Obtaining periarticular tissue samples for culture is an important aspect of the PJI workup. Tissue samples for culture should be obtained in every patient undergoing revision arthroplasty. Three to five tissues and/or fluid samples from the joint should be obtained and processed for culture. A single positive culture is considered a minor criterion in the definition of PJI because it may represent a false-positive scenario and should be interpreted in combination with other test results. In an effort to avoid false-positive cultures, tissue samples should be obtained with a sterile instrument and preferably taken from the implant interface and/or the intramedullary canal.

Anecdotal evidence from the second author's (J.P.) institution suggests that despite all attempts, the infecting organism may not be isolated in up to 28% of patients with PJI. False-negative PJI results may be attributable to administration of antibiotics before the tissue samples were obtained, selection of an inappropriate growth medium for the pathogen, the presence of a biofilm, or a short culture incubation period. Swab cultures from the wound or periprosthetic tissues are discouraged. In an

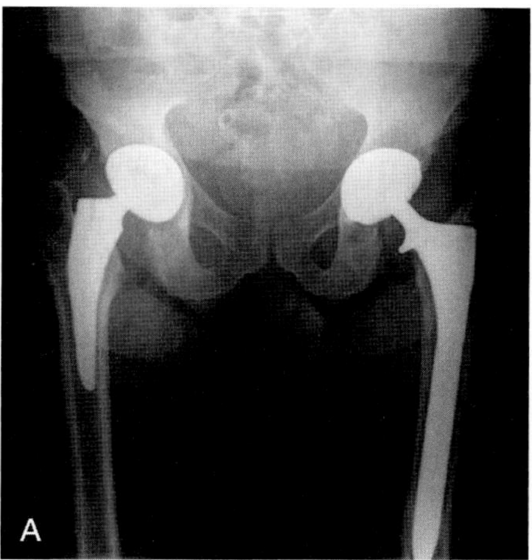

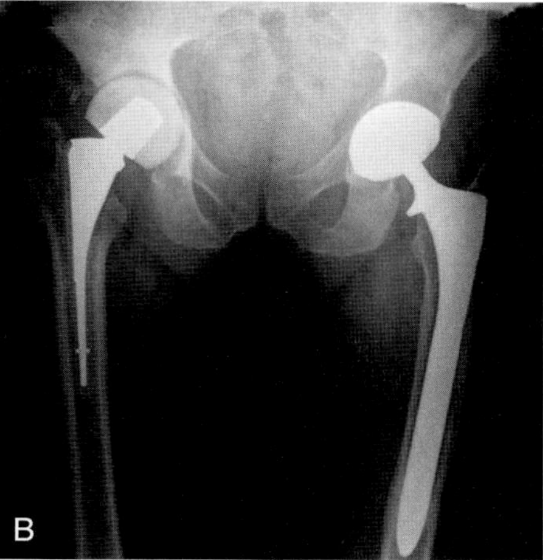

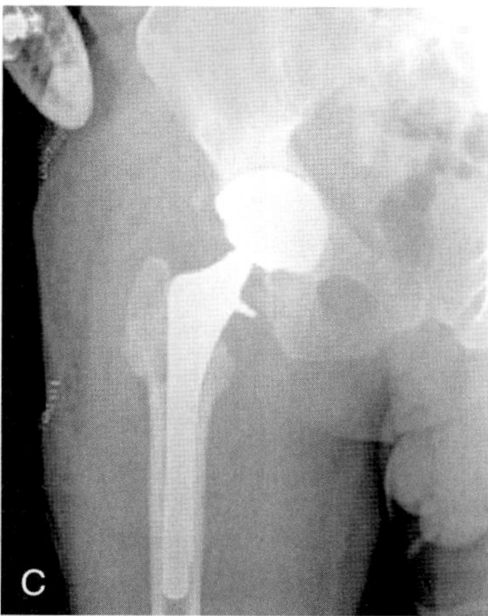

Figure 3 **A,** AP pelvic radiograph demonstrates a severely infected right hip in a 52-year-old man who underwent right total hip arthroplasty 2 years previously. The patient had good results originally, but a pilonidal sinus with severe infection and pain developed in the right hip. The serology was abnormal (erythrocyte sedimentation rate, 43 mm/h; C-reactive protein level, 22 mg/L). Aspiration of the joint revealed a white blood cell count of 2,900 cells/μL and polymorphonuclear neutrophil percentage of 89%. The leukocyte esterase strip test result was ++. Cultures were negative. AP pelvic radiograph (**B**) and AP radiograph of the right hip (**C**) demonstrate the two-stage exchange arthroplasty that was performed. *Staphylococcus aureus* was isolated in cultures obtained intraoperatively.

analysis of 117 revision surgeries, investigators compared three swab cultures with three tissue cultures; the swab cultures had sensitivity and specificity inferior to those of the tissue cultures (70% and 93%, respectively; and 89% and 98%, respectively).

Imaging

Plain radiographs are essential in the investigation of painful prosthetic joints. Although plain radiographs do not confirm PJI, they can reveal signs that raise suspicion of PJI and provide useful information to aid in diagnosis (**Figure 3**). These signs include the presence of focal osteolysis or bone destruction, especially more than 5 years after the index surgical procedure; evidence of loosening of a previously well-fixed implant, especially more than 5 years after the index procedure; periosteal reactions; and an intracortical sinus tract. In addition, plain radiographs can provide valuable information about the etiology of a failed THA.

According to the recommendations of the AAOS and the ICM, bone scan does not accurately diagnose PJI but may be useful in patients with suspected PJI in whom synovial fluid could not be obtained. The AAOS guidelines do not support the use of CT or MRI in the evaluation of patients with suspected PJI of the hip. Because of the presence of metal implants and imaging artifacts, MRI may be of limited use in the diagnosis of PJI. If these tests are ordered, the use of metal-artifact reduction sequence may be helpful.

Joint Aspiration

Aspiration of the joint is an important aspect of the workup of any patient in whom PJI is strongly suspected. Aspiration is not done in patients in whom the presence of a sinus tract definitively indicates PJI unless preoperative identification of the infecting organism is desired, nor is it done in patients with very low suspicion for PJI in whom all serologic markers are normal. Repeat aspiration should be considered in patients with one or two positive minor criteria, patients in whom discordant data points are obtained in synovial fluid analysis, and patients in whom a first attempt at aspiration was unsuccessful.

The AAOS guidelines strongly recommend that aspiration of a joint be attempted when the patient has been off antibiotics for at least 2 weeks. This recommendation is based on level I findings of a false-negative rate of 55% in patients who received antibiotics within the previous 14 days compared with 23% in patients who did not receive antibiotics during that period. The AAOS guidelines also recommend that patients in whom PJI is suspected should not be administered antibiotics before the diagnosis of PJI is reached or refuted.

Histologic Analysis

Although the risk of sampling error is high, histologic analysis of frozen tissue sections may offer a valuable data point in the diagnosis of PJI. However, substantial variability exists between institutions, and no consensus has been reached on appropriate thresholds for the results gleaned from histologic examination of periarticular tissues. According to the MSIS criteria, the threshold to predict PJI is 5 to 10 PMNs per high-power fields (HPFs) in at least 5 HPFs (magnification greater than

×400). A total of 23 PMNs in 10 HPFs seems to have the same accuracy as the MSIS threshold to predict PJI. The use of sharp dissection instead of cautery to obtain samples will decrease the rate of false-positive findings resulting from the entrapment of neutrophils in superficial fibrin.

Analyses Not Included in Diagnosis

Gram stains from periprosthetic tissues or fluids and serum WBC and differential are not useful tests in the diagnosis of PJI. Intraoperative purulence, which was previously a minor criterion, has been removed from the MSIS definition. The major reason for this removal is that cloudy white synovial fluid exists in the joints of many patients with metal particle–induced adverse local tissue reactions, such as those that result from metal-on-metal bearing surfaces, corrosion of the femoral stem taper, or corrosion at the junction of a modular femoral neck and stem.

Management

The appropriate management of confirmed PJI depends on patient characteristics, the acuity of the infection, the type of infecting organism, and other factors that influence the success of treatment and the type of treatment selected. Patient-related factors include overall health status, coexistent comorbidities, duration of symptoms, functional status of the joint, status of the periarticular soft tissue, the patient's expectations and willingness to comply with recommendations, and allergy to antibiotics that may preclude the use of specific antibiotics. Organism-related factors include the virulence and antibiotic susceptibility of the infecting organism. In patients in whom cultures were negative, infections caused by fungi, if undetected, may not be managed with the appropriate antimicrobial agents. Joint-related factors include the status of fixation of the implants, the type of implants (stemmed or nonstemmed), the severity of bone loss, and the status of the soft tissues (abductors) around the joint, which can influence the subsequent functional outcome.

Surgical intervention is the preferred treatment of patients with infected THA. Rarely, the clinician may have no option other than to administer antibiotics despite a lack of evidence supporting nonsurgical treatment of patients solely with suppressive antibiotics. Chronic antibiotic therapy is indicated when surgical treatment would pose a great risk because of the patient's general health condition or in a patient with persistent infection who declines or cannot tolerate additional surgical treatment.

Surgical management of PJI of the hip can consist of irrigation and débridement with retention of the implant, one-stage exchange arthroplasty, or two-stage exchange arthroplasty. In some patients, salvage procedures such as resection arthroplasty or amputation may be considered.

Irrigation and Débridement

Depending on the acuity of the infection, a patient with acute PJI less than 4 weeks after an index arthroplasty or with less than 4 weeks' duration of symptoms may be treated with irrigation and débridement and exchange of modular prosthetic components, followed by antibiotic therapy. The prerequisites for irrigation and débridement and implant retention are acute onset of symptoms, the presence of well-fixed and well-aligned implants, infection with an antibiotic-susceptible organism, and sufficient soft-tissue coverage.

Irrigation and débridement consists of arthrotomy, removal of modular parts (the acetabular liner and the femoral head), thorough débridement of all the infected and necrotic tissues (synovium and periarticular muscles), and irrigation with at least 9 L of fluid. The ICM stresses the importance of surgical technique in irrigation and débridement of a prosthetic joint and provides a detailed account of how the procedure should be performed. According to the ICM, the use of pulsatile lavage with fluids such as dilute povidone-iodine and/or sodium hypochlorite solution (Dakin solution) should be considered. Irrigation and débridement is followed by 4 to 6 weeks of intravenous administration of antibiotics targeting the isolated pathogen. Although irrigation and débridement is an attractive option because of its lower morbidity, the success rate is relatively low at approximately 50%. Higher failure rates of irrigation and débridement are associated with infection by methicillin-resistant *S aureus*, procedures performed more than 2 weeks after presentation of the infection, and infection with gram-negative organisms.

One-Stage Exchange Arthroplasty

One-stage exchange arthroplasty may be considered in the management of acute or chronic PJI. The success of one-stage exchange arthroplasty depends on the technical performance of the procedure. The procedure begins with removal of all implants and foreign material such as cement followed by extensive débridement of the periarticular tissues. To reduce bioburden during the procedure, the initial equipment and instrumentation in the operating room should be replaced with a new set before reimplantation. The operating room personnel should rescrub, and the infected joint should be rescrubbed and re-prepared. Some surgeons recommend the use of antibiotic-impregnated cement or antibiotics mixed with allograft. After the procedure, the patient is placed on antibiotics for 2 to 4 weeks.

Interest in one-stage revision THA has grown worldwide, especially in Europe, because of its cost-effectiveness and average success rate of 85.5%.

Relative and absolute contraindications for one-stage exchange identified by the ICM include the presence of systemic sepsis, inadequate soft-tissue coverage, and culture-negative PJI. Some surgeons also consider PJI with antibiotic-resistant organisms such as methicillin-resistant *S aureus* to be a contraindication to one-stage exchange arthroplasty.

Two-Stage Exchange Arthroplasty

Two-stage exchange arthroplasty is the preferred treatment of patients with chronic PJI of the hip at most institutions in North America. The first stage consists of removal of implants and foreign material, extensive débridement, and placement of an antibiotic-impregnated cement spacer. The patient is treated with 4 to 6 weeks of antibiotics in the interim period, followed by 2 to 3 weeks without administration of antibiotics. After the infection is deemed adequately managed, reimplantation is performed.

One major challenge in two-stage exchange arthroplasty is determining the optimal timing of reimplantation. Currently, no reliable metrics are available to guide the clinician on the timing. The available serologic tests, ESR and serum CRP level, are not reliable markers for determining the timing of reimplantation. Although decreased values of these markers are desired before reimplantation, studies have shown that elevated ESR and CRP level at the time of reimplantation are not predictive of later failure. Aspiration of the joint may be performed before reimplantation, except in patients in whom gross pus is obtained or an infecting organism is isolated. Because thresholds for synovial WBC count and PMN percentage in a joint with a spacer have not been determined, the role of aspiration in guiding the timing of reimplantation remains undefined.

The success of two-stage exchange arthroplasty or of any surgical management of PJI of the hip depends on the definition of success. If a strict definition of success that was reached by the Delphi method is employed, the success rate of two-stage exchange arthroplasty is likely to be much lower than the typically quoted 90% to 95% success rate.

Salvage Procedures

Some patients may require a salvage procedure after failure of multiple reconstructive procedures for the management of PJI. Salvage procedures can consist of Girdlestone resection arthroplasty or hindquarter amputation. Fusion of the hip usually is not a viable option in patients with multiple failed surgical procedures and massive bone loss.

Recent Developments and Ongoing Research

As diagnostic techniques and treatment strategies evolve, clinical practice guidelines will need to be revised and updated. Areas of promising recent research include biomarkers and biofilms.

Synovial biomarkers have shown promise in the detection of PJI. One synovial biomarker, the peptide α-defensin, is secreted into synovial fluid by human cells and exerts an antimicrobial effect via attachment to the cell wall of the pathogen. The α-defensin concentration in synovial fluid is measured with an immunoassay test. The cutoff positive value is 5.2 mg/L. Immunoassay results for α-defensin have been promising. The test has sensitivity and specificity of 100% and is not affected by bloody aspirates, antibiotic therapy, or systemic inflammatory diseases. The synovial biomarkers neutrophil elastase-2, bactericidal/permeability-increasing protein, neutrophil gelatinase-associated lipocalin, and lactoferrin have been found to predict the presence of PJI with 100% sensitivity and specificity. In addition, recent studies have demonstrated the accuracy of synovial CRP level as a predictor of PJI. A threshold of 2.5 mg/L for synovial CRP level has 95.5% sensitivity and 93.3% specificity in the diagnosis of PJI of the hip.

An estimated 80% of infections in humans can be attributed to an infecting organism that exists in a biofilm. Some studies have demonstrated direct clinical evidence of biofilm formation on retrieved infected prostheses with the use of electron or confocal laser scanning microscopy. A high priority in future PJI guidelines may be to consider the role of biofilm in PJI. Because microbial biofilms are not detected by standard culture-based diagnostic measures or addressed in standard treatment strategies, many investigators have aimed to develop novel diagnostic tools and treatment methods. Diagnostics for biofilm-associated PJI include polymerase chain reaction, fluorescence in situ hybridization, and DNA microarrays.

In patients with biofilm-associated PJI, treatment can be supplemented with antibiofilm antibiotics. According to recommendations of the Infectious Diseases Society of America, only rifampin and meropenem have shown consistent antibiofilm activity. Other treatment strategies include quorum quenching, bacteriophages, ultrasonographic therapy, and electrotherapy.

Bibliography

Aggarwal VK, Tischler E, Ghanem E, Parvizi J: Leukocyte esterase from synovial fluid aspirate: A technical note. *J Arthroplasty* 2013;28(1):193-195.

Bedair H, Ting N, Jacovides C, et al: Diagnosis of early postoperative TKA infection using synovial fluid analysis. *Clin Orthop Relat Res* 2011;469(1):34-40.

Bilgen O, Atici T, Durak K, Karaeminoğullari O, Bilgen MS: C-reactive protein values and erythrocyte sedimentation rates after total hip and total knee arthroplasty. *J Int Med Res* 2001;29(1):7-12.

Bozic KJ, Kurtz SM, Lau E, Ong K, Vail TP, Berry DJ: The epidemiology of revision total hip arthroplasty in the United States. *J Bone Joint Surg Am* 2009;91(1):128-133.

Bozic KJ, Ries MD: The impact of infection after total hip arthroplasty on hospital and surgeon resource utilization. *J Bone Joint Surg Am* 2005;87(8):1746-1751.

Chen AF, Heller S, Parvizi J: Prosthetic joint infections. *Surg Clin North Am* 2014;94(6):1265-1281.

Deirmengian C, Kardos K, Kilmartin P, et al: The alpha-defensin test for periprosthetic joint infection outperforms the leukocyte esterase test strip. *Clin Orthop Relat Res* 2015;473(1):198-203.

Deirmengian C, Kardos K, Kilmartin P, Cameron A, Schiller K, Parvizi J: Diagnosing periprosthetic joint infection: Has the era of the biomarker arrived? *Clin Orthop Relat Res* 2014;472(11):3254-3262.

Della Valle C, Parvizi J, Bauer TW, et al; American Academy of Orthopaedic Surgeons: Diagnosis of periprosthetic joint infections of the hip and knee. *J Am Acad Orthop Surg* 2010;18(12):760-770.

Diaz-Ledezma C, Higuera CA, Parvizi J: Success after treatment of periprosthetic joint infection: A Delphi-based international multidisciplinary consensus. *Clin Orthop Relat Res* 2013;471(7):2374-2382.

Gehrke T, Parvizi J; International Consensus Group: Proceedings of the International Consensus Meeting on Periprosthetic Joint Infection. Philadelphia, PA, 2013. Available at: https://www.efort.org/wp-content/uploads/2013/10/Philadelphia_Consensus.pdf. Accessed September 19, 2016.

Ghanem E, Azzam K, Seeley M, Joshi A, Parvizi J: Staged revision for knee arthroplasty infection: What is the role of serologic tests before reimplantation? *Clin Orthop Relat Res* 2009;467(7):1699-1705.

Ghanem E, Houssock C, Pulido L, Han S, Jaberi FM, Parvizi J: Determining "true" leukocytosis in bloody joint aspiration. *J Arthroplasty* 2008;23(2):182-187.

Haasper C, Buttaro M, Hozack W, et al: Irrigation and debridement. *J Orthop Res* 2014;32(suppl 1):S130-S135.

Krenn V, Morawietz L, Perino G, et al: Revised histopathological consensus classification of joint implant related pathology. *Pathol Res Pract* 2014;210(12):779-786.

Kurtz SM, Lau E, Schmier J, Ong KL, Zhao K, Parvizi J: Infection burden for hip and knee arthroplasty in the United States. *J Arthroplasty* 2008;23(7):984-991.

Kusuma SK, Ward J, Jacofsky M, Sporer SM, Della Valle CJ: What is the role of serological testing between stages of two-stage reconstruction of the infected prosthetic knee? *Clin Orthop Relat Res* 2011;469(4):1002-1008.

Omar M, Ettinger M, Reichling M, et al: Synovial C-reactive protein as a marker for chronic periprosthetic infection in total hip arthroplasty. *Bone Joint J* 2015;97-B(2):173-176.

Ong KL, Kurtz SM, Lau E, Bozic KJ, Berry DJ, Parvizi J: Prosthetic joint infection risk after total hip arthroplasty in the Medicare population. *J Arthroplasty* 2009;24(suppl 6):105-109.

Parvizi J, Adeli B, Zmistowski B, Restrepo C, Greenwald AS: Management of periprosthetic joint infection: The current knowledge. *J Bone Joint Surg Am* 2012;94(14):e104.

Parvizi J, Jacovides C, Antoci V, Ghanem E: Diagnosis of periprosthetic joint infection: The utility of a simple yet unappreciated enzyme. *J Bone Joint Surg Am* 2011;93(24):2242-2248.

Parvizi J, Zmistowski B, Berbari EF, et al: New definition for periprosthetic joint infection: From the Workgroup of the Musculoskeletal Infection Society. *Clin Orthop Relat Res* 2011;469(11):2992-2994.

Toossi N, Adeli B, Rasouli MR, Huang R, Parvizi J: Serum white blood cell count and differential do not have a role in the diagnosis of periprosthetic joint infection. *J Arthroplasty* 2012;27(suppl 8):51-54.e1.

Trampuz A, Piper KE, Jacobson MJ, et al: Sonication of removed hip and knee prostheses for diagnosis of infection. *N Engl J Med* 2007;357(7):654-663.

Tzeng A, Tzeng TH, Vasdev S, et al: Treating periprosthetic joint infections as biofilms: Key diagnosis and management strategies. *Diagn Microbiol Infect Dis* 2015;81(3):192-200.

Vanhegan IS, Malik AK, Jayakumar P, Ul Islam S, Haddad FS: A financial analysis of revision hip arthroplasty: The economic burden in relation to the national tariff. *J Bone Joint Surg Br* 2012;94(5):619-623.

Zmistowski B, Della Valle C, Bauer TW, et al: Diagnosis of periprosthetic joint infection. *J Arthroplasty* 2014;29(suppl 2):77-83.

Zmistowski B, Karam JA, Durinka JB, Casper DS, Parvizi J: Periprosthetic joint infection increases the risk of one-year mortality. *J Bone Joint Surg Am* 2013;95(24):2177-2184.

Chapter 35
Management of the Infected Total Hip Arthroplasty

Matthew P. Abdel, MD
Arlen D. Hanssen, MD

Indications

The primary etiologies of a painful total hip arthroplasty (THA) include infection, aseptic loosening, synovitis secondary to wear debris, periarticular soft-tissue inflammation, and referred pain from the lumbar spine. Occasionally, infected hips are evidenced by a draining sinus tract and associated cellulitis. However, because of the large soft-tissue envelope surrounding the hip joint, most patients have well-healed incisions, making detection of swelling or a joint effusion difficult. Although some patients may have painful and restricted range of motion, many patients experience a small increase in aggravated pain during the hip joint examination.

Pain at rest is the most common presenting symptom. Persistent pain suggests the possibility of infection. Other indications include prolonged wound drainage or antibiotic treatment for wound healing difficulties. Purulent drainage, although rare, confirms the presence of infection. Formal débridement of a draining wound to obtain deep tissue cultures occasionally is required to diagnose infection. Subacute or chronic infections are often insidious, and systemic signs of infection are usually absent. Laboratory tests are recommended to diagnose chronic infection-associated pain.

The first step in treatment is to establish and classify the infection according to symptom onset and duration. The four infection categories are positive intraoperative culture, early postoperative infection, acute hematogenous infection, and late chronic infection. Patients with positive intraoperative cultures are best treated with 4 to 6 weeks of intravenous antibiotics. Some patients with early postoperative or late hematogenous infections may be treated with open débridement and prosthesis retention. Patients with late chronic infection generally require removal of the infected implant, unless they cannot undergo further surgery. No laboratory test is completely sensitive to and specific for a diagnosis of infection. A white blood cell count is not helpful in identifying infection. An erythrocyte sedimentation rate (ESR) higher than 30 to 35 mm/h and a C-reactive protein (CRP) level higher than 10 mg/L are abnormal and warrant further investigation. A patient's CRP level returns to normal much faster than his or her ESR; thus, a patient's CRP level is a more sensitive indicator of infection, particularly in the early postoperative period. In the early postoperative period, an ESR of 65 mm/h and a CRP level higher than 90 mg/L are worrisome and warrant further investigation.

Routine aspiration of a painful THA is not indicated, although it should be used selectively in patients with a history of wound healing difficulties, radiographic changes, and an elevated ESR or CRP level. Aspiration is among the best preoperative tools available to document the presence of infection because it identifies any offending organisms, thus allowing more specific direction of the antibiotics used in the cement spacers and administered parenterally in the immediate postoperative period. Similar to an elevated CRP level and ESR in the early postoperative period, an aspiration is helpful because a synovial fluid white blood cell count higher than 12,500 cells/µL (with greater than 85% neutrophils) is concerning for infection.

Plain radiographs are usually normal in patients with late hematogenous infection. However, obtaining radiographs is essential because the status of prosthesis fixation is an important variable in the management decision process. Additional imaging studies are rarely required to diagnose an infected THA. A technetium Tc 99m bone scan has been recommended as an initial screening tool because of its sensitivity; however, it is nonspecific for the diagnosis of infection. A negative technetium Tc

Dr. Abdel or an immediate family member serves as a board member, owner, officer, or committee member of the Minnesota Orthopaedic Society. Dr. Hanssen or an immediate family member has received royalties and research or institutional support from Stryker, and serves as a board member, owner, officer, or committee member of the International Congress for Joint Reconstruction.

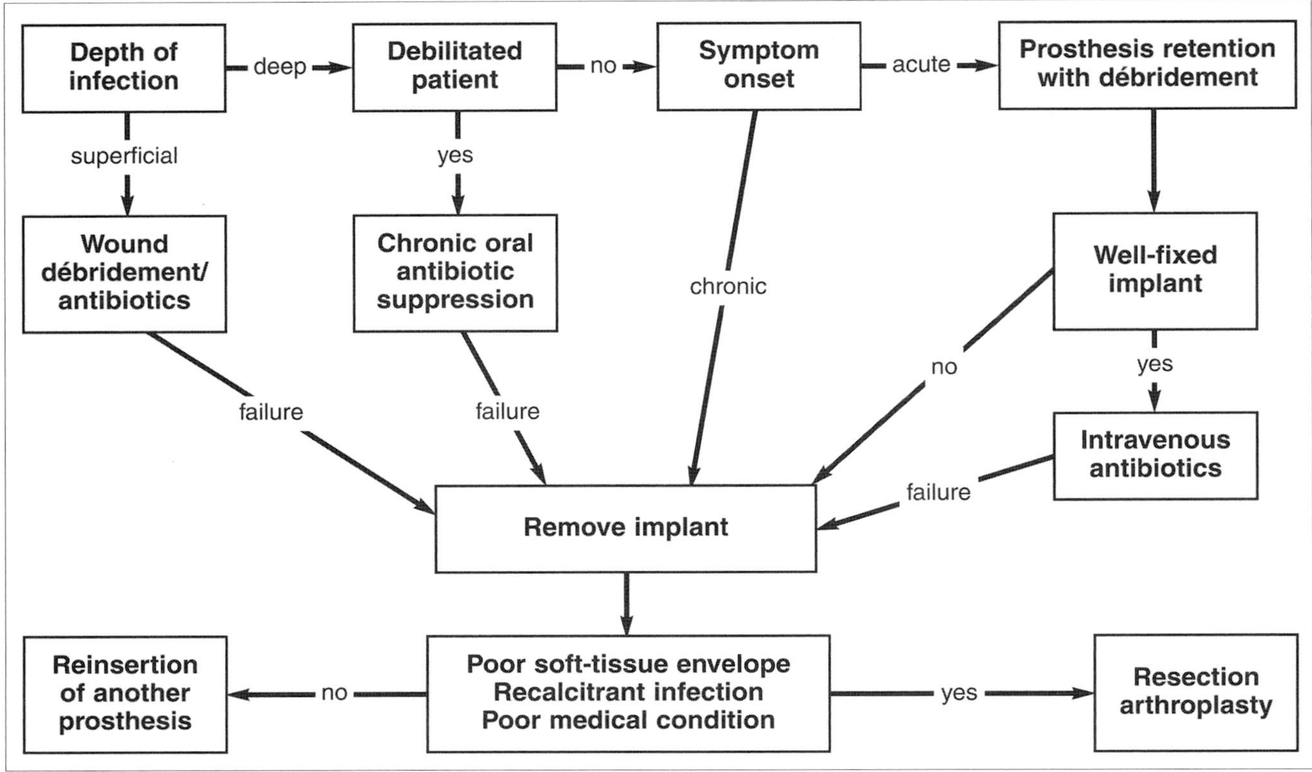

Figure 1 Treatment algorithm for management of an infected total hip arthroplasty. (Reproduced from Hanssen AD: Management of the infected total hip arthroplasty, in Lieberman JR, Berry DJ, eds: *Advanced Reconstruction: Hip*. Rosemont, IL, American Academy of Orthopaedic Surgeons, 2005, pp 233-239.)

99m bone scan suggests that infection is unlikely, but a positive technetium Tc 99m bone scan may indicate that additional bone scintigraphy studies should be ordered.

Contraindications

In patients with chronic infection, débridement with retention of the prosthesis has a very low success rate. Resection arthroplasty is a better choice for most patients who have had multiple failed reimplantations. Although some surgeons advocate use of a direct exchange technique, the authors of this chapter prefer a two-stage procedure for most patients, particularly those with resistant organisms.

Implantation of a new prosthesis is the most desirable method of treatment for most patients. The potential for improved functional outcomes with a new prosthesis must be carefully balanced against the disadvantage of a higher reinfection rate compared with a definitive resection arthroplasty. Contraindications to reimplantation include persistent or recalcitrant infection, medical conditions that preclude multiple reconstructive procedures, severe local soft-tissue damage, and systemic conditions that predispose a patient to reinfection.

Alternative Treatments

Basic treatment objectives include eradicating the infection, alleviating pain, and restoring function. The six basic treatment options available are antibiotic suppression, open débridement, resection arthroplasty, implantation of another prosthesis, arthrodesis, and hip disarticulation, although arthrodesis and hip disarticulation are rarely done. A summary of approaches for managing an infected THA is shown in **Figure 1**.

Antibiotic suppression is rarely indicated and should be used only when prosthesis removal is not feasible (usually because a medical condition precludes surgery), when the microorganism is susceptible to an oral antibiotic that the patient can tolerate without serious toxicity, and when the prosthesis is well fixed and functional.

Débridement with prosthesis retention is indicated for acute fulminant infection in the immediate postoperative period or for late hematogenous infection of a securely fixed and previously functional prosthesis. Débridement is usually not successful if performed more than 2 to 4 weeks after the onset of symptoms, and débridement is rarely indicated in patients with chronic infection. Implants should be well fixed, and any causative organisms should be susceptible to antibiotics that the patient can tolerate. Prosthesis removal is generally required in the presence of organisms such as methicillin-resistant staphylococci.

Girdlestone resection arthroplasty is a highly successful method of eradicating infection and usually provides pain relief. However, most patients undergoing this procedure require use of ambulatory aids, have a Trendelenburg gait, fatigue easily, and have a substantial limb-length discrepancy.

Implantation of another prosthesis after a failed THA provides a patient with markedly better functional recovery. Two-stage reimplantation protocols allow observation of patient response to treatment and assessment for recurring infection after antibiotics are discontinued. The disadvantages of this approach include the hardships experienced by patients during the interval without a prosthesis, the costs of a second surgical procedure, and the technical difficulties associated with delayed prosthesis implantation. Direct exchange techniques are usually precluded by the magnitude of bone loss and the increasing prevalence of drug-resistant organisms. Although direct exchange has a lower success rate than two-stage reimplantation, some surgeons still advocate this technique, and it is commonly used outside the United States. The indications, as outlined by advocates of the technique, include an organism sensitive to antibiotics, a well-vascularized soft-tissue envelope, and minimal bone loss.

Hip arthrodesis for the infected THA is rarely indicated. Hip disarticulation is indicated for life-threatening infection, severe loss of soft tissue and bone stock, and vascular injury. Its use in the management of an infected hip is rare.

Results

A success rate of 85% to 90% generally can be expected after primary two-stage reconstruction (**Table 1**). Unpublished data from the Mayo Clinic have shown that success rates are markedly decreased after a previously failed two-stage exchange.

Technique

Setup/Exposure

- Many aspects of surgical débridement are similar, regardless of treatment approach. In general, previous incisions are used to expose the hip. If the prior incision is invaginated, it is usually advisable to excise the scar and any adjacent sinus tracts so that the skin and subcutaneous tissue layers are well vascularized and will heal readily (**Figure 2**).
- Antibiotics are withheld until tissue specimens are obtained from the pseudocapsule and the bone-prosthetic interfaces of both components.
- The goal of débridement is to remove all necrotic tissue and foreign material yet maintain the vascular supply of the bone and associated soft tissues.
- If possible, it is advisable to use the previous surgical approach to facilitate suture removal and minimize additional devascularization.
- The use of extensile surgical exposures, such as extended trochanteric osteotomy (**Figure 3**), is increasingly common and facilitates removal of well-fixed implants while helping to maintain vascularity of the proximal femur.
- Sonication of the removed implants at the institution of the authors of this chapter has markedly increased the ability to identify an organism, especially if antibiotics were administered within 14 days before the resection.

Procedure

BONE PREPARATION

- A thorough resection of the pseudocapsule is necessary to expose the acetabulum, and the surgeon must carefully look for retained cement if either the existing or prior cup was cemented. This step is accomplished by reaming the acetabulum and carefully looking for cement fragments, particularly in the inferior aspect of the foveal region.
- Intraoperative radiographs can help identify and localize cement fragments.
- For noncemented cups with screws, a burr can be inserted into previous screw holes to débride the screw tracts (**Figure 4**).
- After implant removal and débridement, a decision regarding reimplantation is made. Reimplantation is possible in most patients.

PROSTHESIS IMPLANTATION

- A construct that will deliver high-dose local antibiotics is usually advised.
- Using antibiotic-loaded cement beads is strongly discouraged because removing these beads from the femoral canal or the periacetabular region can be extremely difficult.
- Structural antibiotic-loaded cement spacers can be fabricated in a variety of ways. For patients with substantial bone loss or history of recurrent instability, the authors of this chapter prefer to use a standard cement gun and create a gently tapered dowel that can be easily extracted from the femoral canal

Table 1 Results of One- and Two-Stage Procedures for the Management of Infected Total Hip Arthroplasty

Authors (Year)	Number of Hips	Procedure and Fixation Type	Mean Patient Age in Years (Range)	Mean Follow-up in Years (Range)	Success Rate (%)[a]	Results
Raut et al (1994)	57	One-stage: cemented[b]	66 (17-81)	7.3 (2-12.6)	86	7 patients required rerevision surgery Infection was managed in 49 patients
Mulcahy et al (1996)	15	One-stage: noncemented	64 (49-82)[c]	4.4 (2-7)	100	No recurrence of infection, but these were the healthiest of patients, with good local tissue beds 4 other patients in the series underwent an excisional arthroplasty
Raut et al (1996)	15	One-stage: cemented (13),[b] cemented (2)	65 (52-79)	8 (1-13)	93	2 hips without ALBC had reinfection
Younger et al (1997)	48	Two-stage: cemented[b]	67 (36-90)	3.6 (2-5.25)	94	Reinfection occurred in 3 patients (2 with different organisms and 1 with the same organism)
Younger et al (1998)	28 (27 patients)	Two-stage: cemented[b]	71 (51-88)[d]	3.9 (2-9.5)	96	2 patients died of unrelated causes
Callaghan et al (1999)	24	One-stage: cemented[b]	65.3 (37-86)	9.1 (1-14)	92	At 10-yr follow-up, 12 patients had died and 2 patients had experienced reinfection
Haddad et al (2000)	50	Two-stage: cemented[b]	60 (24-81)	5.8 (2-8.7)	92	Two patients required another two-stage revision
Sanchez-Sotelo et al (2009)	169 (168 patients)	Two-stage: cemented (121 hips),[b] noncemented (48 hips)	67 (32-89)	7 (2-16)	93	12 hips had reinfection
Oussedik et al (2010)	50	One-stage: cemented (11)[b] Two-stage: varied components and fixation types (39)	65 (48-87)	6.8 (5.5-8.8)	One-stage: 100 Two-stage: 95	2 hips from the two-stage group had reinfection Patients in the one-stage group were hyperselected based on host and local tissue grades

ALBC = antibiotic-loaded bone cement.

[a] Success is defined as eradication of infection.

[b] Antibiotic-loaded bone cement was used.

[c] Mean patient age based on original cohort of 19 hips.

[d] Mean patient age based on original cohort of 30 hips (29 patients).

at reimplantation. Such dowels are used in patients with moderate femoral bone loss. This method is preferred primarily because, in the presence of these dowels and in the absence of patient weight bearing, the endosteal surface of the femur undergoes a process of bony spicule formation and cancellization that facilitates the use of antibiotic-loaded cement for femoral fixation.

- Occasionally, a Rush rod is used if a concurrent fracture is present (**Figure 5**).

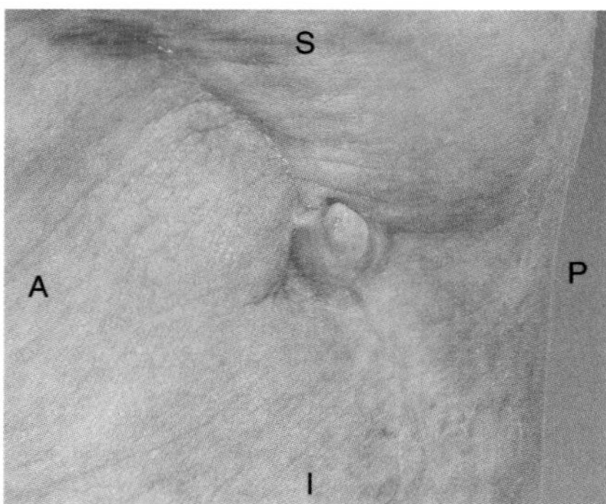

Figure 2 Clinical photograph shows invaginated incisions and adjacent sinus tracts that must be excised for the management of an infected total hip arthroplasty. A = anterior, I = inferior, P = posterior, S = superior.

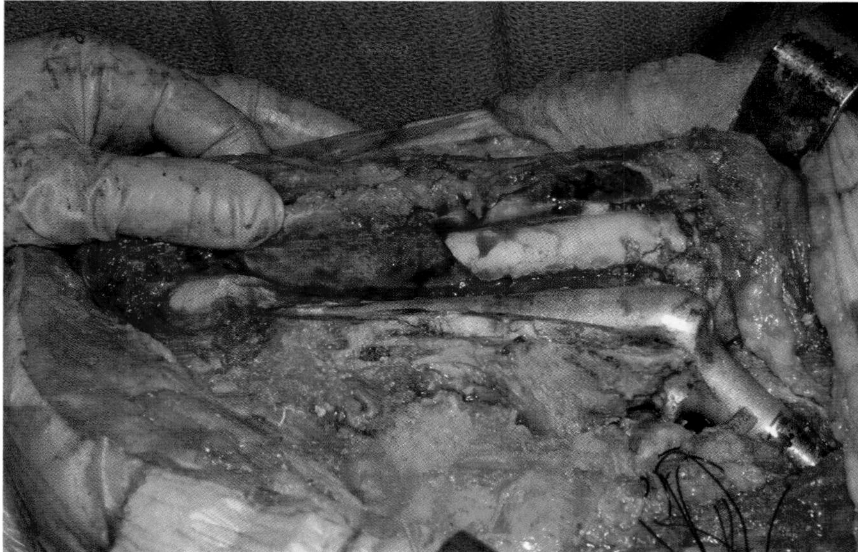

Figure 3 Intraoperative photograph shows extended trochanteric osteotomy, which often is helpful for removal of femoral implants and for adequate débridement (particularly with cemented stems).

- For most patients with preserved bone stock (including those with most contemporary proximal ingrowth femoral components that can be removed without an osteotomy), the authors of this chapter prefer to use a PROSTALAC (prosthesis of antibiotic-loaded acrylic cement, DePuy Synthes) implant (**Figure 6**).
- This hip prosthesis facsimile has a modular stainless steel femoral endoskeleton coated with antibiotic-loaded cement and serves as a local antibiotic delivery system while maintaining limb length and anatomic relationships. This prosthesis prevents contracture of the soft tissues and facilitates safe exposure at reimplantation. However, because of the sclerotic endosteal surface of the femoral canal that forms around these implants, use of a noncemented femoral implant is recommended at the time of reconstruction.
- In the presence of good acetabular bone stock, hip instability can be reduced with a snap-fit articulation between the temporary femoral prosthesis and temporary acetabular polyethylene. The authors of this chapter typically mix 3 g of vancomycin and 3.6 g of gentamicin per 40 g of bone cement to create the dowel or PROSTALAC, and the same amount of cement and antibiotics to cement a PROSTALAC cup in place or to create a cup spacer for the acetabular fossa (**Figure 7**).
- If a nonarticulating spacer is chosen, the use of the acetabular spacer markedly eases exposure of the acetabulum at the time of reimplantation.

Wound Closure

- When performing an extended trochanteric osteotomy, several 18-gauge cerclage wires are used to stabilize the osteotomy at wound closure because the use of large sutures results in insufficient fixation.
- Cables are not recommended because of their increased surface area, which affords more opportunities for infection to develop.

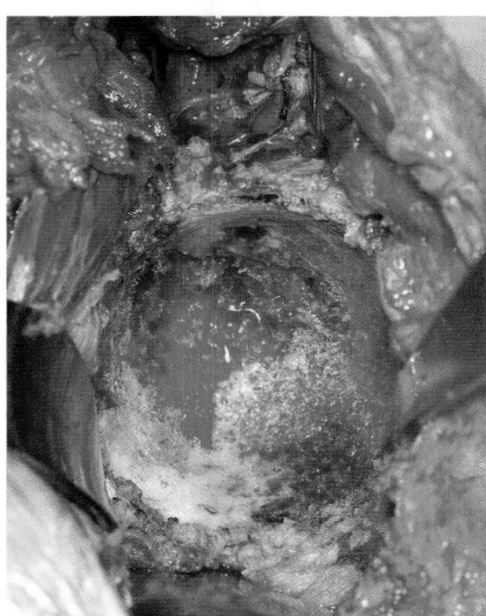

Figure 4 Intraoperative photograph of a hip joint after the acetabular component was removed with minimal bone loss, the screw tracks from the previous surgery were burred, and the socket was reamed to the level of bleeding bone to remove any necrotic bone and tissue.

Reimplantation

- At the time of reimplantation, good intraoperative judgment is required, and consultation with an experienced pathologist to determine whether reimplantation is safe can be valuable.
- A host of femoral implants can be used during the reimplantation. If a

patient is young (usually 65 years or younger; however, physiologic age and comorbidities must be taken into consideration) and has good bone stock, a noncemented stem is preferred.

- Recently, modular fluted tapered stems have gained popularity because they provide immediate axial and rotational control in combination with proximal modularity.
- If a cemented stem is chosen based on patient factors and remaining bone stock, the authors of this chapter use a cemented femoral component fixed with antibiotic-loaded bone cement, using 1 g of vancomycin and 1.2 g of gentamicin per 40 g of acrylic cement. Noncemented hemispheric shells usually can be used on the acetabular side in most patients.

Postoperative Regimen

Patients are mobilized postoperatively as soon as possible. After intravenous

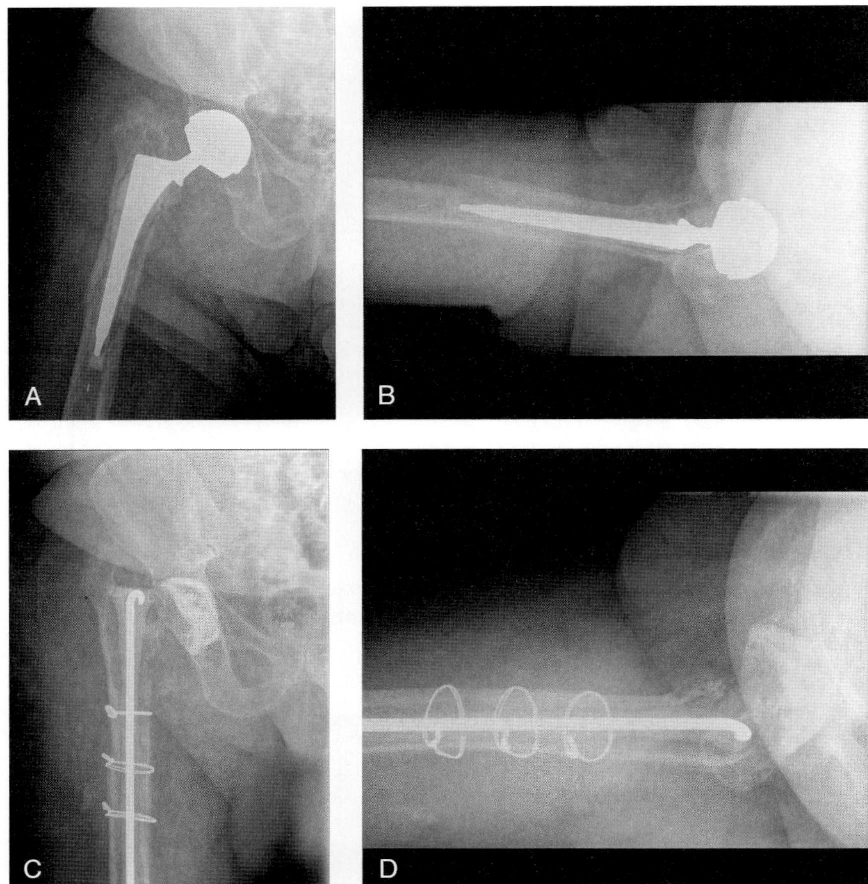

Figure 5 Radiographs of the right hip of a 70-year-old man. AP (**A**) and lateral (**B**) views demonstrate an infected metal-on-metal total hip arthroplasty with a Vancouver type B3 fracture (loose implant with inadequate bone stock). AP (**C**) and lateral (**D**) views demonstrate placement of a static spacer to address the bone loss and fracture.

Figure 6 AP (**A**) and lateral (**B**) radiographs of the right hip of a 65-year-old woman treated with an articulating spacer for a chronic deep periprosthetic infection.

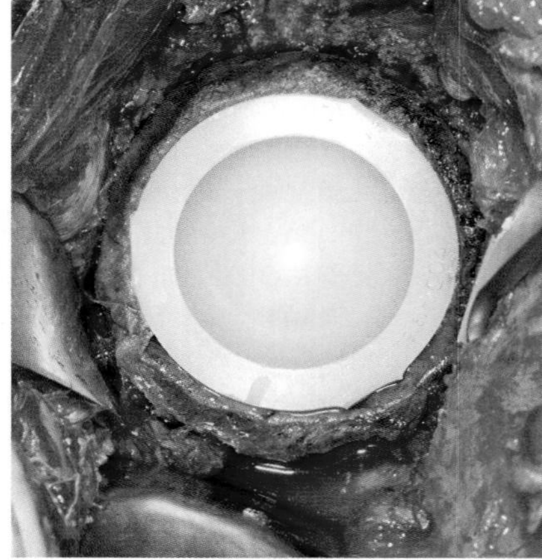

Figure 7 Intraoperative photograph shows the method preferred by the authors of this chapter for placing a semiconstrained acetabular liner with antibiotic-loaded bone cement and methylene blue in preparation for an articulating spacer.

antibiotic therapy is completed, the authors of this chapter prefer to wait 6 to 8 weeks to assess a patient's response to treatment. No antibiotics are administered during this time. A patient's ESR and CRP level are monitored at 6 and 12 weeks postoperatively, respectively. If hematologic parameters have improved, the authors of this chapter proceed with reimplantation at 3 months postoperatively without preoperative aspiration or other imaging modalities. The use of an abduction brace postoperatively is recommended because hip instability is a substantial problem for these patients. If the abductors are deficient, consideration can be given to a dual-mobility construct or use of a constrained liner in patients with challenging circumstances.

Avoiding Pitfalls and Complications

Intraoperative frozen tissue sections are a valuable tool for diagnosing infection and are most useful if preoperative results are unclear. Tissue samples should be obtained from the most inflamed areas and examined by a pathologist who is experienced in the interpretation of such specimens. Gram stain should not be used in intraoperative decision making because it is often more confusing than helpful.

If implants are cemented, antibiotic-loaded cement is recommended to minimize the risk of reinfection. The use of high-dose antibiotic-loaded cement spacers also is helpful and has allowed successful noncemented fixation at the time of reimplantation. Although the optimal duration of management with intravenous antibiotics for infected THA has not been definitively established, 4 to 6 weeks of intravenous antibiotics are recommended.

Identification of the infecting organism and thorough débridement are critical to successful management of an infected THA. Thorough débridement is essential but difficult to quantify and assess. In the presence of good acetabular bone stock, hip instability can be reduced with a snap-fit articulation between the temporary femoral prosthesis and temporary acetabular polyethylene.

Bibliography

Callaghan JJ, Katz RP, Johnston RC: One-stage revision surgery of the infected hip: A minimum 10-year followup study. *Clin Orthop Relat Res* 1999;(369):139-143.

Fehring KA, Abdel MP, Ollivier M, Mabry TM, Hanssen AD: Repeat two-stage exchange arthroplasty for periprosthetic knee infection is dependent on host grade. *J Bone Joint Surg Am*, forthcoming.

Garvin KL, Hanssen AD: Infection after total hip arthroplasty: Past, present, and future. *J Bone Joint Surg Am* 1995;77(10):1576-1588.

Haddad FS, Muirhead-Allwood SK, Manktelow AR, Bacarese-Hamilton I: Two-stage uncemented revision hip arthroplasty for infection. *J Bone Joint Surg Br* 2000;82(5):689-694.

Hanssen AD: Management of the infected total hip arthroplasty, in Lieberman JR, Berry DJ, eds: *Advanced Reconstruction: Hip*. Rosemont, IL, American Academy of Orthopaedic Surgeons, 2005, pp 233-240.

Kalra KP, Lin KK, Bozic KJ, Ries MD: Repeat 2-stage revision for recurrent infection of total hip arthroplasty. *J Arthroplasty* 2010;25(6):880-884.

Masterson EL, Masri BA, Duncan CP: Treatment of infection at the site of total hip replacement. *Instr Course Lect* 1998;47:297-306.

Mulcahy DM, O'Byrne JM, Fenelon GE: One stage surgical management of deep infection of total hip arthroplasty. *Ir J Med Sci* 1996;165(1):17-19.

Oussedik SI, Dodd MB, Haddad FS: Outcomes of revision total hip replacement for infection after grading according to a standard protocol. *J Bone Joint Surg Br* 2010;92(9):1222-1226.

Raut VV, Orth MS, Orth MC, Siney PD, Wroblewski BM: One stage revision arthroplasty of the hip for deep gram negative infection. *Int Orthop* 1996;20(1):12-14.

Raut VV, Siney PD, Wroblewski BM: One-stage revision of infected total hip replacements with discharging sinuses. *J Bone Joint Surg Br* 1994;76(5):721-724.

Sanchez-Sotelo J, Berry DJ, Hanssen AD, Cabanela ME: Midterm to long-term followup of staged reimplantation for infected hip arthroplasty. *Clin Orthop Relat Res* 2009;467(1):219-224.

Spangehl MJ, Younger AS, Masri BA, Duncan CP: Diagnosis of infection following total hip arthroplasty. *Instr Course Lect* 1998;47:285-295.

Trampuz A, Piper KE, Jacobson MJ, et al: Sonication of removed hip and knee prostheses for diagnosis of infection. *N Engl J Med* 2007;357(7):654-663.

Tsukayama DT, Estrada R, Gustilo RB: Infection after total hip arthroplasty: A study of the treatment of one hundred and six infections. *J Bone Joint Surg Am* 1996;78(4):512-523.

Ure KJ, Amstutz HC, Nasser S, Schmalzried TP: Direct-exchange arthroplasty for the treatment of infection after total hip replacement: An average ten-year follow-up. *J Bone Joint Surg Am* 1998;80(7):961-968.

Yi PH, Cross MB, Moric M, Sporer SM, Berger RA, Della Valle CJ: The 2013 Frank Stinchfield Award: Diagnosis of infection in the early postoperative period after total hip arthroplasty. *Clin Orthop Relat Res* 2014;472(2):424-429.

Younger AS, Duncan CP, Masri BA: Treatment of infection associated with segmental bone loss in the proximal part of the femur in two stages with use of an antibiotic-loaded interval prosthesis. *J Bone Joint Surg Am* 1998;80(1):60-69.

Younger AS, Duncan CP, Masri BA, McGraw RW: The outcome of two-stage arthroplasty using a custom-made interval spacer to treat the infected hip. *J Arthroplasty* 1997;12(6):615-623.

Chapter 36

Management of Peripheral Nerve and Vascular Injuries Associated With Total Hip Arthroplasty

Thomas P. Schmalzried, MD
Der-Chen Timothy Huang, MD

Nerve Injury

Prevalence

Nerve injuries are uncommon in total hip arthroplasty (THA), and the mechanism of injury is generally unknown. In an analysis of 34,335 THA procedures (primary and revision), researchers identified 359 nerve palsies for an overall prevalence of 1%. The prevalence of nerve palsy was 0.9% in primary THA and 2.6% in revision THA, suggesting that the risk of nerve injury in revision THA is nearly three times that in primary THA. The overall prevalence of nerve palsy associated with THA was higher in women than in men (1.5% and 0.77%, respectively; $P = 0.005$). That this difference was significant suggests that the risk of nerve palsy associated with THA in women is nearly twice that in men. However, this analysis does not account for any potential confounding variables, such as the etiology of hip disease (such as developmental dysplasia of the hip [DDH]), or any differences in the prevalence of primary and revision surgery among men and women.

Patients with DDH are at increased risk of nerve palsy when undergoing THA. A prevalence of nerve palsy as high as 5.2% has been reported in this patient population. Limb lengthening may account for a portion of the increased prevalence. However, even without substantial limb lengthening, the prevalence of nerve palsy in patients with DDH was reported to be nearly double that in patients with osteoarthritis.

The most commonly injured nerve is the sciatic nerve, specifically its peroneal division. In one review, this injury accounted for 79% of all nerve palsies (**Table 1**). Isolated femoral palsies accounted for 13% of nerve injuries, and obturator palsies accounted for 1.6% of nerve injuries. However, obturator nerve palsy is clinically less obvious than other nerve palsies and thus may be underreported. Simultaneous injury of both the sciatic and femoral nerves represented 5.8% of nerve injuries in that study. The true prevalence of superior gluteal nerve injury is unclear, but the injury has been associated with the Hardinge (transgluteal), transtrochanteric, and modified lateral approaches. These injuries can be functionally difficult to distinguish from partial avulsion or other injury of the gluteus medius and/or gluteus minimus. In several studies, electrical evidence of superior gluteal nerve injury during THA was identified in 14% to 70% of patients. The prevalence of clinical neuropathy is less well documented.

Sensory nerves known to be at risk of injury include the lateral femoral cutaneous nerve, which is at risk in the direct anterior approach. Studies have demonstrated rates of injury ranging from 1% to 5%; however, in a recent survey, 81% of patients reported sensory deficits in the distribution of the lateral femoral cutaneous nerve with a mean severity score of 2.3 on a 10-point scale. Injury to this sensory nerve can range from temporary neurapraxia to painful neuroma with symptoms similar to meralgia paresthetica. In most patients, this phenomenon is similar to the lateral knee numbness that some patients experience after total knee arthroplasty (as a result of transection of the infrapatellar branch of the saphenous nerve) in that the condition does not result in functional limitation.

The rate of injury to the sciatic nerve during hip resurfacing has been reported to be 1.7% to 2.1%, twice as

---

Dr. Schmalzried or an immediate family member has received royalties from DePuy Synthes and Stryker; is a member of a speakers' bureau or has made paid presentations on behalf of Stryker; serves as a paid consultant to Stryker; has stock or stock options held in DePuy Synthes and Stryker; and serves as a board member, owner, officer, or committee member of the Orthopaedic Research and Education Foundation. Neither Dr. Huang nor any immediate family member has received anything of value from or has stock or stock options held in a commercial company or institution related directly or indirectly to the subject of this chapter.

Table 1 Nerves or Nerve Combinations Injured in Association With Total Hip Arthroplasty in an Analysis of 24,469 Procedures

Nerve or Nerve Combination	Prevalence
Peroneal	0.52%
Sciatic	0.27%
Femoral	0.13%
Sciatic and femoral	0.057%
Obturator	0.016%
Tibial	0.004%

Adapted with permission from Schmalzried TP, Noordin S, Amstutz HC: Update on nerve palsy associated with total hip replacement. *Clin Orthop Relat Res* 1997;(344):188-206.

high as that reported in THA. This increased rate of sciatic nerve injury may be related to the increased complexity of the procedure, which includes a more extensive exposure and longer surgical time. With increased surgeon experience, the risk of nerve injury decreases.

Injury to the contralateral limb has been reported in rare instances. Case reports of contralateral femoral and sciatic palsy, rhabdomyolysis, and popliteal artery occlusion necessitating amputation have been reported. Careful padding and patient positioning are required to avoid contralateral limb injury, particularly if extended surgical time is expected. Upper extremity brachial plexus, axillary, ulnar, and median nerve injuries have been reported. Specific recommendations include padding around the abdomen and ankle, use of an axillary roll to protect the brachial plexus, and padding beneath the decubitus knee to protect the peroneal nerve around the fibular head.

Etiology

In most patients the mechanism of nerve injury is unknown. In one study, electromyographic (EMG) evidence of nerve injury was found in 70% of patients after THA. Clinical assessment alone has been found to underestimate the incidence of nerve injury associated with THA. Although frank neuropathy is rare, subclinical injury is common.

Peripheral nerves have unique attributes that make them susceptible to injury. The blood supply to peripheral nerves derives from two integrated but functionally independent microvascular systems. The extrinsic microvascular system is composed of segmentally arranged vessels originating from adjacent muscular and periosteal vessels. They usually are tortuous, with the coiled structure allowing for substantial length and position changes before blood flow is impaired. The local nutrient vessels divide within the epineurium and anastomose intraneurally with the epineurial, perineurial, and endoneurial plexus. This intrinsic microvascular system consists of microvessels that run longitudinally within the endoneurium, which may supply the nerve with critical blood flow when the microvessels are mobilized from their surrounding tissue. The intrinsic system may be more susceptible to external mechanical pressure than the extrinsic system.

Researchers have studied the temporal effects of ischemia on recovery of function after nerve injury. In a rabbit model, peripheral nerve function recovery was complete until 8 hours of pure ischemia was induced, at which time endoneurial edema (the hallmark of irreversible nerve injury) was observed and no recovery of nerve function was seen. In a study of nerve ischemia and compression underneath tourniquets, increased endoneurial vascular permeability and edema were accompanied by irreversible nerve injury after only 2 to 4 hours of compression. Thus, local compression has a much more detrimental effect and is associated with a greater risk of nerve injury than pure ischemia does.

Experimental models have demonstrated that peripheral nerves are particularly sensitive to compression. The susceptibility of large-diameter motor nerve fibers to compression has been attributed to a mechanical process that involves the Laplace law. The disproportionate occurrence of peroneal distribution deficits in patients with sciatic nerve palsy may be partially explained by this compressive effect. In the area of the hip joint, the peroneal division of the sciatic nerve has more tightly packed fascicles and less connective tissue than the tibial division has, which makes it more susceptible to compressive injury (**Figure 1**). The lateral position of this nerve may also make it more vulnerable to surgical trauma than other nerves. In patients undergoing revision surgery, scar tissue from prior surgical treatment can alter the mobility and blood supply to the nerve. Scarring may decrease the capacity of the nerve to accommodate tension and compression and can affect the capacity for regeneration.

Metabolic diseases can alter the inherent characteristics of nerves. Diabetes can increase endoneurial edema via increased aldose reductase and can increase nerve stiffness as a result of the glycosylation of collagen fibers within the nerve. Furthermore, diabetes has been shown to slow antegrade axoplasmic flow. Thyroid disorders can also alter nerve physiology. Hypothyroidism has been known to cause segmental demyelination and decreased nerve conduction velocity.

Nerves around the hip joint are at risk of injury because of their anatomic location (**Figure 2**). The femoral nerve lies on the iliopsoas muscle and courses

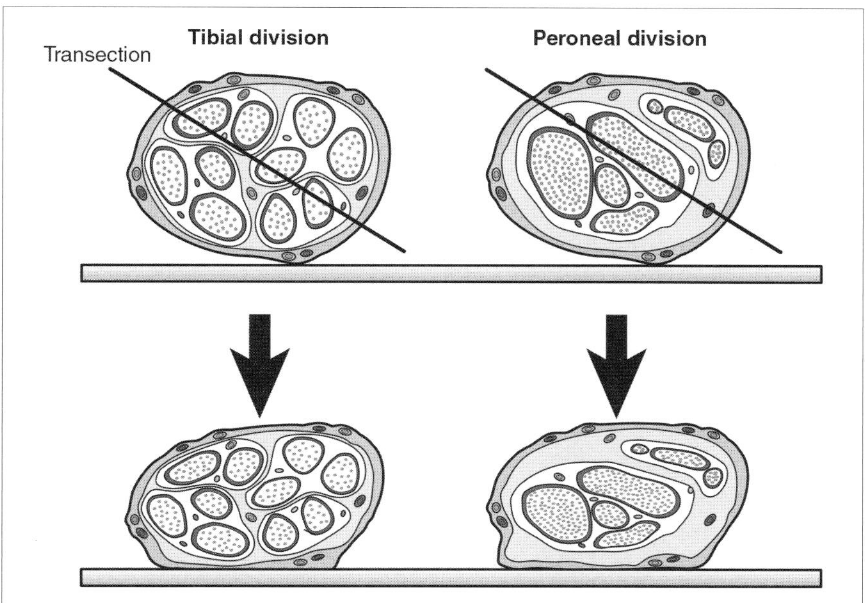

Figure 1 Illustrations depict transection and compression of the sciatic nerve. Multifascicular nerves with abundant connective tissue (such as those in the tibial division) are less vulnerable to injury as a result of transection or compression (indicated by arrows) than are nerves with tightly packed fascicles (such as those in the peroneal division).

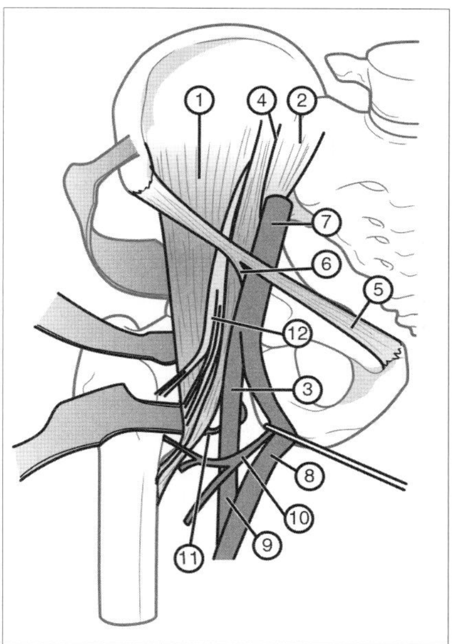

Figure 3 Illustration of the femoral triangle depicts the proximity and vulnerability of the femoral nerve to anterior acetabular retractors. Structures depicted include the iliacus muscle (1), psoas major and minor muscle (2 and 4), deep femoral artery (3 and 9), inguinal ligament (5), iliopectineal arch (6), femoral artery (7 and 8), lateral circumflex femoral artery (10), medial circumflex femoral artery (11), and femoral nerve (12).

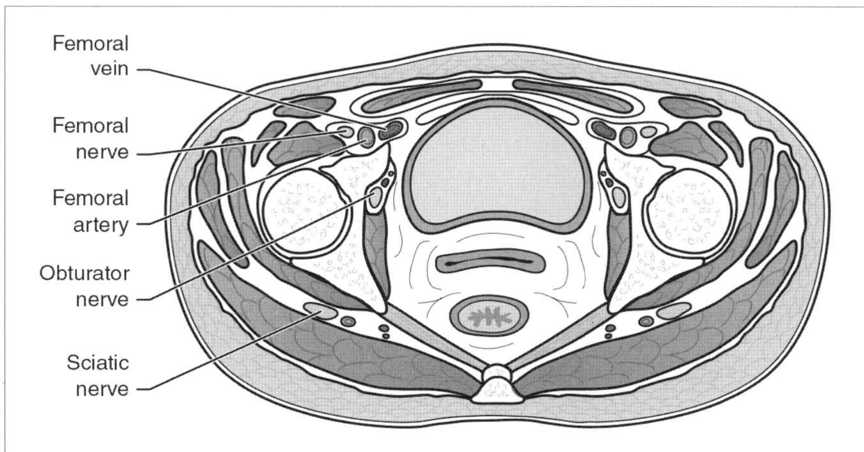

Figure 2 Cross-sectional illustration of the pelvis at the level of the hip joint depicts the location of the obturator, femoral, and sciatic nerves.

in front of the acetabulum. It is farthest (2.65 cm) from retractors placed at the 12 o'clock position on the acetabulum and is closest to the acetabulum (0.95 cm) and most susceptible to injury at the inferior portion just above the superior pubic ramus. Direct anterior retractors (at the 3 o'clock position in the right hip) have been shown to be approximately 2.1 cm from the femoral neurovascular bundle. Pressure on the direct anterior retractor consistently increases pressure in the area of the femoral nerve. Anterior retractors should be placed more proximally to avoid injury to the femoral nerve, but care must be taken to avoid compressing the nerve against the inguinal ligament (**Figure 3**).

The sciatic nerve has a variable course as it exits the pelvis around the piriformis muscle. In most patients, both the peroneal and tibial divisions of the sciatic nerve exit anterior to and below the piriformis, but anatomic variations exist in 1.5% to 35.8% of the population. Variations include the entire sciatic nerve exiting above and posterior to the piriformis muscle, one division of the nerve exiting above and the other division exiting through the piriformis muscle, and the entire nerve exiting through the piriformis muscle. Tenotomy of this tendon and retraction of the piriformis may cause sciatic nerve compression and increase the risk of postarthroplasty sciatica. Around the acetabulum, direct posterior retractors (at the 9 o'clock position in the right hip) have been shown to be, on average,

1.75 cm from the sciatic nerve. As the sciatic nerve courses down the posterior thigh, it is closest to the surgical field around the level of the ischial tuberosity. Additionally, the peroneal division of the sciatic nerve is tethered at the level of the sciatic notch and fibular head. This tethering limits its mobility and may make it more susceptible to stretch injury than the untethered tibial division is.

Intraoperative nerve injuries can result from a variety of mechanisms. Direct penetration or laceration may occur with use of a scalpel, electrocautery, reamers, saws, or sutures and during placement of screws and cerclage wires. Bone fragments can also damage nerves. Compression-type injuries can occur as a result of retractor placement, intraoperative limb manipulation, and positioning. Postoperative surgical dressings and splints may contribute to compression neuropathy. Cement extrusion can cause both compressive and thermal injury to nearby nerves.

Wound hematoma is another potential cause of compression injury. Anticoagulation therapy is generally indicated after THA to prevent deep vein thrombosis, but patients may become more susceptible to a bleeding diathesis. Hematomas have been reported to cause neuropathy as many as 3 weeks after hip arthroplasty. A patient with a clinically relevant wound hematoma usually reports increasing buttock and/or thigh pain. Nerve palsy may not be apparent on initial physical examination but may develop over 12 to 24 hours depending on the degree of compression. In patients with buttock and/or thigh pain associated with a hematoma, monitoring for systemic indications of crush syndrome is necessary. The hematoma creates pressure that can damage the sciatic nerve and disrupt blood flow to the muscles in the gluteal region, resulting in rhabdomyolysis, myoglobinuria, and decreased renal function. Other delayed compression-type neuropathies may occur months to years after THA, with compression caused by pseudotumor formation, osteolysis and wear debris, or, in rare instances, migration of implants.

Nerves are also susceptible to stretch injury during THA. Stretch injury can occur during limb positioning, manipulation, dislocation, and relocation maneuvers. Stretching also may result from lengthening of the limb or increased offset. The authors of a study of limb lengthening reported no significant correlation of nerve palsy with the amount of lengthening. In their review of 1,284 arthroplasty procedures, lengthening ranged from 0.4 to 4 cm in primary THA and from 0.04 to 5.8 cm in revision THA. Only one case of sciatic nerve palsy was reported, and the cause was direct intraoperative laceration of the nerve. The authors of the study recommended reservation when attributing nerve palsy to excessive tension from limb lengthening. In animal models, nerve microcirculation can be affected by stretching of 4% to 6%, with stretching of 8% to 15% demonstrating measurably decreased flow in vessels as tension increases, and with conduction failure occurring with stretching of approximately 25%. This finding makes ischemia secondary to lengthening alone unlikely; however, most experts continue to recommend care when limb lengthening greater than 4 cm is planned. Unfortunately, no definitive guidelines have been established to allow prediction of a safe amount of lengthening.

The Seddon classification of peripheral nerve injury is based on the degree of anatomic disruption. Neurapraxia is a failure of neural conduction resulting from altered nerve physiology in a patient with an intact neurologic structure. Among types of nerve injury, neurapraxia has the best prognosis for recovery. Patients with axonotmesis have some disruption of axons and distal degeneration of myelin (wallerian degeneration), but the endoneurial tube remains intact in these patients. Neurotmesis consists of complete disruption of the nerve and is associated with the poorest prognosis for recovery. The Sunderland classification further subdivides nerve injury into five degrees, with first-degree injury consisting of neurapraxia and fifth-degree injury consisting of neurotmesis. In this classification, axonotmesis is divided into three subcategories of injury, in which second-degree injury is characterized by disruption of axons without scarring, third-degree injury consists of partial endoneurial scarring, and fourth-degree injury denotes nerve continuity but complete scarring across the axon (neuroma in continuity). Both third- and fourth-degree injuries have an unpredictable prognosis for ultimate recovery.

Preoperative Evaluation

Risk factors such as DDH, diabetes mellitus, thyroid disorders, other metabolic disorders, and prior surgery can be identified in preoperative evaluation. Physical examination can reveal any baseline strength and/or sensory deficits. Both limbs should be examined and compared for asymmetry. Examination of reflexes may be help the surgeon discern concurrent spinal issues. In patients with substantial spinal disease, decompression may be warranted. Clinical judgment should be used because no studies are available to guide preoperative decompression. If the spine is the greater issue, decompression may be considered before THA. In this manner, a double crush nerve injury may be prevented. Abnormal preoperative examination findings should be clearly documented to avoid confusion during the postoperative examination.

When preoperative motor deficits suggest neuropathy, the surgeon may consider further investigation with an EMG study or neurologic consultation. Detailed evaluation may help diagnose a systemic disease or localize compressive lesions, and may also help identify deficits that are spinal in origin. Preoperative EMG studies have demonstrated abnormal denervation and reinnervation within the abductor musculature, suggesting that prior nerve pathology can exist preoperatively. To date, no clinical association between EMG changes and clinically relevant abductor weakness (Trendelenburg gait) has been identified. Consequently, a clear role of routine preoperative EMG study has not been established.

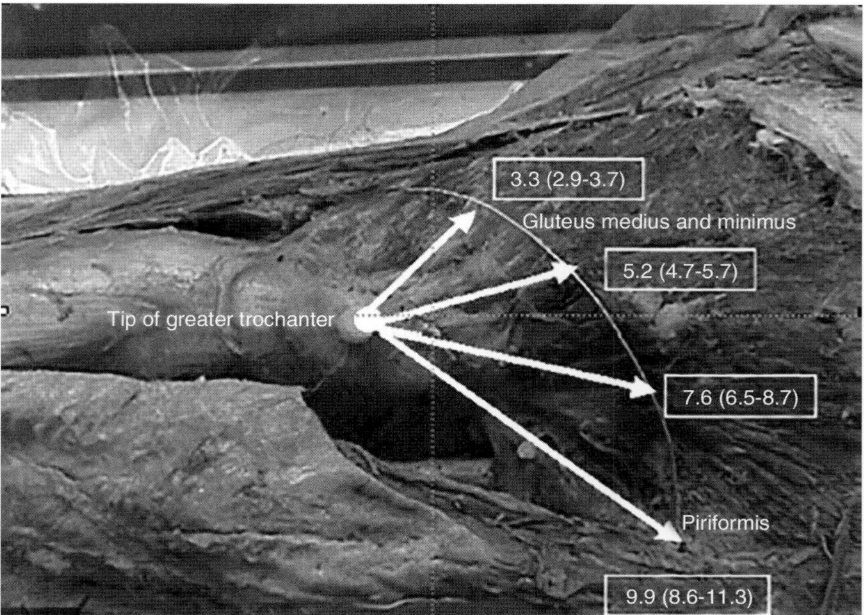

Figure 4 Photograph of a cadaver model depicts the trajectory of the superior gluteal neurovascular bundle (SGNVB) as encountered during acetabular exposure. The wire shows the anatomic path of the SGNVB. The arrows show the means and ranges, in centimeters, of the distances measured in all hemipelvic specimens to four locations over the SGNVB. From bottom, the arrows indicate (1) a line from the tip of the greater trochanter to the SGNVB as it passes the superior border of the piriformis and (2) three lines that separate the gluteus medius into fourths. (Adapted with permission from Lavernia CJ, Cook CC, Hernandez RA, Sierra RJ, Rossi MD: Neurovascular injuries in acetabular reconstruction cage surgery: An anatomical study. *J Arthroplasty* 2007;22[1]:124-132.)

Role of Surgical Technique

APPROACH AND EXPOSURE

The neurovascular structures must be protected intraoperatively. Care must be taken during acetabular exposure. When retractors are placed around the acetabular rim, the femoral nerve is closest to the anterior retractor just above the superior rami, and the sciatic nerve is directly behind the posterior retractor. Assistants also must be aware of how much force they are placing on the adjacent soft tissue when retracting because excessive force can cause compressive or tensile injury to nerves.

Each surgical approach places different nerves at risk of injury. In the posterior approach, the sciatic nerve is at increased risk. Posterior retractors must be placed with care, and attention must be paid to limb positioning throughout the procedure (such as with avoidance of hip flexion during acetabular preparation when a posterior retractor is in place). At the level of the ischium, the tendinous portion of the gluteus maximus may become taut during limb manipulation. Pressure studies around the gluteal sling have shown that substantial compression of the sciatic nerve occurs during preparation of the femoral canal in THA procedures and during acetabular preparation in hip resurfacing procedures. Some authors have recommended completely releasing the tendinous portion of the gluteus maximus during posterior hip arthroplasty procedures to prevent compression of the sciatic nerve, but this technique is not standard practice for most surgeons.

With a posterior approach, the location of the nerve can be assessed to avoid injury, which is especially helpful in revision procedures with compromise of the posterior wall or column. Often, the nerve can be localized by means of finger palpation where the nerve crosses the ischium. In patients with substantial scarring around the nerve, limited neurolysis may be indicated to increase nerve mobility and decrease tension. Because mobilization of the nerve disrupts the extrinsic vascular supply, dissection should be limited to approximately 14 cm. Excessive dissection can result in nerve injury.

When an anterior approach is used, the risk of sciatic nerve injury is lower. However, the femoral nerve and the lateral femoral cutaneous nerve are at risk of injury. When an anterolateral or lateral approach is used, both the femoral nerve and the superior gluteal nerve are at risk of injury. On the basis of anatomic dissections, researchers have generally accepted that limiting dissection to a zone adjacent to the tip of the greater trochanter can prevent injury to the superior gluteal nerve. This safe zone around the greater trochanter starts approximately 5 cm posteriorly and narrows to 3 cm anteriorly (**Figure 4**). Injury to the superior gluteal nerve may result in abductor weakness and a positive Trendelenburg sign or gait. In clinical practice, this guideline appears to be adequate; however, subclinical injury to the nerve may still occur.

INTRAOPERATIVE MONITORING

In several studies, intraoperative cortical somatosensory-evoked potential (SSEP) monitoring of sciatic nerve function during THA has not been demonstrated to reduce the prevalence of nerve palsy. The advantage of spontaneous EMG over cortical SSEP monitoring is that spontaneous EMG involves continuous recording of muscle activity, allowing the surgeon to take immediate corrective action, whereas cortical SSEP monitoring involves recording of a mean impulse over a specified interval. Spontaneous EMG is more specific in patients with certain kinds of trauma, such as direct trauma with cautery, but is not sensitive to changes that occur over time, such as stretching. The efficacy of these techniques for avoiding nerve injury in hip arthroplasty has not been established.

Multimodal intraoperative monitoring consisting of EMG study, monitoring of motor-evoked potentials, and SSEP monitoring has also been suggested to avoid injury to nerves during complex reconstruction procedures. This method is commonly used during spinal surgery and requires the expertise of a neurophysiologist to interpret changes in the recorded data. In one study, researchers reported the results of multimodal monitoring in 69 complex pelvic reconstruction procedures over a 10-year period. They were alerted to possible injury in 35% of patients, and the surgeon was able to modify the technique to prevent nerve injury in all but one patient. In total, the authors of the study reported one true-positive case of injury during attempted limb lengthening in a patient with DDH, and no false-positive or false-negative results, resulting in sensitivity and specificity of 100%. They concluded that it is possible to use multimodal techniques to monitor for nerve injury during complex reconstruction procedures.

Management

Most nerve injuries associated with hip arthroplasty are unrecognized intraoperatively. In the rare event of a recognized direct injury such as laceration, transaction, or cauterization, an acute repair should be performed. Ideally, this repair should be performed at the time of the arthroplasty procedure or within 72 hours because the nerve endings can retract and make primary repair difficult or impossible. If the nerve is damaged and healthy nerve endings cannot be approximated, segmental excision and nerve grafting should be performed. If nerves are entrapped by wire or suture, the offending agent should be removed. If excessive limb lengthening is suspected, revision shortening may be considered. Although shortening has not been shown to be detrimental, it is not guaranteed to improve symptoms in all patients.

Postoperatively, all patients should be examined for motor function, strength, and sensory function. Usually, the diagnosis of substantial nerve injury is not challenging; however, subtle injury can progress, and injury of more notable severity may be noted on subsequent examinations. To test the femoral nerve, the surgeon asks the patient to push the knee posteriorly into the bed and observes the function of the quadriceps. To test the peroneal branch of the sciatic nerve, the surgeon asks the patient to extend the great toe and dorsiflex the ankle. The tibial nerve is tested with active ankle plantar flexion. If an injury is identified, worsening mechanical impairment of sciatic nerve function may be lessened in the acute stage by keeping the hip extended and the knee flexed over the side of the bed to reduce tension on the nerve. The opposite position is used in patients with femoral neuropathy. Minimizing edema is of theoretic benefit, but the efficacy of the use of steroids or osmotic agents in this circumstance has not been documented.

The surgeon should discuss the nerve injury thoroughly with the patient as soon as possible after the diagnosis is made. An educated patient is the best ally in maximizing recovery. The nursing staff and therapists should be advised of the nerve injury, and additional exercises should be prescribed to strengthen weakened muscles and stretch uninjured antagonists to prevent joint contracture. The use of appropriate orthoses should be initiated promptly so that the patient can begin physical therapy. The use of a knee immobilizer or similar removable brace to hold the knee in extension will allow safe ambulation in patients with femoral neuropathy. In patients with sciatic neuropathy, the use of an ankle-foot orthosis can aid in ambulation. The patient should also learn to examine sensory-impaired skin regions daily. If dysesthesia is present, some benefit may result from sensory stimulation, sympathetic nerve blockade, and treatment with a tricyclic antidepressant or tetracyclic antidepressant, although associated orthostatic hypotension or other anticholinergic side effects may outweigh the benefits in patients with occasional dysesthesia.

Surgical wounds should be examined for hematoma formation because many patients who undergo hip arthroplasty are placed on chemical anticoagulation therapy, and an expanding hematoma has been known to cause compression neuropathy. Currently, no absolute indications have been established for secondary surgery to evacuate a hematoma. Good outcomes have been reported with both surgical and nonsurgical management. However, surgical exploration of the hip is appropriate when the patient has progressive neuromuscular deterioration with evidence of a wound hematoma. In such patients, prompt evacuation (within 6 hours) is preferred to minimize nerve injury. Moreover, pain in the distribution of the affected nerve suggests ongoing insult to the nerve. In patients with painful nerve palsies, urgent exploration is recommended.

When a nerve palsy is identified, neurologic consultation can be helpful. The neurologist can validate the physical findings, assist in localization of the nerve injury (often through electrodiagnostic studies), and assist in identifying any causes of peripheral neuropathy that can be managed. A thorough electrodiagnostic evaluation includes recording from the short head of the biceps femoris, which is the only thigh muscle innervated by the peroneal division of the sciatic nerve. Denervation of this muscle indicates nerve injury in the proximal thigh in patients who may otherwise appear to have a peroneal nerve injury at or below the knee.

A neurologist may also be able to help determine nonarthroplasty sources of nerve dysfunction. Coexisting spinal stenosis may increase the risk of symptomatic nerve injury associated with THA. In a study of 21 patients with high-grade spinal stenosis who had foot drop after THA, 12 of 16 patients who underwent surgery improved, and 6 patients had complete recovery. No improvement was observed in the five patients who did not undergo surgery. In general, management of any coexisting causes of peripheral neuropathy would be of theoretic benefit.

In addition to neurologic consultation and EMG study, certain imaging modalities can assist in identifying the location and nature of the injury. Plain radiographs can be used to evaluate implant position, screw placement, limb length, and offset. Screws occasionally can appear to be placed in bone when in fact they are incorrectly placed in a different plane. CT is better than radiography for assessment of implant position and screw placement. MRI is another imaging modality available at most institutions. Although the presence of metal can interfere with image quality, the increase in magnet strength and improvement in imaging sequences with metal artifact subtraction can yield information about the neural structures around orthopaedic implants. In one study, researchers used a 3-T magnet and pulse sequencing to perform magnetic resonance neurography. The sequencing technique was modified to increase the image quality to visualize nerve fascicles and localize lesions of the sciatic nerve. However, metal artifact still exists, and image quality remains admittedly poor in the peritrochanteric region, in which metal is most dense. Both CT and MRI can detect hematoma formation and localized compression, and the use of these modalities is reasonable to consider in the search for a cause of neuropathy that can be managed. Despite the technologic advances, the cause of most nerve injuries is still not readily identifiable.

If no identifiable cause of injury or insult to the nerve is determined, nonsurgical management with serial examinations is acceptable. If the patient demonstrates no improvement, an EMG study should be performed at 4 to 8 weeks postoperatively (most authors recommend 6 weeks). Fibrillations are a poor prognostic indicator. If present, they suggest the discontinuity of axons and the denervation of muscle. If evidence of neural regeneration is present, continued observation is reasonable. The Tinel sign denotes at least partial nerve continuity, and an advancing Tinel sign suggests recovery. Clinically, the Tinel sign may progress until the nerve encounters a secondary site of compression (the fibular head for the peroneal nerve and medial/lateral plantar tunnels for the tibial nerve). If nerve recovery does not progress, surgical decompression of these secondary sites is warranted. A follow-up EMG study should be performed at 3 months postoperatively. If the EMG study at 3 months does not reveal a pattern of regeneration, the surgeon can assume that scarring is present around the nerve and should consider performing neurolysis at the site where injury is most likely to have occurred.

Neurolysis has been shown not to have a detrimental effect and should be performed within the first year after injury for maximal improvement. However, even late neurolysis has been demonstrated to improve pain. Although the benefit is unpredictable, most patients (82% in one study) gain relief from neuropathic pain. Ultimately, the physician must consider all the factors and individualize treatment based on the clinical course of the disorder and the relative risks and benefits of exploration, decompression, neurolysis and/or nerve grafting, and revision surgery.

Outcomes

The degree of injury and the distance between the site of injury and the affected organ determine the prognosis for neurologic recovery. In adults, axon sprouts grow distally at a rate of approximately 1 mm/day. Motor end plates and muscle fascicles can atrophy before regenerated axons reach them, and the Schwann cell basement membrane undergoes degeneration with time, which may result in the possibility that axon sprouts will no longer have a tubular guide. Irreversible muscle fibrosis and motor end plate degeneration typically occur by 24 months after injury. This physiology is the basis for the guarded prognosis of a high-degree injury (axonotmesis or neurotmesis) of the sciatic nerve near the hip, which has the longest regeneration pathway in the body. Conversely, the shorter regeneration pathway of femoral nerve injuries is associated with a more favorable prognosis.

Good prognostic indicators include neurapraxic and partial or incomplete injury of the nerve. Maintenance of sensory function and early return of motor function are good prognostic signs. In general, patients in whom some motor function is maintained or is recovered within 2 weeks after injury have good outcomes. Poor prognostic indicators include the presence of painful dysesthesia and complete motor and sensory loss with no return within the first 2 weeks after injury. Despite these prognostic indicators, the amount of recovery in the early period of injury cannot be predicted, and a large portion of patients will not regain their preinjury status.

In a review of 223 sciatic nerve injuries, 41% of patients had complete or essentially complete recovery, a mild deficit remained in 44%, and weakness that restricted ambulation and/or persistent dysesthesia occurred in 15%. In a study of 27 sciatic nerve injuries, 29% of patients had full recovery, 25% had fair or partial recovery, and 44% had considerable disability. The authors of the study observed that most people with sciatic nerve injury who demonstrate recovery do so by 7 months after injury. However, because of the length of nerve regeneration, improvement may not be readily apparent, and 1 year may pass before initial motor recovery is observed. Clinical improvements can be seen up to 2 or 3 years postoperatively. The prognosis is better in patients with isolated peroneal division injuries than in patients with complete sciatic palsy.

Femoral nerve injury is associated with a good prognosis. Most of these injuries are subtle in presentation, and patients have a shorter period of disability. Hematoma decompression and neurolysis can improve pain and functional recovery. Superior gluteal and obturator nerve injuries tend to be of less functional consequence and may be underrecognized and underreported. In a limited number of patients with obturator palsy, the removal of an identifiable cause of the neuropathy has been associated with resolution of the neuropathy.

In a study of nerve palsies (femoral, sciatic, and superior gluteal) associated with THA, at 8 years postoperatively 91% of patients with mild nerve injury (motor grade 3 to 4 on a 5-point scale) had achieved full recovery within 2 years, and 43% of patients with severe (motor grade 0 to 2 on a 5-point scale) injuries had full recovery within 2 years. One patient had no improvement, and the rest of the patients demonstrated partial improvement. In the study, a correlation appeared to exist between initial preservation of motor function and the potential for recovery from injury. Moreover, patients with initial preservation of motor function were also observed to have recovery of nerve function at 2 years after injury.

Vascular Injury

Prevalence

Vascular injury is an uncommon complication of THA. The incidence of injury has been reported to be approximately 0.2% to 0.3%. The difference in incidence of injury between primary and revision surgery has not been shown to be significant. As with nerve injury, vascular injury is twice as likely to occur in women as in men. Curiously, left hips are twice as likely to be involved as right hips are. Vascular injury most commonly affects the external iliac artery or the femoral artery (48% and 23%, respectively). Thromboembolic events have been shown to account for 46% of vascular injuries, followed by lacerations (26%), pseudoaneurysms (25%), and arteriovenous fistulas (3%). Most of these injuries require vascular surgical intervention in the form of bypass grafting, primary repair, thrombectomy, embolectomy, and/or ligation.

Etiology

Vascular injuries can occur via multiple mechanisms of injury. Direct injury can occur via penetration, transection, or trauma from pressure resulting from retractor placement. Indirect injury can result from elongation or torsion during positioning, dislocation, and relocation maneuvers. During the cementing process, vessels have been known to be compressed, damaged via thermal injury, and even incarcerated. Cement spicules have been known to erode through and perforate arteries, resulting in pseudoaneurysms and arteriovenous fistulas. Acute thrombus formation can manifest intraoperatively or postoperatively and cause arterial ischemia.

Certain risk factors predispose patients to vascular injury. One risk factor is prior vascular surgery. Often these patients already have some arterial ischemia, and their blood vessels may have intrinsic compromise in the form of atherosclerosis and decreased elasticity. These patients are also at high risk of plaque embolization and occlusion of distal vessels. Another common risk factor is prior pelvic orthopaedic surgery. Revision surgery around prior hip implants can pose a surgical challenge. The inherent difficulty of surgical dissection through scar tissue and obliterated tissue planes puts neurovascular structures at risk. Despite the technical difficulties of revision surgery, several studies have shown equal risk of vascular injury in primary and revision hip arthroplasty.

Other risk factors are related to anatomic abnormalities such as acetabular dysplasia; congenital dislocation; acetabular protrusion, particularly with implant migration medial to the Köhler line (**Figure 5**); pelvic fractures; Paget disease; muscle wasting; and scar formation. One potentially underrecognized risk factor pertains to revision of an infected THA. The inflammatory process that occurs with infection makes the perivascular tissues more friable and more likely to sustain injury. Infection in combination with acetabular protrusion has been found to increase the risk of vascular injury.

Preoperative Evaluation

Physical examination should include palpation of the distal pulses and observation for arterial/venous insufficiency. When insufficiency is suspected, the ankle-brachial index (ABI) may help determine the need for further workup.

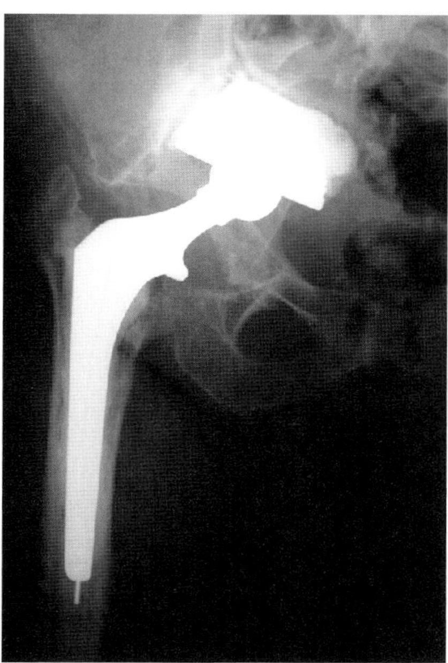

Figure 5 AP radiograph of a right hip demonstrates a cemented acetabular implant that has migrated medial to the Köhler line.

Vascular consultation has been recommended for patients with ABI less than 0.5, and CT angiography has been recommended for patients with ABI less than 0.4. In addition to its use in risk stratification, preoperative arteriography can minimize the duration of acute ischemia by documenting distal arteries that a vascular surgeon can use in bypass procedures. In general, when claudication exists in conjunction with osteoarthritis, preemptive revascularization is performed before orthopaedic procedures only in patients who experience pain when at rest.

In planning for revision surgery, CT angiography has been recommended in some patients with acetabular protrusion, especially when acetabular implants have migrated medial to the Köhler line, and particularly if the acetabular implant was cemented. CT angiography allows the surgeon to identify the relative proximity of the external iliac vessels and to determine whether the vessels have been incarcerated in cement. Also, if the implants are located immediately adjacent to major vessels, removal through a retroperitoneal approach with exposure of the external iliac vessels before extraction of the implant may be safer. Communication and consultation with a vascular surgeon is recommended before THA is performed in patients at high risk of vascular injury.

Role of Surgical Technique

Many surgical approaches to the hip joint are available. Vascular injury can occur through each of these approaches as a result of retractor placement, direct laceration, and intraoperative limb manipulation. Extrapelvic vessels at risk are primarily the common femoral vessels, the deep femoral vessels and their branches, the medial and lateral circumflex arteries, and the obturator artery. Most vascular injuries sustained during THA involve the external iliac and common femoral arteries. Knowledge of the relevant anatomy surrounding the hip joint is paramount to avoiding injury.

Manipulation of the hip with dislocation and relocation maneuvers can cause trauma to atherosclerotic vessels. In a published case report from the Mayo Clinic, positioning of the leg during THA caused acute thrombosis in a patient with an iliofemoral stent. Although a rare occurrence, the hammering involved in the placement of press-fit acetabular and femoral implants may stress atherosclerotic vessels and can dislodge plaques or even cause wall rupture or intimal tears. Care must be taken during cementation of acetabular implants because cement extrusion into the pelvis may cause thermal injury to the external iliac vessels and predispose them to tears, pseudoaneurysms, or fistula formation. Also, when a strut allograft is used, care must be taken to avoid incarceration of vessels when wires or cables are passed around the femur. Even with good surgical technique, constrictive fascial bands may cause indirect tethering and occlusion of vessels that may necessitate secondary surgery.

The placement of acetabular fixation screws poses a known risk of vascular injury. A quadrant system has been developed to help the surgeon intraoperatively identify safe zones for screw placement (**Figure 6, A**). In this system, the acetabulum is divided into anterior and posterior halves by a line originating from the anterior superior iliac spine. A perpendicular line divides each half into superior and inferior quadrants. The intrapelvic structures adjacent to the anterior quadrants include the external iliac vessels and the obturator vessels. The inferior gluteal and the internal pudendal vessels are located adjacent to the posterior inferior quadrant. The posterior superior quadrant is considered the safest zone for screw placement because it has the highest bone depth for secure screw fixation (**Figure 6, B** and **C**). However, the superior gluteal vessels and the sciatic nerve are located beyond this quadrant. Although the quadrant system is an effective method to determine a safe zone for screw placement, the distorted anatomy and deficient bone frequently associated with revision surgery often requires placement of screws outside this zone, with special care taken to keep the drills and screws contained in bone.

Management

Pulsatile bleeding and uncontrolled hemorrhage within the surgical field are unmistakable. If immediate access to the bleeding vessel is available, the vessel should be ligated. Otherwise, the problem may be managed temporarily with local compression, until adequate exposure is attained. Intrapelvic bleeding may occur after acetabular screw placement and may not be visibly apparent, but should be suspected if the patient's hemodynamic status changes. Immediate volume and blood replacement should be undertaken and the patient closely monitored. It is never too early to request the help of a general or vascular surgeon. If the patient demonstrates

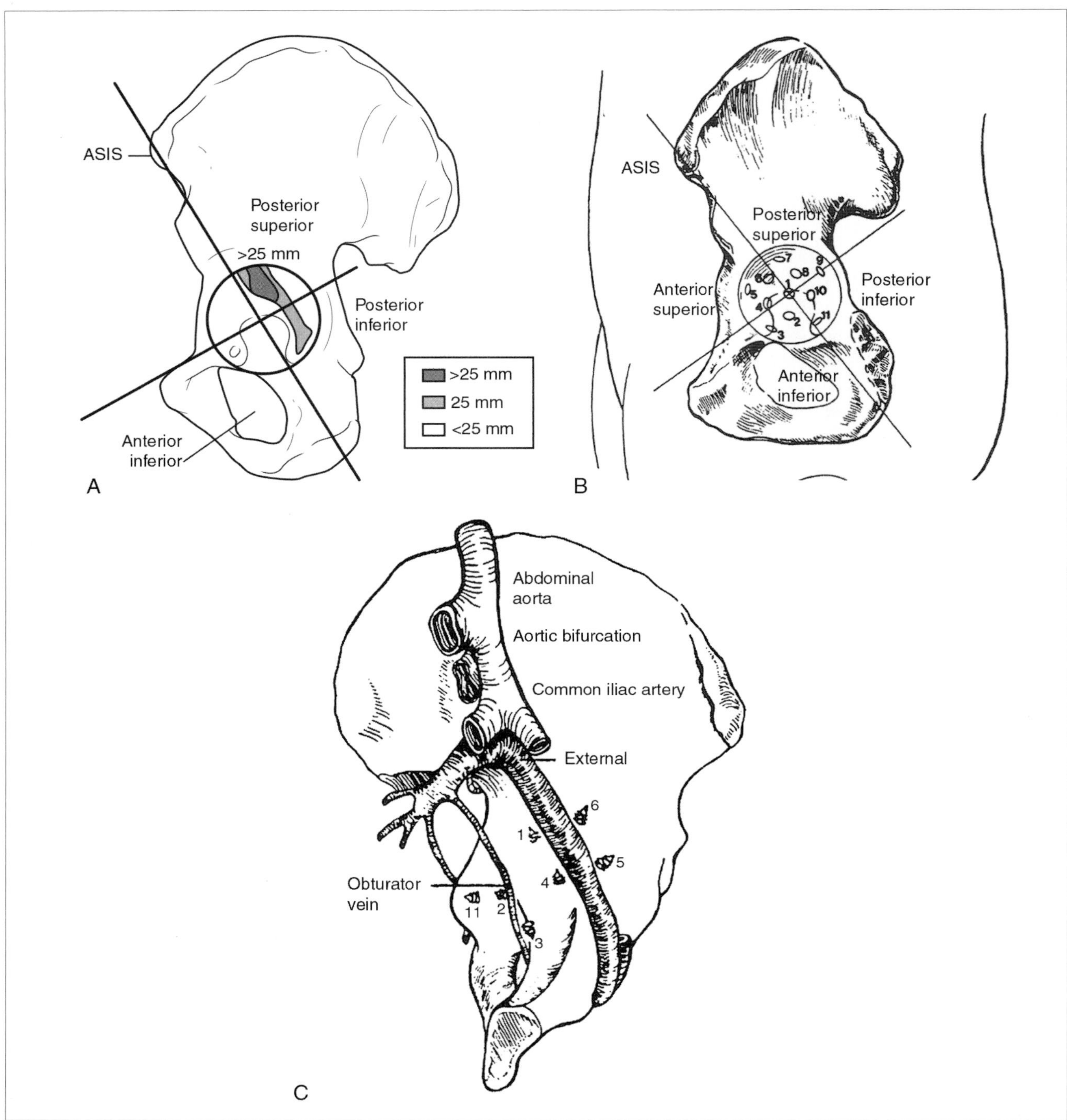

Figure 6 A and **B,** Illustrations depict the acetabular quadrant system that can be used to identify safe zones for placement of acetabular screws. ASIS = anterior superior iliac spine. **A,** Measurements indicate the length of screw that is typically safe to use in the corresponding zone. **B,** The acetabular origin of the screws (numbered 1 through 11). **C,** Illustration depicts the corresponding location of the screws on the quadrilateral intrapelvic surface relative to the iliac venous system. Screws 1, 4, 5, and 6 are near the external iliac vein; their acetabular origin is in the anterior superior quadrant. Screws 2 and 3 are near the obturator vein; their acetabular origin is in the anterior inferior quadrant. (Panels B and C adapted with permission from Wasielewski RC, Cooperstein LA, Kruger MP, Rubash HE: Acetabular anatomy and the transacetabular fixation of screws in total hip arthroplasty. *J Bone Joint Surg Am* 1990;72[4]:501-508.)

hemodynamic instability, immediate laparotomy should be performed with an approach to the iliac vessels because rapid exsanguination may occur. The immediate goal of the orthopaedic surgeon is to apply local compression to minimize the bleeding.

After the wounds are closed and the patient has left the operating room, vessel injury can be present and difficult to diagnose. If continued blood loss occurs, angiography with transcatheter embolization may be necessary. Postoperative examination is crucial to the diagnosis and management of vessel injury. Diminished or absent pedal pulses, cyanosis, or a cold extremity can suggest an arterial injury. Alternatively, edema and swelling out of proportion to the procedure can be a sign of venous injury or a developing hematoma. If palpation does not reveal pulses, a portable Doppler ultrasonographic unit is used for further assessment.

When pulses cannot be detected by Doppler ultrasonography, urgent vascular consultation and angiography are indicated. Ideally, a vascular specialist would perform the angiography so that treatment can be initiated promptly after diagnosis of vessel injury. Interventions available to the vascular surgeon or interventional radiologist include intravascular thrombectomy, stenting, ablation, and coiling. Open vascular management with primary repair, end-to-end anastomosis, or bypass grafting may also be used to reestablish perfusion. Fasciotomies may be necessary to manage or prevent reperfusion-induced compartment syndrome in the distal limb.

Pseudoaneurysms may also occur after hip arthroplasty. These subtle injuries have a mean time to diagnosis of 29 months. Most pseudoaneurysms involve the external iliac artery or the common femoral artery (65% and 18%, respectively). These injuries are thought to be either cement related or caused by retraction during the procedure. A less common cause of pseudoaneurysm is intrapelvic migration of the acetabular implant. Prompt referral to a vascular surgeon after establishment of the diagnosis is paramount to successful treatment. Depending on the vessel involved, treatment options include bypass grafting, primary repair, and/or ligation.

Outcomes

Vascular injury during THA is rare but potentially devastating. Prompt diagnosis and consultation with a vascular specialist have been demonstrated to improve outcomes. The overall mortality rate has been reported to be 7%, with a 15% incidence of major amputation (above the ankle joint) and a 4% incidence of minor amputation (a portion of the foot). Emergent vascular surgery intervention is required in greater than 40% of vessel injuries, with most of these injuries involving the external iliac artery or the common femoral artery. In a study in which a preoperative high-risk patient screening protocol was used and aggressive vascular intervention was performed when injury was identified, limb salvage was achieved in all patients. The authors of the study concluded that thrombectomy alone, which had a 28% success rate, may not be sufficient. More often, bypass was necessary for revascularization. The authors of the study also advocated a completion arteriography after bypass to rule out any underlying intimal flap, suggesting that this step is essential in preventing recurrent thrombosis and that the previous lack of this examination may explain higher historical amputation rates.

Orthopaedic vascular injuries often result in legal action, with approximately 50% of patients initiating litigation against the surgeon. Despite the rare incidence of vascular injury, the consequences are severe enough that they should be discussed in the informed consent process. If an injury occurs, the surgeon should discuss the nature of the injury with the patient, obtain appropriate consultations, and communicate the treatment plan promptly and effectively to the patient.

Summary

Nerve injuries are uncommon in patients who undergo THA, and the mechanism of injury is generally unknown. Evaluation can include electrodiagnostic and imaging studies to identify the location of injury. Ultimately, the physician must weigh all the factors and individualize treatment on the basis of the clinical course of the patient and the relative risks and benefits of exploration, decompression, neurolysis, and/or nerve grafting in each specific patient. Recovery typically depends on the degree of nerve injury and the length of the regeneration pathway (for higher-degree injuries). Femoral, obturator, and superior gluteal nerve injuries have a relatively favorable prognosis, whereas the prognosis is worse in patients with injuries involving the sciatic nerve. Delayed neurolysis has been demonstrated to improve outcomes in some patients, and recovery can occur even more than 2 years after injury.

Vascular injuries are an uncommon complication of THA. Knowledge of risk factors and relevant anatomy can help prevent vascular injury. Arteriography and consultation with a vascular surgeon is recommended for patients with ABI less than 0.4, and advanced imaging (CT scan or CT angiography) is recommended in patients with very aberrant anatomy, extensive intrapelvic cement, or implant migration. Avoidance of excessive traction and rotation maneuvers, careful placement of retractors, and awareness of relevant surgical anatomy can minimize the risk of vascular injury. Despite appropriate preparation and technique, injury may still occur. Prompt recognition of the injury, control of bleeding, fluid replacement, vascular evaluation, and treatment can result in improved outcomes and limb salvage.

Bibliography

Adamson TE, Bunch WH, Baldwin DC Jr, Oppenberg A: The virtuous orthopaedist has fewer malpractice suits. *Clin Orthop Relat Res* 2000;378:104-109.

Baker AS, Bitounis VC: Abductor function after total hip replacement: An electromyographic and clinical review. *J Bone Joint Surg Br* 1989;71(1):47-50.

Barrack RL, Butler RA: Avoidance and management of neurovascular injuries in total hip arthroplasty. *Instr Course Lect* 2003;52:267-274.

Black DL, Reckling FW, Porter SS: Somatosensory-evoked potential monitored during total hip arthroplasty. *Clin Orthop Relat Res* 1991;262:170-177.

Calligaro KD, Dougherty MJ, Ryan S, Booth RE: Acute arterial complications associated with total hip and knee arthroplasty. *J Vasc Surg* 2003;38(6):1170-1177.

DeHart MM, Riley LH Jr: Nerve injuries in total hip arthroplasty. *J Am Acad Orthop Surg* 1999;7(2):101-111.

Goulding K, Beaulé PE, Kim PR, Fazekas A: Incidence of lateral femoral cutaneous nerve neuropraxia after anterior approach hip arthroplasty. *Clin Orthop Relat Res* 2010;468(9):2397-2404.

Hurd JL, Potter HG, Dua V, Ranawat CS: Sciatic nerve palsy after primary total hip arthroplasty: A new perspective. *J Arthroplasty* 2006;21(6):796-802.

Kenny P, O'Brien CP, Synnott K, Walsh MG: Damage to the superior gluteal nerve after two different approaches to the hip. *J Bone Joint Surg Br* 1999;81(6):979-981.

Kohan L, Field CJ, Kerr DR: Early complications of hip resurfacing. *J Arthroplasty* 2012;27(6):997-1002.

Kyriacou S, Pastides PS, Singh VK, Jeyaseelan L, Sinisi M, Fox M: Exploration and neurolysis for the treatment of neuropathic pain in patients with a sciatic nerve palsy after total hip replacement. *Bone Joint J* 2013;95-B(1):20-22.

Lavernia CJ, Cook CC, Hernandez RA, Sierra RJ, Rossi MD: Neurovascular injuries in acetabular reconstruction cage surgery: An anatomical study. *J Arthroplasty* 2007;22(1):124-132.

Lewallen DG: Neurovascular injury associated with hip arthroplasty. *Instr Course Lect* 1998;47:275-283.

Lundborg G: Structure and function of the intraneural microvessels as related to trauma, edema formation, and nerve function. *J Bone Joint Surg Am* 1975;57(7):938-948.

Montgomery AS, Birch R, Malone A: Sciatic neurostenalgia: Caused by total hip arthroplasty, cured by late neurolysis. *J Bone Joint Surg Br* 2005;87(3):410-411.

Navarro RA, Schmalzried TP, Amstutz HC, Dorey FJ: Surgical approach and nerve palsy in total hip arthroplasty. *J Arthroplasty* 1995;10(1):1-5.

Nercessian OA, Piccoluga F, Eftekhar NS: Postoperative sciatic and femoral nerve palsy with reference to leg lengthening and medialization/lateralization of the hip joint following total hip arthroplasty. *Clin Orthop Relat Res* 1994;304:165-171.

Nuwer MR, Schmalzried TP: Nerve palsy: Etiology, prognosis, and prevention, in Amstutz HC, ed: *Hip Arthroplasty.* New York, NY, Churchill Livingstone, 1991, pp 415-427.

Parvizi J, Pulido L, Slenker N, Macgibeny M, Purtill JJ, Rothman RH: Vascular injuries after total joint arthroplasty. *J Arthroplasty* 2008;23(8):1115-1121.

Pekkarinen J, Alho A, Puusa A, Paavilainen T: Recovery of sciatic nerve injuries in association with total hip arthroplasty in 27 patients. *J Arthroplasty* 1999;14(3):305-311.

Pritchett JW: Lumbar decompression to treat foot drop after hip arthroplasty. *Clin Orthop Relat Res* 1994;303:173-177.

Riouallon G, Zilber S, Allain J: Common femoral artery intimal injury following total hip replacement: A case report and literature review. *Orthop Traumatol Surg Res* 2009;95(2):154-158.

Satcher RL, Noss RS, Yingling CD, Ressler J, Ries M: The use of motor-evoked potentials to monitor sciatic nerve status during revision total hip arthroplasty. *J Arthroplasty* 2003;18(3):329-332.

Schmalzried TP, Amstutz HC, Dorey FJ: Nerve palsy associated with total hip replacement: Risk factors and prognosis. *J Bone Joint Surg Am* 1991;73(7):1074-1080.

Schmalzried TP, Neal WC, Eckardt JJ: Gluteal compartment and crush syndromes: Report of three cases and review of the literature. *Clin Orthop Relat Res* 1992;277:161-165.

Schmalzried TP, Noordin S, Amstutz HC: Update on nerve palsy associated with total hip replacement. *Clin Orthop Relat Res* 1997;344:188-206.

Sethuraman V, Hozack WJ, Sharkey PF, Rothman RH: Pseudoaneurysm of femoral artery after revision total hip arthroplasty with a constrained cup. *J Arthroplasty* 2000;15(4):531-534.

Shoenfeld NA, Stuchin SA, Pearl R, Haveson S: The management of vascular injuries associated with total hip arthroplasty. *J Vasc Surg* 1990;11(4):549-555.

Shubert D, Madoff S, Millillo R, Nandi S: Neurovascular structure proximity to acetabular retractors in total hip arthroplasty. *J Arthroplasty* 2015;30(1):145-148.

Solheim LF, Hagen R: Femoral and sciatic neuropathies after total hip arthroplasty. *Acta Orthop Scand* 1980;51(3):531-534.

Sunderland S: A classification of peripheral nerve injuries producing loss of function. *Brain* 1951;74(4):491-516.

Sutherland CJ, Miller DH, Owen JH: Use of spontaneous electromyography during revision and complex total hip arthroplasty. *J Arthroplasty* 1996;11(2):206-209.

Sutter M, Hersche O, Leunig M, Guggi T, Dvorak J, Eggspuehler A: Use of multimodal intra-operative monitoring in averting nerve injury during complex hip surgery. *J Bone Joint Surg Br* 2012;94(2):179-184.

Trousdale RT, Donnelly RS, Hallett JW: Thrombosis of an aortobifemoral bypass graft after total hip arthroplasty. *J Arthroplasty* 1999;14(3):386-390.

Uskova AA, Plakseychuk A, Chelly JE: The role of surgery in postoperative nerve injuries following total hip replacement. *J Clin Anesth* 2010;22(4):285-293.

Wasielewski RC, Cooperstein LA, Kruger MP, Rubash HE: Acetabular anatomy and the transacetabular fixation of screws in total hip arthroplasty. *J Bone Joint Surg Am* 1990;72(4):501-508.

Weale AE, Newman P, Ferguson IT, Bannister GC: Nerve injury after posterior and direct lateral approaches for hip replacement: A clinical and electrophysiological study. *J Bone Joint Surg Br* 1996;78(6):899-902.

Weber ER, Daube JR, Coventry MB: Peripheral neuropathies associated with total hip arthroplasty. *J Bone Joint Surg Am* 1976;58(1):66-69.

Wera GD, Ting NT, Della Valle CJ, Sporer SM: External iliac artery injury complicating prosthetic hip resection for infection. *J Arthroplasty* 2010;25(4):660.e1-660.e4.

Wolf M, Bäumer P, Pedro M, et al: Sciatic nerve injury related to hip replacement surgery: Imaging detection by MR neurography despite susceptibility artifacts. *PLoS One* 2014;9(2):e89154.

Zappe B, Glauser PM, Majewski M, Stöckli HR, Ochsner PE: Long-term prognosis of nerve palsy after total hip arthroplasty: Results of two-year-follow-ups and long-term results after a mean time of 8 years. *Arch Orthop Trauma Surg* 2014;134(10):1477-1482.

Chapter 37
Management of Periprosthetic Femoral Fractures

Nicholas J. Lash, MBChB, FRACS
Donald S. Garbuz, MD, FRCSC
Bassam A. Masri, MD, FRCSC
Clive P. Duncan, MD, MSc, FRCSC

Classification and Management

The Vancouver classification system has been validated in several studies and is the most widely used classification of periprosthetic fractures (**Figure 1**). Fracture types are classified according to the site of the fracture in relation to the prosthesis, implant stability, and available bone stock around the implant. The original Vancouver classification has been expanded in a recently published classification, the Unified Classification System, which describes additional fracture types.

Type A fractures are located within the trochanteric region of the femur. Lesser and greater trochanteric fractures are designated A_L and A_G, respectively. Type B fractures are located around the femoral stem or just distal to the tip of the femoral stem. Type C fractures occur well below the tip of the femoral stem.

Type A fractures can be considered stable or unstable but are not assigned a numeric qualifier. Stability of a type A fracture is defined by whether surgical fixation is deemed necessary. Type B1 designates a fracture around a well-fixed femoral stem, whereas types B2 and B3 designate fractures around loose stems or fractures that have caused loosening of the stem. Type C fractures are distant from the femoral implant and are by nature fractures with stable implants.

Type B fractures are subclassified on the basis of quality of bone stock. In type B1 and B2 fractures, the bone stock is adequate. Type B3 fractures are characterized by inadequate bone stock resulting from severe comminution, advanced osteoporosis, or extensive osteolysis, resulting in implant instability. Periprosthetic fractures around hip implants can be difficult to manage. Type A fractures require surgical management when they are displaced or cause pain. The authors of this chapter prefer to use trochanteric plating for the management of type A_G fractures and cerclage wiring for the management of type A_L fractures. Type B fractures often require surgical management. Type B1 fractures require plate fixation. The authors of this chapter recommend locking plates with either open reduction or minimally invasive techniques, depending on the fracture pattern. The authors of this chapter no longer routinely use strut allografts. Type B2 fractures require implantation of a revision stem. Modern tapered, fluted titanium stems are reliable and are the chapter authors' preference. Historically, type B3 fractures in physiologically young patients were managed with allograft-prosthetic composites (APCs). Currently, type B3 fractures are often managed with tapered titanium stems, and the authors of this chapter add allograft struts as necessary. If the femur is unreconstructable in elderly patients, the authors of this chapter use proximal femoral replacement. Type C fractures are considered femoral fractures, and the authors of this chapter advise plating them with minimally invasive techniques and the use of a lateral locked plate.

Dr. Garbuz or an immediate family member serves as a paid consultant to or is an employee of Zimmer Biomet; has received research or institutional support from DePuy Synthes and Zimmer Biomet; and serves as a board member, owner, officer, or committee member of the M. E. Müller Foundation of North America. Dr. Masri or an immediate family member serves as a board member, owner, officer, or committee member of the Canadian Orthopaedic Association. Dr. Duncan or an immediate family member is a member of a speakers' bureau or has made paid presentations on behalf of Zimmer Biomet. Neither Dr. Lash nor any immediate family member has received anything of value from or has stock or stock options held in a commercial company or institution related directly or indirectly to the subject of this chapter.

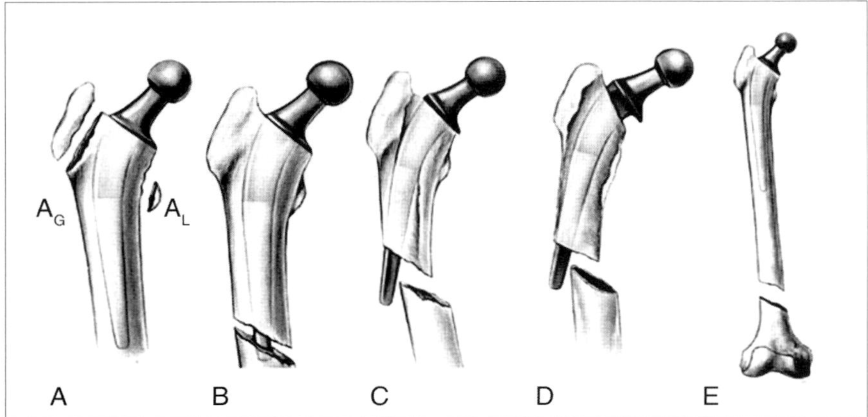

Figure 1 Illustrations depict the Vancouver classification of periprosthetic femoral fractures. **A,** Type A, trochanteric fracture involving the greater trochanter (A_G) or lesser trochanter (A_L). **B** through **D,** Type B, diaphyseal fracture at the level of or just distal to the implant. **B,** Type B1 fractures are characterized by a stable implant. **C,** Type B2 fractures are associated with a loose implant and adequate bone stock. **D,** Type B3 fractures have a loose implant with inadequate bone stock. **E,** Type C, diaphyseal fracture well distal to the tip of the implant. (Adapted from Archibeck MJ, Rosenberg AG, Berger RA, Silverton CD: Trochanteric osteotomy and fixation during total hip arthroplasty. *J Am Acad Orthop Surg* 2003;11[3]:163-173.)

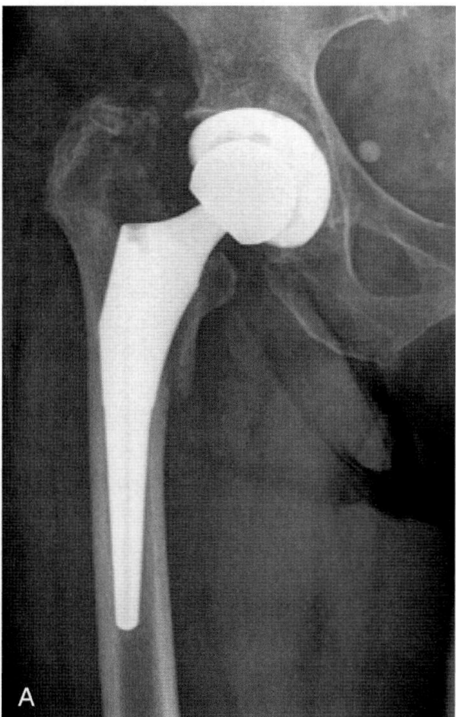

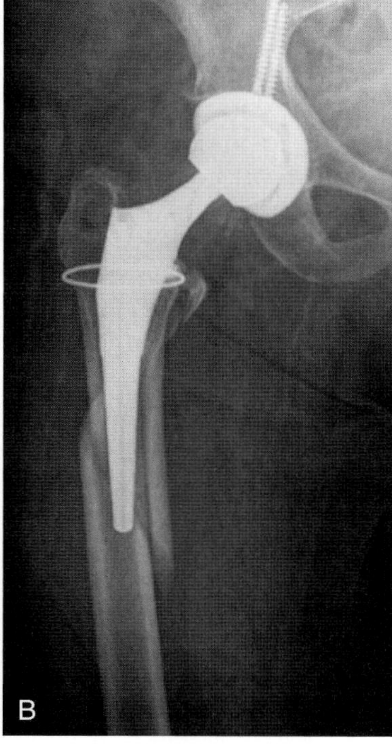

Figure 2 **A,** AP radiograph of a right hip demonstrates an apparent Vancouver type A_L fracture that on further investigation was identified as a type B2 fracture around a noncemented femoral stem. **B,** AP radiograph of a right hip from a different patient demonstrates displacement of an unrecognized B2 fracture on weight bearing. Initial fixation was performed with a single cerclage cable.

Type A_L Fractures

Type A_L fractures make up a small proportion of periprosthetic femoral fractures. They rarely occur in isolation and usually occur in conjunction with type B2 or B3 fractures. True type A_L fractures can be associated with osteolytic lesions in the medial calcar region and can occur with an avulsion fracture resulting from the pull of the psoas muscle. They tend to be associated with osteolysis, requiring attention to the underlying cause of the osteolysis. In patients with good bone quality, the surgeon must take care to ensure that a fracture of type B2 is not missed. Fracture patterns that involve the medial cortex of the femur can appear to involve the lesser trochanter, whereas the extension of the fracture can be underappreciated and a type B2 fracture can exist (**Figure 2**). This scenario is particularly common in patients with tapered, wedge-shaped noncemented stems.

Indications

When a true A_L fracture occurs early in the postoperative period, the possibility of a loose femoral stem should be considered. If preoperative investigation indicates instability of the stem, the fracture is by definition type B2 and requires surgical management. If a true A_L fracture exists and the patient is symptomatic, surgical management is warranted.

Contraindications

An A_L fracture that is an avulsion fracture, usually in the presence of osteolysis, can be managed nonsurgically, provided that the femoral stem is not loose.

Alternative Treatments

Nonsurgical treatment is indicated for most patients with true A_L fractures. A period of protected weight bearing with crutches and analgesia is recommended. Monitoring of the fracture with serial radiographs is critical to ensure detection of any extension of the fracture or the presence of a type B2 fracture. Alternative surgical treatments include revision of metaphyseal-loading femoral stems to diaphyseal-loading stems, calcar-replacement prostheses, and proximal femoral replacement devices. However, if these options are being considered, then the supposed type A_L fracture is likely a type B2 fracture.

Techniques

SETUP/EXPOSURE

- A cerclage wire or cable fixation technique is used for the surgical management of type A_L fractures.
- Lateral positioning is sufficient in most patients and is familiar to most hip surgeons.
- Exposure can be performed using the previous surgical approach, which in most patients is an anterolateral, lateral, or posterior approach.
- The lesser trochanter is identified through the previous approach, with attention paid to relevant neurovascular anatomy.

INSTRUMENTS/EQUIPMENT/IMPLANTS REQUIRED

- Large reduction forceps, wires or cables, a wire or cable passer, and a wire cutter are necessary.
- A drill is used.

PROCEDURE

- Bone grafting of osteolytic defects is performed before reduction of the fracture if the bone stock is deemed to be insufficient.
- Reduction of the lesser trochanter is performed in an open manner to ensure that it is brought back to its original location adjacent to the femoral prosthesis.
- The lesser trochanter is secured with the use of smooth 16- to 18-gauge stainless-steel surgical wire, Luque wires, or braided stainless-steel surgical cables.
- The wire or cables can be used to effect the reduction if placed accurately around the fragment.
- Otherwise, large reduction forceps can be used to clamp the lesser trochanter, reducing it back to the femoral stem and native femoral bone.
- The wire-passing device is passed from posterior to anterior to avoid passing the wire or cable around the sciatic nerve.
- Careful opening of the lateral intermuscular septum at its insertion to the linea aspera will help the surgeon identify perforating branches of the profunda femoris artery.
- The wire passer is manipulated through the intermuscular septum at its attachment to the linea aspera. This step is facilitated by blunt or sharp perforation of the septum.
- The wire passer is kept closely apposed to the posterior femur to avoid entrapping the sciatic nerve and other tissues under the wire or cable.
- The wire or cable is passed and retrieved as it appears in the anterior vastus lateralis muscle fibers.
- If the fragment is large, the use of two wires or cables is recommended. One is placed proximal to the lesser trochanter to resist the pull of the psoas muscle, and one is placed distal to or through the lesser trochanter (through an appropriately sized drill hole).
- The wires or cables are tightened, with the cut ends placed posteriorly to avoid irritation of soft tissues.

WOUND CLOSURE

- The wound is closed in standard manner with No. 1 or No. 2 absorbable sutures for the fascia and 2-0 absorbable sutures for the subcutaneous tissues and skin (to provide a good surface area for the staples), according to the surgeon's preferred method.
- The authors of this chapter do not use drains. A highly absorbent all-in-one foam dressing with a waterproof membrane is used.

Postoperative Regimen

The patient is allowed to bear weight with crutches for protection. Active hip flexion exercises and straight leg raises should be avoided for the first 6 weeks postoperatively.

Avoiding Pitfalls and Complications

Placement of a wire or cable through the lesser trochanter resists proximal migration from the pull of the psoas muscle. Passage of the wire or cable from posterior to anterior protects the sciatic nerve. Ligation of the perforating arteries at the intermuscular septum will reduce hemorrhage.

Type A_G Fractures

Fractures of the greater trochanter can occur intraoperatively during implant removal, during transposition of the femur for access, as a result of errant retractor placement, during femoral bone preparation, and on insertion of trial or final femoral implants in an underprepared or insufficiently cleared proximal femur. Postoperative fractures typically occur as a result of a traumatic fall but can occur with minimal trauma in patients with osteolysis.

Indications

Surgical management of a type A_G fracture is indicated when the fracture is detected intraoperatively, even if nondisplaced, to prevent further displacement on mobilization. This requirement is largely because the surgical exposure around the trochanter can render it less stable than it would be after a postoperative fracture, in which the soft-tissue envelope can impart stability to the fracture. For this reason, fractures sustained well into the postoperative period may not displace substantially. However, if the displacement is greater than 1 cm, fixation is indicated to avoid lateral hip pain, nonunion, abductor dysfunction, limp, or instability of an underlying total hip arthroplasty (THA).

Contraindications

Extreme osteolysis with insufficient bone stock to allow union of the fracture is a relative contraindication. Some surgeons have reported the use of bone grafting to achieve union.

Alternative Treatments

Nondisplaced fractures can be managed with protected weight bearing with crutches and avoidance of active abduction for 10 to 12 weeks. The patient should be monitored radiographically for trochanteric escape. If trochanteric escape is detected, intervention is required. Nonsurgical management of displaced fractures can be considered if symptoms are minimal or well tolerated. Fixation with 14-gauge wire is an alternative to the cable-plate fixation method recommended by the authors of this chapter. If wires are used, they are placed from anterior to posterior through the bone of the trochanteric fragment. The wires are secured distally to a cerclage wire to resist the pull of the abductors. The trochanteric fragment is compressed into its bone bed by wires placed from lateral to medial, distal to the lesser trochanter, again to resist the pull of the abductors. Very small bone fragments that cannot be secured with plates or wires can be excised and the remaining abductor tendon sutured to the bone bed at which the fragment originated.

Results

Results of surgical management of type A_G fractures are reported in **Table 1**. The few relevant studies that exist report greater than 90% rates of union of acute fracture. In patients in whom concurrent osteolytic defects are present, simultaneous fixation and bone grafting also results in high rates of union. With high union rates, patient-reported outcomes similarly improve greatly.

Techniques

- The authors of this chapter recommend cable-plate fixation of type A_G fractures.
- The cable plate fixation technique requires open reduction of the fragment. The fracture is secured with a premade trochanteric plate with claw fixation into the proximal fragment and distal fixation to the femoral shaft. The aim is to secure the fragment to its original location and resist the pull of the abductor musculature. The design of the plate facilitates the passage of cables and allows both proximal and distal fixation.

SETUP/EXPOSURE

- Lateral positioning is sufficient in most patients and is familiar to most hip surgeons.
- Exposure can be performed using the previous approach, which in most patients is an anterolateral, lateral, or posterior approach.
- Extensile exposure from the tip of the trochanter to the vastus lateralis musculature may be required.
- Hip abduction on a covered Mayo table may aid reduction.
- Access to the posterior aspect of the femur is obtained with elevation of the vastus lateralis muscle. The cable plate can be tunneled in a submuscular manner without complete elevation of the vastus.

INSTRUMENTS/EQUIPMENT/ IMPLANTS REQUIRED

- A cable-plate device, large reduction forceps, a cable passer, cables, a tensioner, and a wire cutter are necessary.
- A crimping compressor may be needed.

PROCEDURE

- The greater trochanteric fragment is examined for reduction. If it is reduced, then it is secured in situ.
- If the fracture remains displaced, reduction is performed with large reduction forceps placed proximally at the tip and distally on the femoral metaphysis.
- Substantial osteolysis can be grafted with autograft or allograft particulate cancellous bone graft. Curettage of polyethylene disease and firm packing of the bone graft are performed. Containment of the graft in the osteolytic defect can be challenging.
- The epimysium of the vastus lateralis is opened, and the cable plate is tunneled under the muscle distally.
- The plate is progressively moved down the femur until the proximal claw becomes engaged in the trochanteric fragment.
- Posterior dissection is performed at the level of the lesser trochanter through the lateral intermuscular septum to allow passage of the cable.
- The cable is passed through the prefashioned holes in the plate, around the femur distal to the lesser trochanter, and anteriorly back to the plate, completing a full cerclage of the femur.
- Distal fixation of the plate is performed, either with bicortical screw fixation or with a second cable passed in the same fashion as the first.
- Cables are tensioned, secured via crimping or grub interference screw fixation, and cut short.
- The hip is moved through a gentle range of motion to ensure that the trochanteric fragment does not have undue mobility, which may indicate inadequate tensioning of

Table 1 Results of Management of Periprosthetic Femoral Fracture

Authors (Year)	Fracture Type	Number	Procedure or Approach	Mean Patient Age in Years (Range)	Mean Follow-up (Range)	Results
Wang et al (2006)	A_G	19 patients	Morselized bone allograft and wire fixation	NR	3.8 yr (0-8 yr)	Mean HHS improved from 32.5 to 91.2 Union rate, 95%
Zarin et al (2009)	A_G	31 patients (8 periprosthetic fractures, 7 trochanteric osteotomies, 16 nonunions of fracture of the greater trochanters)	Trochanteric claw plate	68 (45-86)	2.2 yr (0.5-5.9 yr)	Median HHS improved from 47 to 92 ($P < 0.0001$) No patient had a Trendelenburg sign postoperatively 24 patients were pain free postoperatively and 7 patients had mild pain It is unknown whether the 3 patients whose fracture failed to achieve union were in the acute fracture or osteotomy/past nonunion group Union rate, 90%
Siegmeth et al (1998)	B1	42 fractures	ORIF with plate fixation	69 (NR)	36 mo (NR)	10% failure rate, with loosening in 3 fractures and varus failure in 1 fracture Union rate, 90%
Buttaro et al (2007)	B1	14 patients	ORIF with locking plate, with or without strut allograft	68 (34-88)	20 mo (10-30 mo)	8 fractures united at a mean follow-up of 5.4 mo 5 of the 6 fractures that did not unite were not managed with strut allograft Union rate, 57%
Chakravarthy et al (2007)	B1 or C	12 patients (6 type B1, 6 type C)	ORIF with a locking plate	84 (72-86)	14 mo (12-18 mo)	Mean time to union was 4.8 mo 2 failures occurred: 1 before union and 1 after Union rate, 83%
Bryant et al (2009)	B1	10 patients	ORIF with a locking plate	77 (60-89)	27 wk (14-97 wk)	Fractures united in all patients by a mean follow-up of 17 wk Union rate, 100%
Jukkala-Partio et al (1998)	B1, B2, or B3	75 fractures	Revision stem (40), ORIF with plate fixation (35)	NR	20 mo[a] (12-96 mo)	In the revision stem group, there were 5 nonunions and 15 additional reoperations for other reasons In the ORIF group with plate fixation, there were 9 nonunions and 18 additional reoperations for other reasons When revision surgery was performed, high union rates were achieved, with 98% and 97% of fractures uniting for revision femoral stem and revision fixation, respectively Initial union rate for fractures requiring revision arthroplasty, 88% Initial union rate for fractures requiring fixation/ORIF, 74%

HHS = Harris Hip score, NR = not reported, ORIF = open reduction and internal fixation, WOMAC = Western Ontario and McMaster Universities Osteoarthritis Index.
[a] Median value.

Table 1 Results of Management of Periprosthetic Femoral Fracture (*continued*)

Authors (Year)	Fracture Type	Number	Procedure or Approach	Mean Patient Age in Years (Range)	Mean Follow-up (Range)	Results
Lewallen and Berry (1998)	B2 or B3	97 fractures	Cemented, proximally porous-coated noncemented, or extensively porous-coated noncemented	NR	5 yr (2-14 yr)	85% rate of fracture union Stable fixation of revision femoral stem was achieved in 50% of revision cases 33% of hips had a loose femoral stem with pain Union rate with a well-fixed stem, 50%
Springer et al (2003)	B2 or B3	118 hips	Cemented (42), noncemented (58), or allograft-prosthesis composite (18)	65 (37-91)	65 mo (2-185 mo)	Fully porous-coated noncemented femoral stems had the highest survivorship rate of all revision types (77% at a mean follow-up of 42 mo) Revision-free survivorship of 90% at 5 yr, 80% at 10 yr, and 58% at 15 yr
Tsiridis et al (2004)	B2 and B3	106 patients	Cemented revisions with impaction grafting (89), cemented revisions without impaction grafting (17)	68 (39-91)	NR	Union was achieved in 66 of 75 fractures managed with long-stem revision and impaction grafting and in 8 of 14 fractures managed with a short-stem prosthesis and impaction grafting (88% and 57%, respectively; odds ratio, 5.5; $P = 0.009$) Union was achieved in 74 of the 89 fractures treated with impaction grafting and in 11 of the 17 fractures treated only with cemented revision (83% and 64%, respectively; odds ratio, 2.7; $P = 0.09$) Overall union rate, 80%
Corten et al (2012)	B2	31 patients	Long cemented	82 (56-93)	33 mo (0-132 mo)	Survival rate based on the 16 patients who survived and were available for follow-up 2 patients experienced pain-free nonunion Mean HHS, 77.5 Diaphyseal union achieved in all patients
Neumann et al (2012)	B2 or B3	55 patients	Fluted tapered modular stem (curved)	74 (45-84)	67 mo (60-144 mo)	53 hips available for follow-up Mean HHS, 72 100% union rate 2 hips were revised for painful subsidence of >5 mm Chronic infection developed in 1 hip Revision-free survivorship rate, 96%
Abdel et al (2014)	B2 or B3	44 patients (25 B2, 19 B3)	Fluted tapered modular stem, with additional strut allograft used in 18 patients	72 (34-92)	4.5 yr (2-8 yr)	1 patient experienced aseptic loosening 1 patient experienced stem subsidence >5 mm 11% dislocation rate Mean HHS, 83 Revision-free survivorship rate, 98%

HHS = Harris Hip score, NR = not reported, ORIF = open reduction and internal fixation, WOMAC = Western Ontario and McMaster Universities Osteoarthritis Index.
[a] Median value.

Table 1 Results of Management of Periprosthetic Femoral Fracture (*continued*)

Authors (Year)	Fracture Type	Number	Procedure or Approach	Mean Patient Age in Years (Range)	Mean Follow-up (Range)	Results
Munro et al (2014)	B2 or B3	47 patients	Fluted tapered modular stem	72 (44-93)	54 mo (24-143 mo)	1 patient was lost to follow-up 1 nonunion occurred, and 2 patients experienced subsidence of >10 mm Bone stock was maintained or improved in 89% of patients Mean WOMAC, 76 Revision-free survivorship, 96%
Klein et al (2005)	B3	21 patients	Proximal femoral replacement	78.3 (52-90)	3.2 yr (2-7 yr)	Mean HHS, 71 Dislocation occurred in 2 patients: 1 dislocation was managed nonsurgically and 1 required a constrained acetabular device 1 patient experienced acetabular loosening and underwent resection arthroplasty Revision-free survivorship at last follow-up, 90%
Maury et al (2006)	B3	24 patients (25 fractures)	Allograft prosthetic composite	70.2 (60-81)	5.1 yr (2-12.7 yr)	Mean HHS, 70.8 Nonunion at the host bone–allograft junction occurred in 4 hips (16%) Loosening >3 mm occurred in 3 hips (12%) 21 patients experienced little or no pain postoperatively Union rate at host bone–allograft junction, 84%

HHS = Harris Hip score, NR = not reported, ORIF = open reduction and internal fixation, WOMAC = Western Ontario and McMaster Universities Osteoarthritis Index.
[a] Median value.

the cables. Inadequate tensioning can result in fragment escape. Excessive mobility also can result in fibrous nonunion.

WOUND CLOSURE

- The wound is closed in a standard manner, following the same protocol as for type A_L fractures.

Postoperative Regimen

Postoperative management includes partial weight bearing with crutches and no active abduction for 3 months. The authors of this chapter do not routinely use a hip abduction orthosis. However, an orthosis can be used as an extra precaution. Although trochanteric plates have an excellent ability to control fracture reduction, they are bulkier than wire fixation. Soft-tissue irritation can occur around the lateral hip, which requires plate removal after fracture union is achieved.

Avoiding Pitfalls and Complications

Ensuring adequate fixation of the greater trochanteric fragment is important. Creating two small incisions in the abductor tendon will allow the claw aspect of the plate to obtain better purchase in the bone. If these incisions are not made, the thick abductor tendon can hold the claw off the bone. The passage of the first cable distal to or through the lesser trochanter resists the vector force of the abductor muscles. Avoiding anterior and superior placement of the fragment will help avoid host bone-on-bone impingement that could result in instability of the hip. Passage of the cables from posterior to anterior prevents the sciatic nerve from becoming entrapped under the cable. If osteolytic defects are grafted, care must be taken during impaction of the morcellized graft. Containing the graft can be challenging, and care should be taken to avoid debris around the joint space. When osteolysis exists, substantial polyethylene wear may be present, in which case liner exchange is required. If radiographs suggest extensive osteolysis, full revision should be considered.

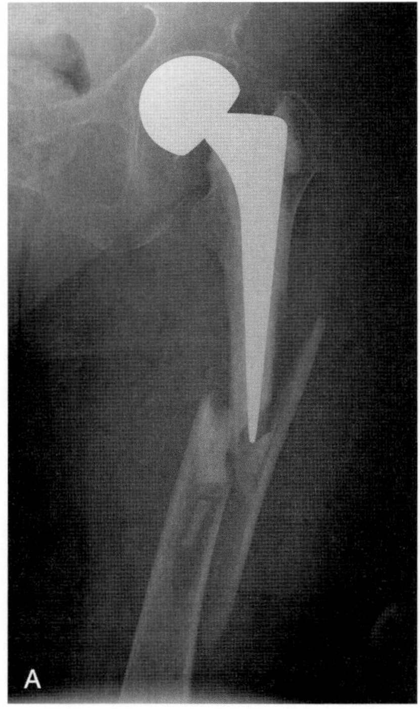

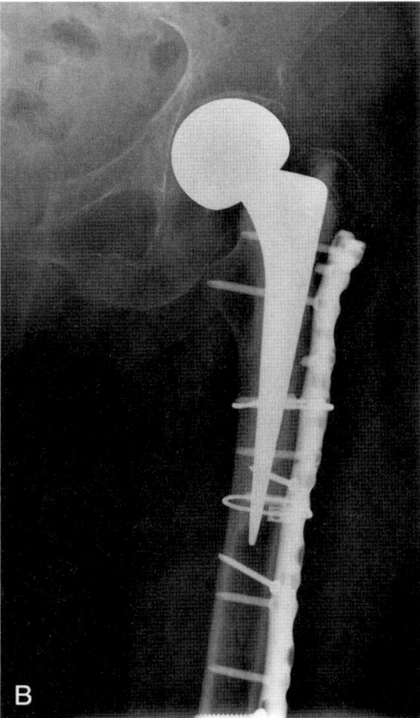

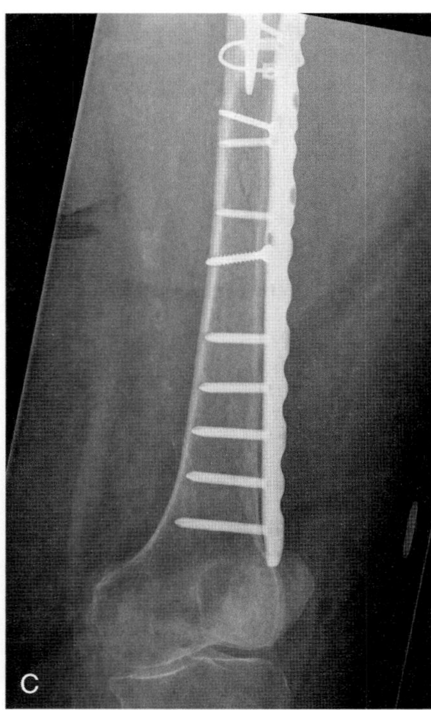

Figure 3 **A,** AP radiograph of a left hip demonstrates a Vancouver type B1 fracture around a well-fixed cemented hemiarthroplasty. Postoperative AP hip (**B**) and AP femoral (**C**) radiographs of the same patient demonstrate fixation with a long polyaxial locking plate.

In patients with fracture displacement or hardware failure, fibrous union can still be achieved; therefore, a period of observation may be indicated.

Type B1 Fractures

By definition, type B1 fractures occur around a well-fixed, stable femoral implant (**Figure 3, A**). In most patients, open reduction and internal fixation (ORIF) is required (**Figure 3, B** and **C**). The surgeon must be prepared for all eventualities. If the fracture has been misdiagnosed and an unstable femoral implant exists, a different approach to reconstruction will be required. Preoperative planning must include preparation for placement of a new femoral stem. As in any hip reconstruction, if the femoral prosthesis is changed, the surgeon also must be prepared to revise the acetabular implants. Internal fixation with plates or cortical allograft strut has been the mainstay of fixation of type B1 fractures. Regardless of whether a plate or allograft strut is used, the reduction and fixation is performed with cerclage wires and screw fixation where appropriate.

Indications

The indication for ORIF of a type B1 fracture is a displaced fracture around a femoral stem that requires additional bone support to allow patient mobility and prevent cantilever stress that may result in premature failure or loosening of the prosthesis. The type of femoral prosthesis should be considered. Diaphyseal press-fit stems that have substantial ingrowth distal to the fracture may be able to withstand axial forces, thereby allowing consideration of nonsurgical management. Femoral stems with predominantly metaphyseal fixation may have little fixation remaining around the fracture fragments; therefore, nonsurgical management would carry the risk of implant loosening or further displacement of the fracture.

The authors of this chapter prefer to perform ORIF with locking plates in patients with type B1 fractures. Cortical strut allografts are reserved for patients who have diminished bone stock that can be addressed with allograft. Careful soft-tissue dissection is necessary to keep the fracture fragments viable and allow fracture union. Knowledge of the existing implants is necessary in case revision of one or more implants is required.

Contraindications

Contraindications to fixation of type B1 fractures are few. Displaced fractures often require fixation to allow stabilization and early mobility. Nondisplaced fractures can be managed with protected weight bearing and close monitoring of the fracture with radiographs.

Alternative Treatments

Nonsurgical treatments include mobilization with protected weight bearing; traction techniques; and the use of a cast brace, hip spica cast, or orthosis. Protected weight bearing is useful for nondisplaced fractures. A cast brace, hip spica cast, or orthosis can be used by patients who cannot undergo the physiologic stress of surgical treatment. Hip spica casts and orthoses are cumbersome, make hygiene care difficult, require increased assistance for transfers, and limit the patient's mobility. With these techniques, controlling the fracture, obtaining reasonable alignment, and achieving fracture union can be challenging. Traction techniques carry risks and introduce the comorbidities of prolonged bed rest.

Results

Results of surgical management of type B1 fractures are reported in **Table 1**. Type B1 fractures require fixation. Because of the inherent stability of the femoral stem, the procedure is performed to achieve fracture union. As a result, union rates rather than survivorship of the prosthesis are commonly reported. Supplemental bone grafting may or may not be used, and type of fixation device varies. In general, reported union rates range from 50% to 100%. Some authors recommend the use of allograft struts to enhance union; however, with the use of newer locked plate designs, other authors recommend the use of locked plates alone, which are associated with high rates of union.

Video 37.1 Periprosthetic Fracture Fixation with Cable Plate and Strut Allograft. Aaron Nauth, MD; Patrick Henry, MD; Emil H. Schemitsch, MD (7 min)

Techniques

SETUP/EXPOSURE

- The patient is placed in the lateral decubitus position.
- Stability of the patient on the table is necessary.
- The pelvis should be oriented at a right angle to the flat surface of the surgical table. This position will be necessary if revision of the acetabular implant is needed.
- Previous skin incisions are used unless the location is not compatible with lateral exposure of the femur. Most previous hip incisions are extensile down the length of the femur.
- After the fascia lata is incised, deep dissection exposes the epimysium of the vastus lateralis muscle.
- The epimysium is split longitudinally, and the fracture fragments are carefully palpated.
- In many patients, the fracture will spiral around the femoral prosthesis, with the fracture line located medially toward the lesser trochanter.
- Evacuation of hematoma and fibrous material is performed.
- The muscle fibers of the vastus lateralis are gently elevated from the fracture margins to allow visualization of the fracture for accurate reduction.

INSTRUMENTS/EQUIPMENT/IMPLANTS REQUIRED

- The procedure requires 4.5-mm large fragment locking compression plates and a cable set including cable passer, tensioner, and wire cutter.
- Reduction forceps, including pointed and Verbrugge clamps, are needed.
- Trochanteric cable-plate devices should be available.
- Femoral stem revision sets should be available.
- A high-speed burr and oscillating saw may be necessary for osteotomy of the femur if revision of the femoral implant is required.

PROCEDURE

- The fracture fragments are mobilized apart from each other with a Cobb elevator to allow inspection of the femoral prosthesis.
- A clamp is placed on the exposed femoral prosthesis, and a proximal distraction force is applied to test axial stability and fixation.
- Alternatively, the distal femur can be pulled distally for assessment. If the prosthesis can be telescoped in and out of the intact distal femur, or if bubbles are present in the hematoma surrounding the interface of the femoral implant and femoral bone, then the implant is loose and femoral revision is required. Sometimes the movement of the femoral implant in and out of the intact distal femur produces an audible sucking noise.
- If the femoral implant is stable and the prosthesis has no articulation problems, opening of the joint with an arthrotomy is not required.
- The fracture fragments are reduced with large reduction forceps. Hematoma or bone comminution may obstruct this maneuver and should be inspected for if accurate reduction is not achieved.
- After reduction is achieved, a plate of sufficient length is placed. The plate should span the fracture, and a longer rather than shorter working length is recommended. Type B1 fractures do not extend past the tip of the prosthesis; therefore, adequate bone will be present down to the flare of the distal metaphysis unless the femoral stem is a long revision-type stem.
- If the femoral stem is long and the distal intact bone is metaphyseal, the use of a precontoured distal femoral condylar plate is recommended. The metaphysis flares from a relatively flat lateral femur to a curved surface proximally at the trochanteric ridge. Proximal contouring of the plate to match the metaphyseal flare of the proximal femur will allow

better apposition of the plate to the femur.

- Fixation of the plate to the femur at the tip of the stem and more distally can be performed with screw fixation in a unicortical or bicortical manner. The authors of this chapter recommend bicortical screw fixation and standard cortical screws because they can be angled around the tip of the femoral stem.
- Locking screws can be used but cannot be angled around the prosthesis in most plate types. Newer plate designs have variable-axis locking technology that allows the surgeon to place locking screws at an angle.
- Some surgeons have suggested that locking screws can create a construct that is too stiff to allow callus formation. The most appropriate screw type to maximize fracture union continues to be debated.
- The authors of this chapter recommend the use of a near-far strategy for the insertion of screws into the plate. Screws are placed close to the fracture and farther away at the extent of the plate to allow flexibility in the construct. Filling every hole in the plate with screws can create excessive stiffness, which can inhibit callus formation.
- Proximal fixation often requires the use of cables. Cables are passed as described for type A_L and A_G fractures from posterior to anterior through a perforation in the lateral intermuscular septum at the linea aspera. The cables are secured to the plate through small capture devices that are placed or screwed into the plate.
- Alternatively, if bone stock is sufficient, screws can be angled around the femoral stem if the prosthesis does not completely fill the canal.
- Some manufacturers have additional periprosthetic plates that can be attached to the main fixation plate. These plates allow the placement of fixed-angle locking screws around the femoral stem into the cortical bone on either side of the prosthesis.
- A strut allograft is not routinely used. However, if the patient has discrete areas of bone deficiency that may result in failure of the femoral stem, a strut allograft can be added to the femoral fixation.
- Because the plate is located on the lateral surface of the femur, the strut allograft usually is placed on the anterior surface. The anterior quadriceps muscle is elevated partially, not completely to the periosteum. Ideally, a small amount of muscle fibers remains on the femoral bone to encourage incorporation of the strut allograft.
- The strut allograft is placed before any cables are applied proximally. Additional cables are required to secure the graft. Typically, the graft is approximately 200 mm long, and four or five cables are required for adequate fixation.

WOUND CLOSURE

- The wound is closed in the same manner as for the previously discussed fractures mentioned.
- Accurate closure of the vastus lateralis epimysium and fascia lata as separate layers is necessary to maintain mobility of the soft tissues and to prevent wound drainage.

Postoperative Regimen

Toe-touch weight bearing is maintained for a minimum of 6 weeks postoperatively. Radiographs are obtained after the procedure and at 6 weeks postoperatively to monitor fracture healing. The authors of this chapter do not routinely use an abduction orthosis; however, it may be considered if the greater trochanter is substantially involved in the fracture pattern. In such patients, limitation of active abduction of the hip for 6 to 12 weeks postoperatively may be necessary to protect the trochanter.

Avoiding Pitfalls and Complications

A major pitfall is misdiagnosing a fracture as type B1 and discovering intraoperatively that the femoral prosthesis is loose. Having the necessary equipment when beginning the procedure as well as the necessary surgical expertise to perform revision arthroplasty is essential. Careful soft-tissue handling is required to maximize the chance of achieving fracture union. Excessive periosteal elevation is discouraged, and periosteal elevation should be limited to the fracture margin for visualization of fracture reduction. Additionally, if a cortical strut graft is used, careful elevation of muscle only, not the periosteum, will aid in graft incorporation.

Type B2 Fractures

Indications

Because type B2 fractures involve a displaced and loose femoral stem (**Figure 4**), surgical management of these injuries is almost always indicated. The procedure requires revision of the femoral prosthesis and therefore is considered a revision hip arthroplasty.

The authors of this chapter prefer to use long tapered, fluted titanium stems for femoral revision in patients with type B2 fractures because of familiarity, good reported outcomes, and the suggestion in some studies that these stems can preserve and occasionally increase proximal femoral bone stock. Although these stems are available with proximal body modularity, the authors of this chapter now use nonmodular varieties because of the ease of insertion and the need for less assembly. The issues of proximal body fretting and fracture of modular stems are less common than previously reported but remain possible.

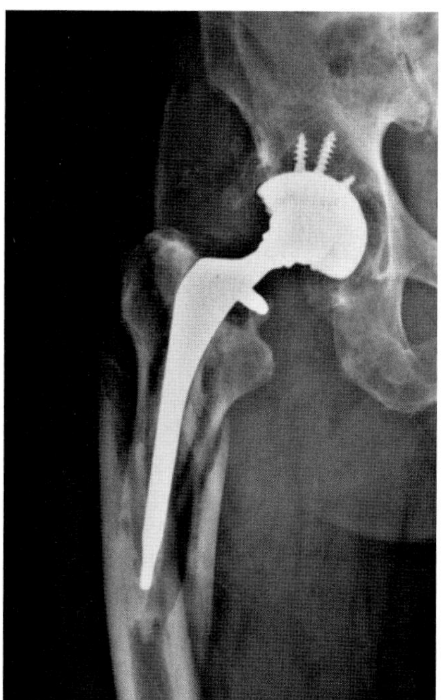

Figure 4 AP radiograph of a right hip demonstrates a Vancouver type B2 fracture around a cemented femoral stem.

Preparation for potential acetabular revision is mandatory. Therefore, thorough knowledge of the existing implants is critical. The ability to change acetabular liners, increase head diameter and offset, or adjust the constraint may be necessary to achieve a stable reconstruction.

Regardless of the technique used for femoral preparation, the authors of this chapter prefer to use large femoral heads (36 to 40 mm) with liner exchange to accommodate these sizes, when possible. Strut allografts are not routinely used; however, in patients who have poor bone stock in isolated areas, a strut can be added to increase bone stock and enhance fracture stability. Additional soft-tissue exposure is required, and devitalization of the fracture fragments should be avoided. This scenario occurs more often in patients with type B3 fractures than in patients with type B2 fractures.

Contraindications

Because a loose femoral stem requires revision surgery, sterile conditions are required. Active infection around a femoral stem is an absolute contraindication for revision directly to a new femoral prosthesis. In such patients, staged procedures with antibiotic-loaded prostheses are required, and formal revision can be performed only when the infection is brought under control.

If inspection of the distal bone quality reveals that the distal diaphyseal segment is too short (that is, the fracture extends beyond the isthmus of the femur), sufficient bone may not be available for a noncemented stem reconstruction. The literature on revision THA recommends 4 cm of diaphyseal bone for fixation of a noncemented stem. This recommendation applies to cylindric coated stems, and its validity with tapered fluted stems has not been established. If sufficient bone stock is not present, cemented stems may offer a better solution. However, to allow cemented revision, stable reconstruction of the fracture must first be achieved, usually with multiple cables. If the femur cannot be reconstructed because of bone deficiency or excessive comminution, cemented revision also is contraindicated.

Alternative Treatments

Because surgical treatment is almost always necessary, alternative treatments revolve around the options for reconstruction. The authors of this chapter prefer noncemented tapered, fluted titanium stems; however, options include cylindric porous-coated stems and long cemented stems. The potential benefits of cylindric porous-coated stems are familiarity and stiffness. Stress shielding is a potential issue with these designs, and some motion in the fracture segments can promote callus formation. The benefit of revision with a cemented stem is immediate weight bearing. However, as noted, reconstruction of the cylindric geometry of the femur is necessary to allow appropriate cementation and insertion. The use of impaction bone grafting with long-stem cemented revision for type B2 and B3 fractures has been reported, although this technique is not commonly used in North America.

Results

Results of surgical management of type B2 fractures are reported in **Table 1**. Most studies report outcomes of revision-free survivorship, but fracture union usually is reported as well. Patient functional outcomes are increasingly reported. Initial studies reported relatively low rates of union and revision-free survivorship (50%). However, more recent studies have reported acceptable results after long-stem cemented revision with impaction grafting and long, noncemented porous-coated or tapered fluted stems. Union rates of greater than 90% and high survivorship rates have been reported with all these treatment options.

Techniques

SETUP/EXPOSURE

- The patient is prepped and draped from the rib cage to the ankle.
- Patient stability on the surgical table is necessary.
- The pelvis is oriented at a right angle to the flat surface of the surgical table. This position is necessary if revision of the acetabular implant is required.
- A padded Mayo table is useful as an assistive device on which to rest the affected leg.
- Management of perioperative blood loss is important. A cell saver is useful to minimize the need for allogeneic blood transfusions.
- Exposure is performed using the previous incision if it is compatible with the proposed approach.
- The authors of this chapter prefer the posterior approach to the hip for revision because it allows

extensile exposure of the femur and acetabulum.

- Anterolateral and direct lateral approaches can be used as alternatives.
- The skin and fascia are incised at a point centered over the greater trochanter. The gluteus maximus muscle is split toward the posterior superior iliac spine.
- The fascia is split down the femur to 10 cm beyond the extent of the fracture.
- Because removal of the femoral stem is planned, arthrotomy is required.
- The posterior border of the gluteus medius muscle is identified and retracted superolaterally to allow identification of the piriformis tendon passing from the greater sciatic notch to its insertion on the tip of the greater trochanter.
- Proximal to the piriformis tendon, the gluteus minimus muscle is elevated off the outer ilium with a Cobb elevator.
- The piriformis and short external rotators are dissected off the posterior proximal femur together with the underlying capsule as a composite flap, which is tagged with a suture for later repair.
- After the capsule is retracted, neocapsular fibrous tissue is excised to expose the femoral neck and head.
- After the fibrous tissue is sufficiently cleared, the femoral head is dislocated.

INSTRUMENTS/EQUIPMENT/IMPLANTS REQUIRED

- Full revision trays including cement and flexible osteotomes are necessary.
- An acetabular cup removal system (Explant; Zimmer Biomet) and curved osteotomes are needed if acetabular extraction is required.
- High-speed burrs and oscillating saws are useful for implant extraction if residual fixation requires an extended trochanteric osteotomy.
- A variety of pointed and Verbrugge clamps is needed for reduction of the fracture.
- Revision implants are required, including femoral stems of varied lengths and offsets. The ability to convert to a cemented stem is useful.
- Acetabular components to match the existing acetabular implant, including liners of different internal diameters and obliquities for stability, must be available. Matching femoral heads with varied offset also are needed.
- New acetabular components, including constrained liners, may be necessary.
- Cables and cable-plate sets, including tensioners and cutters, are required.
- Strut allografts are not typically needed in the management of type B2 fractures.

PROCEDURE

- The femoral prosthesis is removed from the canal with a clamp or pliers.
- Occasionally, a noncemented stem may retain partial fixation to some or all of the fracture fragments, but fixation may be insufficient to allow plate fixation (which would make it a type B1 fracture). In this scenario, attempts to extract the stem without appropriate preparation may cause further damage to the host bone. The fracture fragments are opened to allow access to the implant-bone interface. After the implant-bone interface is exposed, flexible osteotomes are used to free any final bony ingrowth to allow the stem to be extracted. The authors of this chapter use a pencil-tipped high-speed burr to free small areas of ingrowth without causing extensive damage to the host bone.
- After removal of the loose stem, the fracture fragments are mobilized sufficiently to allow access to the intact diaphysis to prepare the femur for a revision stem.
- Careful soft-tissue handling is necessary to avoid destroying the blood supply to fracture fragments or rendering them unstable, thereby making reconstruction more difficult (**Figure 5, A**).
- Care is taken during removal of the stem to ensure that the greater trochanter is not fractured by a prominent shoulder of the prosthesis or by cement overlying the shoulder. Cement over the shoulder of the prosthesis can be removed with careful use of an osteotome or a high-speed burr.
- With exposure of the fracture fragments for removal of cement or a partially fixed noncemented stem, the femoral diaphysis is visible for femoral preparation.
- The authors of this chapter typically place a prophylactic cable distal to the extent of the fracture to prevent fracture propagation during femoral preparation (**Figure 5, A**).
- With the use of tapered conical reamers, the femoral canal is prepared to accept a stem of appropriate diameter.
- Radiographs of the contralateral femur or prefracture radiographs of the affected femur can help guide determination of the diameter, lateral offset, and length of the prosthesis.
- If a modular stem will be used, the distal trial implant is inserted and an appropriately sized modular proximal body is placed (**Figure 5, B**).
- The construct is assessed for rotational and longitudinal stability.
- Attention is paid to acetabular orientation and the presence of liner wear that may contribute to instability. The surgeon should be

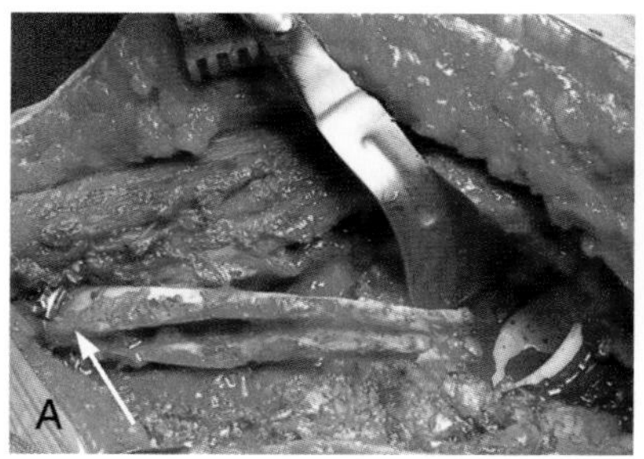

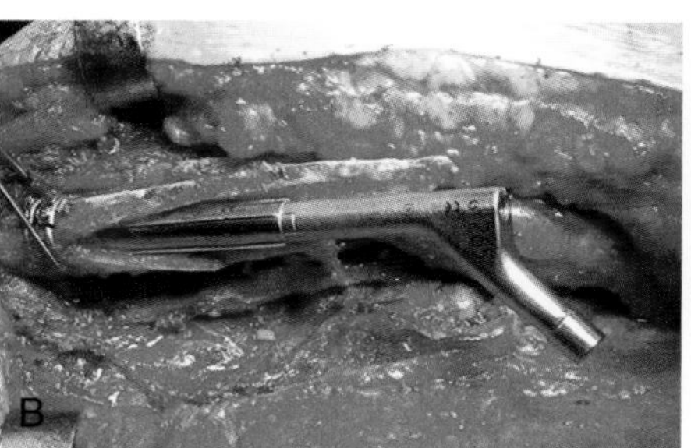

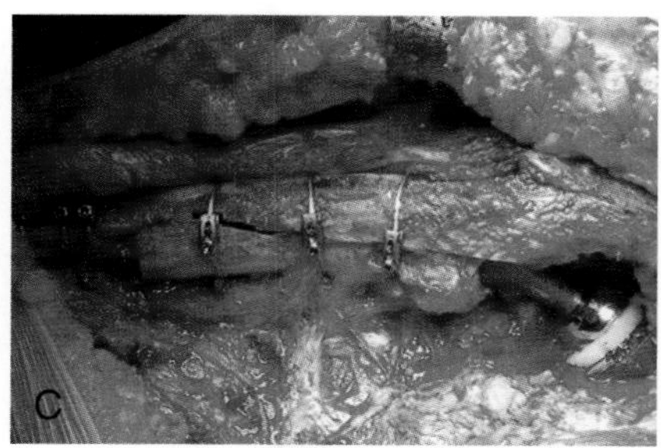

Figure 5 **A,** Intraoperative photograph shows exposed fracture fragments in a patient with a Vancouver type B2 fracture requiring treatment with a revision femoral stem. Note the prophylactic cable distal to the fracture margin (arrow). **B,** Intraoperative photograph shows insertion of a trial femoral stem for assessment of length and stability. **C,** Intraoperative photograph shows reduction and fixation of the fracture fragments with sequential cables. The proximal cable is placed distal to the lesser trochanter to resist pull of the abductor muscles.

prepared to change one or more of the acetabular implants to aid in creating a stable construct.

- After a stable combination of distal and proximal femoral body and femoral head has been achieved, orientation is marked on the host bone for anteversion and length.
- The authors of this chapter recommend that the cables or Luque wires used for fixation of the fracture be placed while the bone fragments are mobile and the soft tissues are lax. This method facilitates passage of the cables, and passing the cables before the definitive prosthesis is placed makes it easier to maintain reduction of the fracture while tightening the cables or wires.
- The authors of this chapter recommend the use of enough cables or wires spaced 3 cm apart to adequately control the fracture fragments.
- The most proximal cable or wire should be placed distal to the lesser trochanter to resist the pull of the abductor muscles. This cable or wire can be passed through a drill hole in the lesser trochanter or just distal to it to help prevent it from slipping.
- The authors of this chapter recommend impacting the distal portion of the stem before the proximal portion.
- The modular proximal femoral body is trialed and appropriate anteversion established.
- After a stable reduction is achieved, the final proximal femoral body is impacted, re-creating the appropriate anteversion.
- Trial femoral heads of varying offset are placed to assess joint stability.
- The appropriate femoral head is impacted and the hip relocated.
- The fracture fragments are reduced and held with tenaculum reduction forceps.
- The previously placed cables or wires are sequentially tightened from distal to proximal (**Figure 5, C**).
- Any gaps in the reduction are packed with femoral reamings.

ALTERNATIVE PROCEDURE

- An alternative, less invasive technique is to perform femoral preparation through the fracture fragments, which are left undisturbed, without soft-tissue stripping.
- This technique can be used only when a noncemented stem (**Figure 6, A**) is removed without the need to open the fracture fragments.
- A prophylactic cable or wire is passed distal to the fracture site as previously described, with minimal elevation of the vastus lateralis if necessary (**Figure 6, B**).
- A guidewire is used to identify the distal femoral canal, which is prepared with conical reamers.
- Great care is taken to ensure that the reamers are in the femoral medulla, and attention is paid to the tactile feedback provided by the femoral bone.
- The assistant holding the patient's thigh should note and inform the surgeon of any passage of a guidewire or reamer outside the femur into the soft tissue.
- The femur is prepared according to preoperative templating.
- A trial stem of appropriate size is placed.
- The hip is reduced into the socket without any attempt to reduce the fracture.
- The fracture is reduced with ligamentotaxis using indirect techniques with simple traction.
- The fracture is palpated through the soft tissues.
- If an acceptable yet imperfect reduction is achieved, a small window of the vastus lateralis is elevated to allow the passage of a wire or cable for provisional fracture reduction (**Figure 6, C**).
- An intraoperative radiograph is

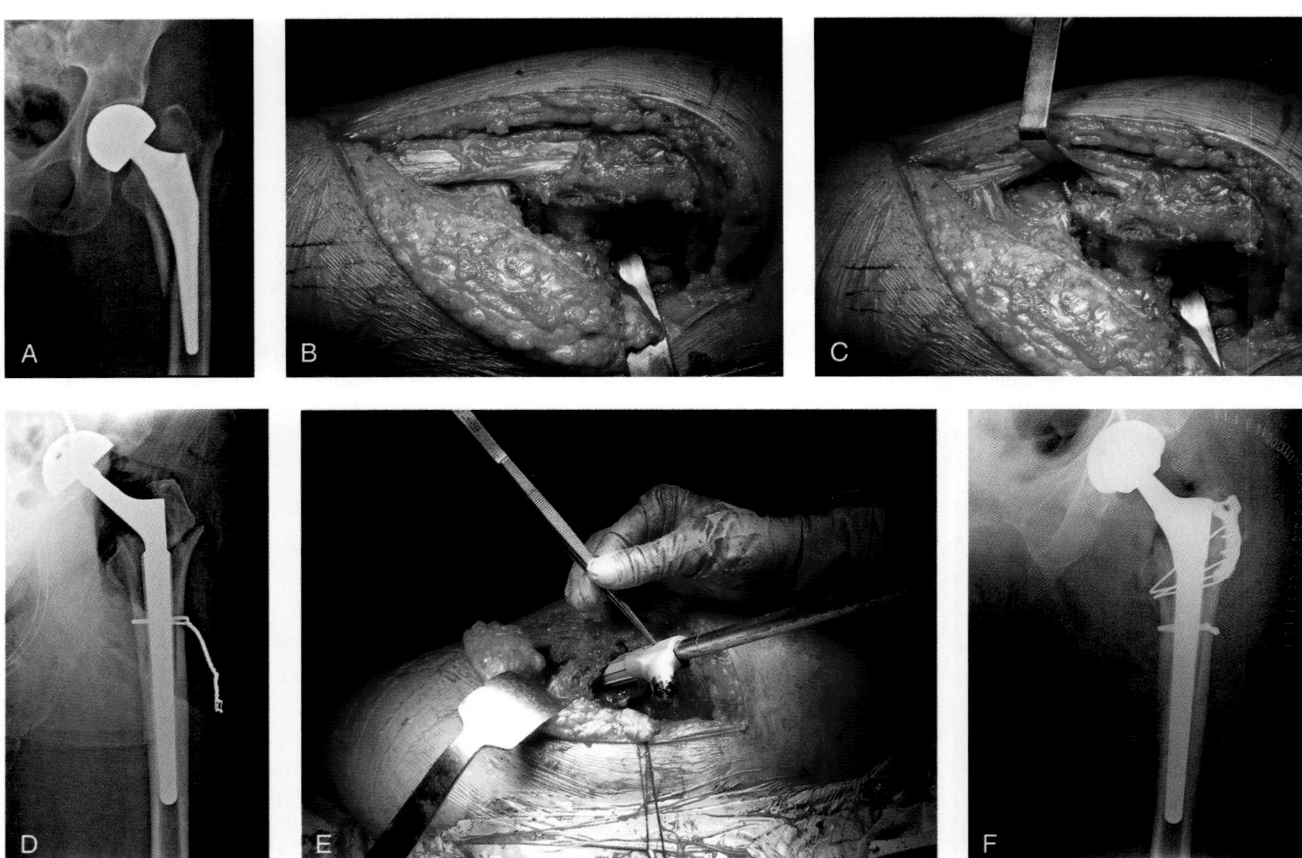

Figure 6 **A,** AP radiograph of a left hip demonstrates a Vancouver type B2 fracture around a loose noncemented hemiarthroplasty with a noncemented femoral stem. **B,** Intraoperative photograph shows exposure of the fracture with minimal soft-tissue stripping of the fracture fragments. **C,** Intraoperative photograph shows placement of temporary cerclage wire fixation with minimal soft-tissue stripping of the fracture fragments. **D,** Intraoperative cross-table radiograph demonstrates placement of the trial femoral stem and provisional reduction of the fracture. Note that ligamentotaxis has reduced the fracture fragments. **E,** Intraoperative photograph shows insertion of the definitive tapered, fluted titanium stem for reconstruction of the fracture. Note the attention to correct anteversion upon insertion. **F,** Postoperative AP radiograph demonstrates reconstruction of the fracture. The trochanteric fragment has been addressed with use of a trochanteric cable plate.

obtained to ensure that the trial implant is within the femur, with satisfactory filling of the canal and satisfactory fracture reduction (**Figure 6, D**).

- After appropriate longitudinal and rotational stability is achieved, the definitive stem is impacted, recreating the length and anteversion necessary (**Figure 6, E**).
- The major advantage of this technique is that the fracture fragments are not opened, reducing blood loss, and soft-tissue attachments are maintained, allowing rapid healing of the fracture and achieving a stable hip (**Figure 6, F**).

WOUND CLOSURE

- The wound is closed in the same manner as in type B1 fractures.

Postoperative Regimen

Toe-touch weight bearing is maintained for 6 to 12 weeks postoperatively depending on radiographic evidence of healing. The patient should avoid active abduction for 8 to 12 weeks postoperatively to prevent loss of reduction and allow fracture healing.

Avoiding Pitfalls and Complications

As noted, careful soft-tissue dissection will facilitate rapid union. The authors of this chapter prefer to use the less invasive technique. However, in many patients, opening of the fracture fragments is necessary for cement or implant removal. In this scenario, care must be taken not to cause further damage to host bone. The aim is to create a stable THA. Placement of a prophylactic cable distal to the extent of the fracture can help avoid fracture propagation and the potential difficulty of obtaining distal fixation.

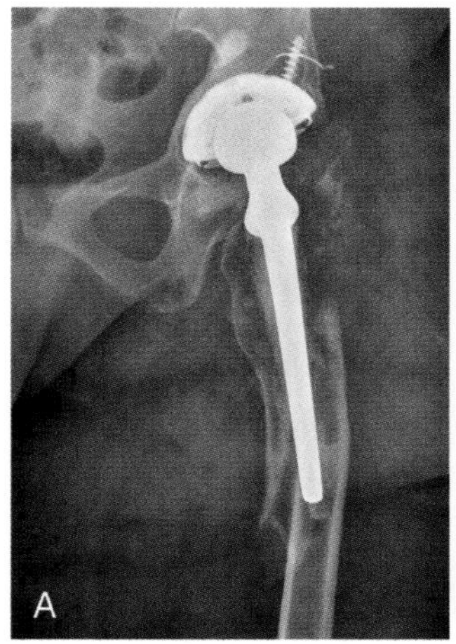

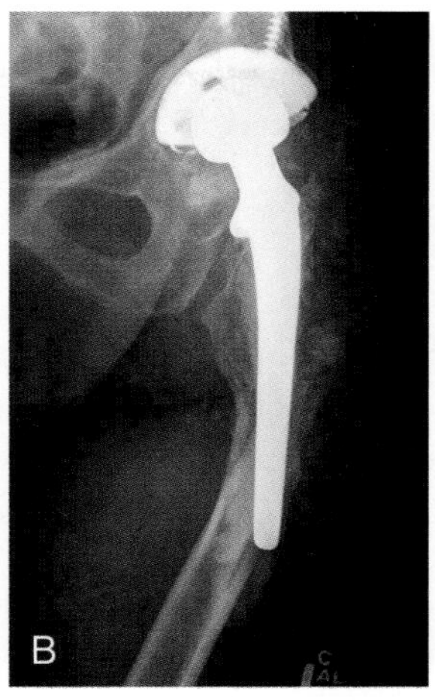

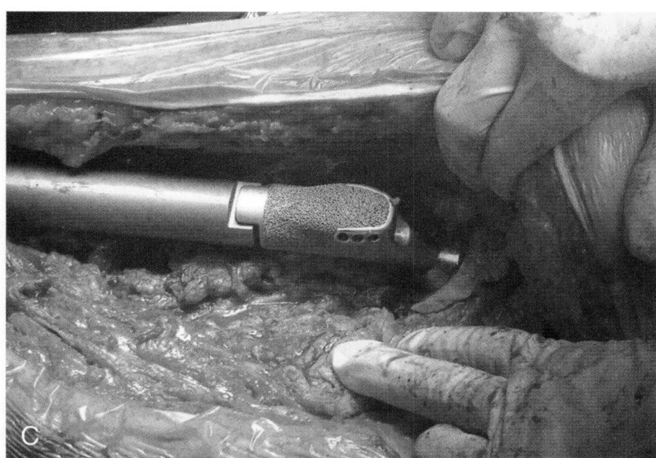

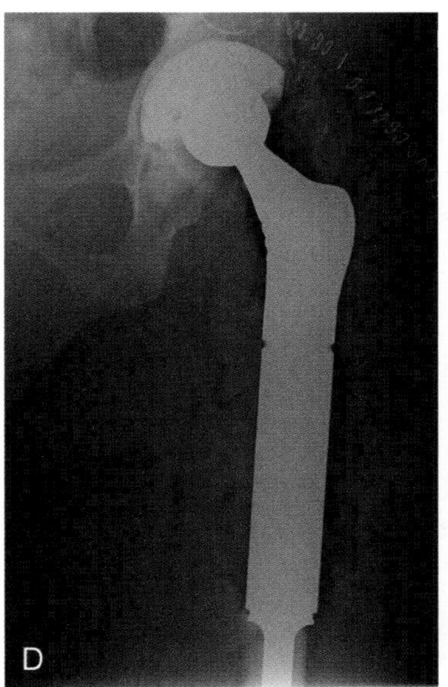

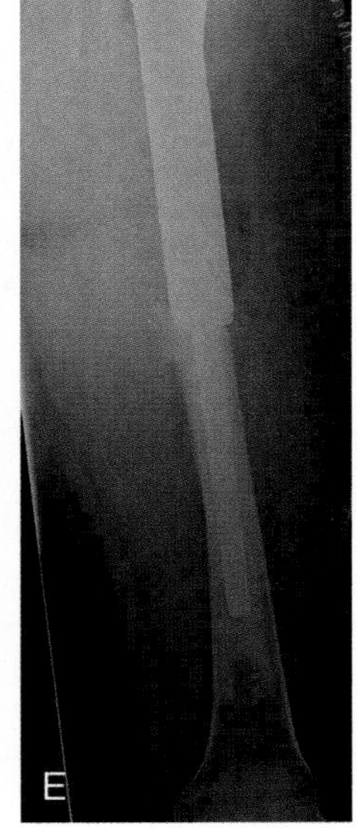

Figure 7 AP (**A**) and anterolateral (**B**) radiographs demonstrate a Vancouver type B3 fracture. Poor bone quality is evident surrounding the cemented femoral stem of the total hip replacement. **C,** Intraoperative photograph shows a segmental modular proximal femoral replacement. The porous surface and suture passage holes at the shoulder of the large endoprosthesis allow soft-tissue repair to the implant. **D** and **E,** Postoperative AP radiographs demonstrate a cemented proximal femoral replacement implant. The poor-quality bone was excised and the soft tissues, particularly the gluteal muscles, were sutured to the endoprosthesis. Typically, the authors of this chapter retain bone fragments to enhance soft-tissue repair where possible.

Cables or wires should be placed around the fracture fragments before placement of the definitive stem because the soft tissues will be lax, making placement of the cables or wires easier. Increasing the femoral head size can help achieve hip stability. The authors of this chapter routinely have acetabular implants available to allow the femoral head size to be changed to maximize stability.

Type B3 Fractures

Indications

The indications for surgical management of type B3 fractures are the same as those for type B2 fractures. In most patients, surgical treatment is required to allow early mobilization. The patient may have poor bone stock secondary to a failing prosthesis, previous loosening of the stem, or substantial fracture comminution (**Figure 7, A** and **B**). The authors of this chapter prefer to revise the femoral prosthesis with tapered, fluted titanium stems with the addition of strut allografts when necessary.

Contraindications

The only absolute contraindication to surgical management is active infection. Active infection can cause periarticular bone loss, and the presence of weakened bone around a prosthesis could represent infection. Appropriate laboratory values including erythrocyte sedimentation rate and C-reactive protein level should be obtained. Aspiration of the joint articulation should be obtained, and if available, pre-fracture radiographs should be reviewed. If the index of suspicion for infection is high, the surgeon should be prepared to obtain intraoperative tissue samples for frozen section and to place an antibiotic-loaded spacer if the results are positive.

Relative contraindications can include age-related health comorbidities, which may be present in patients with a long-standing THA. These factors are a substantial part of the decision-making process and will influence the choice of procedure to manage the fracture.

Alternative Treatments

Alternatives to femoral revision with a distally fixed femoral stem should be considered in patients with poor bone stock either proximally or distally. If severe osteolysis is present around the existing femoral stem, several options are available to improve proximal bone stock. The first is to supplement the femoral revision with strut allografts in focal areas of osteolysis. The second is to perform allograft impaction grafting and revision with a long, cemented stem, which is a complex procedure requiring a certain skill set. If bone stock is severely deficient, an APC technique, consisting of replacement of the proximal femur with a bulk allograft into which a long, cemented stem is placed, is an option. The final alternative, in which improving local bone stock is not a goal, is proximal femoral replacement with a large endoprosthesis (**Figure 7, C**). This option can use press-fit fixation when distal bone is preserved or can use cemented fixation when the diaphysis is ectatic and the use of a press-fit device would be less appropriate (**Figure 7, D** and **E**).

Results

Results of surgical management of type B3 fractures are reported in **Table 1**. Type B3 fractures often are reported as a single cohort with B2 fractures; as a result, treatment results are similar. Femoral stem revision performed with noncemented or cemented long-stem revision results in fracture union and revision-free prosthesis survivorship. High rates of union and survivorship (greater than 90%) are reported. The rate of union between the allograft and host bone junction is greater than 80% after APC reconstruction. This particular issue of union is mitigated when a large endoprosthesis (proximal femoral replacement) is used. However, with endoprosthesis use, acetabular implant failure and dislocation events become more prominent.

Techniques

SETUP/EXPOSURE

- The patient is placed in a lateral position.
- Exposure is achieved through a lateral or posterior approach.
- The authors of this chapter prefer the posterior approach because it is extensile and can provide excellent exposure of the acetabulum when full revision is necessary.

INSTRUMENTS/EQUIPMENT/IMPLANTS REQUIRED

- The authors of this chapter prefer to use distally fixed tapered, fluted titanium stems. Ideally, the distal femoral bone should have at least 4 cm of intact isthmus into which a tapered stem can be impacted.
- The advantage of using a nonmodular stem is the lack of a modular junction that can lead to fretting or that can result in fracture through the prosthesis if cantilever stresses are present, which can occur in patients with substantial proximal femoral bone deficiency.
- Tapered stems come in a variety of taper degrees. Because a stem with a higher taper angle typically engages the remaining bone with greater purchase than a stem with a lower taper angle would, a stem with a larger taper angle may be useful in patients with limited distal bone stock.
- Strut allografts should be available.
- A cable set is necessary to secure the graft and fracture fragments.
- In patients with insufficient distal bone integrity to allow revision with a noncemented femoral stem, an alternative reconstruction method is required. In physiologically robust patients with substantial life expectancy, and higher activity demands, the authors of this chapter prefer to use an APC. This method requires advance planning to obtain a proximal femoral allograft matched to the patient's side, size, and femoral geometry through a suitable tissue bank. In patients with a reduced life expectancy or lower activity demands, the authors of this chapter prefer to perform a cemented proximal femoral replacement, which allows rapid mobilization and does not rely on noncemented stem ingrowth or fracture union.

PROCEDURE

- The technique for surgical management of type B3 fractures is the same as that described for type B2 fractures, with the addition of strut allograft as necessary. The strut allograft application technique is the same as that described for type B1 fractures, with the location of the strut dictated by the area of bone loss.
- Femoral preparation and implantation of a tapered fluted stem is performed as described for type B2 fractures.
- Delivery of the distal femur is necessary to allow the surgeon to assess the bone quality and select an appropriate stem. For this reason, the less invasive alternative technique described for type B2 fractures cannot be used in patients with type B3 fractures.
- If 4 cm of intact isthmus exists, reconstruction with a nonmodular tapered, fluted stem is performed as described.
- If the distal bone is deficient, the authors of this chapter use either an APC or a proximal femoral replacement. The soft-tissue exposure for both of these alternatives requires bivalving of the remnant host femoral bone, which is wrapped

around either the APC or the femoral implant.

- If a proximal femoral allograft is used, the distal femur is delivered and prepared for insertion of the allograft, which has been prepared to accept a long, cemented stem. Cementation of stem into the allograft as a separate step is recommended.
- A step cut of 5 to 6 cm can be made in the lateral aspect of the allograft to provide rotational stability and a broader surface area for graft incorporation.
- Conversely, a transverse cut can be performed and a derotational unicortical plate applied for compression and stability.
- If a proximal femoral replacement is used, a transverse osteotomy is performed in the distal femoral bone below the level of the fracture and existing implant. Segmental trials are placed to restore length and tissue tension. After this is achieved, the distal coupling stem is cemented and segmental trials are placed on the coupling to restore length.
- In both techniques, rotation of the implant at the time of distal cementation is important to re-create appropriate anteversion depending on the surgical approach used (posterior or lateral).
- After the distal cementation is performed, the host bone is wrapped around the allograft or femoral implant for vascularization or soft-tissue reconstruction to re-create the abductor muscle insertion.
- The host bone is secured with cables, Luque wires, and/or surgical tape of appropriate number or amount depending on the amount of bone remaining.

WOUND CLOSURE

- The wound is closed in the same manner as in type B1 fractures.

Postoperative Regimen

If reconstruction with a tapered, fluted titanium stem is performed, toe-touch weight bearing is maintained for 6 to 12 weeks postoperatively with monitoring of fracture union and stem subsidence. If an APC or femoral replacement is used, immediate weight bearing is allowed; however, an abduction prosthesis is used for 6 weeks postoperatively to allow healing of the host bone and reconstitution of the abductor muscle insertion.

Avoiding Pitfalls and Complications

The management of type B3 fractures is challenging, and each reconstruction presents difficulties. When reconstruction is performed with a tapered fluted stem, achieving union of the fracture with sufficient bone stock around the stem to support the stem proximally and avoid fracture of the stem is difficult. Careful soft-tissue dissection must be performed to allow union of the fracture or placement of strut allografts. APC reconstruction and femoral replacement require attention to rotational and axial alignment to achieve appropriate femoral anteversion and ensure stability of the hip joint. Because of the differing alternatives available, the surgeon must be prepared with the appropriate stems or implants and allograft bone.

Type C Fractures

Indications

The indications for surgical management of type C fractures (**Figure 8, A** and **B**) are the same as those for surgical management of native femoral fractures, and it is not necessary to revise the femoral stem. Surgical management is indicated unless the fracture can be aligned and stabilized with closed methods (cast brace, hip spica cast, hip orthosis, skeletal traction). In patients with displaced type C fractures, surgical treatment is often required to restore alignment and stabilize the fracture. The presence of a canal-filling femoral prosthesis makes certain surgical options less optimal than others. Plate fixation is the mainstay of surgical management and is preferred by the authors of this chapter. The authors use minimally invasive percutaneous fixation if possible but perform ORIF with a lateral locking plate when necessary, as described later.

Contraindications

Nondisplaced fractures can be managed with closed techniques and close observation with radiographs. Open fractures require staged management. After the fracture site is clean and sterile, plate fixation can be performed.

Alternative Treatments

Closed reduction and splinting is an option. Retrograde femoral nails are shorter than those used in the management of native femoral fractures and create an interprosthetic region of stress concentration. External fixation is possible, but this option is less attractive because of the need for pin site management, the cumbersome nature of mobilization with a frame, and the short working distances for placement of pins without crossing the knee joint. Revision of the femoral stem is not indicated unless the femoral prosthesis is loose above the fracture.

Results

Results of surgical management of type C fractures are reported in **Table 1**. Type C fractures are distant to the femoral stem; therefore, the goal of the procedure is fracture union. Both type C and type B1 fractures require fixation, and published studies often report management results for both types. Reported union rates are high, and time to union is consistent between the types.

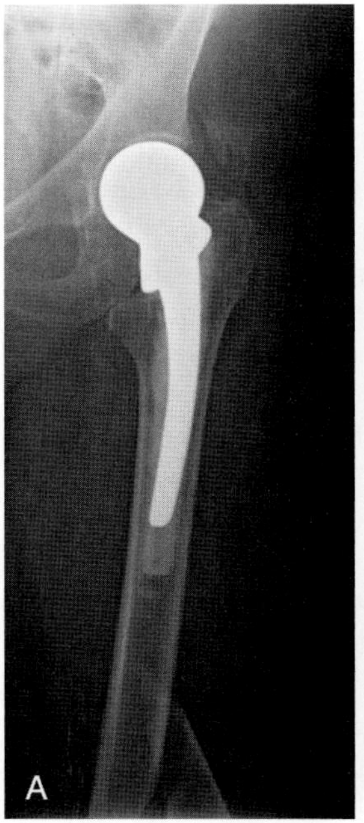

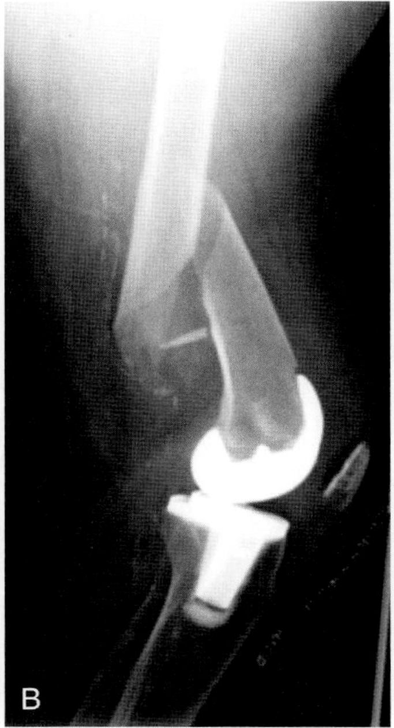

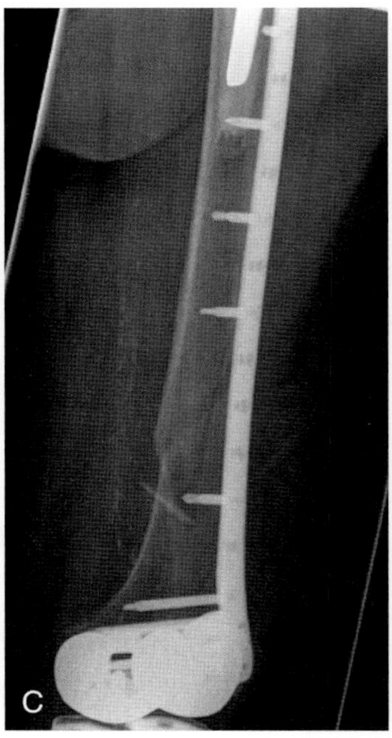

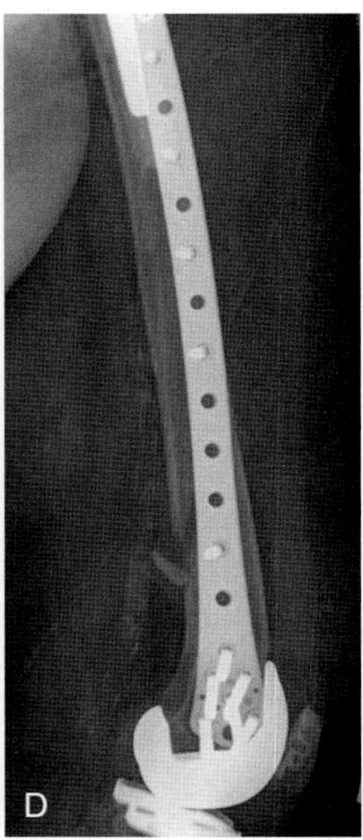

Figure 8 Preoperative AP left hip (**A**) and lateral view distal femoral (**B**) radiographs demonstrate a rotated Vancouver type C fracture. Postoperative AP (**C**) and lateral (**D**) femoral radiographs demonstrate fixation with a long lateral locking plate.

Techniques

SETUP/EXPOSURE

- The setup requires a radiolucent surgical table so that intraoperative fluoroscopy can be used.
- The patient is placed in a supine position, which allows assessment of lower limb length and rotational alignment.
- Alternatively, the patient can be placed in a lateral decubitus position or a fracture traction table can be used.
- The range of motion of the contralateral limb is examined preoperatively, with particular attention to tibial torsion and the foot progression angle.
- Exposure begins with a distal incision measuring 6 to 8 cm at the metaphyseal flare of the femur.
- The fascia lata is incised.
- A straight, large fragment locking compression plate is tunneled under the vastus lateralis muscle.
- The length of the plate should span the tip of the femoral stem to avoid a concentration of stress between the plate and stem.
- If the fracture is closer to the knee joint, a condylar locking plate can be used. In that scenario, the incision should be placed more distally at the knee joint.

INSTRUMENTS/EQUIPMENT/ IMPLANTS REQUIRED

- A large fragment locking compression plate is used. However, if the patient has a low type C fracture, a condylar locking plate is used.
- Bone reduction clamps, large threaded pins, pointed pushers, and a cable set are required.

PROCEDURE

- Fracture reduction can be achieved through a variety of means.
- Indirect reduction consists of application of a plate and reduction of the bone fragments to the plate. Reduction is achieved with percutaneous pointed clamps, percutaneous threaded pins or pointed pushers, nonlocking screws, and the use of locking plate–specific reduction tools (such as push-pull reduction device).
- Alternatively, when alignment cannot be achieved via closed, indirect methods, a limited incision is made at the level of the fracture.
- The authors of this chapter advise minimal muscle fiber stripping to prevent devascularization of the fracture ends.
- A pointed reduction tenaculum is used to hold the reduction while allowing the plate to be tunneled under the tines of the clamp.
- Fluoroscopy is used to confirm appropriate reduction and plate placement.
- Screws are placed through stab incisions or 4- to 5-cm incisions at varying intervals along the plate, allowing placement of several screws at a time.
- The plate is secured with bicortical screws.
- Two locking screws are placed

distally in a near-far configuration, with one above and one below but close to the fracture line.

- Proximally, screw placement can be done in a similar manner. However, it is important not to fill all screw holes with locking screws because doing so could cause over-stiffening of the fixation construct, resulting in nonunion or plate fracture.
- If the amount of bone available for screw fixation is limited, fixation around the stem is required.
- Fixation can be achieved around the stem by placing standard cortical screws around the femoral stem, by using unicortical locking screws, or by passing cables through a limited incision (**Figure 8, C** and **D**).

WOUND CLOSURE

- The wound is closed in the same manner as in type B fractures.
- To avoid herniation of the vastus lateralis muscle, the fascia lata is accurately repaired at each incision that is larger in magnitude than a percutaneous stab incision.

Postoperative Regimen

Weight bearing postoperatively is determined by the fracture pattern and fixation integrity. Most patients can tolerate toe-touch weight bearing with crutches immediately postoperatively. Splinting the knee is not required.

Avoiding Pitfalls and Complications

A long plate length is important for force transmission to intact bone far from the fracture site. The authors of this chapter attempt to achieve fixation that should span the femoral stem along greater than 50% of the length of the stem. Surgical exposure is minimized when possible. Accurate reduction is necessary to re-create anatomic femoral alignment. Placement of screws around the femoral stem can be difficult. Polyaxial locking screws are helpful; however, the authors of this chapter recommend the use of a limited, minimally invasive incision to allow passage of cerclage cables when screw fixation would be unicortical at best.

Bibliography

Abdel MP, Lewallen DG, Berry DJ: Periprosthetic femur fractures treated with modular fluted, tapered stems. *Clin Orthop Relat Res* 2014;472(2):599-603.

Brady OH, Garbuz DS, Masri BA, Duncan CP: Classification of the hip. *Orthop Clin North Am* 1999;30(2):215-220.

Bryant GK, Morshed S, Agel J, et al: Isolated locked compression plating for Vancouver type B1 periprosthetic femoral fractures. *Injury* 2009;40(11):1180-1186.

Buttaro MA, Farfalli G, Paredes Núñez M, Comba F, Piccaluga F: Locking compression plate fixation of Vancouver type-B1 periprosthetic femoral fractures. *J Bone Joint Surg Am* 2007;89(9):1964-1969.

Chakravarthy J, Bansal R, Cooper J: Locking plate osteosynthesis for Vancouver type B1 and type C periprosthetic fractures of femur: A report on 12 patients. *Injury* 2007;38(6):725-733.

Corten K, MacDonald SJ, McCalden RW, Bourne RB, Naudie DD: Results of cemented femoral revisions for periprosthetic femoral fractures in the elderly. *J Arthroplasty* 2012;27(2):220-225.

Duncan CP, Haddad FS: The Unified Classification System (UCS): Improving our understanding of periprosthetic fractures. *Bone Joint J* 2014;96-B(6):713-716.

Jukkala-Partio K, Partio EK, Solovieva S, Paavilainen T, Hirvensalo E, Alho A: Treatment of periprosthetic fractures in association with total hip arthroplasty: A retrospective comparison between revision stem and plate fixation. *Ann Chir Gynaecol* 1998;87(3):229-235.

Klein GR, Parvizi J, Rapuri V, et al: Proximal femoral replacement for the treatment of periprosthetic fractures. *J Bone Joint Surg Am* 2005;87(8):1777-1781.

Lewallen DG, Berry DJ: Periprosthetic fracture of the femur after total hip arthroplasty: Treatment and results to date. *Instr Course Lect* 1998;47:243-249.

Maury AC, Pressman A, Cayen B, Zalzal P, Backstein D, Gross A: Proximal femoral allograft treatment of Vancouver type-B3 periprosthetic femoral fractures after total hip arthroplasty. *J Bone Joint Surg Am* 2006;88(5):953-958.

Munro JT, Garbuz DS, Masri BA, Duncan CP: Tapered fluted titanium stems in the management of Vancouver B2 and B3 periprosthetic femoral fractures. *Clin Orthop Relat Res* 2014;472(2):590-598.

Neumann D, Thaler C, Dorn U: Management of Vancouver B2 and B3 femoral periprosthetic fractures using a modular cementless stem without allografting. *Int Orthop* 2012;36(5):1045-1050.

Siegmeth A, Menth-Chiari W, Wozasek GE, Vécsei V: Periprosthetic femur shaft fracture: Indications and outcome in 51 patients [German]. *Unfallchirurg* 1998;101(12):901-906.

Springer BD, Berry DJ, Lewallen DG: Treatment of periprosthetic femoral fractures following total hip arthroplasty with femoral component revision. *J Bone Joint Surg Am* 2003;85(11):2156-2162.

Tsiridis E, Narvani AA, Haddad FS, Timperley JA, Gie GA: Impaction femoral allografting and cemented revision for periprosthetic femoral fractures. *J Bone Joint Surg Br* 2004;86(8):1124-1132.

Wang JW, Chen LK, Chen CE: Surgical treatment of fractures of the greater trochanter associated with osteolytic lesions: Surgical technique. *J Bone Joint Surg Am* 2006;88(suppl 1 pt 2):250-258.

Zarin JS, Zurakowski D, Burke DW: Claw plate fixation of the greater trochanter in revision total hip arthroplasty. *J Arthroplasty* 2009;24(2):272-280.

Video Reference

Nauth A, Henry P, Schemitsch EH: Video. *Periprosthetic Fracture Fixation with Cable Plate and Strut Allograft*. Toronto, ON, Canada, 2014.

Chapter 38

Management of Fracture of the Greater Trochanter or Deficiency of the Abductor Mechanism After Total Hip Arthroplasty

Mathias P. G. Bostrom, MD
Liza Osagie-Clouard, MBBS

Indications

Abductor Mechanism Deficiency

The abductor mechanism, which consists of the primary and accessory muscles of abduction, is integral to gait and overall hip stability. This mechanism counterbalances lateral tilt during the single-leg stance, maintaining the upright position of the trunk. Deficiency of the abductor mechanism can result in a Trendelenburg gait and substantial patient morbidity. Studies report that the rate of abductor tears or avulsions after total hip arthroplasty (THA) may be as high as 50% with lateral or anterolateral approaches. These tears or avulsions negatively affect patient function and satisfaction but often remain undiagnosed.

Abductor deficiency after THA typically has one of two clinical presentations. It often occurs in patients who have undergone elective THA for the management of osteoarthritis. In these patients, abductor deficiency that was asymptomatic preoperatively may become symptomatic postoperatively, necessitating repair or reconstruction (**Figure 1**). Avulsion of the trochanter or failure of the tendon repair, particularly in patients who have undergone THA using an anterolateral, direct lateral, or transgluteal approach, also may result in symptomatic deficiency requiring intervention. Therefore, the presence of abductor pathology should be considered in a patient who has lateral trochanteric pain, limp, a positive Trendelenburg sign, and weakness with resisted abduction after THA. MRI with artifact suppression typically demonstrates abductor pathology (**Figure 2**).

Abductor dysfunction after THA also can result from superior gluteal neurovascular damage. In multiple studies, abductor weakness has been associated with surgical approaches that require splitting or release of the tendon, which may compromise the neurovascular bundle. Therefore, the risk of iatrogenic injury to the superior gluteal vessels leading to pathology is thought to be increased when a direct lateral, anterolateral, or transgluteal approach is used. Nerve transection typically requires muscle transfer to replace the denervated muscle group.

Chronic tears of the abductor mechanism, which most commonly occur in women 65 years and older, result from a pathologic process similar to that seen in chronic rotator cuff tears of the shoulder. These tears of the abductor mechanism often are referred to as rotator cuff tears of the hip and can be managed with surgical repair.

Tears of the abductor mechanism can be categorized according to the four-part Milwaukee classification (**Figure 3**). In the left hip, the insertion point corresponds to the 9-o'clock position, and the extent of the tear is counted toward the 1-o'clock position. Tears range from grade I, equaling 1 hour on the clock face, to grade IV, which are nearly complete tears or detachments (a so-called bald trochanter). Although this classification delineates the location and size of tears, the size of the injury does not always correspond to the severity of disability, because a small tear may result in substantial functional deficits. Therefore, when a tear of any size is identified on MRI and substantial patient morbidity is observed, especially in the presence of a well-fixed and noninfected prosthesis, surgical abductor repair should be considered.

Intraoperative Fracture of the Greater Trochanter

Intraoperative fractures of the greater trochanter occur in up to 6% of primary THA procedures, with an incidence up

Dr. Bostrom or an immediate family member serves as a paid consultant to Smith & Nephew; has received research or institutional support from Bone Support and Smith & Nephew; and serves as a board member, owner, officer, or committee member of the Orthopaedic Research Society. Neither Dr. Osagie-Clouard nor any immediate family member has received anything of value from or has stock or stock options held in a commercial company or institution related directly or indirectly to the subject of this chapter.

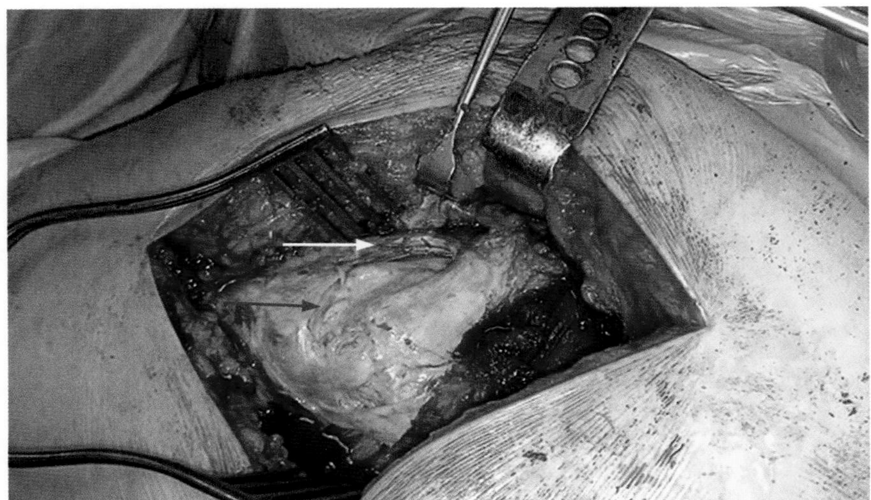

Figure 1 Intraoperative photograph of a right hip shows retraction of the combined tendon of the gluteus medius and minimus (white arrow), resulting in exposure of a bare area of the greater trochanter (blue arrow). (Reproduced with permission from Rao BM, Kamal TT, Vafaye J, Taylor L: Surgical repair of hip abductors: A new technique using Graft Jacket allograft acellular human dermal matrix. *Int Orthop* 2012;36[10]:2049-2053.)

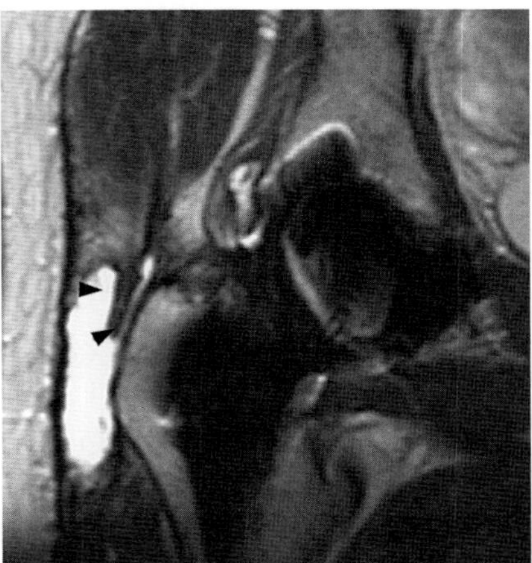

Figure 2 T2-weighted coronal MRI demonstrates rupture of the insertion of the gluteus medius, which is identified by the retracted tendon (between the black arrowheads) and surrounding high-signal defect. (Reproduced with permission from Miozzari HH, Dora C, Clark JM, Nötzli HP: Late repair of abductor avulsion after the transgluteal approach for hip arthroplasty. *J Arthroplasty* 2010;25[3]:450-457.e1.)

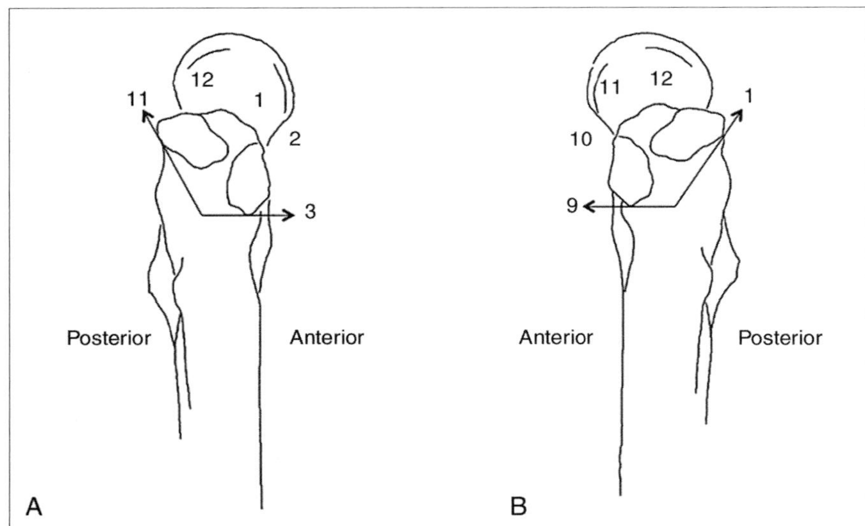

Figure 3 Illustrations depict the Milwaukee classification of tears of the hip abductors, in which grade I involves 1 hour on the clock, grade II involves 2 hours, grade III involves 3 hours, and grade IV consists of nearly complete tear or detachment of the tendons. **A,** Clock-face view of a right hip, in which the insertion point of the abductor mechanism tear begins at the 3-o'clock position and the extent of the tear is counted toward the 11-o'clock position. **B,** Clock-face view of a left hip, in which the insertion point of the abductor mechanism tear begins at the 9-o'clock position and the extent of the tear is counted toward the 1-o'clock position. (Reproduced with permission from Davies JF, Stiehl JB, Davies JA, Geiger PB: Surgical treatment of hip abductor tendon tears. *J Bone Joint Surg Am* 2013;95[15]:1420-1425.)

to 22% during revision arthroplasties. These iatrogenic fractures occur more frequently in noncemented arthroplasty procedures, in procedures using anterolateral and minimally invasive approaches, and in women. Because of the increased incidence in these scenarios, extra care in templating and extra vigilance during broaching and femoral impaction are required in these patients. The index of suspicion must be raised in the event of a sudden change in resistance during stem insertion, which may indicate propagation of a trochanteric fracture into the femoral shaft. Preferred management strategies are determined on the basis of the Vancouver classification of intraoperative periprosthetic fractures, which is distinct from the Vancouver classification of postoperative fractures but is based on similar concepts of implant stability. Intraoperative greater trochanter fractures (type A_G), which typically are classified as subtype 1 (cortical perforation) or subtype 2 (undisplaced fracture), are less likely to affect implant biomechanics. Subtype 3 fractures, which are fully displaced and can include larger trochanteric fragments, may propagate and displace further. Fractures that displace widely and violate the function of the gluteus medius can have a detrimental effect on outcomes and implant survivorship and should be repaired at the time of identification.

For the management of nondisplaced intraoperative fractures of the greater trochanter, the authors of this chapter recommend the use of tension-band wiring or a cable-claw plate configuration before the femoral stem is inserted. This recommendation is particularly important if a surgeon is using an approach in which the greater trochanter is stripped of its soft-tissue envelope, which may hinder union. If appropriate attention is paid to the posterior neurovascular structures, such additions carry limited increased morbidity. If the intraoperative fracture is thought to affect implant insertion or stability, the authors of this chapter recommend changing the implant to a diaphyseal-fitting porous-coated stem that will bypass the metaphyseal deficiency. If the use of a cemented stem is still planned, particular care must be taken to avoid the elution of cement from the breached cortex into surrounding soft tissues because this may hinder reduction of the trochanteric fragment.

Postoperative Fracture of the Greater Trochanter

The incidence of postoperative fractures of the greater trochanter is varied. However, these fractures, particularly those associated with osteolysis resulting from particulate debris and osteoporotic fractures resulting from minor trauma, are increasingly common. The risk factors for postoperative fracture are similar to those for intraoperative fracture and include female sex, older age, revision surgery, arthroplasty for reasons other than osteoarthritis (such as rheumatoid arthritis and congenital dysplasia), osteoporosis, implant loosening, periprosthetic osteolysis, and use of noncemented implants. Intervention typically is considered if the abductor mechanism is affected as a result of fragment displacement (typically greater than 2.0 cm) or if surgical management is thought to have a reasonable likelihood of success.

In patients who have postoperative fractures of the greater trochanter that require surgical intervention, the treatment method depends on the stability of the prosthesis. If the implant is stable (**Figure 4**), osteosynthesis is achieved with the use of cerclage wires, tension-band wiring, or cable-claw plates. In the rarer patient in whom the stability of the implant is jeopardized, a revision procedure may be required.

In patients who have fracture secondary to osteolytic lesions and polyethylene wear, the authors of this chapter advocate revision to remove the particle-generating implant, with concurrent bone grafting and wire fixation. In patients who have multifragmentary fractures or chronic trochanteric nonunion, the tension-band technique cannot be used. In these patients, fixation with a claw plate is more appropriate.

Contraindications

Most patients with a stable implant and a postoperative fracture of the greater trochanter can be treated with protected weight bearing and analgesia. Multiple series have demonstrated that many patients regain most of their prefracture function without surgical intervention.

Little is known about the natural progression of abductor mechanism tears without greater trochanter fracture. Consensus suggests that in patients in whom function is severely impeded, surgical management may be beneficial. Neither patient age nor body mass index have been demonstrated to impede

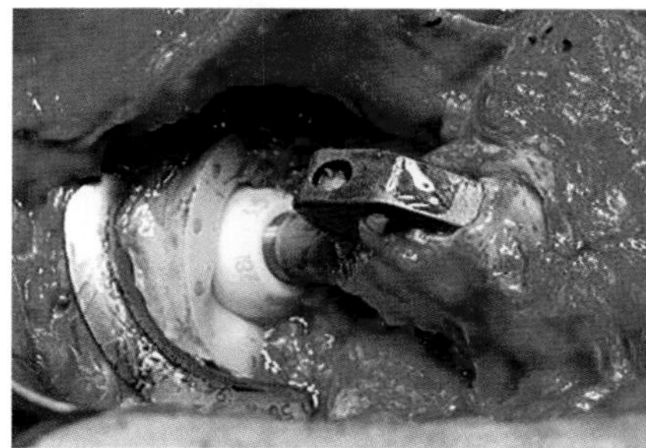

Figure 4 Intraoperative photograph shows absence of the greater trochanter. The implant is visible, and a short stump of the gluteus medius remains proximally. (Reproduced with permission from Kohl S, Evangelopoulos DS, Siebenrock KA, Beck M: Hip abductor defect repair by means of a vastus lateralis muscle shift. *J Arthroplasty* 2012;27[4]:625-629.)

successful surgical management, although slightly improved outcomes have been seen in patients with body mass index less than 30.

Radiographic and MRI findings have identified tears and muscle atrophy in up to 50% of patients at 1 year after THA; however, these findings do not correlate directly with function or satisfaction. Thus, although MRI is the most sensitive modality for the identification of abductor pathology, surgical intervention is not warranted in the absence of symptoms; instead, judicious follow-up is advocated. Similarly, in patients in whom abductor pathology is the result of traction neurapraxia of the superior gluteal nerve, eventual recovery of function is common, and thus, surgical intervention usually is not warranted in these patients.

Results

Multiple series suggest that nondisplaced and minimally displaced intraoperative fractures that are managed effectively with cables, tension-band wiring, or claw plates have no midterm to long-term effects on implant survivorship. However, although survivorship is not

Table 1 Results of Case Series of Abductor Mechanism Repair or Reconstruction After Total Hip Arthroplasty

Author(s) (Year)	Number of Patients	Procedure or Approach	Mean Patient Age in Years (Range)	Mean Follow-up in Months (Range)	Results
Weber and Berry (1997)	9	Direct open repair	66 (59-77)	57.6 (25-162)	75% of patients had improved gait and hip stability 20% of patients had improved pain scores
Lübbeke et al (2008)	19	Direct open repair	68 (51-89)	38 (12-62)	33% of patients had repeat rupture observed on MRI 66% of patients had an improved limp 75% overall patient satisfaction rate Time to repair was the most positively correlated predictor of satisfactory results
Fehm et al (2010)	7	Achilles tendon allograft	73 (63-81)	24 (24-48)	Mean Harris hip score improved from 34.7 to 85.9 Minimal improvements in postoperative pain
Miozzari et al (2010)	12	Direct open repair	62 (35-76)	27.6 (13-54)	40% of patients had repeat rupture observed on MRI Mean Harris hip score improved from 38.8 to 75.1 75% overall patient satisfaction rate
Whiteside (2012)	11	Gluteus maximus transfer	67 (52-73)	33 (16-42)	9 patients regained good abductor function against gravity and had gait improvement and negative Trendelenburg sign

affected, the surgeon must be aware of the risk of neurovascular damage during wiring and the increased incidence of postoperative lateral trochanteric thigh pain. The nonunion and escape rates of surgically fixed Vancouver type A_G fractures are as high as 31%, and these complications can result in a persistent Trendelenburg gait. Therefore, fixation must be secure to withstand vertical, anteroposterior, and rotational forces. Cable-claw systems have been used to reduce and retain the bony fragment, although early systems had high rates of breakage, cable fraying, and nonunion. Improved systems that used polyfilament cables that were oriented transversely and conformed to the anatomy, thus delivering uniform cable compression and more consistent tightening and retightening, have performed much better.

Although many surgeons have studied methods of reconstruction and/or repair of solitary abductor mechanism tears/detachments, there is no true consensus or algorithm for management. Retrospective case series have outlined repair techniques and their corresponding outcomes (**Table 1**). Rates of re-rupture after the management of chronic tears remain variable, with poor outcomes in up to 40% of patients. Re-rupture or fatty muscular degeneration after surgical intervention does not always correspond with a recurrence of symptoms, with reports highlighting a 75% patient satisfaction rate despite recurrent pathology observed in 33% of postoperative MRI studies.

Alternative Treatments

Most solitary Vancouver type A_G postoperative fractures can be managed nonsurgically with protected weight bearing and no active abduction for 8 weeks. This nonsurgical management typically results in return to preinjury function. Surgical intervention typically is warranted only in patients who have gross displacement affecting the abductor arm, intractable pain, and/or concurrent proximal femoral osteolysis.

In patients who have abductor deficiency and no greater trochanter fracture, initial short-term use of NSAIDs and physical therapy may provide some relief of symptoms and improve abductor strength. Persistent pain and abductor dysfunction may warrant surgical intervention for definitive remediation.

Techniques

Fracture of the Greater Trochanter

BONE GRAFTING AND TENSION-BAND WIRING

- In patients with postoperative fracture secondary to osteolysis, the approach used for the primary

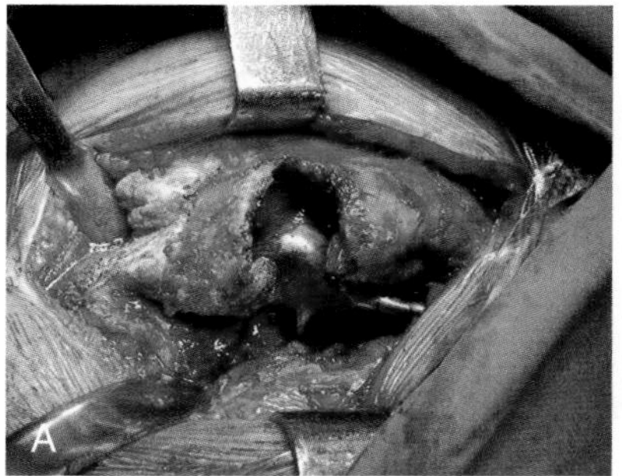

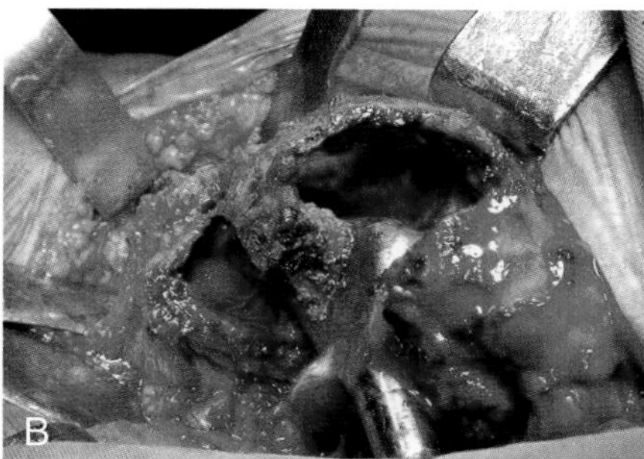

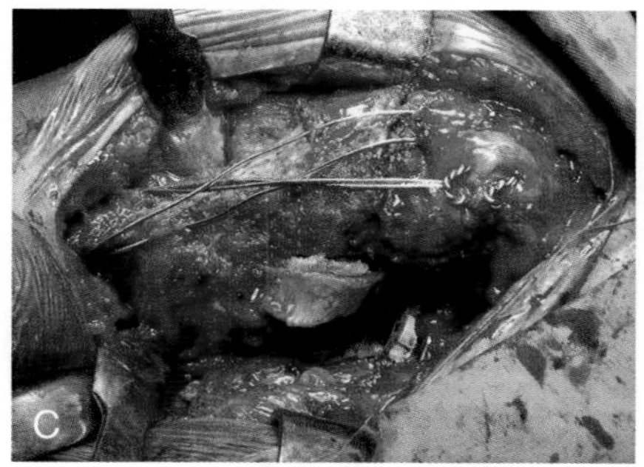

Figure 5 Intraoperative photographs show management of a fracture of the greater trochanter with a large osteolytic lesion. **A,** The fracture and associated large osteolytic lesion are identified. **B,** The lesion is packed with morcellized bone graft. **C,** Fracture reduction and fixation is achieved with tension-band wires. (Reproduced with permission from Wang JW, Chen LK, Chen CE: Surgical treatment of fractures of the greater trochanter associated with osteolytic lesions: Surgical technique. *J Bone Joint Surg Am* 2006;88 [suppl 1 pt 2]:250-258.)

procedure typically is used again.

- Prophylactic antibiotics are administered on induction of anesthesia.
- The subtrochanteric region is exposed.
- An inverted L-shaped incision is made in the vastus lateralis.
- The fragment is detached from its fibers to allow visualization of the osteolytic lesion.
- The lesion is débrided down to a bleeding inner cortex.
- Two 2.6-mm holes are drilled from anterior to posterior through the lateral femoral cortex, 1 cm distal to the fracture.
- A monofilament stainless-steel wire is passed through each hole.
- The wires are configured in a figure-of-8 pattern over the tip of the greater trochanter.
- In patients with intraoperative fracture, or in patients who do not have osteolytic lesions but in whom tension-band wiring is planned, the morcellized femoral head can be used to augment any defects at the fracture site. Alternatively, in patients undergoing fixation of a postoperative fracture of the greater trochanter, morcellized bone graft can be used to fill defects.
- After any defects are filled, the tension-band fixation is completed with the two points of the first and second wires (**Figure 5**).
- In patients with larger fragments, multiple wires may be used for fixation.
- Layered wound closure is done in the standard manner.
- Local anesthetic is injected into the wound.

CABLE-CLAW SYSTEM FIXATION

- The joint is approached through the incision that was used for the original procedure.
- Prophylactic antibiotics are administered on induction of anesthesia.
- Dissection is performed to expose both sides of the gluteus medius.
- In patients with nonunion, the fragment is débrided and cleaned of fibrous tissues and sclerotic bone to leave a bleeding cancellous bed.
- Reduction is maintained with a clamp with the hip in abduction and internal rotation.
- Adjunctive allograft can be used to fill bony defects.
- The claw is placed over the greater trochanter, and light mallet blows are used to embed the hooks.
- Cables are passed through the implant and around the femur. The initial cables are placed in the central portion of the claw plate, thus maintaining appropriate tensioning until maximum torque is achieved.
- The remaining cables are applied and tightened or retightened as necessary.
- The first cable that was passed may be loose and require retightening after the subsequent cables have been passed.
- Layered wound closure is done in the standard manner.
- Local anesthetic is injected into the wound.

Abductor Mechanism Deficiency

DIRECT REPAIR

- The choice of approach depends on the approach used in the patient's previous surgeries. The patient is positioned appropriately for the chosen approach.
- Routine antibiotic prophylaxis is administered at the time of induction of anesthesia.
- Preparation and draping are completed per standard protocol.
- Tissues are dissected to reveal the avulsed tendon and the entire greater trochanter, with care taken to carefully dissect the iliotibial band from the gluteus medius and the vastus lateralis.
- In patients with chronic injuries, tissues often are markedly retracted, scarred, and avascular, and full mobilization is difficult. In these

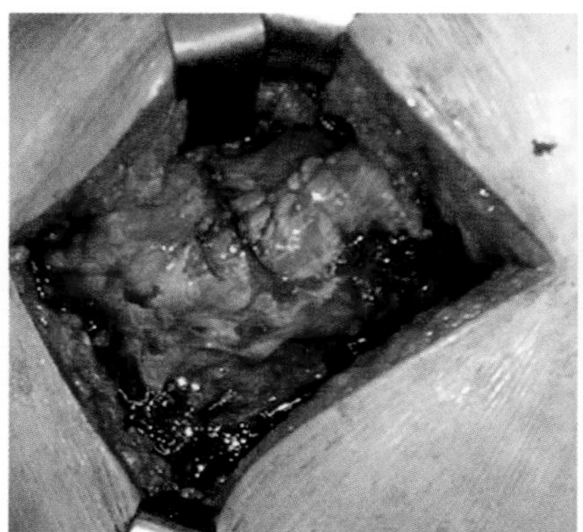

Figure 6 Intraoperative photograph shows the gluteus medius and gluteus minimus attached to the greater trochanter through transosseous tunnels. (Reproduced with permission from Rao BM, Kamal TT, Vafaye J, Taylor L: Surgical repair of hip abductors: A new technique using Graft Jacket allograft acellular human dermal matrix. *Int Orthop* 2012;36[10]:2049-2053.)

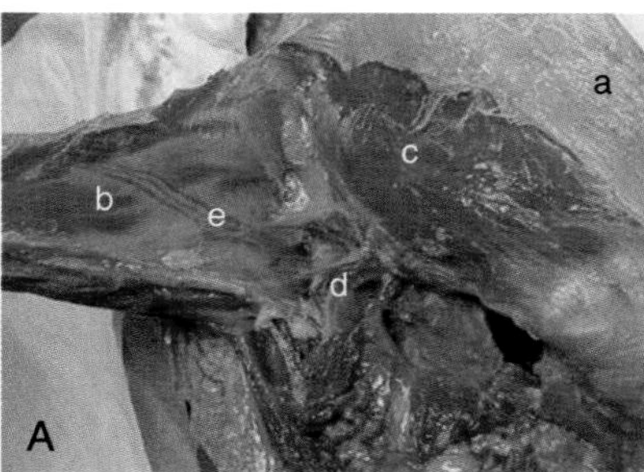

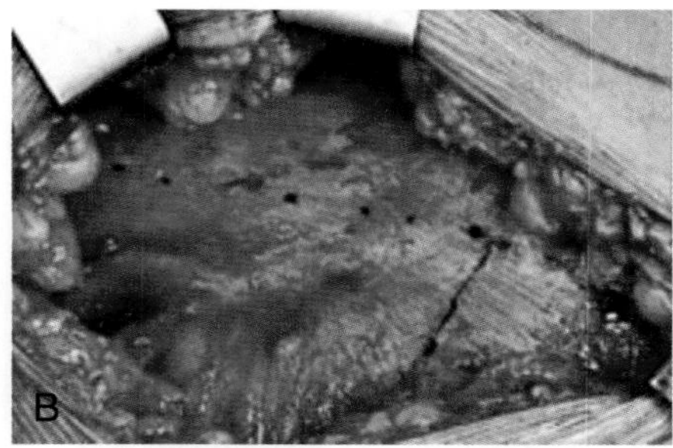

Figure 7 **A,** Photograph shows a cadaver section. The fascia lata (a) has been divided up to the iliac crest, and the anterior gluteus maximus flap (b) has been elevated to expose the gluteus medius (c). Inferior gluteal neurovasculature enters the muscle proximally, running along the undersurface (d, e). **B,** Intraoperative photograph shows marking of the fascial incisions during a gluteus maximus transfer, with a transverse incision and a longitudinal incision. (Panel A reproduced with permission from Whiteside LA: Surgical technique: Gluteus maximus and tensor fascia lata transfer for primary deficiency of the abductors of the hip. *Clin Orthop Relat Res* 2014;472[2]:645-653. Panel B reproduced with permission from Wuerz TH, Bhatia S, Chalmers PN, Nho SJ: A 77-year-old woman with left hip pain and weakness. *Orthopedics Today* 2014; Sep. http://www.healio.com/orthopedics/sports-medicine/news/print/orthopedics-today/%7B98d1167e-194c-4b13-9d00-5841c4da8132%7D/a-77-year-old-woman-with-left-hip-pain-and-weakness?page=1. Accessed March 15, 2015.)

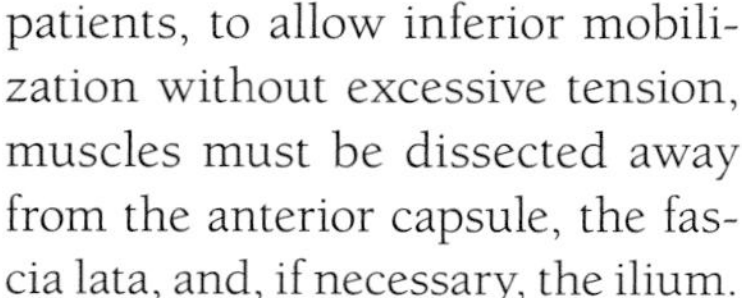

patients, to allow inferior mobilization without excessive tension, muscles must be dissected away from the anterior capsule, the fascia lata, and, if necessary, the ilium.

- Using a periosteal elevator, the plane between the bone and the gluteus minimus is developed anterosuperiorly from its capsular origin. To avoid injury to the superior gluteal vessels, particular care must be taken when working more than 3 cm superiorly.
- Any heterotopic bone that has formed at the capsule or within muscle is excised.
- If the greater trochanter is sclerotic with osteophytes, the osteophytes are removed, and the surface of the greater trochanter is débrided of remaining tissue with a high-speed burr, which also creates a bleeding surface for tendon adhesion.
- A 2.5-mm drill is used to create four or five transosseous tunnels.
- Four or five 5-0 nonabsorbable braided sutures are passed into the tendon.
- The authors of this chapter recommend the use of a Bunnell suture technique to fully anchor the suture within the tendon.
- With the hip in abduction on the surgical stand or abducted to at least 20° with sterile bolsters, the sutures are passed through the tunnels and secured using a Mason-Allen knot (**Figure 6**).
- The edges of the repaired tendon are opposed with an absorbable 3-0 braided absorbable running suture. Concurrent tears in the fascia lata are repaired with a similar continuous suture.
- Tension on the repair is assessed with the hip in adduction to ensure that the tendon is not overtightened.
- The affected hip is placed in an abduction splint, typically at 20° to 25° of abduction and 10° of external rotation.

GLUTEUS MAXIMUS TRANSFER

- Because the gluteus maximus is innervated by the inferior gluteal nerve, it serves as an effective replacement in patients in whom abductor deficiency is caused by denervation or in whom the muscles are severely atrophied as a result of chronic detachment, making direct repair impossible. The anterior gluteus maximus runs parallel with the femoral shaft and can be raised on a pedicle with the fascia lata to serve as a muscular transfer flap. The patient must have an intact and fully innervated gluteus maximus confirmed by MRI and preoperative electromyography.
- A standard posterior approach is used.
- Prophylactic antibiotics are administered on induction of anesthesia.
- The anterior gluteus maximus flap is fashioned by means of deep dissection to expose the muscle, and the flap is elevated with sharp dissection.
- The fascia lata is split in line with its fibers distal to the attachment of the gluteus maximus.
- A triangular flap that consists predominantly of fascia lata distally is raised. The anterior fascial edge

is transected down to muscle to allow appropriate tensioning (**Figure 7**).

- In patients in whom stability of the prosthesis is also compromised by a deficient posterior capsule and/or pathology of the short external rotators, a posterior gluteus maximus flap can be raised to provide further stability to the joint.
- From the posterior gluteus maximus, approximately 2 cm of the distal fascial attachment is elevated. Dissection is continued proximally halfway up the length of the muscle to create a triangular flap that mirrors the anterior flap.
- The anterior capsule is sutured to the posterior flap in a figure-of-8 configuration using 5-0 braided nonabsorbable sutures. The flap is mobilized across the femoral neck and secured to the capsule and the anterior face of the greater trochanter.
- Transosseous sutures through the greater trochanter can be used to reinforce the reconstruction.
- To secure the anterior flap, holes are drilled in the lateral aspect of the greater trochanter as described for the direct repair.
- With the hip abducted on the surgical table, the anterior flap is anchored with 5-0 braided nonabsorbable sutures through the transosseous tunnels in the greater trochanter.
- The remaining corner of the anterior flap is secured beneath the detached vastus lateralis fibers with absorbable 2-0 braided sutures. The vastus lateralis is sutured back to its attachment on the proximal femur.
- After the stability of the reconstruction is confirmed, the anterior and posterior flaps are sutured together.
- The anterior and posterior portions of the fascia lata are secured over the flap transfers.
- The wound is closed.

TENSOR FASCIA LATA TRANSFER

- In patients with chronic disruption and, thus, severe atrophy of the gluteus medius and minimus, in whom tears are not reconstructible, complete substitution of the muscle group can restore hip stability. The tensor fascia lata (TFL) does not depend on any other muscle group; therefore, transfer of this muscle is effective when the gluteus maximus is also damaged or denervated.
- Typically, a posterolateral approach is used.
- Prophylactic antibiotics are administered on induction of anesthesia.
- The TFL is dissected transversely from its fascial attachment and mobilized with sharp dissection.
- The TFL is attached with suture anchors to the bed of the greater trochanter via transosseous tunnels.
- The posterior portion of the muscle is sutured to the anterior portion of the greater trochanter with transosseous sutures.
- Assessment of integrity and closure are the same as described for the direct repair.

ACHILLES TENDON ALLOGRAFT

- The use of Achilles tendon allograft is effective in the management of avulsions at the musculotendinous portion of the abductor mechanism in patients who have adequate remaining muscle quality but tears that are not reconstructible because of retraction.
- Preoperative electromyography must demonstrate contractility of the remaining muscle as a precondition for allograft reconstruction.
- Preoperative MRI analysis of the abductor defect is necessary to delineate the exact location of the avulsion.
- Fresh-frozen Achilles tendon allograft is used. The attached calcaneal bone block is contoured with the use of an oscillating saw.
- The bone block is beveled to be no larger than 2 cm long and 1 cm wide so that it will be the appropriate size to slot into the greater trochanter.
- The approach and exposure are as previously described for direct repair.
- The nonfunctional tissue is débrided to create a vascular bed.
- Using an oscillating saw, a trough is made in the greater trochanter approximately 1 cm distal to the vastus ridge to receive the bone block (**Figure 8**).
- Ideally, a plane is developed between the gluteus medius and the gluteus minimus. However, in patients with avulsion of the gluteus minimus, a plane is developed between the gluteus minimus and the joint capsule. Approximately one-third of patients have tears involving both the gluteus medius and the gluteus minimus.
- The tendinous portion of the graft is looped through the mobilized gluteus minimus 2 to 3 cm proximal to the ruptured end, with the hip in abduction on the surgical stand.
- During the remainder of the procedure, the hip remains in abduction on the surgical stand.
- The allograft bone block is press-fit into the greater trochanter and secured with cable or 16-gauge wire.
- The allograft is sutured to the remaining gluteus medius, anterior capsule, and gluteus minimus with a Krackow stitch.
- The graft is looped back and secured anteriorly to the gluteus minimus and anterior capsule and posteriorly to the gluteus medius and posterior capsule.
- The wound is closed with the hip in abduction as previously described.

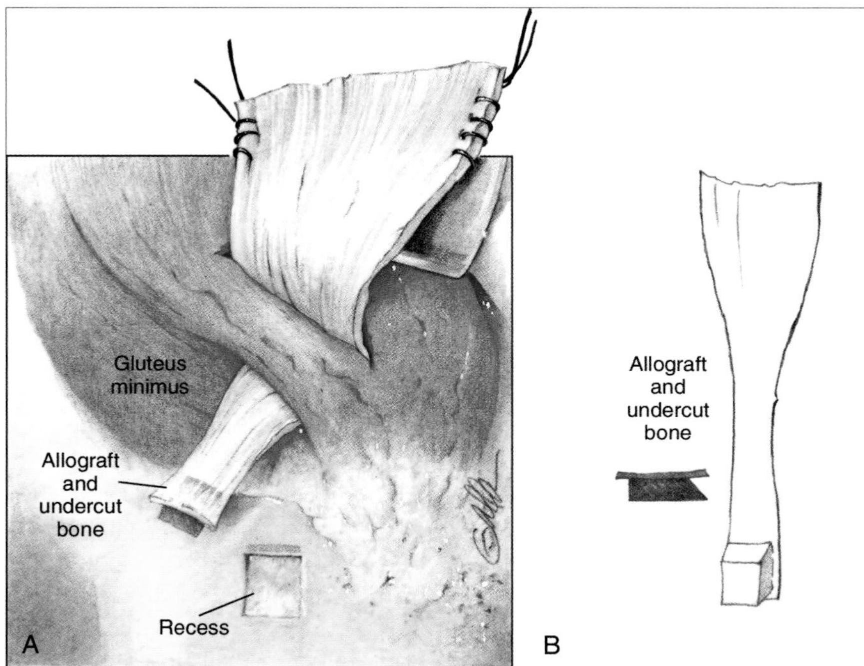

Figure 8 Illustrations depict abductor mechanism repair with Achilles tendon allograft. **A,** The graft is tunneled through the intact gluteus medius muscle. **B,** The bone block is contoured to fit into the greater trochanter. (Reproduced with permission from Fehm MN, Huddleston JI, Burke DW, Geller JA, Malchau H: Repair of a deficient abductor mechanism with Achilles tendon allograft after total hip replacement. *J Bone Joint Surg Am* 2010;92[13]:2305-2311.)

Postoperative Regimen

After repair of a greater trochanter fracture with tension-band wiring, protected weight bearing with restricted abduction is advised for up to 8 weeks postoperatively. Radiographic monitoring is necessary during this period to ensure that no further displacement occurs. After repair with a cable-claw system, patients typically are limited to toe-touch weight bearing without active abduction for 8 to 10 weeks postoperatively, after which weight bearing is progressively increased.

Multiple regimens for postoperative rehabilitation after abductor repair have been suggested. The authors of this chapter advocate the use of an abduction splint on completion of the procedure. If the patient can adhere to precautions, the splint can be removed before the patient is discharged from the hospital. Strict precautions must be followed, with active abduction, passive flexion beyond 60°, and external rotation prohibited for 8 to 10 weeks postoperatively. If these precautions cannot be followed, the authors of this chapter advocate full-time use of a brace during this period. If an Achilles tendon allograft is used, a 2-week non–weight-bearing period is advised, followed by 6 to 8 weeks of toe-touch weight bearing. If a graft is not used, toe-touch weight bearing is permitted immediately postoperatively. After abductor repair with or without grafting, physical therapy, including abductor strengthening exercises, is begun at 8 to 10 weeks postoperatively.

Avoiding Pitfalls and Complications

Fracture of the Greater Trochanter

If tension-band wiring is used for the management of osteolytic lesions, the drill holes should be distal to the osteolytic lesions to avoid screw cutout, whereas the superior wires must be deep to the tip of the greater trochanter. Adjunctive cerclage wires can be used to secure large fragments. Postoperatively, prolonged protected weight bearing with restricted abduction is necessary.

Abductor Mechanism Deficiency

In addition to the general complications of hip surgery, re-rupture is the most substantial risk to the repair or reconstruction. If re-rupture occurs, the patient may not experience resolution of the limp or may have only a slightly improved gait. Early surgical intervention after confirmed abductor deficiency results in improved pain relief and function. With delayed surgical treatment, further atrophy of the tendon occurs, making it more difficult to mobilize for repair or reconstruction.

In patients who have preoperative recurrent dislocation and/or signs of hip instability, the incorporation of a posterior gluteal muscle flap may be considered, both to improve stability and overcome capsular insufficiency. If raising a posterior gluteus maximus flap will expose the sciatic nerve, this nerve should be identified and protected throughout the procedure.

When the transosseous sutures are tensioned, it is crucial to use only enough force to approximate the tendon to bone to avoid strangulating the tendon or graft or cutting through the drilled tunnel.

When the posterior edge of the TFL is dissected for transfer, dissection should predominantly occur on the distal one-half of the muscle because dissection of the proximal one-half places the neurovascular bundle at risk and does not aid the transfer.

If the muscle transfer technique is used, pie-crust incisions are often made in the overlying fascia of the flap to improve vascularity and, thus, survival of the flap.

Appropriate postoperative mobilization and rehabilitation are critically important to the long-term integrity of the repair. Avoidance of active abduction for 8 to 10 weeks postoperatively is vital to avoid early re-rupture. A period of non–weight bearing or toe-touch weight bearing will reduce the risk of complications.

Bibliography

Berry DJ: Epidemiology: Hip and knee. *Orthop Clin North Am* 1999;30(2):183-190.

Bucher TA, Darcy P, Ebert JR, Smith A, Janes G: Gluteal tendon repair augmented with a synthetic ligament: Surgical technique and a case series. *Hip Int* 2014;24(2):187-193.

Cook RE, Jenkins PJ, Walmsley PJ, Patton JT, Robinson CM: Risk factors for periprosthetic fractures of the hip: A survivorship analysis. *Clin Orthop Relat Res* 2008;466(7):1652-1656.

Davies JF, Stiehl JB, Davies JA, Geiger PB: Surgical treatment of hip abductor tendon tears. *J Bone Joint Surg Am* 2013;95(15):1420-1425.

Davies H, Zhaeentan S, Tavakkolizadeh A, Janes G: Surgical repair of chronic tears of the hip abductor mechanism. *Hip Int* 2009;19(4):372-376.

Fehm MN, Huddleston JI, Burke DW, Geller JA, Malchau H: Repair of a deficient abductor mechanism with Achilles tendon allograft after total hip replacement. *J Bone Joint Surg Am* 2010;92(13):2305-2311.

Kohl S, Evangelopoulos DS, Siebenrock KA, Beck M: Hip abductor defect repair by means of a vastus lateralis muscle shift. *J Arthroplasty* 2012;27(4):625-629.

Lindahl H, Malchau H, Herberts P, Garellick G: Periprosthetic femoral fractures: Classification and demographics of 1049 periprosthetic femoral fractures from the Swedish National Hip Arthroplasty Register. *J Arthroplasty* 2005;20(7):857-865.

Lübbeke A, Kampfen S, Stern R, Hoffmeyer P: Results of surgical repair of abductor avulsion after primary total hip arthroplasty. *J Arthroplasty* 2008;23(5):694-698.

Masonis JL, Bourne RB: Surgical approach, abductor function, and total hip arthroplasty dislocation. *Clin Orthop Relat Res* 2002;(405):46-53.

Masri BA, Meek RM, Duncan CP: Periprosthetic fractures evaluation and treatment. *Clin Orthop Relat Res* 2004;(420):80-95.

Miozzari HH, Dora C, Clark JM, Nötzli HP: Late repair of abductor avulsion after the transgluteal approach for hip arthroplasty. *J Arthroplasty* 2010;25(3):450-457.e1.

Odak S, Ivory J: Management of abductor mechanism deficiency following total hip replacement. *Bone Joint J* 2013;95-B(3):343-347.

Rao BM, Kamal TT, Vafaye J, Taylor L: Surgical repair of hip abductors: A new technique using Graft Jacket allograft acellular human dermal matrix. *Int Orthop* 2012;36(10):2049-2053.

Weber M, Berry DJ: Abductor avulsion after primary total hip arthroplasty: Results of repair. *J Arthroplasty* 1997;12(2):202-206.

Whiteside LA: Surgical technique: Transfer of the anterior portion of the gluteus maximus muscle for abductor deficiency of the hip. *Clin Orthop Relat Res* 2012;470(2):503-510.

Chapter 39

Venous Thromboembolic Disease Prophylaxis After Total Hip Arthroplasty

Jay R. Lieberman, MD
Nathanael Heckmann, MD

Indications and Contraindications

One of the most serious complications after total hip arthroplasty (THA) is venous thromboembolic (VTE) disease, which can consist of pulmonary embolism (PE) and/or deep vein thrombosis (DVT). According to Medicare data, the all-cause death rates in the first 90 days after primary and revision THA are 0.95% and 2.56%, respectively, with corresponding PE rates of 0.93% and 0.78%.

All patients undergoing primary and revision THA, including patients with blood dyscrasias and coagulopathies, should receive VTE prophylaxis. No absolute contraindications to VTE prophylaxis exist. On the basis of current evidence, no single prophylactic regimen is considered ideal. Most authors agree that VTE prophylaxis should be used for 14 days or more after THA, and data are available to support the use of prophylaxis for up to 35 days. VTE prophylaxis should be based on individual patient risk factors to balance efficacy and safety.

Guidelines for VTE Prophylaxis

In 2011 the American Academy of Orthopaedic Surgeons (AAOS) published a revised guideline on VTE prophylaxis for patients undergoing THA or total knee arthroplasty. The guideline was based on a systematic review of current publications with a focus on symptomatic events and high-quality studies. On the basis of the available data, the AAOS published 10 recommendations and assigned a grade to indicate the strength of each recommendation (strong, moderate, limited, inconclusive, or consensus; **Table 1**). The AAOS did not recommend a specific prophylactic regimen or duration of prophylaxis because of the lack of studies assessing symptomatic VTE events after THA.

In 2012, the American College of Chest Physicians (ACCP) released the ninth edition of its guidelines for VTE prophylaxis in orthopaedic patients (**Table 2**). Prior versions of the ACCP guidelines were criticized for stressing efficacy at the expense of safety. The new guidelines departed from prior recommendations by placing more emphasis on complications such as bleeding. The ACCP guidelines consist of nine recommendations graded based on certainty (grade 1) or uncertainty (grade 2) and the quality of studies used to make the recommendation (A for high-quality randomization, B for low-quality randomization, and C for observational or nonrandomized studies). In these ACCP guidelines, a variety of prophylactic agents are recommended over no prophylaxis, including low-molecular-weight heparins (LMWHs), vitamin K antagonists, aspirin, fondaparinux, rivaroxaban, dabigatran, apixaban, and portable mechanical compression. The guidelines suggest that chemoprophylaxis be combined with mechanical compression in the hospital and that prophylaxis be continued for up to 35 days postoperatively.

Treatments and Results

Pharmacologic Prophylaxis

A thorough understanding of VTE prophylaxis requires knowledge of the coagulation cascade and the distinct pharmacologic targets of VTE prophylaxis (**Figure 1**). Pharmacologic agents for VTE prophylaxis can be divided into six classes: vitamin K antagonists, LMWHs, direct thrombin inhibitors,

Dr. Lieberman or an immediate family member has received royalties from DePuy Synthes; serves as a paid consultant to Arthrex and DePuy Synthes; has stock or stock options held in Hip Innovation Technology; has received research or institutional support from Arthrex; and serves as a board member, owner, officer, or committee member of the American Academy of Orthopaedic Surgeons and the Western Orthopaedic Association. Neither Dr. Heckmann nor any immediate family member has received anything of value from or has stock or stock options held in a commercial company or institution related directly or indirectly to the subject of this chapter.

Table 1 American Academy of Orthopaedic Surgeons Clinical Practice Guideline: Preventing Venous Thromboembolic Disease in Patients Undergoing Elective Hip and Knee Arthroplasty

No.	Recommendation	Grade
1	We recommend against routine postoperative duplex ultrasonography screening of patients who undergo elective hip or knee arthroplasty.	Strong
2	Patients undergoing elective hip or knee arthroplasty are already at high risk for venous thromboembolism. The practitioner might further assess the risk of venous thromboembolism by determining whether these patients had a previous venous thromboembolism.	Limited
	Current evidence is not clear about whether factors other than a history of previous venous thromboembolism increase the risk of venous thromboembolism in patients undergoing elective hip or knee arthroplasty and, therefore, we cannot recommend for or against routinely assessing these patients for these factors.	Inconclusive
3	Patients undergoing elective hip or knee arthroplasty are at risk for bleeding and bleeding-associated complications. In the absence of reliable evidence, it is the opinion of this work group that patients be assessed for known bleeding disorders like hemophilia and for the presence of active liver disease, which further increase the risk for bleeding and bleeding-associated complications.	Consensus
	Current evidence is not clear about whether factors other than the presence of a known bleeding disorder or active liver disease increase the chance of bleeding in these patients and, therefore, we are unable to recommend for or against using them to assess a patient's risk of bleeding.	Inconclusive
4	We suggest that patients discontinue antiplatelet agents (eg, aspirin, clopidogrel) before undergoing elective hip or knee arthroplasty.	Moderate
5	We suggest the use of pharmacologic agents and/or mechanical compressive devices for the prevention of venous thromboembolism in patients undergoing elective hip or knee arthroplasty, and who are not at elevated risk beyond that of the surgery itself for venous thromboembolism or bleeding.	Moderate
	Current evidence is unclear about which prophylactic strategy (or strategies) is/are optimal or suboptimal. Therefore, we are unable to recommend for or against specific prophylactics in these patients.	Inconclusive
	In the absence of reliable evidence about how long to employ these prophylactic strategies, it is the opinion of this work group that patients and physicians discuss the duration of prophylaxis.	Consensus
6	In the absence of reliable evidence, it is the opinion of this work group that patients undergoing elective hip or knee arthroplasty, and who have also had a previous venous thromboembolism receive pharmacologic prophylaxis and use mechanical compressive devices.	Consensus
7	In the absence of reliable evidence, it is the opinion of this work group that patients undergoing elective hip or knee arthroplasty, and who also have a known bleeding disorder (eg, hemophilia) and/or active liver disease, use mechanical compressive devices for preventing venous thromboembolism.	Consensus
8	In the absence of reliable evidence, it is the opinion of this work group that patients undergo early mobilization following elective hip and knee arthroplasty. Early mobilization is of low cost, minimal risk to the patient, and consistent with current practice.	Consensus
9	We suggest the use of neuraxial (such as intrathecal, epidural, and spinal) anesthesia for patients undergoing elective hip or knee arthroplasty to help limit blood loss, even though evidence suggests that neuraxial anesthesia does not affect the occurrence of venous thromboembolic disease.	Moderate
10	Current evidence does not provide clear guidance about whether inferior vena cava (IVC) filters prevent pulmonary embolism in patients undergoing elective hip and knee arthroplasty who also have a contraindication to chemoprophylaxis and/or known residual venous thromboembolic disease. Therefore, we are unable to recommend for or against the use of such filters.	Inconclusive

Adapted from American Academy of Orthopaedic Surgeons: *Preventing Venous Thromboembolic Disease in Patients Undergoing Elective Hip and Knee Arthroplasty: Evidence-Based Guideline and Evidence Report*. Rosemont, IL, American Academy of Orthopaedic Surgeons, 2011. Available at: http://www.aaos.org/research/guidelines/VTE/VTE_full_guideline.pdf. Accessed August 16, 2016.

Table 2 Highlights of the American College of Chest Physicians Guidelines for the Prevention of Venous Thromboembolism in Orthopaedic Patients

No.	Recommendation[a]
2.1.1	In patients undergoing THA or TKA, we recommend use of one of the following for a minimum of 10 to 14 d rather than no antithrombotic prophylaxis: LMWH, fondaparinux, apixaban, dabigatran, rivaroxaban, low-dose unfractionated heparin, adjusted-dose vitamin K antagonist, aspirin (all grade 1B), or an IPCD (grade 1C).
2.2	For patients undergoing major orthopaedic surgery (THA, TKA, hip fracture surgery) and receiving LMWH as thromboprophylaxis, we recommend starting either 12 h or more preoperatively or 12 hr or more postoperatively rather than within 4 h or less preoperatively or 4 hr or less postoperatively (grade 1B).
2.3.1	In patients undergoing THA or TKA, irrespective of the concomitant use of an IPCD or length of treatment, we suggest the use of LMWH in preference to the other agents we have recommended as alternatives: fondaparinux, apixaban, dabigatran, rivaroxaban, low-dose unfractionated heparin (all grade 2B), adjusted-dose vitamin K antagonist, or aspirin (all grade 2C).
2.4	For patients undergoing major orthopaedic surgery, we suggest extending thromboprophylaxis in the outpatient period for up to 35 d from the day of surgery rather than for only 10 to 14 d (grade 2B).
2.5	In patients undergoing major orthopaedic surgery, we suggest using dual prophylaxis with an antithrombotic agent and an IPCD during the hospital stay (grade 2C).
2.6	In patients undergoing major orthopaedic surgery who have an increased risk of bleeding, we suggest using an IPCD or no prophylaxis rather than pharmacologic treatment (grade 2C).
2.7	In patients undergoing major orthopaedic surgery and who decline or are uncooperative with injections or an IPCD, we recommend using apixaban or dabigatran (alternatively, rivaroxaban or adjusted-dose vitamin K antagonist if apixaban or dabigatran are unavailable) rather than alternative forms of prophylaxis (grade 1B).
2.8	In patients undergoing major orthopaedic surgery, we suggest against using inferior vena cava filter placement for primary prevention over no thromboprophylaxis in patients with an increased bleeding risk or contraindications to both pharmacologic and mechanical thromboprophylaxis (grade 2C).
2.9	For asymptomatic patients following major orthopaedic surgery, we recommend against Doppler (or duplex) ultrasound screening before hospital discharge (grade 1B).

IPCD = intermittent pneumatic compression device, LMWH = low-molecular-weight heparin, THA = total hip arthroplasty, TKA = total knee arthroplasty.

[a] Grades are based on certainty (grade 1) or uncertainty (grade 2) and the quality of studies used to make the recommendation (A for high-quality randomization, B for low-quality randomization, and C for observational or nonrandomized studies).

Adapted from Lieberman JR: Guest Editorial: American College of Chest Physicians evidence-based guidelines for venous thromboembolic prophylaxis: The guideline wars are over. *J Am Acad Orthop Surg* 2012;20(6):333-335.

activated thrombin inhibitors, pentasaccharides, and antiplatelet agents. Each of these classes has strengths and weaknesses, as well as limitations in data (**Table 3** and **Table 4**).

LOW-MOLECULAR-WEIGHT HEPARINS

LMWHs act by binding to antithrombin III, which induces a conformational change allowing antithrombin III to inactivate thrombin and factor Xa. Several trials have examined the efficacy of LMWHs in THA patients. The authors of one study evaluated the symptomatic PE and DVT rates in 3,011 patients undergoing THA who were randomized to receive either enoxaparin or warfarin. The rates of symptomatic DVT (warfarin 2.9% versus enoxaparin 2.6%) and symptomatic PE (warfarin 0.6% versus enoxaparin 0.4%) were similar in the two groups. However, the enoxaparin group had a higher rate of minor bleeding (warfarin 7.1% versus enoxaparin 9.4%; $P = 0.021$) and a higher rate of major bleeding that was not significant (warfarin 0.5% versus enoxaparin 1.2%; $P = 0.055$).

The advantage of LMWHs is that they do not require routine monitoring. However, LMWHs have several disadvantages: they require daily or twice daily injections and are associated with higher bleeding rates. LMWHs are administered via different doses and regimens. The most popular LMWH (enoxaparin) is administered as a daily 40-mg dose starting 12 hours preoperatively (European regimen) or as a 30-mg twice-daily dose beginning 12 to 24 hours postoperatively (North American regimen).

VITAMIN K ANTAGONISTS

Warfarin is commonly used by orthopaedic surgeons because of its historic track record and well-established efficacy in preventing VTE events in patients undergoing THA. Warfarin acts by preventing the carboxylation of glutamic acid residues on clotting factors II, VII, IX, and X and proteins C and S, thereby rendering them ineffective. Warfarin is administered orally and monitored through serial serum international normalized ratio (INR) values, with a target INR of 1.8 to 2.2. In general, warfarin is as effective as LMWH in preventing PE and death but has lower bleeding complication rates. However, warfarin is associated with numerous drug interactions and requires frequent monitoring.

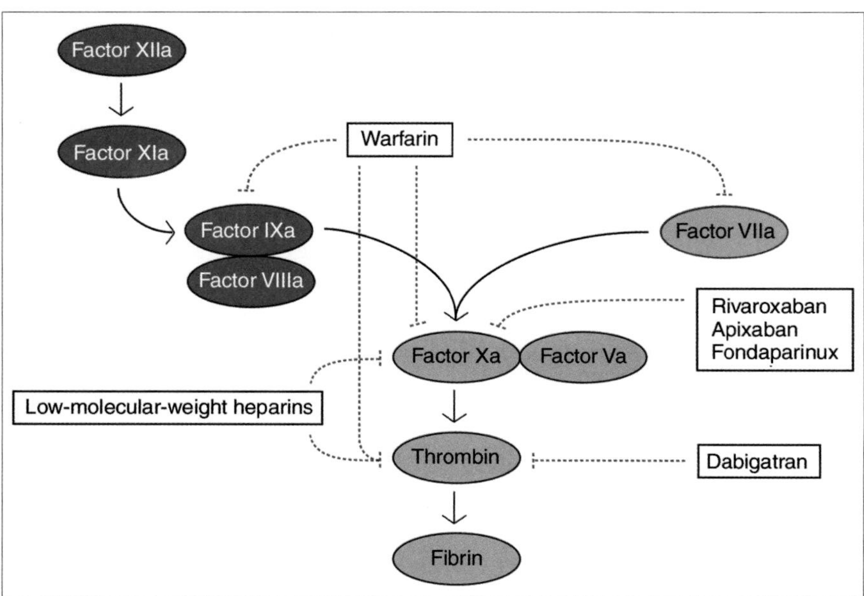

Figure 1 Diagram depicts the coagulation cascade and the pharmacologic targets of venous thromboembolic disease prophylaxis.

FACTOR XA ANTAGONISTS

Factor Xa antagonists have the advantage of not requiring routine blood monitoring or daily injections. Two factor Xa antagonists are approved for VTE prophylaxis in the United States: rivaroxaban and apixaban. A third agent, edoxaban, was recently approved by the FDA for the treatment of DVT and PE; however, phase III trials of this agent for VTE prophylaxis in THA patients have not been completed.

In one trial, 4,541 patients undergoing THA were randomized to receive rivaroxaban or enoxaparin. The composite end point, which consisted of symptomatic and asymptomatic DVT, nonfatal PE, and death from any cause, was observed in 1.1% of patients in the rivaroxaban group and 3.7% of patients in the enoxaparin group ($P <$ 0.001). No differences were found in minor bleeding events (5.8% for both) or major bleeding events (rivaroxaban 0.3% versus enoxaparin 0.1%). In a related study, 2,509 patients undergoing THA were randomized receive to a short course of enoxaparin (10 to 14 days) or an extended course of rivaroxaban (31 to 39 days). The composite end point of symptomatic and asymptomatic DVT, nonfatal PE, and death was observed in 2.0% of patients in the rivaroxaban group and 9.3% of patients in the enoxaparin group ($P < 0.0001$), with no significant differences in minor bleeding (rivaroxaban 6.5% versus enoxaparin 5.5%) or major bleeding (less than 0.1% for both).

In a different trial, 1,949 patients undergoing THA were randomized to receive apixaban or enoxaparin. The composite end point of symptomatic and asymptomatic DVT, nonfatal PE, and death was observed in 1.4% of patients in the apixaban group and 3.9% of patients in the enoxaparin group ($P < 0.001$), with no significant differences in minor bleeding (apixaban 4.1% versus enoxaparin 4.5%) or major bleeding (apixaban 0.8% versus enoxaparin 0.7%) observed.

The advantage of these two agents is that they can be ingested orally and do not require blood monitoring. However, the potential disadvantages include an increased risk of bleeding complications. For this reason, these agents usually are administered in an off-label fashion 18 to 24 hours postoperatively to reduce the risk of bleeding.

DIRECT THROMBIN INHIBITORS

Dabigatran is the only direct thrombin inhibitor available in the United States for the treatment of DVT and PE and for prophylaxis for primary THA. Dabigatran is also approved for the prevention of recurrent VTE in patients who have previously been treated for VTE. Like factor Xa inhibitors, direct thrombin inhibitors have the advantage of not requiring routine blood monitoring or daily injections.

Two large, multicenter trials assessing the efficacy and safety of dabigatran for VTE prophylaxis in patients undergoing THA have been published. One trial randomized 3,494 patients undergoing THA into groups treated with high-dose dabigatran (220 mg), low-dose dabigatran (150 mg), or enoxaparin. The rates of symptomatic VTE or PE events were 0.9% in the two dabigatran groups but only 0.4% in the enoxaparin group; however, this difference was not significant. Furthermore, no differences were found among the three groups in minor bleeding events (high-dose dabigatran, 6.1%; low-dose dabigatran, 6.2%; enoxaparin, 6.4%) or major bleeding events (high-dose dabigatran, 2.0%; low-dose dabigatran, 1.3%; enoxaparin, 1.6%). However, the study was not powered to detect symptomatic PE and DVT events. A subsequent trial randomized 2,055 patients undergoing THA into enoxaparin and oral dabigatran groups. Clinically relevant VTE events and death caused by VTE occurred in 2.2% of patients in the dabigatran group and 4.2% of patients in the enoxaparin group ($P = 0.03$). No significant differences were found in minor bleeding events (dabigatran 2.3% versus enoxaparin 2.0%) or major bleeding events (dabigatran 0.9% versus enoxaparin 1.4%) between the two groups.

Table 3 Summary of Anticoagulation Trials

Study (Authors; Year)	Agent	Duration (d)	Symptomatic Venous Thromboembolism (%)	Total Deep Vein Thrombosis (%)	Total Pulmonary Embolism (%)	Major Bleeding (%)
Colwell et al (1999)	Enoxaparin (30 mg bid)	7.5	3.6	3.2	1.0	1.2[a]
	Warfarin[b]	7	3.7	3.1	0.8	0.5[a]
RECORD 1 (Eriksson et al; 2008)	Enoxaparin (40 mg daily)	35	0.7	3.4[a]	0.1	0.1
	Rivaroxaban (10 mg daily)	35	0.3	0.8[a]	0.3	0.3
RECORD 2 (Kakkar et al; 2008)	Enoxaparin (40 mg daily)	10-14	1.2[a]	8.2[a]	0.5	<0.1
	Rivaroxaban (10 mg daily)	31-39	0.2[a]	1.6[a]	0.1	<0.1
ADVANCE 3 (Lassen et al; 2010)	Enoxaparin (40 mg daily)	35	0.4	3.6[a]	0.2	0.7
	Apixaban (2.5 mg bid)	35	0.1	1.1[a]	0.1	0.8
RE-NOVATE (Eriksson et al; 2007)	Enoxaparin (40 mg daily)	28-35	0.4	6.3	0.3	1.6
	Dabigatran (220 mg daily)	28-35	0.9	4.6	0.4	2.0
	Dabigatran (150 mg daily)	28-35	0.9	7.2	0.1	1.3
RE-NOVATE II (Eriksson et al; 2011)	Enoxaparin (40 mg daily)	28-35	0.6	8.6	0.2	0.9
	Dabigatran (220 mg daily)	28-35	0.1	7.6	0.1	1.4
EPHESUS (Lassen et al; 2002)	Enoxaparin (40 mg daily)	5-9	0.3	9.0[a]	0.2	2.6
	Fondaparinux (2.5 mg daily)	5-9	0.4	4.0[a]	0.2	4.1
PENTATHLON (Turpie et al; 2002)	Enoxaparin (30 mg bid)	5-9	0.1[a]	8.2[a]	0.1	1.0
	Fondaparinux (2.5 mg daily)	5-9	1.0[a]	5.6[a]	0.4	1.8

bid = twice per day.
[a] Significant difference.
[b] Dosing of warfarin with an international normalized ratio goal of 2 to 3.

Table 4 Dosing Regimens of Chemoprophylactic Agents

Drug	Dose	Route	Frequency
Warfarin	INR goal of 1.8-2.2	PO	Daily
Enoxaparin	30 or 40 mg	SC	Daily (40 mg) or bid (30 mg)
Rivaroxaban	10 mg	PO	Daily
Apixaban	2.5 mg	PO	bid
Dabigatran	150 mg	PO	bid
Fondaparinux	2.5 mg	SC	Daily
Aspirin	81 or 325 mg	PO	Daily or bid

bid = twice per day, INR = international normalized ratio, PO = orally, SC = subcutaneous.

PENTASACCHARIDES

Fondaparinux is a synthetic pentasaccharide that is an indirect inhibitor of factor Xa. Fondaparinux binds to antithrombin III, which enhances the ability of antithrombin III to limit factor Xa activity. In one trial, 2,309 patients undergoing THA were randomized to receive fondaparinux or enoxaparin. Mandatory venography was performed in every patient. A significant reduction in VTE events was observed in the fondaparinux group (fondaparinux 4% versus enoxaparin 9%; $P < 0.0001$). However, no significant differences were found in symptomatic DVT (fondaparinux 0.3% versus enoxaparin 0.1%) or PE (fondaparinux 0.2% versus enoxaparin 0.2%). Furthermore, no differences were found in major bleeding events (fondaparinux 4.1% versus enoxaparin 2.6%). In a different study, 2,275 patients were randomized to receive fondaparinux 2.5 mg daily or enoxaparin 30 mg twice daily. Significantly more symptomatic VTE events occurred in the fondaparinux group compared with the enoxaparin group (fondaparinux 1% versus enoxaparin 0.1%; $P < 0.0062$), but no difference was found in rates of minor bleeding (fondaparinux 1.5% versus enoxaparin 2.1%) or major bleeding (fondaparinux 1.8% versus enoxaparin 1.0%). Fondaparinux is FDA approved for use in the treatment of patients with hip fractures, but concerns regarding bleeding have limited its use in total joint arthroplasty patients.

ANTIPLATELET AGENTS

Aspirin is an oral agent that is commonly used for VTE prophylaxis after THA. In one trial, 13,356 patients with hip fractures and 4,088 patients undergoing elective hip or knee arthroplasty (2,648 hips and 1,440 knees) were randomized receive to aspirin or placebo in addition to standard VTE prophylaxis. The authors of the study observed a 34% decrease in DVTs and PEs in the aspirin group in pooled analysis, but subgroup analysis of elective arthroplasty patients did not demonstrate a benefit. The two groups had equivalent rates of DVT (aspirin 0.7% versus placebo 0.9%) and PE (0.4% in both groups). In a recent noninferiority trial, 786 patients undergoing THA were randomized to receive aspirin or dalteparin for 28 days after an initial 10-day course of dalteparin. The authors of the study did not observe a significant difference between the two groups in the incidence of VTE (aspirin 0.3% versus dalteparin 1.3%) or in the rates of minor bleeding (aspirin 2.1% versus dalteparin 4.5%) and major bleeding (aspirin 0.0% versus dalteparin 0.3%). However, enrollment in the study was terminated early, and thus it was inadequately powered to detect significant differences in VTE and bleeding rates.

Aspirin is probably a less powerful anticoagulant than other chemoprophylactic agents; however, it seems to be associated with a lower bleeding rate. Many THA patients may be appropriately treated with less intensive anticoagulation. The selection of a prophylactic agent requires a balance of efficacy and safety. Large, randomized trials evaluating symptomatic events and associated complications are needed to further assess the efficacy and safety of aspirin. Currently, aspirin should be combined with the use of mechanical compression devices while the patient is in the hospital.

Nonpharmacologic Prophylaxis

INTERMITTENT PNEUMATIC COMPRESSION DEVICES

Arthroplasty surgeons commonly use intermittent pneumatic compression devices (IPCDs) as an adjunct to chemoprophylaxis. The use of IPCDs as a solitary mode of VTE prophylaxis has seen renewed interest. IPCDs act by reducing venous stasis and increasing systemic fibrinolytic activity. Within 3 hours of application, IPCD use is associated with a substantial increase in systemic fibrinolytic activity. Types of IPCDs include thigh-high or knee-high devices and foot pumps. No difference in fibrinolytic activity has been observed among the various IPCDs. In addition, the pattern and type of compression vary among devices, and no consensus has been reached on the optimal compression system.

In a registry study, researchers evaluated the rates of symptomatic VTE events in 3,060 total knee arthroplasty and THA patients treated for at least 10 days with a mobile IPCD with or without aspirin (that is, aspirin was given at the surgeon's discretion). In the THA cohort, the observed DVT incidence was 0.33%, and the incidence of PE was 0.20%. The authors of the study compared the data with published results of studies evaluating agents such as warfarin, enoxaparin, rivaroxaban, and dabigatran and concluded that the mobile IPCD was noninferior.

In the most recent ACCP guidelines, mobile IPCDs were recommended as a sole method of VTE prophylaxis provided that they could be worn for at least 18 hours per day. The advantage of mobile compression is that it can be used while the patient is ambulating and can continue after the patient is discharged from the hospital. Concerns related to mobile IPCDs include patient compliance and device cost. In addition, the efficacy of these devices without aspirin supplementation has not been established.

OTHER NONPHARMACOLOGIC METHODS

Data are insufficient to support the routine use of inferior vena cava filters in patients undergoing THA. However, inferior vena cava filters are an option, particularly for patients with relative contraindications to chemoprophylaxis.

Regional anesthesia can be used to reduce the risk of blood loss. However, current evidence suggests that regional anesthesia does not reduce the risk of VTE events compared with general anesthesia.

Avoiding Pitfalls and Complications

Patients undergoing THA require VTE prophylaxis. Several safe and effective options are available. The orthopaedic surgeon should choose a regimen that prevents symptomatic VTE while limiting the risk of bleeding. Risk stratification is paramount because not all patients require the same degree of anticoagulation. Although risk stratification of patients requires further study, the general consensus is that patients with a history of DVT and PE require more intense anticoagulation and a prolonged duration of prophylaxis. The LMWHs rivaroxaban, apixaban, and dabigatran provide intense coagulation, and many surgeons will delay administration of these drugs until 18 to 24 hours after surgery. Warfarin has a delayed onset of action, and it is usually started the evening of the procedure. Aspirin use has increased since its acceptance in the ACCP guideline. Surgeons are interested in aspirin as a prophylaxis agent because it is an oral agent that requires no monitoring and it seems to have low bleeding rates. Additional study of aspirin is needed in randomized trials to determine its true efficacy with respect to the prevention of symptomatic VTE.

Bibliography

American Academy of Orthopaedic Surgeons: Preventing Venous Thromboembolic Disease in Patients Undergoing Elective Hip and Knee Arthroplasty: Evidence-Based Guideline and Evidence Report. Rosemont, IL, American Academy of Orthopaedic Surgeons, 2011. Available at: http://www.aaos.org/research/guidelines/VTE/VTE_guideline.asp. Accessed August 16, 2016.

Anderson DR, Dunbar MJ, Bohm ER, et al: Aspirin versus low-molecular-weight heparin for extended venous thromboembolism prophylaxis after total hip arthroplasty: A randomized trial. *Ann Intern Med* 2013;158(11):800-806.

Colwell CW Jr, Collis DK, Paulson R, et al: Comparison of enoxaparin and warfarin for the prevention of venous thromboembolic disease after total hip arthroplasty: Evaluation during hospitalization and three months after discharge. *J Bone Joint Surg Am* 1999;81(7):932-940.

Colwell CW Jr, Froimson MI, Anseth SD, et al: A mobile compression device for thrombosis prevention in hip and knee arthroplasty. *J Bone Joint Surg Am* 2014;96(3):177-183.

Eriksson BI, Borris LC, Friedman RJ, et al; RECORD1 Study Group: Rivaroxaban versus enoxaparin for thromboprophylaxis after hip arthroplasty. *N Engl J Med* 2008;358(26):2765-2775.

Eriksson BI, Dahl OE, Huo MH, et al; RE-NOVATE II Study Group: Oral dabigatran versus enoxaparin for thromboprophylaxis after primary total hip arthroplasty (RE-NOVATE II*): A randomised, double-blind, non-inferiority trial. *Thromb Haemost* 2011;105(4):721-729.

Eriksson BI, Dahl OE, Rosencher N, et al; RE-NOVATE Study Group: Dabigatran etexilate versus enoxaparin for prevention of venous thromboembolism after total hip replacement: A randomised, double-blind, non-inferiority trial. *Lancet* 2007;370(9591):949-956.

Falck-Ytter Y, Francis CW, Johanson NA, et al; American College of Chest Physicians: Prevention of VTE in orthopedic surgery patients: Antithrombotic therapy and prevention of thrombosis, 9th ed: American College of Chest Physicians evidence-based clinical practice guidelines. *Chest* 2012;141(2 suppl):e278S-e325S.

Kakkar AK, Brenner B, Dahl OE, et al; RECORD2 Investigators: Extended duration rivaroxaban versus short-term enoxaparin for the prevention of venous thromboembolism after total hip arthroplasty: A double-blind, randomised controlled trial. *Lancet* 2008;372(9632):31-39.

Lassen MR, Bauer KA, Eriksson BI, Turpie AG; European Pentasaccharide Elective Surgery Study (EPHESUS) Steering Committee: Postoperative fondaparinux versus preoperative enoxaparin for prevention of venous thromboembolism in elective hip-replacement surgery: A randomised double-blind comparison. *Lancet* 2002;359(9319):1715-1720.

Lassen MR, Gallus A, Raskob GE, Pineo G, Chen D, Ramirez LM; ADVANCE-3 Investigators: Apixaban versus enoxaparin for thromboprophylaxis after hip replacement. *N Engl J Med* 2010;363(26):2487-2498.

Lieberman JR: Editorial: American College of Chest Physicians evidence-based guidelines for venous thromboembolic prophylaxis: The guideline wars are over. *J Am Acad Orthop Surg* 2012;20(6):333-335.

Lieberman JR, Pensak MJ: Prevention of venous thromboembolic disease after total hip and knee arthroplasty. *J Bone Joint Surg Am* 2013;95(19):1801-1811.

Prevention of pulmonary embolism and deep vein thrombosis with low dose aspirin: Pulmonary Embolism Prevention (PEP) trial. *Lancet* 2000;355(9212):1295-1302.

Turpie AG, Bauer KA, Eriksson BI, Lassen MR; PENTATHLON 2000 Study Steering Committee: Postoperative fondaparinux versus postoperative enoxaparin for prevention of venous thromboembolism after elective hip-replacement surgery: A randomised double-blind trial. *Lancet* 2002;359(9319):1721-1726.

SECTION 4
Revision Total Hip Arthroplasty
Jay R. Lieberman, MD

Chapter 40
Revision Total Hip Arthroplasty: Indications and Contraindications

Craig J. Della Valle, MD
Erdan Kayupov, MSE
Aaron G. Rosenberg, MD

Indications

The term indications carries a sense of certainty rarely present in surgical scenarios. Particularly in revision surgery, indications represent the end point of a complex decision-making process that involves both the surgeon and the patient. Currently, the most common indications for revision total hip arthroplasty (THA) in the United States are recurrent instability, aseptic implant loosening, and periprosthetic joint infection. Other common reasons for revision surgery are osteolysis, bearing surface wear, and periprosthetic fracture. Recently, an increasing number of patients seek treatment for failed implants, recalled implants, or pain secondary to metal-on-metal bearings and corrosion-related problems. Familiarity with the nuances of these diagnoses is critical for surgeons who perform revision THA.

The first step in determining whether a revision procedure is indicated is establishing a clear diagnosis and mode of failure. In some patients the diagnosis may be obvious, whereas in other patients establishing a firm diagnosis can be challenging. The surgeon should make every effort to determine a clear diagnosis before surgical treatment and avoid exploratory surgery. A clear diagnosis and understanding of the mechanism of failure will greatly facilitate planning for the revision THA and increase the likelihood of a successful outcome.

In some patients, the severity of the symptoms and the extent of the identified pathology guide the decision-making process. This situation is particularly true in patients with bearing surface wear and/or osteolysis, in whom decision making can be complex. The age and activity level of a patient and the track record of the existing implants are important considerations.

Aseptic Loosening

Aseptic loosening can pose challenges in determining appropriate indications for revision THA. The principal indication for revision THA in a patient with aseptic loosening is pain. Pain associated with loosening usually occurs with weight bearing and often is particularly intense when a patient stands from a resting position and begins to walk (start-up pain). Loose acetabular implants typically cause groin or buttock pain, whereas loose stems usually cause thigh pain. However, these findings are not absolute. A patient must understand that revision THA may not relieve all hip pain from a failed THA. Additionally, marked bone loss, particularly progressive bone loss or bone loss occurring in locations that predispose a patient to periprosthetic fracture, is a strong indication for revision THA.

Aseptic loosening can create functional disability related to pain or altered biomechanics of a failed implant, which may be an indication for revision THA. Hip biomechanics can be adversely affected when loose implants migrate, leading to poorer abductor function or limb shortening. However, a patient must be counseled that precise restoration of leg lengths may not occur in revision THA and that improvements in gait may require extended time,

Dr. Della Valle or an immediate family member has received royalties from Zimmer Biomet; serves as a paid consultant to DePuy Synthes, Smith & Nephew, and Zimmer Biomet; has stock or stock options held in CD Diagnostics; has received research or institutional support from CD Diagnostics, Smith & Nephew, Stryker, and Zimmer Biomet; and serves as a board member, owner, officer, or committee member of the American Association of Hip and Knee Surgeons, the Arthritis Foundation, The Hip Society, The Knee Society, and the Mid-America Orthopaedic Association. Dr. Rosenberg or an immediate family member has received royalties from, is a member of a speakers' bureau or has made paid presentations on behalf of, serves as a paid consultant to, and has stock or stock options held in Zimmer Biomet. Neither Mr. Kayupov nor any immediate family member has received anything of value from or has stock or stock options held in a commercial company or institution related directly or indirectly to the subject of this chapter.

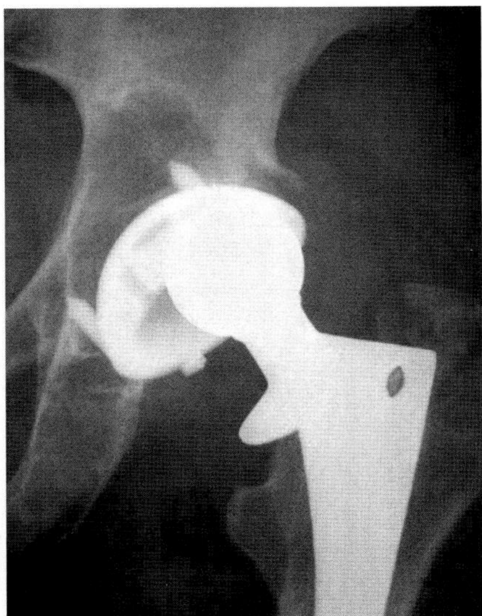

Figure 1 AP radiograph of a left hip demonstrates severe polyethylene wear and associated osteolysis.

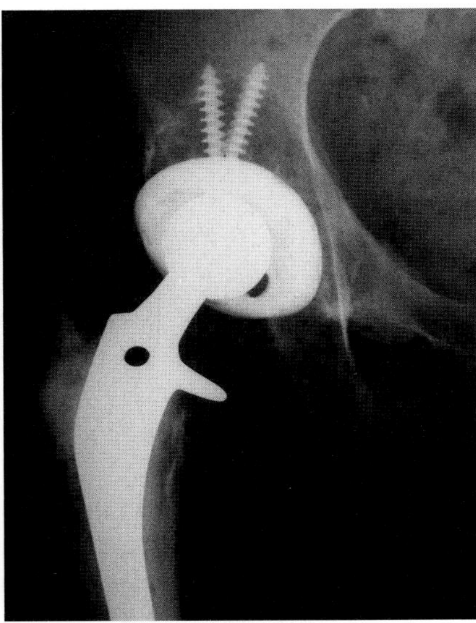

Figure 2 AP radiograph of the right hip of an 86-year-old woman with a 2-month history of groin pain obtained 6 months after total hip arthroplasty demonstrates a healing stress fracture of the superior pubic ramus.

particularly if abductor muscle strength is poor preoperatively.

Bone loss associated with aseptic loosening also can be an indication for revision. Aseptic loosening often causes bone loss as a result of mechanical bone erosion or particulate debris–induced osteolysis. Bone loss associated with implant loosening tends to be progressive, but the rate at which the bone loss occurs varies. Grossly loose sockets tend to cause relatively rapid acetabular bone erosion, and rough surface finish stems that debond from cement have been reported to cause more rapid osteolysis. Conversely, bone loss usually is slow in patients with loose, noncemented stems. Regardless of the rate at which bone loss occurs, bone loss may be an indication for revision THA, depending on a patient's specific circumstances.

Bearing Surface Complications

The decision-making process in the management of bearing surface wear and osteolysis can be complex. Specifically, in younger patients with severe wear and osteolysis (**Figure 1**), the decision to perform revision THA is relatively straightforward. In older and less active patients, particularly those with milder wear and osteolysis, the decision making can be far more complex. In general, the authors of this chapter attempt to educate patients regarding the risks and benefits of intervention to allow them to assist in the decision-making process.

Diagnosis and treatment decisions are even more complex in the common scenario in which a patient has osteolysis associated with well-fixed implants but does not have substantial hip pain. Pain is thought to be attributable to a painful effusion and synovitis or, in some patients, related to a periacetabular or peritrochanteric stress fracture through an osteolytic lesion. Decision making may be further complicated if radiographically evident bearing surface wear is not associated with osteolysis. In general, impending wear through or fracture of the polyethylene bearing surface should prompt consideration of revision THA within a relatively short time frame (approximately 6 months), and full-thickness wear through or fracture of the polyethylene liner should prompt an urgent revision THA to avoid secondary metallosis.

Similarly, breakage of a ceramic head or liner should prompt an urgent revision THA to avoid dispersion of the ceramic particles throughout the hip joint and secondary damage to the femoral implant taper. In patients in whom breakage of a ceramic head or liner has occurred, strong consideration should be given to removal of the acetabular implant to facilitate debris removal. Removal of the femoral implant should be considered if gross damage to the modular taper is encountered. Even if performed correctly by a highly experienced surgeon, revision THA after fracture of a ceramic head or liner tends to result in poor outcomes.

Decision making in patients with a failed metal-on-metal bearing or modular junction corrosion can be complex. Damage to the surrounding soft tissues, particularly the abductor musculature, should be avoided at all costs, and early revision THA should be strongly considered to avoid this situation. Similarly, even apparently mild periarticular osteolysis should be evaluated thoroughly because it may be a harbinger of an aggressive process.

Evaluation

In evaluating a patient with a painful THA, the surgeon should consider diagnoses both intrinsic and extrinsic to the hip joint. The most common intrinsic etiologies include infection, implant loosening, and problems related to the bearing surface. Extrinsic etiologies include stress fractures of the pubic ramus and local problems such as soft-tissue bursitis or tendinitis (**Figure 2**). Remote extrinsic causes of hip pain include lumbar spine disease, peripheral nerve entrapment (such as meralgia paresthetica, which can occur with anterior approaches to the hip), vascular claudication, hernias, and pain referred from intra-abdominal or pelvic pathology.

History and Physical Examination

Evaluation should begin with a thorough history and physical examination. The history should include an assessment of pain severity and the frequency and degree of disability resulting from the pain. In addition, a thorough understanding of the activities that cause and relieve the pain should be sought. The surgeon must obtain an assessment of a patient's risk factors for deep infection, including a history of wound-healing problems, antibiotic administration, or returns to the operating room. An important question that may help guide the evaluation is whether the existing pain is the same as or different from the pain the patient experienced before THA was performed.

The physical examination should include an assessment of previous incisions and the quality of the surrounding skin. Hip range of motion and maneuvers that provoke pain are important to note. Evaluation should include gait, abductor strength, relative leg length, and a general assessment of the lumbar spine and the neurovascular status of the extremity to help identify extrinsic causes of pain. Careful palpation around the hip may yield important clues by suggesting diagnoses such as bursitis and tendinitis; pain with resisted motion may confirm the diagnosis. A cursory examination of the abdomen and groin is helpful. Quantifying functional disability can be more complex, and functional problems are less often associated with reliable indications for revision THA. These problems include hip stiffness, limb-length discrepancy, and persistent limp.

Radiography

Obtaining plain radiographs is the next step in evaluation. The surgeon also should review radiographs obtained before THA. Evidence of minimal pathology suggests either an incorrect diagnosis that led to the original THA or a patient who may tend to be dissatisfied with surgical outcomes. Specifically, patients who exhibit minimal preoperative pathology may have high expectations that cannot be met or a lower pain threshold, or the amount of incremental improvement possible with THA may not be enough to lead to satisfaction. These patients also may have underlying soft-tissue disorders, such as fibromyalgia, or may have depression or other psychosocial disorders that may affect their response to surgical intervention.

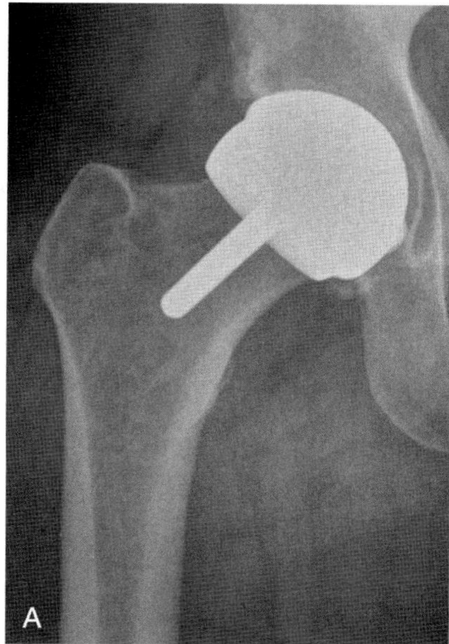

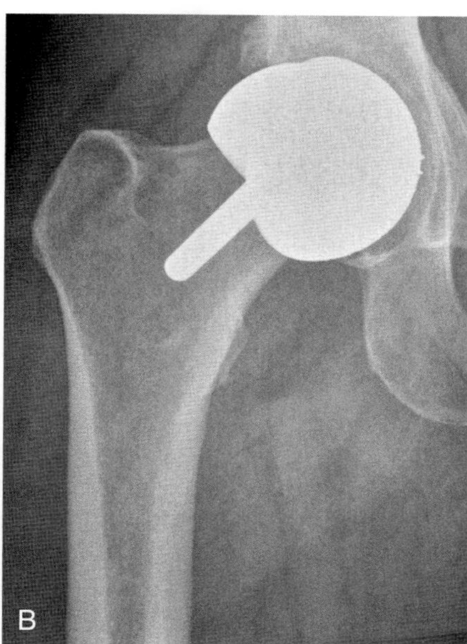

Figure 3 AP radiographs of the right hip of a patient with a painful hip resurfacing obtained 6 weeks (**A**) and 9 months (**B**) postoperatively demonstrate clear migration of the acetabular implant, which is consistent with loosening.

Careful review of plain radiographs is important for identification of implant loosening. Although definitive signs of loosening, such as obvious implant migration; breakage; or, in patients with cemented implants, cement fracture, may be obvious, the use of sequential radiographs, particularly comparison of current radiographs with an immediate or early postoperative radiograph, is typically most useful (**Figure 3**). Plain radiographs also are useful for identifying osteolysis; however, comparison over time and with the initial postoperative radiographs is important because arthritic cysts can mimic areas of osteolysis (**Figure 4**). Periprosthetic fractures and fractures of the trochanter or pubis also can be recognized. Although periosteal changes are unusual, in some patients periosteal changes may suggest chronic periprosthetic infection.

Assessment of implant positioning is an important step in evaluation. In some patients, implant malposition is obvious and points clearly to the diagnosis (**Figure 5**). In other patients, malposition may be more subtle. Specifically, appropriate acetabular implant anteversion can be difficult to differentiate from retroversion unless a shoot-through lateral radiograph is obtained (**Figure 6**). CT can help confirm the anteversion of the cup and stem. This evaluation can be useful because preoperative identification of the need for revision of the femoral implant can greatly change the surgical plan owing to the complexity of removing most well-fixed stems.

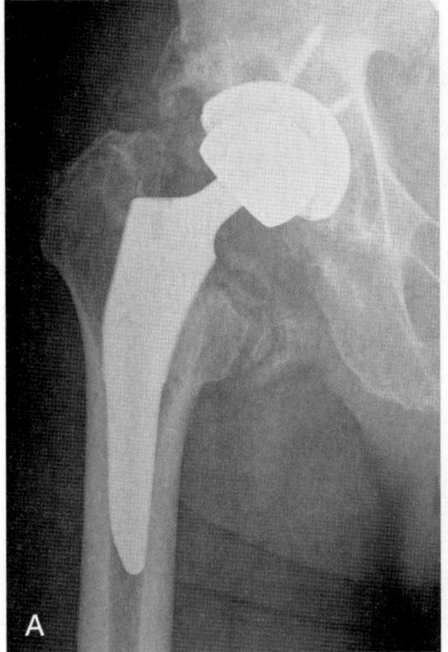

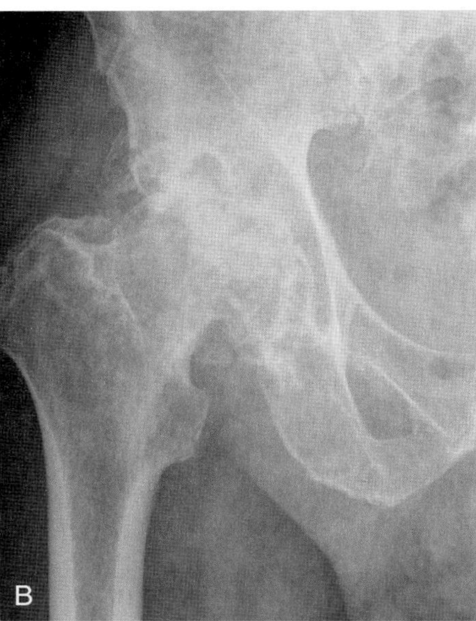

Figure 4 AP radiographs of the right hip of a 63-year-old man. **A,** Radiograph obtained 5 years after total hip arthroplasty (THA) demonstrates that an area of osteolysis may be present in the dome of the acetabulum. However, a preoperative radiograph demonstrates that the patient had an arthritic cyst before he underwent THA (**B**).

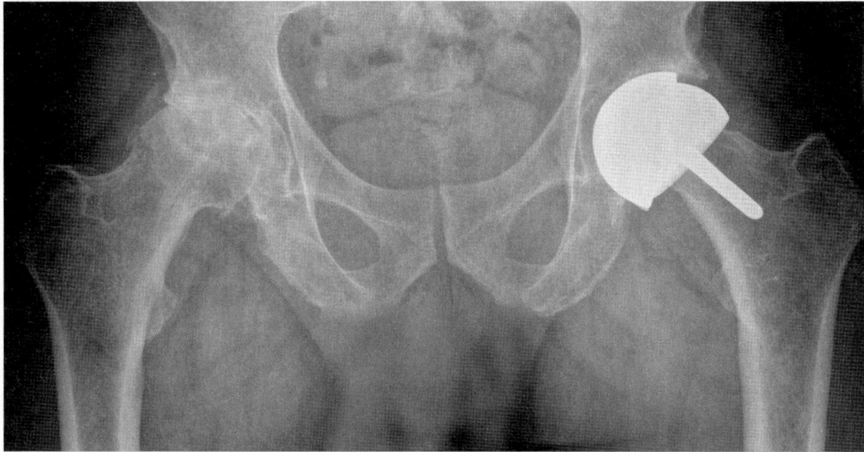

Figure 5 AP pelvic radiograph demonstrates a vertical acetabular implant in a patient who experienced pain after hip resurfacing. This finding raised suspicion for accelerated wear of the metal-on-metal bearing surface and an adverse local tissue reaction.

Acetabular retroversion may predispose a patient to not only instability but also iliopsoas impingement; iliopsoas impingement may be managed effectively with acetabular implant revision.

Serum Laboratory Testing

In general, initial laboratory testing is limited to assessment of the erythrocyte sedimentation rate and C-reactive protein level as an initial screen for infection. If these values are abnormal or if the clinical suspicion for infection is high, the hip should be aspirated and the fluid sent for analysis of synovial white blood cell count and polymorphonuclear neutrophil percentage and for culture. Other relevant laboratory testing may include determination of serum metal levels if failure of a metal-on-metal bearing or corrosion is suspected. Serum metal testing is complex, and the use of a reliable laboratory is critical. Serum metal levels must be evaluated in the context of the entire clinical scenario and rarely should be relied on as the sole indication for revision THA.

An assessment of a patient's general health also is important in deciding whether revision surgery is advisable. Elective surgery may be unwise in patients who have severe metabolic abnormalities. For example, uncontrolled diabetes mellitus, evidenced by elevated serum glucose and/or elevated hemoglobin A1C levels, may increase a patient's risk for periprosthetic joint infection and thromboembolic events, and a clinician may suggest that glucose control be improved before elective surgery is performed. Malnutrition, evidenced by hypoalbuminemia, an abnormal transferrin, or total lymphocyte count, greatly increased the risk of periprosthetic joint infection after aseptic revision procedures in one recent study, and a clinician may consider delaying surgical treatment until these values are normalized. Anemia can be a harbinger of poor health and increase a patient's risk for several perioperative complications. Evaluation of the cause of preoperative anemia may help mitigate risk.

Advanced Imaging

In some patients, advanced imaging studies may help determine the diagnosis or guide management. CT is commonly used to evaluate the presence and extent of osteolysis. In most patients, the surgeon can assume that osteolysis present on plain radiographs will appear more extensive on a CT scan. CT often is useful to confirm the anteversion of an acetabular cup, which can be difficult to objectively assess intraoperatively. The anteversion of a stem can be determined by obtaining a CT scan of the epicondylar axis of the ipsilateral knee, which is overlaid on the measured version of the femoral implant (**Figure 7**). Because postoperative instability is the most common complication of THA, precise knowledge of implant version is extremely helpful for preoperative decision making and planning in not only patients with hip instability but also patients with wear and osteolysis. Although femoral version can be determined intraoperatively with relative ease, acetabular implant positioning can be much more difficult to determine.

CT may be useful for preoperative planning in patients requiring complex revision procedures, such as those in whom pelvic discontinuity is suspected. Three-dimensional reconstruction can be helpful in patients in whom pelvic discontinuity is suspected, although shoot-through lateral radiographs also can be helpful in determining the integrity of the posterior column (as can other radiographic indicators of pelvic discontinuity, including the presence of a transverse fracture line and asymmetry of the obturator foramen on AP pelvic radiographs). Although the use of CT to determine if an implant that is loose has been reported, these results have not been reproduced; therefore, CT is not recommended for this purpose. Similarly, no data have been published on the utility of CT for the diagnosis of periprosthetic joint infection.

Advances in computer software have enabled the routine use of metal-artifact reduction sequence (MARS) MRI at many institutions, allowing for soft-tissue visualization around a THA prosthesis. MARS MRI has been used most extensively for evaluating adverse local tissue reactions associated with metal-on-metal bearings or corrosion. At some institutions, ultrasonography is used as an alternative. Soft-tissue destruction, particularly of the abductor musculature, is a strong indication for timely revision THA to prevent additional irreversible damage to the abductor musculature, which would likely have long-term consequences on a patient's gait pattern, ability to ambulate, and risk for dislocation. MARS MRI also has been used for evaluation of disorders such as iliopsoas tendinitis, with ultrasonography again used as an alternative. Little evidence supports MRI as a useful tool for evaluating infection.

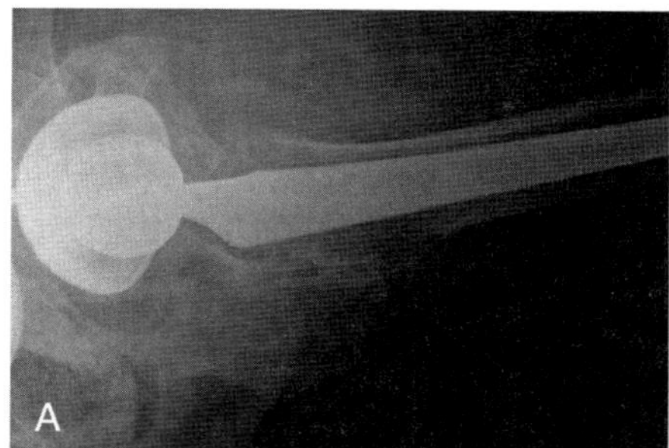

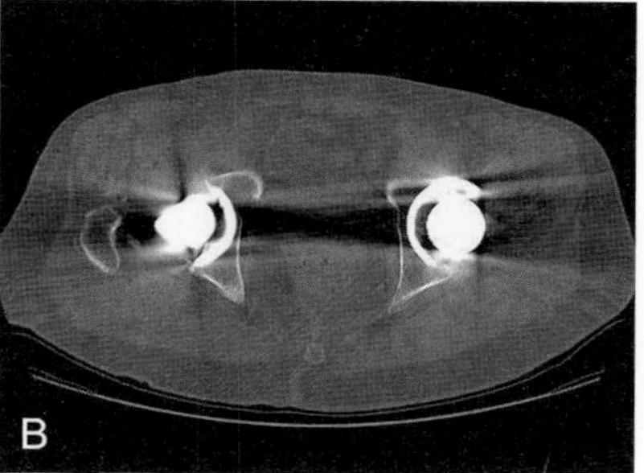

Figure 6 Images of the hip of a patient who sustained several posterior dislocations. **A,** Shoot-through lateral radiograph suggests retroversion of the acetabular implant. **B,** Axial CT scan confirms retroversion of the acetabular cup.

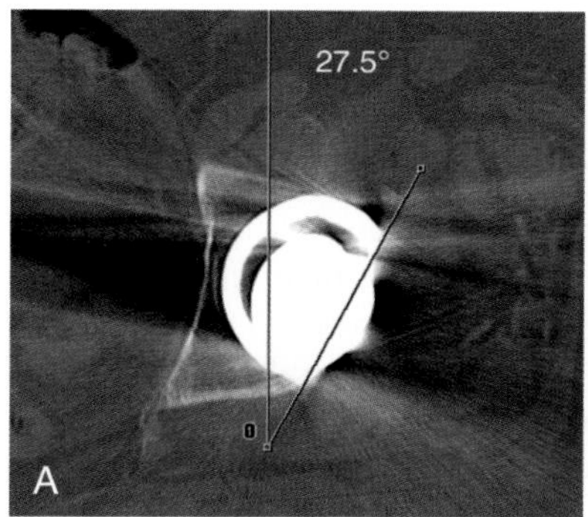

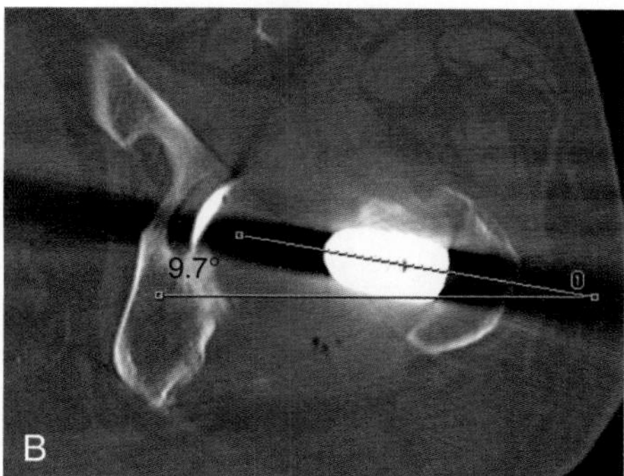

Figure 7 **A,** Axial CT scan of a hip demonstrates retroversion of the acetabular implant. **B,** Axial CT scan of the same hip demonstrates appropriate anteversion of the femoral stem by overlaying the epicondylar axis of the knee onto the image.

Historically, nuclear medicine studies were used extensively, but they have a more limited role in contemporary practice. The most commonly used test is technetium Tc-99m bone scanning, with increased periprosthetic activity suggestive of implant loosening. Bone scanning is useful in the diagnosis of stress fractures (such as of the pubic symphysis), which can be a cause of groin pain after THA. However, this test is nonspecific, most likely is not reliable within 2 years postoperatively, and cannot differentiate septic from aseptic failure. If infection is suspected, an indium In-111–labeled leukocyte scan is most commonly used; however, this test is susceptible to false-positive results, and, therefore, a negative result is most useful. Aspiration of the hip joint has overall better diagnostic utility because of the ability to obtain cultures and synovial fluid white blood cell count and differential. Therefore, indium In-111–labeled leukocyte scanning is rarely used and only in patients in whom aspiration was unsuccessful.

Periarticular Injections

Periarticular injections with a local anesthetic agent can help determine if revision THA is warranted in a patient who has pain after THA. Often, soft-tissue conditions, such as trochanteric bursitis, can cause lateral hip pain. In most patients, this common postoperative

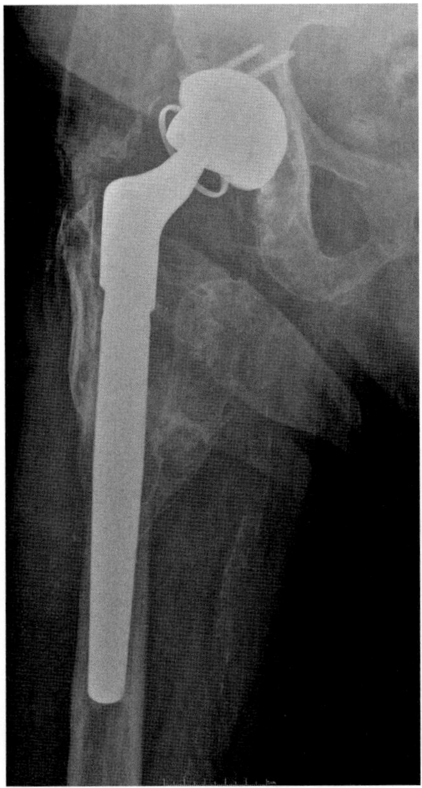

Figure 8 AP radiograph of the right hip of an elderly patient who underwent multiple prior revision total hip arthroplasties. Because of the complexity of removing the well-fixed implant and the challenges of attempting another reconstruction, nonsurgical management of her periprosthetic joint infection was attempted.

complaint responds to nonsurgical management. An injection into the area often can confirm the diagnosis, which is suspected based on reports of lateral hip pain combined with physical examination findings of pain on direct palpation at the base of the trochanter and with resisted hip abduction.

Similarly, iliopsoas tendinitis can cause groin pain and is suggested by reproduction of the pain with resisted hip flexion. In most patients with iliopsoas tendinitis, the condition occurs 6 months to 2 years postoperatively and typically responds to nonsurgical management. However, in some patients iliopsoas tendinitis is recalcitrant and may require release, or it is associated with contact between the iliopsoas tendon and a retroverted or oversized acetabular implant that overhangs the anterior wall of the acetabulum. In patients who have iliopsoas tendinitis, revision THA and reorientation of the acetabular implant to lie behind the anterior wall of the acetabulum may be indicated.

An intra-articular local anesthetic injection can potentially be used to differentiate intra-articular pathology (such as implant loosening) from extra-articular pathology that would not benefit from revision THA. In theory, an intra-articular local anesthetic injection should temporarily relieve an intra-articular cause of pain. Although intra-articular local anesthetic injection is more common after total knee arthroplasty than after THA and its use has little support in the literature, the authors of this chapter have found it to occasionally be useful in practice.

Contraindications

Revision THA usually is not indicated unless a specific problem that can be solved with revision THA is identified. Exploratory surgery is discouraged, and the revision surgeon should seek an appropriate diagnosis and devise a specific strategy and surgical plan to remedy the problem. Revision THA is contraindicated if a patient has medical comorbidities that would make an elective procedure unreasonably risky. In some patients, the orthopaedic risks of revision THA may outweigh the potential benefits, although these situations are rare. One example from the authors' experience is an elderly patient who underwent multiple prior THA revisions and had a Paprosky type 4 femur with a well-fixed stem and a constrained liner that became infected (**Figure 8**). Removal of the implant would have been risky for the patient in terms of extended surgical time and blood loss, and additional reconstruction would have been exceedingly difficult. In patients in whom elective orthopaedic surgery would be risky because of the presence of medical comorbidities, a trial of attempted antibiotic suppression and close observation may be a better course of action than revision THA.

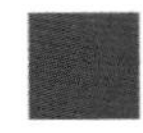

Alternative Treatments

The main alternative to revision THA is ongoing observation. Oral analgesic agents and gait aids can reduce pain and improve function in some patients sufficiently to avoid the need for revision THA. Nonsurgical management of a failing THA should not be considered if further bone loss, functional disability, and a reduced likelihood of successful revision THA are potential sequelae.

Decision Making

Medical decision making requires consideration of the potential risks and benefits of a particular intervention followed by comparisons with other potential courses of action. A simple risk-benefit ratio can be considered by evaluating the sum of all potential medical and surgical risks faced by a patient. Medical risks are best determined by a patient's internist, who is likely to be familiar with the physiologic burden that would be imposed on the patient by revision THA. In some situations, a surgeon must describe these burdens so that an internist can accurately assess the medical risks involved. The general and specific surgical risks, accounting for the specific features of the pathology, the required reconstruction, and the skills of the surgical team, are added to the medical risks.

The presence of substantial comorbidities may preclude surgical intervention in all but the most incapacitated of patients. The risks of perioperative mortality must be carefully weighed against the expected functional improvement and pain relief that can be expected with any type of surgical intervention.

An underlying assumption in most surgical decision making, predicated on the relative unpredictability of surgical outcomes, particularly in the elective setting, is that nonsurgical treatment should be attempted first. Nonsurgical treatment may consist of assistive devices for ambulation, weight loss, systemic or local medications, and physical therapy and activity modification in an effort to make symptoms more tolerable.

Although the degree of functional disability, level of activity, and associated symptoms vary by patient and diagnosis, assessment of these factors can help determine whether revision THA has the potential to eliminate or minimize symptoms. In some patients, the symptoms, physical findings, and radiographic changes are severe enough that revision THA is indicated. If revision THA is indicated for currently asymptomatic problems (eg, progressive osteolysis or accelerated polyethylene wear), the surgeon must explain to the patient why surgical treatment is recommended even though it will not relieve symptoms or improve function and carries substantial potential risks and complications. All interventions must be evaluated in the context of a patient's overall health and expectations.

Bibliography

Abernathy CM, Hamm RM: *Surgical Intuition: What It Is and How to Get It.* Philadelphia, PA, Hanley & Belfus, 1995.

Baron J: *Thinking and Deciding,* ed 3. Cambridge, United Kingdom, Cambridge University Press, 2000.

Bozic KJ, Kurtz SM, Lau E, Ong K, Vail TP, Berry DJ: The epidemiology of revision total hip arthroplasty in the United States. *J Bone Joint Surg Am* 2009;91(1):128-133.

Bozic KJ, Rubash HE: The painful total hip replacement. *Clin Orthop Relat Res* 2004;(420):18-25.

Della Valle C, Parvizi J, Bauer TW, et al; American Academy of Orthopaedic Surgeons: American Academy of Orthopaedic Surgeons clinical practice guideline on the diagnosis of periprosthetic joint infections of the hip and knee. *J Bone Joint Surg Am* 2011;93(14):1355-1357.

Eddy DM: *Clinical Decision Making: From Theory to Practice. A Collection of Essays from the Journal of the American Medical Association.* Sudbury, MA, Jones & Bartlett, 1996.

Mahomed NN, Barrett JA, Katz JN, et al: Rates and outcomes of primary and revision total hip replacement in the United States Medicare population. *J Bone Joint Surg Am* 2003;85(1):27-32.

Riegelman RK: *Minimizing Medical Mistakes: The Art of Medical Decision Making.* Boston, MA, Little, Brown, 1991.

Schwartz S, Griffin T: *Medical Thinking: The Psychology of Medical Judgment and Decision Making.* New York, NY, Springer-Verlag, 1986.

Wera GD, Ting NT, Moric M, Paprosky WG, Sporer SM, Della Valle CJ: Classification and management of the unstable total hip arthroplasty. *J Arthroplasty* 2012;27(5):710-715.

Yi PH, Frank RM, Vann E, Sonn KA, Moric M, Della Valle CJ: Is potential malnutrition associated with septic failure and acute infection after revision total joint arthroplasty? *Clin Orthop Relat Res* 2015;473(1):175-182.

Chapter 41
Revision Total Hip Arthroplasty: Preoperative Planning

Jay R. Lieberman, MD
Daniel J. Berry, MD

Preoperative planning is essential to the success of revision total hip arthroplasty (THA). These complex procedures require the surgeon to know what implants are in place, have the proper extraction instruments available for use if the implants will be removed, and have compatible matching trial and final implants available for use. Preoperative planning helps the surgeon evaluate patterns of bone loss, anticipate the need for special implants or bone grafts, and anticipate whether alternative implants and materials might be needed as a result of intraoperative findings. Perhaps most importantly, good preoperative planning involves a mental rehearsal of the proposed procedure by the surgeon; this rehearsal can help the surgeon work efficiently after the procedure begins. Numerous important considerations should be included in preoperative planning for revision THA. A preoperative checklist or worksheet for revision THA can help the surgeon organize surgical needs.

1. Ensure that the patient has undergone adequate medical evaluation.
   Does the patient's medical status allow a major reconstructive procedure?
   Does the patient have a history of deep vein thrombosis or pulmonary embolism?
   Is the patient being treated with an anticoagulant or an antiplatelet agent on a chronic basis?
   Has the anticoagulant been stopped and has the patient's coagulation status normalized sufficiently for surgical treatment? Should the antiplatelet agent be stopped, and if so, when?

2. Understand the mechanism(s) by which the previous hip arthroplasty failed.
   Will correction of the problem that led to failure of the previous hip arthroplasty be possible?

3. Determine whether the arthroplasty is infected.
   Are the erythrocyte sedimentation rate and C-reactive protein level normal? If not, has the hip joint been aspirated?
   What are the results of hip aspiration?
   What are the cell count and percentage of neutrophils?
   What are the culture results?

4. Understand what implants are in place and determine their design and size.
   Have you reviewed the previous surgical reports?
   Do you have copies of the implant labels that were placed in the medical record at the time of the patient's previous surgical procedure(s)?

Dr. Lieberman or an immediate family member has received royalties from DePuy Synthes; serves as a paid consultant to or is an employee of Arthrex and DePuy Synthes; has stock or stock options held in Hip Innovation Technology; has received research or institutional support from Arthrex; and serves as a board member, owner, officer, or committee member of the American Academy of Orthopaedic Surgeons and the Western Orthopaedic Association. Dr. Berry or an immediate family member has received royalties from DePuy Synthes; serves as a paid consultant to DePuy Synthes; has received research or institutional support from DePuy Synthes; and serves as a board member, owner, officer, or committee member of the American Joint Replacement Registry, the Hip Society, and the Mayo Clinic.

5. Ensure that adequate, good-quality radiographs are available.
   Do the radiographs show enough of the femur?
   Are any special radiographs (Judet views) or three-dimensional imaging studies such as CT or MRI needed?

6. Template the hip radiographs.
   Do you know the magnification of the hip radiographs?
   What type of socket do you plan to place? What socket diameter?
   What type of femoral implant do you plan to place? Do you need a modular stem? What stem diameter and stem length are needed?

7. Ensure that optimal perioperative systemic and local-delivery antibiotics are available.
   Do you have optimal antibiotics for systemic perioperative coverage, with the patient's allergies or any previous infections taken into account?
   Do you have antibiotic-loaded cement available for use if needed?

8. Consider which implants will be removed and which will be retained; determine what compatible implants may be needed.
   If the metal socket will be retained, do you have compatible liners available?
   Will you cement a different liner into a retained metal socket?
   If the socket and femoral implant will be retained, do you have compatible femoral head sizes available to match the socket?
   If the femoral implant will be retained, do you have compatible modular heads and trial heads available to match it?
   If you plan to place a ceramic femoral head on an existing taper, do you have compatible ceramic heads with a titanium adapter sleeve?

9. Consider the surgical approach.
   What exposure will help you best remove the implant and cement?
   What exposure will you need to place new implants?
   What exposure will optimize hip stability?
   Will an osteotomy be required? Do you have wires or cables available to repair the osteotomy site?

10. Consider what special instruments are needed for implant or cement removal.
    Do you need special curved gouges of specific sizes to remove a noncemented socket?
    Do you have hand instruments available for cement removal?
    Do you need special power instruments? Metal-cutting instruments? Trephines? High-speed burrs? Ultrasonic cement-removal instruments?
    Do you need manufacturer-specific or implant-specific extraction devices for the acetabular polyethylene liner, the acetabular screws, the acetabular implant, and the femoral implant?

11. Consider what your options will be in the event that the first choice of implants cannot be used intraoperatively.
    What are your first and second alternative choices for acetabular reconstruction?
    What are your first and second alternative choices for femoral reconstruction?

12. Consider what options will be available for use in case of intraoperative complications.
    Do you have implants to manage unexpected bone fracture?

13. Evaluate bone loss and management.
    Do you anticipate the need for porous metal augments?
    Will a cage or cup-cage construct be needed?
    Do you anticipate needing acetabular bone grafts? Particulate grafts? Bulk grafts?
    Do you anticipate needing femoral bone grafts? Strut grafts? Particulate grafts? Large-segment grafts?
    Do you have all potentially necessary bone grafts readily available?

14. Evaluate the need for internal fixation devices.
    Is there evidence of pelvic discontinuity?
    Will pelvic reconstruction plates be needed for the management of pelvic discontinuity?
    Will screws be needed to fix a bulk acetabular graft?
    Will cables or wires be needed for femoral cerclage?
    Will femoral plates be needed?
    Will you need special trochanteric fixation devices? Claw plates? Hook plates? Wire mesh?

15. Consider how you will manage intraoperative hip instability if it is present.
    Do you need extra-large-diameter femoral heads and matching acetabular liners of extra-large inside diameter?
    Do you need constrained acetabular implants or dual-mobility implants?

16. Consider blood replacement needs.
    Would intraoperative blood salvage be of value?

17. Will a postoperative abduction brace be necessary?

18. What type venous thromboembolism prophylaxis will be used? What will be the duration?

19. Consider the patient's postoperative needs.
    Do you need to arrange a bed in the intensive care unit?
    Do you need social services for postdischarge planning?

Revision Total Hip Arthroplasty (THA) Checklist

1. Patient Name: ______________________ 2. Patient ID Number: ______________

3. Sex: M F 4. Date of Birth: ____________ 5. Date of Planned Procedure: ____________

6. Primary Diagnosis (Original THA): ______________________

7. Secondary Diagnosis (Planned Procedure): ______________________

8. Procedure: Acetabulum: ______________________

Femur: ______________________

9. Implants in Place: Acetabulum: ______________________

Type/Company: ______________________

Femur: ______________________

Type/Company: ______________________

10. Acetabular Shell Revision: Yes No

If no: Polyethylene Liner Exchange: Option 1: ______________________

Type/Company: ______________________

Option 2: ______________________

Type/Company: ______________________

If yes: Procedure: ______________________

Implant Selection: Option 1: ______________________

Type/Company: ______________________

Option 2: ______________________

Type/Company: ______________________

Option 3: ______________________

Type/Company: ______________________

Porous metal augments: Yes No Type/Company: ______________________

Bone Grafts Morcellized: Yes No

Structural Graft: Yes No

Structural Graft Options:

Distal Femur: Yes No

Femoral Head: Yes No

Other: ______________________

Cage: Yes No Type/Company: ______________________

Cemented cup: Yes No Type/Company: ______________________

11. Femoral Stem Revision: Yes No

If No: Femoral Head Exchange (Type/Company): ______________________

If Yes: Procedure: ______________________

Implant selection: Option 1: ______________________

Type/Company: ______________________

Option 2: ______________________

Type/Company: ______________________

Option 3: ______________________

Type/Company: ______________________

Cemented Implant? Yes No

Option 1: ______________________

Type/Company: ______________________

Option 2: ______________________

Type/Company: ______________________

Bone Graft Morcellized: Yes No

Femoral Strut: Yes No

Proximal Femur: Yes No

Other: ______________________

12. Special Equipment: High-speed Burrs: Yes No

Ultrasonic Cement-Removal Instruments: Yes No

Type/Company: ______________________

Cables: Yes No

Type/Company: ______________________

Trephine: Yes No

Abduction Brace: Yes No

Cell Saver: Yes No

Other: ______________________

Other: ______________________

Chapter 42
Surgical Approaches for Revision Total Hip Arthroplasty

Nicholas J. Lash, MBChB, FRACS
Donald S. Garbuz, MD, FRCSC
Bassam A. Masri, MD, FRCSC
Clive P. Duncan, MD, MSc, FRCSC

Introduction

Total hip arthroplasty (THA) is a highly successful strategy for the management of numerous hip disorders, and increasing numbers of THAs are being performed. However, failure of THA and the need for revision can result from osteolysis and polyethylene wear, implant dissociation, implant fracture, instability, infection, and periprosthetic fracture. In most revision hip surgery, one of the standard hip approaches is used with the addition of soft-tissue extensile maneuvers or an osteotomy. The goals of revision THA are to address the reason for revision and achieve a comfortable, stable THA that will allow mobilization with optimal hip mechanics and functional outcomes. One major cause of failure to achieve these desired results is the inability to access the hip sufficiently to perform the revision and avoid intraoperative complications. Therefore, any surgeon performing revision THA must understand and have experience performing the standard soft-tissue exposures and adjunct extensile exposures of the hip.

Surgical approaches to the hip are generally categorized according to the direction from which the joint is approached or the relationship of the surgical corridor to an anatomic landmark, such as the anterolateral approach (in front of the gluteus medius), the lateral or transgluteal approach (through the gluteus medius), and the posterolateral approach (behind the gluteus medius). Variations include the use of the anterior corridor (between the sartorius and the tensor fascia lata [TFL]); transosseous approaches, such as a trochanteric osteotomy; or, uncommonly, the use of a femoral canal access window. Abundant information on these approaches and their modification for revision hip arthroplasty is available in the published literature.

Because revision THA procedures vary in magnitude, the degree of exposure required also varies. Simpler procedures, such as acetabular liner exchange, may require only a standard, nonextensile approach to the hip. More complex scenarios, such as the presence of bone defects, material or implants that are retained or difficult to remove, or extensive soft-tissue stiffness, may require an extensile approach. An osteotomy of the femur can be used to gain access to the proximal femur and can be extended into the diaphysis at the surgeon's discretion. Several femoral or trochanteric osteotomies can be performed with different hip approaches (**Figure 1**). Preoperative planning will aid in determining the length of the osteotomy required to access the desired level.

Results

The results of the extensile approaches to the hip for revision hip arthroplasty vary (**Table 1**), with wide variation in rates of complications and adverse events, time to union, and functional outcome scores both in studies comparing different techniques and in studies of patients undergoing revision with a single technique. The variation in results can be attributed to the fact that both

Dr. Garbuz or an immediate family member serves as a paid consultant to or is an employee of Zimmer Biomet; has received research or institutional support from DePuy Synthes and Zimmer Biomet; and serves as a board member, owner, officer, or committee member of the M. E. Müller Foundation of North America. Dr. Masri or an immediate family member serves as a board member, owner, officer, or committee member of the Canadian Orthopaedic Association. Dr. Duncan or an immediate family member is a member of a speakers' bureau or has made paid presentations on behalf of Zimmer Biomet. Neither Dr. Lash nor any immediate family member has received anything of value from or has stock or stock options held in a commercial company or institution related directly or indirectly to the subject of this chapter.

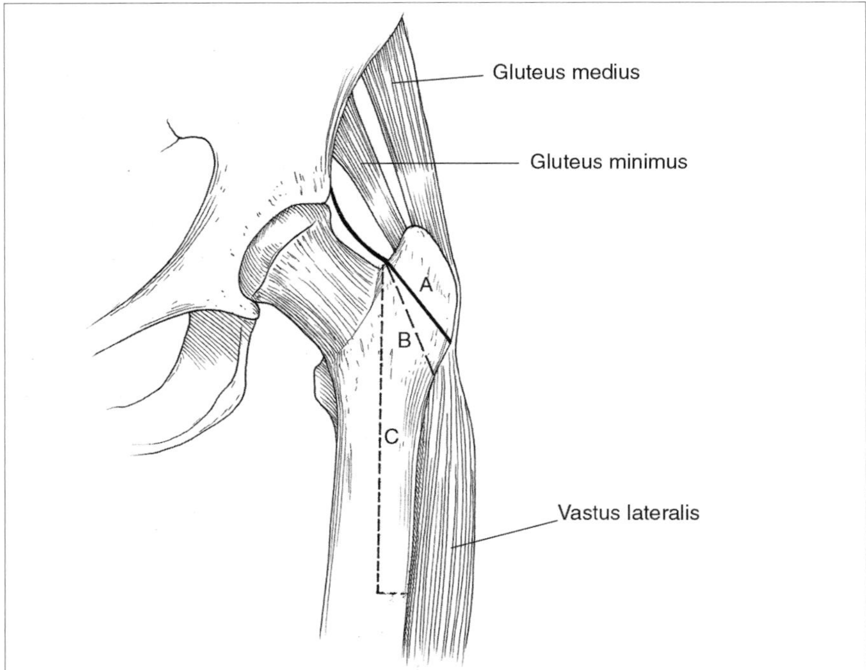

Figure 1 Illustration depicts the paths of the standard trochanteric osteotomy (**A**), the trochanteric slide osteotomy (**B**), and the extended trochanteric osteotomy (**C**). The trochanteric slide osteotomy and the extended trochanteric osteotomy incorporate the origin of the vastus lateralis muscle, whereas the standard trochanteric osteotomy does not. (Reproduced from Archibeck MJ, Rosenberg AG, Berger RA, Silverton CD: Trochanteric osteotomy and fixation during total hip arthroplasty. *J Am Acad Orthop Surg* 2003;11[3]:163-173.)

the revision procedures and the extensile maneuvers differ in magnitude.

Subvastus Exposure (Vastus Slide)

Indications

The vastus slide is an extensile soft-tissue exposure that is used in conjunction with a direct lateral approach to the hip. It offers the advantages of the direct lateral approach and affords additional exposure of the femoral diaphysis. In revision hip surgery, the vastus slide allows controlled medullary exposure via a window corticotomy, exposure of the femur for the management of iatrogenic fracture during femoral preparation, or reduction of periprosthetic fracture fragments around a previously placed fixed femoral stem. The extra exposure also allows removal of previous internal fixation devices and assists in implant or cement removal. The addition of the vastus slide to a direct lateral approach is ideal in straightforward revision scenarios.

Contraindications

In patients requiring extensive intramedullary exposure for extraction of a cement mantle or for removal of a well-fixed femoral implant, an extended trochanteric osteotomy (ETO) may be a better strategy.

Alternative Treatments

The ETO is the main alternative to a vastus slide for complete exposure of the femoral canal. However, the ETO has the disadvantage of requiring union to re-create continuity of the hip abductors and the femur.

Techniques

SETUP

- Typically, the patient is placed in the lateral decubitus position for the direct lateral approach.
- A standard surgical table is used. The patient is secured with padded bolsters with the pelvis positioned vertically to facilitate accurate acetabular implantation.
- All bony prominences are padded to avoid pressure injury and neurapraxia.
- The authors of this chapter prefer to use alcoholic iodine or chlorhexidine skin disinfectant and disposable drapes with a rubberized aperture, secured with bio-occlusive drapes to exclude the groin from the surgical field.
- A padded Mayo table facilitates internal rotation, abduction, and extension of the surgical hip intraoperatively.

INSTRUMENTS/EQUIPMENT/IMPLANTS REQUIRED

- Standard hip revision retractors are used.
- Suture ligatures and/or surgical vascular clips may be used to control bleeding from perforating vessels arising from the deep femoral artery.

PROCEDURE

- A skin and deep fascial incision is performed for the direct lateral approach.
- The anterior one-third of the abductors is released, with a cuff of tendon left for later repair (**Figure 2, A**).
- The muscle fibers are split proximally to within 5 cm of the greater trochanter or 4 cm from the superior margin of the acetabulum. Care is taken to protect the superior gluteal nerve and vessels.
- The abductor release is continued distally into the fascia/epimysium

Table 1 Results of the Extensile Approaches to the Hip for Revision Hip Arthroplasty

Authors (Year)	Number of Patients (Exposures/ Cases)	Approach	Mean Patient Age in Years (Range)	Mean Follow-up in Months (Range)	Results
Glassman et al (1987)	86 (90)	TSO	NR	NR	Broken wires and proximal migration (mean, 7 mm [range, 2-26 mm]) occurred in 7 patients 28% of all patients had a positive Trendelenburg test or lurch Union rate, 90%
Schutzer and Harris (1988)	177 (188)	Trochanteric osteotomy (71 with three-wire fixation; 94 with four-wire fixation; 23 with two horizontal wires only) 141 had supplementary mesh fixation 115 were distalized	57 (17-87)	≤24	Union rate, 97% Of the 3% that failed or were slow to unite, one or more vertical wires broke early (<12 wk postoperatively Overall, 27% of wires broke, but most breakage occurred after the osteotomy had united
Peters et al (1993)	21 (21)	ETO (12), ETO with strut allograft (9)	NR	NR	4 patients in the ETO group had delayed union but had united at 6 mo postoperatively The 9 patients who underwent ETO with strut allograft achieved union at a mean of 12 mo postoperatively Union rate, 100% at final follow-up (NR)
Younger et al (1995)	20 (20)	ETO (17), ETO with strut allograft (3)	64.5 (32-81)	18.2 (15-24)	All 17 ETO patients had union at 3 mo postoperatively All 3 ETO with strut allograft patients had union at 12 mo postoperatively No migration of any ETO with or without strut allograft >2 mm Union rate, 100% at final follow-up (mean, 18.2 mo)
Chen et al (2000)	45 (46)	ETO (29), ETO with strut allograft (17)	66.3 (36-84)	44 (18-88)	Mean time to union of 4.3 mo after ETO and 6.1 mo after ETO with allograft Time to union was not related to bone quality 1 patient had migration of 5 mm and achieved union at 6 mo postoperatively Union rate, 98%
Miner et al (2001)	152 (166)	ETO	65.8 (26-84)	45 (36-90)	2 patients had migration of the ETO >2 mm 18 (10.8%) of 166 hips had femoral cracks at the time of insertion of the trial implant or stem; all healed No stems had subsidence or failure of ingrowth Union rate, 98.8% at 3 mo
Langlais et al (2003)	94 (94)	TSO at lateral aspect of prosthesis; four-wire fixation	NR	NR	92 patients were followed for >12 mo 36 patients were available for follow-up at 60 mo Mean Merle d'Aubigné score at last follow-up was 16 (on 18-point scale) Union rate of 96% for the entire cohort

ETO = extended trochanteric osteotomy, HHS = Harris hip score, LFCN = lateral femoral cutaneous nerve, NA = not applicable, NR = not reported, TSO = trochanteric slide osteotomy, WOMAC = Western Ontario and McMaster Universities Osteoarthritis Index.

Table 1 Results of the Extensile Approaches to the Hip for Revision Hip Arthroplasty (*continued*)

Authors (Year)	Number of Patients (Exposures/ Cases)	Approach	Mean Patient Age in Years (Range)	Mean Follow-up in Months (Range)	Results
Goodman et al (2004)	57 (57)	TSO (27 standard TSO dividing the posterior capsule and short external rotators; 30 modified TSO performed lateral to the posterior tissues)	Standard TSO: 63 (NR) Modified TSO: 64 (NR)	≤12 mo (NR)	14% dislocation rate after standard TSO 3% dislocation rate after modified TSO
Kennon et al (2004)	458 (468)	Direct anterior	68 (25-92)	NR	3% dislocation rate No patient had LFCN palsy at 6 mo postoperatively 10% of patients experienced femoral fracture, 57% of which required fixation
Mardones et al (2005)	73 (75)	ETO (57), ETO with strut allograft (18)	67.9 (39-88)	36 (12-60)	1 hip had migration >5 mm requiring revision 1 nonunion 9 femoral cracks at osteotomy junction (8 healed spontaneously; 1 required revision for stem loosening) Union rate without additional intervention, 97%
Morshed et al (2005)	13 (13)	ETO for removal of infected THA implant, with fixation of the ETO at the time of placement of second-stage implant	52.6 (40-82)	39 (24-68)	Mean time to union, 3.9 mo 3 intraoperative fractures occurred (all healed) Mean HHS improved from 25 to 68 2 patients had >5 mm subsidence 3 patients had recurrent infection Union rate, 100% at final follow-up (mean, 39 mo)
Park et al (2007)	62 hips	ETO (19), ETO with strut allograft (13), control group without ETO (30)	60 (36-80)	50 (24-144)	Mean postoperative HHS for ETO with or without allograft was 88.8, compared with 85.7 for the control group ($P = 0.23$) 2 intraoperative femoral fractures occurred No hips with ETO had perforation or subsidence >5 mm, which was significant compared with the control group ($P = 0.49$) Union rate, 100% at a mean 4 mo postoperatively
Mast and Laude (2011)	51 (51)	Direct anterior (21 patients had acetabular revision only; 21 patients had combined femoral and acetabular revision; 32 patients had previously undergone procedures with a direct anterior approach)	61 (33-88)	55 (8-160)	Mean postoperative WOMAC score, 83 Union rate NR

ETO = extended trochanteric osteotomy, HHS = Harris hip score, LFCN = lateral femoral cutaneous nerve, NA = not applicable, NR = not reported, TSO = trochanteric slide osteotomy, WOMAC = Western Ontario and McMaster Universities Osteoarthritis Index.

of the vastus lateralis (**Figure 2, A**).

- The line of the incision into the vastus fascia curves posteriorly toward the intermuscular septum.
- The fibers of the vasti muscles are elevated in the same manner as for an ETO (described later in this chapter).
- The perforating vessels are

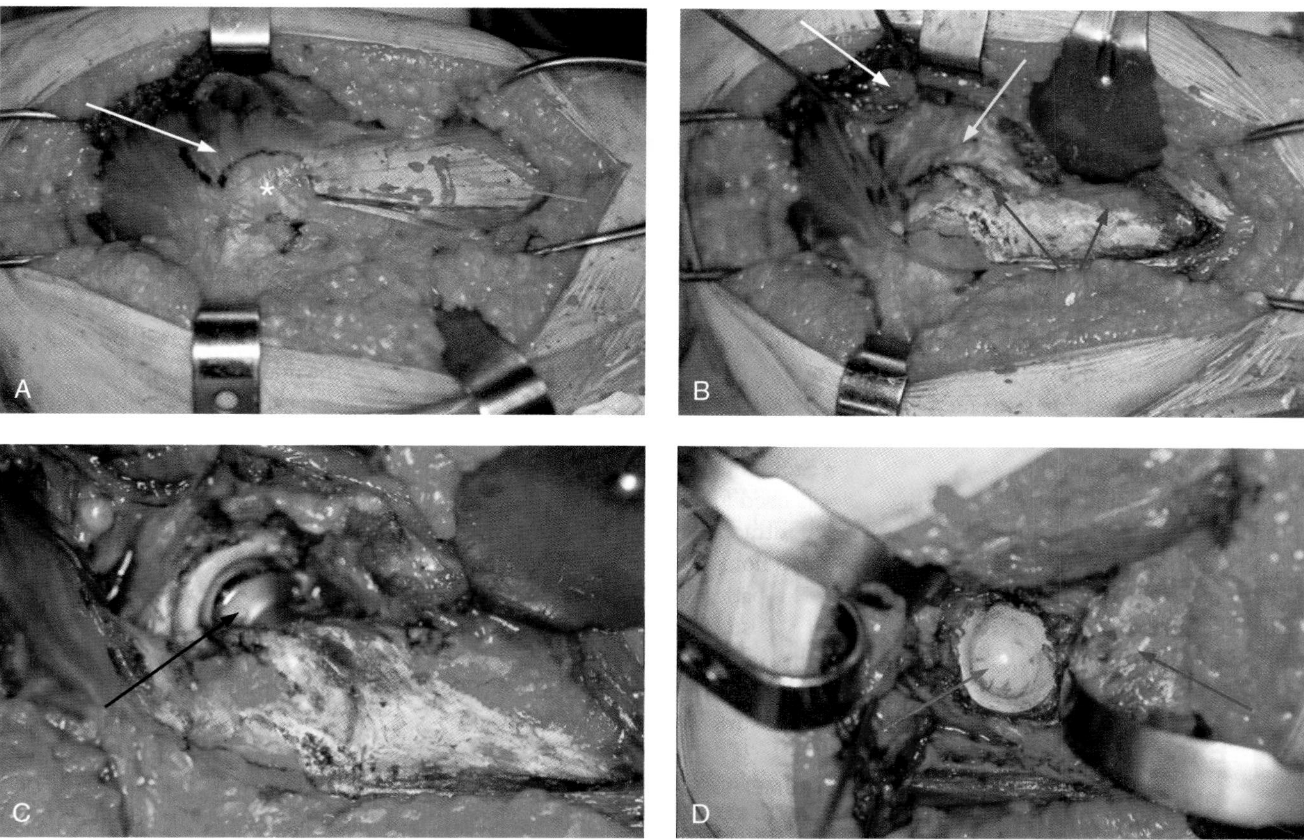

Figure 2 Intraoperative photographs show the subvastus exposure (vastus slide). **A,** The anterior halves of the glutei (white arrow) are elevated from the greater trochanter (asterisk), and the vasti muscles (green arrow) are elevated from the femur. **B,** The anterior halves of the glutei (white arrow) are retracted exposing the anterior capsule (yellow arrow). The vasti muscles are reflected anteriorly, exposing the anterior femoral neck and femoral shaft (blue arrows). **C,** A capsulectomy has been performed, exposing the femoral head (arrow). **D,** The femur (blue arrow) is retracted posteroinferiorly, allowing wide exposure of the acetabulum (green arrow).

addressed and ligated before they retract and cause hemorrhage.

- The distal extent of elevation of the vasti muscles depends on the length of exposure required.
- Release of the gluteus medius and minimus in continuity with the vastus lateralis elevation, draws these structures anteriorly to expose the hip joint and femur (**Figure 2, B**).
- The exposure affords good access to the hip joint and, via an anterior capsulectomy or capsulotomy, to the proximal femur and anterolateral femur (**Figure 2, C**). The posterior wall and column remain difficult to access because of obstruction by the femur.
- Division of the medial and posterior capsular attachments of the proximal femur can increase the mobility of the femur, allowing it to be positioned more advantageously for acetabular preparation (**Figure 2, D**).

WOUND CLOSURE

- As with any transgluteal approach, accurate and meticulous repair of the gluteus medius and minimus back to the proximal femur is performed.
- If possible, the hip abductors are secured transosseously. If that is not possible, the abductor tendons are repaired to the remaining cuff of tendon on the femur. Regardless of the repair, absorbable No. 1 or No. 2 sutures are used.
- No. 1 absorbable sutures are used for the fascia.
- The subcutaneous tissues are closed with 2-0 absorbable sutures.
- The skin can be closed with staples, according to the surgeon's preferred method.
- The authors of this chapter prefer to not use any drains.
- A highly absorbent all-in-one foam dressing with a waterproof membrane is used.

Postoperative Regimen

Patients who undergo a vastus slide do not usually require any postoperative

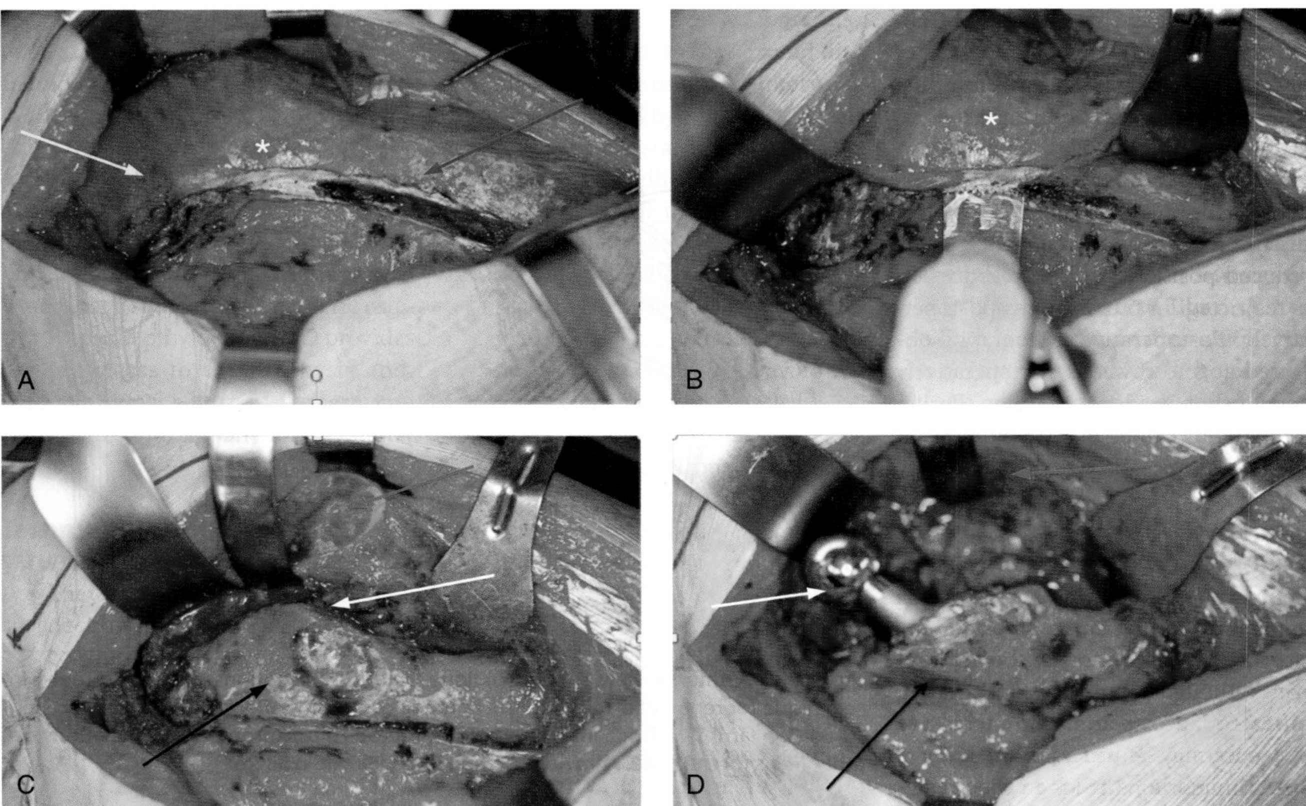

Figure 4 Intraoperative photographs show the trochanteric slide osteotomy. **A,** The gluteus medius and minimus (yellow arrow) and vasti muscles (blue arrow) are elevated slightly from the pelvis and femur, but are left attached to the greater trochanter (asterisk). **B,** A shallow trochanteric osteotomy is performed from posterior to anterior through the greater trochanter (asterisk) with a thin broad saw blade. **C,** The trochanteric fragment (green arrow) is reflected anteriorly with the glutei and vasti muscles attached. The anterior capsule (white arrow) is exposed. The trochanteric bed (black arrow) remains intact for reattachment. **D,** The femoral head and neck (white arrow) is dislocated anteriorly after the capsulectomy. The trochanteric fragment (green arrow) remains retracted anteriorly, and the trochanteric bed (black arrow) is rotated posteriorly as the hip is dislocated.

Alternative Treatments

Although a standard trochanteric osteotomy will afford the same exposure, the trochanteric slide osteotomy has greater inherent stability because of the combined proximal and distal soft-tissue attachments. With the fascia of the vastus lateralis muscle counteracting the pull of the hip abductors, trochanteric escape is not a concern. If trochanteric bone stock is poor, an ETO should be considered to allow the reapproximation of the osteotomy to be performed in the diaphyseal region, where bone stock can more readily accommodate the repair.

Techniques

SETUP

- Preoperative radiographic analysis is performed to assess the quality of the greater trochanter and ensure the presence of adequate bone for the osteotomy and its subsequent fixation.
- The patient is placed in a standard lateral decubitus position.

INSTRUMENTS/EQUIPMENT/ IMPLANTS REQUIRED

- A powered oscillating saw with a broad, thin blade is needed.
- Cerclage wires, wire passers, a cable plate and/or trochanteric claw, small and large fragment screws, and appropriate drills should be available for repair of the trochanteric fragment.

PROCEDURE

- Skin and fascial incisions for a posterolateral approach are made as described, with the use of either a standard Kocher incision or a modified Gibson interval.
- When the fascial opening is retracted and the posterolateral aspect of the hip is exposed, visualization of the confluence of the gluteus

medius muscle and tendon, the greater trochanter, and the vastus lateralis muscle is critical (**Figure 4, A**).

- The surrounding anatomy, including the proximity of the sciatic nerve and the short external rotators, is observed.
- After the interval between the piriformis and the vastus lateralis, gluteus medius, and gluteus minimus is developed, the vastus lateralis muscle is elevated off the metaphysis of the femur, and the gluteus medius and minimus are elevated slightly off the outer table of the pelvis (**Figure 4, A**). This step creates the digastric myofascial flap that will contain the trochanter.
- An osteotomy fragment 10 to 15 mm deep is created with the passage of a thin-blade oscillating saw from posterior to anterior in the sagittal plane (**Figure 4, B**). Care is taken to initiate the cut just lateral to the insertion of the external rotators so that the external rotators and the capsule remain attached to the femur.
- To mobilize the osteotomized fragment anteriorly, it is translated forward with the gluteus medius and minimus and the vasti muscles attached (**Figure 4, C**). Simultaneous external rotation of the distal femur facilitates this maneuver.
- The plane between these muscles and the anterior capsule is developed. Gradual flexion and external rotation of the femur facilitates this step.
- After exposure is obtained, a capsulectomy is performed and the hip joint is dislocated anteriorly (**Figure 4, D**).
- The femur can be further mobilized by performing a full circumferential release of the capsular insertions and retracting the proximal femur in a posteroinferior direction. This mobilization is particularly useful if retention of the stem is planned.
- If access to the posterior column is required, delayed release of the posterior capsule and external rotators can be considered.
- Although the gluteus maximus insertion is not routinely released, it can be released to allow further femoral mobilization.
- After the reconstruction is complete, anatomic reduction and secure fixation of the trochanter is accomplished with the use of Luque wires, cables, a cable grip, or a cable hook plate.
- If desirable, the trochanter can be advanced to dynamize the hip after a lateral bleeding bed is created on the cortex of the proximal femur just below the original trochanteric bed.

WOUND CLOSURE

- The deep layers are closed with No. 1 absorbable suture.
- The superficial layers are closed with 2-0 absorbable suture.
- Skin closure is done per the surgeon's preferred method.

Postoperative Regimen

As with other trochanteric osteotomies, active hip abduction should be avoided for 6 to 8 weeks postoperatively to allow time for initial union of the osteotomy fragment.

Avoiding Pitfalls and Complications

Preoperative templating is important to ensure that the bone stock is adequate to allow union of the osteotomy. The use of a thin blade on the osteotomy saw will minimize the bone loss that occurs during the osteotomy. Irrigation of the saw blade during the cutting process will minimize thermal damage to the bone. The fragment should be at least 10 mm thick to avoid fracture during the revision surgery. Cutting most of the osteotomy with the saw and completing the cut with an osteotome is safer and creates small irregularities in the opposing bone surfaces that enhance stability at repair. To avoid the risk of trochanteric escape, maintaining the continuity of the abductor and vastus lateralis insertions on the greater trochanter fragment is crucial. Flexion, adduction, and external rotation will aid in opening the osteotomy and exposing the underlying gluteus minimus and capsule.

Extended Trochanteric Osteotomy

Indications

The ETO was developed primarily to provide efficient and safe access to the femoral medullary canal to facilitate removal of well-fixed implants or cement and to address deformity of the femoral shaft (**Figure 1**). It has since evolved into a reproducible technique. The ETO can be advanced slightly, after removal of a small amount of distal bone from the fragment, to tension the abductors and dynamize the hip during closure. If properly mobilized, with its soft tissues attached, an ETO can facilitate wider exposure of the acetabulum. However, the presence of a soft-tissue hinge imparts partial stability to the fragment and maintains crucial blood supply, enhancing union of the osteotomy. An intact blood supply is of paramount importance in patients undergoing revision for infection because soft-tissue stripping and devascularization of the bone in these patients would increase the risk of persistence of infection.

Careful preoperative planning is necessary to optimize results. The length of the ETO is decided during preoperative planning on the basis of the length needed to accomplish the primary goal of the osteotomy and the need to preserve bone stock and the femoral isthmus. In a patient who has a short, well-integrated stem or well-fixed cemented stem, the

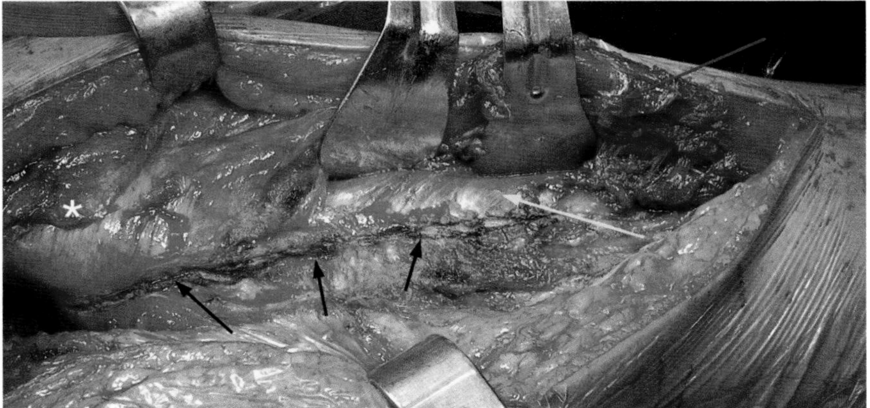

Figure 5 Intraoperative photograph shows an extended trochanteric osteotomy. The cephalad direction is to the left. The asterisk indicates the greater trochanter. The vastus lateralis (blue arrow) has been judiciously elevated to expose the femur. The planned osteotomy is outlined with cautery (black arrows). Soft tissues, including nonviolated periosteum (yellow arrow), remain attached to the osteotomy fragment.

ETO generally is done to the lower level of the stem, leaving adequate bone distally to facilitate fixation of the revision stem. If the existing implant is long or the cement mantle is extensive, treatment is more challenging. Two options are available, and experts disagree as to which should be favored: (1) extend the osteotomy as distally as necessary and perform reconstruction as needed or (2) extend the osteotomy only partway down the stem, divide the stem if it is noncemented, and trephine out the distal segment with specialized tools designed for that purpose. In a patient in whom an extensive cement column is present, the second option requires removal of the remaining distal cement through the osteotomy site with specialized tools, including ultrasonic devices if necessary. The major advantage of the second option is retention of more diaphyseal bone for the femoral reconstruction.

Contraindications

As with other trochanteric osteotomies, abductor deficiency and a bald trochanter are contraindications to ETO. Severe bone deficiency in the region of the metadiaphysis or diaphysis is a relative contraindication because it would hinder adequate fixation; therefore, an ETO should be used judiciously in patients in whom such deficiency is seen.

Alternative Treatments

An alternative to the use of an ETO is the use of any other hip approach that provides access to the acetabulum and proximal femur, in combination with a window corticotomy (described later in this chapter).

Techniques

SETUP/EXPOSURE

- A posterolateral or direct lateral approach is used, depending on the surgeon's expertise and preference.
- The patient is placed in the lateral decubitus position for either the posterolateral or lateral approach.

INSTRUMENTS/EQUIPMENT/IMPLANTS REQUIRED

- A powered oscillating saw with thin blades and a Gigli saw are used.
- Luque/cerclage wires, wire passers and tensioners, stainless-steel surgical cables, and a trochanteric cable plate and claw should be available for fixation.

PROCEDURE

ETO in a Posterolateral Approach

- The patient is secured in the lateral decubitus position, with care taken to orient the coronal plane of the pelvis perpendicular to the floor.
- An incision is made for a standard posterolateral approach, incorporating previous scars if possible. The length of the incision depends on the planned distal extent of the ETO.
- The incision is carried through the superficial and deep tissues.
- The sciatic nerve is identified and protected. If the sciatic nerve is not easily identified, the surgeon can avoid it by passing directly down to the posterolateral edge of the greater trochanter, carefully raising a composite flap of the external rotators and posterior capsule, and using the flap as a buffer or soft-tissue cuff to protect the nerve.
- Alternatively, the nerve can be identified in more normal tissue, such as deep to the gluteus maximus tendon, and followed proximally with careful dissection to minimize the risk of nerve damage.
- After specimens are harvested for bacteriologic and histologic analysis, the proximal femur is further mobilized using circumferential dissection and is dislocated posteriorly.
- An exit channel for the stem is created in the medial surface of the greater trochanter to avoid fracture during extraction. The stem is removed if it can be easily extracted.
- If substantial acetabular reconstruction is required, the femur can be left intact at this time and osteotomized later in the procedure. This method will reduce blood loss and protect the femur from injury during retraction.
- In preparation for the ETO, the posterior surface of the trochanter is defined. The vasti muscles are

raised from the lateral intermuscular septum for a short width, exposing the posterior cortex lateral to the linea aspera, to the distal extent planned preoperatively (**Figure 5**). This distance can be measured from the tip of the greater trochanter or by other means, such as with the use of the extracted stem as a ruler if it was used as a reference point in preoperative templating.

- An oscillating saw with a thin blade is used to cut through the greater trochanter and cortical bone from back to front, including the cement mantle if present.
- At the planned distal extent of the ETO, the blade is angled proximally 45° to the axis of the femur to appropriately bevel the exit track.
- Osteotomes are used to gently open the ETO and elevate it off the underlying bone and contents of the medullary canal (**Figure 6**).
- If the stem could not be easily extracted and remains within the canal, the osteotomy technique must be modified because the saw blade cannot traverse the canal to open the bone with sufficient width. In this circumstance, after the posterior bone has been divided and the distal exit site prepared, a series of osteotomes are teased through the belly of the vasti muscles down to the desired location on the anterior surface of the femur where the osteotomy will exit, and the osteotomes are used to perforate the bone in that location. The osteotomes are advanced up the cortex in a stepwise manner, with each osteotome acting as a marker for the next, to weaken the anterior bone where required. When the ETO is gently opened through the posterior surface, it will also open through the sites where the anterior surface was weakened by the osteotomes.
- In either of the preceding techniques (the direct anteroposterior osteotomy across an empty canal or the modification described for use in the presence of a canal-filling stem), care is taken to expose only a short width of the posterolateral cortex and to leave the vasti muscles attached to the ETO. Similarly, the periosteum is not elevated (**Figure 5**).
- The location and orientation of the osteotomy should allow the surgeon to elevate the lateral one-third of the femur, leaving the remaining two-thirds medially. As the femur flares and broadens proximally, the line of the osteotomy must follow the flare of the femur to avoid cutting into the greater trochanter.
- A prophylactic cable is placed just below the exit site of the distal extent of the osteotomy. This is done to avoid the risk of uncontrolled fracture initiation at that site during implant extraction, femoral preparation, or insertion of the new stem.
- Well-fixed noncemented stems or retained cement can be removed (**Figure 7**).
- The femur is prepared, and an appropriate-size trial implant is placed and assessed for length and stability (**Figure 8**).
- With the trial femoral stem in place, the osteotomy is reduced with internal rotation of the femur and reduction of the fragment with a tenaculum or other bone reduction forceps.
- If the osteotomy does not reduce, the internal surface of the fragment is examined for retained cement or bone that is impinging on the trial implant. It is common for bone to prevent reduction at the shoulder of the prosthesis.
- Prominent bone can be removed with the use of rongeurs or a high-speed burr to allow the osteotomy to seat properly. However, an incomplete reduction is preferable to an iatrogenic fracture.
- The fixation cables or wires are passed from posterior to anterior to protect the sciatic nerve from entrapment. The cables or wires are evenly spaced, with the total number depending on the length of the osteotomy (**Figure 9**).
- The proximal cable or wire is passed distal to the lesser trochanter to counteract the pull of the abductors. It can be passed through a drill hole in the lesser trochanter for additional security.

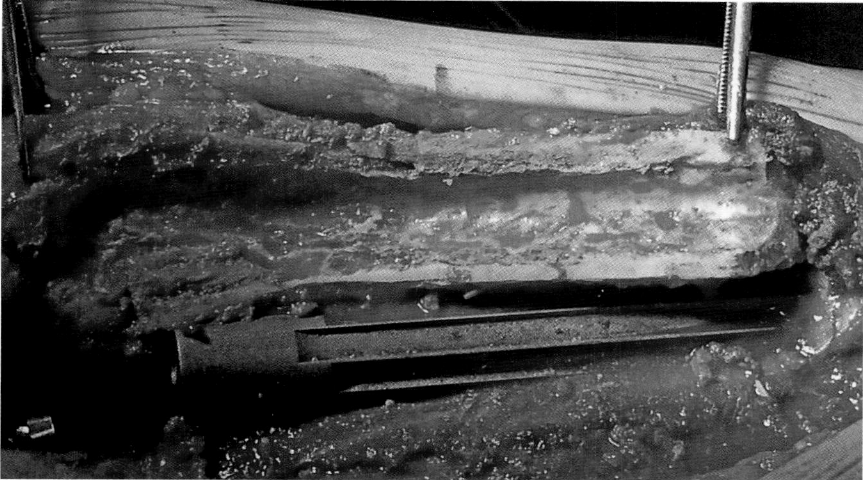

Figure 6 Intraoperative photograph shows the raised extended trochanteric osteotomy fragment. It is bleeding because the soft tissues remain attached.

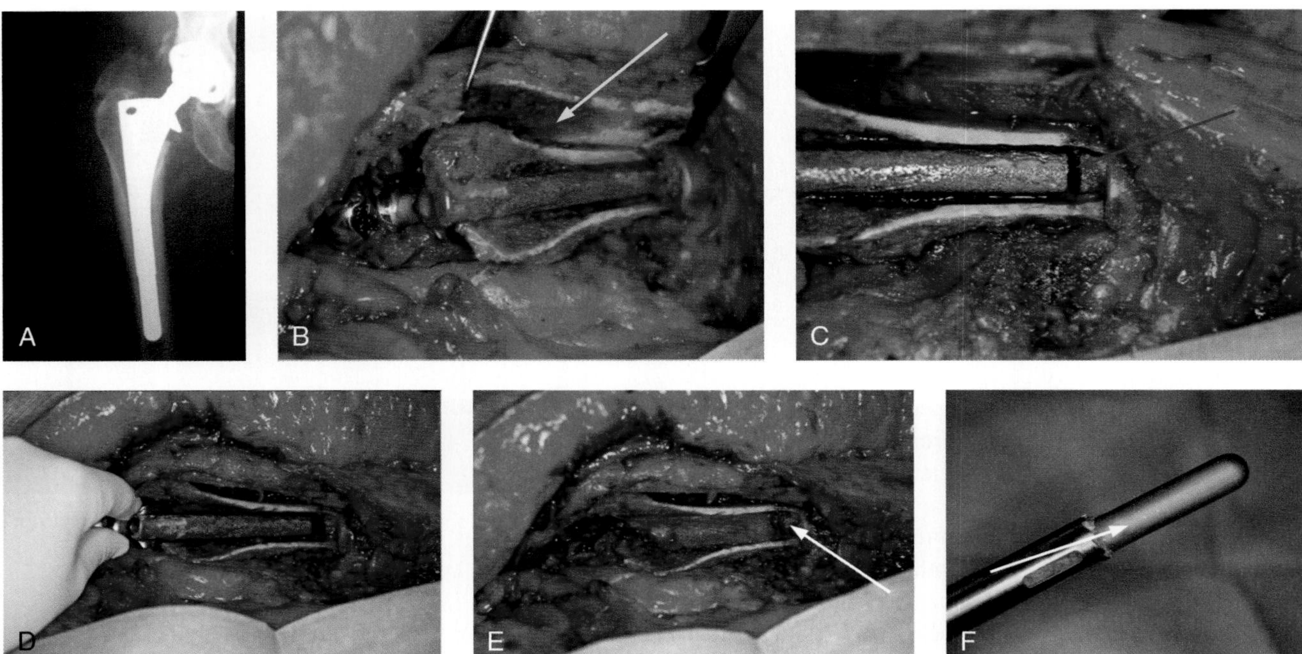

Figure 7 **A,** AP hip radiograph of a right hip demonstrates a well-fixed noncemented femoral stem with late infection. **B,** Intraoperative photograph shows an extended trochanteric osteotomy with the trochanteric fragment (arrow) transposed anteriorly. **C** and **D,** Intraoperative photographs show removal of the proximal part of the femoral stem after division of the stem (blue arrow) with a metal-cutting burr. **E,** After the proximal portion of the femoral prosthesis has been removed, the remaining distal portion of the prosthesis (arrow) is removed with a trephine. **F,** Photograph shows the distal stem (arrow), which was removed with a trephine.

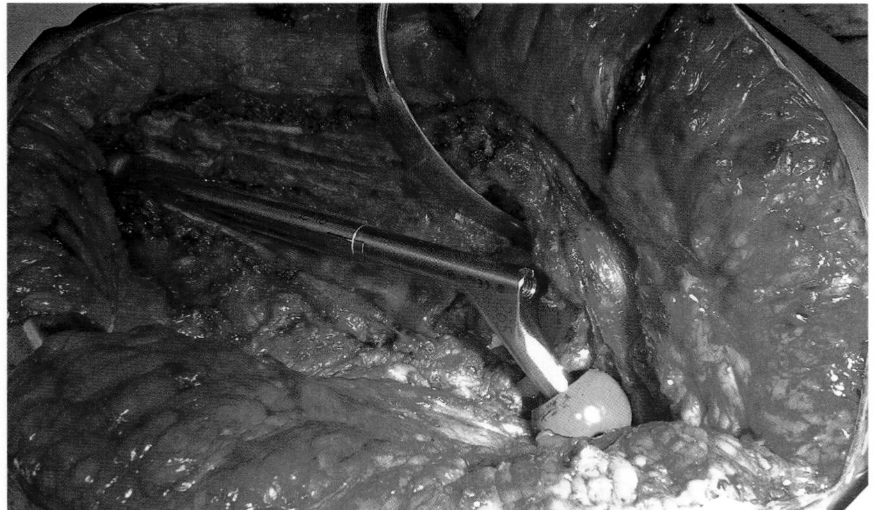

Figure 8 Intraoperative photograph shows an extended trochanteric osteotomy with a trial femoral stem placed for assessment of limb length and stability.

Additionally, cables can be passed after removal of the trial implant but before placement of the definitive femoral prosthesis, while the respective ETO and diaphysis remain more mobile to facilitate cable passage.

- The final prosthesis is inserted to the level of and in the same version as the trial.
- The ETO is reduced and cables are tightened and crimped.
- If necessary, the fixation of the osteotomy is augmented with bone graft consisting of reamings from the acetabular preparation or, in patients who have weak and deficient cortical bone, with a cortical onlay allograft, which also acts as a hard platform to prevent cables from cutting through the underlying weak bone. A disadvantage of the use of an onlay allograft is that soft-tissue elevation or stripping of the lateral cortex is required to place the allograft strut. Therefore, this method is not commonly used.

ETO in a Lateral Approach

- The principles and techniques of the ETO in a lateral approach are the same as those in a posterolateral approach. However, the local anatomy requires several differences in the procedure.

- With the patient in the lateral position, a linear skin incision centered over the greater trochanter is made. The distal extent of the incision is over the femur, and the length of the incision must accommodate the planned osteotomy.
- The deep fascia is incised in line with the skin incision.
- The gluteus medius muscle is exposed with dissection and placement of deep retractors.
- The anterior one-third of the fibers of the gluteus medius are detached from the anterior facet of the greater trochanter.
- The underlying gluteus minimus is detached separately or with the medius fibers.
- A cuff of tendon is left attached to the muscle for repair to the trochanteric bone later in the procedure. Elevation of the tendons together with a wafer of bone also can assist in reattachment.
- To avoid injury to the superior gluteal neurovascular bundle, the detached gluteus medius muscle fibers are split in line up to 5 cm proximal to the tip of the greater trochanter.
- The vastus lateralis muscle is split in the midsubstance of the muscle belly, and this incision is extended proximally to connect with the released inferior edge of the glutei.
- The released gluteal muscles are retracted anteriorly to expose the anterior capsule. The fibers of the vastus lateralis are elevated carefully to allow identification of the femur but avoid stripping the periosteum. The muscle is elevated in its midsubstance to facilitate creation of the anterior line of the osteotomy.
- As in the technique described for ETO using a posterolateral approach, a cut is made in the sagittal plane with an oscillating saw or burr. However, in this approach the cut is made from anterior to posterior. A posterior soft-tissue hinge is maintained.
- The distal cut is made as described previously for the posterolateral approach, angled at 45° to create a rounded and beveled distal portion of the osteotomy.
- The posterior portion of the osteotomy can be completed with the saw through the anterior cut. Alternatively, it can be completed through the muscle belly with osteotomes as previously described; however, this maneuver carries some risk of damage to the perforating vessels and resultant blood loss.
- After the three cuts are completed, the osteotomy is opened with sequential osteotomes.
- A prophylactic cable is placed just below the exit site of the distal extent of the osteotomy. This is done to avoid the risk of uncontrolled fracture initiation at that site during implant extraction, femoral preparation, or insertion of the new stem.
- The surgeon proceeds with the preparation of the femoral canal and insertion of the new femoral stem as previously described for ETO using a posterolateral approach.
- Closure of the osteotomy is performed as described previously.

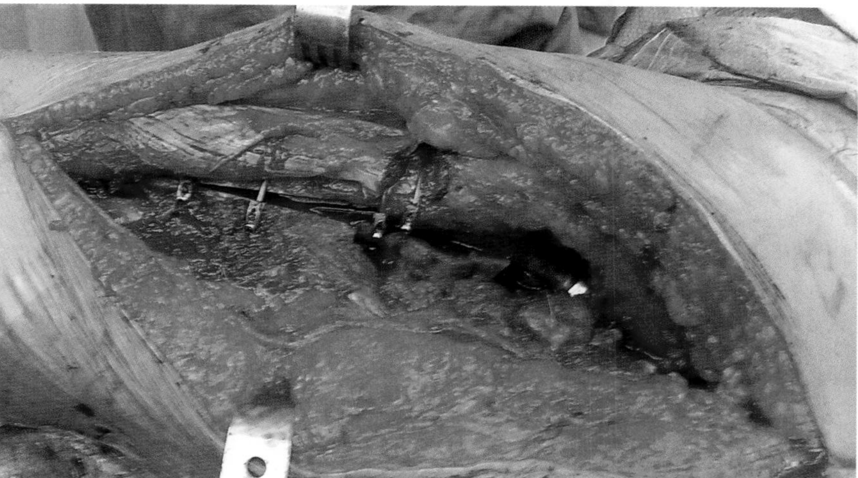

Figure 9 Intraoperative photograph shows fixation of an extended trochanteric osteotomy. The osteotomy fragments have been closed with satisfactory but not anatomic reduction. Soft tissue remains attached to the fragments, providing blood supply.

WOUND CLOSURE

- The deep fascia is closed using No. 1 absorbable suture.
- The superficial adipose tissue is closed using 2-0 absorbable suture.
- The skin is closed according to the surgeon's preferred method.

Postoperative Regimen

As with the other trochanteric osteotomies, active hip abduction is avoided for 6 to 8 weeks postoperatively.

Avoiding Pitfalls and Complications

Accurate templating of the length of the osteotomy to access the relevant parts of the femur is crucial. The presence of deformity should be noted to allow the surgeon to plan for a double osteotomy if necessary. Whether the ETO is used in conjunction with a posterolateral or direct lateral approach, maintenance of the muscular attachment is important for vitality of the osteotomy and stability of the hip. Placement of a prophylactic cable or wire distal to the end of the osteotomy will help prevent fracture propagation from any irregular bone at

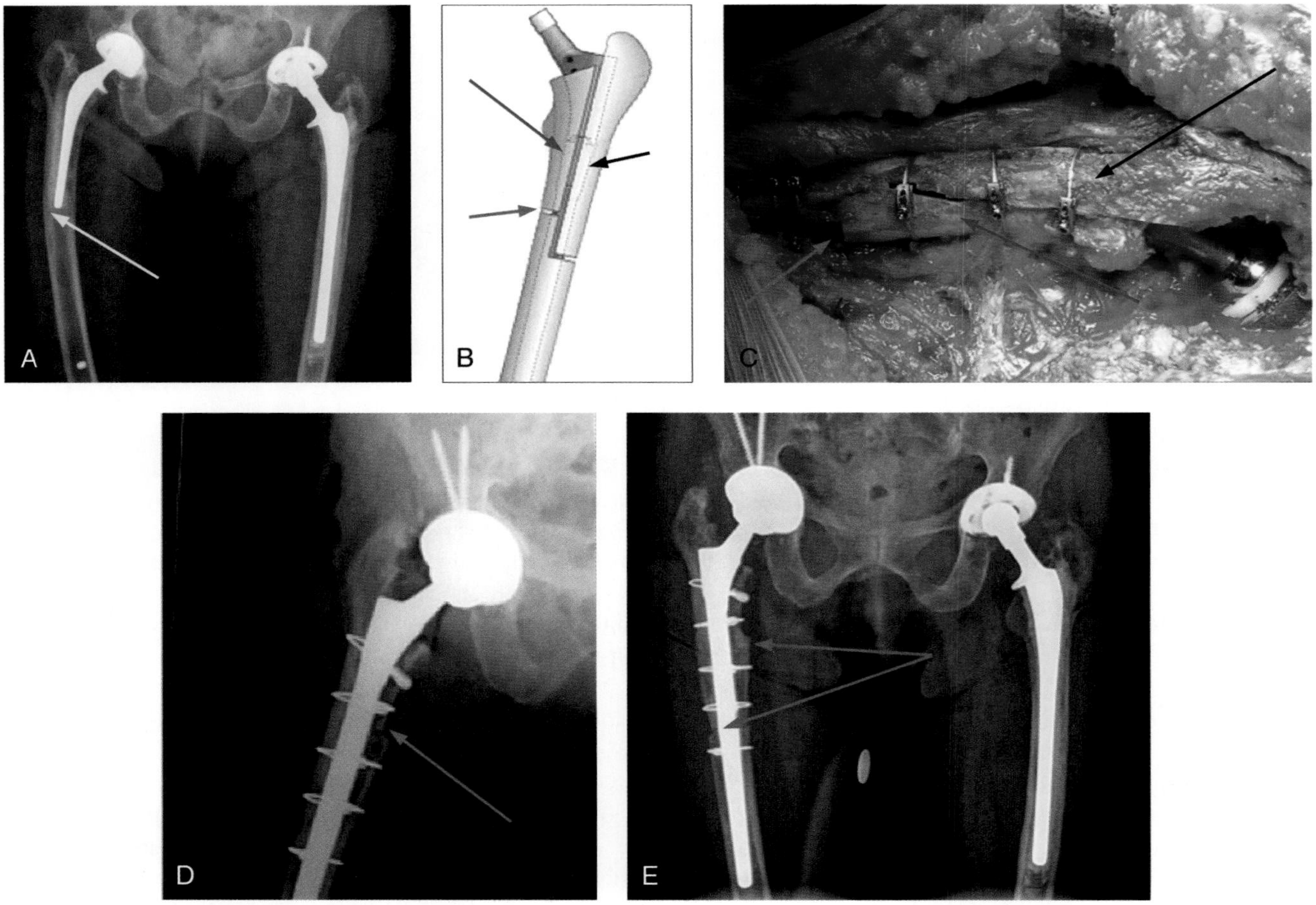

Figure 10 **A,** Preoperative AP pelvic radiograph demonstrates varus remodeling (arrow) in the right hip. Templating suggests that a double osteotomy will be required. **B,** Illustration depicts the planned double osteotomy. An extended trochanteric osteotomy (ETO) is performed (black arrow). The medial osteotomy (green arrow) is done late in the procedure and is located 5 cm above the exit site of the lateral osteotomy to create a step-cut junction and accommodate two cables. This leaves a medially based proximal fragment (blue arrow) that is drawn laterally onto the femoral prosthesis as the cables are tightened. **C,** Intraoperative photograph shows closure of the double osteotomy. Two cables have been placed at the step cut. The arrows point to the respective osteotomies and proximal fragment represented in panel B. **D,** Early postoperative AP radiograph of the right hip demonstrates reduction of the osteotomy, with the medial osteotomy (green arrow) allowing apposition of the medial fragment to the femoral stem. **E,** AP pelvic radiograph obtained 6 months postoperatively demonstrates union at both the ETO and the medial osteotomy (green arrows).

the distal extent of the osteotomy. Placement of the cables or wires for osteotomy fixation after the trial femoral implant is removed but before the definitive prosthesis is placed will allow easier passage of the cables or wires because the bone fragments will not be under tension. Passage of the cables or wires from posterior to anterior will reduce the risk to the sciatic nerve. In patients in whom bone stock is diminished, the use of a strut allograft is optional. Published studies report a longer time to union and a higher nonunion rate when a strut allograft is used, probably because of the poor bone stock that prompted the use of the graft and the additional soft-tissue stripping that is required to place the graft.

Double Osteotomy

Indications

In some patients who have severe varus remodeling or pronounced anterior femoral bowing, deformity in the nonosteotomized medial cortex can preclude safe or accurate placement of a long revision femoral stem (**Figure 10, A**). Additionally, it may not be possible to achieve sufficient reduction of the ETO because of the residual gap between the medial two-thirds and the lateral one-third of the femur. In this infrequent circumstance, a second osteotomy may be necessary. The second osteotomy is done through the medial cortex so that the proximal femur can be closed around the proximal stem and the two osteotomy fragments apposed (**Figure 10, B**). Rarely, a double osteotomy is done to allow coaptation in the presence of a markedly ectatic proximal femur. In that scenario, one or two vertical osteotomies are completed after insertion of the final stem, with or without removal of a narrow V-shaped segment of bone. The femur is collapsed or coapted onto the underlying stem, with some fragment overlap, with the use of bone reduction forceps or the force of the cerclage cable tensioners. Care is taken to minimize the amount of soft-tissue stripping or devascularization.

Contraindications
The use of double osteotomy as an adjunct to an ETO has no absolute contraindications.

Alternative Treatments
To compensate for femoral deformity, a bone-replacing stem can be used. This strategy typically is used in the patient who has substantial osteolysis and remodeling around a failed stem because an ETO would be unlikely to heal to the remaining inadequate bone stock. A tumor endoprosthesis may be used in these patients.

Some commercially available curved revision stems can negate small amounts of anterior bowing resulting from the presence of a failed femoral stem.

Techniques
SETUP/EXPOSURE
- Setup and exposure are the same as for the ETO.

INSTRUMENTS/EQUIPMENT/IMPLANTS REQUIRED
- Instruments and equipment are the same as for the ETO.

PROCEDURE
- The potential need for a double osteotomy will be recognized during preoperative templating (**Figure 10, A**). The second osteotomy is delayed until late in the procedure and is done if the need for it is confirmed after insertion of the trial stem.
- The second (medial) osteotomy site is placed 5 cm proximal to the lateral osteotomy exit site so that the final configuration will be a step-cut osteotomy and will accommodate two cables across the step-cut configuration to enhance interfragmentary fixation (**Figure 10, B** and **C**).
- The second (medial) osteotomy can be initiated with multiple drill holes before the final stem is inserted, and the constricting force of bone reduction forceps or tightening of the fixation cables can be used to complete the medial osteotomy.
- Alternatively, the second osteotomy can be delayed until after stem insertion and completed with a Gigli saw. If this method is used, the Gigli saw is passed in the same manner as a fixation cable. Passage of the Gigli saw is easiest when the trial stem has not been placed and the soft tissues are not under tension. With the Gigli saw in place and the fixation cables passed, the trial stem is introduced, and the hip is assessed for limb length and stability. The definitive stem is placed, and the double osteotomy is completed. The cables are tightened, resulting in apposition of the osteotomy fragments to the stem and to each other (**Figure 10, D** and **E**).

WOUND CLOSURE
- The deep fascia is closed using No. 1 absorbable suture.
- The superficial adipose tissue is closed using 2-0 absorbable suture.
- The skin is closed according to the surgeon's preferred method.

Postoperative Regimen
As with the ETO, active hip abduction is avoided for 6 to 8 weeks postoperatively.

Avoiding Pitfalls and Complications
Preoperative planning is essential to ensure that the lateral extent of the ETO is at the apex of the varus deformity. The second (medial) osteotomy is done at a level that is proximal to the lateral extent of the ETO to create a step cut. This step-cut configuration reduces the stress at the osteotomy site and allows placement of several cables at the zone at which the medial and lateral bone overlap. If a Gigli saw is used, it should be put into place before stem placement, when the soft tissues are not under tension.

Controlled Perforation or Window Corticotomy

Indications
In select patients, a controlled perforation or cortical window in the femur can be used instead of an ETO. This technique permits better access to the canal for the management of a discrete retained cement mantle, a bony pedestal, or broken implants, and it offers improved illumination and irrigation. A series of 9-mm in-line drill holes can be made in the femoral cortex to access the femoral medulla (**Figure 11**). A more formal cortical osteotomy can be performed for the management of broken femoral stems or a more extensive cement mantle (**Figure 12, A**).

Contraindications
In a patient who has extensive retained obstructions, an ETO may be a more appropriate extensile maneuver to facilitate extraction.

Alternative Treatments
An ETO can be used as an alternative to controlled perforation or window corticotomy.

Techniques

SETUP/EXPOSURE

- A window corticotomy or controlled perforation can be performed in conjunction with any of the standard approaches to the hip. This technique is particularly amenable for use in conjunction with a vastus slide exposure or a posterolateral approach.
- Patient positioning is the same for the primary approach of choice. The skin and deep fascial incision is extended as far distally as required.

INSTRUMENTS/EQUIPMENT/IMPLANTS REQUIRED

- A powered oscillating saw, a drill and drill bits, and a variety of rigid osteotomes are required.

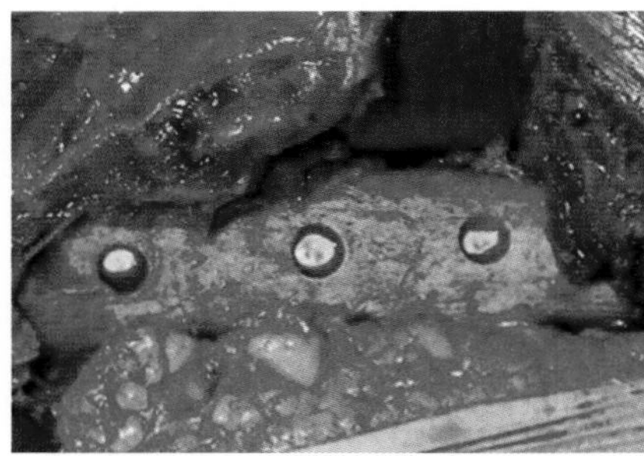

Figure 11 Intraoperative photograph shows subvastus controlled perforations (pilot holes) drilled in the femoral cortex.

- Cables or cerclage wires and passers are needed for reconstruction of the corticotomy.

PROCEDURE

- In the same manner as described for an ETO, the vastus lateralis muscle is elevated proximal and distal to the required location of the cortical window.
- A lateral one-third corticotomy with rounded edges is made using an oscillating saw or high-speed burr. The distal and proximal ends of the osteotomy are created at a 45° angle, generating a rounded edge on the cylindric femur.
- If a posterolateral approach is used, the anterior portion of the corticotomy is created with multiple drill holes with the use of a 4.5-mm drill, or with osteotomes introduced through the vastus muscle.
- The muscular attachment can be preserved by raising the fragment attached to an anterior hinge of soft tissue (**Figure 12, B**). This modification should be seriously considered in patients with proven infection.
- After the retained femoral obstruction is addressed, the window corticotomy is fixed as described for an ETO.

WOUND CLOSURE

- The deep fascia are closed using No. 1 absorbable suture.
- The superficial adipose tissue is closed using 2-0 absorbable suture.
- The skin is closed according to the surgeon's preferred method.

Postoperative Regimen

Depending on the reconstruction, the patient is routinely allowed to bear weight and resume activity as tolerated immediately after surgery.

Avoiding Pitfalls and Complications

Templating to identify the exact location of the corticotomy is important. Choosing obvious landmarks, such as the tip of the greater trochanter, will aid in accuracy. The surgeon should be prepared to achieve control of hemorrhage that may occur from the perforating branches of the deep femoral artery. The muscular and periosteal attachment to the so-called hinge of the cortical window is important to maintain stability and blood supply of the cortical fragment. Beveling of the edges of the cortical window will reduce the risk of fracture propagation when distal reaming is performed. To reduce the risk of periprosthetic fracture, the femoral stem should bypass the area of the cortical window.

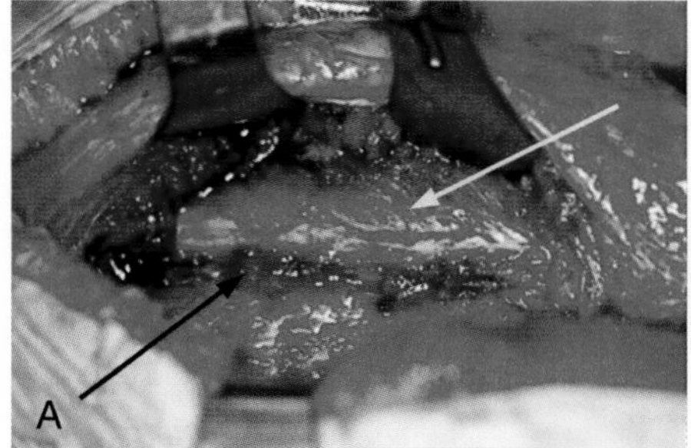

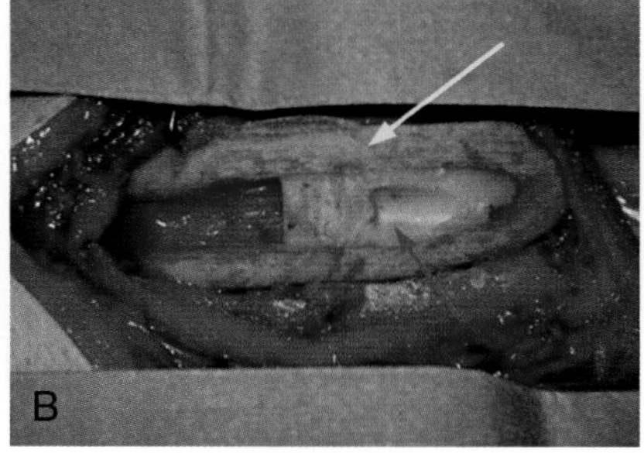

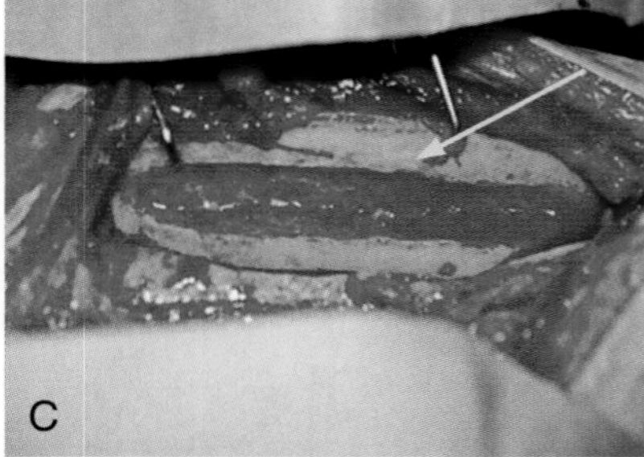

Figure 12 **A,** Intraoperative photograph shows planned window corticotomy (black arrow) with attached soft tissues to planned window corticotomy fragment (yellow arrow). **B,** Intraoperative photograph shows the use of an elevated vascularized window corticotomy (yellow arrow) to gain access to the femoral canal for the extraction of retained cement (green arrow). **C,** The window corticotomy fragment (arrow) is bleeding as the result of the maintenance of soft tissues and blood supply.

Bibliography

Charnley J: Total hip replacement by low-friction arthroplasty. *Clin Orthop Relat Res* 1970;(72):7-21.

Chen WM, McAuley JP, Engh CA Jr, Hopper RH Jr, Engh CA: Extended slide trochanteric osteotomy for revision total hip arthroplasty. *J Bone Joint Surg Am* 2000;82(9):1215-1219.

English TA: The trochanteric approach to the hip for prosthetic replacement. *J Bone Joint Surg Am* 1975;57(8):1128-1133.

Glassman AH, Engh CA, Bobyn JD: A technique of extensile exposure for total hip arthroplasty. *J Arthroplasty* 1987;2(1):11-21.

Goodman S, Pressman A, Saastamoinen H, Gross A: Modified sliding trochanteric osteotomy in revision total hip arthroplasty. *J Arthroplasty* 2004;19(8):1039-1041.

Kennon R, Keggi J, Zatorski LE, Keggi KJ: Anterior approach for total hip arthroplasty: Beyond the minimally invasive technique. *J Bone Joint Surg Am* 2004;86(suppl 2):91-97.

Langlais F, Lambotte JC, Collin P, Langlois F, Fontaine JW, Thomazeau H: Trochanteric slide osteotomy in revision total hip arthroplasty for loosening. *J Bone Joint Surg Br* 2003;85(4):510-516.

Levine MA: A treatment of central fractures of the acetabulum: A case report. *J Bone Joint Surg Am* 1943;25:902-906.

Mardones R, Gonzalez C, Cabanela ME, Trousdale RT, Berry DJ: Extended femoral osteotomy for revision of hip arthroplasty: Results and complications. *J Arthroplasty* 2005;20(1):79-83.

Masri BA, Campbell DG, Garbuz DS, Duncan CP: Seven specialized exposures for revision hip and knee replacement. *Orthop Clin North Am* 1998;29(2):229-240.

Mast NH, Laude F: Revision total hip arthroplasty performed through the Hueter interval. *J Bone Joint Surg Am* 2011;93(suppl 2):143-148.

Miner TM, Momberger NG, Chong D, Paprosky WL: The extended trochanteric osteotomy in revision hip arthroplasty: A critical review of 166 cases at mean 3-year, 9-month follow-up. *J Arthroplasty* 2001;16(8 suppl 1):188-194.

Moreland JR, Marder R, Anspach WE Jr: The window technique for the removal of broken femoral stems in total hip replacement. *Clin Orthop Relat Res* 1986;(212):245-249.

Morshed S, Huffman GR, Ries MD: Extended trochanteric osteotomy for 2-stage revision of infected total hip arthroplasty. *J Arthroplasty* 2005;20(3):294-301.

Park YS, Moon YW, Lim SJ: Revision total hip arthroplasty using a fluted and tapered modular distal fixation stem with and without extended trochanteric osteotomy. *J Arthroplasty* 2007;22(7):993-999.

Peters PC Jr, Head WC, Emerson RH Jr: An extended trochanteric osteotomy for revision total hip replacement. *J Bone Joint Surg Br* 1993;75(1):158-159.

Schutzer SF, Harris WH: Trochanteric osteotomy for revision total hip arthroplasty: 97% union rate using a comprehensive approach. *Clin Orthop Relat Res* 1988;(227):172-183.

Sydney SV, Mallory TH: Controlled perforation: A safe method of cement removal from the femoral canal. *Clin Orthop Relat Res* 1990;(253):168-172.

Younger TI, Bradford MS, Magnus RE, Paprosky WG: Extended proximal femoral osteotomy: A new technique for femoral revision arthroplasty. *J Arthroplasty* 1995;10(3):329-338.

Chapter 43
The Evaluation of Metal-on-Metal Total Hip Arthroplasty

Kevin I. Perry, MD
Steven J. MacDonald, MD, FRCSC

Introduction

Total hip arthroplasty (THA) implants with metal-on-metal (MoM) bearings were introduced in 1938 and first became popular in the 1960s, with the McKee-Farrar prosthesis being the most common. Potential advantages of MoM bearings over conventional metal-on-polyethylene articulations include decreased volumetric wear, increased fracture toughness, and the ability to use larger femoral heads to decrease postoperative instability. Despite the popularity of MoM bearings in the 1960s and 1970s, they were quickly overtaken by metal-on-polyethylene designs because of higher loosening rates and concern regarding metal sensitivities. However, growing concerns regarding polyethylene wear and osteolysis sparked the introduction of a second-generation MoM THA implant in 1988. The popularity of MoM articulations continued to rise through the 1990s and 2000s. In 2005, 35% of all hip arthroplasties performed in the United States used MoM articulations. Estimates suggest that more than 1,000,000 MoM articulations have been implanted since 1996.

Although many early studies regarding MoM bearings were generally favorable, numerous unforeseen complications have been elucidated, including early osteolysis and adverse soft-tissue reactions (pseudotumors) likely related to a delayed-type hypersensitivity response. MoM bearings have a higher incidence of pain after THA or hip resurfacing than any other bearing type. Therefore, these implants are under close scrutiny and in some instances have been recalled from the market. Because of the large (and growing) number of complications surrounding these implants, most surgeons in North America have abandoned their use. Current indications for implantation of MoM bearings are limited. Their use should be restricted to hip resurfacing in men younger than 65 years.

Although many patients with MoM hip arthroplasties have asymptomatic hips in which the implant will likely last a lifetime, all patients should undergo surveillance to evaluate for indicators of potential impending failure of the implants or soft-tissue reaction to metal wear particles. Information gathered in the evaluation of these patients should be used to assess whether each patient is at low, intermediate, or high risk of implant failure. On the basis of this risk assessment, the surgeon will be able to determine whether each patient with a MoM THA or hip resurfacing should be offered routine follow-up, closer monitoring, or revision hip arthroplasty.

History

Evaluation of a patient with a MoM hip arthroplasty should start with a detailed history. To begin, the surgeon should determine whether the patient is currently symptomatic. Although the absence of symptoms does not guarantee that the implants are functioning well, the evaluation of asymptomatic patients differs from that of symptomatic patients.

Patients who are symptomatic at the time of evaluation should undergo a more thorough history than is necessary in asymptomatic patients. Specifically, patients should be asked whether they experienced improvement after the index arthroplasty. In patients who did

Dr. MacDonald or an immediate family member has received royalties from and serves as a paid consultant to or is an employee of DePuy Synthes; has stock or stock options held in Hip Innovation Technology and JointVue; has received research or institutional support from DePuy Synthes, Smith & Nephew, and Stryker; and serves as a board member, owner, officer, or committee member of The Knee Society. Neither Dr. Perry nor any immediate family member has received anything of value from or has stock or stock options held in a commercial company or institution related directly or indirectly to the subject of this chapter.

Table 1 Intrinsic and Extrinsic Causes of Hip Pain

Intrinsic to the hip
Implant-related causes
Infection
Loosening
Instability
Periprosthetic fracture
Impingement
Adverse soft-tissue reaction (pseudotumor)
Extra-capsular causes
Trochanteric bursitis
Iliopsoas tendinitis
Extrinsic to the hip
Spinal stenosis
Disk herniation
Peripheral vascular disease
Hernias
Peripheral nerve injury
Malignancy or metastases
Metabolic bone disease (eg, Paget disease, osteopetrosis, osteomalacia)

Adapted with permission from Kwon YM, Fehring TK, Lombardi AV, Barnes CL, Cabanela ME, Jacobs JJ: Risk stratification algorithm for management of patients with dual modular taper total hip arthroplasty: Consensus statement of the American Association of Hip and Knee Surgeons, the American Academy of Orthopaedic Surgeons and the Hip Society. *J Arthroplasty* 2014;29(11):2060-2064.

not experience a period of pain relief, the indication for the initial arthroplasty should be questioned and the surgeon should look for alternative sources of the pain. Conversely, if the patient experienced a period of pain relief after the index arthroplasty, careful evaluation of the arthroplasty is paramount.

Pain after MoM hip arthroplasty can be classified as arising from sources that are intrinsic or extrinsic to the arthroplasty (**Table 1**). Sources of pain intrinsic to the arthroplasty include acute or chronic infection, aseptic loosening of the implants, instability, fracture, impingement, and adverse soft-tissue reaction (pseudotumor) related to a lymphocytic host-tissue response to metal wear particles (aseptic, lymphocyte-dominated, vasculitis-associated lesion). Sources of pain extrinsic to the arthroplasty include spinal stenosis, disk herniation, peripheral vascular disease, hernias, peripheral nerve injury, malignancy or metastases, and metabolic bone disease (eg, Paget disease, osteopetrosis, osteomalacia).

The painful MoM THA or hip resurfacing should be evaluated as to the onset, duration, severity, location, and character of the pain, because these factors can all be indicators of specific pathology. For example, buttock pain can indicate pathology in the lower back, pain occurring over the lateral aspect of the hip can indicate trochanteric bursitis, and deep-seated groin pain can indicate intra-articular pathology. MoM implants have been associated with a higher incidence of groin pain than other articulations. Pain at rest can indicate inflammation or infection, pain with the first few steps taken can indicate loose implants, and pain on stair climbing or hip flexion can indicate psoas tendon pathology. As in any patient with a painful THA, infection should always be high on the list of possible diagnoses, and the patient should be asked about recent illnesses, infection at other sites, and wound drainage. Patient perception of any soft-tissue masses or fluid collections may be an indicator of an adverse soft-tissue reaction to the metal wear particles.

If intra-articular pathology seems unlikely on the basis of the history, other causes of pain, including low back pathology and disk herniation, should be evaluated. These sources can often be differentiated from hip pathology by the fact that the pain typically occurs in the buttock or lower back and often radiates down the leg below the level of the knee.

The surgical report from the index arthroplasty should be obtained, if possible, to assess the specific implants in place. First, the surgeon should determine if the acetabular implant is monoblock or modular because monoblock implants have been associated with increased rates of failure after MoM arthroplasty. Second, the cup should be assessed to see if it is hemispheric because nonhemispheric cups have been associated with increased failures and increased metal ion levels. The femoral head diameter should be noted because larger diameters are associated with greater metal ion levels than are smaller diameters. Modularity of the neck of the femoral implant should be noted because modular femoral implants have been associated with a failure rate higher than that of femoral implants without a modular neck.

Physical Examination

After completion of the history, the patient should undergo a thorough physical examination, starting with careful inspection of the hip. Specific attention to the location of the scar can indicate the approach used for the index arthroplasty. Inspection of the skin can reveal evidence of possible infection, including a draining sinus or erythema surrounding the hip. Palpation of the soft tissues surrounding the hip can provide evidence of any fluid accumulation or soft-tissue masses in the area. Pain with palpation of the soft tissues around the greater trochanter can indicate trochanteric bursitis.

The patient's gait should be carefully assessed for signs of a Trendelenburg gait, which can indicate abductor insufficiency or tearing. Any changes in the patient's gait from previous assessments should be noted because changes can suggest the extent of soft-tissue damage resulting from pseudotumor or hypersensitivity reaction. The hip should be taken through a range of motion including internal and external rotation and hip adduction and abduction. Pain with these maneuvers suggests intra-articular pathology. Specifically, pain at the extremes of motion suggests loosening of the implants or impingement, whereas pain throughout the arc of motion is indicative of active inflammation or infection. Pain with resisted flexion and passive extension of the hip can indicate psoas tendon pathology, which is more common in patients with the large femoral heads used in many MoM hip arthroplasties.

Radiographic Evaluation

Routine screening of all MoM hip arthroplasties should include an AP pelvic radiograph as well as AP and lateral hip radiographs. The radiographs should be scrutinized for evidence of osteolysis of the bone surrounding the prosthesis and loosening of the femoral or acetabular implant (**Figure 1**). Radiographic evaluation of the hip in conjunction with the patient's history can reliably provide evidence of implant loosening. Evidence of a soft-tissue shadow can be indicative of soft-tissue masses or fluid collections.

The position of the implants should be carefully evaluated. Specifically, an increase in acetabular implant abduction angle (>55°) has been associated with increased metal ion levels and increased failures of MoM hip arthroplasty. Both excessive and insufficient cup anteversion have been associated with increased serum metal ion levels. Larger femoral heads are more likely to lead to increased groin pain as well as psoas tendon pathology and irritation than are smaller femoral heads. If modularity was not previously determined, the femoral implant should be assessed for the presence of a modular neck because modular implants have been associated with increased rates of failure and revision.

Laboratory Analysis and Aspiration of the Hip

Patients with MoM arthroplasties have substantially elevated serum and urine levels of metal ions compared with patients with metal-on-polyethylene bearings, even with a well-functioning arthroplasty. Elevation of serum metal ion levels in an asymptomatic patient has been associated with pseudotumor formation. As a result, most North American surgeons agree that although routine laboratory screening of patients with MoM THA at every visit is not indicated, the surgeon should obtain a baseline level in asymptomatic patients who have other risk factors (excessive cup abduction angle, an implant with a poor track record) and in all symptomatic patients. In asymptomatic patients in whom evaluation is indicated, at a minimum, cobalt and chromium levels should be obtained. In symptomatic patients, the white blood cell (WBC) count, erythrocyte sedimentation rate (ESR), C-reactive protein (CRP) level, and cobalt and chromium levels should be tested to evaluate for possible infection and possible metal reaction.

Multiple cutoff values for serum cobalt and chromium levels have been proposed with varying sensitivities and specificities. Initially, cutoff values of 7 parts per billion (ppb) of cobalt or chromium were described. Because of the low sensitivity of the test, some authors have recommended lowering the cutoff value to 5 ppb. With either cutoff value, serum cobalt levels seem to be most specific and sensitive for abnormal functioning of the MoM articulation. Nevertheless, metal ion levels should be evaluated in the context of the overall clinical assessment of the patient and should not be relied on as the sole determinant of the need for revision surgery. Metal ion levels can be helpful but are not specifically diagnostic.

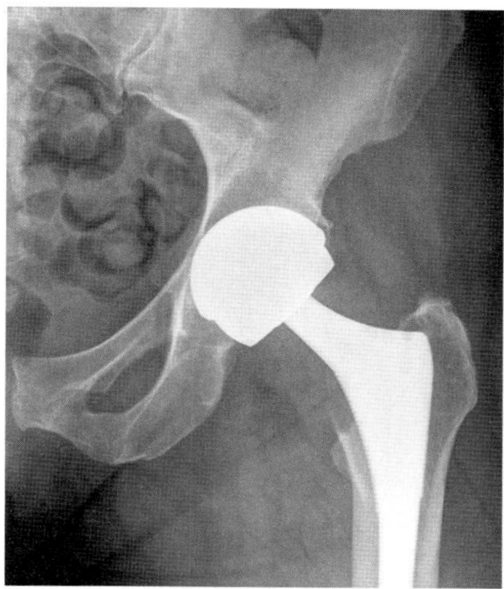

Figure 1 AP radiograph of a metal-on-metal total hip arthroplasty in a left hip demonstrates osteolysis of the calcar, which is concerning for metal-on-metal reaction.

Aspiration of the hip should be considered in patients with elevated metal ion levels, WBC count, ESR, or CRP level because it can aid in diagnosing infection. Nevertheless, the surgeon must use caution when interpreting serum and synovial values in patients with MoM hip arthroplasties. Several studies have shown that metal reaction can mimic infection, and no consensus exists on the best tests to diagnose periprosthetic joint infection in patients with MoM arthroplasty. The surgeon should order a manual WBC count instead of an automated count because tissue debris in suspension (from metal reaction) can result in falsely elevated automated cell counts.

One study demonstrated that serum ESR and CRP and synovial WBC all have low specificity and sensitivity for the diagnosis of infection in patients with MoM hip arthroplasties. Thus, the authors of the study recommended using the neutrophil percentage from the synovial fluid analysis instead. All patients with MoM THA and infection in that study had a synovial neutrophil percentage greater than 80%. However,

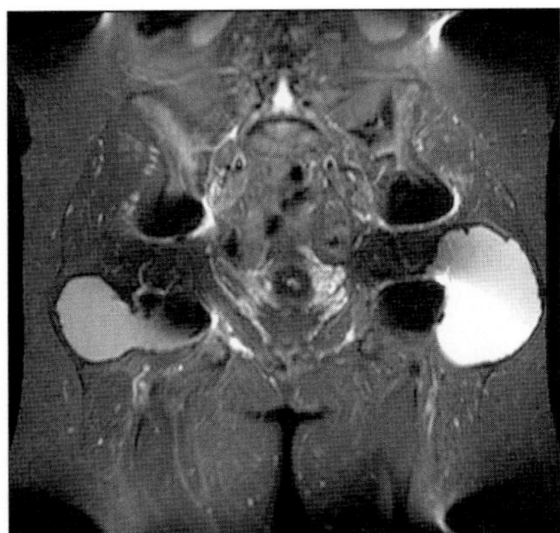

Figure 2 Coronal metal-artifact reduction sequence (MARS) MRI demonstrates pseudotumors surrounding bilateral metal-on-metal hip resurfacings.

the authors of a different study reviewed 150 patients undergoing revision of MoM hip arthroplasties (of which 19 were found to be infected according to Musculoskeletal Infection Society criteria) and found that the synovial WBC count was the best test to diagnose periprosthetic joint infection. They determined that an absolute synovial WBC count of 4,350 cells/µL in the synovial fluid was an effective cutoff to rule infection in or out. In that study, the ESR and CRP level both had good sensitivity, at 83% and 94%, respectively.

Advanced Imaging

In patients with an obvious soft-tissue mass on examination, elevated serum metal ion levels (cobalt or chromium), or unexplained pain after implantation of a MoM articulation, advanced imaging of the arthroplasty may be helpful. Several studies have shown that ultrasonography is a useful and effective screening modality for detecting adverse soft-tissue reactions surrounding hip arthroplasty implants. Advantages of ultrasonography include its availability at most institutions, its low cost, and the lack of image distortion from metal artifact around the implants. Disadvantages include its lower sensitivity than that of metal-artifact reduction sequence (MARS) MRI.

MARS MRI has been shown to be highly sensitive and specific for the detection of adverse soft-tissue reaction and pseudotumor (**Figure 2**). With MARS MRI, the size of the pseudotumor, the capsular wall thickness, and involvement of muscle can be delineated. In a study of 68 failed MoM hip arthroplasties, MARS MRI had sensitivity of 94% and specificity of 87% for detecting adverse soft-tissue reactions. The authors of the study also reported 90% sensitivity and 86% specificity of MARS MRI for quantifying intraoperative tissue damage. Advantages of MRI include its high specificity and sensitivity as well as its ability to detect and quantify the extent of soft-tissue damage. Disadvantages of MRI include expense and the limited availability of MARS MRI in some institutions.

Not all pseudotumors identified on ultrasonography or MARS MRI warrant revision surgery. A subset of patients who have evidence of pseudotumor will remain asymptomatic and do not require revision. Therefore, surgeons should not rely too heavily on one specific test; rather, the entire clinical presentation should be examined before deciding to revise an implant. Some pseudotumors will decrease in size over time in patients who are asymptomatic. Characteristic findings on MARS MRI that suggest the need for revision surgery include a progressive increase in size of the pseudotumor, muscle involvement, and substantial bony destruction.

Individual Patient Assessment

Patients with an existing MoM THA or hip resurfacing implant should be carefully and routinely screened for evidence of potential failure or soft-tissue reaction to these implants. All patients should be assessed individually and the risk of impending failure (and need for revision) of the implants established (**Table 2**). For patients deemed low risk, the authors of this chapter recommend follow-up on a yearly basis with at least radiographic and physical evaluation. If any changes from the previous examination are noted, the surgeon should consider repeat testing of metal ion levels and the use of advanced imaging. For patients at intermediate risk of implant failure, the authors of this chapter recommend follow-up in 6 months to ensure that no substantial changes in symptoms, radiographic appearance, or metal ion levels have occurred. In patients at high risk of implant failure, revision arthroplasty should be considered.

Summary

The number of complications reported after MoM hip arthroplasties has resulted in a drastic reduction in the use of such implants in North America. Patients in whom MoM bearings were previously implanted must be monitored for signs of impending failure and reaction to metal wear particles. Thorough patient history and physical examination as well as routine radiographic screening are warranted. A baseline laboratory analysis should be obtained for comparison with any subsequent analyses required to evaluate for elevated serum and urine levels of metal ions. Hip aspiration may be done to evaluate for infection. Ultrasonography may be useful for detecting adverse soft-tissue reactions about MoM implants. MARS MRI may be obtained in patients with suspected adverse soft-tissue reaction and pseudotumor.

Table 2 Patient Risk Stratification

Factor	Risk: Low	Risk: Moderate	Risk: High
Patient	Low activity level	Male or female Dysplasia (for hip resurfacing) Moderate activity level	Female with dysplasia (for hip resurfacing) High activity level
Symptoms	Asymptomatic (including no systemic or mechanical symptoms)	Mild local hip symptoms (eg, pain, mechanical symptoms) No systemic symptoms	Severe local hip and/or mechanical symptoms Systemic symptoms
Clinical examination	No change in gait (ie, no limp) No abductor weakness No swelling	Change in gait (ie, limp) No abductor weakness No swelling	Change in gait (ie, limp or Trendelenburg gait) Abductor weakness Swelling
Implant type	Small-diameter femoral head (<36 mm) modular MoM THA Hip resurfacing in men age <50 yr with osteoarthritis	Large-diameter femoral head (>36 mm) modular or nonmodular MoM THA Recalled MoM implant Hip resurfacing with risk factors (as in female patients or patients with dysplasia) Implant with modular femoral neck	Large-diameter femoral head (>36 mm) modular or nonmodular MoM THA Recalled MoM implant Hip resurfacing (in female patients with dysplasia)
Radiographs	Optimal acetabular cup orientation (40° ± 10° inclination for hip resurfacing) No implant osteolysis/loosening	Optimal acetabular cup orientation No implant osteolysis/loosening	Suboptimal acetabular cup orientation Implant osteolysis/loosening
Infection workup	Within normal limits	Erythrocyte sedimentation rate and C-reactive protein level, with or without hip aspiration, within normal limits	Within normal limits
Metal ion level test	Low (<3 ppb)	Moderately elevated (3-10 ppb)	High (>10 ppb)
Cross-sectional imaging	Within normal limits	Presence of abnormal tissue reactions without involvement of surrounding muscles and/or bone Simple cystic lesions or small cystic lesions without thickened wall	Presence of abnormal tissue reactions with involvement of surrounding muscles and/or bone Solid lesions Cystic lesions with thickened wall Mixed solid and cystic lesions
Management recommendation	Annual follow-up	Follow-up in 6 mo Consider revision surgery	Consider revision surgery

MoM = metal-on-metal, ppb = parts per billion, THA = total hip arthroplasty.

Adapted with permission from Kwon YM, Fehring TK, Lombardi AV, Barnes CL, Cabanela ME, Jacobs JJ: Risk stratification algorithm for management of patients with dual modular taper total hip arthroplasty: Consensus statement of the American Association of Hip and Knee Surgeons, the American Academy of Orthopaedic Surgeons and the Hip Society. *J Arthroplasty* 2014;29(11):2060-2064.

Bibliography

Bartelt RB, Yuan BJ, Trousdale RT, Sierra RJ: The prevalence of groin pain after metal-on-metal total hip arthroplasty and total hip resurfacing. *Clin Orthop Relat Res* 2010;468(9):2346-2356.

Benson MK, Goodwin PG, Brostoff J: Metal sensitivity in patients with joint replacement arthroplasties. *Br Med J* 1975;4(5993):374-375.

Bozic KJ, Browne J, Dangles CJ, et al: Modern metal-on-metal hip implants. *J Am Acad Orthop Surg* 2012;20(6):402-406.

Bozic KJ, Kurtz S, Lau E, et al: The epidemiology of bearing surface usage in total hip arthroplasty in the United States. *J Bone Joint Surg Am* 2009;91(7):1614-1620.

Clarke MT, Lee PT, Arora A, Villar RN: Levels of metal ions after small- and large-diameter metal-on-metal hip arthroplasty. *J Bone Joint Surg Br* 2003;85(6):913-917.

Daniel J, Pynsent PB, McMinn DJ: Metal-on-metal resurfacing of the hip in patients under the age of 55 years with osteoarthritis. *J Bone Joint Surg Br* 2004;86(2):177-184.

De Haan R, Pattyn C, Gill HS, Murray DW, Campbell PA, De Smet K: Correlation between inclination of the acetabular component and metal ion levels in metal-on-metal hip resurfacing replacement. *J Bone Joint Surg Br* 2008;90(10):1291-1297.

Delaunay CP: Metal-on-metal bearings in cementless primary total hip arthroplasty. *J Arthroplasty* 2004;19(8 suppl 3):35-40.

Forster-Horvath C, Egloff C, Valderrabano V, Nowakowski AM: The painful primary hip replacement: Review of the literature. *Swiss Med Wkly* 2014;144:w13974.

Glyn-Jones S, Pandit H, Kwon YM, Doll H, Gill HS, Murray DW: Risk factors for inflammatory pseudotumour formation following hip resurfacing. *J Bone Joint Surg Br* 2009;91(12):1566-1574.

Hart AJ, Buddhdev P, Winship P, Faria N, Powell JJ, Skinner JA: Cup inclination angle of greater than 50 degrees increases whole blood concentrations of cobalt and chromium ions after metal-on-metal hip resurfacing. *Hip Int* 2008;18(3):212-219.

Hart AJ, Skinner JA, Henckel J, Sampson B, Gordon F: Insufficient acetabular version increases blood metal ion levels after metal-on-metal hip resurfacing. *Clin Orthop Relat Res* 2011;469(9):2590-2597.

Judd KT, Noiseux N: Concomitant infection and local metal reaction in patients undergoing revision of metal on metal total hip arthroplasty. *Iowa Orthop J* 2011;31:59-63.

Kwon YM, Fehring TK, Lombardi AV, Barnes CL, Cabanela ME, Jacobs JJ: Risk stratification algorithm for management of patients with dual modular taper total hip arthroplasty: Consensus statement of the American Association of Hip and Knee Surgeons, the American Academy of Orthopaedic Surgeons and the Hip Society. *J Arthroplasty* 2014;29(11):2060-2064.

Kwon YM, Ostlere SJ, McLardy-Smith P, Athanasou NA, Gill HS, Murray DW: "Asymptomatic" pseudotumors after metal-on-metal hip resurfacing arthroplasty: Prevalence and metal ion study. *J Arthroplasty* 2011;26(4):511-518.

Lavigne M, Laffosse JM, Ganapathi M, Girard J, Vendittoli P: Residual groin pain at a minimum of two years after metal-on-metal THA with a twenty-eight-millimeter femoral head, THA with a large-diameter femoral head, and hip resurfacing. *J Bone Joint Surg Am* 2011;93(suppl 2):93-98.

Lehil MS, Bozic KJ: Trends in total hip arthroplasty implant utilization in the United States. *J Arthroplasty* 2014;29(10):1915-1918.

Long WT, Dorr LD, Gendelman V: An American experience with metal-on-metal total hip arthroplasties: A 7-year follow-up study. *J Arthroplasty* 2004;19(8 suppl 3):29-34.

MacDonald SJ, McCalden RW, Chess DG, et al: Metal-on-metal versus polyethylene in hip arthroplasty: A randomized clinical trial. *Clin Orthop Relat Res* 2003;(406):282-296.

McKee GK, Watson-Farrar J: Replacement of arthritic hips by the McKee-Farrar prosthesis. *J Bone Joint Surg Br* 1966;48(2):245-259.

Mikhael MM, Hanssen AD, Sierra RJ: Failure of metal-on-metal total hip arthroplasty mimicking hip infection: A report of two cases. *J Bone Joint Surg Am* 2009;91(2):443-446.

Muraoka K, Naito M, Nakamura Y, Hagio T, Takano K: Usefulness of ultrasonography for detection of pseudotumors after metal-on-metal total hip arthroplasty. *J Arthroplasty* 2015;30(5):879-884.

Nawabi DH, Gold S, Lyman S, Fields K, Padgett DE, Potter HG: MRI predicts ALVAL and tissue damage in metal-on-metal hip arthroplasty. *Clin Orthop Relat Res* 2014;472(2):471-481.

Nishii T, Sakai T, Takao M, Yoshikawa H, Sugano N: Is ultrasound screening reliable for adverse local tissue reaction after hip arthroplasty? *J Arthroplasty* 2014;29(12):2239-2244.

Sidaginamale RP, Joyce TJ, Lord JK, et al: Blood metal ion testing is an effective screening tool to identify poorly performing metal-on-metal bearing surfaces. *Bone Joint Res* 2013;2(5):84-95.

Siddiqui IA, Sabah SA, Satchithananda K, et al: A comparison of the diagnostic accuracy of MARS MRI and ultrasound of the painful metal-on-metal hip arthroplasty. *Acta Orthop* 2014;85(4):375-382.

Wyles CC, Larson DR, Houdek MT, Sierra RJ, Trousdale RT: Utility of synovial fluid aspirations in failed metal-on-metal total hip arthroplasty. *J Arthroplasty* 2013;28(5):818-823.

Yi PH, Cross MB, Moric M, et al: Do serologic and synovial tests help diagnose infection in revision hip arthroplasty with metal-on-metal bearings or corrosion? *Clin Orthop Relat Res* 2015;473(2):498-505.

Chapter 44

Revision of Metal-on-Metal Hip Implants

Christopher Pomeroy, MD
Thomas K. Fehring, MD

Indications

Metal-on-metal (MoM) bearings gained popularity in total hip arthroplasty (THA) when issues of polyethylene wear, late instability, and osteolysis associated with the use of metal-on-polyethylene bearings became apparent. The lower volumetric wear rates and improved stability with the use of larger-diameter femoral head sizes caused many surgeons in the United States to change their implant preference. By 2006, nearly 33% of all primary THA procedures performed in the United States had MoM bearing surfaces. In patients younger than 65 years, nearly 42% of primary THAs had MoM bearings by 2006.

The initial laboratory testing of MoM bearings was promising. However, expanded clinical data provided in national joint registries have shown a two- to threefold increase in failure of MoM bearings compared with that of non-MoM bearings in THA. Increased failure with MoM bearings primarily occurs with femoral heads at least 36 mm in diameter. Femoral heads of up to 32 mm in diameter in MoM THAs perform similarly to traditional metal-on-polyethylene bearing surfaces. With many of the larger MoM femoral head sizes, the use of a monoblock acetabular cup is necessary. Evidence suggests that monoblock MoM implants fail at a higher rate than modular MoM implants do. The first FDA recall of a monoblock MoM acetabular implant occurred in 2008 and was followed shortly thereafter by the recall of a second monoblock implant in 2010. The primary design flaws of monoblock shells include fixation problems, cup deformation on implantation, and a functional articular surface less than a hemisphere in size. These factors place monoblock MoM implants at high risk of failure.

A MoM hip arthroplasty implant can fail by one of several mechanisms. Many of these mechanisms, such as infection, aseptic loosening, instability, and periprosthetic fracture, are not specific to MoM implants but occur with all bearing surfaces. Modes of failure specific to MoM implants include femoral neck fractures in resurfacing procedures, early loosening of monoblock acetabular implants, and adverse local tissue reactions (ALTRs) or metallosis. The combination of these modes of failure accounts for the higher rate of revision of MoM hip arthroplasties. Because of increasing awareness of implant design, the advent of ALTRs, and the large number of patients with MoM THA implants, a systematic approach to monitoring these patients is important.

When evaluating a patient with a painful MoM THA, the surgeon should rule out other causes of pain before attributing the problem to the bearing. A thorough physical examination must be performed to rule out an extrinsic etiology of the hip pain. Physical examination should include assessment for spine disease, peripheral nerve injury, and malignancy. Intrinsic factors including infection, loosening, instability, fracture, and bursitis or tendinitis around the hip must also be considered. After ruling out these possibilities, the MoM bearing can be considered the source of pain.

When determining whether revision of a MoM THA implant is required, the surgeon should stratify each patient as low, medium, or high risk according to the risk stratification algorithm of the American Association of Hip and Knee Surgeons, the American Academy of Orthopaedic Surgeons, and The Hip Society. Clinical factors considered in risk stratification of a patient with

Dr. Fehring or an immediate family member has received royalties from, is a member of a speakers' bureau or has made paid presentations on behalf of, serves as a paid consultant to, has received research or institutional support from, and has received nonincome support (such as equipment or services), commercially derived honoraria, or other non–research-related funding (such as paid travel) from DePuy Synthes and serves as a board member, owner, officer, or committee member of the American Association of Hip and Knee Surgeons and The Knee Society. Neither Dr. Pomeroy nor any immediate family member has received anything of value from or has stock or stock options held in a commercial company or institution related directly or indirectly to the subject of this chapter.

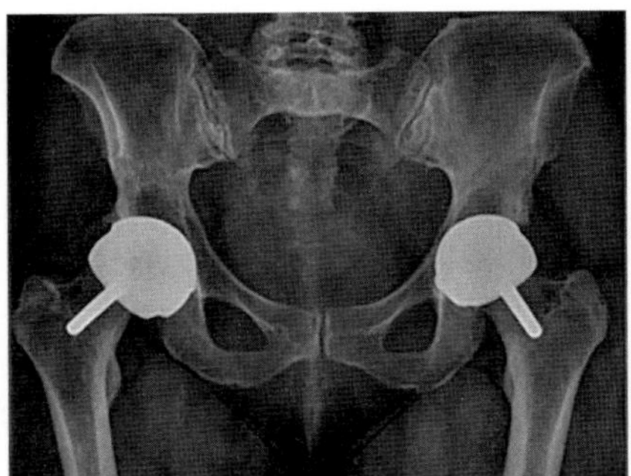

Figure 1 AP pelvic radiograph from a patient with bilateral metal-on-metal bearings demonstrates large amounts of osteolysis behind the acetabular implants. Osteolysis is greater on the right side than the left. Bone loss less than 30% is not evident on plain radiographs.

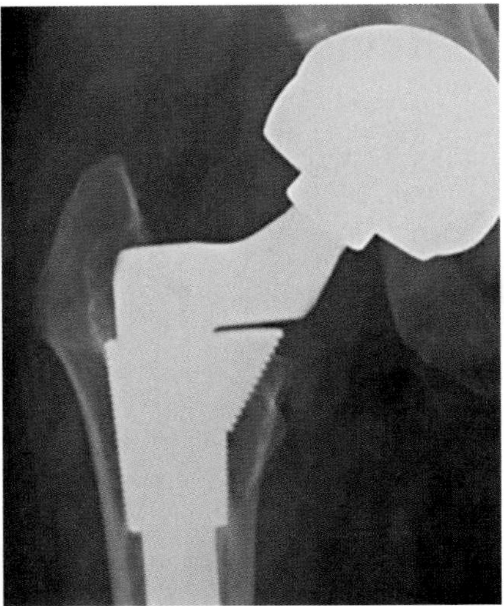

Figure 2 AP radiograph of a right hip demonstrates subtle signs of loosening with osteolysis in the greater trochanter adjacent to the femoral implant.

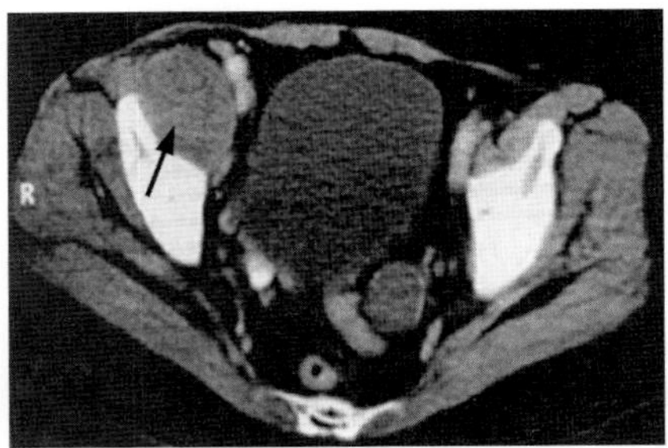

Figure 3 Axial metal-artifact reduction sequence MRI demonstrates a large soft-tissue adverse local tissue reaction anterior to the right hip (arrow).

MoM hip arthroplasty include pain, abductor weakness, mechanical symptoms, implant position, implant type, metal ion levels, cross-sectional imaging findings (metal-artifact reduction sequence [MARS] MRI), and systemic findings. Any one of these factors may put a patient at risk, but none of them alone should be used to make the decision for revision. When evaluating a painful MoM hip, the surgeon should first obtain radiographs and critically assess them for implant position, implant type, and possible osteolysis surrounding the implants. MARS MRI can be used to evaluate soft-tissue integrity and the presence or absence of ALTRs. Metal ion levels should be obtained and used as an objective monitoring marker. Serum metal ion levels will be lower for hip resurfacing compared with MoM THA because of the additional implant surfaces, such as the femoral trunnion, in THA. A direct comparison of metal ion levels between hip resurfacing and MoM THA cannot be made because of dissimilar implant designs. The findings from a thorough physical examination to evaluate the abductor mechanism and these advanced imaging and laboratory markers are used to decide whether to revise a painful MoM hip.

After deciding to proceed with revision, preoperative planning is essential. AP pelvic and lateral hip radiographs should be obtained and carefully inspected for signs of osteolysis. In patients with MoM implants, subtle osteolysis is a poor prognostic factor (**Figures 1** and **2**). Because 30% bone loss is necessary to visualize osteolysis on plain radiographs, the amount of osteolysis is usually much worse than radiographs alone would suggest. MARS MRI should be evaluated closely for fluid collection, solid masses, or intrapelvic extension of the ALTR (**Figure 3**). The amount of bone loss is likely to be more severe than initially expected on the basis of preoperative radiographs. If the amount of osteolysis is moderate or severe on radiographs, CT is warranted. If necessary, three-dimensional CT modeling can be used to help plan the reconstruction.

The patient's preoperative abductor strength is important for diagnosis. If an anterolateral approach was used in the index procedure, it may be difficult to differentiate abductor insufficiency owing to a pathologic source from that resulting from a repair failure. MRI can help assess the integrity of the abductors. If the patient has any signs of weakness regardless of cause, a constrained implant should be available at the time of revision. The previous surgical note should be obtained when possible. Identifying the current implants and knowing what options are available if part of the THA implant is retained will limit surprises intraoperatively.

Contraindications

Revision of a MoM implant should not be performed if other possible causes of hip pain have not been ruled out. After potentially confounding intrinsic and extrinsic etiologies of the hip pain have been considered, the patient should be stratified as low, medium, or high risk. If the patient has a well-positioned, nonrecalled implant with low levels of metal ions and negative cross-sectional imaging for ALTRs, revision surgery should not be performed. A study of the Australian Orthopaedic Association National Joint Replacement Registry demonstrated that the revision rate for MoM implants is nearly twice that of other bearing surfaces; however, approximately 90% of MoM implants are well functioning at 8-year follow-up, regardless of femoral

Table 1 Results of Revision Surgery for the Management of Failed Metal-on-Metal Implants

Authors (Year)	Number of Hips	Reason for Revision	Mean Patient Age in Years (Range)	Mean Follow-up in Years (Range)	Results
Gross and Liu (2014)	58	Acetabular loosening, femoral neck fracture, femoral loosening, ALTR	50 (12-65)	5.2 (2-11.4)	2 hips (3%) had complications 2 of 16 patients (13%) revised for acetabular loosening underwent rerevision
Matharu et al (2014)	64	ALTR	57.8 (31-78.8)	4.5 (1.0-14.6)	8 hips (12.5%) underwent rerevision (2 for recurrent dislocation, 2 for recurrent ALTR, 1 for deep infection, 1 for impingement, 1 for acetabular loosening, 1 for unexplained pain) 13 hips (20.3%) had complications
Munro et al (2014)	32	ALTR, infection, aseptic loosening of the acetabular cup	57.5 (46-76)	2.1 (0.8-4.0)	28% dislocated 13% had failure of ingrowth 22% underwent rerevision 12 hips (38%) had complications
Wyles et al (2014)	37	Aseptic loosening, ALTR, periprosthetic fracture, impingement, dislocation	55.2 (29-76)[a]	2.75 (2.0-6.75)	8% underwent two-stage repeat revision for the management of deep infection 95% survivorship free of rerevision at 2-yr follow-up 3 hips (8%) underwent rerevision
Stryker et al (2015)	114	Metallosis, aseptic loosening, infection, pain, malposition, instability, impingement, periprosthetic fracture	60 (17-84)	1.2 (0-10.2)	18 hips (16%) underwent rerevision (6% aseptic loosening, 6% deep infection, 4% dislocation, 3% acetabular fracture) 23 hips (20%) had complications

ALTR = adverse local tissue reaction.

[a] Age at the time of the primary procedure.

head size. Although the accessibility of information via social media and the Internet may lead many patients with MoM implants to inquire about revision surgery, some patients may need only routine follow-up visits with careful monitoring of previously noted factors.

Alternative Treatments

If the painful MoM hip does not meet requirements for revision, it should be monitored. There are no alternative treatment options for the painful MoM hip that meet revision criteria.

Results

Revision surgery for the management of failed MoM implants has a high rate of complications in recent reports with limited numbers of patients (**Table 1**). The authors of one study reported major complications including dislocation, failure of ingrowth to the acetabular cup, and recurrent ALTR in 12 of 32 revisions of MoM implants (38%). In a different study, researchers found an 8% postoperative infection rate after revision of MoM implants in 37 patients. In a study of 58 revisions of hip resurfacing arthroplasty, 2 of 16 patients (13%) who underwent revision for acetabular loosening required rerevision for failure of acetabular fixation. In a study of revision for ALTR in patients with MoM bearings, postoperative complications occurred in 20.3% of the revisions, and 12.5% required rerevision. The authors of a study of 114 revisions of monoblock MoM THA reported a 20% complication rate, and 18 of 114 revisions (16%) required a secondary procedure. The most common complications in that study were aseptic loosening, deep infection, dislocation, and acetabular fracture. In a study evaluating the survivorship of 86 THA implants with femoral head-neck taper corrosion, no difference in survivorship was found between the 32 implants with high-grade corrosion and the 54 implants with low-grade corrosion.

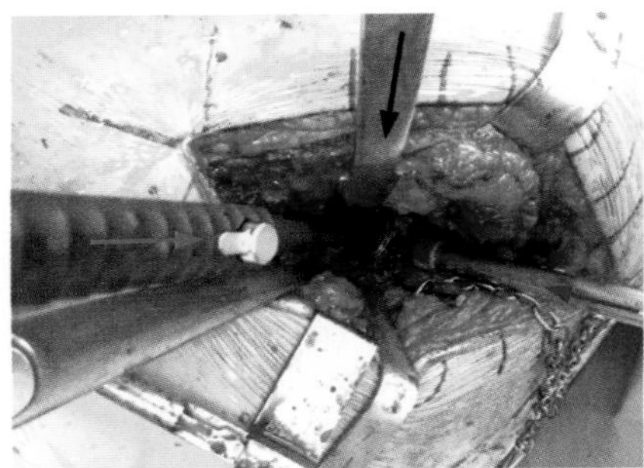

Figure 4 Intraoperative photograph shows placement of a retractor anteriorly (black arrow) to allow translation of the femur for three-column inspection of the acetabulum. With proper exposure, a suction device (red arrow) is applied to the modular liner for gentle traction while the edge of the cup is tapped with a 3-lb mallet and tamp (blue arrow) at different frequencies to dissociate the liner.

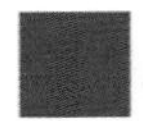

Techniques

Setup/Exposure

- The senior author of this chapter (T.K.F.) prefers a posterior approach because it is the most versatile and facilitates complex acetabular revision, including a trochanteric slide or flip osteotomy if necessary for exposure.
- If an isolated acetabular revision is performed, the femoral trunnion should be protected by creating a pouch in the anterolateral supra-acetabular region for placement of the prosthetic femoral neck. The femur is then translated anteriorly with a Mueller retractor to allow three-column inspection of the acetabulum (**Figure 4**).

Instruments/Equipment/ Implants Required

- Because most MoM revisions involve the acetabular implant, a cup extraction system and acetabular gouges should be readily available (**Figure 5**).
- Manufacturer-specific instrumentation to remove the femoral implant should be available for use if the femoral implant appears loose or malrotated.
- In routine revisions, a porous metal acetabular implant should be used because ingrowth is a common problem in revision of MoM implants.
- Reconstruction plates should be available because extraction fractures or unrecognized preoperative fractures are common.
- A cup-cage system and conventional cages should be available for use in patients with severe bone deficiency.
- Alternatively, a custom triflange implant can be used to span severe acetabular defects in patients with severe bone loss.

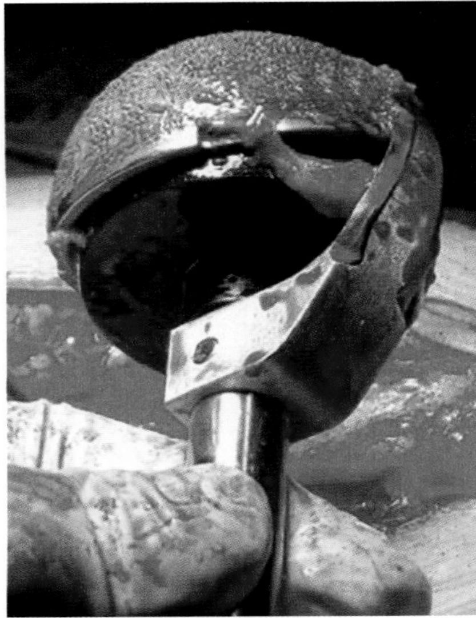

Figure 5 Intraoperative photograph shows an extraction device that facilitates acetabular cup removal with minimal associated bone loss. (Courtesy of Innomed, Savannah, GA.)

Procedure

INSPECTION OF THE FEMORAL IMPLANT

- After exposure is achieved, the femoral implant is inspected closely for signs of loosening.
- The rotational stability of the femoral implant is tested, which can be done using an implant-specific extraction device that threads into the femoral implant.
- The trunnion is inspected.
- A small amount of corrosion is not an indication for revision of the femoral implant. Only if the trunnion is severely damaged or cracked should a well-fixed femoral implant be revised.
- Revision ceramic femoral heads or metal femoral heads should be available for reimplantation on a well-fixed retained femoral trunnion.

REVISION OF A MONOBLOCK ACETABULAR IMPLANT

- Because of their poor survivorship, monoblock acetabular cups should be revised regardless of their position.
- Although some surgeons place dual-mobility polyethylene heads while retaining the existing metal shell, the authors of this chapter do not endorse this technique because objective data are not available to support its use. The rims of many monoblock implants have sharp edges that may shred the polyethylene (**Figure 6**).

REVISION OF A MODULAR ACETABULAR IMPLANT

- Implants with acceptable survivorship may be more amenable to liner exchange than those fraught with complications would be.
- The screws of the modular implant are removed to test implant stability. To facilitate removal of these screws, the metal liner is extracted.
- To dissociate the liner, a 3-lb mallet and tamp are used to tap the side of the implant at different frequencies while slight axial traction is applied to the liner with a suction device (**Figure 4**). After the liner is removed, the screws will be visible for removal.
- If the modular implant is not well fixed, it should be removed.

- If the implant is well fixed, is well oriented, and has a successful history, modular acetabular revision with a polyethylene liner may be sufficient.

REAMING

- If the acetabular implant will be exchanged, conservative reaming should be performed, as in all acetabular implant revisions.
- If osteonecrosis is noted, reaming continues until viable bleeding bone is encountered.
- Aseptic loosening of the acetabular implant after revision of MoM implants is common. Therefore, if bleeding bone is not encountered with a moderate amount of reaming, the use of a cup-cage construct or conventional cage should be considered.

IMPLANTATION OF THE REVISION IMPLANT

- After a good bleeding bed has been established, the new acetabular implant is placed.
- A porous metal implant is preferred because it will maximize bony ingrowth, which can help prevent early aseptic loosening of the revision cup.
- If the abductors are deficient but present, the use of a dual-mobility implant, or at least an implant with a good constrained option, should be considered for stability.
- If the abductors are severely compromised or soft-tissue tension cannot be established, a constrained implant is used.

Wound Closure

- If a posterior approach was used, the posterior capsule or soft-tissue sleeve is repaired to help maximize stability. Dislocation can occur after revision of a MoM implant because the large MoM femoral head size is often decreased with exchange to a polyethylene liner.
- Thorough soft-tissue débridement is performed in a patient with an ALTR (**Figure 7**).
- The wound is closed in standard manner, which includes closure of the posterior capsule, fascia, and superficial tissues.

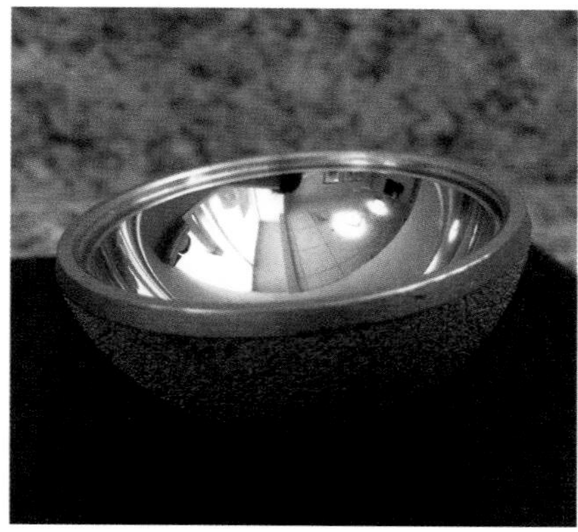

Figure 6 Photograph shows a monoblock acetabular cup (ASR; DePuy Synthes). If the cup is retained and the metal femoral head is exchanged for a dual-mobility implant, the sharp edges of the rim of the cup may shred the polyethylene of the dual-mobility implant.

Postoperative Regimen

The postoperative regimen is determined based on intraoperative findings. If there are any concerns regarding acetabular fixation or bone vascularity, the patient should be limited to touch-down weight bearing for 6 to 8 weeks postoperatively. If the abductor mechanism was repaired during wound closure, the patient should be placed in an abduction brace for 6 weeks postoperatively.

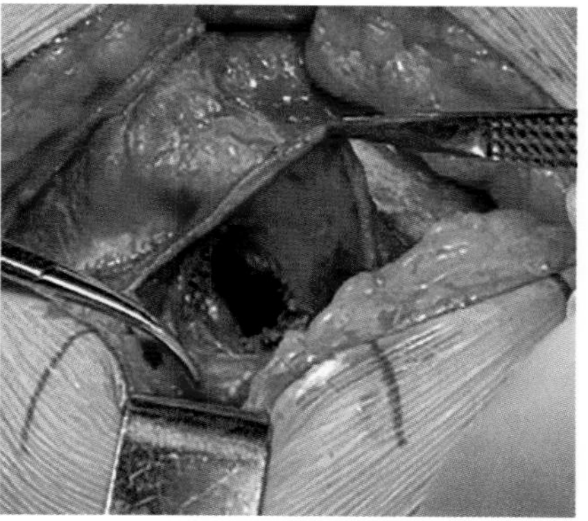

Figure 7 Intraoperative photograph after the arthrotomy via a posterior approach shows a typical adverse local tissue reaction seen in patients with metal-on-metal bearings requiring revision. The soft tissue should be thoroughly débrided before the surgical wound is closed.

Avoiding Pitfalls and Complications

Understanding the history and survivorship of the patient's specific MoM implant is crucial because implants with poor reported results should be scrutinized for their orientation, stability, and need for revision. High complication rates after revision MoM THA have been reported (**Table 1**). Preparation and planning before the revision may help decrease postoperative failures and the need for rerevision. Preoperative radiographs should be examined closely. A patient with severe osteolysis should undergo further evaluation with CT. Three-dimensional models of the hip can help the surgeon accurately identify the location and severity of bone loss. If the abductor mechanism appears to be affected, whether from the previous surgical approach or ALTR, constrained implants should be available. Because aseptic loosening is common, porous metal acetabular implants should be used to encourage bony ingrowth.

Bibliography

Australian Orthopaedic Association: *National Joint Replacement Registry Hip and Knee Arthroplasty: Annual Report 2008*. Adelaide, South Australia, Australian Orthopaedic Association, 2008. Available at: https://aoanjrr.sahmri.com/annual-reports-2008. Accessed August 23, 2016.

Bozic KJ, Kurtz S, Lau E, et al: The epidemiology of bearing surface usage in total hip arthroplasty in the United States. *J Bone Joint Surg Am* 2009;91(7):1614-1620.

Goyal N, Ho H, Fricka KB, Engh CA Jr: Do you have to remove a corroded femoral stem? *J Arthroplasty* 2014; 29(9 suppl):139-142.

Graves SE, Rothwell A, Tucker K, Jacobs JJ, Sedrakyan A: A multinational assessment of metal-on-metal bearings in hip replacement. *J Bone Joint Surg Am* 2011;93(suppl 3):43-47.

Gross TP, Liu F: Outcomes after revision of metal-on-metal hip resurfacing arthroplasty. *J Arthroplasty* 2014; 29(9 suppl):219-223.

Howie DW, Holubowycz OT, Middleton R; Large Articulation Study Group: Large femoral heads decrease the incidence of dislocation after total hip arthroplasty: A randomized controlled trial. *J Bone Joint Surg Am* 2012;94(12):1095-1102.

Kwon YM, Lombardi AV, Jacobs JJ, Fehring TK, Lewis CG, Cabanela ME: Risk stratification algorithm for management of patients with metal-on-metal hip arthroplasty: Consensus statement of the American Association of Hip and Knee Surgeons, the American Academy of Orthopaedic Surgeons, and the Hip Society. *J Bone Joint Surg Am* 2014;96(1):e4.

MacDonald SJ, McCalden RW, Chess DG, et al: Metal-on-metal versus polyethylene in hip arthroplasty: A randomized clinical trial. *Clin Orthop Relat Res* 2003;(406):282-296.

Matharu GS, Pynsent PB, Sumathi VP, et al: Predictors of time to revision and clinical outcomes following revision of metal-on-metal hip replacements for adverse reaction to metal debris. *Bone Joint J* 2014;96-B(12):1600-1609.

Munro JT, Masri BA, Duncan CP, Garbuz DS: High complication rate after revision of large-head metal-on-metal total hip arthroplasty. *Clin Orthop Relat Res* 2014;472(2):523-528.

National Joint Registry for England, Wales, and Northern Ireland: *5th Annual Report*: *2008*. Hemel Hempstead, England, National Joint Registry, 2008.Available at: http://www.njrcentre.org.uk/NjrCentre/Portals/0/Documents/England/Reports/5th%20Annual.pdf. Accessed August 23, 2016.

Stryker LS, Odum SM, Fehring TK, Springer BD: Revisions of monoblock metal-on-metal THAs have high early complication rates. *Clin Orthop Relat Res* 2015;473(2):469-474.

Wyles CC, Van Demark RE III, Sierra RJ, Trousdale RT: High rate of infection after aseptic revision of failed metal-on-metal total hip arthroplasty. *Clin Orthop Relat Res* 2014;472(2):509-516.

Chapter 45

Taper Corrosion After Total Hip Arthroplasty: Evaluation and Management

Michael J. Taunton, MD

Derek F. Amanatullah, MD, PhD

Indications

The use of modular implants in total hip arthroplasty (THA) helps reestablish leg length, femoral offset, and femoral anteversion intraoperatively. Femoral head-neck modularity reduces implant inventory and allows a surgeon to make final intraoperative adjustments to femoral offset and leg length that are critical for stability. Metaphyseal-diaphyseal modularity allows a surgeon to attain fixation independent of femoral anteversion and leg length, simplifying revision THA. Dual modular systems with both head-neck and neck-stem modularity allow a surgeon to implant the stem into the femoral metadiaphysis and independently position the femoral neck (varus or valgus and anteversion or retroversion) to more accurately correct or match a patient's anatomy. However, modularity is associated with radiolucent lines, early aseptic loosening, and increased osteolysis. The necessity of modularity in THA has come under increasing scrutiny, with the recognition of mechanically assisted taper corrosion and the voluntary recall of certain dual modular femoral implants. Mechanically assisted taper corrosion is not limited to dual modular femoral stem designs but also occurs at head-neck and metaphyseal-diaphyseal junctions. Mechanically assisted taper corrosion leads to the production of metal ions and can result in failure via implant fracture.

The management of modular junction corrosion in THA requires an algorithmic approach (**Figure 1**). Patients with a symptomatic metal-on-metal (MoM) articulation or modular junction usually report hip and/or groin pain as the chief complaint. Patients with metal reaction often have good results in the immediate postoperative period, with symptoms developing over time, sometimes as early as 3 months postoperatively. These symptoms may mimic infection or loosening. Patients may have a palpable mass or fluid collection near the hip with or without loss of hip abduction. Because catching, locking, and crepitus are common, assessment of hip range of motion is imperative. Patients may also be asymptomatic and have normal imaging of a recalled implant but have substantially elevated serum chromium and cobalt levels.

Dr. Taunton or an immediate family member serves as a paid consultant to or is an employee of DJO; has received research or institutional support from Stryker; and serves as a board member, owner, officer, or committee member of the American Academy of Orthopaedic Surgeons and the Minnesota Orthopaedic Society. Dr. Amanatullah or an immediate family member serves as a paid consultant to Sanofi; has stock or stock options held in BlueJay Mobile Health; and has received research or institutional support from Acumed.

Mechanisms of Failure

CORROSION

Corrosion of orthopaedic implants was first described in 1956. The corrosive process occurs via several modes, including galvanic corrosion, fretting corrosion, crevice corrosion, pitting corrosion, and intergranular corrosion (**Table 1**). Surface oxidation protects metals from corrosion. The process of surface oxidation is known as passivation. If the passivation layer is disrupted, the underlying metal oxidizes to reestablish a passivation layer. However, re-passivation is not always possible at a modular junction, leading to mechanically assisted taper corrosion.

Modular junctions are particularly susceptible to crevice corrosion. Crevice corrosion is a local version of galvanic corrosion caused by subtle changes in the chemical microenvironment at the surface of a metal. A crevice is created because modular junctions have very tight tolerances but may have a small gap between the two surfaces. This small, isolated gap (that is, crevice) may have insufficient oxygen to re-passivate the surface metal, and, thus, the passivation layer is disrupted. This environmental microisolation results in crevice corrosion. Crevice corrosion is initiated by the difference in oxygen concentration outside the crevice (that is, the cathode) and inside the crevice (that is, the anode), which establishes a galvanic

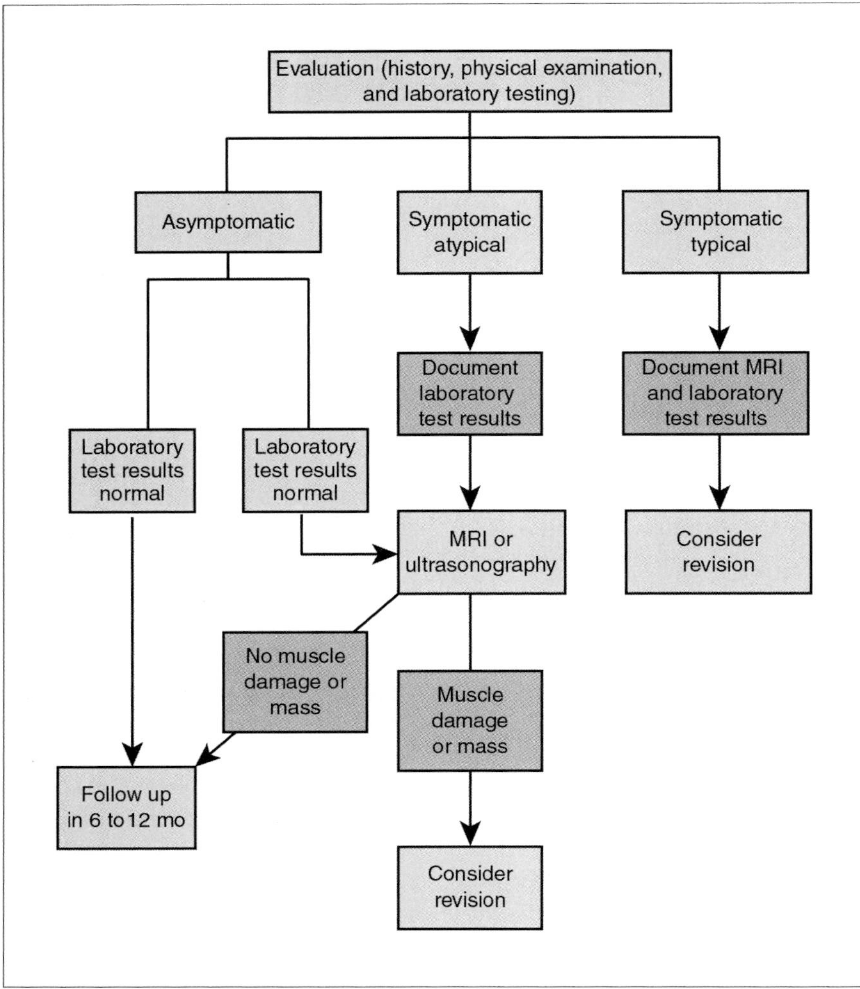

Figure 1 Algorithm shows the management of metal-related hip arthroplasty implant failure.

Table 1 Modes of Corrosion

Mode of Corrosion	Cause	Solution
Galvanic	Dissimilar metals	Avoidance of dissimilar metals Passivation layer
Fretting	Micromotion	Avoidance of micromotion
Crevice[a]	Microscopic isolation	Improved tolerances Passivation layer
Pitting[a]	Surface defects	Polishing of surfaces Passivation layer
Intergranular	Carbide-grain boundaries	Molybdenum alloys Low-carbon alloys

[a] Crevice and pitting corrosion are local versions of galvanic corrosion caused by subtle changes in the chemical microenvironment at the surface of the metal and occur between similar metals or the same metal.

circuit (**Figure 2**). At the cathode, the concentration of oxygen is high and that of hydrogen ions and chloride ions is low. At the anode, the concentration of oxygen is low and that of hydrogen ions and chloride ions (that is, hydrochloric acid) is high. The concentration of chloride and hydrogen ions inside the crevice leads to the liberation of metal ions such as cobalt and chromium. The liberated chromium ions interact with organic phosphate ions, forming a chromium(III) phosphate precipitate on the interface surface (**Figure 3**). Therefore, corrosion at a modular junction results in differential elevation of serum cobalt ions compared with that of serum chromium ions. Crevice corrosion has been reported in more than 30% of mixed-alloy femoral head-neck junctions, less than 10% of all-titanium-alloy modular implants, and less than 6% of all-cobalt-alloy devices.

Modular junctions are particularly susceptible to fretting corrosion. Micromotion at the taper junction can physically damage the underlying metal, disrupt the passivation layer, liberate metal ions, and facilitate crevice corrosion. The amount of fretting corrosion changes with taper design, taper geometry, neck rigidity, metal alloy combination, mechanical environment, and material performance.

No standardization exists in the taper designs offered by device manufacturers. A study of the three-dimensional topography of 11 common tapers demonstrated that 64% had varying threaded surface textures that consisted of repetitive peaks and troughs, whereas 36% had smooth surface textures. Increased taper roughness and decreased taper length have been associated with greater corrosion. The flexural rigidity of the femoral neck is inversely proportional to the amount of fretting corrosion. The offset of the femoral head affects fretting corrosion. Neutral-offset femoral heads piston on the trunnion, whereas femoral heads with increased offset tend to

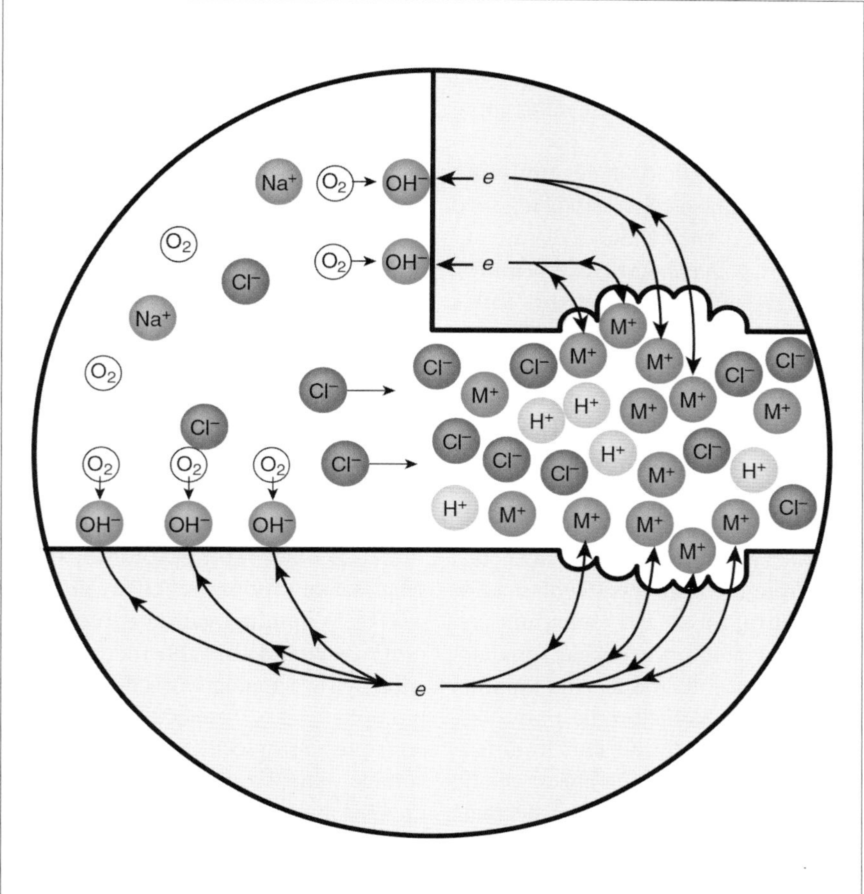

Figure 2 Simplified illustration shows an oxygen gradient between a crevice and the surrounding environment. The oxygen gradient establishes the potential for transfer of electrons (*e*) from the metal to oxygen (O_2), resulting in the formation of hydroxide ions (OH^-) in the presence of water, accumulation of positively charged metal ions (M^+) within the crevice, disassociation of sodium chloride (Na^+, Cl^-), lowering of the pH (H^+) in the crevice, and degradation of the implant.

rock on the trunnion and increase the amount of fretting corrosion. Increased femoral offset results in greater frictional torque at the articulation and fretting corrosion. The amount of micromotion at a taper is subject to the manufacturing tolerance of the trunnion.

Taper assembly affects fretting. Dry taper assembly does not prevent fretting-induced wear but increases the load required to initiate micromotion at the interface. Off-axis loading causes the conical bore of the femoral head to tip with respect to the trunnion and double the amount of micromotion with a given force. Fretting corrosion has been reported in 4% of head-neck junctions and 94% of dual modular junctions. The authors of this chapter recommend carefully cleaning and drying the femoral trunnion and impacting it with strong blows delivered directly in line with the femoral neck, rather than at an offset angle.

Conflicting data exist regarding the relationship of femoral head size to mechanically assisted corrosion. Some studies reported no relationship between femoral head size and serum metal ion levels. Other studies reported increased serum metal ion levels with 28-mm femoral heads compared with 36-mm femoral heads. A study of data from the Australian Orthopaedic

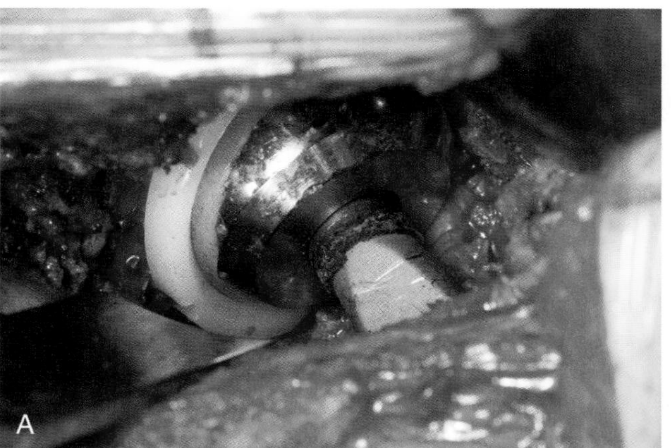

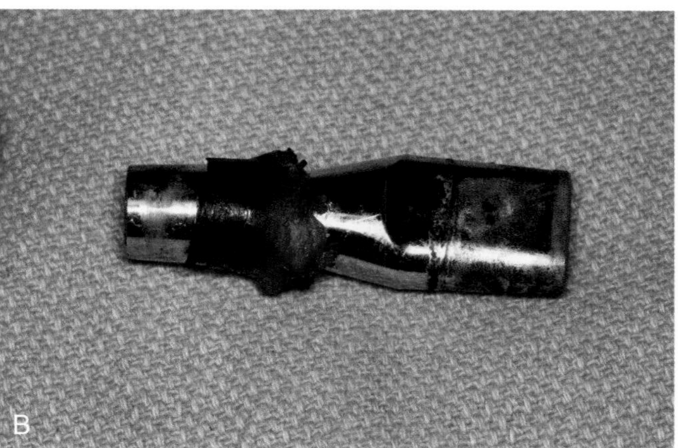

Figure 3 Intraoperative (**A**) and clinical (**B**) photographs of a total hip implant show the deposition of chromium(III) phosphate as a result of fretting and crevice corrosion at the femoral head-neck junction (**A**) and the neck-stem junction (**B**).

Association National Joint Replacement Registry reported an increased failure rate with femoral head sizes larger than 32 mm. Modular metal-on-polyethylene THA implants with 36-mm heads have greater corrosion damage to the head-neck trunnion compared with THA implants with 28-mm heads. Metal ion production is increased in MoM THA implants with large femoral heads and short taper lengths. Anecdotal evidence from the institution of the authors of this chapter suggests an increased risk of ion production with larger femoral heads and with increased offset of the femoral head.

All modular junctions (head-neck, dual modular, and metaphyseal-diaphyseal) are susceptible to mechanically assisted corrosion via the mechanisms of fretting and crevice corrosion. Fretting and crevice corrosion have been associated with catastrophic implant fracture, especially in patients with titanium dual modular stems.

BIOLOGIC REACTION TO METAL IONS

Cobalt and chromium ions are considered toxic at high concentrations, with ionic valence playing an important role in the extent of toxicity. Specifically, the Cr^{6+} ion causes pulmonary epithelial cancer after inhalation, whereas the Cr^{3+} ion, which is released from orthopaedic implants, is much less harmful. Cobalt is considerably more toxic, with systemic effects including severe neurologic and cardiac manifestations. Overall, cobalt and chromium particles pose three main threats to human cells: genotoxicity, cytotoxicity, and hypersensitivity.

Both cobalt and chromium are genotoxic, with chromium being slightly more so than cobalt. The DNA damage is induced via oxidation. Additionally, cobalt and chromium inhibit DNA repair, and cobalt inhibits topoisomerase II. The leukocytes of patients with a MoM implant have a significant increase in the number of chromosomal translocations and aneuploid cells compared with the leukocytes of patients without a MoM implant. Even at concentrations considered less than toxic, cobalt and chromium ions can cause substantial DNA damage. However, the clinical effect of genotoxicity is currently unknown. A Finnish cohort study reported no increase in the incidence of any cancer type in patients with MoM bearings. In fact, the mortality of patients with a MoM articulation is equivalent to that of the general population.

Cobalt and chromium particles are cytotoxic, but cobalt is substantially more cytotoxic than chromium. Cobalt induces a hypoxic-like state with oxidative stress and upregulation of hypoxia-regulated gene products. Neither cobalt nor chromium inhibits osteoblast activity. In vitro, cobalt and chromium particles generated using a wear simulator were reported to reduce the viability of histiocytes and fibroblasts by 97% and 95%, respectively. This finding is in sharp contrast to the effects of alumina ceramic particles, which decrease the viability of histiocytes by only 18% and have no effect on the viability of fibroblasts. A retrieval study supports these results, with the authors of the study reporting a reaction similar to tumoral calcinosis, along with necrosis and necrobiosis, in their observation of histiocytes that had taken up metal debris surrounding MoM implants.

The term hypersensitivity refers to an overreaction of a specific immune system to an allergen. On the skin, this reaction is characterized by the wheal and flare reaction. Metal hypersensitivity is a well-known, common condition affecting approximately 10% to 15% of the general population. Nickel, which is used in cobalt-chromium alloys, followed by cobalt and chromium, are the most common and potent immunologic sensitizing metals. Metal ions themselves are too small to stimulate an immune response. Metal ions react with protein carriers, such as albumin, to denature the protein and form a hapten (that is, the complex between the metal ion and the carrier). Haptens are antigens and are large enough to create a robust immune response.

Patients who are sensitive to nickel often have cross-reactivity with cobalt and chromium. This reactivity is attributable to the fact that when a patient reacts to a hapten, such as chromium-albumin or cobalt-albumin, the allergic response that is elicited is actually in response to the denatured carrier, in this case albumin. Nickel, cobalt, and chromium denature carrier proteins in similar ways and, therefore, cause cross-reaction. A cell-mediated type IV hypersensitivity reaction occurs when nickel, cobalt, and chromium particles form immunoreactive haptens. $CD4^+$ T lymphocytes are presented with a hapten through their interaction with a major histocompatibility complex class II molecule on an antigen-presenting cell, such as a macrophage. The hapten-sensitized $CD4^+$ T lymphocytes release interferon-γ. Interferon-γ activates macrophages to secrete cytokines (granulocyte/-macrophage-colony stimulating factor, tumor necrosis factor, and interleukins) and recruit cytotoxic T lymphocytes involved in the cell-mediated type IV hypersensitivity reaction. A higher incidence of hypersensitivity to nickel, as quantified by lymphocyte transformation testing, has been reported in patients with MoM THA implants compared with control subjects. MoM THA function was independent of nickel hypersensitivity. Interestingly, the risk of revision THA also is independent of metal hypersensitivity.

ADVERSE LOCAL TISSUE REACTION

Adverse local tissue reaction (ALTR), which also is called adverse reaction to metal debris, is the adverse clinical manifestation that results from the presence of metal wear debris and the production of metal ions. How ALTR correlates with the biologic issues of genotoxicity,

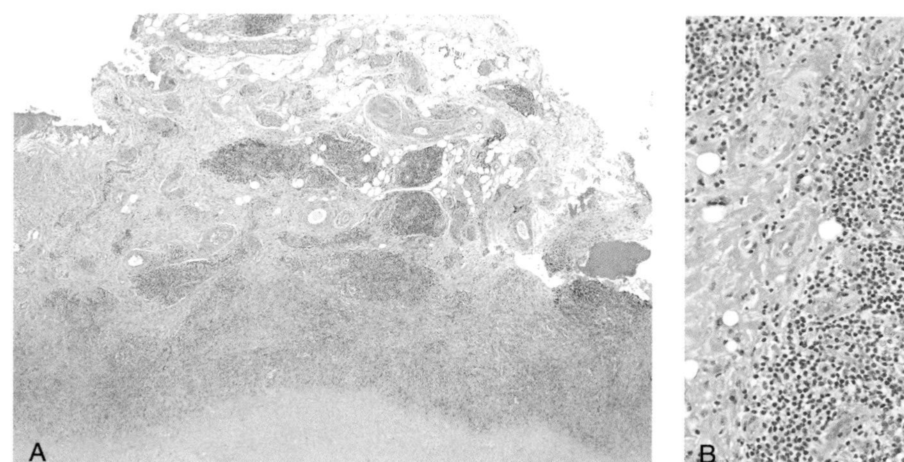

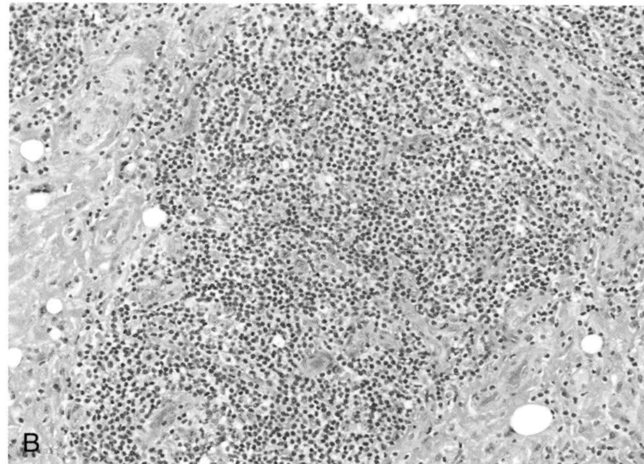

Figure 4 Hematoxylin-eosin, magnification ×5 (**A**) and hematoxylin-eosin, magnification ×20 (**B**) photomicrographs show the diffuse perivascular infiltrates of T- and B-lymphocytes along with plasma cells and macrophages with or without metal debris. These findings are characteristic of aseptic lymphocyte-dominated vasculitis-associated lesions.

cytotoxicity, and hypersensitivity is unknown.

ALTR includes two major subgroups: soft-tissue reactions and bony reactions. Soft-tissue reactions also are referred to as aseptic lymphocyte-dominated vasculitis-associated lesions (ALVALs). An ALVAL is a histologic diagnosis used to describe the clinical appearance of soft-tissue necrosis and abnormal joint fluid at the time of revision THA. Tissue samples obtained at the time of revision THA in patients with MoM implants who had persistent symptoms or early recurrence of preoperative symptoms showed diffuse perivascular infiltrates of T and B lymphocytes and plasma cells and an accumulation of macrophages with or without metal debris (**Figure 4**). Notably, tissues involved in an ALVAL that contain lymphocytes have a significantly higher mean metal content than ALVAL-like tissues that contain macrophages.

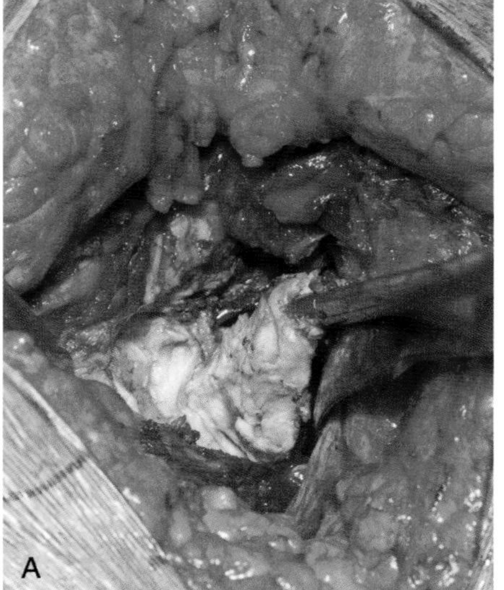

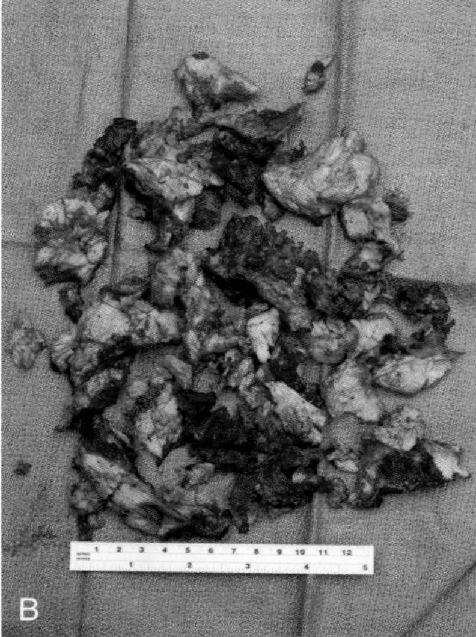

Figure 5 **A,** Intraoperative photograph shows a pseudotumor in the abductor musculature surrounding a modular total hip implant with a cobalt-chromium neck, titanium stem, and ceramic-on-polyethylene bearing. **B,** Photograph shows resected tissue as a gross specimen.

The term pseudotumor describes a large cystic lesion in patients who have previously undergone THA with a MoM articulation or junction (**Figure 5**). The histologic appearance of these lesions is very similar to that of ALVALs; however, the lymphocytic infiltrate is more diffuse and the areas of connective tissue necrosis are more extensive. Pseudotumors can be large and have a varied presentation, including pain, nerve palsy, spontaneous dislocation, and a palpable mass. The prevalence of pseudotumors varies greatly, with studies reporting rates as high as 32% to 61% in asymptomatic patients. A study of patients with cobalt-chromium dual modular tapers revealed pseudotumors in 45% of asymptomatic hips and elevated cobalt-to-chromium ratios. A pseudotumor may compromise the abductor musculature and necessitate abductor reconstruction (with vastus lateralis, gluteus maximus, or Achilles tendon allograft) or the use of a constrained liner at the time of revision THA.

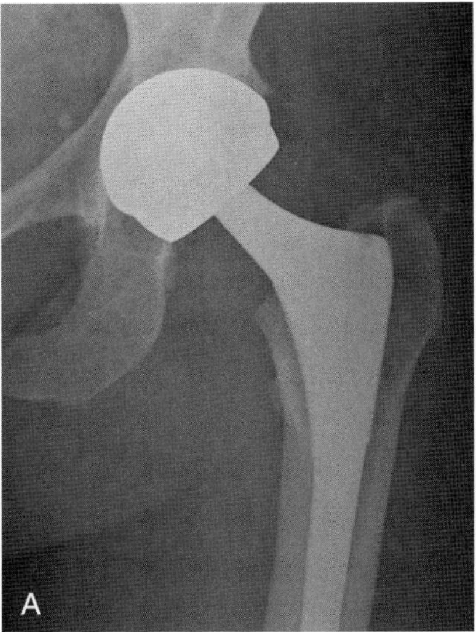

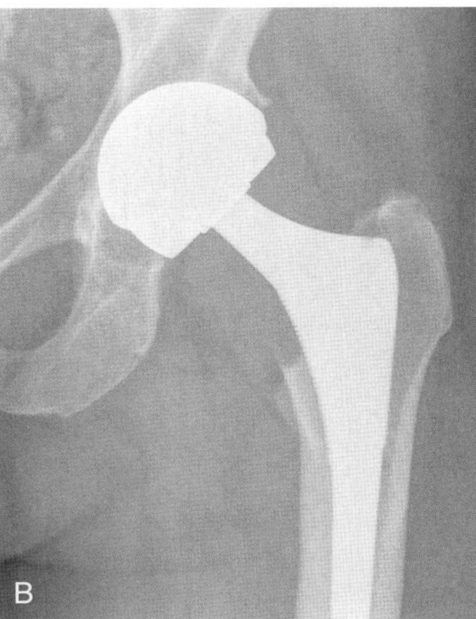

Figure 6 AP radiographs of a left hip demonstrate metal-on-metal total hip arthroplasty with a large femoral head immediately postoperatively (**A**) and 5 years postoperatively, with severe osteolysis of the calcar (**B**).

Osteolysis is bone loss resulting from stimulated osteoclast resorption of bone. Osteolysis appears as cystic lesions or radiolucent regions near the femoral and acetabular implants on plain radiographs (**Figure 6**). The histologic appearance of tissue from patients with failed MoM implants secondary to osteolysis and aseptic loosening is similar to that of ALVALs. Perivascular lymphoplasmacytic infiltrates and metal debris suggest that osteolysis is the bony counterpart of ALVALs. Erosion of the medial calcar is often an early finding of osteolysis in the presence of metal reaction (**Figure 6**). This finding may be the result of greater exposure of the calcar to synovial fluid compared with that of other parts of the bone, which usually are covered with soft tissue. Additionally, the calcar is closest in proximity to the modular head-neck and neck-stem junctions.

Evaluation

After an appropriate history and inventory of symptoms, a complete physical examination is necessary. Range of motion should be assessed, and any pain, catching, or grinding should be noted. Palpation for fluid or solid masses may indicate a pseudotumor. A careful examination of neurologic function may reveal subtle nerve involvement. Although nerve palsies are uncommon, assessment of the neurovascular status of the limb is essential in any musculoskeletal examination. The authors of this chapter have found a previously undocumented sciatic nerve palsy secondary to necrosis around the sciatic nerve on two separate occasions. Likewise, the notation of muscle strength is key. Placement of patients on their side for both palpation and assessment of abductor function may reveal local muscle involvement. In the experience of the authors of this chapter, the abductor musculature is the primary muscle group affected by modular taper corrosion because of its proximity to the hip and the potential use of the anterolateral approach.

A radiographic evaluation should begin with AP pelvic and cross-table lateral hip radiographs. The surgeon should evaluate the radiographs, comparing them first with the immediate postoperative radiographs. Taking the time to obtain these radiographs from an outside institution, if necessary, may make a difference in the diagnosis. Comparison of current radiographs with preoperative radiographs aids in the assessment of implant subsidence, implant loosening, and early-onset osteolysis. An assessment of overall leg length, implant position, and bone quality should be performed. As noted, erosion of the medial calcar is often an early finding of osteolysis in patients with metal reaction (**Figure 6**).

The possibility of infection should always be considered in these patients, and appropriate laboratory markers must be evaluated. A patient's synovial white blood cell (WBC) count, serum erythrocyte sedimentation rate, and serum C-reactive protein level are poor diagnostic markers of infection if symptomatic MoM articulations or modular junction corrosion is present. Aspiration of the joint is more helpful. A neutrophil percentage greater than 80% indicates infection. A patient's WBC count should be done manually because the presence of metal ions can lead to an overestimation of the WBC count if the cell count is performed by a machine.

Serum cobalt and chromium ion concentrations are used for screening and diagnosis; however, mixed results have been reported regarding formal cutoff levels. In a retrospective study of serum cobalt and chromium ion levels for the prediction of failure of MoM articulations, the cutoff of 7 parts per billion (ppb) that was set by the United Kingdom Medicine and Healthcare Products Regulatory Agency in 2010 had 89% specificity and 52% sensitivity for the detection of unexplained failure of a MoM articulation. However, the optimal cutoff for serum cobalt and chromium levels was 5 ppb, which has a 63% specificity and 85% sensitivity for the detection of unexplained failure of a MoM articulation.

In patients with modular junction corrosion, the liberated chromium ions interact with organic phosphate ions, forming a chromium(III) phosphate precipitate that causes differential elevation of serum cobalt ions and serum chromium ions (**Figure 3**). This differential elevation of serum cobalt above serum chromium is not typically observed in patients with failure of a MoM articulation. Additionally, whole blood testing may be quicker and provide a more accurate representation of systemic exposure to metal ions compared with serum testing. If a patient's serum metal ion levels are elevated, radiographs should be scrutinized for osteolysis and implant malpositioning. If either is present, revision THA should be strongly considered. In asymptomatic patients without osteolysis and with appropriately oriented implants, careful monitoring of serum metal ion levels every 6 to 12 months is recommended. In symptomatic patients, the clinical track record of the implant should be considered, with revision THA considered in patients with recalled implants or implants voluntarily taken off the market. Observation should be considered only in asymptomatic patients in whom serum cobalt and chromium ion levels remain constant, regardless whether the patient has a simple cyst identified on metal-artifact reduction sequence (MARS) MRI or ultrasonography. Yearly observation is suggested because cyst progression in less than 6 months has not been observed on MARS MRI or ultrasonographic studies.

The presence of fluid or a soft-tissue mass is a strong indication for revision THA. Although measurement of serum metal ion levels is an important part of the standard diagnostic algorithm, serum metal ion levels are poor predictors of soft-tissue damage and the need for revision THA. MRI has emerged as a powerful diagnostic tool for patients with ALTR or pseudotumor (**Figure 7**). Early signs of metal reaction on MARS MRI often include joint effusion, capsular thickening, or synovitis. Edema also may be noted in the pericapsular musculature, especially if a capsular rent is present. In patients with advanced reaction, tissue involvement may include the presence of complex cystic or solid masses with muscle destruction, tendon rupture, and bony erosion. The amount of implant artifact observed on standard MRI is substantial. Adjusting the matrix and receiver bandwidth of an MRI can reduce 90% of the artifact from the implant. In a study in which MARS MRI was used to prospectively evaluate 31 patients with painful hip implants, researchers reported fluid collections, severe muscle atrophy, and muscular edema. MARS MRI is useful for diagnosing and monitoring soft-tissue damage in patients with hip implants at risk for revision THA. However, a more recent case-control study reported that although fluid collection, or pseudotumors, can readily be found in patients with MoM articulations, no difference was found between patients with a well-functioning implant and patients with a painful implant. Similar results have been reported in the radiology literature, in which conventional sequences using 1.5-T clinical imaging demonstrated no correlation between the presence or size of a pseudotumor and pain. Ultrasonography is a cost-effective imaging modality for the detection of soft-tissue changes surrounding hip implants but may be user dependent. The presence of a complex cyst or mass on MARS MRI or ultrasonography necessitates revision THA because it suggests that implant failure is occurring in a symptomatic patient and impending in an asymptomatic patient. Although serum metal ion levels do not correlate with symptoms, emerging evidence suggests that serum metal ions may correlate with pseudotumor formation.

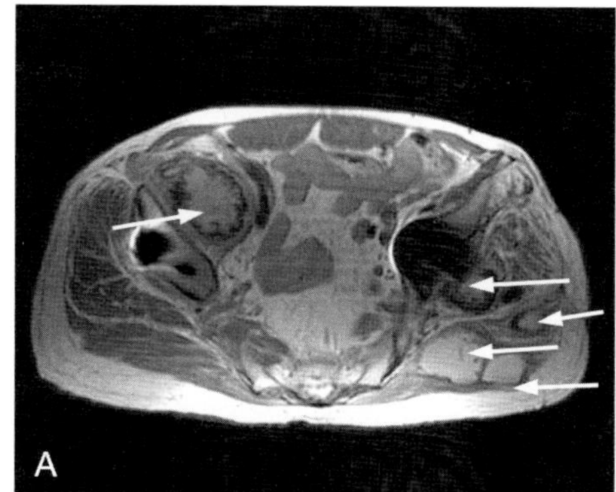

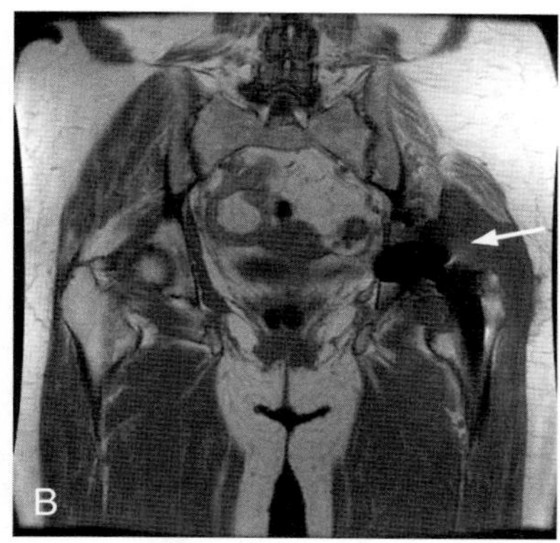

Figure 7 **A,** Axial T1-weighted metal-artifact reduction sequence MRI of a pelvis demonstrates bilateral pseudotumors (arrows) involving the gluteus maximus muscle in the left hip and the iliopsoas muscle in the right hip. **B,** Coronal T1-weighted metal-artifact reduction sequence MRI of the pelvis of a patient who underwent total hip arthroplasty with a modular cobalt-chromium neck, titanium stem, and ceramic-on-polyethylene bearing demonstrates a pseudotumor (arrow) encompassing the entire left hip capsule, with detachment of the abductor musculature.

Decision Making

An implant recall does not always necessitate revision THA. If a modular junction is present but a patient is asymptomatic and has no evidence of soft-tissue damage or elevated serum metal ion levels, the implant does not require revision THA. Complications associated with revision THA include infection, fracture, dislocation, and other medical complications related to the surgical procedure. Therefore, a complete understanding of the risks, benefits, and alternatives and a discussion of these factors with the patient is of the utmost importance in this situation. After the decision has been made to revise a symptomatic or failing modular implant, a critical review of the implants should be undertaken. The clinical track record of the implant, prior voluntary or involuntary recalls, and the positioning of the implant will influence the final decision to revise the implant and the extent of the revision THA.

Although the focus of this chapter is on the management of corrosion of the modular femoral junction, a brief comment on acetabular implant management is warranted. Acetabular implants that are out of the safe zone (>50° of abduction), particularly nonhemispheric metal acetabular implants, should be considered for revision THA. Acetabular implant revision may be indicated if the implant is insufficiently anteverted or if the combined anteversion causes concern for instability after revision THA. The presence of severe soft-tissue necrosis or abductor disruption may decrease the threshold for acetabular revision to optimize implant positioning and use implants that allow for dual-mobility or constrained acetabular inserts.

Contraindications

There are no contraindications.

Alternative Treatments

There are no alternative treatments.

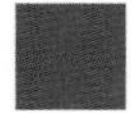

Results

Most of the current studies discussing clinical scenarios, ion levels, imaging findings, and revision THA rates involve implants that have been recalled (**Table 2**). Therefore, the findings of these studies likely represent the highest rates of complication. A retrospective evaluation of 118 hips with a Rejuvenate (Stryker) dual modular femoral implant reported pseudotumors in 74% of symptomatic patients and 45% of asymptomatic patients. Similar to many other studies, a substantial difference was reported between serum chromium and cobalt ion levels (2.0 and 9.5 µg/L, respectively). The rate of revision THA in this study was 31%. Similarly, a retrospective review of 17 hips with the ABG II (Stryker) dual modular femoral implant reported a revision rate of 41%, and all of the hips demonstrated ALTR on MARS MRI. Another large series of ABG II dual modular femoral implants reported similar differential elevation in serum chromium and cobalt ion levels (1.26 and 4.64 µg/L, respectively).

Infection in patients with ALTR requires two-stage revision THA. Direct exchange is contraindicated in patients with soft-tissue necrosis because retention of implants will likely fail. Thus, resection of all implants, placement of a high-dose antibiotic cement spacer, and subsequent ceramic-on-polyethylene revision THA is the best option. In anecdotal evidence from the institution of the authors of this chapter, a small number of hips in a series of revision MoM THAs had acute, delayed, or late joint infection. The rate of infection observed in patients with metal implant failure was four times higher compared with that of a historical cohort from the same institution.

Techniques

Setup/Exposure

- Any approach may be used for revision THA; however, the authors of this chapter prefer to use a posterior approach for revision THA.
- Use of the prior incision may be preferred to facilitate débridement.

Procedure

- If the femoral implant has been recalled, removal is usually warranted.
- Strong consideration should be given to revising any dual modular implant with taper corrosion.
- Well-fixed nonmodular femoral implants with head-neck junction corrosion should be assessed on a patient-by-patient basis. Most surgeons agree that cleaning the trunnion with saline and a clean towel is warranted. Further mechanical débridement with abrasive materials is controversial.
- If gross metal loss has occurred at the trunnion or a new head cannot be securely attached to the trunnion, the femoral implant should be revised.
- If a titanium-alloy stem is retained, the new femoral head placed on the retained trunnion usually consists of a ceramic head with a titanium sleeve.
- If a cobalt-chromium alloy stem is retained, revision to a ceramic head with a titanium sleeve is controversial. Some authors have speculated that deformation of the titanium sleeve against the retained trunnion provides a more favorable interface compared with a cobalt-chromium alloy taper; however, scant data on this point are available.
- In both cases, revision to a ceramic head without a titanium sleeve is not recommended by any manufacturer. In either situation, the retained trunnion will continue to be subject to fretting and crevice corrosion, raising concerns for late implant failure despite early reports of success with titanium sleeves and ceramic heads.
- If the femoral implant will be revised, the implant removal technique depends on the stem design and the surgeon's experience.
- If a femoral stem is well fixed, particularly in the case of a taper stem design, a pencil-tipped burr can be passed around the proximal stem,

Table 2 Results of Revision Total Hip Arthroplasty for Modular Femoral Implants

Authors (Year)	Number of Hips	Type of Modular Femoral Implant	Mean Patient Age at Revision in Years	Time to Revision	Results[a]
Cooper et al (2013)	12	Rejuvenate (Stryker)	60	Mean, 15 mo	All hips were revised for metal reaction Serum chromium, 0.6 ng/mL Serum cobalt, 6.0 ng/mL 89% rate of pseudotumor
Meftah et al (2014)	123	Rejuvenate	64	≤2 yr	28% revision rate for metal reaction Serum cobalt, 5.4 µg/L Serum chromium, 2.1 µg/L 9% rate of pseudotumor
Molloy et al (2014)	17	ABG II (Stryker)	64	NA	41% revision rate for metal reaction Chromium range, 1.3-11.26 ppb Cobalt range, 0.52-1.92 ppb MRI demonstrated adverse local tissue reaction in all patients with grade 2 or grade 3 calcar erosion
Pivec et al (2014)	166	ABG II	NA	NA	12% revision for metal reaction Serum chromium, 1.26 µg/L Serum cobalt, 4.64 µg/L 17% rate of pseudotumor
Ghanem et al (2015)	109	Rejuvenate	60	Mean, 24.1 mo	31% revision for metal reaction Serum chromium, 2.0 µg/L Serum cobalt, 9.5 µg/L 74% rate of pseudotumor in symptomatic patients, 45% rate of pseudotumor in asymptomatic patients

NA = not available.

[a] All results are mean values unless otherwise indicated.

and multiple osteotomes can be passed around the stem.

- Use of an extraction device designed for the particular stem is helpful.
- If an extraction device is unavailable, a vice-grip back-slapping extractor is used.
- If extraction attempts are unsuccessful, quick and judicious use of an extended osteotomy is done to facilitate removal of the femoral stem and proper placement of a revision THA implant.
- Wires and/or cables are placed to reinforce the diaphysis and close the extended osteotomy.
- The authors of this chapter avoid the placement of cables above the lesser trochanter specifically to avoid corrosion and further metal debris in the joint. Instead, doubled Luque wires are used above the lesser trochanter.
- Management of the necrotic tissue and pseudotumor is often complicated. The authors of this chapter recommend careful and complete débridement of the necrotic tissue. Débridement requires patience because dissection around nerves and near vascular structures may be required to properly remove the necrotic tissue. The assistance of a neurosurgeon skilled in peripheral nerve management may be required if extensive neurolysis is required. The assistance of a vascular surgeon can be helpful if extensive pseudotumor involvement of the femoral vascular structures is present.
- Tissue necrosis should elicit strong suspicion of underlying low-grade infection. Therefore, the authors of this chapter usually obtain at least three tissue samples for culture.
- Because of the extensive removal of capsule, muscle, bone, and tendon, instability after revision THA for metal reaction is common. Careful assessment of stability at the end of the procedure is important.
- The use of a large (36- or 40-mm)

titanium-sleeved ceramic revision head helps provide stability. The use of a dual-mobility or constrained acetabular implant should be considered if necessary.

Wound Closure

- Wound closure is performed in layers based on surgeon preference.

Postoperative Regimen

Patients are mobilized postoperatively as soon as possible with appropriate weight bearing. Patients who underwent femoral head and acetabular liner exchanges may be mobilized with weight bearing as tolerated. If implants were revised, weight bearing is modified based on fixation. In patients with severe soft-tissue compromise, especially those who underwent removal of a massive pseudotumor, a careful consideration of dislocation precautions is necessary. The use of a knee immobilizer, hip abduction brace, or hip spica cast may be considered.

Infection that occurs weeks after a revision THA for metal reaction is a newly recognized phenomenon that occurs much more frequently after revision THA for metal reaction than after other revision THAs. Standard prophylactic intravenous antibiotics are administered for 24 hours postoperatively, and a first-generation oral cephalosporin is administered for 7 days postoperatively or until initial cultures are negative. If postoperative cultures demonstrate infection, the patient should remain on broad-spectrum antibiotics, an infectious disease specialist should be consulted, and the species of bacteria and its antibiotic susceptibilities should be determined. Often, a 6-week course of an appropriate intravenous antibiotic, possibly followed by oral suppression antibiotic treatment, is recommended.

At 3 months postoperatively, radiographs are obtained, serum chromium and cobalt ion levels are tested, and the erythrocyte sedimentation rate and C-reactive protein level are measured. These findings are used to confirm resolution of the metal reaction and can serve as a new baseline in case of future infection.

Avoiding Pitfalls and Complications

Modularity reduces inventory and simplifies surgical procedures but can result in mechanically assisted taper corrosion. Surgeons should consider reducing modularity if possible. In addition, surgeons should decrease the factors that may increase a modular implant's risk of failure by cleaning the taper, ensuring forceful impaction of the femoral head, and avoiding off-axis impaction. Surgeons should be aware of the presentation of a failing modular junction, understand the ramifications of failure, and implement the emerging management algorithm in these challenging scenarios.

Bibliography

Bernstein M, Walsh A, Petit A, Zukor DJ, Huk OL, Antoniou J: Femoral head size does not affect ion values in metal-on-metal total hips. *Clin Orthop Relat Res* 2011;469(6):1642-1650.

Collier JP, Mayor MB, Williams IR, Surprenant VA, Surprenant HP, Currier BH: The tradeoffs associated with modular hip prostheses. *Clin Orthop Relat Res* 1995;(311):91-101.

Cooper HJ, Urban RM, Wixson RL, Meneghini RM, Jacobs JJ: Adverse local tissue reaction arising from corrosion at the femoral neck-body junction in a dual-taper stem with a cobalt-chromium modular neck. *J Bone Joint Surg Am* 2013;95(10):865-872.

de Steiger RN, Hang JR, Miller LN, Graves SE, Davidson DC: Five-year results of the ASR XL Acetabular System and the ASR Hip Resurfacing System: An analysis from the Australian Orthopaedic Association National Joint Replacement Registry. *J Bone Joint Surg Am* 2011;93(24):2287-2293.

Donaldson FE, Coburn JC, Siegel KL: Total hip arthroplasty head-neck contact mechanics: A stochastic investigation of key parameters. *J Biomech* 2014;47(7):1634-1641.

Dyrkacz RM, Brandt JM, Ojo OA, Turgeon TR, Wyss UP: The influence of head size on corrosion and fretting behaviour at the head-neck interface of artificial hip joints. *J Arthroplasty* 2013;28(6):1036-1040.

Engh CA, MacDonald SJ, Sritulanondha S, Korczak A, Naudie D, Engh C: Metal ion levels after metal-on-metal total hip arthroplasty: A five-year, prospective randomized trial. *J Bone Joint Surg Am* 2014;96(6):448-455.

Fricka KB, Ho H, Peace WJ, Engh CA Jr: Metal-on-metal local tissue reaction is associated with corrosion of the head taper junction. *J Arthroplasty* 2012;27(suppl 8):26-31.e1.

Ghanem E, Ward DM, Robbins CE, Nandi S, Bono JV, Talmo CT: Corrosion and adverse local tissue reaction in one type of modular neck stem. *J Arthroplasty* 2015;30(10):1787-1793.

Gilbert JL, Buckley CA, Jacobs JJ: In vivo corrosion of modular hip prosthesis components in mixed and similar metal combinations: The effect of crevice, stress, motion, and alloy coupling. *J Biomed Mater Res* 1993;27(12):1533-1544.

Gilbert JL, Mehta M, Pinder B: Fretting crevice corrosion of stainless steel stem-CoCr femoral head connections: Comparisons of materials, initial moisture, and offset length. *J Biomed Mater Res B Appl Biomater* 2009;88(1):162-173.

Goldberg JR, Gilbert JL: In vitro corrosion testing of modular hip tapers. *J Biomed Mater Res B Appl Biomater* 2003;64(2):78-93.

Goldberg JR, Gilbert JL, Jacobs JJ, Bauer TW, Paprosky W, Leurgans S: A multicenter retrieval study of the taper interfaces of modular hip prostheses. *Clin Orthop Relat Res* 2002;(401):149-161.

Kop AM, Swarts E: Corrosion of a hip stem with a modular neck taper junction: A retrieval study of 16 cases. *J Arthroplasty* 2009;24(7):1019-1023.

Mathew MT, Abbey S, Hallab NJ, Hall DJ, Sukotjo C, Wimmer MA: Influence of pH on the tribocorrosion behavior of CpTi in the oral environment: Synergistic interactions of wear and corrosion. *J Biomed Mater Res B Appl Biomater* 2012;100(6):1662-1671.

Meftah M, Haleem AM, Burn MB, Smith KM, Incavo SJ: Early corrosion-related failure of the Rejuvenate modular total hip replacement. *J Bone Joint Surg Am* 2014;96(6):481-487.

Meyer H, Mueller T, Goldau G, Chamaon K, Ruetschi M, Lohmann CH: Corrosion at the cone/taper interface leads to failure of large-diameter metal-on-metal total hip arthroplasties. *Clin Orthop Relat Res* 2012;470(11):3101-3108.

Molloy DO, Munir S, Jack CM, Cross MB, Walter WL, Walter WK Sr: Fretting and corrosion in modular-neck total hip arthroplasty femoral stems. *J Bone Joint Surg Am* 2014;96(6):488-493.

Pivec R, Meneghini RM, Hozack WJ, Westrich GH, Mont MA: Modular taper junction corrosion and failure: How to approach a recalled total hip arthroplasty implant. *J Arthroplasty* 2014;29(1):1-6.

Shareef N, Levine D: Effect of manufacturing tolerances on the micromotion at the Morse taper interface in modular hip implants using the finite element technique. *Biomaterials* 1996;17(6):623-630.

Chapter 46
Acetabular Revision: Implant Removal

Kevin J. Bozic, MD, MBA
Jonathan L. Berliner, MD

 Indications

Because of the projected increase in demand for revision total hip arthroplasty (THA) procedures in the United States, arthroplasty surgeons must have a comprehensive understanding of the indications for removal of an acetabular implant. Indications for removal include mechanical loosening, chronic periprosthetic joint infection, polyethylene wear in a nonmodular cup, implant malpositioning resulting in instability, and bony or soft-tissue impingement. Periacetabular osteolysis may require acetabular implant removal if the implant is loose or damaged, or if access to the osteolytic lesion is difficult without removal of the cup.

Although aseptic loosening is the most common reason for revision of both femoral and acetabular implants, instability is the most common indication for isolated acetabular revision. Revision for instability secondary to implant malposition represents approximately 33% of isolated acetabular implant revision procedures. Mechanical loosening is the second most common reason for isolated acetabular revision, accounting for 24.2% of these procedures.

The decision to remove the acetabular implant at the time of femoral implant revision or modular implant exchange is controversial. Typically, the acetabular implant is retained if it meets the following criteria: it is well fixed, demonstrated by careful intraoperative testing after all screws have been removed; it is well positioned; it is of adequate size to contain a new liner that accommodates a femoral head of reasonable size; the locking mechanism is functional; and a stable construct, demonstrated by intraoperative stability testing, can be achieved.

Acetabular implant removal can be a technically challenging and time-consuming process. Proficiency in the basic techniques of implant removal facilitates an efficient procedure in which risk to the patient is minimized and host bone stock is preserved. It is essential that the posterior column and superior dome of the pelvis be preserved in order to obtain durable fixation of the revision acetabular component. Limiting periacetabular bone loss during implant removal can be challenging due to the relative osteopenia of adjacent bone. Ultimately, the manner in which the acetabular component is extracted dictates the possible reconstructive options.

Because of the complexity of most revision THA procedures, preoperative planning is indispensable for a successful outcome. The tools and techniques selected preoperatively for removal of the acetabular implant can have a substantial effect on the revision implant options and the ultimate strength of fixation. Critical aspects of preoperative planning include determining the preexisting implant design, the type and status of the current fixation, and selecting the appropriate tools and instrumentation necessary for implant removal and reimplantation. The procedure requires a team effort from the entire operating room staff, who should be informed preoperatively of all necessary equipment. All previous surgical reports should be reviewed to identify the exact manufacturer, type, and size of the existing THA implants. A thorough understanding of the existing implants allows the surgeon to prepare for special circumstances such as the presence of implant fixation augmentation (screws, fixation pegs) or acetabular cups for which device-specific extraction tools are available from the manufacturer.

Preoperative serial radiographs are essential and allow the surgeon to detect loosening, osteolysis, heterotopic ossification, a broken cement mantle, or implant migration. Surgeons must determine whether the implant is either well fixed or loose because this finding influences the method of implant extraction.

Dr. Bozic or an immediate family member serves as a paid consultant to the Institute for Healthcare Improvement, and serves as a board member, owner, officer, or committee member of the American Academy of Orthopaedic Surgeons, the American Association of Hip and Knee Surgeons, and the Orthopaedic Research and Education Foundation. Neither Dr. Berliner nor any immediate family member has received anything of value from or has stock or stock options held in a commercial company or institution related directly or indirectly to the subject of this chapter.

Advanced imaging may be considered in patients with intrapelvic implant migration, osteolysis, or concerning bone loss. The use of CT can more accurately define periacetabular bone stock and the position of the implant in relation to other pelvic structures. In patients with substantial acetabular implant protrusio, the use of CT with arterial infusion may be prudent to help determine the position of important anatomic structures such as the iliac vessels, the pelvic nerves, and the ureter.

Contraindications

Removal of the acetabular implant should be performed only if warranted according to the previously mentioned indications. Implant retention should be considered for well-fixed, well-positioned cups for which a new liner with adequate inside cup diameter can be locked or cemented into the existing component. Implant removal has numerous disadvantages, with the primary disadvantage being the potential for substantial bone loss, which can result in a difficult and compromised reconstruction. When revising a well-fixed implant, there is always a risk that the revision implant will fail to achieve stability through bony ingrowth. Other potential drawbacks include increased cost, procedure time, blood loss, and physiologic stress on the patient.

Alternative Treatments

Because of the potential consequences of acetabular implant removal, the decision to remove the cup should be questioned in every patient. The reconstruction may ultimately be less durable than the alternative with shell retention. Patients with stable osteolysis, demonstrated by serial radiographs, and asymptomatic loosening can be followed closely. However, a symptomatic patient with evidence of progressive osteolysis requires surgical intervention. During revision for osteolysis, failure of the polyethylene liner within a modular implant does not always necessitate complete acetabular revision. Well-fixed, well-positioned acetabular shells may be retained during revision for osteolysis if a new polyethylene liner of acceptable thickness can be implanted and the osteolytic defect can be accessed for débridement and bone grafting. Several techniques to access the retroacetabular osteolytic granuloma have been described. In the presence of an acetabular implant containing screw holes, both débridement of the lesion and bone grafting of the defect may be performed through the screw holes. If this method is not possible, the osteolytic defect may be accessed through a small cortical window in the lateral ilium. However, care must be taken to preserve the bony stability of the acetabular implant, which may be tenuous because of osteolytic bone loss. Surgeons must confirm preoperatively that a new liner of sufficient thickness that also allows for a femoral head of reasonable size is available, especially for cups with a diameter of less than 50 mm. In addition, cup retention has limitations, including the inability to optimize cup orientation or to increase the size of the acetabular implant. These factors are important considerations in preventing postoperative instability, which is the most common complication after exchange of modular implants.

Simple liner exchange may not be possible in modular acetabular shells with a damaged locking mechanism or in shells with interior damage. In these patients, a reasonable alternative is to cement a new polyethylene liner into the original shell. Numerous studies suggest that the strength of this construct may exceed that of the original locking mechanism. Done correctly, this technique can provide a lasting solution without the need for cup removal. The size of the liner should be decreased to allow a 2-mm cement mantle, and the back surface of the polyethylene should be roughened with the use of a high-speed burr to prevent failure at the polyethylene-cement interface.

Results

The authors of this chapter are not aware of any studies that have compared the efficacy or outcomes of specific techniques or instruments for removing the acetabular implant during revision surgery. For multiple reasons, such a study would be difficult to perform or would be clinically irrelevant. Often, more than one technique or device is used simultaneously during a revision procedure. As discussed later in this chapter, improved tools and techniques have been developed to remove both acetabular and femoral implants, with the goal of preserving bone stock and limiting damage to surrounding structures. However, similar tools and techniques used by different surgeons do not necessarily work in a similarly effective manner. Surgeons who perform revision THA must become familiar with a multitude of options and become proficient with the tools and techniques that best suit their skill set.

Techniques

Setup/Exposure

- In most revision hip procedures, the original incision should be used if possible and extended as needed to allow implant extraction and implantation without undue tension on the superficial tissues.
- Surgeon preference and anticipated bony defects may influence the specific exposure used.
- Historically, most revision THA procedures were performed through either a posterior or direct lateral

approach. With increasing popularity of the direct anterior approach, a growing number of surgeons are choosing to perform revision procedures through an anteriorly based exposure. Each approach has advantages and drawbacks.

- Although anterior exposures may provide easier access to the acetabulum, the implant extraction and reimplantation procedure, especially on the femoral side, can be technically demanding. Therefore, this approach should be reserved for surgeons who have extensive experience with anteriorly based approaches and who feel comfortable performing the approach in an extensile manner.
- The posterior approach can be used after any previous approach and can be easily extended to improve femoral exposure. Often, an extensile exposure with soft-tissue releases is required to visualize and reconstruct the acetabulum. However, the posterior approach does not provide reliable access to anterior pelvic or anterior column defects.
- Regardless of the surgical approach selected, an unobstructed circumferential view of the acetabulum is necessary, whether for a simple liner exchange or extensive reconstruction.
- For patients in whom the femoral implant must be retained, removing the modular femoral head will facilitate acetabular exposure and can be performed as necessary.
- An unobstructed circumferential view of the acetabular implant allows for unhindered disruption of the prosthetic fixation, thereby minimizing unintended bone loss and other associated complications such as pelvic fracture or discontinuity. It also allows for efficient removal of a modular liner and unobstructed locking of the newly implanted liner.

Instruments/Equipment/ Implants Required

- A requisite of preoperative planning includes determination of the instrumentation and equipment necessary for a successful acetabular implant extraction. This extremely important element of revision THA must not be overlooked.
- A diverse set of hand tools, including non–implant-specific tools such as universal extractors, modular implant separators, vice grips, and slap hammers, should be accessible.
- A wide range of osteotomes and gouges, including curved acetabular and U-shaped osteotomes, will facilitate cup extraction (**Figure 1**).
- A broken-screw removal set and trephines should be readily available.
- Implant-specific extractors can be extremely valuable and reduce surgical time considerably. Examples include polyethylene liner extractors, cup extractors, and screwdrivers with unique tip designs. Implant-specific cup extractors allow safe penetration at the bone-implant interface, thereby minimizing associated periacetabular bone loss.
- In more demanding patients, power tools or ultrasonic devices can help break up implant interfaces, remove cement, or cut metal or polyethylene implants into pieces for removal. Frequently used power tools include high-speed burrs with various tip options and sagittal or reciprocating saws.

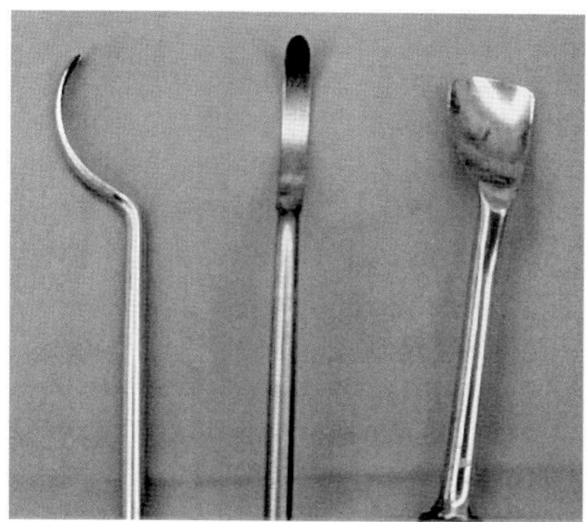

Figure 1 Photograph shows curved acetabular osteotomes, which are available in varying depths and are used to disrupt the bone-prosthesis or cement-prosthesis interface around the acetabular implant. Inadvertent periacetabular bone loss is minimized by initiating the process with the shortest osteotome and progressively increasing the length of the osteotome until the cup is free. (Reproduced with permission from Masri BA, Mitchell PA, Duncan CP: Removal of solidly fixed implants during revision hip and knee arthroplasty. *J Am Acad Orthop Surg* 2005;13[1]:18-27.)

Procedure

ISOLATED MODULAR LINER EXCHANGE

- After a thorough preoperative assessment has confirmed that liner exchange is a viable option, the specific type and size of the existing implants is determined.
- Locking mechanisms differ for each implant. Depending on the manufacturer, an implant-specific extraction device may be necessary to remove the liner.
- To facilitate liner removal, the entire perimeter of the acetabular implant is fully exposed with removal of soft tissue and bony overgrowth that may impede liner removal.
- After the liner is removed, the orientation of the acetabular implant is assessed.
- If the cup is malpositioned, the surgeon should strongly consider full acetabular implant revision because of the increased incidence of postoperative instability after liner exchange.
- Trialing of implants and a thorough assessment of hip stability are essential, even in simple liner exchange procedures.
- To further minimize the risk of postoperative instability, femoral head size should be increased during the revision procedure. This method requires a modular

liner that can accommodate a larger head size. Numerous studies have demonstrated the benefit of an increased femoral head-to-neck ratio, which increases both the range of motion of the joint and the jump distance required for dislocation.

- Although removal of cup screws at the time of liner exchange is controversial, it is often warranted to confirm solid fixation of the acetabular shell. Any motion detected during testing indicates a loose implant that should be revised.
- Acetabular liner options for modular noncemented implants include polyethylene, metal, and ceramic. Each requires different methods for successful exchange.

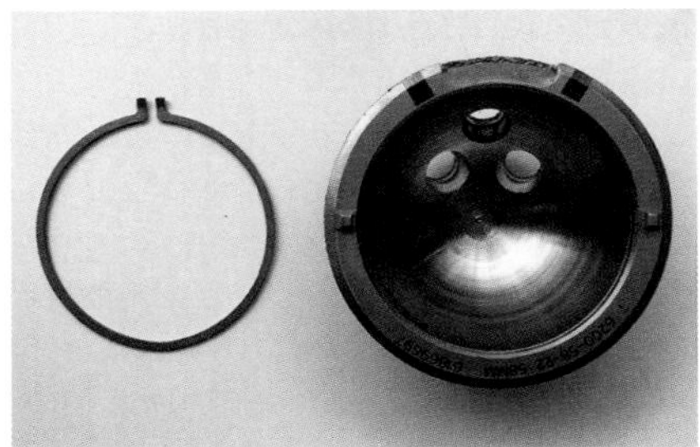

Figure 2 In modular acetabular implants, the polyethylene liner can be secured in place with the type of metal ring locking mechanism shown in this clinical photograph. Forceful extraction of the liner can result in damage to the ring, in which case the ring should be replaced. A replacement locking mechanism should always be available at the time of revision surgery.

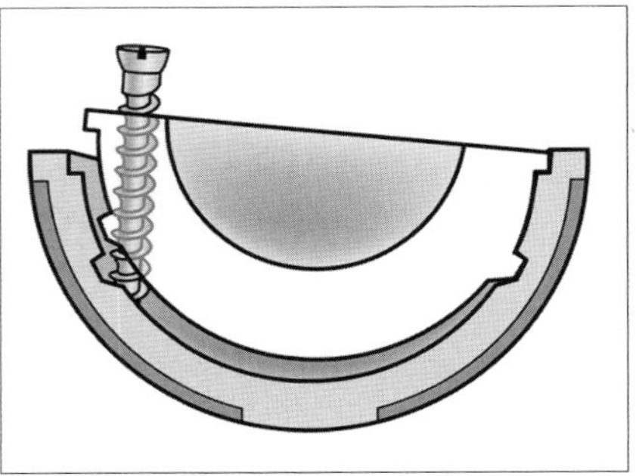

Figure 3 Illustration shows insertion of an acetabular fixation screw through a drill hole near the periphery of the polyethylene liner, which facilitates component removal. The advancing screw contacts the interface between the liner and the shell, creating a levering force that dislodges the liner from its engaged position.

POLYETHYLENE LINER REMOVAL

- The implant-specific locking mechanism often determines how easily a modular polyethylene liner can be removed at the time of revision.
- If the liner is grossly loose, it can be easily removed by grasping the rim of the liner with a clamp and pulling it from the acetabular shell.
- Some polyethylene liners are held in place by a wire or ring that is frequently damaged during extraction.
- In all patients, a damaged locking mechanism should be replaced. Therefore, a replacement locking mechanism should always be available at the time of the procedure (**Figure 2**).
- Polyethylene liners held in place by a metal locking ring may require an implant-specific extractor for removal.
- Implant-specific tools have the lowest likelihood of damaging the locking mechanism and, therefore, should be used if available.
- If an implant-specific extraction tool is not available, most polyethylene liners that are properly engaged within the locking mechanism can be removed by simply

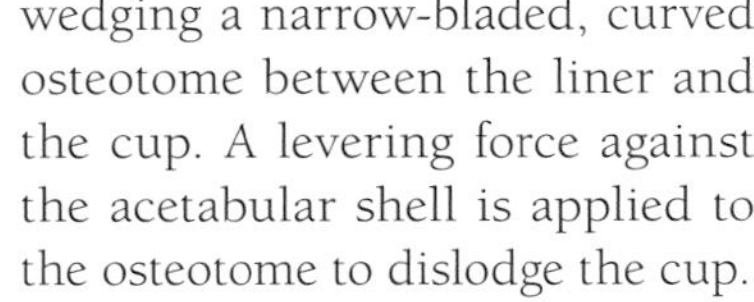

wedging a narrow-bladed, curved osteotome between the liner and the cup. A levering force against the acetabular shell is applied to the osteotome to dislodge the cup.

- An alternative method is to use an acetabular fixation screw. A drill hole is made in the polyethylene liner near its perimeter. A screw is then inserted through the liner. The advancing screw contacts the interface between the liner and shell, eventually levering the liner from its engaged position (**Figure 3**). If the acetabular implant contains screw holes, care is taken to avoid penetrating the cup and entering the bone. Excessive damage to the shell must be avoided because it can eventually contribute to backside wear of the new liner.
- Polyethylene-insert extraction devices employ a similar strategy (**Figure 4**). After a drill hole is placed into the center of the liner, the extracting device is threaded into the polyethylene. The extraction device is advanced through the polyethylene until the threaded portion of the instrument contacts the metal acetabular implant, resulting in eventual dislodgement of the liner.
- If all else fails, a high-speed burr can be used to divide the polyethylene liner into multiple fragments that can be individually removed with a clamp. Afterward, the wound should be thoroughly lavaged to remove as much of the polyethyelene debris as possible.
- Despite preoperative planning, unforeseen circumstances may prohibit the implantation of a new polyethylene liner. The necessary liner may not be available, the existing mechanism may be irreparably broken, or the interior of the shell may be damaged. In these patients, a new polyethylene liner can be cemented into place if the existing acetabular shell is well fixed and well positioned.

METAL OR CERAMIC LINER REMOVAL

- Most ceramic or metal modular liners are fixed directly to the metal shell with a taper lock mechanism.
- As with polyethylene liners, if an implant-specific extractor is available from the manufacturer, it should be used. Typically, these devices contact the peripheral rim of the acetabular cup. When an

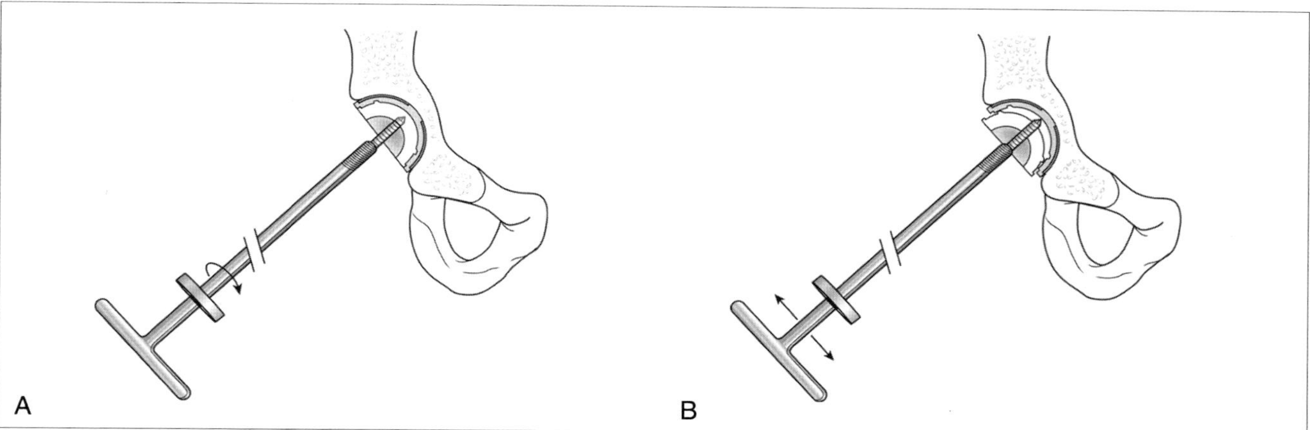

Figure 4 **A,** Illustration depicts threading (curved arrow) of a polyethylene-insert extractor into a drill hole centered in the polyethylene liner. **B,** Illustration shows that the extractor is advanced, eventually contacting the metal acetabular implant and levering the modular liner out of position (arrows).

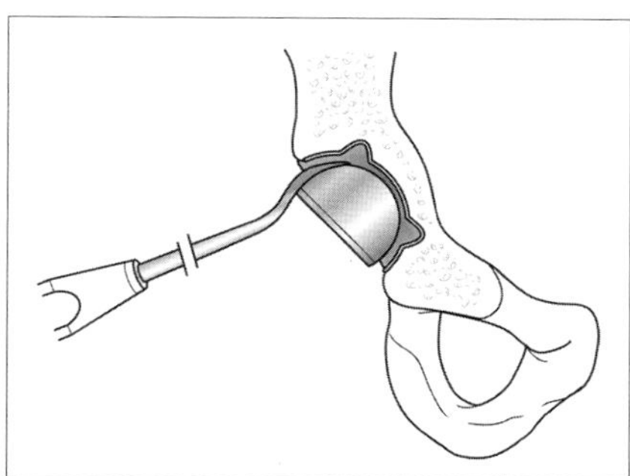

Figure 5 Illustration depicts an acetabular gouge specifically designed to fit around a hemispheric acetabular implant. Although the instrument is preferentially inserted into the cement-prosthesis interface as shown here, it also can be carefully inserted at the bone-cement interface to loosen cement from the underlying acetabular bone.

impaction force is applied to the extractor, a vibratory force disrupts the taper lock of the metal or ceramic bearing.

- If an implant-specific extractor is not available, a bone tamp is applied to the peripheral rim of the shell and impacted with a mallet. The impaction will create a vibratory force that disrupts the taper lock, thereby dislodging the liner.
- Fractured ceramic liners pose a unique challenge because cracks within the implant often allow the vibratory forces to dissipate before the taper lock is disrupted. If necessary, the fragmented liner can be directly impacted with a bone tamp or osteotome to dislodge it. The multiple fragments are then individually removed. If this technique is used, the wound is thoroughly irrigated to remove all debris, which if left in place can contribute to third-body wear of the new bearing surface.

LOOSE IMPLANT REMOVAL

- Careful study of serial preoperative radiographs should reveal whether the acetabular implant is loose or well fixed.
- Subtle loosening that is not obvious on preoperative imaging can be detected by observing the fixation surface while a force is applied to the rim of the acetabular implant. If movement or fluid extravasation at the fixation interface is observed, the implant should be presumed to be loose.
- Failure of ingrowth into a modern, noncemented acetabular implant is rare and should heighten clinical suspicion for infection.
- Grossly loose acetabular implants typically can be removed with a clamp.
- Porous acetabular implants that appear loose on preoperative imaging may appear well fixed during intraoperative stability testing because of fibrous ingrowth. These acetabular implants should be removed as described later in this chapter.
- Before the implant is extracted, all acetabular screws are removed to prevent inadvertent periacetabular bone loss.

CEMENTED ACETABULAR IMPLANT REMOVAL

- Removal of a well-fixed, cemented acetabular implant requires 360° disruption of the bone-cement interface. During this process, every effort must be made to preserve the maximum amount of periacetabular bone.
- The safest method to accomplish this goal is to first disrupt the cement-prosthesis interface (**Figure 5**). Damage to surrounding bone is more likely to occur with attempted disruption of the cement-bone interface than with disruption of the cement-prosthesis interface.
- The cement-prosthesis interface

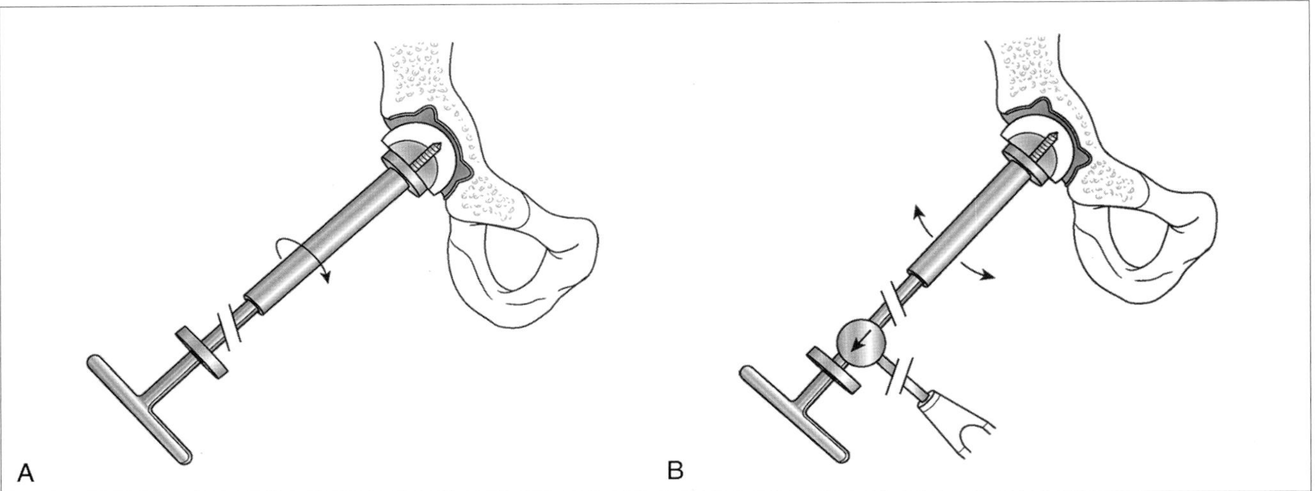

Figure 6 **A,** Illustration depicts an acetabular implant extractor threaded into the all-polyethylene acetabular implant after a drill hole is placed into the center of the implant with a drill bit. An outer sleeve is then lowered down the shaft of the extractor and tightened (curved arrow) against the rim of the implant. **B,** Illustration shows that after the extractor has been securely threaded into the polyethylene component, a rocking motion (curved arrows) creates a gentle extraction force that should dislodge the implant. To assist with extraction, a mallet is used to apply a gentle axial force (straight arrow) to the instrument. Use of a mallet is not always necessary.

typically is disrupted with the use of curved osteotomes or acetabular gouges specifically designed to fit around the acetabular implant (**Figure 5**). The osteotome or gouge that most closely contours the radius of curvature of the cup is selected. Starting with a short gouge, the more superficial cement-prosthesis interface is disrupted followed by progressively longer gouges until the implant is dislodged.

- For cemented acetabular cups with an impenetrable cement-prosthesis interface, alternative techniques have been devised for implant removal. However, they may increase the risk of inadvertent bone loss.
- A threaded acetabular implant extractor can be an effective instrument for removing all-polyethylene cemented implants (**Figure 6**). The tool is initially threaded into a hole drilled into the center of the polyethylene implant. An outer sleeve is lowered onto the rim of the implant, which helps to distribute the levering force. After the device is properly secured, the acetabular implant is removed with a gentle levering force that should disrupt the cement-prosthesis or cement-bone interface. The cement-prosthesis interface should, at least in part, be initially disrupted with gouges or osteotomes in order to limit bone loss as the component is levered or malleted out of position.
- An alternative method involves the use of a small acetabular reamer that fits into the polyethylene implant to ream the interior of the cup. Reaming is carried down to the level of the prosthesis-cement interface. The remaining polyethylene is divided with the use of an osteotome, a saw blade, or a high-speed burr.
- Cemented polyethylene implants also can be removed with the use of multiple screws placed through the periphery of the implant. After a 2.5-mm drill is used to create multiple holes throughout the implant, 4.5-mm cortical screws are inserted and removed sequentially to fragment the cement mantle until the entirety of the cement-prosthesis interface is disrupted.
- As a last resort, the polyethylene implant can be sectioned with the use of a high-speed burr and removed in pieces. However, this process creates substantial polyethylene debris that must be carefully removed.
- After the acetabular implant has been successfully removed, the next step is to meticulously extricate all cement from the acetabular bed.
- The residual cement, which is often poorly fixed to bone, can frequently be removed with the use of a curette.
- Cement that is strongly fixed to bone should be divided into small fragments and removed in a piecemeal fashion. This method limits the risk of bone loss, which can occur inadvertently when large pieces of cement are removed.
- If the cement mantle is too thick for this process, it should first be thinned with a high-speed burr. Drill holes also can be placed throughout the cement mantle to create stress risers.

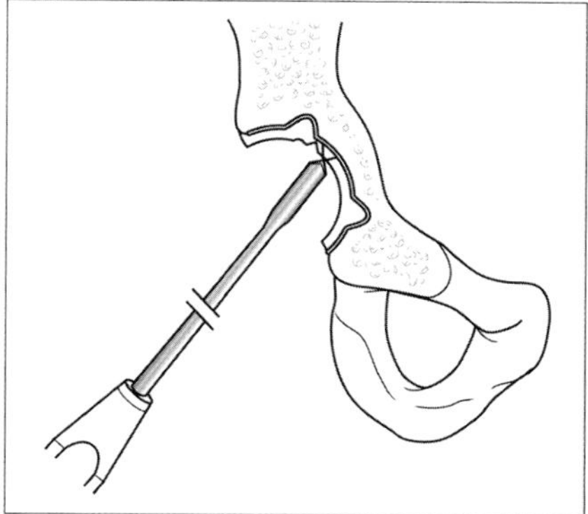

Figure 7 Illustration depicts the use of a pointed osteotome to create stress risers within the cement to facilitate cement fragmentation. Fragmented cement is subsequently freed with a curet.

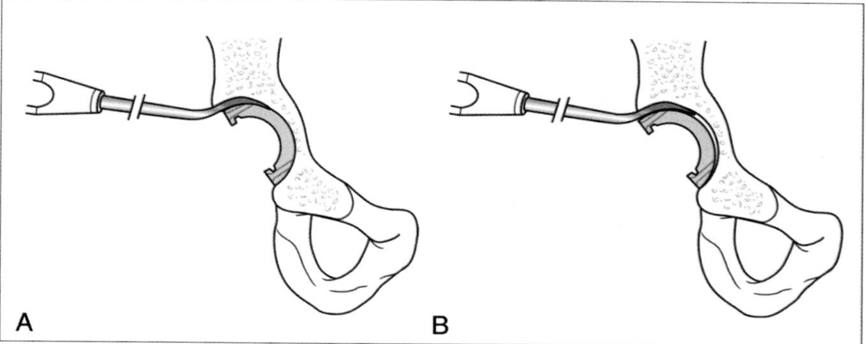

Figure 8 Illustrations depict the use of hand-guided, curved osteotomes to disrupt the bone-prosthesis interface around a well-fixed press-fit acetabular implant. **A,** A short osteotome is introduced into the fixation interface around the circumference of the implant. **B,** The process is repeated with progressively longer osteotomes until the cup is freed from the underlying bone.

- When the remaining cement mantle is of reasonable thickness, narrow, sharp osteotomes, such as pointed Moreland osteotomes, can be used to create stress risers that fracture the cement (**Figure 7**).
- All cement, including anchoring-hole cement, if present, must be meticulously removed from the acetabular bed to allow unobstructed acetabular reaming in preparation for reconstruction. Failure to remove anchoring-hole cement can result in pelvic fracture or additional bone loss during reaming.
- The only exception is cement fragments that have migrated into the pelvis. Intrapelvic cement may adhere to vascular structures that potentially could be damaged with cement removal.
- Intraosseous cement pegs often can be removed with curettage or, if necessary, fragmentation with an osteotome followed by removal with a curette. A high-speed burr also can be used to thin the cement pegs prior to removal.

NONCEMENTED ACETABULAR IMPLANT REMOVAL

- Well-fixed noncemented acetabular implants can be difficult to extract. Therefore, careful consideration should be made as to the necessity of implant removal. Despite meticulous technique, extensive bone loss is always a risk.
- As discussed, complete exposure of the acetabular implant is indispensable for a successful extraction. Often, bony overgrowth obscures the peripheral margin of the porous-coated shell. Bony overgrowth should be removed with a high-speed burr or with hand tools such as osteotomes.
- For the successful removal of a well-fixed noncemented cup with supplemental screw fixation, the modular liner is first removed as described previously.
- Even if acetabular screws are not present, liner removal often can be helpful because it may allow better visualization of the bone-prosthesis interface to assist with extraction.
- Acetabular screws should be identified on preoperative imaging so that the required screwdrivers will be available. Flexible screwdrivers often facilitate the removal of screws in areas that are difficult to reach.
- If the necessary screwdrivers are not available or if the screw becomes stripped or is inaccessible with a screwdriver, the screw head can be removed with a high-speed, carbide-tipped burr. Later, after the acetabular implant is removed, the remaining broken screws are extracted with a broken-screw removal set, trephines, or vice grips.
- After all supplemental fixation is removed and an unobstructed view of the acetabular metal shell margin is achieved, the bone-prosthesis interface can be disrupted with the use of a series of hand-guided, curved acetabular osteotomes, such as Moreland osteotomes or Aufranc acetabular gouges. This process requires patience and precise targeting of the bone-prosthesis interface to limit unnecessary damage to the surrounding bone.
- First, with a relatively short osteotome, the superficial interface is disrupted around the entire periphery of the implant. Progressively longer osteotomes are used to disrupt the bony ingrowth around the perimeter of the cup until it is freed (**Figure 8**).
- Care is taken to stay as close to the prosthesis as possible throughout its depth and to avoid levering with the tools.
- To avoid fractures of the acetabular rim and surrounding bone,

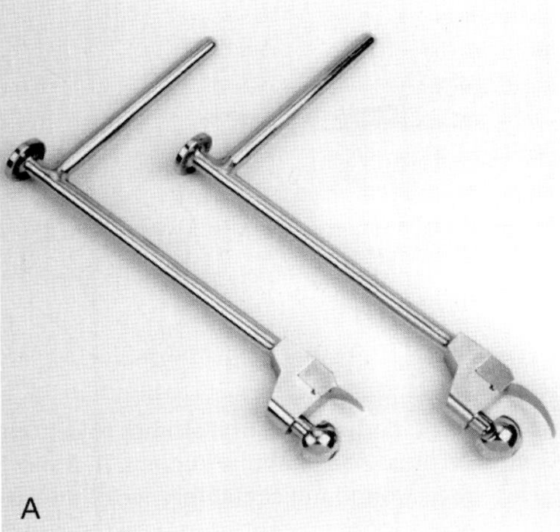

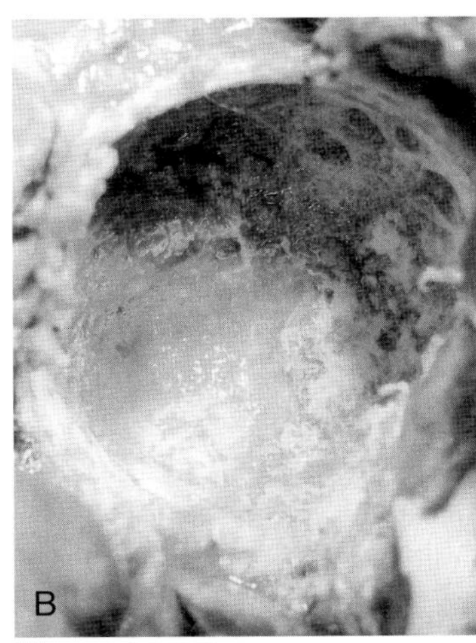

Figure 9 **A,** Photograph shows guided curved osteotome systems, which have a hemispheric head and a curved size-specific blade designed to contour and match the outside diameter of the metal acetabular implant. With progressive lengthening of the modular blade, the bone-prosthesis interface is efficiently disrupted with minimal bone loss. **B,** Intraoperative photograph shows the typical appearance of the host bone after removal of a solidly fixed, noncemented acetabular implant with a size-specific curved osteotome system. (Reproduced with permission from Masri BA, Mitchell PA, Duncan CP: Removal of solidly fixed implants during revision hip and knee arthroplasty. *J Am Acad Orthop Surg* 2005;13[1]:18-27.)

disruption of the bone-prosthesis interface should begin in areas in which the underlying bone stock is thickest, such as the ilium, ischium, and pubic ramus. Eventually, the osteotomes are introduced into thinner areas, such as the anterior and posterior rim.

- Particular care is taken to preserve the posterior and superior periacetabular bone because this bone stock is essential for fixation and stability of the revision acetabular implant.
- The use of a guided curved osteotome system has been shown to be an efficient and bone-preserving method of removing press-fit acetabular implants (**Figure 9**).
- The instrument consists of a hemispheric head that centers the tool within the acetabular cup and thin, curved osteotome-like blades that are designed to contour the metal shell on the basis of its size. Therefore, the inside diameter of the liner and the outside diameter of the cup should be determined preoperatively.
- The acetabular implant removal system is centered within the acetabular implant by placing an appropriately sized hemispheric head into either the existing modular liner or a trial liner.
- The modular blades of the removal instrument are thin, match the exact radius of the cup, and are progressively lengthened during extraction of the cup.
- Spiked acetabular shells require a different procedure because it is impossible to completely disrupt the bone-implant interface with the use of curved acetabular osteotomes or an acetabular implant removal system. In patients with these shells, care must be taken to disrupt the maximum portion of the fixation interface before the cup is levered out of the acetabulum. Even so, spikes are often sites of substantial bony ingrowth at which large defects can occur if the cup is forcefully removed.
- An alternative option that may reduce periacetabular bone loss in patients with spiked acetabular shells is to use a targeting template provided by the implant manufacturer, if available. The template identifies the location of all spikes, allowing the surgeon to separate the spikes from the shell with the use of a high-speed, carbide-tipped burr.
- If all efforts to disrupt the bone-prosthesis interface fail, the cup can be cut in situ with a high-speed burr. This technique also can be considered in patients with acetabular implants that are substantially medialized. Cups that approach the Köhler line pose a substantial risk to the pelvic columns.
- After the bone-prosthesis interface is completely disrupted and the metal shell is clearly loose, the implant is extracted with the use of a clamp, pliers, or a universal acetabular extraction device.
- The universal acetabular extraction device binds to the cup by engaging the groove of the cup's locking mechanism (**Figure 10**). The long handle of the extractor affords additional torque to facilitate removal of the cup.

INTRAPELVIC CEMENT AND IMPLANTS

- Implants medial to the iliopectineal or ilioischial lines are considered intrapelvic in location and deserve special consideration and preoperative planning, including CT angiography to assess the proximity of vascular structures.
- Most intrapelvic cement and implants can be extracted through a standard hip incision with the use of careful dissection to free the implant from its fibrous capsule.
- To avoid substantial risk to vital intrapelvic structures, an intrapelvic

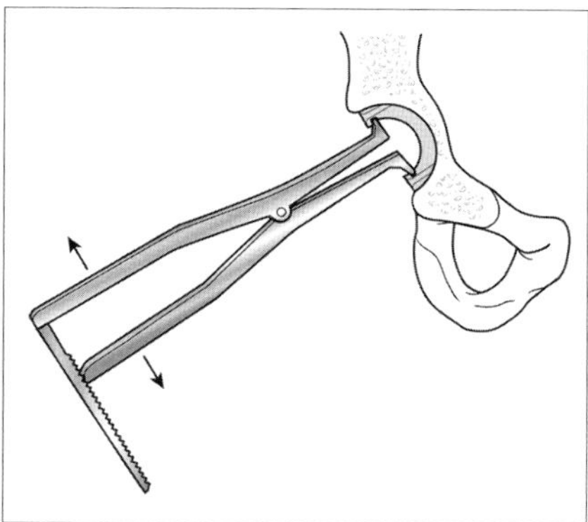

Figure 10 Illustration depicts the use of an acetabular implant extraction device, which binds to the interior of the cup by engaging the groove of the locking mechanism. After the device is secured to the cup, the long handle provides additional torque to facilitate removal of the implant.

implant should never be removed forcefully or in haste.

- Cement that extrudes through a small medial acetabular defect into the intrapelvic space cannot be removed through a standard hip incision.
- As previously discussed, preoperative advanced imaging is indicated in patients with intrapelvic cement and implants. The implant may be intimately associated with large vascular structures, posing a substantial risk during removal. One option is to leave the cement in place if infection is not present.
- If removal is indicated, cement or intrapelvic implants not accessible through a standard hip incision can be removed with the use of a variation of the ilioinguinal, retroperitoneal approach.
- A general or vascular surgeon should be available to assist with the approach and implant removal as needed.

Wound Closure

- Thorough cleansing of the wound is necessary before closure because many of the techniques described in this chapter can result in considerable debris within the wound. The debris must be removed in order to limit third-body wear and minimize the risk of an adverse soft-tissue reaction.
- Wound closure depends on the surgeon's preference and the approach used.

Postoperative Regimen

The postoperative regimen depends on multiple factors, including the type of implants used for the reconstruction, the specific approach used, any intraoperative complications, the patient's bone quality, and the surgeon's confidence in the rigidity of intraoperative fixation of the new acetabular implant. Most patients are restricted to protected weight bearing for 6 to 8 weeks postoperatively and then gradually progress to full weight bearing. Physical therapy should begin as soon as tolerated, typically on the day of the procedure or on the first postoperative day. Because of the risk of postoperative instability, patients who undergo acetabular implant revision should be restricted with hip precautions specific to the approach used. If an extended trochanteric osteotomy is required for implant removal, hip abduction should be limited until sufficient bone healing has occurred, and the use of a hip abduction orthosis should be considered.

Avoiding Pitfalls and Complications

Because of the complex nature of revision hip arthroplasty, the outcome of the procedure depends on adequate preparation. Preoperative planning begins with the decision to remove or retain the acetabular implant. Because of the inherent risks of the procedure, the need for implant removal should always be questioned. Thorough preoperative planning ensures that the surgeon is well prepared for both anticipated and unforeseen difficulties. The primary goal during acetabular implant extraction is to preserve the maximum amount of periacetabular bone, which will afford the greatest number of reconstructive options.

Intraoperatively, it is important to follow the preoperative plan in a stepwise, logical progression. Implant removal can be tedious, and patience is essential. Undue haste can result in catastrophic bone loss. Adequate exposure of the acetabular implant, meticulous disruption of the fixation interfaces, and avoidance of excessive force will minimize the risk of fracture and inadvertent damage to periacetabular bone. A thorough understanding of the key principles and techniques of the procedure will result in efficient acetabular implant removal and, ultimately, reduced risk for complications and improved outcomes for the patient.

Bibliography

Boucher HR, Lynch C, Young AM, Engh CA Jr, Engh C Sr: Dislocation after polyethylene liner exchange in total hip arthroplasty. *J Arthroplasty* 2003;18(5):654-657.

Bozic KJ, Kurtz SM, Lau E, Ong K, Vail TP, Berry DJ: The epidemiology of revision total hip arthroplasty in the United States. *J Bone Joint Surg Am* 2009;91(1):128-133.

Burstein G, Yoon P, Saleh KJ: Component removal in revision total hip arthroplasty. *Clin Orthop Relat Res* 2004;(420):48-54.

Della Valle CJ, Stuchin SA: A novel technique for the removal of well-fixed, porous-coated acetabular components with spike fixation. *J Arthroplasty* 2001;16(8):1081-1083.

de Thomasson E, Mazel C, Gagna G, Guingand O: A simple technique to remove well-fixed, all-polyethylene cemented acetabular component in revision hip arthroplasty. *J Arthroplasty* 2001;16(4):538-540.

Haft GF, Heiner AD, Dorr LD, Brown TD, Callaghan JJ: A biomechanical analysis of polyethylene liner cementation into a fixed metal acetabular shell. *J Bone Joint Surg Am* 2003;85(6):1100-1110.

Haidukewych GJ: Osteolysis in the well-fixed socket: Cup retention or revision? *J Bone Joint Surg Br* 2012; 94(11 suppl A):65-69.

Kostensalo I, Junnila M, Virolainen P, et al: Effect of femoral head size on risk of revision for dislocation after total hip arthroplasty: A population-based analysis of 42,379 primary procedures from the Finnish Arthroplasty Register. *Acta Orthop* 2013;84(4):342-347.

Lombardi AV Jr, Berend KR: Isolated acetabular liner exchange. *J Am Acad Orthop Surg* 2008;16(5):243-248.

Maloney WJ, Paprosky W, Engh CA, Rubash H: Surgical treatment of pelvic osteolysis. *Clin Orthop Relat Res* 2001;(393):78-84.

Maloney WJ, Wadey VM: Removal of well-fixed cementless components. *Instr Course Lect* 2006;55:257-261.

Mitchell PA, Masri BA, Garbuz DS, Greidanus NV, Wilson D, Duncan CP: Removal of well-fixed, cementless, acetabular components in revision hip arthroplasty. *J Bone Joint Surg Br* 2003;85(7):949-952.

Paprosky WG, Weeden SH, Bowling JW Jr: Component removal in revision total hip arthroplasty. *Clin Orthop Relat Res* 2001;(393):181-193.

Schmalzried TP, Fowble VA, Amstutz HC: The fate of pelvic osteolysis after reoperation: No recurrence with lesional treatment. *Clin Orthop Relat Res* 1998;(350):128-137.

Chapter 47
Acetabular Revision: Overview and Strategy

Stuart B. Goodman, MD, PhD, FRCSC, FACS

Indications

Revision of the acetabular implant after total hip arthroplasty (THA) was performed for different reasons in previous decades than in the present. First, before the introduction of cross-linked polyethylene, wear of the polyethylene liner with periprosthetic osteolysis was frequently seen after many years of in vivo prosthesis use, necessitating revision surgery. Second, although not commonly used in the United States, cemented cups often required revision after 10 years because of late aseptic loosening. Third, suboptimal acetabular implant position and the use of smaller femoral heads were associated with a higher incidence of recurrent dislocation, which necessitated revision of the entire acetabular implant. Fourth, infection of cemented or noncemented THA implants required excision arthroplasty and reimplantation, with the challenge of surgical reconstruction associated with major acetabular bone loss rather than excision arthroplasty as the final stage.

Currently, many prostheses with conventional polyethylene continue to be revised because they are in their second or third decade of use. Acetabular implants, especially those with more modern designs and additional screw fixation, usually have bony integration and rarely become loose; however, early-generation locking mechanisms and the use of conventional polyethylene predispose these cups to failure. Periprosthetic infection is increasing in incidence, in part because indications for hip arthroplasty have become more widespread, especially in elderly or immunocompromised patients. Finally, the use of metal-on-metal articulations has led to an increased incidence of pain, instability, and infection and has created unique indications for socket revision, such as the need to change the bearing surfaces.

Because the loosening process is generally insidious, loose cemented acetabular implants often are not painful. Periprosthetic osteolysis results from cement fragmentation and loss of mechanical fixation, or from polyethylene wear and centripetal osteolysis, which undermines the cement-bone interface. The diagnosis of acetabular loosening of cemented cups is made in patients reporting new onset of vague groin pain and limp. Radiographs demonstrate progressive acetabular migration with a complete circumferential radiolucent line greater than 2 mm in diameter. Cement fractures and conventional polyethylene wear with eccentricity of the femoral head and acetabular osteolysis may be noted.

Loose noncemented acetabular implants are almost always painful because of movement and abrasion of the stiff, metallic acetabular shell directly on bone. Periprosthetic radiolucent lines, screw breakage, progressive cup migration, or complete displacement of the cup from the acetabular bone bed may be noted. These findings usually are associated with sudden pain in the groin and buttock, often of a high intensity.

Rarely, substantial, progressive wear-associated osteolysis is associated with acute fracture of the acetabulum or with progressive neurologic or vascular deficit resulting from the mass effect of the foreign-body reaction to byproducts of wear. These findings are more common in patients with a failed metal-on-metal articulation than in those with metal-on-plastic articulations

---

Dr. Goodman or an immediate family member serves as a paid consultant to Integra LifeSciences; serves as an unpaid consultant to Accelalox and Biomimedica; has stock or stock options held in Accelalox, Biomimedica, and RegenMed Systems; has received research or institutional support from Baxter and DJO; and serves as a board member, owner, officer, or committee member of the American Academy of Orthopaedic Surgeons and the Society for Biomaterials.

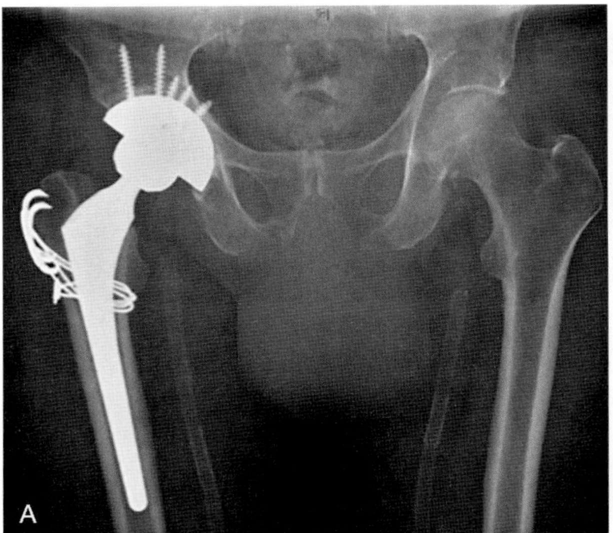

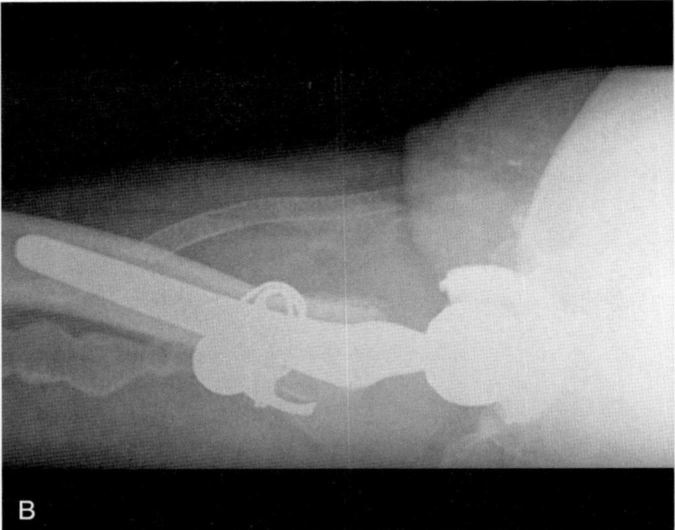

Figure 1 **A,** AP pelvic radiograph demonstrates satisfactory acetabular cup inclination in a patient who had an unstable right total hip arthroplasty and recurrent posterior dislocation. **B,** The cross-table lateral radiograph demonstrates retroversion of the cup. The patient subsequently underwent revision of the entire socket.

because of the toxic effects of metal byproducts.

Evaluation

History and physical examination are important in the diagnosis of acetabular cup problems. Pain resulting from loose implants usually is located in the groin and buttock and is related to activity. Unremitting postoperative pain may be the result of failure to achieve bony integration of a noncemented cup. Pain that progresses over time may be the result of cup migration. Wound-healing problems, continued postoperative drainage, and systemic symptoms (fever, chills, malaise) suggest a diagnosis of deep infection. Wear and osteolysis are generally asymptomatic until chronic synovitis and microfractures occur, at which time groin or buttock pain becomes more noticeable. Catastrophic socket failure resulting from aseptic loosening and cup migration, polyethylene liner dislodgement, major fracture through an osteolytic lesion, or hip dislocation is associated with acute, severe pain and loss of function.

The physical examination should include assessment of the patient's gait; the position of the affected limb while the patient is supine; and the location of tender points around the hip girdle, pelvis, and spine. The incision should be inspected for redness and drainage. The range of motion (ROM), including the presence of instability and pain, should be documented. A quick spinal assessment, including a basic neurologic examination consisting of documentation of sensation to touch or pinprick and strength testing, should be performed. Sciatic and femoral nerve function should be documented. The lateral femoral cutaneous nerve may be abnormal, especially in patients in whom anterior surgical approaches to the hip were used.

Radiography should include, at a minimum, an AP pelvic radiograph (which the author of this chapter prefers to a hip radiograph) and a cross-table lateral radiograph of the hip (which is especially helpful to assess for cup anteversion; **Figure 1**). Judet views often are useful to view occult fractures and more fully assess osteolytic lesions. In some patients, metal-artifact reduction CT is helpful to visualize structural bone deficits. Metal-artifact reduction sequence MRI will help demonstrate synovitis, osteolytic lesions, pseudotumors, and the integrity of soft tissues such as the hip abductors and the neurovascular bundle.

To help rule out infection, the patient's complete blood count, erythrocyte sedimentation rate, and C-reactive protein level should be obtained. If any of these values are out of the normal range, hip aspiration should be ordered to examine the cell counts; determine the percentage of neutrophils; and obtain a culture for aerobic and anaerobic bacteria and, in immunocompromised patients, a culture for fungi and tuberculosis (**Figure 2**). Routine cultures should be kept for several weeks to allow isolation of slow-growing organisms such as *Propionibacterium acnes*. Synovial fluid assessment, such as the use of a urinary strip test for leukocyte esterase and an immunoassay test for α-defensin, can help rule out infection.

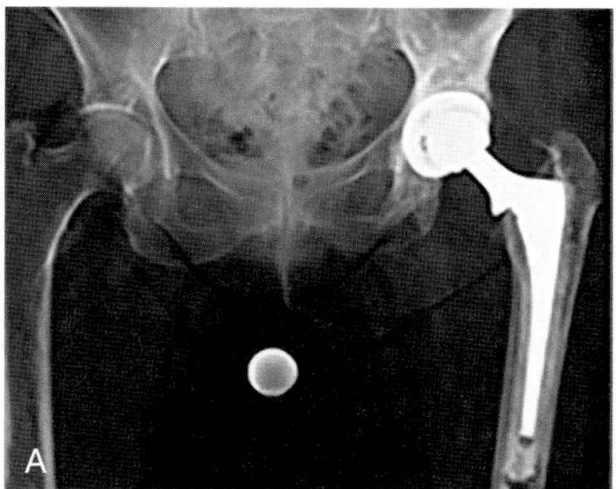

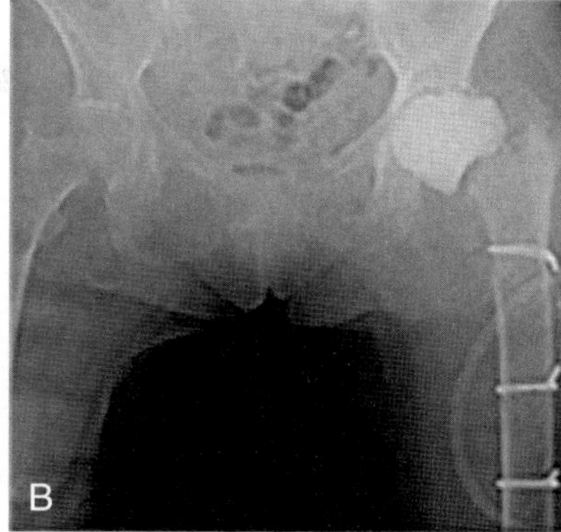

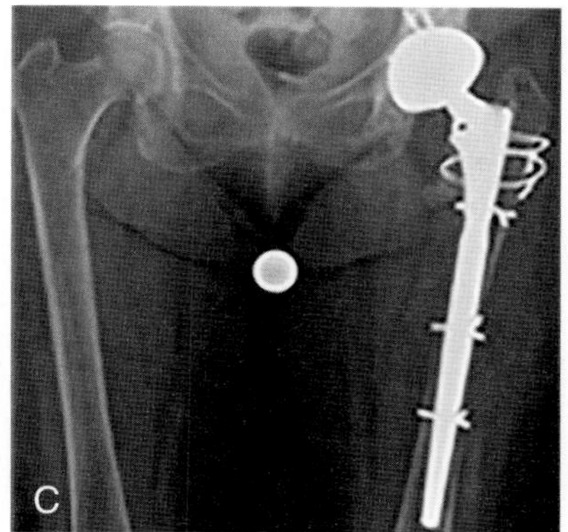

Figure 2 **A,** AP pelvic radiograph demonstrates a painful, infected hybrid left total hip arthroplasty. Subsequent workup showed that the erythrocyte sedimentation rate and C-reactive protein level were both elevated. Hip aspiration cultures grew *Staphylococcus aureus*. **B,** AP pelvic radiograph demonstrates excision of the hip arthroplasty implant with an extended trochanteric osteotomy and placement of an antibiotic-laden spacer. **C,** AP pelvic radiograph demonstrates reimplantation of a noncemented cup and noncemented tapered stem after inflammatory markers normalized and a negative hip aspiration result was obtained.

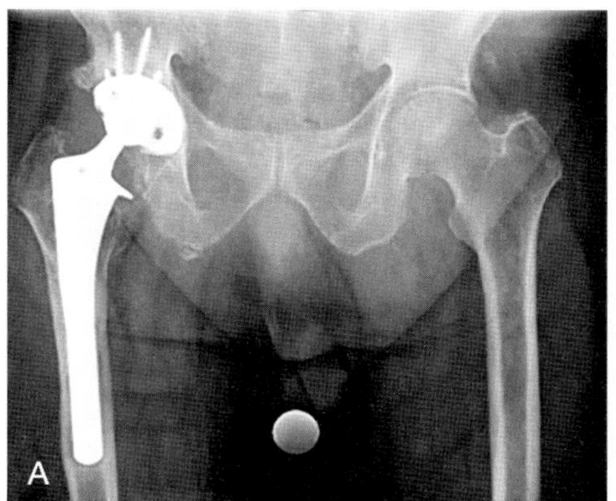

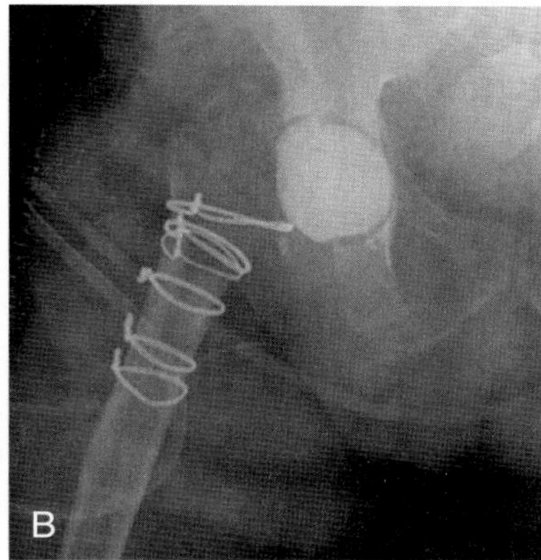

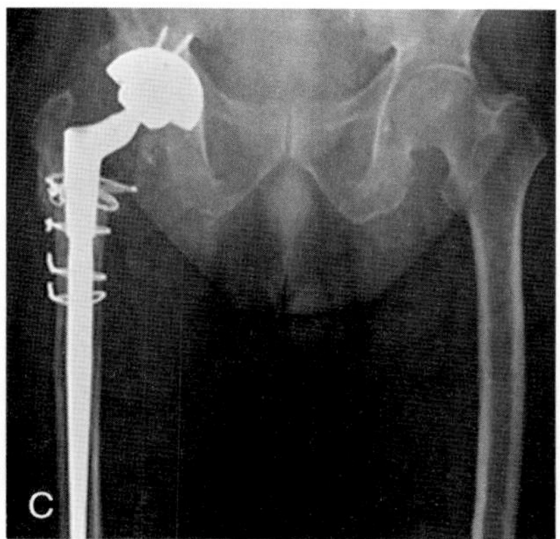

Figure 3 **A,** AP pelvic radiograph demonstrates an infected noncemented total hip arthroplasty with polyethylene wear. Radiolucent lines are present around the cup and stem. The cup and stem were suspected to be loose, and the polyethylene wear was thought to have caused osteolysis as a result of particle disease. Subsequent workup demonstrated infection. Two-stage revision arthroplasty was performed. **B,** AP radiograph of the left hip demonstrates resection arthroplasty with the use of an extended trochanteric osteotomy to aid in extraction of the stem. An antibiotic-laden cement spacer was placed. **C,** AP pelvic radiograph demonstrates the final reconstruction with noncemented implants and impaction grafting of the acetabular bed.

Classification

Several classifications of acetabular bone loss are available. The most useful classifications are highly descriptive, are progressive in terms of bone loss, are easily identifiable both preoperatively (radiographically) and intraoperatively, and guide the surgeon on the optimal method of reconstruction. The Paprosky classification is widely used and has been shown to be valid and reliable. A Paprosky type I defect has the least bone loss. In a type I defect, the acetabulum has a supportive rim and does not demonstrate substantial osteolysis of the teardrop or ischium. Type II acetabular bone loss is more extensive than type I, with loss of bone superiorly in the dome and moderate bone loss in the ischium and the inferior teardrop. The acetabular rim is still capable of providing support for a metallic shell. Subtypes denote the direction of cup migration: superomedial (type IIA), superolateral (type IIB), or directly medial (type IIC; **Figure 3**). Type III defects are the most extensive. In these defects, bone loss has destroyed the dome superiorly such that cup migration is greater than 3 cm. In type IIIA defects, bone loss superiorly and in the ischium inferiorly is extensive, such that the rim cannot support an acetabular shell. Type IIIB defects are even more extensive, with both rim deficiency and the inability to support bony ingrowth. These designations of bone loss can usually be determined on the basis of routine and Judet radiographs or with a CT scan with appropriate reconstruction.

Techniques

When reconstructing the acetabulum, the surgeon should have a clear preoperative plan, sufficient assistance to complete the procedure efficiently and safely (often one assistant is insufficient for difficult procedures), and appropriate implants and a variety of sizes of femoral heads available. The surgeon should have backup plans to allow completion of the procedure because the bone quality and extent of osteolysis are often worse than anticipated. Furthermore, new fractures and discontinuities can be found or can occur intraoperatively, necessitating changes in the original plan. All the necessary hardware, bone grafts, and biologics should be preordered and available.

Anesthesia usually includes both spinal and general anesthesia. Spinal anesthesia will decrease systemic blood pressure and peripheral vascular resistance, leading to decreased blood loss locally in the surgical field. Because many of these procedures are complex and long, general anesthesia keeps the patient comfortably positioned. Intraoperative use of a red blood cell retrieval device will also minimize overall blood loss.

Previous surgical scars need to be assessed for their appropriateness for the anticipated reconstruction. So-called minimally invasive approaches are usually insufficient because they do not allow wide exposure to facilitate 360° visualization of the acetabulum. An anterior or posterior slide osteotomy (which maintains proximal and distal soft-tissue attachments) of the greater trochanter may be required for full visualization; an extended trochanteric osteotomy performed to address the femoral implant accomplishes the same purpose. Capsular tissues should be tagged and preserved when possible for later closure. Three to five deep samples should be taken from the joint fluid and tissues for culture to determine the presence of infection. Experienced surgeons may evaluate intraoperative frozen sections of tissue samples to determine the number of polymorphonuclear leukocytes (PMNs) per high-power field (hpf; >5 PMN/hpf is abnormal).

If a noncemented acetabular cup is well positioned and stable, has a satisfactory locking mechanism, and has a sufficiently large modern polyethylene liner available for the desired head size, acetabular liner wear can be managed with direct exchange of the liner with or without bone grafting of the osteolytic lesion. If the locking mechanism is insufficient or archaic, a liner usually can be cemented into an existing acceptable shell, provided that the desired liner allows enough room circumferentially for an adequate cement mantle of 1 to 2 mm (**Figure 4**). If these conditions cannot be met, or in patients with failed cemented acetabular reconstruction, the entire acetabular implant should be removed.

When the existing acetabular implant is removed, all soft tissue affected by foreign-body reaction and all nonviable bone must be excised. Useful tools to accomplish this task include specialized small and large osteotomes and gouges, such as Aufranc gouges, and commercially available acetabular implant removal systems, in which different sizes and lengths of gouges or blades are attached to a manual rotating device. After excision of all foreign material and inflamed soft tissue, the Paprosky classification of the defect and the presence of fractures or discontinuity should be reassessed. The underlying bone is then freshened with gentle reaming.

Principles of Reconstruction

The following principles are essential for a successful reconstruction. Absolute mechanical stability of the acetabular reconstruction must be obtained intraoperatively. The surgeon should attempt to place the reconstructed acetabular implant as close as possible to the true anatomic hip center to restore normal hip biomechanics. Reconstruction of the hip center in a slightly superior position is acceptable, but implants with longer femoral necks will have to be used to reestablish leg length and avoid impingement.

Contained acetabular defects can be managed successfully with impaction grafting with morcellized cancellous bone if the host bone bed is viable and cup stability can be achieved. This approach is ideal in patients with Paprosky type I defects and many patients with Paprosky type II defects.

The reconstruction needs to withstand physiologic loads. A fully circumferential rim fit is not necessary but is desirable. When a noncemented cup is used, numerous screws or pegs are used to supplement rim fixation (**Figure 5**). Bone ingrowth into porous-coated cups occurs most extensively around these screws or pegs.

In patients with larger defects in whom rim stability cannot be achieved, supplementary devices are needed. This scenario usually occurs in patients with type IIB and type IIIA defects. Supplementary fixation can be achieved with porous metal augments and screws; impaction grafting with the use of a metallic shell, ring, or cage and a cemented polyethylene liner; or the use of a structural corticocancellous bone allograft with a cage and a cemented polyethylene liner. Metal augment devices have largely replaced the previous use of fresh-frozen structural bone allografts; however, in younger patients in whom restoration of bone stock is desirable, allograft techniques can be useful.

Type IIIB defects are extremely challenging to manage. In some patients, these reconstructions need to be staged, with restoration of bone stock before the final reconstruction. Other options include structural allografts with reconstruction rings, cup-cage constructs, and custom large metallic implants such as those typically used in tumor surgery.

In patients with pelvic discontinuity, the failure rate is high if bone grafting

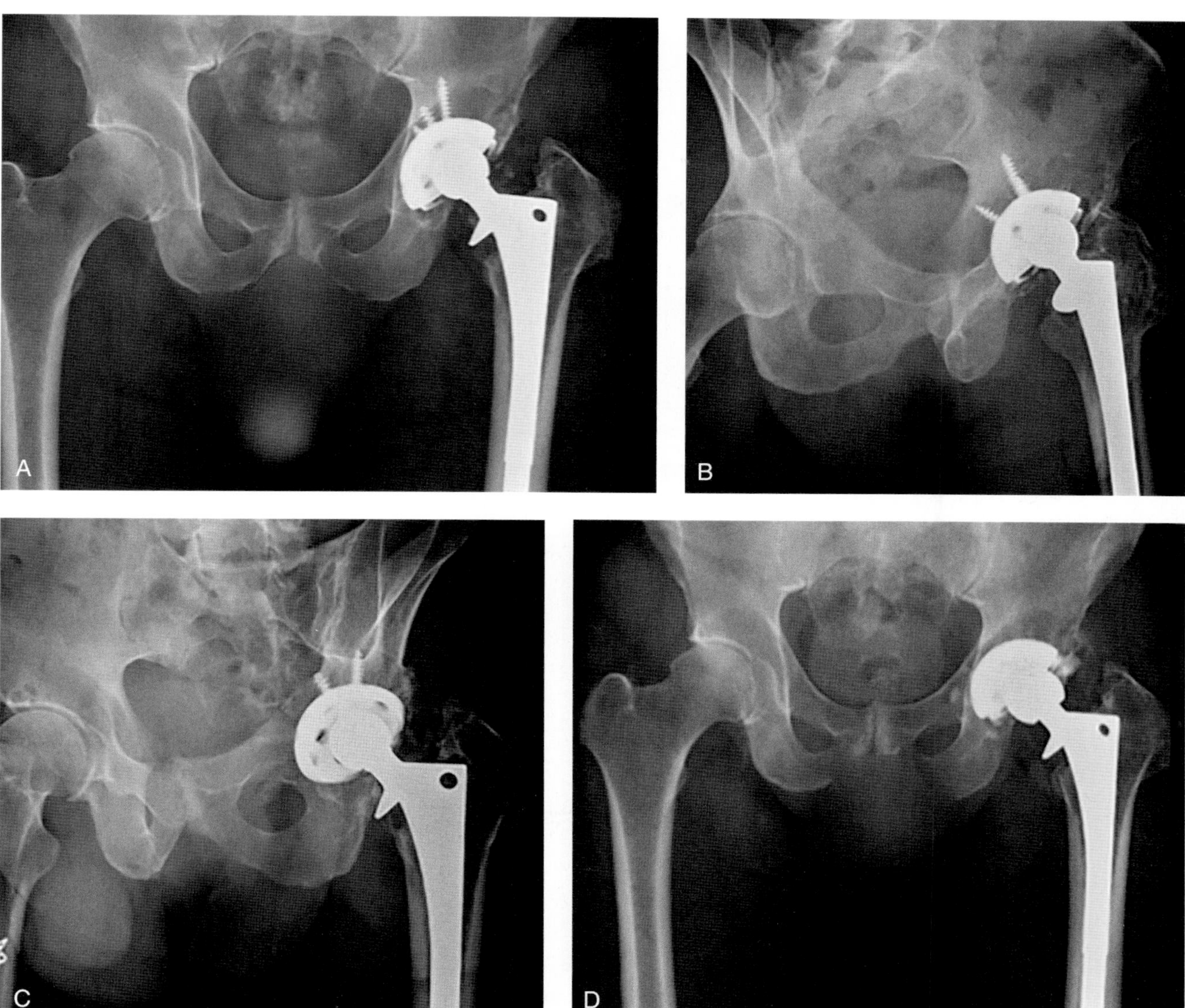

Figure 4 **A,** AP pelvic radiograph demonstrates polyethylene wear with eccentricity of the femoral head within the liner and osteolysis of the proximal femur in a patient with a noncemented left total hip arthroplasty. The cup and stem are stable, but the shell has a first-generation locking mechanism. Iliac (**B**) and obturator (**C**) Judet oblique radiographs further demonstrate the extent of the osteolysis involving the dome and columns of the acetabulum. **D,** Postoperative AP pelvic radiograph demonstrates the revision. The screws have been removed. The cup and stem were found to be stable and well positioned. The area of osteolysis was débrided and grafted with demineralized bone matrix using the screw holes in the cup. A new liner was cemented into the existing acetabular metal shell.

with placement of a standard noncemented cup or ring alone is performed. In such patients, the surgeon can plate the discontinuity and subsequently address the deficient socket according to the Paprosky defect type and the surgical techniques outlined previously. Alternatively, the surgeon can use the acetabular distraction technique to jam a porous metallic cup at the level of the discontinuity to attain stability, and then supplement the reconstruction with screws and bone graft.

Large femoral heads (≥32 mm) give added stability to the hip and extend the ROM. The femoral head size used is dictated in part by the size of the socket (to allow sufficient polyethylene thickness). Impingement during ROM must be avoided. If soft tissues in the hip, especially the abductor musculature, are deficient, the surgeon should consider the use of the largest possible femoral head size, constrained liners, or dual-mobility or tripolar constructs.

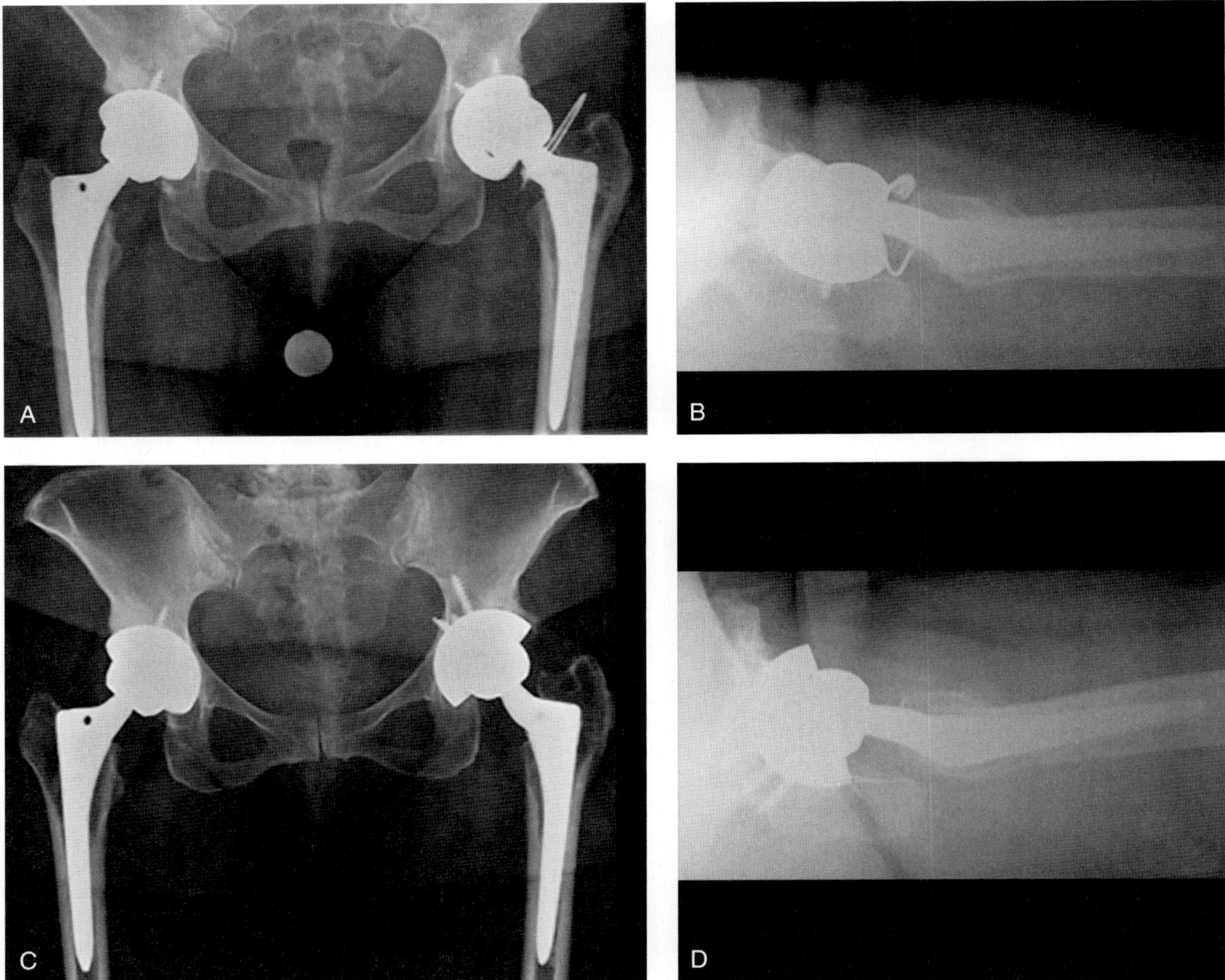

Figure 5 **A,** AP pelvic radiograph demonstrates an unstable left total hip arthroplasty in a patient who had undergone several surgical procedures for the management of instability. The socket is vertically oriented. **B,** Cross-table lateral radiograph demonstrates excessive anteversion of the socket. The dislocations occurred anterosuperiorly. **C,** AP pelvic radiograph demonstrates satisfactory inclination of the cup after revision of the socket. **D,** Cross-table lateral radiograph demonstrates appropriate anteversion of the socket.

Options for Bone Reconstruction

Several options are available for bone reconstruction. Autograft is osteoconductive, osteoinductive, and osteogenic. It provides a scaffold, numerous growth factors, and bone cells. However, supply is limited to local tissues (eg, acetabular reamings) and remote harvesting, usually from the iliac crest. A technique to avoid local morbidity from bone grafting involves aspiration of marrow from the iliac crest and concentration of the osteoprogenitor cells with the use of a centrifuge or other device. The cells are mixed with a scaffold, such as demineralized bone matrix, and applied directly to the defect. This cell grafting technique can also be used to augment osteolytic defects, with the use of a needle and syringe to inject the material, during polyethylene liner exchange procedures in which a well-fixed metallic shell is left in situ. This technique can also be used for grafting around well-fixed cups via a small periacetabular bone window without disturbing the overall stability of the cup.

Freeze-dried cancellous allograft cuboid bone chips are the mainstay of acetabular reconstructions. These grafts are osteoconductive, readily available, and safe. They can be mixed with demineralized bone matrix to increase their osteoinductivity or with acetabular reamings or harvested marrow cells to

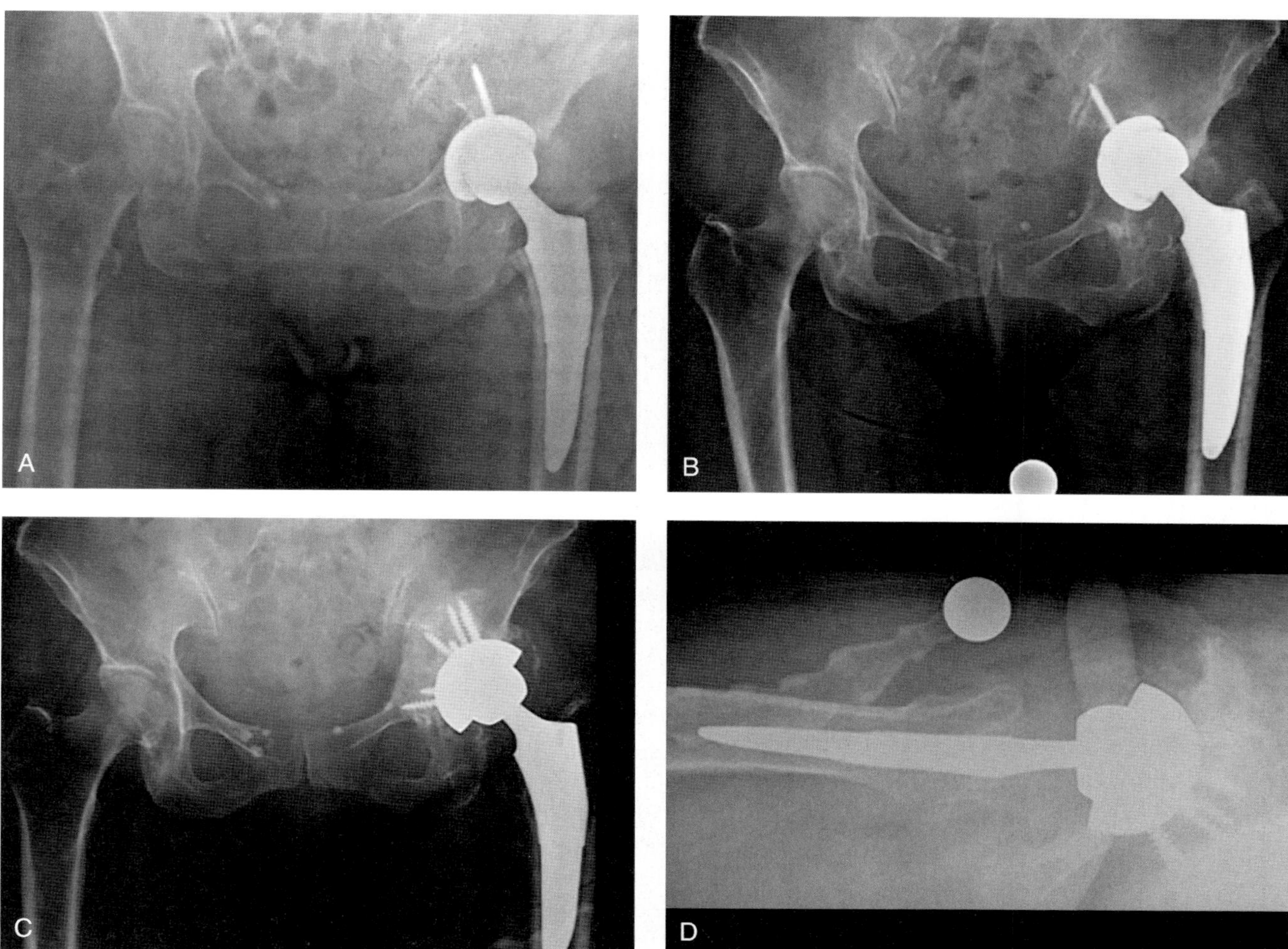

Figure 6 **A,** AP pelvic radiograph demonstrates left total hip arthroplasty in an elderly woman with osteopenia. The procedure was performed through an anterior approach. The acetabulum was overreamed and the cup overmedialized intraoperatively. **B,** AP pelvic radiograph of the same patient obtained 1 month postoperatively demonstrates fracture of the acetabulum and loss of fixation of the cup. The patient did not have pelvic discontinuity. AP pelvic (**C**) and cross-table lateral (**D**) radiographs obtained after extensive impaction bone grafting and placement of a new noncemented cup and numerous screws.

increase their osteogenic ability. Impaction grafting using reverse reaming allows the surgeon to sculpt the graft into the acetabular defect (**Figure 6**). When this technique is used, the resulting acetabular socket is much smaller than the original defect.

Because of the advent of structural porous metallic augments fixed with screws, structural allografts are used less frequently than they previously were. However, in younger patients with a potentially long life span, restoration of bone stock with structural allografts may be useful. Fresh-frozen structural allografts can consist of bone from the femoral head, distal femur, or acetabulum and can be shaped to the particular defect and fixed with screws. Structural allografts must be protected with a ring, a cage, or another device. Although some graft absorption always occurs, structural allografts provide additional bone stock for use if revision is necessary in the future.

Bone void fillers or extenders, such as calcium sulfate or calcium phosphates or carbonates, mimic the mineralized phase of bone. These substances are not commonly used in acetabular reconstruction because they are osteoconductive only and have weak mechanical properties. They can be mixed with other biologics, such as autograft or allograft bone, to fill larger voids. The degradation rate of these substances depends on the particular chemical composition, and the time to degradation ranges from weeks to many years.

Options for Implants

Historically, standard acetabular revision procedures using cemented and noncemented cups have demonstrated reasonably good outcomes. However, cemented revision cups often required supportive metallic mesh or the combination of a roof ring and screw fixation to attain mechanical stability because the bone bed is insufficient to support simple cement fixation. Noncemented cups and screws, with impaction cancellous bone grafting, are currently the mainstay of acetabular revision surgery.

More recently, newer acetabular revision implants have overtaken the marketplace. These robust metallic shells, which have porous coatings with a structure like that of cancellous bone, are rougher and provide more friction resistance at the interface, resulting in improved initial mechanical stability compared with that of earlier shell designs (**Figure 5**). These cups have excellent versatility because they offer multiple holes for screw fixation and, in some cases, the ability to drill through the metal shell for additional screw fixation.

Acetabular augments, which also are made of low-modulus, porous-coated metals that mimic cancellous bone, are based on similar concepts. These augments generally extend the acetabular rim, provide mechanical structural support, or provide internal support. These augments are fixed with screws to the remaining pelvis and often allow additional screw fixation by means of holes drilled directly through the augment. Cement may be placed between the augment and the acetabular shell to unify the construct. In the cup-cage construct, an internal shell, functioning similarly to a structural bone graft, is protected by a reconstruction cage. These constructs have replaced the use of stainless steel roof rings and cages, which often resulted in late failure because of lack of bony integration.

The most difficult Paprosky type III defects require technical skill and ingenuity. Management of these defects may require the use of structural allografts and cages, cup-cage constructs, or custom CT-based acetabular or pelvic implants. As noted, difficult reconstructions may have to be staged, with restoration of bone stock in the first stage and the final acetabular reconstruction in the second stage.

Postoperative Regimen

Postoperative bracing is used by many clinicians because of the increased rate of dislocation after revision THA. Bracing may limit hip ROM and reduce the possibility of dislocation when the patient is out of bed and in potentially precarious situations, such as getting out of a chair or being in a crowd. Bracing usually is continued for 6 weeks postoperatively, but it may be extended if the surrounding soft tissues are pliable or deficient. Weight bearing must be individualized to the initial stability and integrity of the reconstruction and is progressed as bone healing and osseointegration occur.

Avoiding Pitfalls and Complications

Acetabular revision surgery should be carefully planned so that the procedure can proceed smoothly and result in a favorable outcome. Infection needs to be ruled out preoperatively. Intraoperative cultures should be obtained because some patients who appear to require aseptic revision actually have infection. The Paprosky classification of acetabular defects is helpful in planning the reconstruction. Impaction grafting with cancellous allograft cuboid bone chips and the use of a noncemented cup and screws are still the mainstay of acetabular reconstruction and provide a stable reconstruction. Structural allografts, roof rings, and reconstruction rings have been largely replaced by newer acetabular implants with porous metal surfaces like that of cancellous bone, new augments, and custom devices. Occasionally, in the most difficult scenarios in patients with extensive bone loss, a staged reconstruction is necessary.

Bibliography

Batuyong ED, Brock HS, Thiruvengadam N, Maloney WJ, Goodman SB, Huddleston JI: Outcome of porous tantalum acetabular components for Paprosky type 3 and 4 acetabular defects. *J Arthroplasty* 2014;29(6):1318-1322.

Blom AW, Wylde V, Livesey C, et al: Impaction bone grafting of the acetabulum at hip revision using a mix of bone chips and a biphasic porous ceramic bone graft substitute. *Acta Orthop* 2009;80(2):150-154.

Brubaker SM, Brown TE, Manaswi A, Mihalko WM, Cui Q, Saleh KJ: Treatment options and allograft use in revision total hip arthroplasty: The acetabulum. *J Arthroplasty* 2007;22(7 suppl 3):52-56.

Emms NW, Buckley SC, Stockley I, Hamer AJ, Kerry RM: Mid- to long-term results of irradiated allograft in acetabular reconstruction: A follow-up report. *J Bone Joint Surg Br* 2009;91(11):1419-1423.

Gross AE, Goodman S: The current role of structural grafts and cages in revision arthroplasty of the hip. *Clin Orthop Relat Res* 2004;(429):193-200.

Hall A, Eilers M, Hansen R, et al: Advances in acetabular reconstruction in revision total hip arthroplasty: Maximizing function and outcomes after treatment of periacetabular osteolysis around the well-fixed shell. *J Bone Joint Surg Am* 2013;95(18):1709-1718.

Hansen E, Ries MD: Revision total hip arthroplasty for large medial (protrusio) defects with a rim-fit cementless acetabular component. *J Arthroplasty* 2006;21(1):72-79.

Issack PS: Use of porous tantalum for acetabular reconstruction in revision hip arthroplasty. *J Bone Joint Surg Am* 2013;95(21):1981-1987.

Oakes DA, Cabanela ME: Impaction bone grafting for revision hip arthroplasty: Biology and clinical applications. *J Am Acad Orthop Surg* 2006;14(11):620-628.

Ochs BG, Schmid U, Rieth J, Ateschrang A, Weise K, Ochs U: Acetabular bone reconstruction in revision arthroplasty: A comparison of freeze-dried, irradiated and chemically-treated allograft vitalised with autologous marrow versus frozen non-irradiated allograft. *J Bone Joint Surg Br* 2008;90(9):1164-1171.

Sheth NP, Nelson CL, Springer BD, Fehring TK, Paprosky WG: Acetabular bone loss in revision total hip arthroplasty: Evaluation and management. *J Am Acad Orthop Surg* 2013;21(3):128-139.

Sporer SM, Bottros JJ, Hulst JB, Kancherla VK, Moric M, Paprosky WG: Acetabular distraction: An alternative for severe defects with chronic pelvic discontinuity? *Clin Orthop Relat Res* 2012;470(11):3156-3163.

Ullmark G, Sörensen J, Nilsson O: Bone healing of severe acetabular defects after revision arthroplasty. *Acta Orthop* 2009;80(2):179-183.

van Haaren EH, Heyligers IC, Alexander FG, Wuisman PI: High rate of failure of impaction grafting in large acetabular defects. *J Bone Joint Surg Br* 2007;89(3):296-300.

Yu R, Hofstaetter JG, Sullivan T, Costi K, Howie DW, Solomon LB: Validity and reliability of the Paprosky acetabular defect classification. *Clin Orthop Relat Res* 2013;471(7):2259-2265.

Chapter 48
Noncemented Acetabular Revision

Scott M. Sporer, MD
Brett D. Rosenthal, MD
Barrett Steven Boody, MD

Indications

With an aging population, increasing life expectancy, and expanding indications for primary total hip arthroplasty (THA), the number of revision THA procedures has increased in recent years and is projected to continue to increase, despite advances in surgical technique and implant design for primary THA. Revision of the acetabular implant most frequently is performed for the management of dislocation, mechanical loosening, and implant failure. Less common indications include periprosthetic fracture, osteolysis, infection, and wear. In patients with noncemented primary acetabular shells, substantial acetabular bone loss can result from osteolysis and stress shielding before the patient experiences symptoms, further complicating revision procedures.

The goal of acetabular revision is to achieve a durable, stable implant that is oriented and positioned to minimize the risk of dislocation and closely re-create native hip kinematics. The factors that have the greatest influence on implant durability and stability are the method of fixation, the biologic potential of surrounding tissues, and the inherent stability of the implant.

Fixation options include biologic and nonbiologic methods. Biologic fixation methods rely on interdigitating ingrowth from the surrounding bone to create secure fixation at the bone-implant interface. A variety of implants use biologic fixation, including hemispheric noncemented cups with either anatomic or high hip centers, jumbo cups, oblong cups, and modular noncemented implants. Nonbiologic fixation methods rely on adjunct fixation to secure the implant to the acetabulum. Implants that use nonbiologic fixation include cemented polyethylene cups, anti-protrusio cages, impaction grafts, and total acetabular allografts. The focus of this chapter is on biologic noncemented fixation.

Biologic fixation is the preferred method of acetabular revision surgery. The biologic potential of the tissues immediately surrounding an acetabular implant is crucial to the durability of the implant. Successful fixation requires both bony apposition and tissue viability. Bony apposition is critical because a gap greater than 150 µm between the implant and bone prevents bony integration. The importance of tissue viability is demonstrated by evidence suggesting that previously irradiated bone is associated with early implant failure in noncemented acetabular revision surgery.

Even before bony ingrowth has occurred, the stability of a trial implant can be assessed intraoperatively. Poor initial cup fixation is associated with early complications and long-term dysfunction. The inherent stability depends on bone quality, exactness of reaming, and accuracy of cup insertion. A simple classification system can be used to identify the amount of inherent stability. Full inherent stability allows the surgeon to push on the rim of the trial implant and perform a trial reduction without displacing the trial implant. Partial inherent stability allows for the position to be maintained after the trial implant insertion device is removed, but loss of position results from any attempt at reduction or pushing on the rim of the trial implant. Implants without inherent stability have inadequate host bone to maintain trial cup position after removal of the trial implant insertion device. This classification system is useful for intraoperative assessment of the degree to which bone loss may compromise fixation and assists a surgeon in

Dr. Sporer or an immediate family member serves as a paid consultant to Pacira Pharmaceuticals, Smith & Nephew, and Zimmer Biomet; has received research or institutional support from Central DuPage Hospital, Stryker, and Zimmer Biomet; and serves as a board member, owner, officer, or committee member of the American Joint Replacement Registry and The Hip Society. Neither of the following authors nor any immediate family member has received anything of value from or has stock or stock options held in a commercial company or institution related directly or indirectly to the subject of this chapter: Dr. Rosenthal and Dr. Boody.

Table 1 Paprosky Classification of Acetabular Bone Loss

Defect Type	Femoral Head Center Migration	Rim	Columns	Ischial Osteolysis	Köhler Line	Teardrop	Expected Inherent Stability
I	Minimal (<3 cm)	Intact	Supportive	None	Intact	Intact	Full
IIA	Mild (<3 cm)	Distorted	Supportive	Mild	Intact	Intact	Full
IIB	Moderate (<3 cm)	Distorted	Supportive	Mild	Intact	Intact	Full
IIC	Mild (<3 cm)	Distorted	Supportive	Mild	Disrupted	Moderate osteolysis	Full
IIIA	Severe (>3 cm)	Missing	Nonsupportive	Moderate	Intact	Moderate osteolysis	Partial
IIIB	Severe (>3 cm)	Missing	Nonsupportive	Severe	Disrupted	Severe osteolysis	None

determining which strategies are necessary to achieve noncemented biologic fixation.

Preoperative planning facilitates an efficient procedure and helps a surgeon prepare for contingencies should unforeseen issues arise. Before any revision procedure, the patient should be evaluated for infection in the implant. Additional radiographs, including Judet views, may facilitate identification of bone defects and existing implants. In patients with acetabular protrusion, CT angiography and consultation with a vascular surgeon should be completed preoperatively.

Classification

Systematic preoperative interpretation of radiographs can help predict intraoperative stability and postoperative durability of a revision construct. Many classification systems have been proposed to assist with this prediction. The authors of this chapter prefer to use the Paprosky classification of acetabular bone loss (**Table 1**) because it is helpful in preoperative planning for noncemented revision of the acetabular implant. The Paprosky classification is based on the severity of bone loss and a surgeon's ability to attain noncemented fixation with a given pattern of bone loss. The remaining acetabular bone is completely supportive of a revision implant in type I defects, partially supportive in type II defects, and nonsupportive in type III defects. This classification system helps identify inherent stability and the potential for biologic fixation, which are crucial to implant durability and long-term stability.

To determine the type, the Paprosky classification uses four radiographic parameters: superior migration of the hip center, ischial osteolysis, teardrop osteolysis, and the position of the implant relative to the Köhler line. Superior migration of the hip center refers to bone loss in the acetabular dome, which consists of bone stock from the anterior and posterior columns. Superomedial migration suggests greater anterior column bone loss, whereas superolateral migration suggests greater posterior column bone loss. Superior migration is measured relative to the superior obturator line. Ischial osteolysis is bone loss from the inferior aspect of the posterior column and posterior wall. Teardrop osteolysis and disruption of the Köhler line both suggest medial acetabular bone loss.

The goal of acetabular reconstruction in patients with type IIIA defects is to restore full inherent stability intraoperatively so that a noncemented implant can be used. The shape of a type IIIA defect is critical in determining the appropriate treatment option. Spheric defects, which are less common than oblong defects, can be managed with a jumbo hemispheric cup, with excellent results. Oblong defects can be managed with a high hip center noncemented hemispheric cup, a superior number 7 distal femoral structural graft and a noncemented hemispheric cup, or a porous metal cup with superior metal augmentation. Bilobed implants are not recommended in these reconstructions because of their high rate of loosening and increased technical difficulties.

The authors of this chapter prefer to avoid reconstruction with a high hip center in patients with oblong type IIIA defects. In patients with severely deficient bone stock, a superior shift of the hip center can maximize contact between the porous-coated implant and the host bone. Biomechanical analyses to identify alterations in joint kinematics after a superior shift have demonstrated mixed results. Some analyses identified alterations in abductor muscle exertion required to maintain pelvic stabilization, whereas others did not reveal substantial alterations in joint forces. Computer modeling has demonstrated that compensatory increases in the length of the femoral neck can sufficiently restore the abductor moment arm. Without compensatory changes in the femoral neck length, calcar replacement, or trochanteric advancement, the use of a high hip center increases the risk of limb-length discrepancy, dislocation, and altered abductor muscle tensioning. Additionally, the nonanatomic location of the hip center increases the risk of impingement.

The second option for the management of oblong type IIIA defects is a superior number 7 distal femoral structural graft with a hemispheric cup. To obtain a stable construct with restoration of the native hip center, a structural allograft in the shape of the number 7 is added to the superior aspect of the acetabulum to improve initial stability of the noncemented acetabular implant. Because femoral head allograft is insufficient as a structural support, fresh-frozen distal femoral or proximal tibial allograft is preferred. Trabecular patterns of the graft should be oriented parallel to the direction of load to optimize stress transfer. The likelihood of union is increased by meticulously contouring the shape of the allograft to maximize the contact surface area between the graft and host bone. This technique has demonstrated a high rate of clinical and radiographic success at an average follow-up of 10 years in patients with at least 50% host bone support.

The third option for the management of oblong type IIIA defects is the use of a porous metal cup with superior metal augmentation of the acetabular rim. The advantages of metal augmentation over distal femoral allograft are that the metal augments are nonresorbable, are technically easier to use, and do not carry a risk of disease transmission. Additionally, their use does not require extensive stripping of the ilium or mobilization of the abductors. Metal augmentation has demonstrated low rates of loosening, acceptable functional improvements, and pain relief at mean 5-year follow-up.

In patients with Paprosky type IIIB defects, substantial measures must be taken to allow noncemented acetabular revision. If the patient does not have pelvic discontinuity, biologic fixation can be attained with the use of custom triflange implants (not described in this chapter) or porous metal augmentation. The authors of this chapter typically attain initial stability via compression in patients with acute pelvic discontinuity and via distraction in patients with chronic pelvic discontinuity. The use of a cup-cage construct is an emerging strategy for the management of pelvic discontinuity. Midterm studies demonstrate good longevity, with the authors of one study of cup-cage reconstruction reporting survival rates of 93% at 5 years and 85% at 10 years postoperatively, with failure defined as revision for any cause.

Algorithmic Approach

An algorithmic approach to noncemented revision of the acetabular implant is depicted in **Figure 1**. The first decision point is the assessment of the bone stock as indicated by the location of the hip center. If the hip center has not migrated more than 3 cm, a trial implant can be inserted to assess the inherent stability. If the remaining bone stock is adequate and provides press-fit stability of the trial implant, the defect is Paprosky type I or type II, and noncemented fixation of a hemispheric cup likely will be adequate. If disruption of the Köhler line is present on radiographs, the defect is type IIC, which will require rim fixation to support the noncemented hemispheric implant. Medial cancellous allograft may be useful in this situation to lateralize the hip center.

If the hip center has migrated more than 3 cm superiorly, or if the trial implant does not have full press-fit inherent stability, the defect is Paprosky type III. If partial inherent stability is present, the potential for durable biologic fixation exists, and the defect is graded type IIIA. The shape of the defect then dictates the necessary revision implant. As noted previously, in patients with a spheric type IIIA defect, a jumbo hemispheric cup may be beneficial. Oblong defects can be managed with a hemispheric cup with high hip center, a number 7 distal femoral structural graft and a hemispheric cup, or a modular porous metal augment with a hemispheric cup.

If the trial implant demonstrates no inherent stability, the defect is graded type IIIB. In these patients, pelvic discontinuity should be assessed intraoperatively by compressing the anterior and posterior columns with a Cobb elevator and assessing the motion between the superior and inferior hemipelvises. If no pelvic discontinuity exists, treatment options include nonbiologic fixation with impaction allograft and a cage, nonbiologic fixation with structural allograft and a cage, biologic fixation with modular porous metal augmentation, and biologic fixation with a custom triflange implant. If pelvic discontinuity is observed intraoperatively, the potential of the discontinuity to heal must be determined. If the discontinuity appears to have healing potential, it is considered acute; if not, it is considered chronic. Acute pelvic discontinuities are managed with compression plating in addition to one of the aforementioned options for type IIIB defects. Chronic pelvic discontinuities are managed with distraction via the insertion of bone graft into the defect, which enhances initial stability. The distracted defect subsequently is managed with an acetabular transplant and cage, a porous metal implant with a porous metal augment, or a custom triflange implant.

Results

Long-term follow-up data have shown excellent survivorship of noncemented revision acetabular implants (**Table 2**).

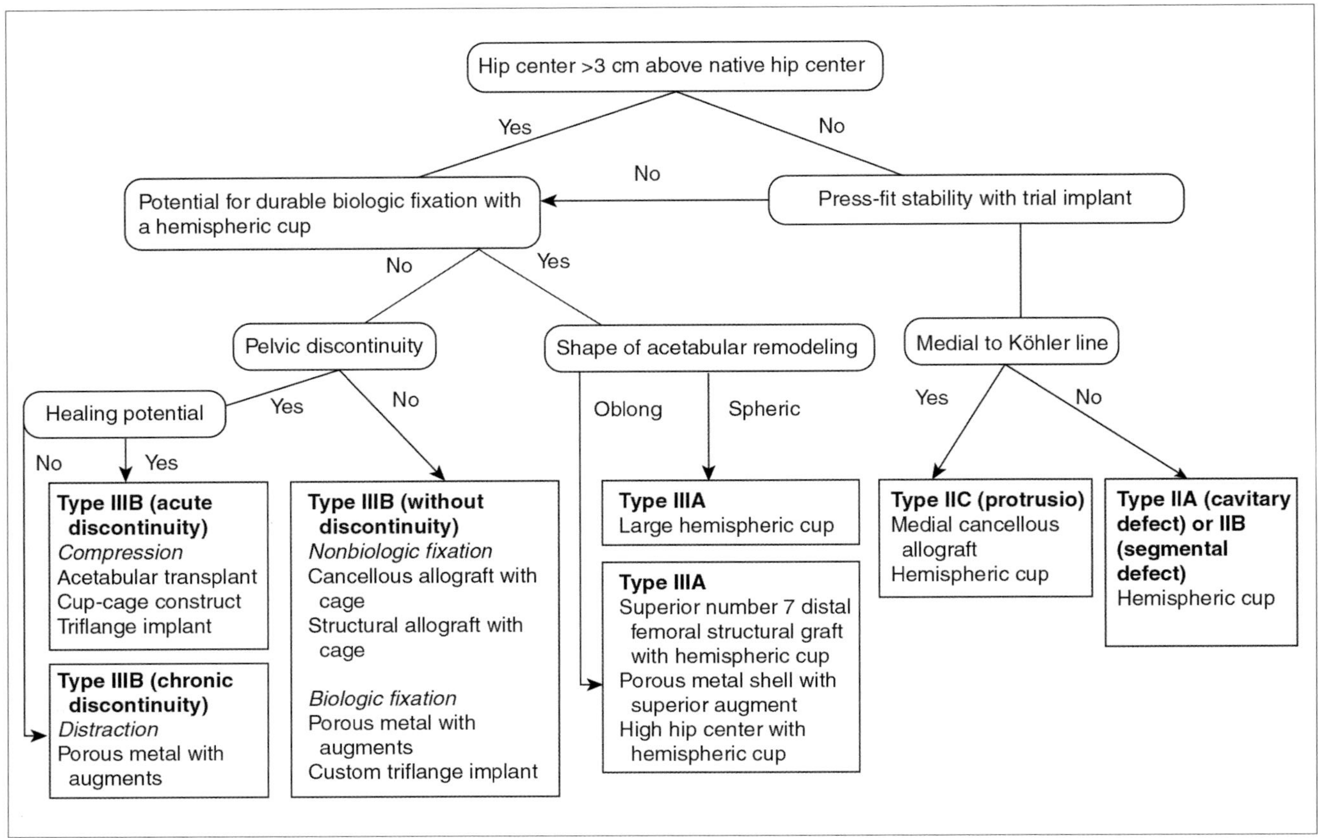

Figure 1 Algorithm shows the decision-making process for noncemented acetabular implant revision.

Several other studies demonstrate similar results. The authors of one study reported a radiographic loosening rate of only 3% at a minimum 20-year follow-up. The author of a different study identified a 1.8% loosening rate at mean 19.4-year follow-up; in that series, the revision rate was 21% for any reason. The rate of failure for aseptic loosening repeatedly has been reported to be less than that of cemented acetabular revision implants. The revision rate of a series of noncemented Harris-Galante implants at a minimum 15-year follow-up was less than that of a series of cemented Charnley implants at a minimum 25-year follow-up (P = 0.0778). Revision hip arthroplasties with noncemented acetabular implants have good functional results even at long-term follow-up. In one study, Harris hip scores initially improved from a mean of 55 points preoperatively to 95 points at 2 years postoperatively. Subsequently, Harris hip scores depreciated slowly, with a mean of 91 points at 6 years postoperatively and a mean of 85 points at 19.4 years postoperatively.

Video 48.1 Stoppa Approach for Removal of the Intrapelvic Cup for Acetabular Revision. Francisco Chana, PhD, MD; Manuel Villanueva, PhD, MD; José Rojo, PhD, MD; María Pérez, MD; José Fernández-Mariño, PhD, MD; Javier Vaquero, PhD, MD (19 min)

Techniques

Setup/Exposure

- An extensile exposure is used to facilitate extraction of the implant. Ideally, the exposure should be an extension of previous incisions to avoid skin bridges and flap necrosis. For the posterior approach, the plane between the iliotibial band and the underlying vastus lateralis may be difficult to redevelop because of scarring.
- Dissection is carried down to the short external rotators in the plane between the capsule and abductors, which are mobilized anteriorly.
- A posterior capsular flap is created subperiosteally from the greater trochanter to the superior aspect of the acetabulum and extended distally along the proximal femur as necessary for visualization of the implant.
- After the posterior capsular flap is retracted, an anterior capsulectomy is performed.

Table 2 Results of Noncemented Acetabular Revision

Author(s) (Year)	Number of Hips	Procedure or Approach	Mean Patient Age in Years (Range)	Mean Follow-up in Years (Range)	Success Rate (%)[a]	Results
Weber et al (1996)	61	Transtrochanteric	68 (39-89)	6.5 (5-8)	100	1.6% radiographically loose
Lachiewicz and Poon (1998)	57	Transtrochanteric (40), posterior (17)	56 (22-82)	7 (5-12)	100	No failures
Chareanchol-vanich et al (1999)	40	Posterior (trochanteric osteotomy in 16)	50 (25-77)	8 (5-11)	87.5	12.5% failure rate
Garcia-Cimbrelo (1999)	65	Lateral (26), posterolateral (20), lateral with trochanteric osteotomy (19)	54.7 (29-77)	8.3 (6-11)	89.2	10.8% failure rate 28% radiographically loose
Leopold et al (1999)	138	Not specified	50 (20-79)	10.5 (7-14)	100	1.8% radiographically loose
Templeton et al (2001)	61	Not specified	67.6 (39-89)	12.9 (11.5-14.3)	100	3.5% radiographically loose

[a] Success is defined as no revision of the acetabular implant for aseptic loosening.

- Subperiosteal dissection of the posterior column and superior aspect of the ilium is performed to improve exposure.
- The acetabular implant is extracted. Retained hardware is removed in a meticulous fashion to minimize bone loss, which can compromise future implant fixation.
- After the polyethylene liner and acetabular fixation screws are removed, the previous acetabular shell is extracted.
- Removal of well-fixed noncemented implants is particularly challenging because of the high risk for bone loss.
- Techniques to minimize bone loss include the use of curved osteotomes, pneumatic impact wrenches, keyhole osteotomies, reciprocating saws, and metal-cutting burrs.
- The authors of this chapter prefer to use an acetabular implant removal device. The device consists of two blades that are attached to a rotating handle and match the outer diameter of the acetabular shell. The center of rotation is maintained with the use of a headpiece that matches the inner diameter of the acetabular shell. The first blade is shorter and used to disrupt the dense peripheral bone and open a passage for the second blade, which is equal in length to the radius of the cup. The second blade functionally frees the dome of the acetabular shell. This technique causes minimal bone loss, allows for time-efficient implant removal, and poses minimal risk.
- If the femoral implant is to be retained, the femoral head is extracted and the stem and femur are translated anteriorly to allow for better visualization of the acetabulum.
- Systematic débridement of interface membrane and granulation tissue improves visualization of the remaining bone stock and allows for improved assessment of pelvic discontinuity.

Procedure

PAPROSKY TYPE I DEFECTS

- As noted previously, a hemispheric noncemented implant likely will have full inherent stability in patients with type I defects.
- The level of the true acetabulum is determined by placing a retractor in the obturator foramen, which is at the level of the inferior border of the acetabulum.
- Acetabular reaming is performed with sequentially larger hemispheric reamers until both the anterior and posterior columns are engaged. In general, sacrifice of anterior acetabular bone poses less risk of causing accidental pelvic discontinuity than does reaming of posterior acetabular bone.
- If the prosthesis is implanted with 45° of abduction and 15° of anteversion, it may be partially uncovered. This incomplete coverage should be tolerated, and the surgeon should resist the temptation to place the

implant more vertically to improve coverage. Substantial deviation from these measures may increase the risk of dislocation and wear.

- Cavitary defects may be packed with local autograft or allograft via reverse running of a reamer 2 mm smaller than the largest reamer that was used.
- Press-fit fixation can be attained if the periphery of the implant is 2 mm larger than the largest hemispheric reamer that was used.
- The use of multiple cancellous screws as supplemental fixation is recommended to reduce micromotion and promote bone ingrowth.

PAPROSKY TYPE IIA DEFECTS

- Aside from the potential need for allograft to fill a cavitary defect, acetabular reconstruction of type IIA defects is similar to that of type I defects.
- A hemispheric noncemented implant is used (**Figure 2**).

PAPROSKY TYPE IIB DEFECTS

- As noted previously, a hemispheric noncemented implant can be used successfully in type IIB defects (**Figure 3**). Most reconstructions of type IIB defects are successful without grafting of the segmental defect.
- If grafting is desired to restore bone stock, the authors of this chapter typically use a number 7 femoral head allograft. This technique involves cutting a femoral head allograft into the shape of the number 7.
- The longitudinal/superior portion of the number 7-shaped graft is placed outside the acetabulum, with the angle of the number 7-shaped graft abutting the superior lip of the acetabulum and the shorter, transverse portion of the number 7-shaped graft lying within the acetabulum.
- Cancellous screws are placed through the long portion of the graft into the iliac bone to provide rigid fixation. This technique is beneficial because it allows for

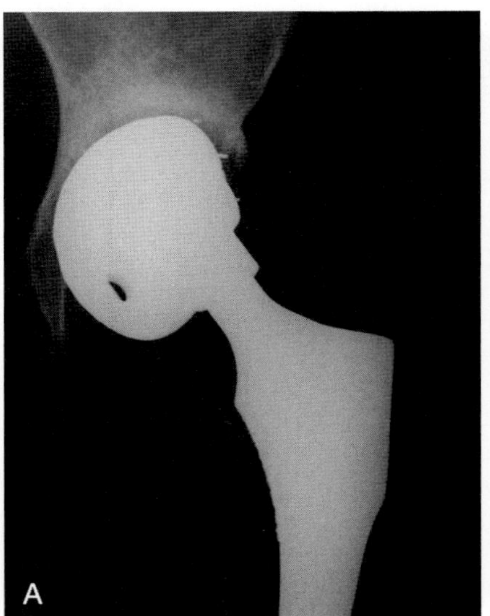

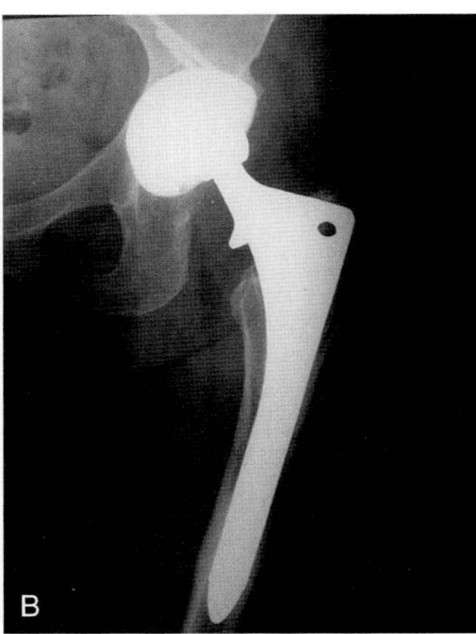

Figure 2 **A,** Preoperative AP hip radiograph demonstrates a Paprosky type IIA defect. Note the acetabular rim distortion and mild ischial osteolysis. **B,** Postoperative AP hip radiograph demonstrates revision with a hemispheric noncemented implant with supplemental acetabular screw fixation.

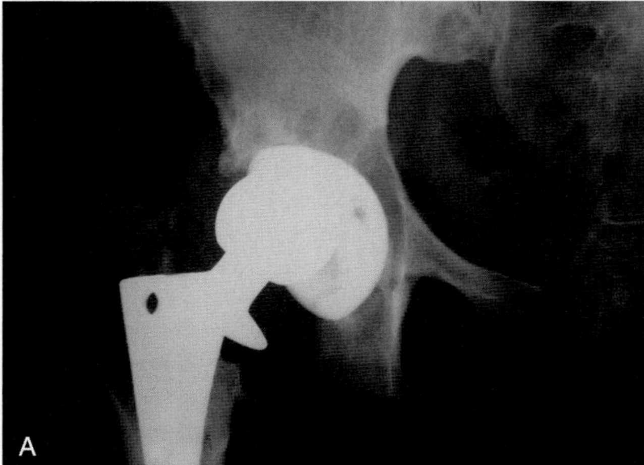

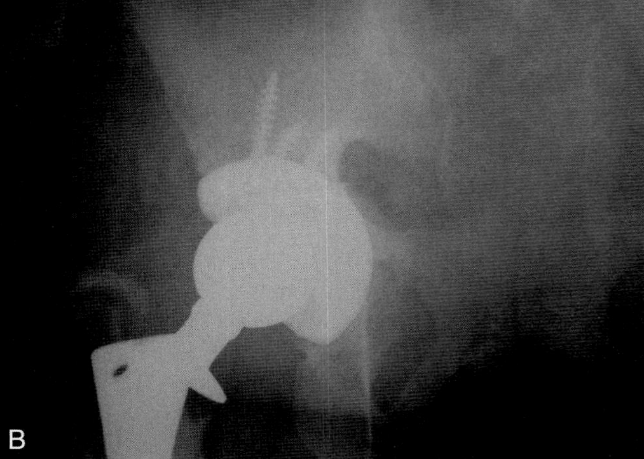

Figure 3 **A,** Preoperative AP hip radiograph demonstrates a Paprosky type IIB defect. Note the segmental bone loss. **B,** Postoperative AP hip radiograph demonstrates revision with a hemispheric noncemented implant with supplemental acetabular screw fixation.

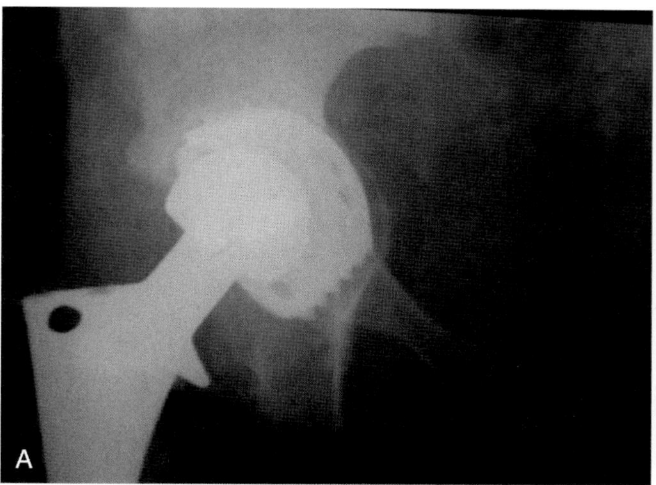

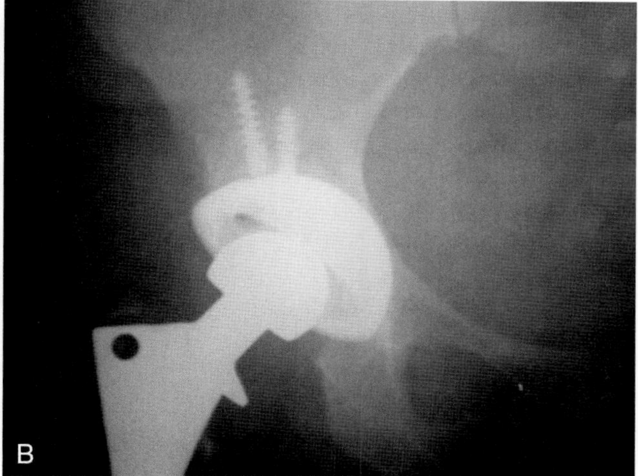

Figure 4 **A,** Preoperative AP hip radiograph demonstrates a Paprosky type IIC defect. Note the disruption of the Köhler line and medialization of the acetabular implant. **B,** Postoperative AP hip radiograph demonstrates revision with a hemispheric noncemented implant with peripheral press-fit fixation and supplemental screw fixation.

graft fixation without interfering with reaming.

- Reaming is performed until the anterior and posterior columns are engaged to allow intrinsic stability of the trial implant. Reaming should be slightly superior to improve coverage of the implant.
- The superior portion of the acetabular implant can be left uncovered.
- To fill cavitary defects, reverse reaming is performed with a reamer 1 to 2 mm smaller than the reamer that engaged the anterior and posterior columns.
- A cup with multiple holes is used. A spiked cup should not be used.

PAPROSKY TYPE IIC DEFECTS

- A hemispheric noncemented implant can be used in patients with type IIC defects (**Figure 4**).
- The hip center is lateralized by impacting particulate bone graft into the defect medially while running reamers in reverse.
- If the medial wall is insufficient to buttress the bone graft, a wafer of femoral head allograft with a diameter greater than that of the defect is used as a buttress.
- If the reamer, running in reverse, contacts the host acetabular rim, the reamer will disengage from its drive shaft. When this occurs, hip center lateralization is sufficient.
- The acetabular implant is placed with 2-mm press-fit fixation. If the acetabulum is between cup sizes, the larger cup size is used. A cup with multiple holes is used.

PAPROSKY TYPE IIIA DEFECTS

- As noted previously, the shape of a type IIIA defect is critical to determining the appropriate treatment option.
- Spheric defects can be managed with a jumbo hemispheric cup.
- Options for the management of oblong defects are a noncemented hemispheric cup with high hip center, a noncemented hemispheric cup and a superior number 7 distal femoral structural graft, or a porous metal cup with superior metal augmentation (**Figure 5**).
- Bilobed implants are not recommended for these reconstructions because of their high rate of loosening and increased technical difficulties.
- As noted, the authors of this chapter prefer not to use a hemispheric cup with high hip center because of the risk of impingement and other potential complications.

Hemispheric Cup With Superior Number 7 Distal Femoral Structural Graft

- Before contouring the graft, the surgeon should assess the patient for pelvic discontinuity.
- If pelvic discontinuity is present, a posterior column plate is applied before allograft reconstruction begins.
- The abductor musculature is elevated with a Taylor retractor to allow for adequate visualization of the iliac wing.
- The desired hip center is identified in relation to either the cotyloid notch or the transverse acetabular ligament.
- Sequentially larger reamers are used at the site of the desired hip center until both columns are engaged.
- The tendency to ream the superior aspect of the acetabulum must be avoided.
- After both columns are engaged, a trial implant is inserted. The trial

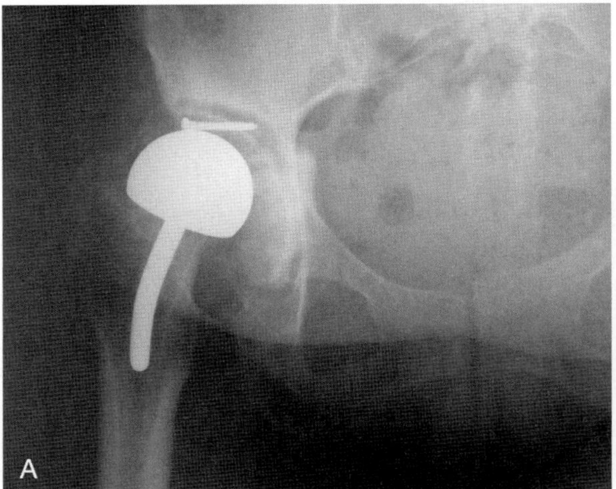

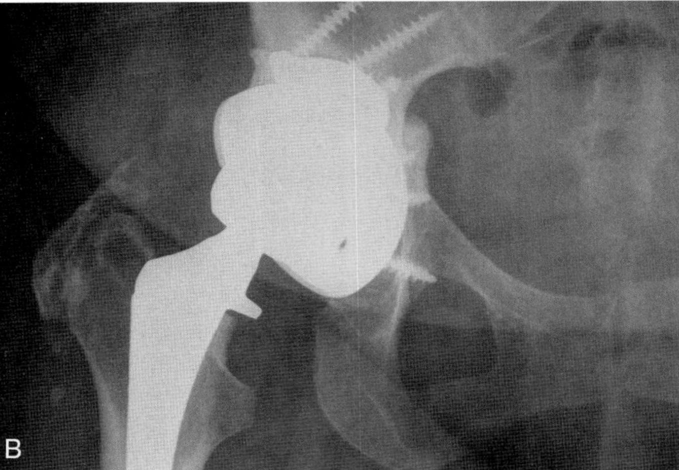

Figure 5 **A,** Preoperative AP hip radiograph demonstrates a Paprosky type IIIA defect. Note the superolateral migration and extensive bone loss. **B,** Postoperative AP hip radiograph demonstrates revision with superior metal augmentation to restore the anatomic hip center.

implant will likely demonstrate partial inherent stability.

- Before the distal femoral allograft is opened, the surgical site is verified to be free of infection.
- The femoral allograft should be cultured before it is inserted into the acetabular defect.
- The use of femoral head allograft should be avoided.
- To begin the contouring of the distal femoral graft, the epicondyles are trimmed so that the medial-to-lateral dimension matches the diameter of the acetabular cavity.
- A female reamer 1 to 2 mm larger than the acetabular cavity is used to ream the distal aspect of the allograft in slight flexion, with care taken to avoid notching of the anterior cortex.
- A coronal cut is made to create the number 7 shape. The longitudinal portion of this cut should be slightly posterior to the midline of the allograft.
- An axial cut is made such that the longitudinal portion of the number 7-shaped graft is 5 to 6 cm in length. The acuity of the cut angle in the coronal plate should be adjusted with a burr to optimize contact between the allograft and the host bone (both ilium and acetabulum). The allograft should be cut at slightly less than 90° to allow intrinsic stability.
- After satisfactory contouring is achieved, the superior/longitudinal limb of the allograft is provisionally secured to the ilium with Steinmann pins.
- Three or four 6.5-mm cancellous screws with washers are used to affix the allograft to the ilium. To minimize the risk of graft fracture, the screw holes should be tapped. The screws should be oriented obliquely into the ilium in the direction of loading with staggered positioning.
- After the allograft is secured, the acetabular cavity is reamed again. Particulate allograft is used to fill any remaining bone defects.
- The implant is placed. Care is taken not to place the implant in excessive abduction and retroversion. The cup should be left uncovered.
- Screws are placed through the cup, allograft, and host bone if possible.

Superior Metal Augmentation With a Porous Metal Cup

- The native hip center is identified by means of the cotyloid notch or transverse acetabular ligament.
- Progressive reaming is performed in anatomic position with sequentially larger reamers until both the anterior and posterior columns are engaged to allow intrinsic stability of the trial acetabular implant.
- With the trial implant in place (with appropriate version and abduction), the superior augment is placed. Metal augments can be placed in any position and orientation to improve initial stability. A barrel burr can be used on either the augment or the host bone to optimize the contact area between the two surfaces. A gap of 1 to 2 mm is left between the cup and the augment for placement of cement.
- A motorized burr is used along the superior dome to fit the host bone to the augment to improve intrinsic stability and maximize bone contact.
- With the trial acetabular implant in place, the augment is fixed with screws.

- The augment is packed with bone graft, with the portion of the augment facing the cup exposed.
- Polymethyl methacrylate cement is placed on the porous revision cup only in areas that will be in contact with the augment. The use of antibiotic-laden cement should be considered.
- To maximize interdigitation of the cup and augment, the cup is inserted after the cement has a doughlike consistency.
- The implant is placed with press-fit fixation. However, multiple screws are recommended to improve initial fixation and minimize micromotion.
- An attempt should be made to place screws in the revision cup before the cement hardens to eliminate motion during final seating of the screws.
- Bone wax is placed in the ends of the screws to facilitate removal of the cup.

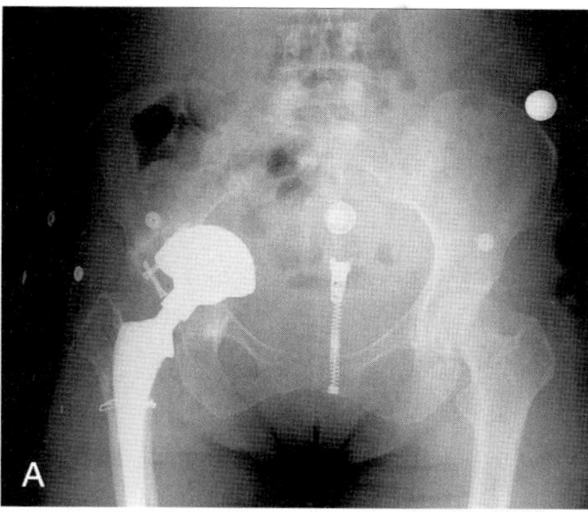

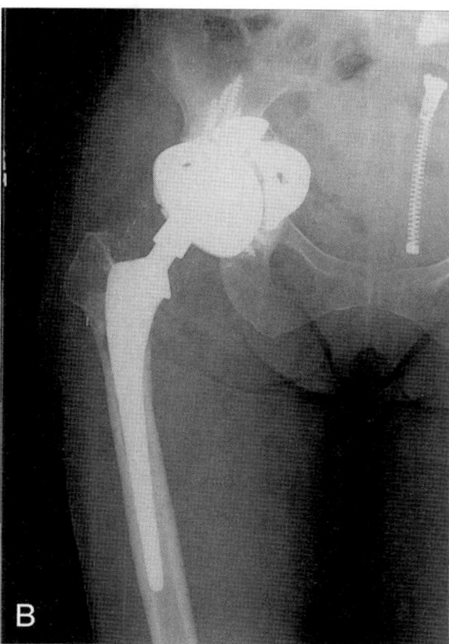

Figure 6 **A,** Preoperative AP pelvic radiograph demonstrates a Paprosky type IIIB defect of the right hip. Note the superomedial migration and extensive bone loss. **B,** Postoperative AP hip radiograph demonstrates revision with metal augmentation to bridge the pelvic discontinuity and increase the stability of the cup after placement.

PAPROSKY TYPE IIIB DEFECTS

- Type IIIB defects require substantial measures to achieve noncemented acetabular revision reconstruction (**Figure 6**).

Type IIIB Defects Without Pelvic Discontinuity

- In patients with type IIIB defects without pelvic discontinuity, nonbiologic augments are used to reconstruct the pelvis.
- All margins of the acetabular defect must be exposed.
- Progressive reaming is performed until two points of fixation (anterior-posterior, anterior-inferior, posterior-inferior) can be achieved.
- The inferior bone stock (ischium) often is minimally involved.
- A trial implant is placed. Attainment of intrinsic stability will be impossible.
- Augments are placed to decrease the acetabular volume and facilitate press-fit fixation between the cup and the augment. Attempts are made to place the augment in direct contact with the revision cup.
- The augment is secured.
- With the augment in place, reverse reaming is performed to pack the augment with bone graft.
- Bone graft is cleared from the exposed host bone to maximize contact of the host bone and the porous revision cup.
- The cup is placed. An attempt is made to place screws inferiorly into the ischium to avoid pullout of the cup.

Type IIIB Defects With Chronic Pelvic Discontinuity

- In patients with type IIIB defects with chronic pelvic discontinuity, a porous acetabular implant is used to reconstruct the pelvis with internal biologic fixation.
- All margins of acetabular defect and discontinuity are thoroughly exposed.
- If gross motion is observed and bone contact is possible, a posterior column plate is used.
- Progressive reaming is performed until two points of fixation (anterior-posterior, anterior-inferior, posterior-inferior) are achieved.
- A trial implant is placed. Attainment of intrinsic stability will be impossible.
- Augments are used to decrease the acetabular volume and facilitate press-fit fixation between the cup and the augment. Attempts are made to place the augment in direct contact with the revision cup.
- The discontinuity is bridged with the augment. Screws are placed cephalad and caudal.
- Fibrous tissue is removed from the discontinuity. The cancellous allograft is placed.
- With the augment in place, reverse reaming is performed to pack the augment with bone graft.
- Bone graft is cleared from the exposed host bone to maximize

contact of the host bone and the revision cup.

- The cup is placed and secured with multiple screws.
- Alternatively, an emerging strategy for the management of pelvic discontinuity is the use of a cup-cage construct. In this method, a porous-coated shell is placed using standard press-fit technique. Screw fixation is used to augment the press-fit stability. An anti-protrusio cage is cemented within the shell. Screw fixation to both the ischium and ilium is achieved. Finally, a polyethylene liner is cemented into the cage in the desired orientation.

Wound Closure

- The deep fascia and subcutaneous tissue are closed in the standard manner.

Postoperative Regimen

The surgical procedures described in this chapter are extremely varied. The postoperative protocol is individualized based on the severity of the defect, the method of fixation, and other medical comorbidities.

Avoiding Pitfalls and Complications

Noncemented acetabular revision often is complicated by bone loss, which compromises both implant fixation and stability. Nonetheless, a noncemented hemispheric implant can be used successfully in most acetabular revision procedures. By following the algorithm presented in this chapter, surgeons can systematically address complex patterns of bone loss and obtain stable intraoperative fixation even in patients with severe bone loss.

Bibliography

Amenabar T, Rahman WA, Hetaimish BM, Kuzyk PR, Safir OA, Gross AE: Promising mid-term results with a cup-cage construct for large acetabular defects and pelvic discontinuity. *Clin Orthop Relat Res* 2016;474(2):408-414.

Chareancholvanich K, Tanchuling A, Seki T, Gustilo RB: Cementless acetabular revision for aseptic failure of cemented hip arthroplasty. *Clin Orthop Relat Res* 1999;(361):140-149.

Del Gaizo DJ, Kancherla V, Sporer SM, Paprosky WG: Tantalum augments for Paprosky IIIA defects remain stable at midterm followup. *Clin Orthop Relat Res* 2012;470(2):395-401.

Gaffey JL, Callaghan JJ, Pedersen DR, Goetz DD, Sullivan PM, Johnston RC: Cementless acetabular fixation at fifteen years: A comparison with the same surgeon's results following acetabular fixation with cement. *J Bone Joint Surg Am* 2004;86(2):257-261.

Garcia-Cimbrelo E: Porous-coated cementless acetabular cups in revision surgery: A 6- to 11-year follow-up study. *J Arthroplasty* 1999;14(4):397-406.

Kim YH: Long-term results of the cementless porous-coated anatomic total hip prosthesis. *J Bone Joint Surg Br* 2005;87(5):623-627.

Lachiewicz PF, Poon ED: Revision of a total hip arthroplasty with a Harris-Galante porous-coated acetabular component inserted without cement: A follow-up note on the results at five to twelve years. *J Bone Joint Surg Am* 1998;80(7):980-984.

Leopold SS, Rosenberg AG, Bhatt RD, Sheinkop MB, Quigley LR, Galante JO: Cementless acetabular revision: Evaluation at an average of 10.5 years. *Clin Orthop Relat Res* 1999;(369):179-186.

Paprosky WG, Perona PG, Lawrence JM: Acetabular defect classification and surgical reconstruction in revision arthroplasty: A 6-year follow-up evaluation. *J Arthroplasty* 1994;9(1):33-44.

Park DK, Della Valle CJ, Quigley L, Moric M, Rosenberg AG, Galante JO: Revision of the acetabular component without cement: A concise follow-up, at twenty to twenty-four years, of a previous report. *J Bone Joint Surg Am* 2009;91(2):350-355.

Sporer SM, O'Rourke M, Chong P, Paprosky WG: The use of structural distal femoral allografts for acetabular reconstruction: Average ten-year follow-up. *J Bone Joint Surg Am* 2005;87(4):760-765.

Sporer SM, Paprosky WG, O'Rourke MR: Managing bone loss in acetabular revision. *Instr Course Lect* 2006;55:287-297.

Templeton JE, Callaghan JJ, Goetz DD, Sullivan PM, Johnston RC: Revision of a cemented acetabular component to a cementless acetabular component: A ten to fourteen-year follow-up study. *J Bone Joint Surg Am* 2001;83(11):1706-1711.

Weber KL, Callaghan JJ, Goetz DD, Johnston RC: Revision of a failed cemented total hip prosthesis with insertion of an acetabular component without cement and a femoral component with cement: A five to eight-year follow-up study. *J Bone Joint Surg Am* 1996;78(7):982-994.

Whaley AL, Berry DJ, Harmsen WS: Extra-large uncemented hemispherical acetabular components for revision total hip arthroplasty. *J Bone Joint Surg Am* 2001;83(9):1352-1357.

Video Reference

Chana F, Villanueva M, Rojo JM, Pérez M, Fernández-Mariño J, Vaquero J: Video. *Stoppa Approach for Removal of the Intrapelvic Cup for Acetabular Revision*. Madrid, Spain, 2013.

Chapter 49

Polyethylene Liner Exchange for Acetabular Osteolysis

Derek F. Amanatullah, MD, PhD
William J. Maloney, MD

Indications

The decision whether to retain or revise an acetabular component is made based on fixation status (**Table 1**). A well-fixed acetabular component (type I) that meets all six criteria noted in **Table 1** can be managed with lesion débridement and polyethylene liner exchange. Use of a three-dimensional ingrowth surface such as tantalum, fiber mesh, or cobalt-chromium beads results in improved retention of acetabular components. Higher loosening rates have been reported with the use of on-growth surfaces (including titanium plasma spray) in patients with acetabular osteolysis. A well-fixed acetabular component (type II) that does not meet all six criteria in **Table 1** should be removed before acetabular reconstruction. An unstable acetabular component (type III) necessitates acetabular reconstruction.

Fixation is assessed radiographically on AP pelvis and cross-table lateral hip views (**Table 2**). The presence of peripheral, noncontinuous, nonprogressive radiolucent lines is not indicative of loosening. Such lines are commonly seen in patients with noncemented acetabular components. The radiographic signs of a well-fixed noncemented acetabular component indicate component ingrowth and include absence of radiolucent lines, presence of a superolateral buttress, medial bone stress-shielding, radial trabeculae, and an inferomedial buttress. In a study of 119 total hip arthroplasties (THAs) that later underwent revision surgery, 97% of noncemented acetabular components with three to five radiographic signs of fixation were well fixed at the time of revision surgery, whereas 83% of the noncemented acetabular components with one or two radiographic signs of fixation demonstrated loosening at the time of revision surgery. Radiographic signs of loosening for noncemented acetabular components include radiolucent lines that initially appeared or progressed after 2 years, a continuous radiolucent line in all three DeLee and Charnley zones, a radiolucent line greater than 2 mm in any DeLee and Charnley zone, or component migration of more than 2 mm. Other than component loosening, none of these radiographic indicators alone is sufficient to determine loosening. Although radiographic examination is helpful in evaluating the stability of noncemented acetabular components, the true measure of stability or instability can only be determined intraoperatively.

Size of osteolytic lesions is often underestimated radiographically. CT offers the greatest accuracy in determining size and location of osteolytic lesions. In one study, fewer than 40% of osteolytic lesions were detected on AP pelvis radiograph alone, and obtaining an iliac oblique view as well improved detection only slightly. However, nearly 90% of lesions were detected on CT scan. Nearly one-half of noncemented acetabular components evaluated on CT scan exhibit osteolysis in asymptomatic patients, thus underscoring the insidious onset of osteolysis.

Contraindications

Severe medical comorbidities precluding surgery, infection, acetabular component loosening, component malposition affecting stability, an acetabular component with a poor track record, a cemented acetabular component, lack of an available highly cross-linked polyethylene liner, or lack of an available

Dr. Amanatullah or an immediate family member serves as a paid consultant to Sanofi; has stock or stock options held in BlueJay Mobile Health; and has received research or institutional support from Acumed. Dr. Maloney or an immediate family member has received royalties from Stryker and Zimmer Biomet; serves as a paid consultant to Flexion Therapeutics and ISTO Technologies; has stock or stock options held in Abbott, Flexion Therapeutics, Gilead Sciences, ISTO Technologies, Johnson & Johnson, Merck, Moximed, Pfizer, Pipeline Orthopaedics, Stemedica, and Total Joint Orthopedics; and serves as a board member, owner, officer, or committee member of the American Academy of Orthopaedic Surgeons, the American Joint Replacement Registry, the American Association of Hip and Knee Surgeons, Flexion Therapeutics, ISTO Technologies, Stemedica, and the Western Orthopaedic Association.

Table 1 Classification of and Treatment Indications for Well-Fixed Noncemented Acetabular Components

Factor	Type I	Type II	Type III
Radiograph	Stable Focal osteolysis	Stable Focal osteolysis	Unstable Component migration Circumferential lucency
Mandatory criteria for head-liner exchange	Well fixed Well positioned Modular noncemented component with a good track record Undamaged acetabular component or component capable of accepting a new liner Adequate liner available for acetabular component (ie, highly cross-linked polyethylene) Component not infected	One or more of the mandatory criteria for head-liner exchange is NOT present	—
Treatment	Component retention Head-liner exchange ± defect grafting	Liner cementation[a] Acetabular revision ± defect grafting	Acetabular revision ± defect grafting

[a] Liner cementation with or without defect grafting is a modification to the Maloney and Rubash algorithm that may be used in type I components that do not have an adequate liner available for the locking mechanism and type II components with damage to the acetabular component and/or locking mechanism that will support cement fixation. Liner cementation cannot compensate for malposition or an acetabular component with a poor track record and is subject to components that can reliably accept cement.

Adapted with permission from Amanatullah D, Maloney W: Techniques to manage osteolysis around well-fixed acetabular components, in Berry DJ, Maloney M, eds: *Master Techniques in Orthopaedic Surgery: The Hip*, ed 3. Philadelphia, PA, Wolters Kluwer, 2016, pp 411-419.

Table 2 Radiographic Signs of a Noncemented Acetabular Component

Loose

Appearance/progression of radiolucent lines >2 yr postoperatively

Continuous radiolucent line in all three DeLee and Charnley zones

Radiolucent line >2 mm in any DeLee and Charnley zone

Component migration >2 mm

Fixed

No radiolucent lines

Superolateral buttress

Inferomedial buttress

Medial stress shielding

Radial trabeculae

Adapted with permission from Amanatullah D, Maloney W: Techniques to manage osteolysis around well-fixed acetabular components, in Berry DJ, Maloney M, eds: *Master Techniques in Orthopaedic Surgery: The Hip*, ed 3. Philadelphia, PA, Wolters Kluwer, 2016, pp 411-419.

femoral head for a modular femoral component are each absolute contraindications to polyethylene liner exchange in the setting of acetabular osteolysis. Damage to the acetabular locking mechanism in a well-fixed acetabular component with a two-dimensional ongrowth surface is a relative contraindication to polyethylene liner exchange in the setting of acetabular osteolysis.

Results

In patients with pelvic osteolysis in whom the acetabular component is well fixed, well positioned, not damaged, and has a good clinical track record, polyethylene liner exchange is a reliable treatment option (**Table 3**). Patients with type I acetabular components retain radiographic stability at short-term (<10-year) follow-up after liner exchange. Studies have shown that regardless whether bone graft is used, approximately one-third of osteolytic defects resolve and two-thirds decrease in size. The rate of acetabular component loosening after polyethylene liner exchange is low. According to data from the Norwegian Arthroplasty Register on revision THAs performed over an 18-year span, polyethylene liner exchange is successful in well-selected patients. Patient selection is optimized with use of

Table 3 Results of Acetabular Component Retention or Revision to Manage Osteolysis

Authors (Year)	Number Treated	Intervention for Managing the Acetabular Component	Mean Patient Age in Years (Range)	Mean Follow-up in Months (Range)	Success Rate (%)[a]	Results	Comments
Schmalzried et al (1998)	21 patients (23 hips)	Retention and grafting (10 hips) Retention, no grafting (5 hips) Revision and grafting (8 hips)	54 (20-73)	40 (25-74)	100	No new osteolytic lesions All hips were well fixed radiographically and no additional reoperation was necessary	15 type I and 8 type II acetabular components Dislocation not reported
Maloney et al (2001)	68 patients	Retention and grafting (29) Retention, no grafting (11) Revision and grafting (28)	NA	42 (24-60)	100	All components were radiographically stable No new osteolytic lesions	40 type I and 28 type II acetabular components Dislocation not reported
Terefenko et al (2002)	10 patients	Retention and grafting (6) Retention, no grafting (4)	47 (30.6-65.7)	74.4 (58.8-98.4)	100	All components were radiographically stable Dislocation occurred in 1 patient who underwent retention without grafting	All type I acetabular components
Boucher et al (2003)	24 patients	Retention ± grafting	59 (NA)	56 (NA)	96	1 patient required re-revision 6 patients experienced dislocation	All type I acetabular components
Griffin et al (2004)	55 patients	Retention and grafting	53.6 (NA)	30 (NA)	95	5 patients experienced multiple dislocations, and 3 of those patients underwent re-revision	All type I acetabular components
Lie et al (2007)[b]	1,649 hips	Retention ± grafting (type I; 318 [liner exchange]) Revision and grafting (type II; 398 [fixed component]) Revision and grafting (type III; 933 [loose component])	60.2 (14-91)	N/A	Retention ± grafting (type I): 84 Revision and grafting (type II): 88 Revision and grafting (type III): 87	Risk of acetabular re-revision was lower after revision and grafting of well-fixed implants and exchange of loose acetabular components when compared with liner exchange alone	60 different types of noncemented acetabular components The risk of re-revision after liner exchange was almost double that for a fixed or loose acetabular component revision Reasons for re-revision included instability (28%), pain (12%), aseptic loosening (11%), infection (9%), and wear (8%) The risk of re-revision for pain was five times less after revision of a well-fixed acetabular component than after liner exchange alone
Restrepo et al (2009)	62 patients (67 hips)	Retention and grafting (36) Revision and grafting (31)	62.4 (31-88)	33.6 (24-60)	Retention and grafting: 92 Revision and grafting: 97	3 of the 36 hips had extensive superior and medial osteolysis 1 of the 31 hips underwent re-revision	36 type I and 31 type II acetabular components Dislocation not reported

NA = not available, N/A = not applicable.

[a] Implant survival constitutes success.

[b] Analysis of revision of primary noncemented acetabular implants results reported to the Norwegian Arthroplasty Register.

the criteria noted in **Table 1**. Of the 1,649 revision THAs performed between 1987 and 2005 and documented in the Norwegian Arthroplasty Register, liner exchange was performed in 318, the acetabular component was fixed in 398, and the acetabular component was loose in 933.

A dislocation rate of 25% has been reported after femoral head and acetabular liner exchange. The surgeon and patient must be vigilant about hip instability intraoperatively and postoperatively. The surgeon should perform a posterior capsular closure if a posterior approach is used, and the patient must adhere to strict precautions regarding posterior hip motion. In addition, the surgeon should give consideration to alternative surgical approaches with lower dislocation rates. Evaluation of preoperative and intraoperative radiographs for component position (impingement, malposition) is necessary to optimize outcomes.

Techniques

Setup/Exposure

- A direct anterior, anterolateral, direct lateral, or posterior approach is used, depending on the surgeon's preference or the approach used for the primary procedure.
- An extended trochanteric osteotomy, trochanteric slide, or standard trochanteric osteotomy may facilitate femoral and/or acetabular exposure in patients with complex pathology.
- All bony prominences are padded and peripheral nerves protected.
- Typically, intravenous prophylactic antibiotics are administered before incision; however, administration can be delayed if deep culture is planned.
- Surgical incisions from primary procedures are incorporated, if possible.

Instruments/Equipment/Implants Required

- A Cobb elevator is used.
- An extraction tool may be used.
- A 3.2-mm drill bit and 6.5-mm cancellous screw are used for liner removal in the single-screw technique.
- Reamers, osteotomes, and/or a high-speed burr may be required for removal of the acetabular polyethylene liner.

Procedure

- The authors of this chapter prefer the posterior approach, which is described here.
- A full-thickness pseudocapsular flap is elevated off the greater trochanter and protected for later use during closure.
- Inside-out débridement of visible granulomatous tissue is performed.
- The hip is dislocated.
- If a modular femoral head was used in the primary surgery, it is removed with an impactor, taking care to protect the femoral trunnion during and after removal of the femoral head.
- If visualization of the acetabulum is compromised by the femur or femoral component, the femur is mobilized to enhance the exposure. A Cobb elevator is used to create a subperiosteal space under the gluteus medius muscle and tuck the femoral trunnion into the anterosuperior corner (if using the posterior approach).
- The femur is mobilized with partial or complete releases. For example, the gluteus maximus tendon insertion may be released if the posterior approach is used. If additional femoral mobilization is required for adequate exposure of the acetabulum, it may be necessary to perform a trochanteric osteotomy or remove the femoral component.
- Circumferential acetabular exposure is attained, and osteophytes and overhanging bone are removed to facilitate visualization of the acetabular component rim.
- The polyethylene liner is removed, taking care not to damage the acetabular component. Use of an extraction tool is recommended, if available. If a single-screw technique is used for liner removal, the polyethylene liner is pierced using a 3.2-mm drill bit (**Figure 1, A**), after which a 6.5-mm cancellous screw is used to engage the liner and back it out of the acetabular component (**Figure 1, B**). If additional pressure is necessary to remove the liner, a second screw can be used as well. It is critical to ensure that the drill engages the metal component, not a screw hole. If the screw technique fails, the polyethylene liner is removed in fragments using reamers, osteotomes, and/or a high-speed burr.
- Damage to the acetabular component during polyethylene liner removal must be avoided because damage to the locking mechanism may necessitate cementation or acetabular component removal and revision.
- All screws are removed from the acetabular component.
- Stability of the acetabular component is assessed intraoperatively with a clamp, heavy needle driver, bone tamp, Cobb elevator, or acetabular component inserter.
- Gross visualization of bone ingrowth is reassuring.
- If there is any motion at the implant-bone interface, the component is removed, lytic lesions débrided and grafted, and a revision component placed.
- The granulomatous tissue from behind the acetabular cup may be removed using the periphery of the acetabular component, screw holes, or a central hole in the acetabular

component (**Figure 2**). A cortical window or trapdoor may be made in the superior or posterior acetabulum if additional exposure to the osteolytic lesion is necessary for adequate débridement. However, if a window or trapdoor is created, the surgeon must take care to prevent acetabular component destabilization.

- Bone ingrowth that is providing acetabular stability must not be disrupted.
- After débridement, the defects are filled with allograft bone, demineralized bone matrix, or bone graft substitute. Typically, defects in the anterior column and pubis are not grafted due to limited access.
- Screws may be reinserted into the acetabular component.
- A trial component is placed, and stability is assessed.
- The decision to impact or cement the new liner in place is based on intraoperative hip stability, liner availability, femoral head availability, acetabular component type, and damage to the locking mechanism or acetabular component.
- If the surgeon elects to use cement, first the inner surface of the acetabular component and the outer surface of the polyethylene liner must be adequately texturized. In addition, to facilitate cementation, the outer diameter of the polyethylene liner should be 2 mm smaller than the inner diameter of the acetabular component. A proud liner is at risk for impingement; thus, it is important to fully seat the cemented liner within the acetabular component.
- The femoral head is impacted into position on axis with the femoral neck for modular stems.
- The hip is reduced.

Wound Closure

- Wound closure is performed in a routine fashion.

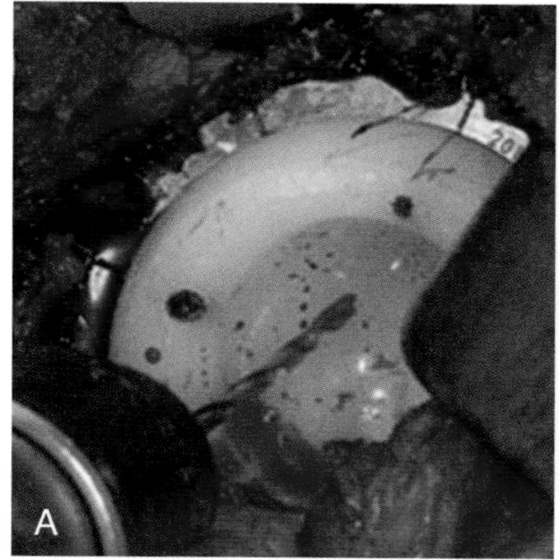

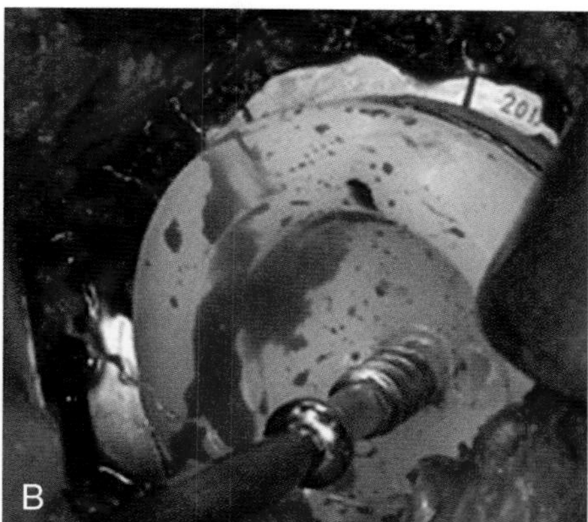

Figure 1 Intraoperative photographs show steps in the single-screw technique for removing an acetabular polyethylene liner. **A,** A 3.2-mm drill bit is used to pierce the polyethylene. **B,** A 6.5-mm cancellous screw is used to engage the polyethylene. After the screw strikes the metal shell of the acetabular cup, the screw is used to back out the polyethylene liner.

- If the posterior approach was used, the pseudocapsular flap elevated at the outset of the procedure is repaired back to the greater trochanter.

Postoperative Regimen

Patients with a well-fixed, retained acetabular component are allowed to bear weight as tolerated postoperatively. The patient's weight-bearing status should be reassessed in the setting of revision of either the femoral or the acetabular component. There is sparse evidence for the use of an abductor brace, abductor pillow, or knee immobilizer while the patient is in bed. Rigorous posterior hip precautions should be observed for at least 3 months postoperatively if a posterior approach was used.

Avoiding Pitfalls and Complications

Preoperative planning is essential, including radiographic evaluation of the position and fixation of the acetabular and femoral components. Osseointegration of the acetabular component, inspection of the supporting bone, and an intact locking mechanism with a good track record after head-liner exchange are prerequisites for survival after head-liner exchange. Several types of acetabular components perform poorly after polyethylene liner exchange. Ongrowth fixation surfaces such as titanium plasma spray or hydroxyapatite coating are predisposed to continued loosening and failure after revision surgery. The Acetabular Cup System (DePuy Synthes) and the Harris-Galante (Zimmer Biomet) acetabular components have locking mechanisms that are predisposed to failure after polyethylene liner exchange. The authors of this chapter recommend revising these components or considering cementing a liner into acetabular components with poor locking mechanisms.

Intraoperatively, the surgeon must restore femoral offset and equalize leg lengths if appropriate. It may be necessary to revise the acetabular component if positioning is suboptimal. Because of the risk for impingement and reduced stability, lipped acetabular liners and skirted femoral heads should not be used, if possible. Even if the acetabular component has the appearance

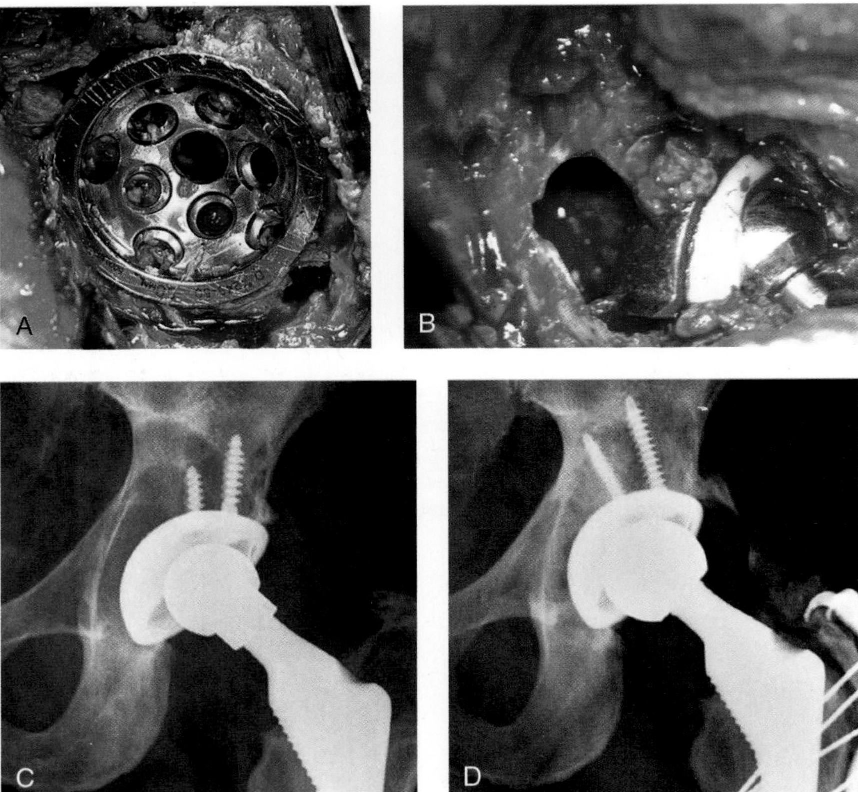

Figure 2 Images show steps in treating osteolytic lesions in patients with severe osteolysis and a retained well-fixed acetabular component. The lesions are accessed through screw holes (**A**) or a cortical window (**B**). After débridement and an assessment of acetabular component stability, osteolytic lesions are grafted through the same screw holes or cortical window shown in panels **A** and **B**, respectively, and a femoral head and acetabular liner exchange is performed. **C,** AP radiograph of a painful noncemented total hip arthroplasty (THA) demonstrates a large osteolytic lesion superior to a well-fixed acetabular component. **D,** AP radiograph of a THA demonstrates bony reconstitution of the defect 5 years after débridement, bone grafting, and liner exchange. (Panels A and B reproduced with permission from Amanatullah D, Maloney W: Techniques to manage osteolysis around well-fixed acetabular components, in Berry DJ, Maloney M, eds: *Master Techniques in Orthopaedic Surgery: The Hip*, ed 3. Philadelphia, PA, Wolters Kluwer, 2016, pp 411-419.)

of radiographic fixation, the surgeon should test the component intraoperatively after removal of the liner and screws. If the single-screw technique is used to remove the polyethylene liner, care should be taken to avoid stripping the polyethylene. Motion of the acetabular component indicates lack of osseointegration, and revision of the acetabular component is required in these patients. In addition, if the acetabular component is so severely damaged that it cannot support cementation or component malposition exists that affects stability, the component should be revised. When using cement to fix a texturized polyethylene liner into an unpolished acetabular component with screw holes, it is important to adequately texturize the two component surfaces to reduce the risk of failure at the cement-liner interface. Texturization prior to cementation provides similar stability to most locking mechanisms, but texturizing the polyethylene liner will decrease the polyethylene thickness available for articulation. For polished nontextured acetabular components without screw holes, the acetabular component should be revised or a metal cutting burr should be used to texturize the inner surface of the acetabular component to prevent failure at the cement-implant interface. Proper seating of the cement liner is essential to preclude cementing the liner proud and increasing the risk of impingement and loosening. Cementing a polyethylene liner with an outer diameter 1 to 2 mm less than the inner diameter of the acetabular component helps avoid improper seating and provides a reasonable cement mantle.

Recovery occurs quickly after polyethylene liner exchange, and patients must be cautioned to adhere to postoperative hip restrictions. In addition, it may be necessary to limit weight bearing postoperatively to avoid premature implant failure.

Bibliography

Amanatullah D, Maloney W: Techniques to manage osteolysis around well-fixed acetabular components, in Berry DJ, Maloney M, eds: *Master Techniques in Orthopaedic Surgery: The Hip,* ed 3. Philadelphia, PA, Wolters Kluwer, 2015, pp 411-419.

Amlie E, Høvik Ø, Reikerås O: Dislocation after total hip arthroplasty with 28 and 32-mm femoral head. *J Orthop Traumatol* 2010;11(2):111-115.

Boucher HR, Lynch C, Young AM, Engh CA Jr, Engh C Sr: Dislocation after polyethylene liner exchange in total hip arthroplasty. *J Arthroplasty* 2003;18(5):654-657.

DeLee JG, Charnley J: Radiological demarcation of cemented sockets in total hip replacement. *Clin Orthop Relat Res* 1976;121:20-32.

Griffin WL, Fehring TK, Mason JB, McCoy TH, Odum S, Terefenko CS: Early morbidity of modular exchange for polyethylene wear and osteolysis. *J Arthroplasty* 2004;19(7 suppl 2):61-66.

Hummel MT, Malkani AL, Yakkanti MR, Baker DL: Decreased dislocation after revision total hip arthroplasty using larger femoral head size and posterior capsular repair. *J Arthroplasty* 2009;24(6 suppl):73-76.

Leung S, Naudie D, Kitamura N, Walde T, Engh CA: Computed tomography in the assessment of periacetabular osteolysis. *J Bone Joint Surg Am* 2005;87(3):592-597.

Lie SA, Hallan G, Furnes O, Havelin LI, Engesaeter LB: Isolated acetabular liner exchange compared with complete acetabular component revision in revision of primary uncemented acetabular components: A study of 1649 revisions from the Norwegian Arthroplasty Register. *J Bone Joint Surg Br* 2007;89(5):591-594.

Lin HC, Chi WM, Ho YJ, Chen JH: Effects of design parameters of total hip components on the impingement angle and determination of the preferred liner skirt shape with an adequate oscillation angle. *Med Biol Eng Comput* 2013;51(4):397-404.

Maloney WJ, Galante JO, Anderson M, et al: Fixation, polyethylene wear, and pelvic osteolysis in primary total hip replacement. *Clin Orthop Relat Res* 1999;(369):157-164.

Maloney WJ, Herzwurm P, Paprosky W, Rubash HE, Engh CA: Treatment of pelvic osteolysis associated with a stable acetabular component inserted without cement as part of a total hip replacement. *J Bone Joint Surg Am* 1997;79(11):1628-1634.

Maloney WJ, Paprosky W, Engh CA, Rubash H: Surgical treatment of pelvic osteolysis. *Clin Orthop Relat Res* 2001;(393):78-84.

Mehin R, Yuan X, Haydon C, et al: Retroacetabular osteolysis: When to operate? *Clin Orthop Relat Res* 2004;(428):247-255.

Moore MS, McAuley JP, Young AM, Engh CA Sr: Radiographic signs of osseointegration in porous-coated acetabular components. *Clin Orthop Relat Res* 2006;(444):176-183.

Moskal JT, Mann JW III: A modified direct lateral approach for primary and revision total hip arthroplasty: A prospective analysis of 453 cases. *J Arthroplasty* 1996;11(3):255-266.

O'Brien JJ, Burnett RS, McCalden RW, MacDonald SJ, Bourne RB, Rorabeck CH: Isolated liner exchange in revision total hip arthroplasty: Clinical results using the direct lateral surgical approach. *J Arthroplasty* 2004;19(4):414-423.

Puri L, Wixson RL, Stern SH, Kohli J, Hendrix RW, Stulberg SD: Use of helical computed tomography for the assessment of acetabular osteolysis after total hip arthroplasty. *J Bone Joint Surg Am* 2002;84-A(4):609-614.

Restrepo C, Ghanem E, Houssock C, Austin M, Parvizi J, Hozack WJ: Isolated polyethylene exchange versus acetabular revision for polyethylene wear. *Clin Orthop Relat Res* 2009;467(1):194-198.

Rubash HE, Sinha RK, Paprosky W, Engh CA, Maloney WJ: A new classification system for the management of acetabular osteolysis after total hip arthroplasty. *Instr Course Lect* 1999;48:37-42.

Schmalzried TP, Fowble VA, Amstutz HC: The fate of pelvic osteolysis after reoperation: No recurrence with lesional treatment. *Clin Orthop Relat Res* 1998;(350):128-137.

Stulberg SD, Wixson RL, Adams AD, Hendrix RW, Bernfield JB: Monitoring pelvic osteolysis following total hip replacement surgery: An algorithm for surveillance. *J Bone Joint Surg Am* 2002;84(suppl 2):116-122.

Terefenko KM, Sychterz CJ, Orishimo K, Engh CA Sr: Polyethylene liner exchange for excessive wear and osteolysis. *J Arthroplasty* 2002;17(6):798-804.

Chapter 50
Acetabular Revision: Structural Grafts and Metal Augments

Tatu J. Mäkinen, MD, PhD, FEBOT
Kevin Koo, MD, FRCSC
Paul Kuzyk, MD, MASc, FRCSC
Oleg A. Safir, MD, MEd, FRCSC
David Backstein, MD, MEd, FRCSC
Allan E. Gross, MD, FRCSC, O.Ont

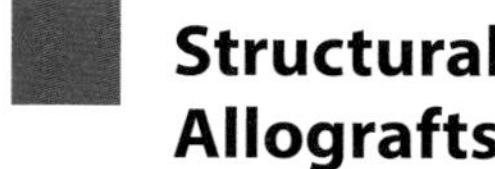

Structural Allografts

Indications

Structural allografts can be used to restore bone stock deficiency in revision total hip arthroplasty (THA). In patients with uncontained (segmental) Gross type III, IV, and V periacetabular bone defects, structural allografts can be used to address the bony defect and increase contact of bone with the acetabular implant (**Table 1**). Although allograft bone can be used in contained and uncontained defects, structural allografts should be reserved for the management of uncontained bone defects in which the host bone contact is less than 70%. In patients with host bone contact between 50% and 70%, a minor column graft is indicated (**Figure 1**). In patients with host bone contact less than 50%, a major column graft should be used with a cage construct to protect the bone graft (**Figure 2**). The goals of the use of structural allografts are to restore bone loss, maintain the anatomic hip center of the revision shell, and improve stability of the acetabular construct. Structural allografts are especially useful in younger patients (age 40 years or younger), in whom restoration of bone stock may help with future repeat revision of the acetabular implant.

Overall, the use of structural allografts in acetabular revision provides a reasonable strategy for addressing bone loss. However, the disadvantages of structural allografts are concerns of allograft resorption, infection, and loosening of the construct. Additionally, incorporating structural allografts into revision surgery is technically demanding and challenging and requires the availability of allograft bone. The ease of use of porous metal augmentation and its wide availability and variability have led to reduced use of structural allograft.

Contraindications

The use of structural allografts is contraindicated in patients with active infection of the hip. Preoperative laboratory studies and/or aspiration and intraoperative frozen sections should be used to rule out any possibility of infection. Structural bone grafts that do not meet the bone donor selection criteria established in the guidelines of the American Association of Tissue Banks should not be used. Metabolic bone disorder is a relative contraindication because it may play a role in abnormal bone resorption or result in difficulty of host-allograft union.

Dr. Kuzyk or an immediate family member serves as a paid consultant to Intellijoint Surgical and has received research or institutional support from Stryker and Zimmer Biomet. Dr. Safir or an immediate family member serves as a paid consultant to Intellijoint Surgical. Dr. Backstein or an immediate family member has received royalties from MicroPort Orthopedics; is a member of a speakers' bureau or has made paid presentations on behalf of MicroPort Orthopedics and Zimmer Biomet; serves as a paid consultant to Avenir Medical, MicroPort Orthopedics, and Zimmer Biomet; has stock or stock options held in Intellijoint Surgical; and has received research or institutional support from Zimmer Biomet. Dr. Gross or an immediate family member has received royalties from, is a member of a speakers' bureau or has made paid presentations on behalf of, and serves as a paid consultant to Zimmer Biomet; has stock or stock options held in Intellijoint Surgical; and serves as a board member, owner, officer, or committee member of the Canadian Orthopaedic Association, The Hip Society, and The Knee Society. Neither of the following authors nor any immediate family member has received anything of value from or has stock or stock options held in a commercial company or institution related directly or indirectly to the subject of this chapter: Dr. Mäkinen and Dr. Koo.

Table 1 Gross Classification of Periacetabular Bone Defects and Options for Management

Type	Defect	Management Options	
		Structural Allograft	**Metal Augment**
I	No substantial loss of bone stock	None	None
II	Contained loss of bone stock	None (use morcellized bone grafting)	None (use morcellized bone grafting), conventional augment for massive superior defect
III	Minor column defect: uncontained loss of bone stock involving <50% of the acetabulum	Minor column graft	Conventional augment (wedge or flying buttress configuration)
IV	Major column defect: uncontained loss of bone stock involving ≥50% of the acetabulum	Major column graft protected with a cage	Anterior, posterior, or straight column buttress augment; triflange cup
V	Pelvic discontinuity with uncontained loss of bone stock	Major column graft protected with a cage	Conventional or buttress augments combined with cup-cage reconstruction

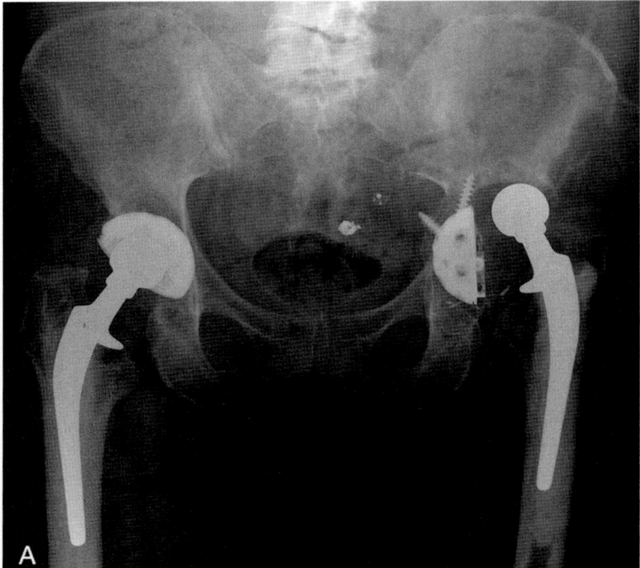

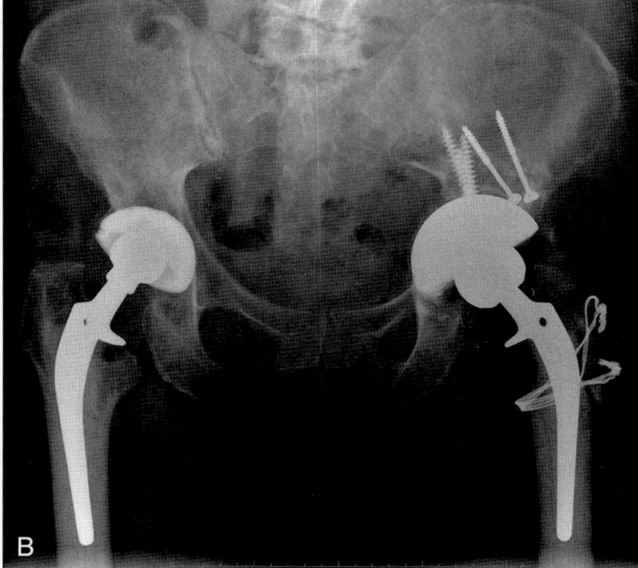

Figure 1 **A,** AP pelvic radiograph demonstrates a loose acetabular implant with associated minor column defect in the left hip. **B,** Postoperative AP pelvic radiograph demonstrates reconstruction with a trabecular metal revision shell and minor column structural allograft (shelf graft).

Alternative Treatments

Porous metal augments are an alternative option for the management of uncontained defects in acetabular revision surgery. The use of metal augments has increased in popularity because it is technically less demanding than the use of structural allografts in terms of preparation and implementation.

In patients with Gross type III defects, alternatives to using structural allografts and metal augments include placing the joint at a higher hip center or using an oblong cup. Neither of these solutions restores bone stock for future surgery. A high hip center results in shortening of the operated leg and may necessitate femoral lengthening. The incidence of loosening is higher with the high hip center technique than with other techniques. Oblong cups restore the hip center; however, results vary among institutions. In patients with type IV defects, an alternative to structural allografts and metal augments is the triflange cup, which is a custom device with inconsistent results.

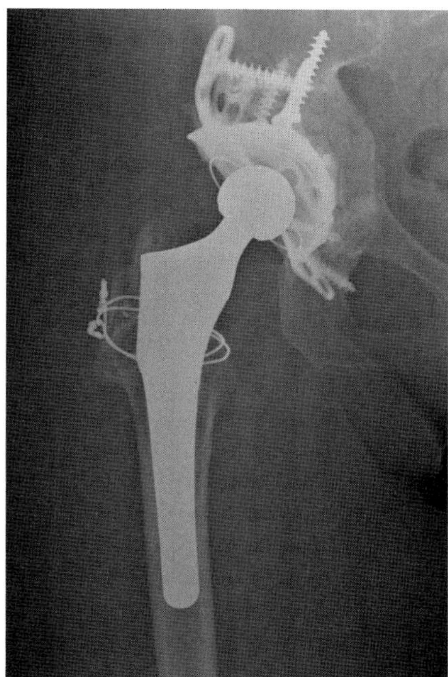

Figure 2 AP radiograph of a right hip demonstrates reconstruction with a cage and major column structural allograft.

Results

The use of structural allograft in addressing bony defects in revision arthroplasty allows restoration of the hip center and leg length, increased stability and bony contact of the acetabular implant, and restoration of bone stock. Early studies of structural allografts showed no difficulties with host-bone union. However, with repeat revision defined as the end point for allograft success, mixed short-term, midterm, and long-term results were obtained (**Table 2**). Three separate studies showed success rates of 55% at mean 7 years, 53% at mean 10 years, and 40% at mean 16.5 years postoperatively. However, two different studies demonstrated superior results, with success rates of approximately 86% at mean 5.1 years and mean 7.1 years postoperatively. An additional study demonstrated 94.1% allograft survivorship and 78.4% cup survivorship at 10 years. The authors of a study with mean 16-year follow-up reported a success rate of 82.4% with a mean time to repeat revision of 6.1 years.

In a study of patients who underwent repeat acetabular revision after a failed previous revision that had been performed using structural allograft, 31 of 50 hips (62%) had restoration of bone stock, and only 9 of 50 hips (18%) had deterioration of bone stock. Moreover, 17 of 50 hips (34%) did not require any allograft (morcellized or structural), augments, rings, or cages. This study showed that the use of structural allograft bone for the management of massive uncontained defects in acetabular revision can effectively restore host bone stock and can facilitate subsequent repeat revision surgery if required.

Techniques

SETUP/EXPOSURE

- Reconstruction of the acetabulum in a THA revision requires good exposure and access to both the anterior and posterior columns.
- Any conventional approach to the hip can be used, provided that the acetabulum can be fully exposed and the severity of the bone loss can be defined and appreciated.
- The authors of this chapter commonly use a trochanteric osteotomy approach.
- For structural defects, a modified trochanteric slide osteotomy is preferred because it decreases the incidence of trochanteric escape and nonunion compared with the classic transverse osteotomy. The trochanteric slide osteotomy maintains a continuous sling of abductor and vastus muscles attached to the greater trochanter and allows an extensile exposure to the acetabulum.
- The authors of this chapter perform the modified trochanteric slide osteotomy by leaving approximately 1 cm of the posterior part of the greater trochanter intact with the femur. This method preserves the external rotators and posterior capsule, reducing the risk of posterior dislocation.

PROCEDURE

- After the acetabular implant is removed, all fibrous tissue is removed from the acetabulum and around the acetabular rim to allow thorough evaluation of the acetabular cavity.
- After the joint is fully débrided, the bony defect is inspected and defined.
- The ilium, the dome, and the anterior and posterior columns are exposed and examined to determine the extent of bone loss and possible pelvic discontinuity.
- Progressive reaming is performed to reach bleeding host bone and to help engage the acetabular rim.
- The location of the ischium and the transverse acetabular ligament, if available, can be used as a guide to determine the location and version of the native acetabulum.
- Reaming is completed with the largest possible reamer.
- A trial cup is placed at the correct anatomic level to define the extent of the bony defect.
- In patients with a contained cavitary defect, bone stock can be restored by using impacted morcellized cancellous allograft bone.
- In patients with segmental bone loss in whom the trial cup cannot be stabilized at the approximately correct anatomic level, structural allograft is indicated.
- To appropriately gauge the size of the structural bone graft required, it is necessary to determine the percentage of the host bone support for the cup.
- If host bone support is between 50% and 70%, a minor column graft is indicated.
- If host bone support is less than 50%, a major column graft is used.
- If the defect is less than 30% of the acetabulum, structural graft usually is not necessary.
- In patients with chronic pelvic

Table 2 Results of the Use of Structural Allografts in the Management of Acetabular Bone Defects

Authors (Year)	No. of Patients (Hips)	Procedure	Mean Patient Age in Years (Range)	Mean Follow-up in Years (Range)	Success Rate (%)[a]	Results
Kwong et al (1993)	28 (30)	Revision with femoral head allografts, minor and major column grafts	51 (NR)	10 (8-13.3)	53	All grafts united 47% of hips had failure of fixation of acetabular implant 33% of hips required revision
Hooten et al (1994)	27 (27)	Revision with structural femoral head allograft (16 hips) or distal femoral allograft (11 hips)	NR	3.8 (NR)	55.6	44% of hips had radiographic loosening at mean 3.8-yr follow-up 18.5% of hips required repeat revision Early failures (<2 yr postoperatively) were the result of technical errors Later failures resulted in gradual migration of the cup into the graft
Paprosky et al (1994)	69 (69)	Revision with structural femoral head; acetabular, proximal tibia, or distal femoral allograft	NR	5.1 (2-10)	85.5	All grafts united 29% of grafts showed partial resorption No failures in 36 hips with type IIIA defects in which distal femoral or proximal tibia allografts were used 3 of 9 hips with type IIIA defects managed with femoral head allograft loosened 17 of 24 hips with type IIIB defects did not fail
Garbuz et al (1996)	32 (33)	Revision with major column grafts and roof-reinforcement ring	60 (32-85)	7 (5-11)	55	All grafts united 21% of hips required revision despite intact allograft 24% of hips required revision with failed allograft
Morsi et al (1996)	28 (29)	Revision with structural minor column allografts	53.2 (32-73)	7.1 (5-12)	86	Grafts united in 96.6% of hips 89.7% of hips had no or minimal graft resorption 14% of hips required revision for deep infection (1 hip) or loosening (3 hips)
Shinar and Harris (1997)	62 (70)	Revision with femoral head autograft and allograft, minor and major column grafts	45.2 (16-69)	16.5 (14.1-21.4)	40	All grafts united 9 of 15 hips with allograft required revision Loosening occurred in 1 of 15 hips (7%) with allograft
Woodgate et al (2000)	47 (51)	Revision with minor column grafts	52 (22-75)	9.9 (5.7-16.3)	Cup survival: 78.4 Allograft survival: 94.1	Grafts united in 98% of hips 22% of hips required revision for loosening 2% of hips had infection Complications included aseptic cup failure (10), late infection (1), recurrent dislocation (3), acute infection (1), posttraumatic loosening (1), intraoperative allograft fracture (1), greater trochanter nonunion (1), and perioperative death (1)
Dewal et al (2003)	13 hips	Revision with femoral head or distal femoral allograft in segmental defects (4 hips) and combined segmental and cavitary defects (9 hips)	52.2 (NR)	6.8 (2.2-10.3)	92.3	15% of hips had radiographic loosening, but none required revision 1 hip was symptomatic, but the patient refused surgical treatment
Lee et al (2010)	74 (85)	Revision with minor column allograft	54 (28-53)	16 (5.3-25)	82.4	15- and 20-yr survivorship rates were 61% and 55% for cups and 78% for grafts with repeat revision as the end point 31.8% of hips required repeat revision for all causes at mean 6.9-yr follow-up 17.6% of hips failed with mean time to repeat revision of 6.1 yr

NR = not reported.

[a] Success is defined as procedures not requiring repeat revision and is based on number of hips.

discontinuity, a cage or cup-cage reconstruction should be considered.
- Allograft bone should conform to the criteria and guidelines established by the American Association of Tissue Banks. The structural allograft can be prepared from acetabular allografts for major column defects and from male femoral heads or distal femurs for minor column defects.
- The acetabular allograft bone graft is prepared by thawing in warm 50% povidone-iodine and saline solution.
- The bone is rinsed with a mixture of one part 3% hydrogen peroxide, two parts normal saline solution, and bacitracin (30,000 units per 1,000 mL of normal saline) before implantation.
- All cartilage is removed from the allograft. The subchondral bone is left intact.
- The allograft bone is appropriately shaped to match the host defect.
- After the structural allograft is shaped and the host joint is prepared, the graft is fixed into the defect with placement of two superomedially directed 4.5- or 6.5-mm cancellous screws with washers into the host bone.
- In patients with minor column bone defects, additional gentle reaming of the inferior aspect of the bone graft can help shape the acetabulum so that the graft comes into close contact with the cup. The acetabular implant can be inserted with or without cement. Additional morcellized graft can be placed superiorly around the host-allograft junction to enhance union and remodeling (**Figure 3**).
- In patients with major column defects, the graft is protected by a cage that spans from the ilium to the ischium. Fixation of the cage can be achieved by slotting the inferior flange into the ischium and placing a minimum of three cancellous screws into the ilium. The cage should fit into the allograft and the host joint. A polyethylene cup 2 to 3 mm smaller than the inner diameter of the cage should be used. A trial cup should be used for trial reduction to evaluate the cup position, leg length, and hip stability. After the desired cup version and inclination is chosen, the cup is cemented directly into the cage (**Figure 4**).
- The trochanteric slide osteotomy is fixed with cerclage wires. The osteotomy is advanced to retension the abductor musculature if necessary.

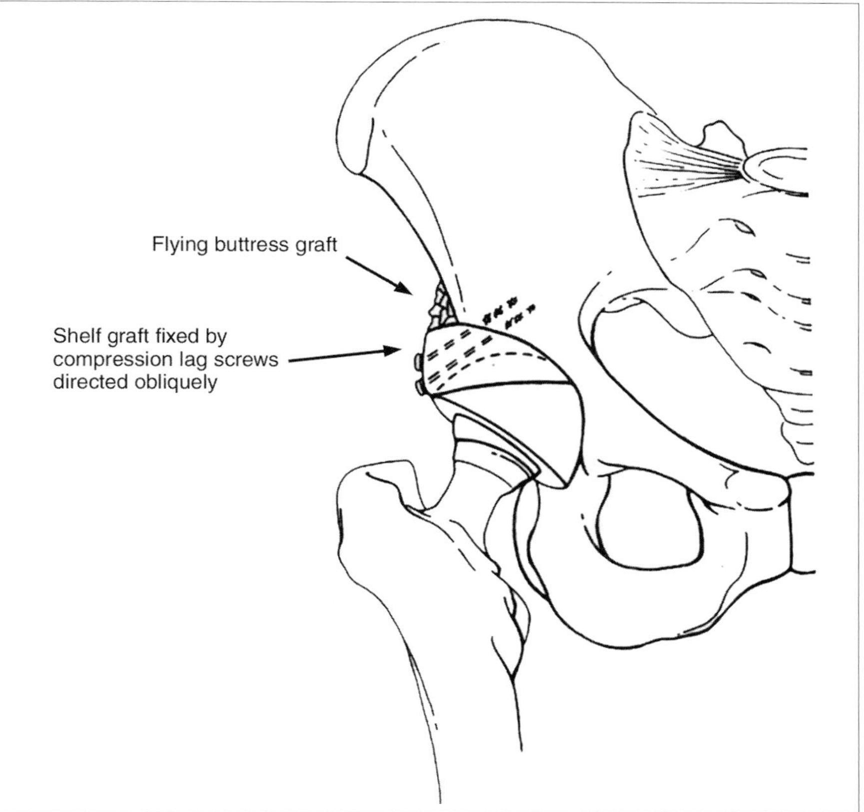

Figure 3 Illustration shows a minor column defect of the acetabulum reconstructed with a shelf graft and a flying buttress graft packed between the ilium and the shelf graft. (Reproduced with permission from Abolghasemian M, Drexler M, Abdelbary H, et al: Revision of the acetabular component in dysplastic hips previously reconstructed with a shelf autograft: Study of the outcome with special assessment of bone-stock changes. *Bone Joint J* 2013;95-B:777-781.)

WOUND CLOSURE
- Meticulous closure is performed with standard absorbable sutures.
- Attempts should be made to close all dead spaces.
- Drains are not routinely used.

Postoperative Regimen

Structural allograft reconstructions are protected with toe-touch weight bearing for the first 6 weeks postoperatively and partial weight bearing for the following 6 weeks. Gradual return to full weight bearing can occur at 3 to 4 months postoperatively. Hip precautions are used for 6 weeks postoperatively. The need for hip precautions depends on the exposure that was used and must also

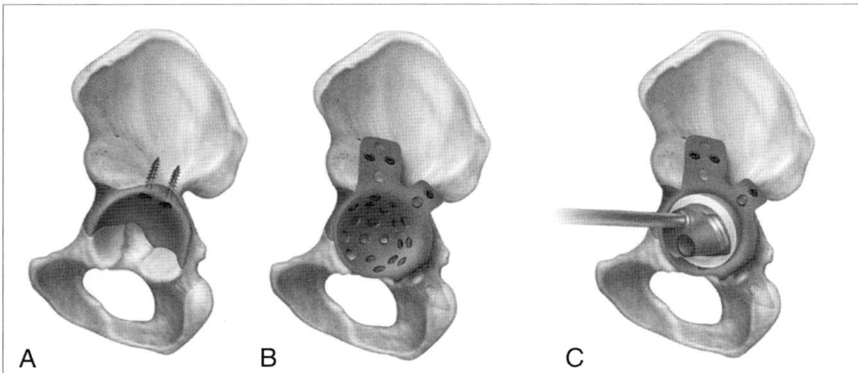

Figure 4 Illustrations depict reconstruction of a major column defect of the acetabulum with a major column graft and a cage. **A,** The major column graft is fixed with two screws. **B,** A cage is implanted on top of the graft to protect it. **C,** The liner is cemented at the desired inclination and anteversion. (Courtesy of Zimmer Biomet, Warsaw, IN.)

take into account the reconstruction performed on the femoral side, if any. Deep vein thrombosis (DVT) prophylaxis should be used in accordance with the institution's DVT prevention strategy. Pharmacologic and/or mechanical prophylaxis against DVT is initiated according to the current guidelines of the American College of Chest Physicians and the American Academy of Orthopaedic Surgeons. Intravenous antibiotics are administered for 5 days postoperatively.

Avoiding Pitfalls and Complications

Every effort should be made to ensure adequate exposure of the acetabulum, the dome, and the ilium so that bone defects can be carefully inspected and identified. A ball-spiked pusher can be used to stress the posterior column to help identify undiagnosed pelvic discontinuity. After the acetabulum is fully reamed, the amount of host bone contact should be accurately identified so that an appropriate allograft (minor or major) can be chosen. A major column graft should be protected with a cage construct to prevent early failures.

The use of structural allograft remains integral to the management of bone loss in younger patients (younger than 40 years) because it helps restore bone stock for future repeat revision. With the wide availability of metal augments, the use of structural allograft in older patients (older than 40 years) has become less popular.

Metal Augments

Indications

The primary indication for the use of porous metal augments during acetabular revision surgery is a loose acetabular implant with an associated bone defect that prevents stable and reliable fixation of a hemispheric acetabular implant at the correct anatomic level. Metal augments can be used to address contained or uncontained bone defects.

The type and degree of acetabular bone deficiency is classified intraoperatively (**Table 1**). A type I defect does not require augmentation and can be managed with hemispheric noncemented implants. Although most type II defects (contained) can be managed with morcellized bone grafting and hemispheric noncemented implants, in patients with a massive contained superior defect, a metal augment can be used as an adjunct to ensure the initial stability of the noncemented implant at the correct hip center. Type III (minor column) and IV (major column) defects usually require acetabular augments to enhance the stability of the noncemented hemispheric implant at the correct anatomic level. In patients with type V defects (pelvic discontinuity), acetabular augments can be used to address the associated uncontained defects, but a cup-cage construct or rigid cage also is needed to prevent medial migration.

Contraindications

The use of metal augments is contraindicated in the presence of active infection. In patients with pelvic discontinuity, the hemispheric shell with metal augments is unlikely to provide a biomechanically valid construct to prevent medial migration. Therefore, a cup-cage construct or a rigid cage with metal augments should be used in patients with pelvic discontinuity.

Alternative Treatments

Structural allografts are preferred in patients younger than 40 years, and reasonable long-term results have been reported. High hip center, oblong cup, and triflange cup have been used, but the results of each of these treatments are inconsistent.

Results

Trabecular metal augments used in conjunction with trabecular metal shells have shown excellent short-term and midterm results. With loosening as an end point, survival of the acetabular shell of 91% to 100% has been reported at up to 9-year follow-up (**Table 3**). The survival of the augments has been even higher because in some patients the augment obtains solid bony integration despite loosening of the shell.

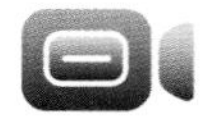

Video 50.1 Acetabular Revision: Structural Grafts and Metal Augments. Allan E. Gross, MD, FRCSC (5 min)

Techniques

SETUP/EXPOSURE

- Several approaches can be used in acetabular revision surgery.
- If metal augmentation of the acetabulum or concomitant stem revision is considered, extensile revision approaches such as a modified trochanteric slide osteotomy or modified extended trochanteric osteotomy (ETO) should be considered.
- Modified trochanteric slide osteotomy was developed to reduce the high dislocation rate associated with trochanteric slide osteotomy. The modified technique maintains the integrity of the external rotators and the posterior capsule by starting anterior to the external rotators, thereby leaving a sleeve of the external rotators and posterior capsule attached to the femur. The trochanteric fragment is moved anteriorly with the gluteus medius and vastus lateralis attached cranially and caudally, respectively.
- The ETO is a particularly useful approach if the femoral stem needs to be addressed in the same procedure. The external rotators and posterior capsule are left intact, attached to the femur. The advantage of the ETO over the modified trochanteric slide osteotomy is the higher union rate resulting from the larger surface area, which allows better bony apposition.

INSTRUMENTS/EQUIPMENT/ IMPLANTS REQUIRED

- Previous surgical reports and implant stickers must be obtained preoperatively to provide data about the stem and the taper.
- Use of the acetabular implant removal system will ease the removal of well-fixed acetabular shells.
- A broken-screw removal set should be available if the previous acetabular implant was secured with screws.
- A complete set of trial implants for trabecular metal revision shells and augments is needed (**Figure 5**).
- A high-speed burr is helpful if the size or shape of the augments or defect needs to be adjusted so that they match.

PROCEDURE

- The acetabulum is exposed through the selected approach.
- The previous implants are removed, with care taken to avoid further compromise of the already defective bone stock.
- After the implants are removed, the fibrous tissue that often forms in patients with a loose implant is removed.
- The medial floor of the acetabulum is exposed.
- Gentle reaming to prepare the bony bed is performed at the correct anatomic level. The authors of this chapter aim to engage the anterior and posterior columns with sequential hemispheric reamers.
- The type and degree of acetabular bone deficiency is classified (**Table 1**). The authors of this chapter use the Gross classification, which is based on the percentage of acetabular bone that is lost.
- After the acetabular bone defect is classified, a hemispheric trial shell is placed at the anatomic hip center.
- The location, type, and size of the augment depend on the bone defect pattern and are chosen through trials of the augment in combination with the acetabular trial implant against the host bone. The aim is to provide maximal support for the final noncemented implant as well as contact of the augment with host bone. The augments can be placed in any position or orientation. Some common scenarios follow.
- In patients with a minor or major column defect (type III or IV) with an intact acetabular rim within 30 mm of the outer perimeter of the trial shell, the defect usually can be managed with the use of one or two conventional augments placed in a wedge-shaped configuration to fill the acetabular defect (**Figure 6**). The diameter of the augment is dictated by the internal diameter of the segmental acetabular defect and typically is equal to or smaller than the diameter of the trial shell.
- In patients with a severe contained medial defect with an intact but thin peripheral acetabular rim, a noncemented revision shell alone would not be sufficient. To provide adequate medial support for the revision shell, a conventional augment is inserted directly into the medial defect (**Figure 7**).
- In patients with a minor column defect with no acetabular rim within 30 mm of the outer diameter of the trial shell but a supportive acetabular bone bed, conventional augments are assembled into a flying buttress configuration. The augments are placed medially against the ilium just above the trial shell and fixed with screws (**Figure 8**). In this type of defect, most forces are transmitted via the supportive acetabular bone bed, and only moderate shear forces are projected onto the augment. To attain the widest possible contact with the host bone, a thicker augment typically is used.
- In patients with a major column defect with no acetabular rim within 30 mm of the outer diameter of the trial shell, the lack of coverage of the acetabular implant is such that conventional augments will be unlikely to resist the shear forces because of limited host bone contact. Therefore, the reconstruction should use buttress augments to maximize the stability

Table 3 Results of Trabecular Metal Augments Used in Conjunction With Trabecular Metal Shells for Acetabular Reconstruction

Authors (Year)	No. of Patients (Hips)	Procedure	Mean Patient Age in Years (Range)	Mean Follow-up in Months (Range)	Success Rate (%)[a]	Results
Nehme et al (2004)	16	Revision with trabecular metal revision shell and trabecular metal augments	63.6 (34-86)	31.9 (24-39)	For loosening: 94 For any acetabular revision: 94 For augment loosening: 100	1 patient underwent revision with cup-cage construct for management of pelvic discontinuity 1 patient had dislocation, managed with closed reduction 1 patient had partial sciatic nerve palsy
Sporer and Paprosky (2006)	28	Revision with trabecular metal revision shell (10) or trabecular metal modular shell and trabecular metal augments (18)	64 (36-89)	37 (12-48)	For loosening: 100 For any revision: 96 For augment loosening: 100	1 patient underwent revision with constrained liner for management of recurrent dislocation
Lingaraj et al (2009)	23 (24)	Revision with trabecular metal revision shell Trabecular metal augments used in 21 hips	67 (38-81)	41 (24-62)	For loosening: 96 For any revision: 91 For augment loosening: NR	1 patient had radiologic loosening and did not undergo revision 2 patients underwent revision with constrained liner or tripolar implant for management of recurrent dislocation 3 patients had sciatic nerve injury 1 patient had superficial infection
Siegmeth et al (2009)	34	Revision with trabecular metal revision shell and trabecular metal augments	64 (37-97)	34 (24-55)	For loosening: 94 For any revision: 91 For augment loosening: 94	1 patient underwent revision with new cup-augment construct for management of acetabular loosening 1 patient was awaiting revision for management of failed augment 1 patient underwent revision with constrained liner for management of recurrent dislocation 1 patient had dislocation managed with closed reduction

NR = not reported.

[a] Success is defined as procedures not requiring repeat revision for the reason specified.

[b] Abolghasemian M, Tangsataporn S, Sternheim A, Backstein D, Safir O, Gross AE: Combined trabecular metal acetabular shell and augment for acetabular revision with substantial bone loss: A mid-term review. *Bone Joint J* 2013;95-B(2):166-172.

Table 3 Results of Trabecular Metal Augments Used in Conjunction With Trabecular Metal Shells for Acetabular Reconstruction (*continued*)

Authors (Year)	No. of Patients (Hips)	Procedure	Mean Patient Age in Years (Range)	Mean Follow-up in Months (Range)	Success Rate (%)[a]	Results
Van Kleunen et al (2009)	90 (97)	Revision with trabecular metal revision shell (75 hips) or trabecular metal modular shell (22 hips) Trabecular metal augments used in 23 hips	59 (27-87)	45 (24-79)	For loosening: 100 For any revision: 83 For augment loosening: NR	10 patients underwent revision with resection arthroplasty or irrigation and débridement and/or chronic antibiotic suppression for management of infection 2 patients underwent revision with liner exchange for management of recurrent dislocation 5 patients had dislocation managed with closed reduction 4 patients had postoperative hematoma managed with incision and drainage 2 patients had liner dislodgment managed with liner exchange 1 patient had liner fracture and recurrent dislocation managed with a constrained liner
Del Gaizo et al (2012)	36 (37)	Revision with trabecular metal revision shell (15 hips) or trabecular metal modular shell (22 hips) and trabecular metal augments	60 (36-80)	60 (26-106)	For loosening: 97 For any revision: 81 For augment loosening: 97	1 patient was awaiting revision for management of acetabular loosening 4 patients underwent revision with constrained liner for management of recurrent dislocation 3 patients had acute infection managed with irrigation and débridement
Abolghasemian et al (2013)[b]	34	Revision with trabecular metal revision shell and trabecular metal augments	69.3 (46-86)	64.5 (27-107)	For loosening: 91 For any revision: 85 For augment loosening: 97	3 patients underwent revision for management of loosening 2 patients underwent revision for management of infection
Whitehouse et al (2015)	56	Primary (3 patients) or revision (53 patients) with trabecular metal revision shell and trabecular metal augments	67 (SD 14.8)	Median, 110 (88-128)	For loosening: 93 For any revision: 89 For augment loosening: 92	3 patients underwent revision for management of acetabular loosening 1 patient underwent revision for management of infection 1 patient had radiologic loosening and did not undergo revision 2 patients underwent revision for management of recurrent dislocation

NR = not reported.

[a] Success is defined as procedures not requiring repeat revision for the reason specified.

[b] Abolghasemian M, Tangsataporn S, Sternheim A, Backstein D, Safir O, Gross AE: Combined trabecular metal acetabular shell and augment for acetabular revision with substantial bone loss: A mid-term review. *Bone Joint J* 2013;95-B(2):166-172.

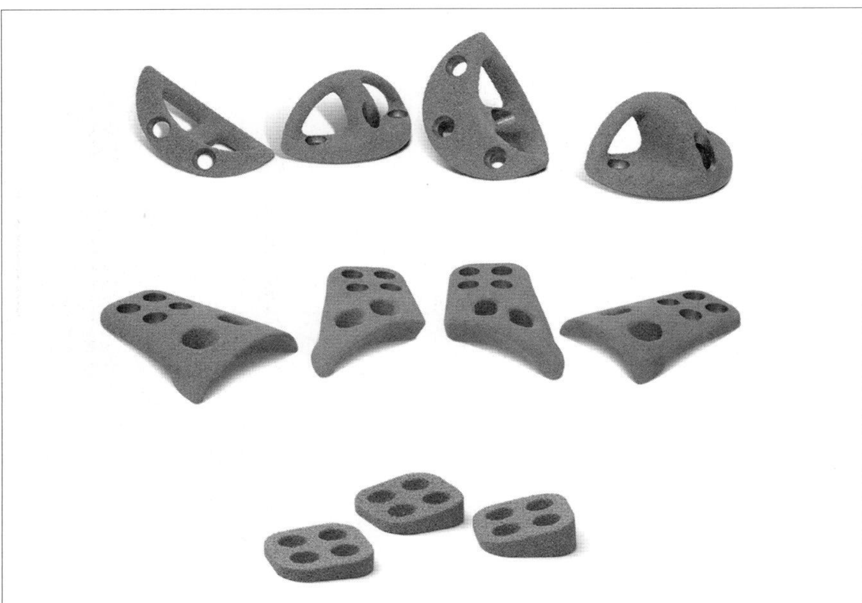

Figure 5 Photograph shows conventional (top row), buttress (middle row), and shim (bottom row) trabecular metal augments.

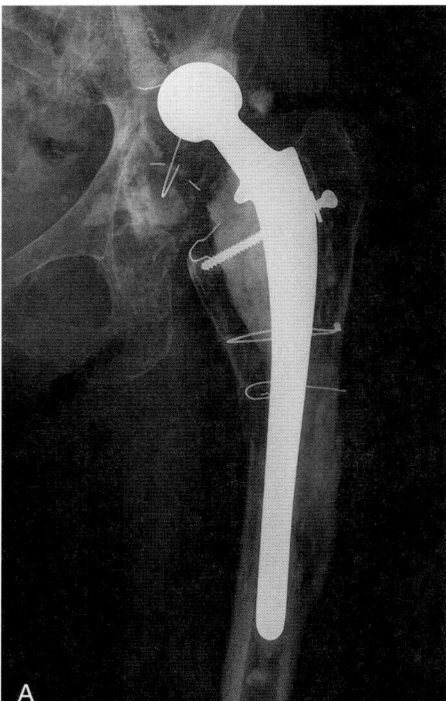

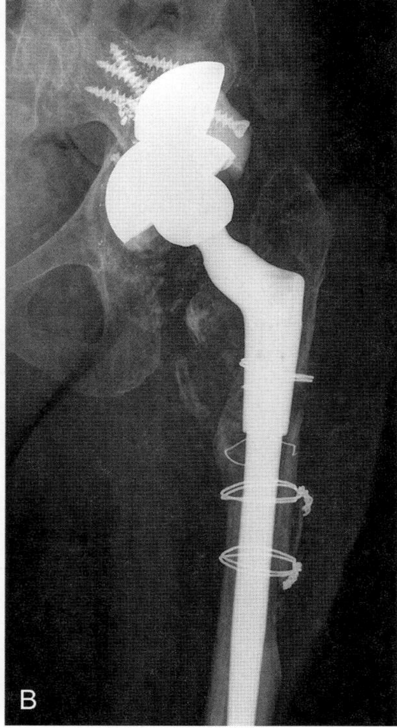

Figure 6 **A,** AP radiograph of a left hip demonstrates a loose polyethylene acetabular implant and associated superior bone defect. **B,** AP hip radiograph obtained after reconstruction with a trabecular metal revision shell and conventional augment in a wedge-shaped configuration. The femoral implant was revised because of its monoblock design.

of the construct by increasing the surface contact between the host bone and the augment (**Figure 9**). Superior defects are addressed with the use of a straight buttress augment (figure-of-7 shape). Defects located anteriorly or posteriorly are addressed with anterior or posterior column buttress augments, respectively. The ilium is exposed cranially to allow seating of the augment. Occasionally, it is necessary to apply shim augments between the buttress augment and the ilium to maximize bone contact.

- The augment that was selected on the basis of the bone defect and acetabular trial is held against the prepared host bone and fixed with two or more 6.5-mm bone screws.
- The trial acetabular shell is held in place during fixation of the augment.
- The augment and any residual contained bone defect are packed with morcellized cancellous allograft. Autograft reamings can also be used when available.
- The final hemispheric shell is impacted against the bleeding acetabular host bone and the augment.
- The authors of this chapter use polymethyl methacrylate cement to cover the interface between the cup and the augments. This technique increases the overall stability of the construct and minimizes the amount of metal debris released if bony integration is delayed.
- In patients with highly deficient bone stock, suboptimal orientation of the final shell (high inclination angle, retroversion) may be necessary to maximize host bone contact and initial fixation. Suboptimal orientation of the final shell is also frequently necessary in cup-cage reconstructions to allow seating of the ischial flange of the cage. However, the orientation of the cemented liner can be adjusted

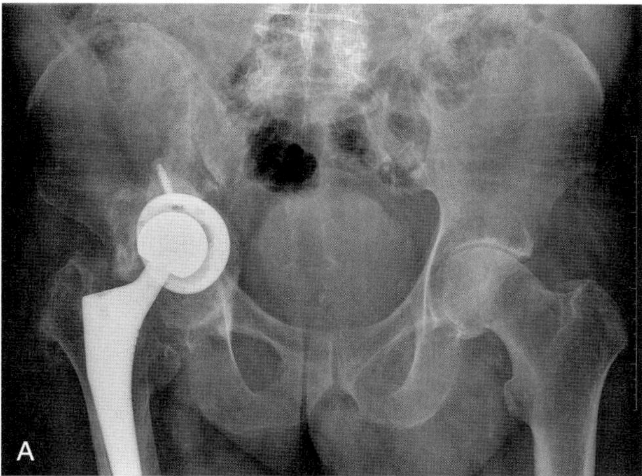

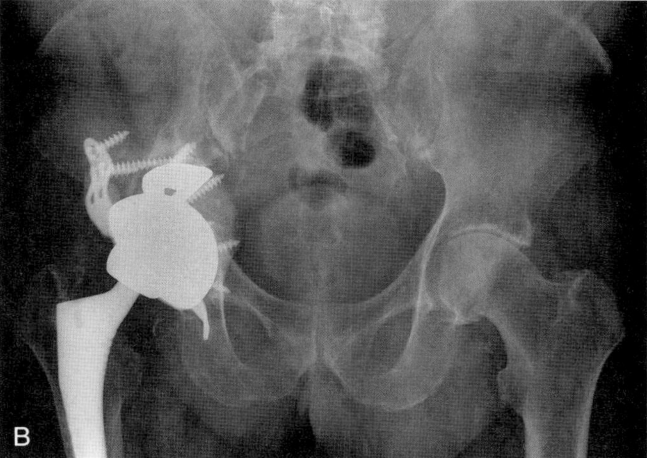

Figure 7 **A,** AP pelvic radiograph demonstrates a migrated acetabular implant. **B,** Postoperative AP pelvic radiograph demonstrates reconstruction with a cup-cage construct and the use of a conventional augment to fill the medial defect.

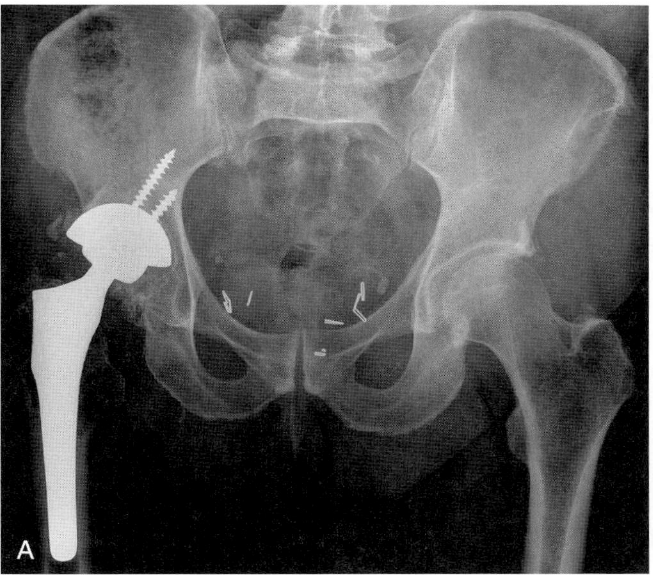

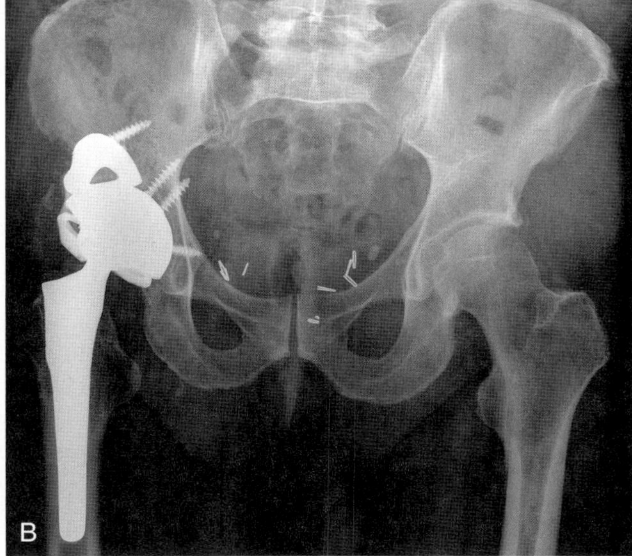

Figure 8 **A,** AP pelvic radiograph demonstrates well-fixed implants. The patient underwent revision for the management of recurrent instability. **B,** Postoperative AP pelvic radiograph demonstrates reconstruction with a trabecular metal revision shell, a conventional augment in flying buttress configuration, and a constrained liner.

to achieve the combined version needed for hip stability.

- The revision shell is anchored to the host bone with multiple screws.
- A trial liner is used to determine the position of the liner.
- The empty screw holes of the shell are covered with bone wax to prevent extrusion of cement into the interface of the host bone and the implant during cementation of the highly cross-linked polyethylene liner.
- The authors of this chapter routinely use liners with an elevated rim to reduce the risk of postoperative instability.
- Constrained liners should be used cautiously because they can increase the torque at the interface of the host bone and the implant before bony ingrowth occurs.

WOUND CLOSURE

- The ETO or trochanteric slide osteotomy is fixed with cerclage wires.
- The osteotomy is advanced to retension the abductor musculature if necessary.
- Drains are not routinely used.

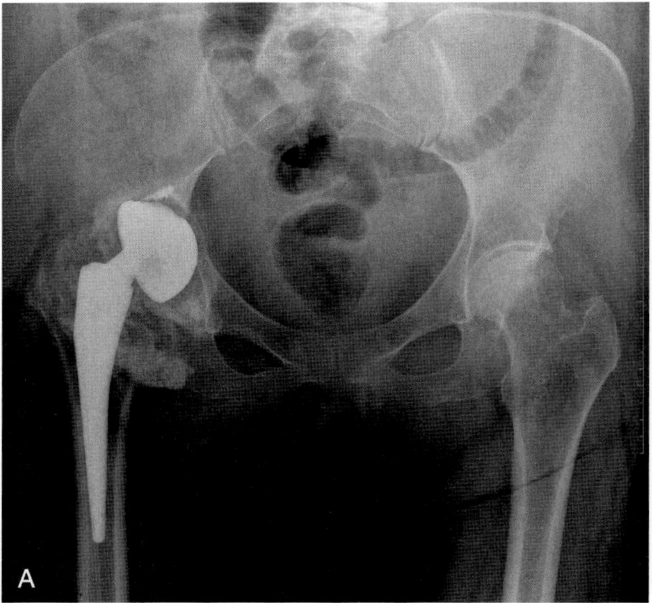

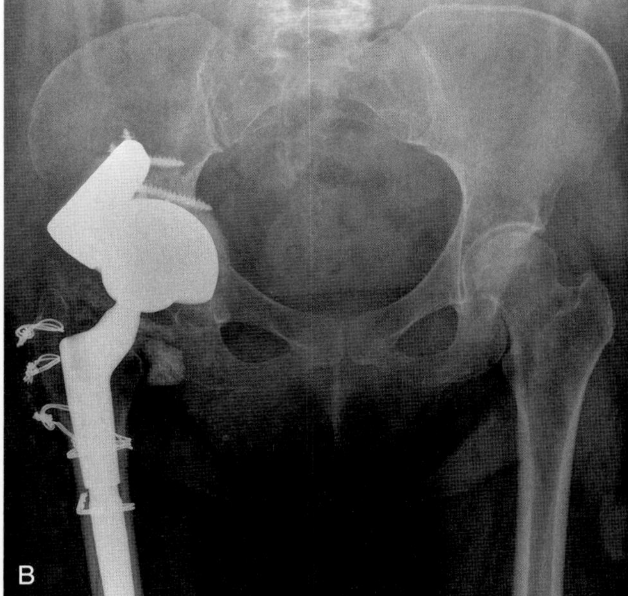

Figure 9 **A,** AP pelvic radiograph demonstrates a fractured ceramic liner and loose acetabular implant. **B,** Postoperative AP pelvic radiograph demonstrates reconstruction with a noncemented hemispheric acetabular implant and a buttress augment.

- The incision is closed in layers.
- Staples are used for skin closure.

Postoperative Regimen

Pharmacologic and/or mechanical prophylaxis against DVT is initiated according to the current guidelines of the American College of Chest Physicians and the American Academy of Orthopaedic Surgeons. Partial weight bearing with the use of a walking aid is maintained for at least 6 weeks postoperatively. Hip precautions depending on the exposure that was used are maintained for 6 weeks postoperatively. In patients with multiple risk factors for hip instability (such as previous dislocations, abductor deficiency, neurologic disorders), the use of an abduction brace is considered.

Avoiding Pitfalls and Complications

Undiagnosed pelvic discontinuity is a potential pitfall in every complex acetabular revision. After the previous implants have been removed and the acetabulum has been débrided, stability of the acetabulum must be carefully evaluated. The posterior column is stressed with a Cobb elevator, and any motion between the superior and inferior pelvis is noted. If discontinuity is present, the hemispheric revision shell is likely to fail by medial migration, even if it is combined with augments. Chronic pelvic discontinuity should be managed with cup-cage reconstruction, the use of a rigid cage, or the use of a pelvic distraction technique with a trabecular metal cup and augments.

Every attempt should be made to obtain adequate stability of the hip intraoperatively. The combined anteversion should be assessed routinely to evaluate the positioning of the implants. When the final liner is cemented to the revision shell, the position can be corrected as much as 20° in one plane. Liners with an elevated rim are used routinely. If acceptable stability cannot be obtained in a patient with an absent abductor mechanism, the use of a constrained liner can be considered. However, constrained liners should be used with caution because they can transmit high torques to the interface of the construct and host bone before bony ingrowth occurs.

Two distinct modes of failure are possible. One mode of failure is loosening of both the augment and the shell; the other is loosening of the shell with the augment ingrown into host bone. The most common reasons for repeat revision are recurrent dislocation and deep infection. Hip instability is a common complication after revision THA. Although the etiology of instability is often multifactorial, it is certainly related to the extent of soft-tissue dissection during exposure and compromised abductor musculature. Additionally, to avoid early failure, constrained liners should be used reluctantly in tenuous acetabular revisions. Trabecular metal implants seem to have inherent properties that allow them to resist the development of deep infection compared with titanium acetabular implants.

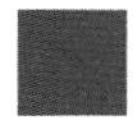

Bibliography

Abolghasemian M, Sadeghi Naini M, Tangsataporn S, et al: Reconstruction of massive uncontained acetabular defects using allograft with cage or ring reinforcement: An assessment of the graft's ability to restore bone stock and its impact on the outcome of re-revision. *Bone Joint J* 2014;96-B(3):319-324.

Abolghasemian M, Tangsataporn S, Sternheim A, Backstein D, Safir O, Gross AE: Combined trabecular metal acetabular shell and augment for acetabular revision with substantial bone loss: A mid-term review. *Bone Joint J* 2013;95-B(2):166-172.

Abolghasemian M, Tangsataporn S, Sternheim A, Backstein DJ, Safir OA, Gross AE: Porous metal augments: Big hopes for big holes. *Bone Joint J* 2013;95-B(11 suppl A):103-108.

Alberton GM, High WA, Morrey BF: Dislocation after revision total hip arthroplasty: An analysis of risk factors and treatment options. *J Bone Joint Surg Am* 2002;84(10):1788-1792.

American Academy of Orthopaedic Surgeons: *Preventing Venous Thromboembolic Disease in Patients Undergoing Elective Hip and Knee Arthroplasty: Evidence-Based Guideline and Evidence Report.* Rosemont, IL, American Academy of Orthopaedic Surgeons, 2011. Available at: http://www.aaos.org/research/guidelines/VTE/VTE_guideline.asp. Accessed August 31, 2016.

DeBoer DK, Christie MJ: Reconstruction of the deficient acetabulum with an oblong prosthesis: Three- to seven-year results. *J Arthroplasty* 1998;13(6):674-680.

DeBoer DK, Christie MJ, Brinson MF, Morrison JC: Revision total hip arthroplasty for pelvic discontinuity. *J Bone Joint Surg Am* 2007;89(4):835-840.

Del Gaizo DJ, Kancherla V, Sporer SM, Paprosky WG: Tantalum augments for Paprosky IIIA defects remain stable at midterm followup. *Clin Orthop Relat Res* 2012;470(2):395-401.

Dennis DA: Management of massive acetabular defects in revision total hip arthroplasty. *J Arthroplasty* 2003;18(3 suppl 1):121-125.

Dewal H, Chen F, Su E, Di Cesare PE: Use of structural bone graft with cementless acetabular cups in total hip arthroplasty. *J Arthroplasty* 2003;18(1):23-28.

Falck-Ytter Y, Francis CW, Johanson NA, et al; American College of Chest Physicians: Prevention of VTE in orthopedic surgery patients: Antithrombotic therapy and prevention of thrombosis, 9th ed: American College of Chest Physicians evidence-based clinical practice guidelines. *Chest* 2012;141(2 suppl):e278S-e325S.

Fawcett KJ, Barr AR, eds: *Tissue Banking.* Arlington, VA, American Association of Blood Banks, 1987.

Garbuz D, Morsi E, Gross AE: Revision of the acetabular component of a total hip arthroplasty with a massive structural allograft: Study with a minimum five-year follow-up. *J Bone Joint Surg Am* 1996;78(5):693-697.

Gross AE: Revision arthroplasty of the acetabulum with restoration of bone stock. *Clin Orthop Relat Res* 1999;(369):198-207.

Gross AE, Goodman S: The current role of structural grafts and cages in revision arthroplasty of the hip. *Clin Orthop Relat Res* 2004;(429):193-200.

Hooten JP Jr, Engh CA Jr, Engh CA: Failure of structural acetabular allografts in cementless revision hip arthroplasty. *J Bone Joint Surg Br* 1994;76(3):419-422.

Köster G, Willert HG, Köhler HP, Döpkens K: An oblong revision cup for large acetabular defects: Design rationale and two- to seven-year follow-up. *J Arthroplasty* 1998;13(5):559-569.

Kwong LM, Jasty M, Harris WH: High failure rate of bulk femoral head allografts in total hip acetabular reconstructions at 10 years. *J Arthroplasty* 1993;8(4):341-346.

Lakstein D, Backstein DJ, Safir O, Kosashvili Y, Gross AE: Modified trochanteric slide for complex hip arthroplasty: Clinical outcomes and complication rates. *J Arthroplasty* 2010;25(3):363-368.

Lee PT, Raz G, Safir OA, Backstein DJ, Gross AE: Long-term results for minor column allografts in revision hip arthroplasty. *Clin Orthop Relat Res* 2010;468(12):3295-3303.

Lingaraj K, Teo YH, Bergman N: The management of severe acetabular bone defects in revision hip arthroplasty using modular porous metal components. *J Bone Joint Surg Br* 2009;91(12):1555-1560.

Morsi E, Garbuz D, Gross AE: Revision total hip arthroplasty with shelf bulk allografts: A long-term follow-up study. *J Arthroplasty* 1996;11(1):86-90.

Nehme A, Lewallen DG, Hanssen AD: Modular porous metal augments for treatment of severe acetabular bone loss during revision hip arthroplasty. *Clin Orthop Relat Res* 2004;(429):201-208.

Oakeshott RD, Morgan DA, Zukor DJ, Rudan JF, Brooks PJ, Gross AE: Revision total hip arthroplasty with osseous allograft reconstruction: A clinical and roentgenographic analysis. *Clin Orthop Relat Res* 1987;(225):37-61.

O'Rourke MR, Paprosky WG, Rosenberg AG: Use of structural allografts in acetabular revision surgery. *Clin Orthop Relat Res* 2004;(420):113-121.

Pagnano W, Hanssen AD, Lewallen DG, Shaughnessy WJ: The effect of superior placement of the acetabular component on the rate of loosening after total hip arthroplasty. *J Bone Joint Surg Am* 1996;78(7):1004-1014.

Paprosky WG, Magnus RE: Principles of bone grafting in revision total hip arthroplasty: Acetabular technique. *Clin Orthop Relat Res* 1994;(298):147-155.

Paprosky WG, Perona PG, Lawrence JM: Acetabular defect classification and surgical reconstruction in revision arthroplasty: A 6-year follow-up evaluation. *J Arthroplasty* 1994;9(1):33-44.

Saleh KJ, Holtzman J, Gafni A, et al: Development, test reliability and validation of a classification for revision hip arthroplasty. *J Orthop Res* 2001;19(1):50-56.

Shinar AA, Harris WH: Bulk structural autogenous grafts and allografts for reconstruction of the acetabulum in total hip arthroplasty: Sixteen-year-average follow-up. *J Bone Joint Surg Am* 1997;79(2):159-168.

Siegmeth A, Duncan CP, Masri BA, Kim WY, Garbuz DS: Modular tantalum augments for acetabular defects in revision hip arthroplasty. *Clin Orthop Relat Res* 2009;467(1):199-205.

Sporer SM, Bottros JJ, Hulst JB, Kancherla VK, Moric M, Paprosky WG: Acetabular distraction: An alternative for severe defects with chronic pelvic discontinuity? *Clin Orthop Relat Res* 2012;470(11):3156-3163.

Sporer SM, Paprosky WG: The use of a trabecular metal acetabular component and trabecular metal augment for severe acetabular defects. *J Arthroplasty* 2006;21(6 suppl 2):83-86.

Stans AA, Pagnano MW, Shaughnessy WJ, Hanssen AD: Results of total hip arthroplasty for Crowe type III developmental hip dysplasia. *Clin Orthop Relat Res* 1998;(348):149-157.

Tokarski AT, Novack TA, Parvizi J: Is tantalum protective against infection in revision total hip arthroplasty? *Bone Joint J* 2015;97-B(1):45-49.

Van Kleunen JP, Lee GC, Lementowski PW, Nelson CL, Garino JP: Acetabular revisions using trabecular metal cups and augments. *J Arthroplasty* 2009;24(6 suppl):64-68.

Whitehouse MR, Masri BA, Duncan CP, Garbuz DS: Continued good results with modular trabecular metal augments for acetabular defects in hip arthroplasty at 7 to 11 years. *Clin Orthop Relat Res* 2015;473(2):521-527.

Woodgate IG, Saleh KJ, Jaroszynski G, Agnidis Z, Woodgate MM, Gross AE: Minor column structural acetabular allografts in revision hip arthroplasty. *Clin Orthop Relat Res* 2000;(371):75-85.

Video Reference

Gross AE: Video. *Acetabular Revision: Structural Grafts and Metal Augments.* Toronto, ON, Canada, 2015.

Chapter 51
Acetabular Bone Impaction Grafting and Cemented Revision

Jean W. M. Gardeniers, MD, PhD, DTHM
Wim H. C. Rijnen, MD, PhD
Tom J. J. H. Slooff, MD, PhD
B. Willem Schreurs, MD, PhD

Indications

Acetabular bone loss can compromise the outcome of both primary and revision total hip arthroplasty (THA). The surgeon should strive for reconstruction of this bone loss because restoration of bone stock is crucial to the success of future revisions. Acetabular bone impaction grafting in hip reconstruction is appealing from a biologic perspective. The method is based on the principle that the lost bone stock should be restored with the use of cancellous bone grafts tightly impacted in contained defects. This method has been used since 1979, and many long-term follow-up studies of patients in every age group are available in the international literature.

Bone impaction grafting, in combination with a cemented polyethylene cup, has been used for complex primary and revision THA. This technique makes replacement of lost bone stock and restoration of normal hip biomechanics and hip function possible with a standard implant. Although the technique works in patients of all ages, it is especially beneficial in patients younger than 50 years who may require future revision procedures. Another group of patients who may benefit from this procedure are patients with rheumatoid arthritis who require acetabular revision. Renewed fixation of a revision cup in patients with rheumatoid arthritis is extremely difficult because these patients have very poor bone quality.

Acetabular bone impaction grafting is suitable for the reconstruction of both simple cavitary bone defects and extensive acetabular bone defects with loss of segmental structures, such as medial wall defects or superolateral rim defects. The technique is reliable but is more demanding in patients with extensive acetabular defects. In patients with acetabular wall defects or acetabular column defects, it is essential to use specially designed metal mesh to convert a combined segmental and cavitary defect into a contained defect. The impacted cancellous grafts adapt to any irregularities of the host bone without forming a gap. Even after tight impaction with the use of a metal impactor and a mallet, the structure of the reconstructed impacted bone bed still facilitates cement penetration of 2 to 3 mm and hence interdigitation into the graft layer. The bone cement must be pressurized using a pressurizer and a seal to optimize cement penetration into the graft. A polyethylene cup is then inserted.

As with most revision techniques in patients with extensive lesions, surgeon-related factors have a marked effect on the outcome of acetabular bone impaction grafting procedures. The authors of this chapter strongly recommend building surgical skills by starting with the use of this technique in patients with relatively simple defects. Bone impaction grafting in simple cavitary defects is technically easy, and favorable long-term results can be expected. Ongoing experience and familiarity with the essentials of the technique will then permit successful reconstruction of more extensive defects.

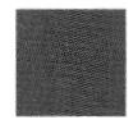

Contraindications

In patients who have untreated infections, a one-stage revision is not recommended. The procedure is contraindicated in patients in whom a large segmental defect, either peripheral or central, cannot be contained; patients

Dr. Gardeniers or an immediate family member has received research or institutional support from Stryker. Dr. Rijnen or an immediate family member serves as a paid consultant to Stryker. Dr. Schreurs or an immediate family member serves as a paid consultant to Stryker. Neither Dr. Slooff nor any immediate family member has received anything of value from or has stock or stock options held in a commercial company or institution related directly or indirectly to the subject of this chapter.

Table 1 Results of Acetabular Bone Impaction Grafting in Acetabular Revision

Authors (Year)	Number of Hips	Patient Group	Mean Patient Age in Years (Range)	Mean Follow-up in Years (Range)	Success Rate (%)[a]
Schreurs, Keurentjes, et al (2009)	62	Patients undergoing consecutive acetabular revisions	59 (23-82)	22 (20-25)	Any reason: 75 Aseptic loosening: 87
Schreurs, Luttjeboer, et al (2009)	35	Patients with rheumatoid arthritis	57 (31-73)	11 (8-19)	Any reason: 80 Aseptic loosening: 85
Busch et al (2011)	42	Patients aged <50 yr	37 (20-49)	23 (20-28)	Any reason: 52 Aseptic loosening: 77
Schreurs et al (2015)[b]	11	Patients requiring repeat acetabular revision	67 (43-83)	10 (5-15)	Any reason: 91 Aseptic loosening: 100

[a] Success is defined as survivorship of the acetabular reconstruction, with the end point defined as revision for the specified reason.

[b] The index acetabular revision procedures performed on these patients were reported on in the study by Schreurs, Keurentjes, et al published in 2009.

with unhealed acetabular fracture or pelvic dissociation; patients who have previously undergone radiation therapy of the affected hip; and elderly patients with multiple associated medical conditions. Reconstruction using bone impaction grafting can be performed in a patient with septic loosening after the infection is managed. Bone impaction grafting after management of infection is performed in a two-stage procedure.

Acetabular revisions can be performed in patients with an acetabular fracture and/or pelvic dissociation, but only after the fracture is stabilized. The bridging of a pelvic dissociation with metal mesh alone will fail because this fixation method is not adequate for management of a fracture.

Bone impaction grafting will be unsuccessful in many patients with loss of bone stock or in patients whose hips have failed as a result of radiation therapy to the pelvis. Nonvital pelvic bone does not provide suitable host bone to allow ingrowth of cancellous bone. In these patients, the infection rate is also unacceptably high.

Satisfactory results of bone impaction grafting cannot be attained without sufficient knowledge of the techniques of acetabular cementation.

Alternative Treatments

Many options exist for acetabular revision. Cement-only reconstruction may be indicated in elderly patients with limited life expectancy. Many techniques and implants for noncemented reconstruction are also available. The use of impacted bone grafts in combination with rigid metal shells, reconstruction rings, and noncemented cups has been described. Although the authors of this chapter do not have extensive experience with these techniques, some studies suggest that acetabular bone impaction grafting can be used successfully with noncemented acetabular implants. However, adverse outcomes of bone impaction grafting have resulted from minor modifications of the bone impaction grafting technique. For example, the use of grafts smaller than 4 mm on the acetabular side or the use of reverse reaming to impact the bone grafts will hamper the outcome.

Results

A review of the literature on outcomes of bone impaction grafting on the acetabular side was recently published. A summary of different studies of acetabular reconstruction using bone impaction grafting from the chapter authors' institution is shown in **Table 1**.

Between 1979 and 1986, four surgeons performed 62 acetabular reconstructions in 56 consecutive patients (13 men, 43 women) for the management of failed hip arthroplasty. The indication for the revision surgery was aseptic loosening in 58 hips and septic loosening in 4 hips. The mean age of the patients at the time of the procedure was 59 years. Defects were cavitary in 39 hips and a combination of cavitary and segmental in 23 hips (10 central defects and 13 defects of the peripheral wall). No hip was lost to follow-up at the last review. The Kaplan-Meier survivorship of the cup with the end point of revision for any reason was 75% at 20 years postoperatively (95% confidence interval [CI], 62% to 88%). Excluding two revisions that were performed for the management of septic

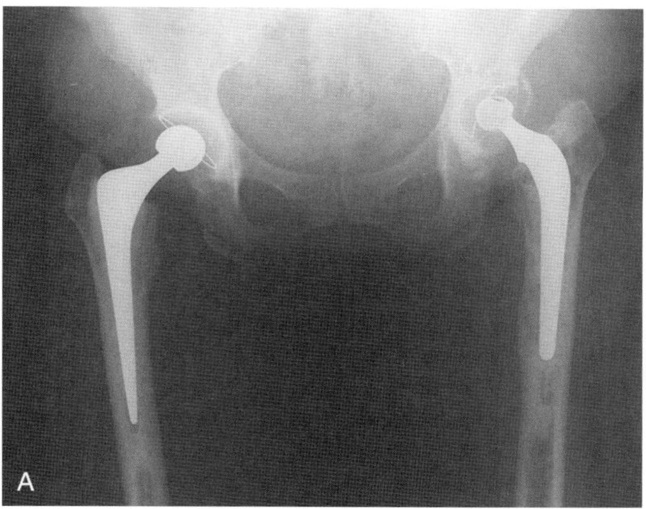

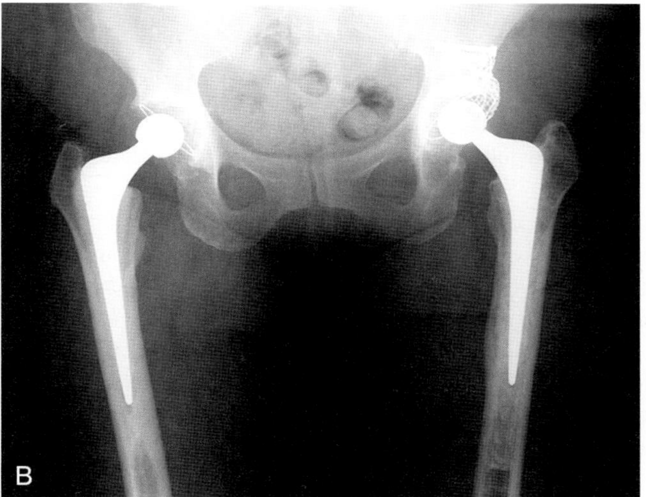

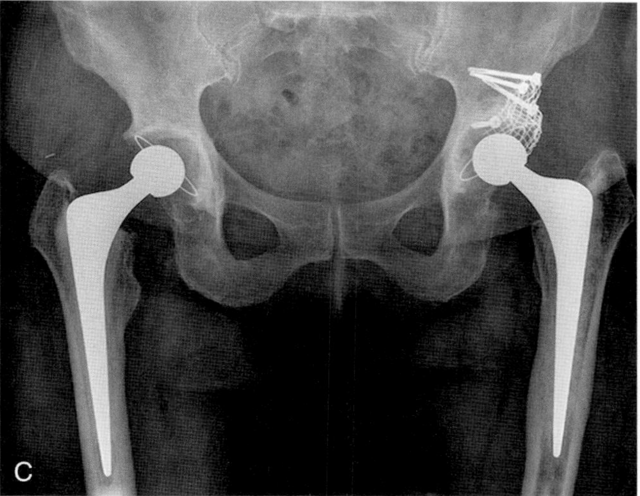

Figure 1 **A,** AP pelvic radiograph demonstrates aseptic loosening of the left cup and stem in a 54-year-old woman 13 years after primary total hip arthroplasty for the management of primary osteoarthritis. **B,** AP pelvic radiograph obtained 6 weeks after revision of the cup and stem. Femoral bone impaction grafting was performed. On the acetabular side, a mesh was placed to reconstruct the superolateral wall of the acetabulum, bone impaction grafting was performed, and a polyethylene cup was cemented into place. **C,** AP pelvic radiograph obtained 11 years after revision of the cup and stem demonstrates complete radiologic incorporation of the bone graft on the acetabular and femoral sides with a stable stem and cup.

loosening at 3 and 6 years postoperatively, survivorship with the end point of aseptic loosening was 87% at 20 years postoperatively (95% CI, 67% to 93%). Most hips had a stable radiologic appearance (**Figure 1**). The reconstructions that failed because of aseptic loosening typically showed radiolucent lines early in the postoperative period. One of the hips that was not revised had radiologic loosening. However, four patients who had radiologic loosening and did not undergo revision because their symptoms were mild died during the follow-up period. Based on the results of this study at long-term follow-up, bone impaction grafting was deemed to be a safe and adequate biologic method of reconstruction of acetabular bone defects in revision surgery for the management of failed acetabular implants.

In a more recent study, the authors evaluated the outcome of the revisions performed for the management of the implant failures in the previous study in an attempt to prove that reconstruction with bone impaction grafting facilitates future revision. This study examined the clinical and radiographic outcomes of 11 consecutive repeat acetabular revisions in 10 patients with repeat bone impaction grafting and a cemented polyethylene cup within the previously reported cohort of 62 acetabular revisions. Data were collected prospectively. The mean follow-up was 10 years after

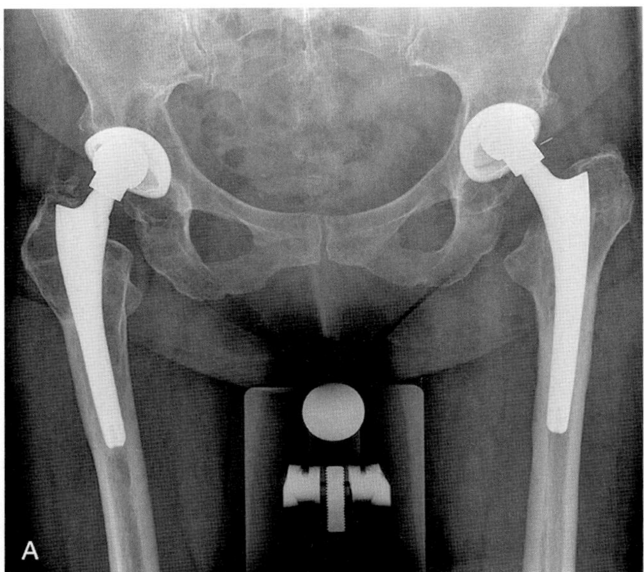

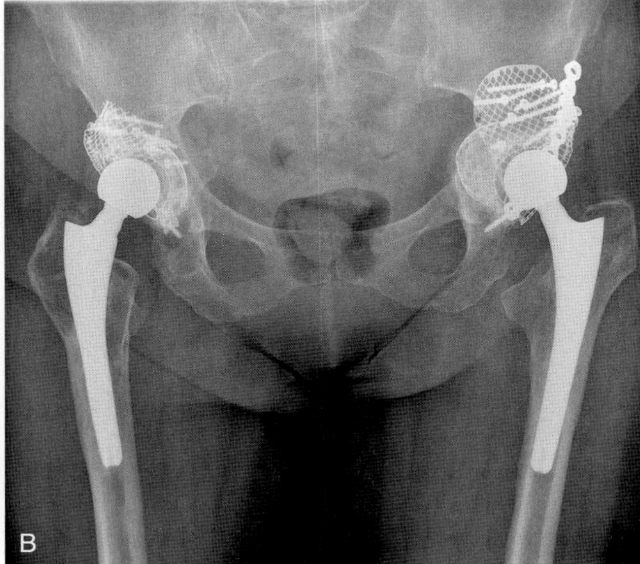

Figure 2 **A,** AP pelvic radiograph demonstrates bilateral aseptic loosening of the acetabular cup and extensive wear of the polyethylene liner. **B,** AP pelvic radiograph obtained 2 years after bilateral acetabular cup revision. In each hip, reconstruction of the medial wall was performed, and a segmental defect of the posterolateral and superolateral wall was reconstructed with the use of a large rim mesh and supported by a plate. Bone impaction grafting was performed, and a polyethylene cup was cemented into place.

repeat revision and 28 years after the primary revision. No patients were lost to follow-up. Kaplan-Meier survivorship analysis demonstrated that survival with further revision of the cup for any reason as the end point was 91% (95% CI, 51% to 99%) at 10 years postoperatively. With the exclusion of one early repeat revision of the cup for malpositioning at 3 weeks postoperatively, survivorship with further cup revision for aseptic loosening as the end point was 100% (95% CI, 37% to 100%) at 10 years postoperatively.

In patients with rheumatoid arthritis, the use of noncemented cups for revision has been shown to have high failure rates at midterm follow-up. The best results cited in the literature have been achieved using simple repeat cementation or bone impaction grafting with a cemented cup. In a study at the chapter authors' institution, 35 consecutive acetabular revisions were performed in 28 patients with rheumatoid arthritis using acetabular bone impaction grafting and a cemented cup. At 8 to 19 years postoperatively, no patient was lost to follow-up, but outcomes were included for 8 patients (10 hips) who died during the follow-up period. Acetabular bone stock defects were cavitary (11 hips) or combined segmental and cavitary (24 hips). At minimum 8-year follow-up, eight hips required repeat revision. With septic loosening excluded, Kaplan-Meier analysis demonstrated a survival rate with aseptic loosening as the end point of 85% (95% CI, 71% to 99%) at 11-year follow-up.

The process of incorporation of impacted bone grafts has been studied in both animal experiments and human biopsies, with nearly complete incorporation of these grafts demonstrated in animal studies. To determine whether incorporation occurs in humans, 24 acetabular bone biopsy specimens were obtained from 20 patients (21 hips) between 3 months and 15 years after acetabular reconstruction in both complex primary procedures and revision procedures. Histologic analysis showed revascularization of the graft followed by osteoclast resorption. Bone formation occurred on the graft, on fibrin accumulations, or in fibrous stroma that invaded the graft. A combination of graft, bone, and fibrin resulted in a new trabecular structure with normal lamellar bone and little remaining graft material. Some patients retained small, localized areas of unincorporated bone graft within fibrous tissue.

Satisfactory outcomes of acetabular bone impaction grafting for the management of cavitary and simple segmental defects in revision procedures have been reported in many studies. However, the limitations of the technique are unclear. This technique has been shown to be effective in Paprosky type IIB, IIIA, and IIIB defects, with 10-year survival of 88% (95% CI, 74% to 100%) with acetabular revision for any reason as the end point. A different study confirmed these data. Because the procedure is technically very demanding, the authors of this chapter recommend the use of this technique in patients with these large defects only by surgeons who have considerable experience in hip revision procedures and bone impaction grafting (**Figure 2**).

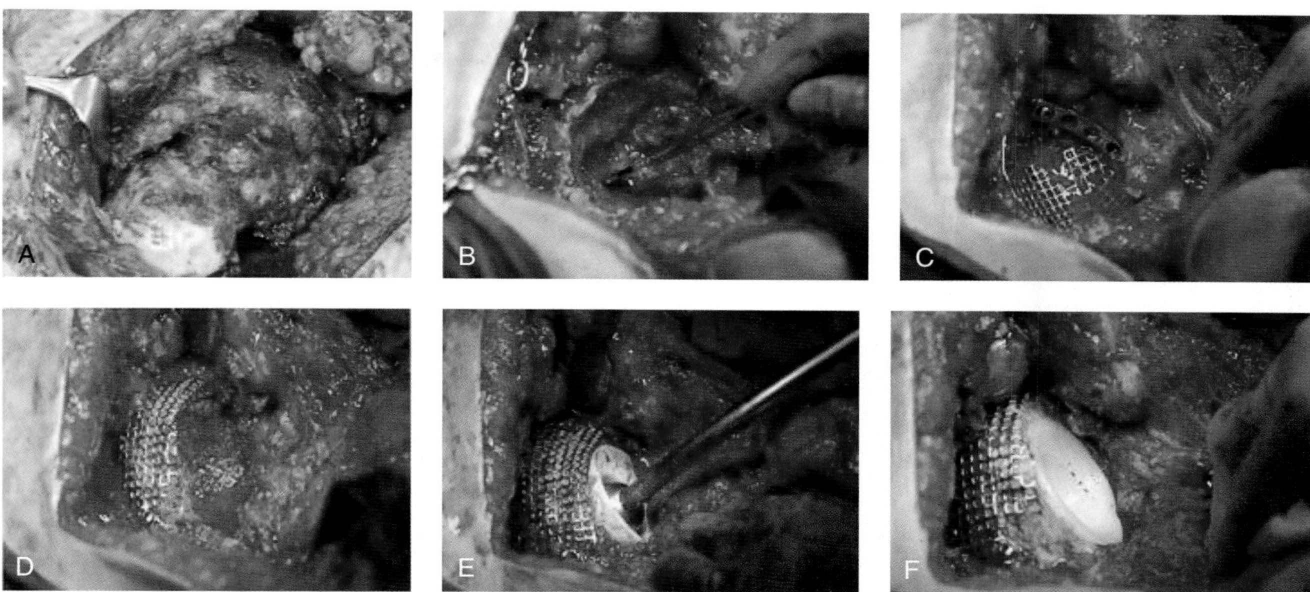

Figure 3 Intraoperative photographs show grafting of a massive acetabular defect. **A,** A massive defect of the rim and medial wall is visible. **B,** Forceps are used to determine the size of the medial wall defect. **C,** The medial wall is reinforced with a pelvic plate and a wire mesh. **D,** The rim mesh is fixed, and the first graft layer is impacted. **E,** A trial prosthesis is placed in the reconstructed acetabulum. **F,** The cup is cemented at the anatomic level.

A promising new development is the use of acetabular impaction grafting in combination with porous metal augments or structural grafts, especially in patients with very large or even massive bone defects. In patients with extensive defects, the use of large mesh alone can result in substantial cup migration and fatigue failure of the mesh. To avoid these complications, the use of a pelvic reconstruction plate or porous metal or structural bone augments can be helpful in large reconstructions (**Figure 3**).

Techniques

Setup/Exposure

- The authors of this chapter generally use the posterolateral approach with the patient placed in a lateral position. Other approaches also can be used.
- Regardless of approach, extensive exposure of the anterior and posterior acetabular walls is mandatory.
- Trochanteric osteotomy is rarely necessary when the posterolateral exposure is used.
- Care must be taken to identify the major landmarks because the previous surgical procedures and the resultant bone loss and scar tissue may have altered the normal anatomy. Landmarks include the transverse ligament, the tip of the greater trochanter, the lesser trochanter, the tendinous part of the gluteus maximus, the lower border of the gluteus medius and minimus, and the sciatic nerve.
- Fluid may be aspirated for white blood cell count and culture before the joint capsule is opened.
- Femoral fracture can be prevented by performing a release of the proximal femoral area before the hip is dislocated.
- Wide exposure of the acetabulum is obtained.
- All scar tissue is removed, and a circumferential capsulotomy is performed.
- The iliopsoas tendon is released if necessary.
- The failed implant is removed, with care taken to preserve as much bone stock as possible.
- Biopsy specimens are obtained from the implant-bone interface for bacterial culture and intraoperative frozen-section analysis.
- Systemic antibiotics are administered after all cultures are obtained and biopsies performed.
- All interface membrane, metal debris, implants, and, if present, bone cement remnants are thoroughly removed from the acetabulum. Spoons and curets are used at the implant-bone interface to lessen the risk of tissue damage.

Instruments/Equipment/Implants Required

- An explant system is used to remove a fixed noncemented cup.
- A reamer is used to remove a polyethylene cup.
- A drill and drill bits are required.

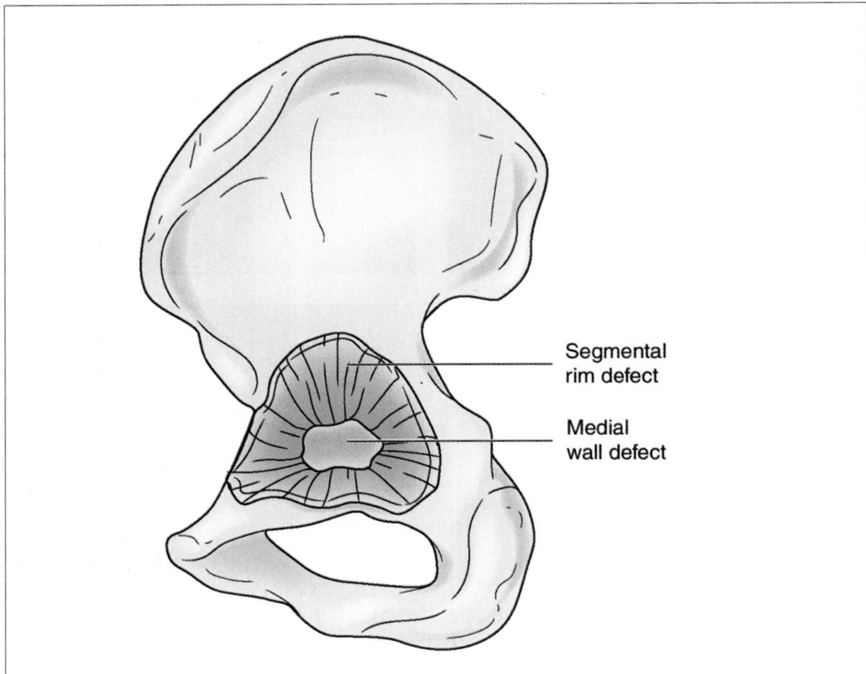

Figure 4 Illustration depicts a combined defect of the medial wall and peripheral segmental rim after removal of a failed acetabular implant and fibrous interface.

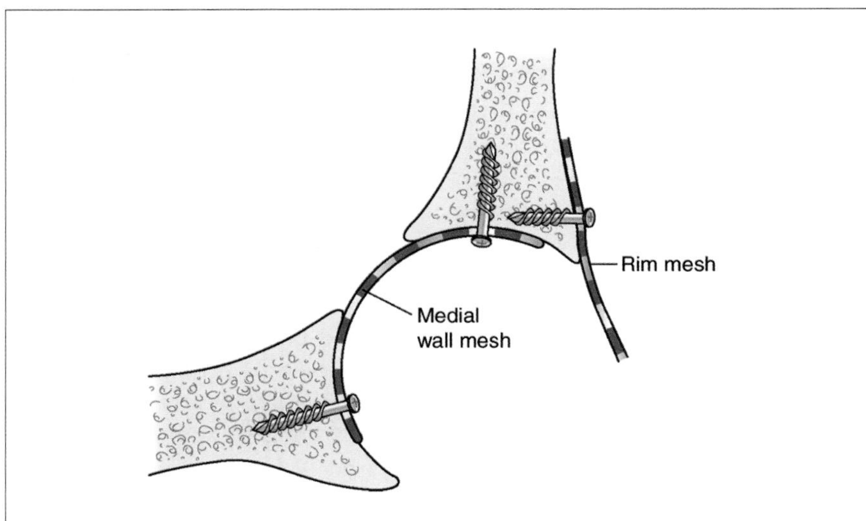

Figure 5 Illustration depicts the use of flexible stainless steel mesh to close a segmental defect of the acetabulum. The rim mesh at the peripheral segmental defect should be fixed rigidly with at least three small screws at 1.5-cm intervals. Screws should be perpendicular to the host bone for better fixation.

- A revision instrument set is required consisting of bone chisels of different sizes, shapes, and lengths.
- Curets and sharp spoons are used.
- A high-speed burr is needed.
- A bone cement removal system is used.

Procedure

BONE PREPARATION

- The entire acetabulum is inspected meticulously to identify bone stock defects (**Figure 4**).
- The transverse ligament, which is nearly always present, is identified and used as a landmark. A retractor beneath this ligament facilitates better exposure.
- A trial cup is positioned against the ligament in the ideal position, facilitating detection of the extent of an existing superolateral rim defect.
- Defects of the peripheral rim and the medial wall are reconstructed with the use of flexible stainless steel mesh. The mesh is trimmed to fit the existing defects with the use of specially designed scissors and pliers.
- Peripheral rim mesh is placed on the anterior and posterior borders of the acetabulum (**Figure 5**).
- The overlying muscles (abductors) are elevated off the pelvic bone with limited risk of neurovascular damage. To achieve correct orientation of the mesh, the trial cup is held in place during this step.
- The peripheral mesh is fixed to the pelvic bone with the use of well-fixed screws every 1.5 cm around the entire edge of the mesh. Self-drilling, self-tapping screws are recommended because they are easier to use, but small-fragment AO screws are sometimes better in patients with large defects or sclerotic host bone.
- Fixation of the anterior and posterior corners of the wire mesh is crucial to prevent micromotion of the mesh, which would hamper stability and ingrowth of the impacted graft.
- To obtain optimal fixation, the screws should be perpendicular to the pelvic bone.
- If medial wall mesh is necessary, the correctly sized piece is placed

to prevent graft penetration into the pelvis during the impaction process. This step is particularly important in patients with weak but intact medial walls.

- In patients with large medial wall defects, reconstruction or reinforcement with a small-fragment pelvic plate is mandatory. Rather than avoiding vigorous impaction to reduce the risk of medial wall fracture, the surgeon instead should reinforce the medial wall.
- If a perfect and stable fit of the medial wall mesh is obtained, screw fixation may not be necessary.
- After the segmental defects in the acetabulum are contained, reconstruction with bone graft is begun.
- Preparation of the host bone bed is essential before grafting.
- Sclerotic acetabular areas are penetrated with multiple small drill holes (approximately 2 mm in diameter and depth). These holes enhance the surface contact between the host bone and the graft and improve revascularization of the graft.

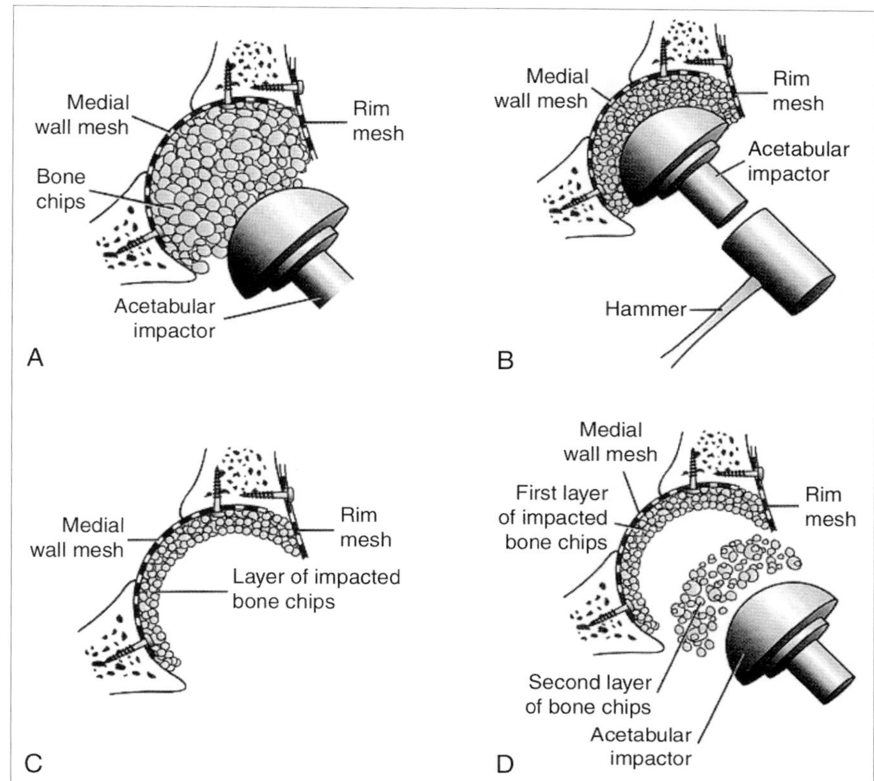

Figure 6 Illustrations depict reconstruction of a cavitary defect. **A,** The appearance of fresh-frozen morcellized bone chips used in acetabular reconstruction before impaction. Metal impactors of several diameters are used. **B,** A hammer is used to compress the bone chips tightly. **C,** After the first impaction, the layer of bone chips is inspected. This layer adheres to the surrounding bone after the impactor is removed. **D,** A second layer of bone chips is impacted on the first layer. The entire defect is reconstructed in layers. (Reproduced from Slooff TJJH, Schreurs BW, Gardeniers JWM: Acetabular revision: Impaction bone grafting and cement, in Lieberman JR, Berry DJ, eds: *Advanced Reconstruction: Hip*. Rosemont, IL, American Academy of Orthopaedic Surgeons, 2005, pp 353-359.)

BONE GRAFT PREPARATION

- Acetabular bone impaction grafting is best performed with pure, cancellous, fresh-frozen bone chips 7 to 10 mm in diameter.
- All soft tissue and cartilage must be removed from the femoral head allograft before the chips are made. Soft-tissue inclusions reduce the stability of the reconstruction and hamper incorporation of the graft.
- Using a rongeur or a bone mill, the substantial cancellous bone chips are cut from the femoral head allograft.
- Even when performed by experienced surgeons, harvesting fresh-frozen trabecular bone chips with the use of a rongeur is tedious and time consuming.
- Although commercial bone mills can be used, most mills produce chips measuring 2 to 5 mm in diameter that are not optimal for the acetabulum. A bone mill that produces chips measuring 7 to 10 mm in diameter and even up to 12 mm is recommended.
- Although the authors of this chapter typically use fresh-frozen cancellous bone grafts harvested from femoral head autograft and allograft, the use of a combination of trabecular and cortical bone or irradiated bone may be necessary. The authors of this chapter have limited experience with the use of freeze-dried bone in bone impaction grafting.

PLACEMENT OF BONE GRAFT AND PROSTHESIS

- The acetabulum is cleaned immediately before graft impaction with the use of pulsatile lavage.
- The contained acetabular defect is packed tightly with bone chips.
- If necessary, small irregular cavities are filled and impacted with the use of small impactors.
- The entire cavitary defect is reconstructed in layers. To begin, the most caudal part of the host bone bed is reconstructed at the level of the transverse ligament (**Figure 6**).
- The graft is impacted with specially designed acetabular impactors and

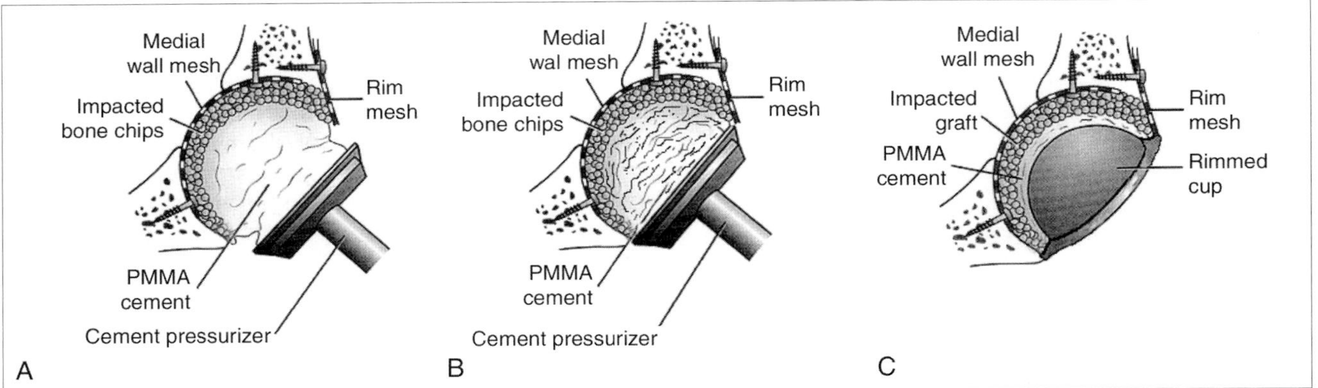

Figure 7 Illustrations depict cementing of the acetabular cup. **A,** The layer of impacted graft should be at least 5 mm thick to prevent penetration of cement through the graft. Bone cement in a relatively viscous state is introduced and pressurized to force the bone cement 2 mm into the compacted graft layer. **B,** The cement is pressurized with the use of a rimmed pressurizer to contain the graft and the cement and allow application of continuous and sufficient pressure. **C,** A rimmed cup is placed at the anatomic level. PMMA = polymethyl methacrylate. (Panels A and C reproduced from Slooff TJJH, Schreurs BW, Gardeniers JWM: Acetabular revision: Impaction bone grafting and cement, in Lieberman JR, Berry DJ, eds: *Advanced Reconstruction: Hip*. Rosemont, IL, American Academy of Orthopaedic Surgeons, 2005, pp 353-359.)

a solid hammer. The graft layer should be at least 5 mm thick; otherwise, cement will intrude through the thin bone layer, enclose the small bone chips, and hamper graft incorporation.

- The last impactor used should be 2 to 4 mm larger than the desired cup diameter to obtain a 2-mm cement layer.
- While the antibiotic-loaded bone cement is being prepared, pressure is maintained on the bone graft with the last impactor that was used.
- Bone cement is inserted and is pressured after insertion with the use of a silicone seal, as in primary cemented hip arthroplasty.
- The cup is inserted when the cement has a doughlike consistency.
- Pressure is maintained on the cup until the cement is fully polymerized (**Figure 7**).

Wound Closure

- After reduction of the hip joint, the surgical area is inspected for substantial bleeding.
- All bone graft remnants and cement particles are removed with intensive pressure lavage.
- If possible, the posterior capsule and the external rotators should be reconstructed.
- The fascia, the subcutaneous layer, and the skin are meticulously closed.

Postoperative Regimen

According to the current protocol, patients remain on bed rest for a maximum of 2 days postoperatively, after which they are mobilized with two crutches and toe-touch weight bearing for 6 weeks postoperatively. Clinical and radiologic recovery are assessed at 6 weeks postoperatively, after which 50% weight bearing with the use of one or two crutches is allowed for the next 6 weeks. Full weight-bearing is allowed at 12 weeks postoperatively. The only exceptions to this postoperative protocol are for patients in whom the medial wall could not be adequately reconstructed (because early weight bearing may cause the reconstruction to migrate medially) and for patients with very extensive reconstruction.

Avoiding Pitfalls and Complications

Reconstruction with acetabular bone impaction grafting for the management of lost acetabular structural integrity and deficient mechanical implant support is based on several principles. First, hip mechanics are repaired by positioning the reconstruction and cup at the level of the anatomic acetabulum (the teardrop). Next, segmental defects are closed with metal wire mesh to achieve containment of the defect. In patients with large defects, extra reinforcement with structural bone grafts and/or metal augments may be considered. Periprosthetic bone loss is addressed by filling the created cavitary defect with allograft bone chips. Stability of the construction is restored with solid impaction of the chips onto the host bone bed and the use of pressurized bone cement.

Although bone mills are an option for producing the bone chips used in the reconstruction, the surgeon should be aware of several pitfalls. First, if fresh-frozen femoral heads are used, all soft tissue and cartilage should be cleaned from the femoral head. Any remaining cartilage particles, if milled and included in the morcellized bone graft, will hamper the mechanical properties of the reconstruction because these particles will not incorporate into the reconstructed bone. Second, as noted previously, commercial bone mills typically produce particles 2 to 5 mm in diameter. These particles are best used on the femoral side, where the dimensions of the graft are limited by the diameter of the femoral canal. For acetabular reconstruction, bone chips 7 to 10 mm in diameter must be used because smaller chips will result in less initial stability.

The impaction should be performed with a solid hammer and specially designed impactors. The use of an acetabular reamer rotating in reverse to compress the graft will substantially reduce the stability of the cup. Researchers have demonstrated greater initial cup migration with reverse reaming than with manual impaction, especially when reverse reaming is performed in combination with the use of slurry grafts (1 to 3 mm in diameter).

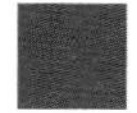

Bibliography

Bolder SB, Schreurs BW, Verdonschot N, van Unen JM, Gardeniers JW, Slooff TJ: Particle size of bone graft and method of impaction affect initial stability of cemented cups: Human cadaveric and synthetic pelvic specimen studies. *Acta Orthop Scand* 2003;74(6):652-657.

Borland WS, Bhattacharya R, Holland JP, Brewster NT: Use of porous trabecular metal augments with impaction bone grafting in management of acetabular bone loss. *Acta Orthop* 2012;83(4):347-352.

Busch VJ, Gardeniers JW, Verdonschot N, Slooff TJ, Schreurs BW: Acetabular reconstruction with impaction bone-grafting and a cemented cup in patients younger than fifty years old: A concise follow-up, at twenty to twenty-eight years, of a previous report. *J Bone Joint Surg Am* 2011;93(4):367-371.

Garcia-Cimbrelo E, Cruz-Pardos A, Garcia-Rey E, Ortega-Chamarro J: The survival and fate of acetabular reconstruction with impaction grafting for large defects. *Clin Orthop Relat Res* 2010;468(12):3304-3313.

Ibrahim MS, Raja S, Haddad FS: Acetabular impaction bone grafting in total hip replacement. *Bone Joint J* 2013; 95-B(11 suppl A):98-102.

Schreurs BW, Keurentjes JC, Gardeniers JW, Verdonschot N, Slooff TJ, Veth RP: Acetabular revision with impacted morsellised cancellous bone grafting and a cemented acetabular component: A 20- to 25-year follow-up. *J Bone Joint Surg Br* 2009;91(9):1148-1153.

Schreurs BW, Luttjeboer J, Thien TM, et al: Acetabular revision with impacted morselized cancellous bone graft and a cemented cup in patients with rheumatoid arthritis: A concise follow-up, at eight to nineteen years, of a previous report. *J Bone Joint Surg Am* 2009;91(3):646-651.

Schreurs BW, Te Stroet MA, Rijnen WH, Gardeniers JW: Acetabular re-revision with impaction bone grafting and a cemented polyethylene cup; a biological option for successive reconstructions. *Hip Int* 2015;25(1):44-49.

Slooff TJ, Huiskes R, van Horn J, Lemmens AJ: Bone grafting in total hip replacement for acetabular protrusion. *Acta Orthop Scand* 1984;55(6):593-596.

van der Donk S, Buma P, Slooff TJ, Gardeniers JW, Schreurs BW: Incorporation of morselized bone grafts: A study of 24 acetabular biopsy specimens. *Clin Orthop Relat Res* 2002;396:131-141.

van Egmond N, De Kam DC, Gardeniers JW, Schreurs BW: Revisions of extensive acetabular defects with impaction grafting and a cement cup. *Clin Orthop Relat Res* 2011;469(2):562-573.

Chapter 52
Acetabular Revision With Triflange Cups

Jason M. Jennings, MD, DPT
Raymond H. Kim, MD
Douglas A. Dennis, MD

Indications

Periacetabular bone loss in patients requiring revision total hip arthroplasty (THA) can be categorized according to the Paprosky classification and the American Academy of Orthopaedic Surgeons classification (**Table 1**). The primary indication for the use of a custom triflange acetabular cup (CTAC) is the presence of massive acetabular bone loss (Paprosky type IIIB [columns intact, superior lateral migration creating a dome defect, migration of the femoral head center less than 3 cm, minimal ischial lysis, Köhler line intact], AAOS types III and IV) that precludes the ability to obtain a stable construct with a standard hemispheric revision implant.

Patients requiring revision with a CTAC typically have undergone multiple previous surgical hip procedures. Therefore, infection must be ruled out preoperatively with laboratory studies (complete blood count, erythrocyte sedimentation rate, and C-reactive protein level). The authors of this chapter routinely perform fluoroscopically guided hip aspiration to obtain fluid for white blood cell count analysis, Gram stain, and cultures.

The decision to use a CTAC must be made preoperatively. Plain radiographs must be obtained and may include oblique pelvic views to assess bone loss (**Figure 1**). If substantial limb-length inequality is present as a result of superior implant migration, full-length orthoradiography may be of value in preoperative planning. In patients who have substantial limb shortening secondary to protrusion of the acetabular implant, especially if the femoral implant is to be retained, an AP radiograph of the pelvis with traction on the affected limb is recommended to help determine where to place the hip center (**Figure 2**). In one such patient in the chapter authors' experience, the surgeon placed the hip center of the CTAC at the true level of the acetabulum. Because of proximal migration of the CTAC and subsequent chronic soft-tissue contracture, relocation of the hip was not possible, and the patient required removal of a well-fixed femoral implant to allow reduction of the hip joint.

Table 1 American Academy of Orthopaedic Surgeons Classification of Acetabular Defects

Type	Description
I	No substantial bone loss
II	Columns and rim intact Contained cavitary loss
III	Columns may be deficient Uncontained defect involving <50% of acetabulum
IV	Columns deficient Uncontained defect involving >50% of acetabulum Pelvic discontinuity may be present

Adapted with permission from Johnson DR, Dennis DA, Kim RH: Acetabular revision: Rings, cages, and custom implants, in Berry DJ, Lieberman JR, eds: *Surgery of the Hip*. Philadelphia, PA, Elsevier Saunders, 2013, pp 1111-1122.

Thin-slice CT is essential to evaluate bone loss and assess for the presence of a pelvic discontinuity. A CT scan with three-dimensional reconstruction and the use of rapid prototyping technology are needed for the design and production of the CTAC. If severe protrusion of the acetabular implant is present, CT angiography is ordered to assess the proximity of intrapelvic vessels to the failed

Dr. Kim or an immediate family member has received royalties from DJO and Innomed; is a member of a speakers' bureau or has made paid presentations on behalf of CeramTec and ConvaTec; serves as a paid consultant to DJO; and serves as a board member, owner, officer, or committee member of the International Congress for Joint Reconstruction. Dr. Dennis or an immediate family member has received royalties from DePuy Synthes and Innomed; is a member of a speakers' bureau or has made paid presentations on behalf of and serves as a paid consultant to DePuy Synthes; has stock or stock options held in Joint Vue; and has received research or institutional support from DePuy Synthes and Porter Adventist Hospital. Neither Dr. Jennings nor any immediate family member has received anything of value from or has stock or stock options held in a commercial company or institution related directly or indirectly to the subject of this chapter.

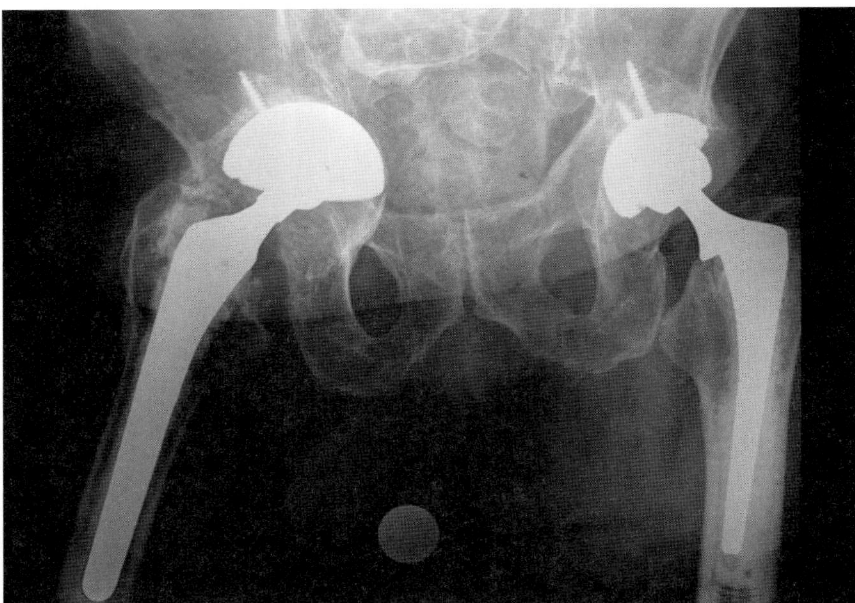

Figure 1 AP pelvic radiograph demonstrates a failed total hip arthroplasty with acetabular implant loosening and massive periacetabular bone loss in the right hip.

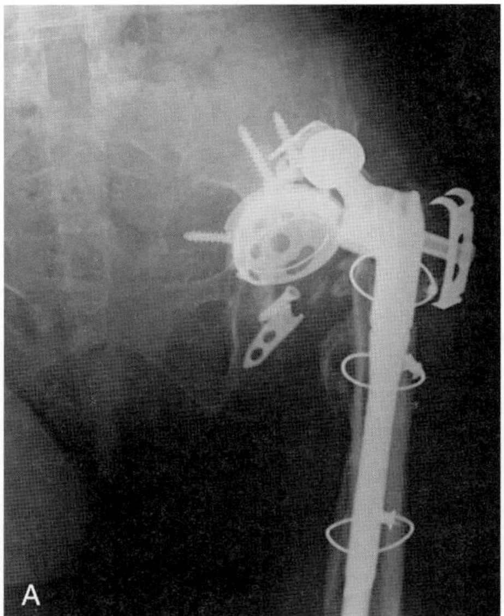

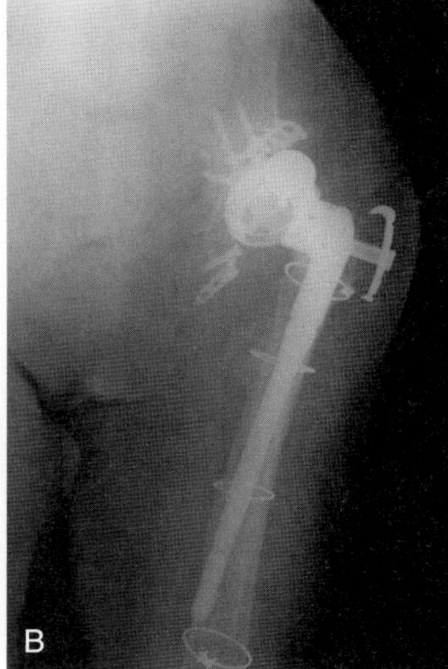

Figure 2 **A,** AP hip radiograph demonstrates a failed total hip arthroplasty with substantial shortening secondary to chronic dislocation. **B,** AP hip radiograph demonstrates a traction view used for preoperative planning of the hip center.

acetabular implant. If vascular structures are at risk, a preoperative evaluation by a vascular surgeon is warranted, and a retroperitoneal exposure may be required to free the intrapelvic structures before removal of the implant.

Contraindications

Absolute contraindications to the use of CTACs in patients with massive acetabular bone loss include persistent infection and the inability to obtain adequate prosthetic fixation because of severe acetabular bone deficiency. In the experience of the authors of this chapter, most failures have occurred in patients with a preoperative pelvic discontinuity in which large gaps (greater than 1 cm) are present between bony surfaces. The inclusion of locking screws in the design of CTACs has substantially improved clinical results in patients with pelvic discontinuity.

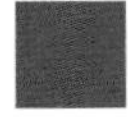

Alternative Treatments

Other methods for the management of these substantial defects include the use of large hemispheric cups with bulk structural allograft with or without column plating, off-the-shelf cup-cage constructs, oblong acetabular implants, and porous-coated or ultraporous metal jumbo acetabular implants with or without porous metal augments. A recent study showed that the costs of a CTAC and a cup-cage construct were equivalent.

Results

A paucity of evidence is available for review because of the rare need to use these custom implants (**Table 2**). Short-term and midterm results have been promising, with reported clinical success rates between 79% and 100%. In addition, radiographic healing of pelvic discontinuities has been reported in 81% to 97% of patients. Mechanical failures have been observed in only a small percentage of patients and appear to be associated with pelvic discontinuities without supplemental posterior column plate or locking screw fixation. The most commonly reported reason for revision surgery is recurrent instability requiring conversion to a constrained liner.

Table 2 Results of Revision Hip Arthroplasty With Custom Triflange Acetabular Cups

Authors (Year)	Number of Hips	Approach	Mean Patient Age in Years (Range)	Mean Follow-up in Years (Range)	Success Rate (%)[a]	Results
Christie et al (2001)	67	Posterior	59 (29-87)	4.5 (2-9)	100	No mechanical failures 15% dislocation rate 8% required revision for instability
Joshi et al (2002)	27	Triradiate transtrochanteric	68 (55-77)	5 (4-6)	100	No mechanical failures 3% required revision for instability 3% required revision for sciatic nerve palsy
Holt and Dennis (2004)	26	Extensile posterior or trochanteric osteotomy	68 (NA)	4.5 (2-7)	88.5	3% had mechanical failure 6% had radiographic loosening without revision 7.8% dislocation rate
DeBoer et al (2007)	20	Posterior	56 (30-77)	10 (7-13)	100	No mechanical failures 30% dislocation rate 25% required revision for instability 5% required revision for sciatica and loose ischial screws
Taunton et al (2012)	57	Posterior	61 (35-81)	5 (2-17)	84	1.8% had mechanical failure 21% dislocation rate 17.4% required revision for instability
Wind et al (2013)	19	Posterior	58 (42-79)	2.6 (1.3-4.9)	79	11% of implants were removed because of failure 16% had postoperative complications 26% dislocation rate 32% rate of secondary surgery for any reason
Berasi et al (2015)	24	Lateral	67 (47-85)	4.8 (2.3-9)	100	17% rate of revision for any reason 8% infection rate 8% had periprosthetic fracture No instability noted

NA = not available.

[a] Success is defined as no radiographic evidence of migration.

Adapted with permission from Johnson DR, Dennis DA, Kim RH: Acetabular revision: Rings, cages, and custom implants, in Berry DJ, Lieberman JR, eds: *Surgery of the Hip*. Philadelphia, PA, Elsevier Saunders, 2013, pp 1111-1122, and Christie MJ, DeBoer DK, Morrison JC: Acetabular revision: Triflange cups, in Lieberman JR, Berry DJ: *Advanced Reconstruction Hip*. Rosemont, IL, American Academy of Orthopaedic Surgeons, 2005, pp 367-374.

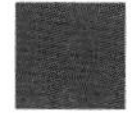

Techniques

Preoperative Planning

- An acrylic model of the hemipelvis or complete pelvis is created from the three-dimensional CT images (**Figure 3**).
- Cup orientation; hip center location; and the length, number, and position of screws are assessed. Locking screws are routinely incorporated into the CTAC design (**Figure 4**). The authors of this chapter prefer to use two rows of three iliac screws (six total) and a minimum of

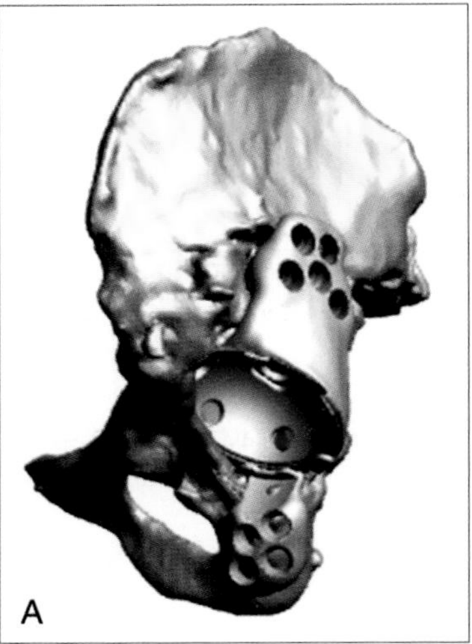

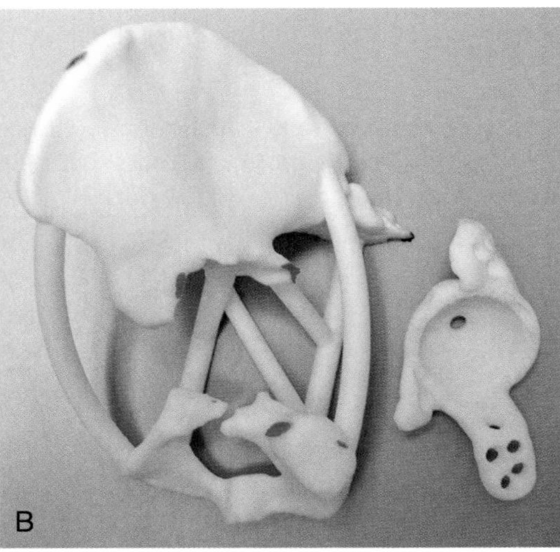

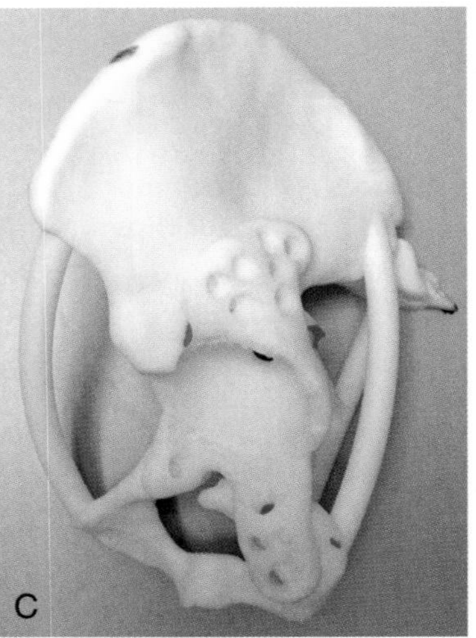

Figure 3 **A,** Three-dimensional CT reconstruction demonstrates a patient's hemipelvis with the proposed acetabular implant in place. The reconstruction is used in conjunction with rapid prototyping technology to design the custom triflange acetabular cup. **B,** Clinical photograph shows the acrylic models of the hemipelvis and acetabular implant generated based on the CT reconstruction. The model demonstrates massive acetabular bone loss. **C,** Clinical photograph shows the acrylic model of the hemipelvis with the model of the acetabular implant positioned in it.

four ischial screws. In the chapter authors' experience, fixation failure of ischial screws has been observed.

- It is critical to ensure that the superior aspect of the dome (cup) portion of the CTAC engages the inferior ridge of the remaining ilium. This design places compressive loads on the ilium and lessens shear stresses on the flange fixation screws.
- Multiple modifications are often necessary and may require extensive communication between the surgeon and the design engineer. This process may take up to 6 weeks to complete.
- In patients with pelvic discontinuity in whom a plate will be used for reduction, the CTAC must be designed to accommodate both the plate and the screws.
- Careful preoperative design of the CTAC is critical because intraoperative changes are not possible.

Setup/Exposure

- The authors of this chapter prefer to use an extensile posterolateral approach, although an extensile anterolateral or transtrochanteric approach may be used.
- The patient is placed in the lateral decubitus position.
- The patient is draped to allow as much exposure as possible for this extensile approach.
- If exposure for placement of the iliac flange of the CTAC would place the superior gluteal nerve at risk for traction injury, a trochanteric osteotomy is recommended to relieve tension on the superior gluteal nerve.
- Use of a trochanteric slide or standard greater trochanteric osteotomy facilitates exposure and hip dislocation and will protect the superior gluteal nerve from excessive tension during exposure of the ilium (**Figure 5**).
- Identification of the sciatic nerve before posterior dissection is imperative. In some patients, substantial scarring of the nerve may require neurolysis. If the surgical planes are difficult to identify, the nerve typically is identified either distally or proximally in preparation for neurolysis.
- Occasionally, release of the iliopsoas and/or gluteus maximus tendons is necessary to allow mobilization of the femoral implant and gain the necessary access to the acetabular region.

Instruments/Equipment/ Implants Required

- The acrylic model of the hemipelvis and the CTAC are sterilized preoperatively and used intraoperatively to help the surgeon understand pelvic orientation and as a trial model to assess implant position and fit.
- Length and position of the locking screws must be confirmed preoperatively on the basis of the preoperative plan.

Procedure

EVALUATION OF THE FEMORAL IMPLANT

- The femoral implant is assessed for signs of failure.
- The version angle should be noted because it may be a potential cause

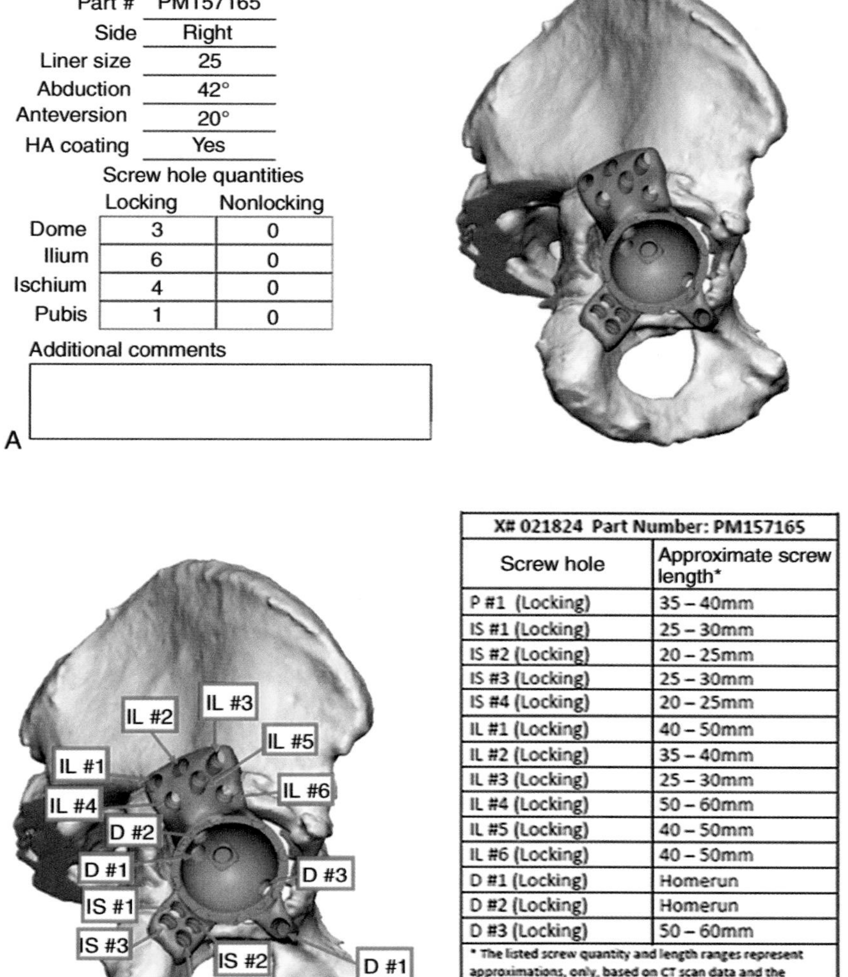

X# 021824 Part Number: PM157165	
Screw hole	Approximate screw length*
P #1 (Locking)	35 – 40mm
IS #1 (Locking)	25 – 30mm
IS #2 (Locking)	20 – 25mm
IS #3 (Locking)	25 – 30mm
IS #4 (Locking)	20 – 25mm
IL #1 (Locking)	40 – 50mm
IL #2 (Locking)	35 – 40mm
IL #3 (Locking)	25 – 30mm
IL #4 (Locking)	50 – 60mm
IL #5 (Locking)	40 – 50mm
IL #6 (Locking)	40 – 50mm
D #1 (Locking)	Homerun
D #2 (Locking)	Homerun
D #3 (Locking)	50 – 60mm

* The listed screw quantity and length ranges represent approximations, only, based on CT scan data and the implant design, and are not meant to replace the intraoperative judgement of the surgeon. Appropriate screw length and quantity must be determined intraoperatively based on patient anatomy.

Figure 4 **A,** Three-dimensional CT reconstruction (right) and list of the final design features (left) of a custom triflange acetabular cup for this particular patient show the preoperative flexibility in the design process. **B,** Schematic diagram of screw placement demonstrates the available options and lengths based on the patient's bone loss and the orientation of the custom triflange acetabular cup. D = dome, HA = hydroxyapatite, IL = iliac screw, IS = ischial screw, P = pubis.

of intraoperative instability requiring removal and revision.

ILIAC EXPOSURE

- Exposure of 3 to 5 cm is typically required to allow placement of the iliac flange of the CTAC.
- As previously discussed, the use of a trochanteric slide or other trochanteric osteotomy during the initial exposure can facilitate exposure of the ilium and decrease tension on the superior gluteal neurovascular pedicle.

ISCHIAL EXPOSURE

- Soft tissues are elevated as a sleeve.
- Keeping the hip in extension and the knee flexed will decrease the tension placed on the sciatic nerve.
- Occasionally, a subperiosteal release of the origin of the hamstring is necessary to facilitate exposure and placement of the ischial flange of the CTAC. This release is most commonly required in patients with a small pelvis to accommodate the placement of four or five ischial screws in the ischial flange.

ACETABULAR EXPOSURE

- Exposure of the acetabulum includes removal of the existing acetabular implant, cement, and membrane to facilitate placement of the CTAC.
- The pelvis is assessed for subtle discontinuity by means of application of traction or rotary torque with the use of bone tenacula placed on the upper and lower aspects of the acetabulum.
- Excess bone is carefully removed in accordance with the preoperative plan to shape the pelvis to accommodate the CTAC.

IMPLANTATION OF THE CTAC

- The acrylic model of the CTAC is initially inserted to assess fit and determine the easiest method of insertion. Occasionally, it may be necessary to remove additional small amounts of acetabular bone to ensure proper placement and seating of the implant.
- The iliac flange is most commonly placed first because this method places less tension on the superior gluteal neurovascular pedicle.
- Placement of the iliac flange is facilitated by translating the lower limb proximally with hip flexion and abduction, which relaxes the abductor musculature.
- The knee is flexed and the hip

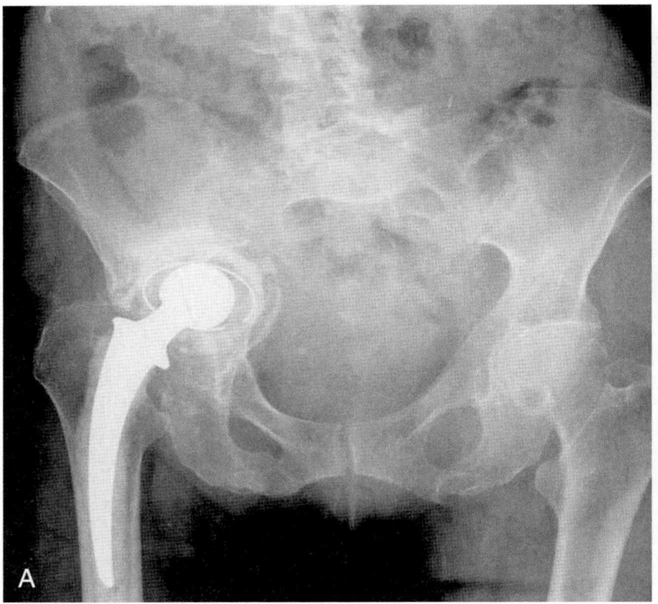

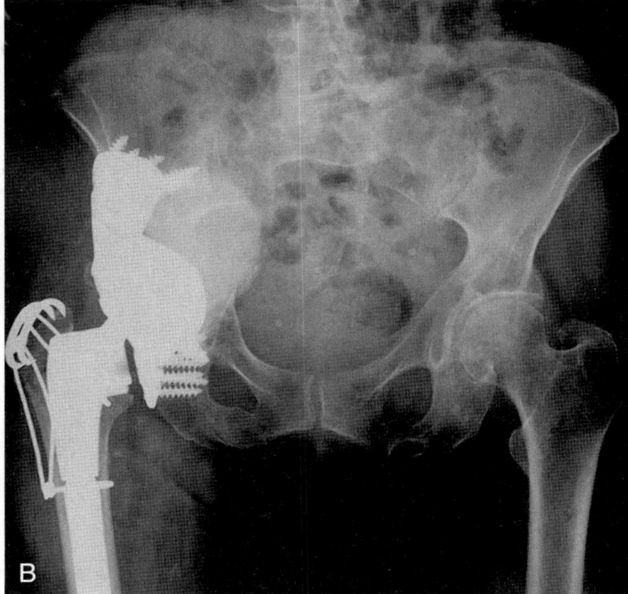

Figure 5 **A,** AP pelvic radiograph demonstrates substantial bone loss and associated protrusion of the femoral implant. **B,** Postoperative AP pelvic radiograph demonstrates placement of a custom triflange acetabular cup. A trochanteric osteotomy was performed to facilitate exposure of the joint and protection of the superior gluteal neurovascular bundle.

extended to relax the posterior soft tissues, facilitating rotation of the pubic and ischial flanges into position.

- The ischial flange is critically assessed for overhang to avoid irritation of the sciatic nerve.
- If necessary, the pelvic model that was created preoperatively is referenced after implantation to ensure that the fit of the implant is similar to the preoperative plan.
- The CTAC is assessed for motion. If the implant is placed appropriately, very little motion should be observed.

FIXATION OF THE CTAC

- One or two locking screws are placed in the ischial bone, which typically is weakened and often is osteolytic. The ischial screws are placed before the iliac screws to avoid superior migration of the implant.
- One or two locking screws are placed in the ilium to allow for provisional fixation.
- Additional screws are inserted to complete the fixation. The authors of this chapter recommend placement of at least four to six locking screws in the ischial bone. In patients with pelvic discontinuity, the CTAC may be placed with or without a planned reduction of the discontinuity.
- Reduction of the discontinuity is chosen if reduction improves bony support of the CTAC and brings the hemipelvic segments into closer contact, enhancing the probability of healing of the discontinuity. Bone grafting is considered in patients with residual defects.
- A disadvantage of reduction is the risk of not being able to obtain a complete reduction as a result of chronic discontinuity. Incomplete reduction results in the inability to properly seat the CTAC, which was designed to fit with the discontinuity properly reduced.
- The reduction technique involves securing the CTAC to the ilium with screw fixation. With a reduction maneuver, the shape of the implant causes the inferior hemipelvis to rotate into position against the implant, which reduces the discontinuity.
- After implantation, a trial reduction is performed.
- An intraoperative AP pelvic radiograph is obtained to ensure adequate positioning of the implant and assess screw lengths.
- Hip stability and limb lengths are assessed.
- If a trochanteric osteotomy or trochanteric slide osteotomy was done, the fragment is repaired with cables, a hook plate, or a claw plate.

Wound Closure

- Closure of the remaining viable posterior capsule structures is attempted.
- The authors of this chapter place a deep subfascial drain in an attempt to avoid postoperative hematoma.
- The fascia is closed with a nonabsorbable suture.

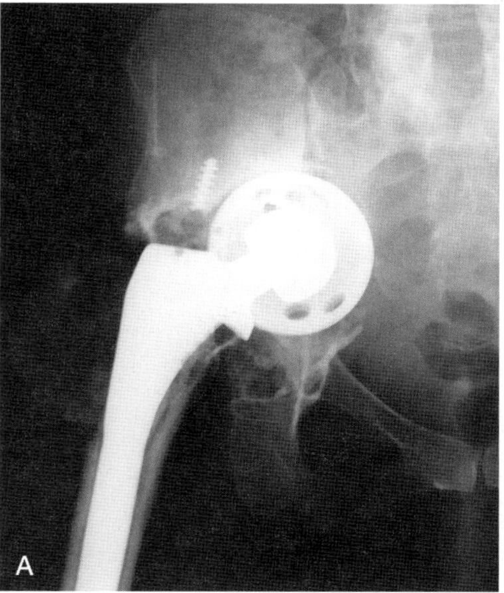

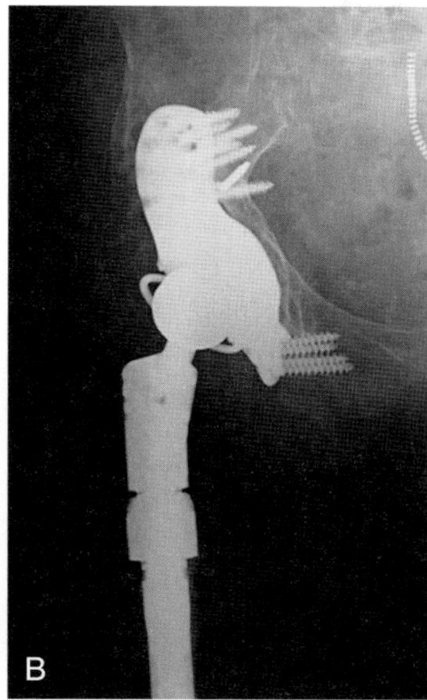

Figure 6 **A,** Preoperative AP radiograph of a right hip demonstrates a failed total hip arthroplasty with massive associated bone loss. **B,** Postoperative AP radiograph obtained 12 years after acetabular reconstruction with a custom triflange acetabular cup demonstrates stable fixation.

- The subcuticular layer is closed with an absorbable suture.
- Skin closure is performed with staples or a nonabsorbable suture.
- Judicious use of vacuum-assisted wound closure may be considered in patients at increased risk for wound complications.

Postoperative Regimen

Risk stratification is used to select an appropriate postoperative anticoagulation strategy. Careful monitoring in the acute period is imperative to avoid a thrombotic event or hematoma formation. The authors of this chapter typically recommend toe-touch weight bearing for 1 to 2 months postoperatively. Progression to partial weight bearing with the assistance of bilateral ambulatory aids continues for another 1 to 2 months. Full weight bearing may begin in most patients 3 to 4 months postoperatively depending on findings from the clinical examination and serial radiographs (**Figure 6**). In patients with pelvic discontinuity, weight-bearing restrictions may be extended until the surgeon is convinced that the posterior column has been reconstituted. A hip abduction orthosis is used for 6 weeks postoperatively in patients thought to be at high risk for dislocation. A hip abduction orthosis also may be used for protection in patients in whom trochanteric osteotomy was performed for exposure.

Avoiding Pitfalls and Complications

Instability, the most common complication, is multifactorial in origin and has an incidence of 3% to 30%. Careful preoperative design of the CTAC is critical to ensure appropriate cup inclination, anteversion, and hip center position. Many patients requiring implantation of a CTAC have associated abductor insufficiency secondary to multiple surgical procedures or insufficiency of the superior gluteal nerve, trochanteric nonunion, or capsular insufficiency, which may explain the higher rates of dislocation. If instability is noted intraoperatively, a thorough assessment is performed to determine any correctable causes of the instability. Often, high-wall, face-changing, or constrained polyethylene liners and larger femoral head diameters are required. If the abductor mechanism is intact, trochanteric advancement can be helpful. If instability is noted postoperatively in a previously stable hip, the possibility of infection in these high-risk patients must be considered.

Sciatic nerve injury occurs in a small percentage of patients. Traction injury is more common than direct injury to the nerve. The extremity should be positioned with the hip in extension and the knee in flexion to decrease tension on the nerve during posterior dissection and placement of the ischial flange. The ischial flange must be properly designed and positioned to avoid overhang of the ischium and subsequent irritation of the sciatic nerve. Careful preoperative assessment is mandatory because the hip center may be medialized with substantial superior migration. Restoring the hip center of rotation in these patients will functionally lengthen the affected limb and may place the nerve at risk after the hip is reduced to its native position. In selected patients, it may be necessary to remove and revise a well-fixed femoral stem to shorten the femur and achieve an acceptable limb length without excessive nerve tension. Intraoperative neurologic monitoring may be used during exposure; however, the authors of this chapter consider the previously mentioned techniques to be sufficient and do not use intraoperative monitoring. After the trial implants are in place, an intraoperative straight leg raise test is performed to assess for excessive tension on the sciatic nerve.

Mechanical failure of the reconstruction can occur. The most common reasons for mechanical problems are failure to obtain mechanical stability of the CTAC intraoperatively and failure to stabilize a pelvic discontinuity. If motion is detected at the time of implantation of the CTAC, failure is imminent. Depending on the patient's specific presentation, a variety of methods can be used to improve implant fixation. Options for enhancement of fixation include use of an increased number of screws, addition of locking screws if not already included in the design, cement augmentation of screws placed into osteolytic bone, application of hydroxyapatite to the CTAC, and posterior column plating of pelvic discontinuities. In patients with pelvic discontinuity, posterior column plating and bone grafting can be considered if the posterior column bone stock allows. The authors of this chapter have used this technique less frequently since the addition of flange locking screws to the CTAC design. As noted, a critical characteristic of the implant design is the creation of a central dome that contacts the remaining ilium superiorly to reduce the shear on the flange fixation screws. This iliac shelf provides a sound structure to prevent further superior migration of the implant even in patients with massive acetabular bone loss or pelvic discontinuity.

Bibliography

Berasi CC IV, Berend KR, Adams JB, Ruh EL, Lombardi AV Jr: Are custom triflange acetabular components effective for reconstruction of catastrophic bone loss? *Clin Orthop Relat Res* 2015;473(2):528-535.

Christie MJ, Barrington SA, Brinson MF, Ruhling ME, DeBoer DK: Bridging massive acetabular defects with the triflange cup: 2- to 9-year results. *Clin Orthop Relat Res* 2001;(393):216-227.

D'Antonio JA, Capello WN, Borden LS, et al: Classification and management of acetabular abnormalities in total hip arthroplasty. *Clin Orthop Relat Res* 1989;(243):126-137.

DeBoer DK, Christie MJ, Brinson MF, Morrison JC: Revision total hip arthroplasty for pelvic discontinuity. *J Bone Joint Surg Am* 2007;89(4):835-840.

Glassman AH, Engh CA, Bobyn JD: A technique of extensile exposure for total hip arthroplasty. *J Arthroplasty* 1987;2(1):11-21.

Holt GE, Dennis DA: Use of custom triflanged acetabular components in revision total hip arthroplasty. *Clin Orthop Relat Res* 2004;(429):209-214.

Joshi AB, Lee J, Christensen C: Results for a custom acetabular component for acetabular deficiency. *J Arthroplasty* 2002;17(5):643-648.

Paprosky WG, Perona PG, Lawrence JM: Acetabular defect classification and surgical reconstruction in revision arthroplasty: A 6-year follow-up evaluation. *J Arthroplasty* 1994;9(1):33-44.

Taunton MJ, Fehring TK, Edwards P, Bernasek T, Holt GE, Christie MJ: Pelvic discontinuity treated with custom triflange component: A reliable option. *Clin Orthop Relat Res* 2012;470(2):428-434.

Wind MA Jr, Swank ML, Sorger JI: Short-term results of a custom triflange acetabular component for massive acetabular bone loss in revision THA. *Orthopedics* 2013;36(3):e260-e265.

Chapter 53
Acetabular Revision With Cup-Cage Constructs

James A. Browne, MD
David G. Lewallen, MD

Indications

In most acetabular reconstructions, a noncemented hemispheric socket with screw fixation provides acceptable initial stability and contact with host bone. These implants are successful in most patients who have supportive host bone and a reliable ingrowth surface. However, there are limitations to the use of hemispheric porous-coated implants. It may not be possible to achieve adequate stability and host bone contact in patients with massive bone loss, pelvic discontinuity, or pathologic bone. Use of a standard hemispheric socket will have a high anticipated failure rate in such patients.

In the early and mid 1990s, many surgeons began using large anti-protrusio cages in patients with massive bone loss, pelvic discontinuity, or pathologic bone. Although these cages often were successful in attaining initial stability, fracture and early loosening occurred in patients in whom the construct was not adequately supported by graft or host bone. In addition, these early devices had no potential for osseointegration, and the lack of biologic fixation often resulted in mechanical failure in the mid- to long-term.

The use of a tantalum cup-cage construct was first reported in 2005. This construct adds biologic fixation to a simple cage in an effort to secure a highly porous, hemispheric metal implant against the maximum amount of native host bone possible and supplement this fixation with a cage (**Figure 1**). After the cup is placed and stabilized with screws, the cage is placed into the socket. The cage is fixed to the ilium with screws and to the ischium through the inferior flange. The polyethylene liner is cemented into the cup-cage construct, which secures the liner and unitizes the cup and cage. The well-fixed cage provides initial stability and offloads the cup to promote bone ingrowth. The stability and offloading provided also allow remodeling of morcellized graft behind the socket. One clear advantage of this technique compared with a traditional cage is the potential for biologic fixation; after ingrowth into the porous tantalum cup has occurred, the cage becomes unnecessary and is unlikely to fail mechanically as a result of fatigue.

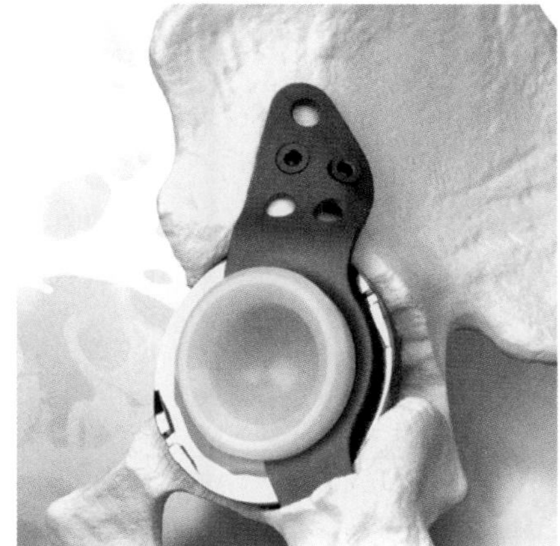

Figure 1 Photograph shows a porous tantalum cup-cage construct with a cemented polyethylene liner. (Courtesy of Zimmer Biomet.)

The authors of this chapter use cup-cage constructs in patients who have severe bone loss with or without pelvic discontinuity (Paprosky type IIIA and IIIB deficiencies), in whom adequate stability and cup-host bone contact cannot be achieved with a hemispheric socket (**Figure 2**). Midterm success also has been achieved with this construct in patients with destructive nonprimary periacetabular tumors (**Figure 3**), in patients with prior pelvic irradiation, and for reconstruction of the native acetabulum after a fracture. Although preoperative planning is important in anticipating the need for a cup-cage construct, the final determination on whether to use this technique can be made intraoperatively.

Dr. Browne or an immediate family member serves as a paid consultant to Biocomposites, DJO Global, and Ethicon. Dr. Lewallen or an immediate family member has received royalties from Stryker, Pipeline Biomedical Holdings, and Zimmer; is a member of a speakers' bureau or has made paid presentations on behalf of Zimmer; serves as a paid consultant to Pipeline Biomedical Holdings and Zimmer; serves as an unpaid consultant to and has stock or stock options held in Ketai Medical Devices; and serves as a board member, owner, officer, or committee member of the American Joint Replacement Registry and the Orthopaedic Research and Education Foundation.

Contraindications

The use of a cup-cage construct is not necessary if simpler methods can be used to achieve a satisfactory result. The authors of this chapter reserve this technique for patients in whom routine noncemented sockets will be unreliable. Typically, patients who have a stable hemispheric cup and greater than 50% cup-host bone contact do not need a cage. As with any revision surgery, the presence of active infection is a relative contraindication to prosthetic reconstruction. Finally, it may be impossible to achieve adequate screw fixation through the cage in patients who have severe bone loss of the ilium and ischium, and alternative methods may be necessary to achieve stability.

Alternative Treatments

The two most suitable alternative treatments to the cup-cage construct are the anti-protrusio cage and the custom triflange cup. The main limitations to traditional rings and anti-protrusio cages were described previously. Although midterm results of cages have been generally satisfactory, the lack of biologic fixation in these constructs resulted in a high rate of long-term failure in many series because of mechanical failure and loosening. Given the concerns for long-term fixation, anti-protrusio cages seem best suited for elderly patients.

The triflange cup is similar to the cup-cage in that the goal is to achieve biologic fixation to the pelvis. In essence, the triflange cup is a monoblock version of the cup-cage that allows bridging of acetabular defects and the potential for rigid fixation in the ilium, ischium, and pubis. However, unlike the cup-cage construct, triflange

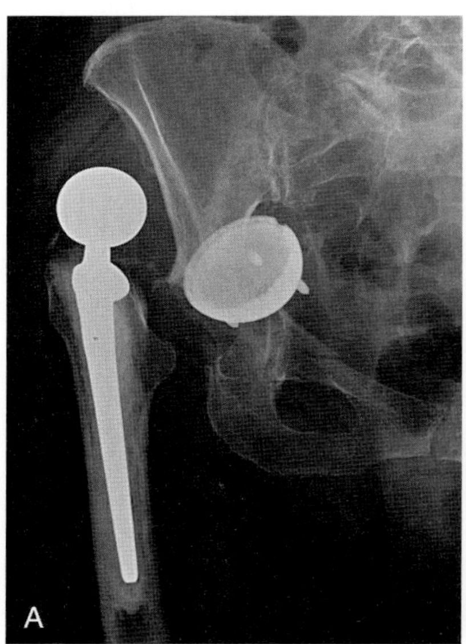

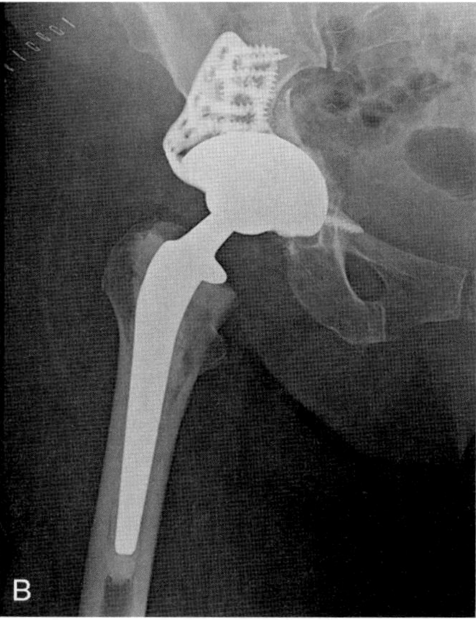

Figure 2 **A,** Preoperative AP radiograph of the right hip in a patient who sustained periacetabular fracture and resulting pelvic discontinuity 1 month after undergoing primary total hip arthroplasty. **B,** Postoperative AP radiograph obtained after cup-cage reconstruction. At the time of revision, the posterior column was found to be severely comminuted and the bone was osteoporotic.

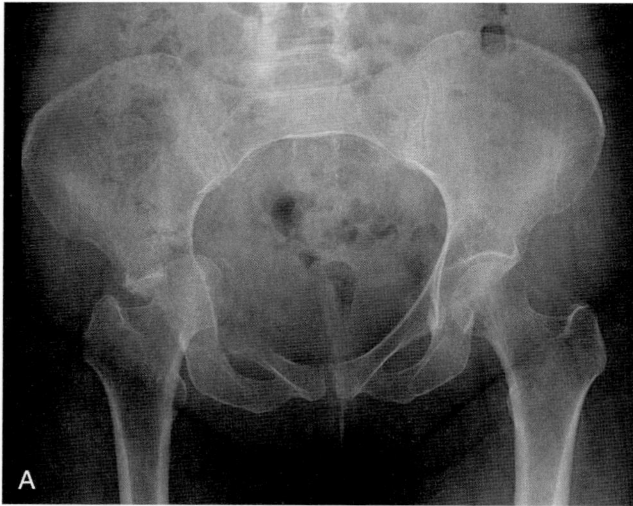

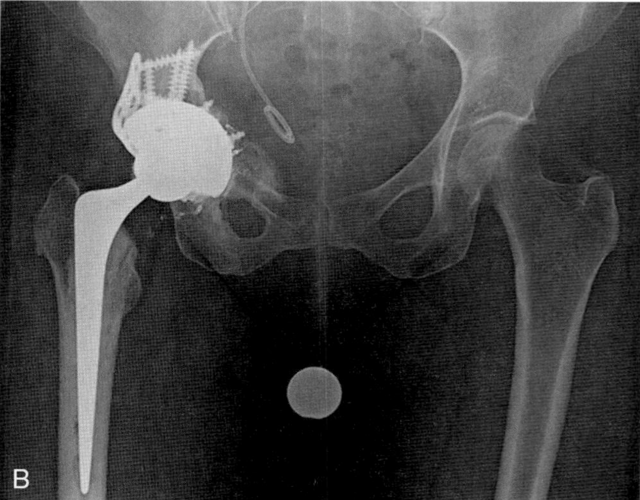

Figure 3 Preoperative (**A**) and 1-year postoperative (**B**) AP pelvic radiographs of a patient who underwent cup-cage reconstruction to manage a pathologic acetabular fracture in the right hip secondary to metastatic endometrial adenocarcinoma.

implants are customized to match an individual patient based on a model generated from a preoperative CT. Advantages of this custom technique include optimization of cup-host bone contact and the potential for biologic ingrowth into the porous- or hydroxyapatite-coated flanges. Disadvantages include the time required to fabricate the custom implant, lack of intraoperative flexibility, and overall cost.

Results

The cup-cage construct is a relatively new technique that has gained in popularity in the past decade. Early and midterm results have been favorable, although long-term follow-up studies are lacking (**Table 1**). Midterm reports have suggested better improvements in outcome compared with conventional cages in patients who have pelvic discontinuity. This construct also has shown promise with difficult reconstructive scenarios including destructive nonprimary periacetabular tumors, previous pelvic irradiation, and acetabular fractures in elderly patients.

Technique

Setup/Exposure

- As in all complex acetabular reconstructions, adequate exposure is necessary for a successful outcome.
- Although any approach that allows visualization of the ilium, pubis, and ischium may be used, selection of approach depends on the status of the femoral implant, bone loss, previous exposures, and surgeon experience and training.
- The posterior approach provides good exposure and is extensile.
- If a lateral transgluteal approach is used, care must be taken to avoid excessive proximal splitting of the gluteus medius muscle to prevent damage to the superior gluteal nerve.
- Femoral osteotomies can further increase exposure. Osteotomy options include trochanteric slide, extended trochanteric, or Wagner.

Instruments/Equipment/Implants Required

- The cup-cage reconstruction uses a revision porous tantalum hemispheric shell in conjunction with an ilioischial cage.
- A metal-cutting burr tip can be helpful in creating additional screw holes through the tantalum cup to enhance screw fixation.
- Different cages are available from different manufacturers.
- The cage should be sized to fit within the cup; cages manufactured from titanium are preferred because they can be contoured to match the patient's anatomy.
- Multiple screw holes in the proximal flange are necessary to achieve fixation to the lateral ilium; different flange lengths are available.
- The ischial flange of the cage may be fixed to the lateral ischium with screws or driven into the ischium through a slot. Occasionally, the ischial flange may be removed with a metal-cutting burr if it is not necessary for stability.
- Cement is necessary to attach the cage to the cup and secure the polyethylene liner into the construct.

Procedure

- After adequate exposure has been achieved and any previous implants removed, fibrous tissue and debris are cleared from the acetabulum.
- The acetabular cavity is gently reamed to accept the largest porous tantalum shell allowed by the local anatomy; shell size typically is limited by the anteroposterior dimension of the acetabulum.
- The cup should be large enough to bridge the ilium to the ischium.
- A trial fenestrated cup is placed into the cavity to help assess cup-host bone contact and bone deficiencies.
- Morcellized autograft or allograft is packed into cavitary defects, whereas modular metal augments may be used in the setting of residual uncontained bone defects.
- The hemispheric cup is placed against as much native host bone as possible.
- The tantalum revision shells have a hemi-ellipsoid geometry with an equatorial diameter 2 mm larger than the polar diameter, which allows an initial 2-mm press-fit with line-to-line reaming.
- Multiple screws are placed through the cup.
- A metal-cutting burr may be used to create additional screw holes in the revision tantalum shell for added fixation.
- Bone wax is placed over screw heads before cementation of the liner to aid in later screw removal should it be necessary in the future.
- If screw fixation or cup-host bone contact is not adequate, then a cage is placed over the top of the cup external to the hemispheric socket (**Figure 4, A**).
- Typically, the cage engages the ischium and ilium. However, in some patients the ischial flange is cut off and screws are placed only into the ilium.
- If used, the ischial notch can be identified by palpation.
- Care is taken to avoid injury to the sciatic nerve during dissection.
- A small osteotome is used to initiate a slot in the ischium to accept the inferior flange of the cage.
- The gluteus minimus and medius muscles must be carefully elevated off the ilium to allow placement of the superior flange.
- A cage provisional may be used to

Table 1 Results of Cup-Cage Reconstructive Hip Surgery for Various Indications

Authors (Year)	Number of Cup-Cage Reconstructions	Indication for Cup-Cage	Mean Patient Age in Years (Range)	Mean Follow-up in Months (Range)	Success Rate (%)	Results
Kosashvili et al (2009)	26	Pelvic discontinuity	64.9 (44-84)	44.6 (24-68)	88.5	23 hips had no clinical or radiographic evidence of loosening Results of 3 hips unknown
Chana-Rodriguez et al (2012)	6	Elderly patients with acetabular fractures	77 (70-85)	25 (24-26)	100	Fractures healed and morcellized graft incorporated
Joglekar et al (2012)[a]	3	Pelvic irradiation for malignancy	71 (57-89)	Minimum, 60	100	No radiographic signs of loosening, even in irradiated bone
Khan et al (2012)	7	Metastatic acetabular tumors	60 (22-80)[b]	56 (26-85)[c]	100	No loosening or implant migration
Rogers et al (2012)[d]	42	Chronic pelvic discontinuity	67.5 (27-88)	35 (24-93)	90.5	4 hips were revised: 2 for instability and 2 for failed reconstruction 86.3% 8-yr survivorship rate
Tangsataporn et al (2013)[e]	7	Failed acetabular reinforcement ring and anti-protrusio cages	61 (27-80)	57 (24-209)	71	2 failures occurred: 1 hip was re-revised and at the time of study publication, 1 hip was awaiting rerevision to manage loosening Use of tantalum constructs provided better results compared with revising to a second acetabular reinforcement ring
Abolghasemian et al (2014)	26	Pelvic discontinuity	65 (44-84)	82 (12-113)	85	4 hips failed because of septic or aseptic loosening 7-yr survivorship rate of 87.2% with a cup-cage construct compared with only 49.9% with a traditional cage

[a] Patient age and follow-up based on original cohort of 29 patients.
[b] Based on original cohort of 20 patients.
[c] Based on the nine surviving patients.
[d] Patient age and follow-up based on original cohort of 62 patients.
[e] Patient age and follow-up based on original cohort of 33 patients.

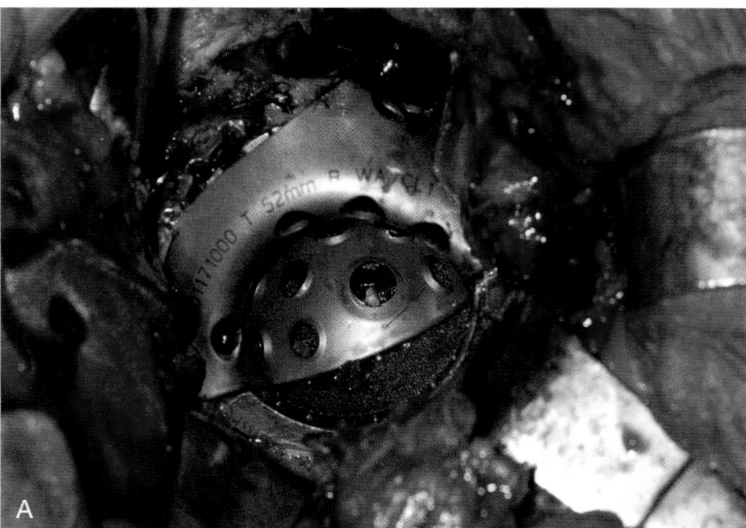

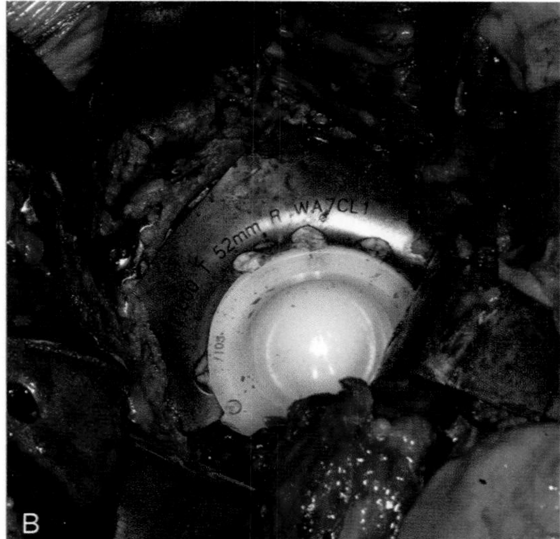

Figure 4 **A,** Intraoperative photograph shows a cage placed into a porous tantalum revision acetabular shell. **B,** Intraoperative photograph shows the polyethylene liner cemented into the cup-cage construct to unitize the cage and cup.

size and contour the construct to achieve optimal fit.

- After the final cage has been contoured, it is implanted into the ilium first with the aid of a spiked ball-pusher with the superior flange subsequently positioned against the lateral portion of the ilium. The cage need not be completely bottomed out against the cup.
- The superior flange is secured to the ilium with multiple screws; this typically provides excellent fixation. At least two bicortical screws are recommended, but four to six screws typically are used.
- The presence of the cage inside the cup reduces the available space for the polyethylene liner. Trials are used to assess the remaining space and select the appropriate-size outer diameter for the polyethylene liner. Revision shell liners designed for cementation are available.
- Alternatively, a burr can be used to roughen the backside of a standard polyethylene liner to ensure good cement fixation.
- Bone wax is placed over the screw heads before cementation to aid in screw removal, should that be required at a later time.
- Cement has been shown to be a durable locking mechanism for the polyethylene liner.
- Bone cement of a doughlike consistency is applied into the dome of the cup-cage and finger-packed to ensure the cement fills the gaps between the cage and cup.
- The polyethylene liner is inserted into the desired position, and the cement is pressurized (**Figure 4, B**).
- Minor adjustments can be made to the version and inclination of the polyethylene liner if cementing, although the surgeon must ensure that the liner is well seated within the cup-cage.
- The cement should interdigitate through the holes in the cup and cage to unitize the construct and prevent motion between the cup and cage.

Wound Closure

- Excess cement is removed before closure.
- Wound closure is performed in a routine manner.

Postoperative Regimen

Patients are restricted to toe-touch weight bearing for 6 weeks postoperatively. A hip abduction brace may be worn during this time. Patients are advanced to partial weight bearing at 6 weeks postoperatively and then to full weight bearing by 12 weeks postoperatively.

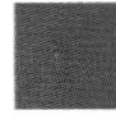

Avoiding Pitfalls and Complications

Cup-cage constructs are used in patients who have challenging reconstructive problems. As with all acetabular revisions, instability is a concern. Dislocation rates of up to 15% have been reported with cup-cage constructions. Carefully mating the cage with the cup to maximize the outer diameter of the cemented polyethylene liner permits the use of larger diameter femoral heads. It may be necessary to revise the femoral implant as well to provide the appropriate combined anteversion and abductor tension. A constrained liner should be considered if the abductors are deficient.

Care also must be taken to avoid neurovascular injury. Careful and adequate exposure reduces the risk for injury. Sciatic nerve injury is a risk if using the inferior flange, and care should be taken to slot the flange into the ischium to keep the flange well away from the nerve. Exposure of the iliac wing can damage the superior gluteal nerve and artery. Care also should be taken to avoid the internal iliac and obturator vessels when placing screws through the superior flange of the cage.

The long-term success of the cup-cage construct depends on biologic fixation into the porous metal hemisphere. For this to occur, the cup must be in contact with host bone. The best possible press-fit against host bone should be attained. Excessive allograft behind the cup must be avoided because it can prevent seating against host bone. Screw fixation through the cup also is critical; even in patients who have massive bone loss, it is typically possible to place at least two screws with good purchase in the dome or posterior column. Additional fixation medially or inferiorly into the ischium and/or pubis also should be attempted if possible. Use of a metal-cutting burr with the revision shell is advantageous because the surgeon can create screw holes where host bone remains in order to achieve maximal screw fixation. The surgeon is not constrained by the hole position provided by the manufacturer.

Bibliography

Abolghasemian M, Tangsaraporn S, Drexler M, et al: The challenge of pelvic discontinuity: Cup-cage reconstruction does better than conventional cages in mid-term. *Bone Joint J* 2014;96-B(2):195-200.

Chana-Rodríguez F, Villanueva-Martínez M, Rojo-Manaute J, Sanz-Ruíz P, Vaquero-Martín J: Cup-cage construct for acute fractures of the acetabulum, re-defining indications. *Injury* 2012;43(suppl 2):S28-S32.

Hanssen AD, Lewallen DG: Modular acetabular augments: Composite void fillers. *Orthopedics* 2005;28(9):971-972.

Joglekar SB, Rose PS, Lewallen DG, Sim FH: Tantalum acetabular cups provide secure fixation in THA after pelvic irradiation at minimum 5-year followup. *Clin Orthop Relat Res* 2012;470(11):3041-3047.

Khan FA, Rose PS, Yanagisawa M, Lewallen DG, Sim FH: Surgical technique: Porous tantalum reconstruction for destructive nonprimary periacetabular tumors. *Clin Orthop Relat Res* 2012;470(2):594-601.

Kosashvili Y, Backstein D, Safir O, Lakstein D, Gross AE: Acetabular revision using an anti-protrusion (ilio-ischial) cage and trabecular metal acetabular component for severe acetabular bone loss associated with pelvic discontinuity. *J Bone Joint Surg Br* 2009;91(7):870-876.

Petrie J, Sassoon A, Haidukewych GJ: Pelvic discontinuity: Current solutions. *Bone Joint J* 2013;95-B(11 suppl A):109-113.

Rogers BA, Whittingham-Jones PM, Mitchell PA, Safir OA, Bircher MD, Gross AE: The reconstruction of periprosthetic pelvic discontinuity. *J Arthroplasty* 2012;27(8):1499-1506.e1.

Sheth NP, Nelson CL, Springer BD, Fehring TK, Paprosky WG: Acetabular bone loss in revision total hip arthroplasty: Evaluation and management. *J Am Acad Orthop Surg* 2013;21(3):128-139.

Tangsataporn S, Abolghasemian M, Kuzyk PR, Backstein DJ, Safir OA, Gross AE: Salvaged failed roof rings and antiprotrusion cages: Surgical options and implant survival. *Hip Int* 2013;23(2):166-172.

Chapter 54
Pelvic Discontinuity

Jeremy M. Gililland, MD
Robert B. Jones, MD
Christopher E. Pelt, MD
Christopher L. Peters, MD

Indications

Pelvic discontinuity is the loss of structural continuity between the ileum and ischiopubic portions of the innominate bone or hemipelvis. Typically, this condition occurs in patients in whom acetabular bone is compromised secondary to osteolysis around a failed acetabular component, secondary to acetabular component loosening and/or migration, or as the result of multiple revisions. In addition, iatrogenic discontinuity can occur in revision hip surgery during either implant removal or revision cup placement, or as a result of an acute acetabular fracture in elderly patients.

As more total hip arthroplasties are performed, and in younger patients, surgeons will increasingly be required to address severe periacetabular bone loss in repeat revisions. Historically, pelvic discontinuity was managed with bone graft or bulk allograft and then stabilized with a revision acetabular component. However, the use of a standard multihole hemispheric acetabular component in a patient who has pelvic discontinuity has not produced acceptable results. Current revision strategies prioritize bridging of the ileum to the ischiopubic segment with highly porous ingrowth materials or custom triflange implants, with augmentation of bone healing potential. Typically, this is accomplished with bone graft substitutes with osteoconductive and osteogenic properties. Successful results rely not only on rigid internal fixation but also on restoration or augmentation of biologic healing potential.

The literature on management of pelvic discontinuity consists of limited numbers of relatively small case series. To achieve pelvic and acetabular implant stability, the intervention selected must adequately address the amount of associated bone loss. Stability is essential because a porous metal implant can be successful only if it is adequately stabilized against host bone to allow ingrowth to occur. Excessive motion (greater than approximately 300 μ) at the bone-implant interface can allow the formation of fibrous tissue, which can lead to eventual failure of the reconstruction.

Preoperative planning is crucial to successful outcome. A complete plain radiographic series including AP, lateral, and oblique pelvic views should be obtained to identify displacement as well as any rotation of the ischiopubic segment. CT scans, often with three-dimensional (3D) reconstructions, help accurately characterize bone loss and pelvic structural integrity (**Figure 1**) and are necessary if custom triflange implants are being considered.

Contraindications

Major reconstructive surgery is contraindicated in patients who have substantial systemic health concerns, local or systemic sepsis, or insufficient bone stock for implant stability or healing.

Dr. Gililland or an immediate family member serves as an unpaid consultant to and has stock or stock options held in OrthoGrid, and has received research or institutional support from Angiotech and Biomet. Dr. Pelt or an immediate family member is a member of a speakers' bureau or has made paid presentations on behalf of, serves as a paid consultant to, and has received research or institutional support from Biomet, and serves as a board member, owner, officer, or committee member of the American Academy of Orthopaedic Surgeons and the American Association of Hip and Knee Surgeons. Dr. Peters or an immediate family member has received royalties from, is a member of a speakers' bureau or has made paid presentations on behalf of, and serves as a paid consultant to Biomet, and serves as a board member, owner, officer, or committee member of the American Academy of Orthopaedic Surgeons and the American Association of Hip and Knee Surgeons. Neither Dr. Jones nor any immediate family member has received anything of value from or has stock or stock options held in a commercial company or institution related directly or indirectly to the subject of this chapter.

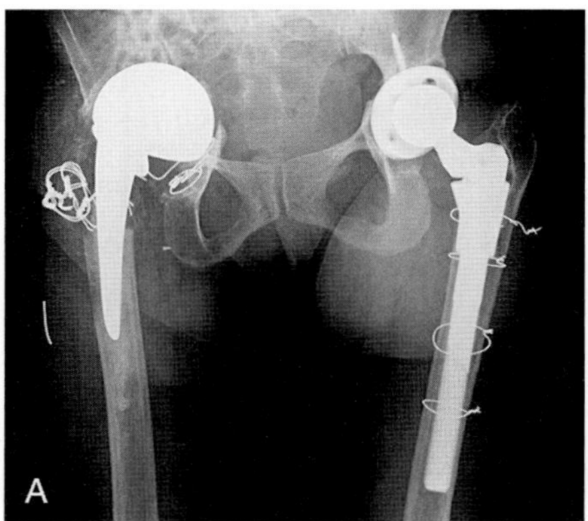

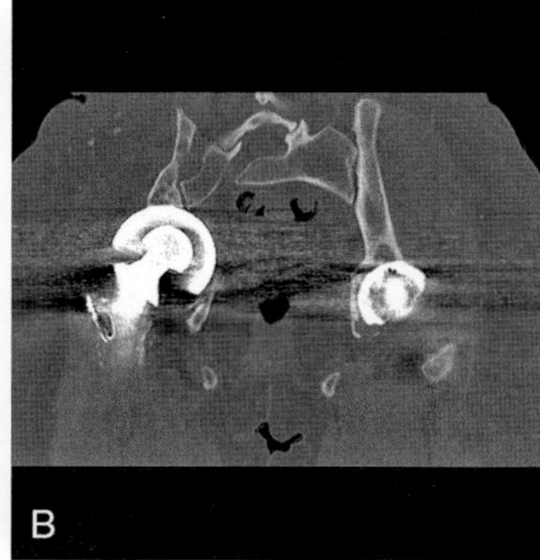

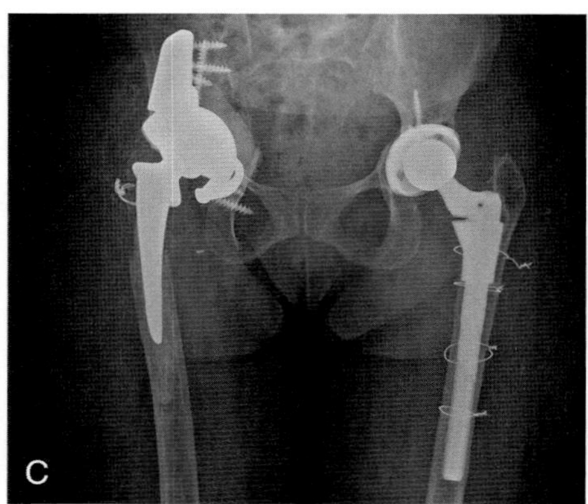

Figure 1 AP pelvic radiograph (**A**) and pelvic CT scan (**B**) demonstrate features of discontinuity in a right hip, including a visible fracture line through the anterior and posterior columns, medial translation of the inferior hemipelvis, and rotation of the inferior hemipelvis as noted by asymmetry of the obturator rings. **C,** AP radiograph obtained after management of discontinuity with a distraction technique using a large porous implant and superior and inferior porous augments.

Alternative Treatments

A variety of surgical procedures exist for managing pelvic discontinuity. Pelvic open reduction and internal fixation with allograft augmentation, cemented and noncemented acetabular component placement, cage reconstruction constructs, custom triflange implants, and jumbo porous metal implants with or without modular augments has been described. Recently, a distraction technique with porous metal implants that can achieve both initial stability and long-term biologic fixation was described. Additional biomechanical stability can be conferred to the reconstruction with additional anterior column fixation. A Girdlestone resection arthroplasty is a pain-relieving option in the most severe cases of discontinuity in elderly patients with low activity demands.

Results

The main objective in surgical management of pelvic discontinuity is to effectively bridge the discontinuity and gain component ingrowth into the ileum and ischiopubic segment. Ideally, component and innominate bone stability will be followed by bony healing of the discontinuity, particularly if biologic supplementation to enhance bone healing is used. The available data are composed of small numbers of patients reported on in larger studies on acetabular revision (**Table 1**). Even without high-powered comparison studies, some conclusions can be drawn. Pelvic discontinuity is a negative prognostic factor for a successful outcome irrespective of the type of reconstructive technique used. Some techniques clearly produce poor results, such as noncemented acetabular components with simple screw augmentation, cemented cup fixation without grafting (even with plate stabilization), and noncemented hemispheric cups with extensive grafting (with or without plates or cages).

Discontinuity associated with minor acetabular bone defects (typically more acute fractures associated with component removal or placement) can be managed by means of posterior column plating, bone grafting, and placement of a noncemented acetabular revision cup with screw augmentation. In these patients, healing of the discontinuity typically ensues when compression can be applied across the discontinuity and biologically capable bone is present.

Isolated large hemispheric jumbo cup placement is appropriate only in patients in whom greater than 50% contact exists between host bone and the acetabular implant. In patients with little available rim support and less than 50% bone-implant contact, augmentation is necessary for implant stability. Structural allografts alone do not reliably deliver long-term stability to either cemented or noncemented acetabular implants, and porous metal augments are increasingly used instead. Porous metal augments can assist in filling bony defects to provide pelvic fixation and more predictable stability of the acetabular implant. Additionally, acetabular reconstruction cages can provide added initial construct stability to foster ingrowth of a noncemented cup in a cup-cage combination (**Figures 2** and **3**). When using the cup-cage technique, it is important for the surgeon to understand that the underlying porous acetabular component is being used more like a bulk augment to bridge the discontinuous defect and the acetabular liner is cemented into the appropriate position into the overlying cage. Because of this, it is necessary to place the underlying acetabular component more vertical and retroverted than typical to facilitate proper placement of the overlying cage.

Table 1 Results of Revision Hip Surgery for Acetabular Discontinuity

Authors (Year)	Number of Hips	Reconstruction Type	Mean Patient Age in Years (Range)	Mean Follow-up in Years (Range)	Success Rate (%)[a]	Results
Berry et al (1999)[b]	27	Anti-protrusio cage, posterior plating, cemented or noncemented cup, some bulk allograft	61 (38-80)	3 (0.2-7)	85	4 hips underwent rerevision for aseptic loosening Another 5 hips underwent rerevision for instability (4) or deep infection (1)
Stiehl et al (2000)[c]	10	Bulk allograft, noncemented cup, posterior plating	73 (53-81)	7 (3.4-11)	80	Extensile triradiate approach was used in 9 hips, and posterior approach was used in 1 hip 40% dislocation rate (4 hips from the extensile approach group) Bulk allograft failure in 2 hips
Goodman et al (2004)	10	Anti-protrusio cage	67.3 (49-77)	3.3	70	Aseptic loosening developed in 3 hips Implant fracture occurred in 2 hips Dislocation occurred in 3 hips
Sporer and Paprosky (2006)	13	Distraction technique, porous metal cup, augments	63 (47-88)	2.6 (1-3)	100	Screw failure and acetabular loosening developed in 1 hip, but rerevision surgery was not necessary
DeBoer et al (2007)	20	Custom triflange	55.8 (30-77)	10.25 (7.4-13.1)	100	30% dislocation rate 6 rerevision surgeries were required: 5 for instability and 1 for loose screws
Kosashvili et al (2009)	26	Porous metal cup-cage	64.9 (44-84)	3.7 (2-5.6)	100	Instability developed in 2 hips 3 hips underwent rerevision surgery to manage component migration
Sporer et al (2012)	20	Distraction technique, porous metal cup, augments	67.5 (43-85)	4.5 (2-7)	95	1 rerevision was performed to manage aseptic loosening Asymptomatic radiographic loosening occurred in 4 hips
Taunton et al (2012)	57	Custom triflange	61 (35-81)	6.3 (2-18)	98	1 hip progressed to aseptic failure 2 hips progressed to septic failure Instability developed in 12 hips: 2 were managed with closed reduction and 10 underwent rerevision surgery

[a] Success rate is defined as procedures not requiring rerevision surgery for aseptic loosening.

[b] Mean patient age and follow-up based on original cohort of 31 hips.

[c] Mean patient age and follow-up based on the 7 surviving patients.

Additionally, the underlying acetabular component must be large enough in diameter to accept a cage. It may not be possible to use the cup-cage technique in patients with very small anatomy.

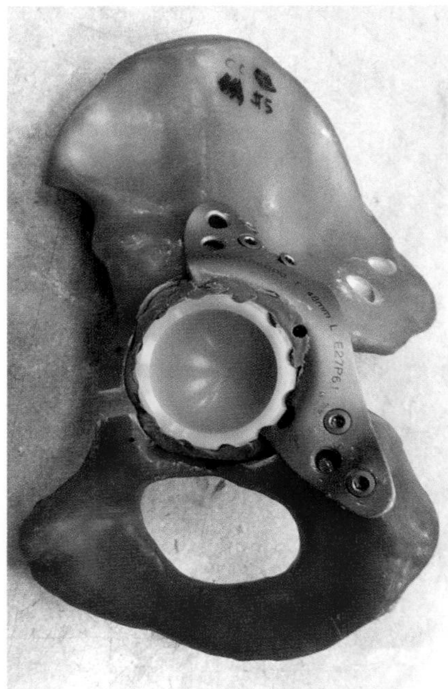

Figure 2 Clinical photograph of a liner cemented into a cup-cage construct spanning a model in which pelvic discontinuity is present.

Distraction techniques are those that bridge large, chronic, discontinuous defects in patients with little or no potential for healing. In these patients, a large hemispheric cup, with or without the addition of porous augments, engages the ilium and ischium and initially uses ligamentotaxis for temporary stabilization. A cup approximately 6 to 8 mm larger than the final reamer is press-fit, providing temporary fixation while multiple screws are placed into the ischium and ilium (**Figure 1, C**). Performing the technique thus distracts the discontinuity and provides increased compression of the bony segments to the distracting porous cup and/or augments. The goal of the distraction technique is to obtain healing of the superior iliac segment and the inferior ischial segment to the porous metal acetabular component without necessarily obtaining bone-to-bone union of these two discontinuous bony segments. The cup-cage construct as described here is an application of the distraction philosophy because the underlying cup is used as a large intervening metal augment between the iliac and ischial bony segments, with the primary goal of healing to the bridging cup rather than healing of the discontinuity itself.

Pelvic reconstruction rings and antiprotrusio cages also may be used in isolation to manage pelvic discontinuity. Rings and cages are sufficiently flexible to allow intraoperative modification, but they may not provide sufficient stability to enhance fracture healing. Additionally, these devices lack ingrowth technology, and these malleable metallic constructs can be prone to fatigue and failure, particularly in the absence of fracture healing. Some surgeons have used porous-coated ingrowth implants with rigid cups and modular malleable flanges, such as the Par5 component (Biomet) in an attempt to solve this problem. However, concerns related to these off-the-shelf implants are similar to those regarding reconstruction cages

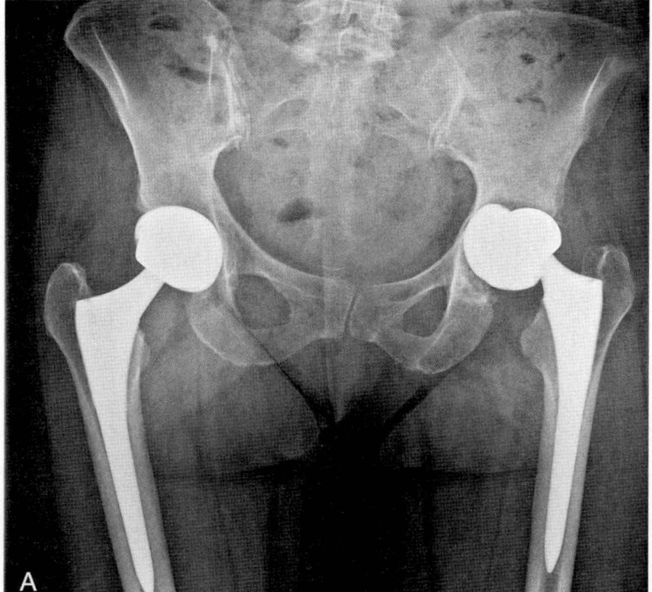

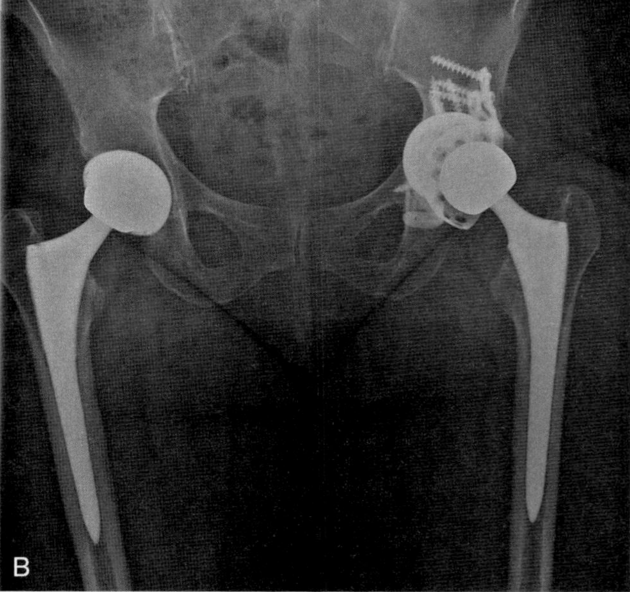

Figure 3 **A,** Preoperative AP pelvic radiograph demonstrates signs of acetabular discontinuity on the left side, including asymmetry of the obturator foramina and a break in the Köhler line. **B,** AP pelvic radiograph obtained after a cup-cage reconstruction with cementation of a liner into the overlying cage. The cage provides temporary stability until ingrowth occurs into the porous metal cup.

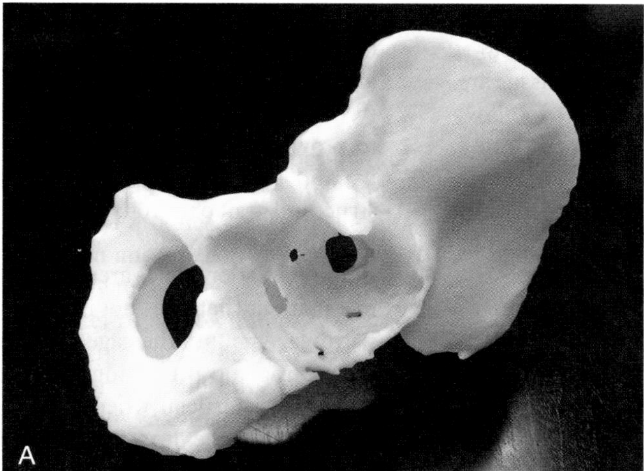
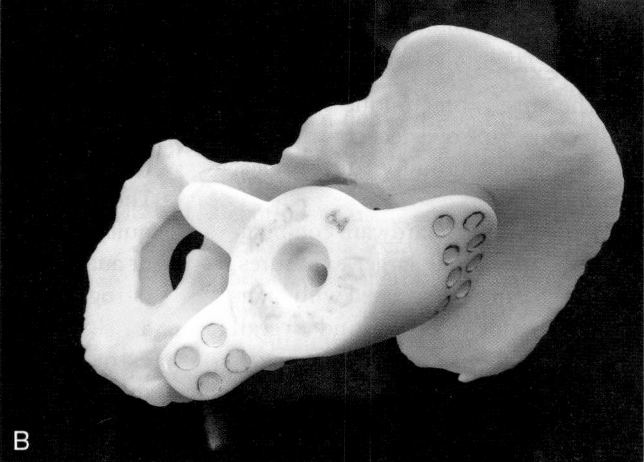

Figure 4 Photographs of a three-dimensional printed model of a hemipelvis generated based on a CT scan. **A,** The model of the hemipelvis defect and remaining pelvic landmarks. **B,** Placement of the custom triflange component modeled from the patient's CT scan. This model is an example of a custom-created triflange component; it does not represent a case of pelvic discontinuity.

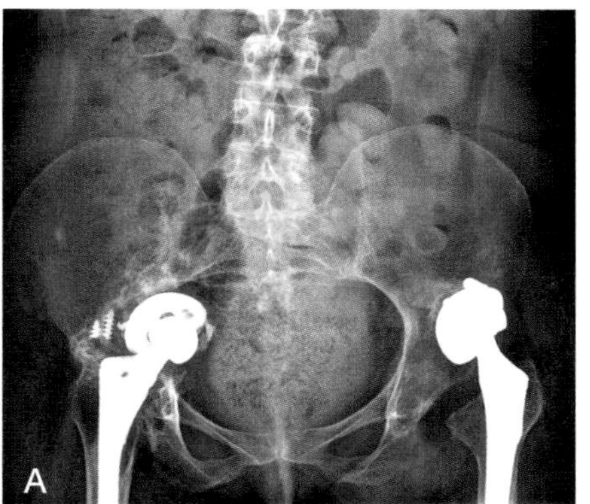
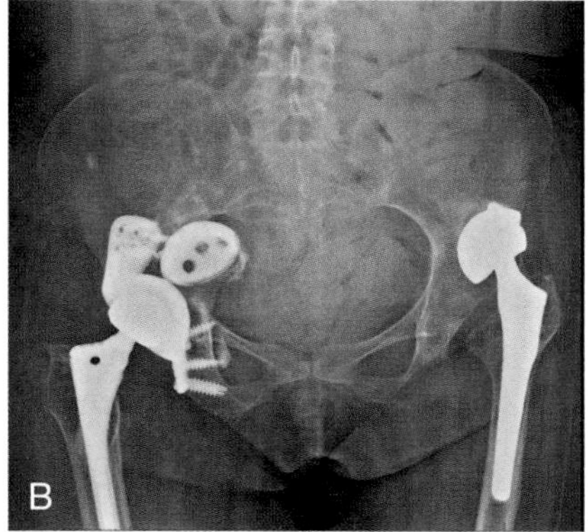
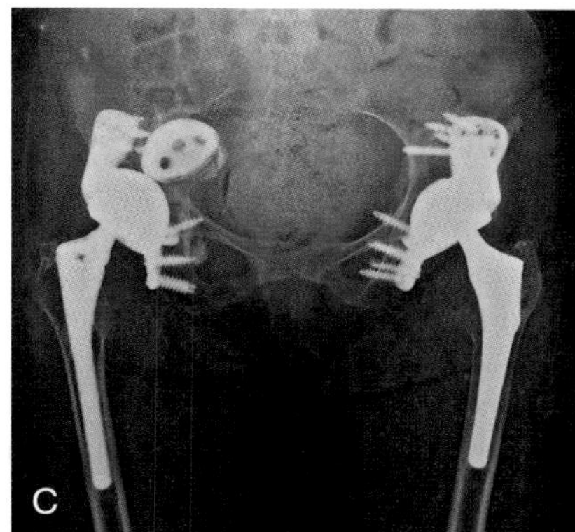

Figure 5 **A,** Preoperative AP pelvic radiograph demonstrates right-side pelvic discontinuity with protrusion of the acetabular component after medial acetabular wall breach. Additionally, a large osteolytic defect was noted in the left hemipelvis with aseptic loosening and superolateral escape of the acetabular component. **B,** AP pelvic radiograph obtained after placement of a right-side custom triflange component. The original intrapelvic acetabular implant was left in situ because the position of the previously placed cup did not preclude placement of the triflange component and because of the high potential of morbidity of removing that implant as a result of considerable scarring and proximity of the iliac vessels. **C,** AP pelvic radiograph obtained after placement of bilateral custom triflange components to restore the anatomic hip centers.

because of the need for relatively thin malleable flanges that can be molded to a variety of bone defects. This malleability makes these devices prone to fatigue failure and precludes the use of coatings that might enhance biologic fixation.

The triflange component is a rigid custom implant that can span massive defects in patients who have little residual bony support. Implant design is finalized preoperatively based on a 3D printed model of a CT reconstruction of the patient's hemipelvis (**Figure 4**). Obtaining purchase in less compromised bone in the ilium and ischium as well as using modern ingrowth/ongrowth surfaces and locking screws can achieve increased stability. Use of a custom implant not only enables bridging of a gap that cannot be accommodated by a jumbo cup but helps reestablish the hip center to a more anatomic position. In a patient with severe chronic protrusio of a prior acetabular component, the triflange can be designed to facilitate retention of the prior acetabular component to avoid injury to the iliac vessels with acetabular component removal (**Figure 5, A** and **B**). The patient shown in **Figure 5** experienced good results with the triflange reconstruction of the chronic pelvic discontinuity on the right, and a triflange reconstruction was later successfully performed to reconstruct the extremely large osteolytic defect in the left hemipelvis (**Figure 5, C**).

DeBoer DK, Christie MJ, Brinson MF, Morrison JC: Revision total hip arthroplasty for pelvic discontinuity. *J Bone Joint Surg Am* 2007;89(4):835-840.

Gililland JM, Anderson LA, Henninger HB, Kubiak EN, Peters CL: Biomechanical analysis of acetabular revision constructs: Is pelvic discontinuity best treated with bicolumnar or traditional unicolumnar fixation? *J Arthroplasty* 2013;28(1):178-186.

Goodman S, Saastamoinen H, Shasha N, Gross A: Complications of ilioischial reconstruction rings in revision total hip arthroplasty. *J Arthroplasty* 2004;19(4):436-446.

Kosashvili Y, Backstein D, Safir O, Lakstein D, Gross AE: Acetabular revision using an anti-protrusion (ilio-ischial) cage and trabecular metal acetabular component for severe acetabular bone loss associated with pelvic discontinuity. *J Bone Joint Surg Br* 2009;91(7):870-876.

Petrie J, Sassoon A, Haidukewych GJ: Pelvic discontinuity: Current solutions. *Bone Joint J* 2013;95-B(11 suppl A):109-113.

Sporer SM, Bottros JJ, Hulst JB, Kancherla VK, Moric M, Paprosky WG: Acetabular distraction: An alternative for severe defects with chronic pelvic discontinuity? *Clin Orthop Relat Res* 2012;470(11):3156-3163.

Sporer SM, Paprosky WG: Acetabular revision using a trabecular metal acetabular component for severe acetabular bone loss associated with a pelvic discontinuity. *J Arthroplasty* 2006;21(6 suppl 2):87-90.

Stiehl JB, Saluja R, Diener T: Reconstruction of major column defects and pelvic discontinuity in revision total hip arthroplasty. *J Arthroplasty* 2000;15(7):849-857.

Taunton MJ, Fehring TK, Edwards P, Bernasek T, Holt GE, Christie MJ: Pelvic discontinuity treated with custom triflange component: A reliable option. *Clin Orthop Relat Res* 2012;470(2):428-434.

Chapter 55
Femoral Revision: Overview and Strategy

John J. Callaghan, MD
Steve S. Liu, MD

Introduction

The success and durability of femoral reconstruction in revision total hip arthroplasty (THA) have improved markedly over the past three to four decades. For optimal results, meticulous preoperative planning, an ability to conceptualize and attain extensile surgical exposure, and a practical understanding of all available options for reconstruction are required. Many femoral options are available for revision THA, and proper implant selection based on the amount of bone loss present at the time of reconstruction is critical to success.

Classification

The Paprosky classification of femoral bone loss is a reliable system that remains applicable decades after its introduction. In a type I defect, both metaphyseal and diaphyseal host bone are preserved, and the femoral bone available for reconstruction is similar to that of primary replacement. In a type II defect, metaphyseal bone is compromised and diaphyseal bone is intact. In a type III defect, the metaphysis is nonsupportive and the diaphysis is partially intact. A type IIIA defect has at least 4 cm of intact femoral isthmus, whereas a type IIIB defect has less than 4 cm of intact isthmus. A type IV defect has no supportive isthmus and only a cortical tube remaining for reconstruction.

Femoral Prosthesis Options

Long-term studies have demonstrated the durability of cemented femoral implants in primary THA. Although use of cemented implants in primary THA is declining in the United States, surgeons in other countries continue to use cemented implants.

High failure rates have been reported with the use of cemented stems in revision arthroplasty, especially in patients who have substantial bone loss. However, the use of a cemented stem (preferably polished) with impaction bone grafting in the femoral canal provides durable results even in patients who have severe femoral bone deficiencies (Paprosky type IV; **Figure 1**). Because of the high rate of delayed femoral fracture after impaction grafting, long stems are recommended for this technique in patients who have diaphyseal bone deficiencies.

Cemented modular or nonmodular proximal femoral replacement implants also can be used in elderly patients who have type IV defects with or without discontinuities of the cortical tube and who have low activity demands. In such patients, the bone defect is excised and replaced proximally with metal, and the stem is cemented into the remaining intact femur (**Figure 2**). In a young patient with proximal bone loss and an intact isthmus, allograft prosthetic composite is a treatment option.

Noncemented Femoral Implants

Noncemented femoral implants used in primary hip arthroplasty also can be used in revision arthroplasty in patients with Paprosky type I defects. Noncemented implants include anatomic stems that match the contour of the proximal femur and straight stems in which the femoral isthmus is machined to provide diaphyseal fixation. The proximal femur is broached to provide the largest metaphyseal triangle possible. Straight implants can be proximally coated or extensively coated. The authors of this chapter prefer extensively coated stems for revision, including in patients who

Dr. Callaghan or an immediate family member has received royalties from and serves as a paid consultant to DePuy Synthes and serves as a board member, owner, officer, or committee member of the International Hip Society, The Knee Society, and the Orthopaedic Research and Education Foundation. Neither Dr. Liu nor any immediate family member has received anything of value from or has stock or stock options held in a commercial company or institution related directly or indirectly to the subject of this chapter.

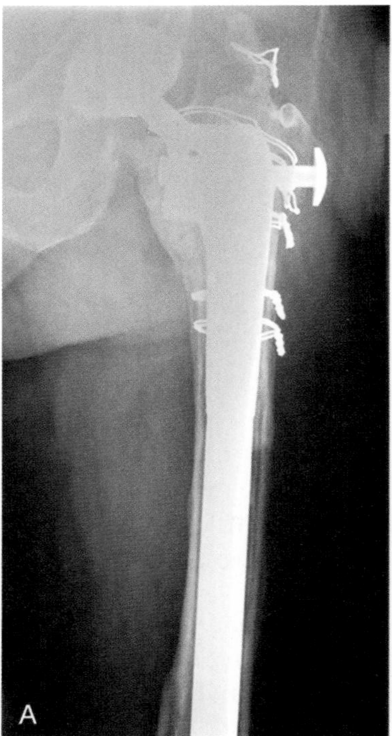

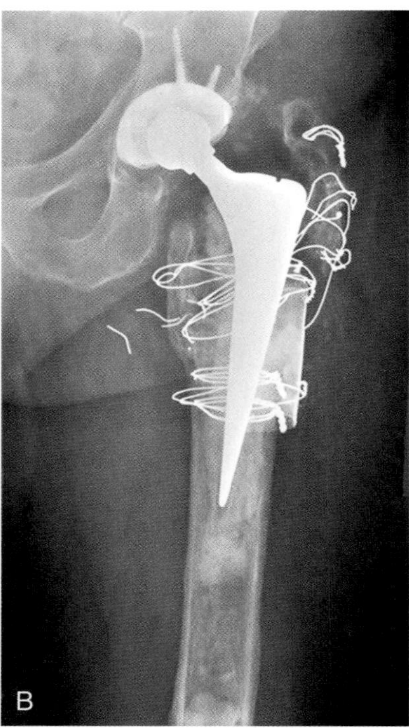

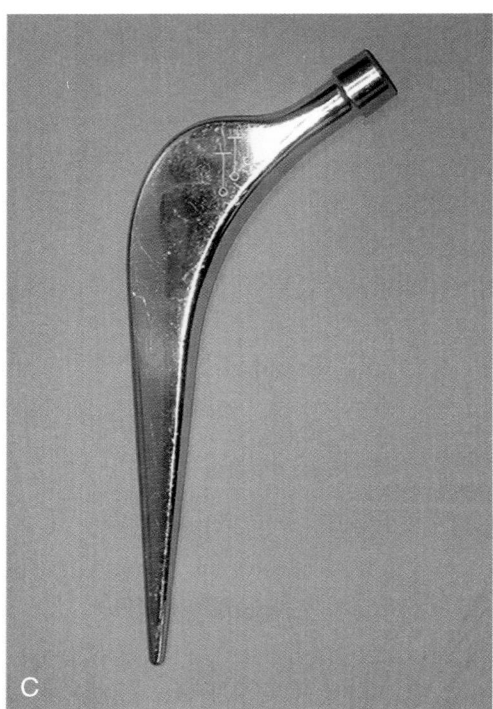

Figure 1 **A,** AP radiograph of a left hip demonstrates a Paprosky type IV femoral defect with a 32-mm-wide tubular bony defect. AP radiograph (**B**) obtained after revision arthroplasty consisting of impaction grafting and insertion of a polished tapered stem. **C,** Photograph shows a polished tapered stem.

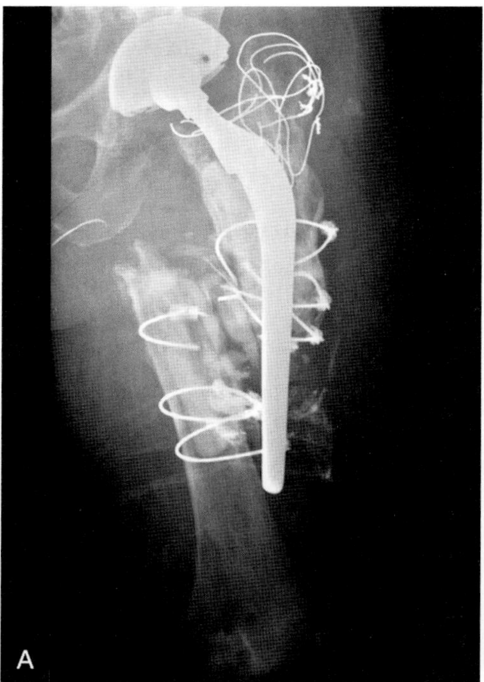

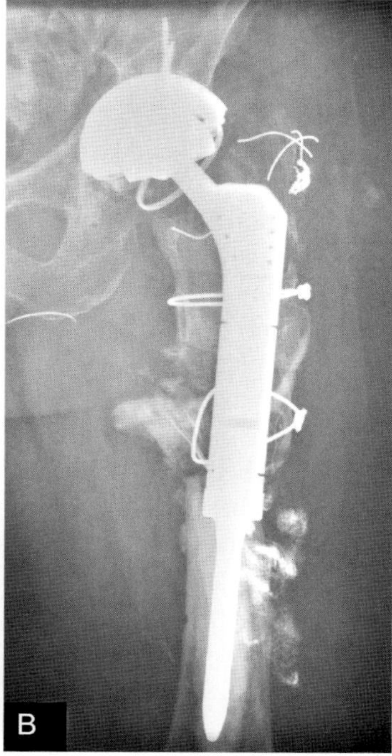

Figure 2 **A,** AP radiograph of the left hip of an 83-year-old patient demonstrates proximal femoral bone loss and wide distal canal around a primary femoral implant. **B,** AP radiograph obtained after revision to a modular proximal femoral implant that was cemented into the distal femur.

have type I defects. Tapered stems with proximal coating (porous, hydroxyapatite, or both) also can be used in patients who have type I defects.

Historically, type II defects were reconstructed with extensively coated stems (typically, 6-inch primary stems) or modular body stems (**Figure 3**). Since approximately 2010, tapered, fluted modular stems also have been used to manage type II defects. First-generation modular fluted stems were associated with a high rate of fracture at the proximal body-stem modular junction; however, improved design has markedly reduced the occurrence of such fracture.

Type III defects also were reconstructed with extensively coated long stems (8 to 10 inches, straight and curved), often in conjunction with an extended trochanteric osteotomy (ETO; 12 to 13 cm distal to the tip of the greater trochanter) to aid in removal of the failed stem and introduction of the revision stem (**Figure 4**). Currently, ETO

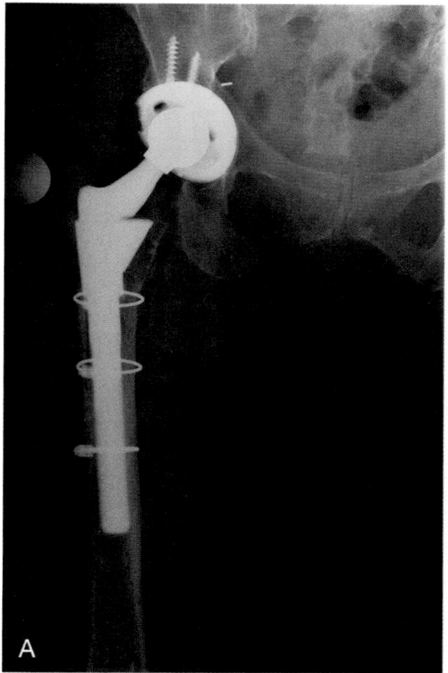

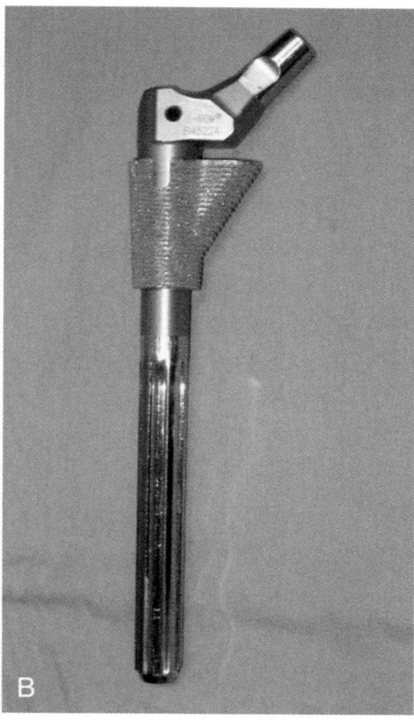

Figure 3 **A,** AP radiograph of a right hip demonstrates a noncemented modular femoral stem used to treat a Paprosky type II defect. **B,** Photograph shows the modular stem.

is done in revisions in which either extensively coated or modular fluted stems are used (**Figure 5**).

The use of fluted stems enables attainment of distal fixation in patients in whom little to no femoral isthmus remains, including most patients with Paprosky type IV defects. However, because of the risk for fractures at the proximal body–fluted stem modular junction, some surgeons have returned to using a monolithic fluted tapered stem popularized by Wagner (**Figure 6**).

Modular Total Femur Systems

If bone loss extends distal to the isthmus, salvage surgery with a total femoral prosthesis can provide reasonable functional results (**Figure 7**). These systems provide a total hip replacement and a

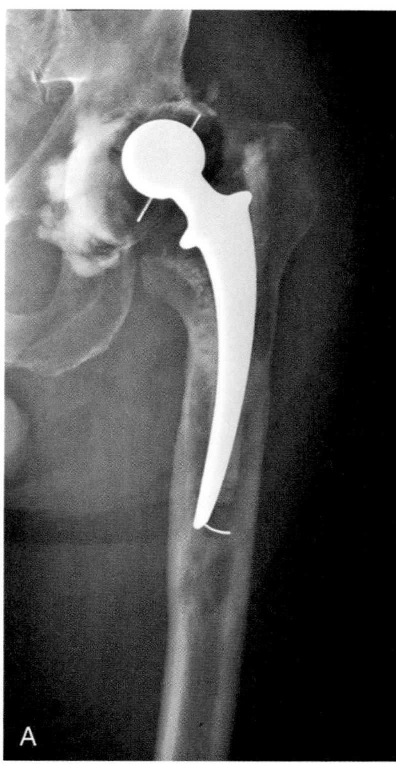

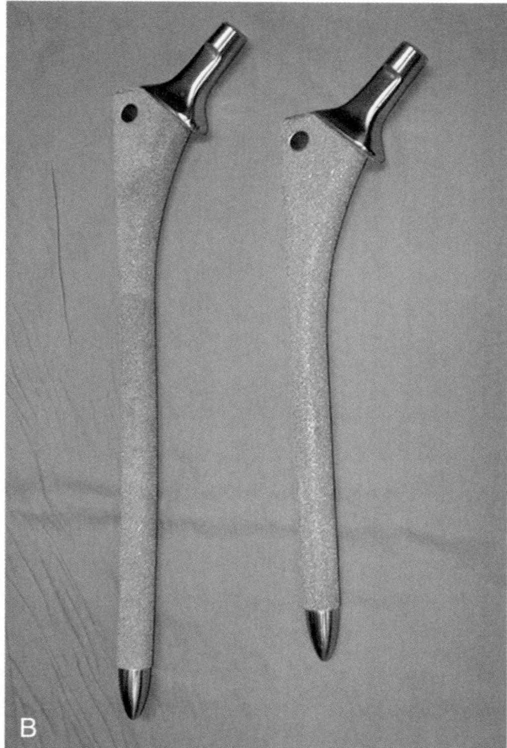

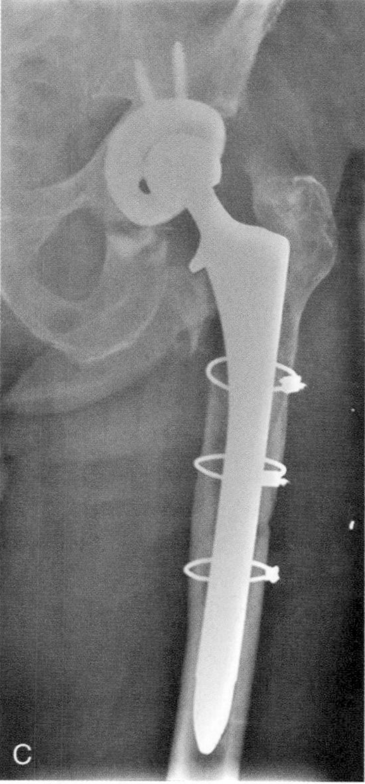

Figure 4 **A,** AP radiograph of a left hip demonstrates Paprosky type IIIA femoral deficiency. **B,** Photograph shows extensively coated stems. **C,** AP radiograph obtained after extended trochanteric osteotomy and insertion of an extensively coated noncemented stem.

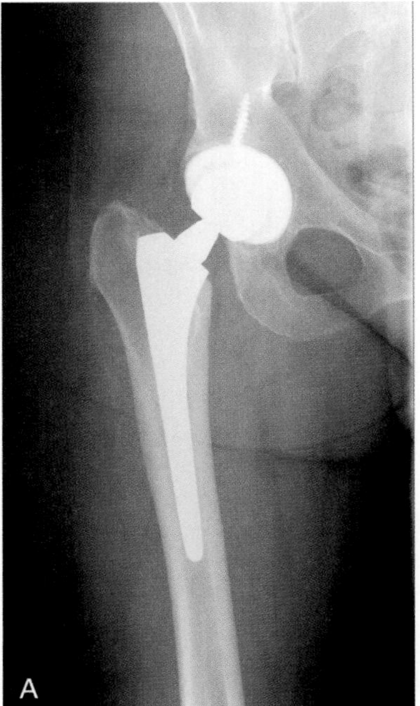

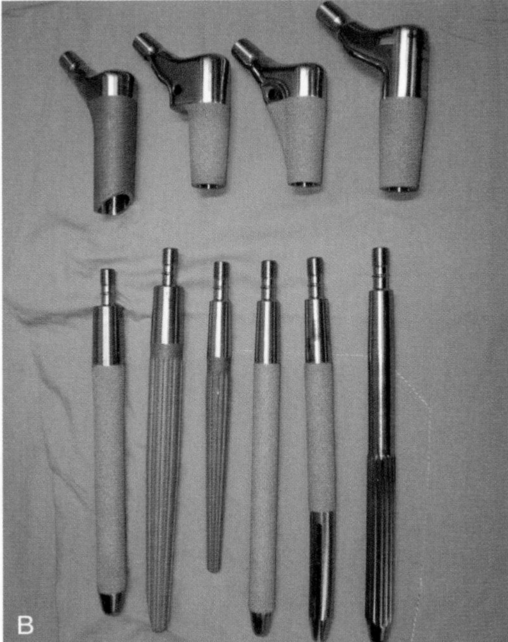

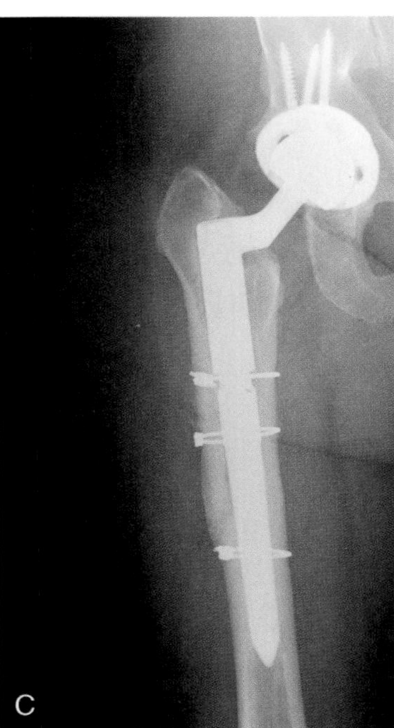

Figure 5 **A,** AP radiograph of a right hip in a patient who experienced adverse local tissue response to the primary femoral implant. **B,** Photograph shows fluted modular stems of different lengths and designs. **C,** AP radiograph obtained after insertion of a fluted modular noncemented stem in conjunction with an extended trochanteric osteotomy.

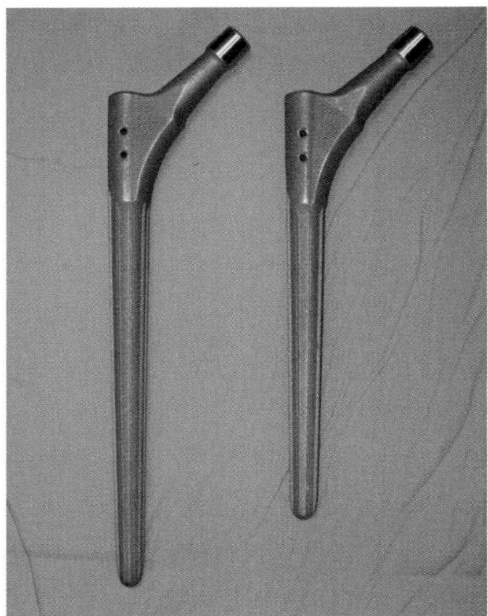

Figure 6 Photograph shows nonmodular fluted, tapered femoral stems.

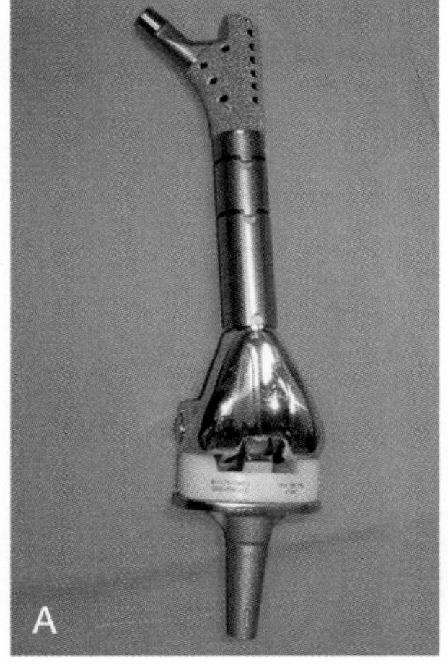

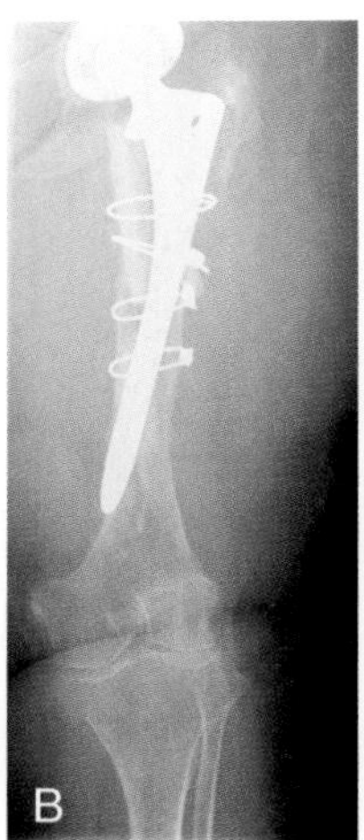

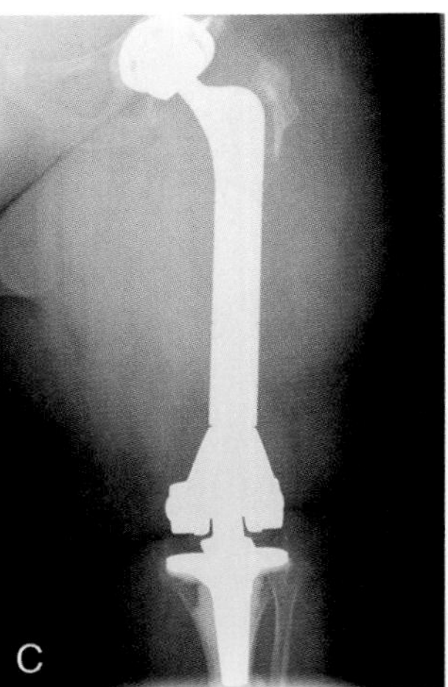

Figure 7 **A,** Photograph shows a modular total femoral prosthesis. **B,** Preoperative AP radiograph of the left hip from a patient who has Paprosky type IV bony deficiency and an arthritic knee. **C,** AP radiograph obtained after revision to a modular total femur prosthesis.

total knee replacement with intercalary modular metal segments. These segments allow the surgeon to modify the length of the construct to fit the specific patient.

Strategy for Reconstruction

Many stem options are available for femoral revision. Surgical exposure must be sufficient to allow removal of the original implant with the least possible disruption of the remaining femoral bone. Adequate exposure also allows preparation and insertion of the selected implant for revision. If an extensile exposure is necessary, ETO is a commonly used option. The surgeon also must recognize the increased risk for instability after revision surgery, and care should be taken to restore leg length, appropriate anteversion of the femoral implant, and adequate reconstruction of the soft tissues around the hip.

Bibliography

Bedard NA, Callaghan JJ, Stefl MD, Liu SS: Systematic review of literature of cemented femoral components: What is the durability at minimum 20 years followup? *Clin Orthop Relat Res* 2015;473(2):563-571.

Callaghan JJ, Bracha P, Liu SS, Piyaworakhun S, Goetz DD, Johnston RC: Survivorship of a Charnley total hip arthroplasty: A concise follow-up, at a minimum of thirty-five years, of previous reports. *J Bone Joint Surg Am* 2009;91(11):2617-2621.

Engh CA Jr, Ellis TJ, Koralewicz LM, McAuley JP, Engh CA Sr: Extensively porous-coated femoral revision for severe femoral bone loss: Minimum 10-year follow-up. *J Arthroplasty* 2002;17(8):955-960.

Fetzer GB, Callaghan JJ, Templeton JE, Goetz DD, Sullivan PM, Johnston RC: Impaction allografting with cement for extensive femoral bone loss in revision hip surgery: A 4- to 8-year follow-up study. *J Arthroplasty* 2001;16(8 suppl 1):195-202.

Halliday BR, English HW, Timperley AJ, Gie GA, Ling RS: Femoral impaction grafting with cement in revision total hip replacement: Evolution of the technique and results. *J Bone Joint Surg Br* 2003;85(6):809-817.

Hook S, Moulder E, Yates PJ, Burston BJ, Whitley E, Bannister GC: The Exeter Universal stem: A minimum ten-year review from an independent centre. *J Bone Joint Surg Br* 2006;88(12):1584-1590.

Konan S, Garbuz DS, Masri BA, Duncan CP: Non-modular tapered fluted titanium stems in hip revision surgery: Gaining attention. *Bone Joint J* 2014;96-B(11 suppl A):56-59.

Miner TM, Momberger NG, Chong D, Paprosky WL: The extended trochanteric osteotomy in revision hip arthroplasty: A critical review of 166 cases at mean 3-year, 9-month follow-up. *J Arthroplasty* 2001;16(8 suppl 1):188-194.

Paprosky WG, Lawrence JM, Cameron HU: Femoral defect classification: Clinical application. *Orthop Rev* 1990;19(9 suppl):9-15.

Tetreault MW, Shukla SK, Yi PH, Sporer SM, Della Valle CJ: Are short fully coated stems adequate for "simple" femoral revisions? *Clin Orthop Relat Res* 2014;472(2):577-583.

Trumm BN, Callaghan JJ, George CA, Liu SS, Goetz DD, Johnston RC: Minimum 20-year follow-up results of revision total hip arthroplasty with improved cementing technique. *J Arthroplasty* 2014;29(1):236-241.

Van Houwelingen AP, Duncan CP, Masri BA, Greidanus NV, Garbuz DS: High survival of modular tapered stems for proximal femoral bone defects at 5 to 10 years followup. *Clin Orthop Relat Res* 2013;471(2):454-462.

Weeden SH, Paprosky WG: Minimal 11-year follow-up of extensively porous-coated stems in femoral revision total hip arthroplasty. *J Arthroplasty* 2002;17(4 suppl 1):134-137.

Chapter 56
Femoral Revision: Implant Removal

Charles L. Nelson, MD
David H. So, MD

Indications

Indications for revision of a femoral implant after total hip arthroplasty (THA) include infection, symptomatic aseptic loosening, implant malposition, hip instability, excessive metallic wear or corrosion, adverse tissue reactions, periprosthetic fracture, implant fracture, failure of modular junctions, and substantial trunnion damage.

Preoperative planning is critical for successful removal of well-fixed femoral implants. The manufacturer, brand, and size of the existing implants should be identified. The implant stickers from the initial surgical record are the most reliable source of this information. These stickers, or copies of the stickers, are usually found in the progress note section of the paper hospital chart, orthopaedic surgical logbook, or electronic medical record. Another possible source of this information is the surgical report, in which many surgeons document the prosthetic device implanted. If these records are unavailable, an experienced orthopaedic surgeon or an industry representative may be able to identify the implants on the basis of plain radiographs. Alternatively, the patient's radiographs can be cross-referenced with images in arthroplasty reference books. Correct identification of the implants can help decrease morbidity, the extent of the surgical procedure, and the surgical time.

Preoperative imaging should include an AP radiograph of the pelvis and AP and lateral radiographs of the femur. These images can help the surgeon identify the implants and determine the mode of fixation. The stability of the stem is determined on the basis of the radiographs. In patients with cemented stems, loosening may be indicated by subsidence of the femoral implant, fracture of the stem or cement, or the presence of a progressive radiolucent line at the interface between the stem and cement that is not present in the immediate postoperative radiographs. In patients with noncemented stems, instability is suggested by progressive reactive lines in the area of the porous coating, implant migration with subsidence, varus or valgus tilting, or late shedding of particles from the porous-coated surface.

To anticipate the site at which the bone-implant interface will have to be disrupted, the surgeon should identify the location of surfaces with bony ingrowth and the extent of ingrowth. Other features of the stem, such as an extraction hole or threaded stem insertion hole in the stem shoulder that may allow the use of a stem-specific or universal extraction device, should be identified. In patients with cemented stems, the quality of the cement mantle, the length of the distal cement column, or cement past the isthmus should be evaluated.

Contraindications

Contraindications to revision THA and implant removal include medical illness or severe comorbidities that preclude major surgery. In patients who have an uninfected, well-positioned implant, it is generally preferable to leave a well-fixed femoral implant in place at the time of acetabular implant revision, particularly if modularity of the implant allows appropriate restoration of limb length and soft-tissue tension.

Alternative Treatments

Alternatives to revision THA depend on the indication for the procedure. Retention of the implant may be considered in patients with periprosthetic joint infection, which can be managed with irrigation and débridement, with or

Dr. Nelson or an immediate family member serves as a paid consultant to Zimmer Biomet, and serves as a board member, owner, officer, or committee member of the American Association of Hip and Knee Surgeons and the J. Robert Gladden Orthopaedic Society. Neither Dr. So nor any immediate family member has received anything of value from or has stock or stock options held in a commercial company or institution related directly or indirectly to the subject of this chapter.

without chronic suppressive antibiotic therapy. Hip spica casting or an abduction orthosis may be used for the management of hip instability. In patients who have periprosthetic femur fractures, alternatives to femoral revision include nonsurgical management of isolated trochanteric fractures or open reduction and internal fixation of fractures in which the femoral implant remains well fixed, such as Vancouver type B1 and C fractures. In patients who have aseptic loosening or osteolysis, alternative management strategies include analgesia, activity modification, and physical therapy. The use of adjunctive ambulatory aids such as canes, crutches, walkers, or wheelchairs should be considered.

Techniques

Setup/Exposure

- The surgical approach is chosen according to the surgeon's preference. The most common approaches are the posterolateral and direct lateral (modified Hardinge) approaches.
- Regardless of the approach used, a wide exposure is necessary to improve mobility of the proximal femur and decrease the risk of intraoperative fracture.
- Removal of the pseudocapsule will allow greater mobility of the proximal femur, reduce the risk of fracture of the greater trochanter, and improve visualization of the acetabulum.
- The posterolateral approach offers better exposure of the posterior acetabular wall and column.
- The standard trochanteric osteotomy, trochanteric slide osteotomy (TSO), Wagner extended osteotomy, and extended trochanteric osteotomy (ETO) provide increasing amounts of exposure, greatly facilitating implant extraction while decreasing the risk of femoral perforation.
- A standard trochanteric osteotomy provides enhanced acetabular exposure and improved abductor tensioning, but only a limited increase in femoral exposure. Trochanteric osteotomy can be complicated by nonunion, fibrous union, fragmentation of the trochanter, proximal migration, and abductor weakness with associated abductor lurch. Soft-tissue irritation is commonly associated with the hardware used for fixation of the osteotomy, such as cerclage cables or a claw plate.
- Alternatively, a TSO may be performed. In this technique, both the abductors and the vastus lateralis are left attached to the trochanteric fragment, preventing superior migration of the trochanteric fragment. The resultant force of the abductors and vastus lateralis muscles results in compression at the osteotomy site. Despite this compression, nonunion and trochanteric escape can occur after TSO. Other disadvantages, including soft-tissue irritation secondary to the presence of the hardware needed for fixation of the osteotomy, are similar to those of the standard trochanteric osteotomy.
- If an anterolateral, direct lateral, or posterior approach to the hip is used, a Wagner extended osteotomy of the proximal femur can be done. The anterior one-third to one-half of the abductors are reflected in continuity with the anterior one-third of the proximal femur. To enable removal of the anterior segment of bone, cuts are made from lateral to medial, resulting in an osteotomy in the coronal plane. This approach is useful in removing well-fixed cemented or noncemented stems.
- Compared with other osteotomies, the ETO offers several advantages. It provides greater exposure for acetabular and femoral implant removal; allows for correction of deformity, especially varus femoral remodeling; offers predictable healing; and allows for abductor advancement and neutral reaming of the femoral canal with decreased risk of cortical perforation.
- Extensively porous-coated noncemented stems and double-tapered, proximally coated stems with osseointegration generally require an ETO for safe removal.
- Most cemented implants can be extracted from the cement mantle without an ETO. However, certain prostheses with an anteroposterior dimension widest in the midsection of the implant occasionally require an ETO for removal.
- An ETO also is indicated in patients with stem fracture; a cement mantle that extends beyond the anterior bow of the femur; or a long, bowed femoral implant.
- Disadvantages of an ETO are the need for cerclage fixation, hardware-related pain, and the risk of intraoperative or postoperative fracture of the osteotomy fragment. Rarely, nonunion with abductor weakness can occur secondary to proximal migration. When cemented femoral revision is planned, with or without impaction grafting, ETO is less optimal because of the risk of cement extrusion from the osteotomy site.

Instruments/Equipment/Implants Required

- After the implant and mode of fixation have been identified, appropriate instrumentation is ordered. A surgeon preparing for a revision hip procedure should be aware of all available options.
- Hand tool sets can be used for implant removal. These tool sets generally have variations for removal of cemented and noncemented implants (**Figure 1**). These

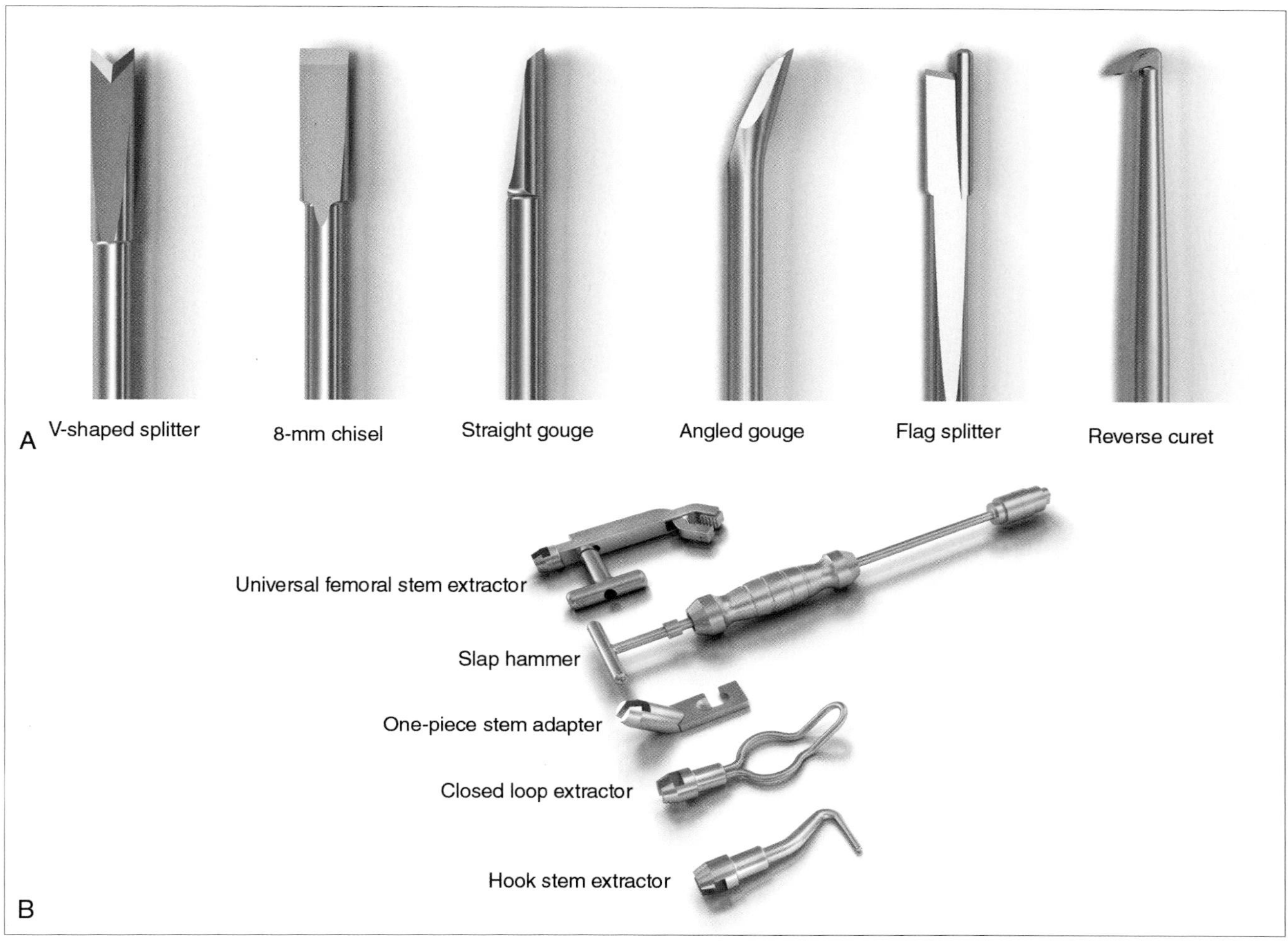

Figure 1 **A,** Photograph shows manual cement removal tools from a cemented revision instrumentation set (DePuy Synthes, Warsaw, IN). **B,** Photograph shows a universal femoral stem extraction handle and attachments allowing removal of modular and nonmodular stems (Zimmer Biomet, Warsaw, IN).

instruments facilitate removal of cement at the bone-cement interface. The surgeon should visualize areas of cement interdigitation to ensure that all cement is removed.

- High-speed burrs facilitate implant extraction and cement removal.
- Although rapid cement removal can be achieved with hand tools, the use of motorized devices is an option. Motorized instruments allow rapid, controlled impact, and some of these devices include fluorescent light sources to improve visualization.
- Ultrasonic devices can be useful for cement removal. The OSCAR 3 (Orthosonics) also includes probes that can be used to disrupt the bone-prosthesis interface in the removal of noncemented femoral implants (**Figure 2**).

Procedure

CEMENTED STEMS

- Extraction of cemented stems consists of two phases: disimpaction of the stem from the cement mantle and removal of cement.

Disimpaction of the Stem

- To disimpact the stem from the cement mantle, the surgeon must clear any bone or cement that may overhang the shoulder of the prosthesis at the medial aspect of the greater trochanter. To avoid fracture of the greater trochanter, a clear path must be available for disimpaction of the implant.
- A high-speed burr is used to remove any overhanging bone and cement. The use of osteotomes is discouraged because they occupy space, and their use can result in trochanteric fracture because of increased hoop stresses.
- To decrease surgical time and reduce the risk of complications, the surgeon should use instruments specifically designed for the

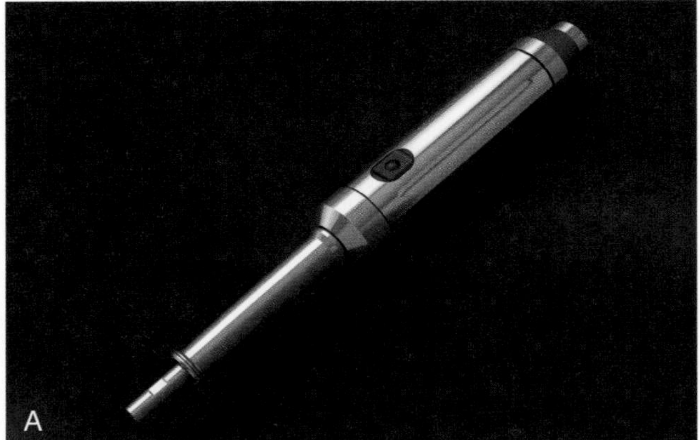

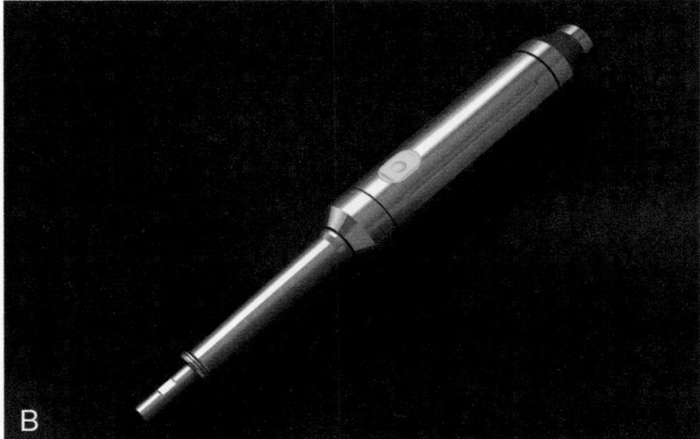

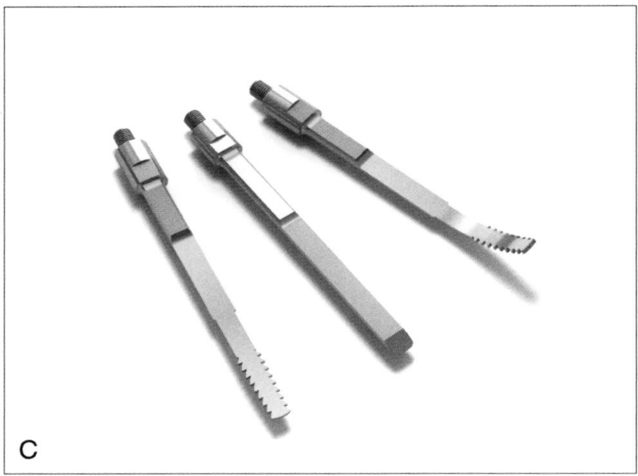

Figure 2 Photographs show OSCAR ultrasonic handles and probes (Orthosonics, Berkshire, United Kingdom) used in the removal of femoral implants. **A,** The handle for probes used in the removal of noncemented stems. **B,** The handle for probes, such as cement piercers and reverse scrapers, used to remove remaining cement after extraction of cemented implants. **C,** Probes used in the removal of noncemented stems.

removal of cemented stems.

- In patients with marked subsidence of the implant, removal of the femoral implant is more difficult. In these patients, a medial collar may have bony overgrowth that must be cleared before the implant can be removed. Subsidence can compromise the attachment of universal extraction devices to the trunnion.
- After the trajectory of the prosthesis is clear, an implant-specific or universal extraction device can be used. When a universal device is used for removal of an implant without a lipped taper, it may be necessary to notch the undersurface of the neck with a metal-cutting burr so that the prosthesis can be firmly grasped with the extraction device.
- Most highly polished or textured stems can be removed with three to five firm, controlled disimpaction blows.
- If these blows do not free the prosthesis, the cement-prosthesis interface can be disrupted with a narrow pencil-tipped burr or thin, flexible osteotomes. After the prosthesis-cement interface has been disrupted, the surgeon can proceed with retrograde disimpaction of the prosthesis. However, because the use of osteotomes can increase the risk of fracture, the authors of this chapter prefer to use an ETO to accomplish difficult extractions. In patients in whom extraction of the stem from the cement mantle is not possible, an ETO may be necessary for removal.

Removal of Cement

- Because cement removal can be challenging, a cement-in-cement technique may be preferable in patients with good bone-cement interdigitation and without infection. In this technique, the existing cement mantle is roughened and textured with burrs or ultrasonic tools to create space for the new prosthesis and enhance cement-to-cement bonding.
- In patients with loose implants, the surgeon may be able to remove the cement mantle and distal cement column en masse by drilling a hole and threading a tap into the cement mantle and disimpacting the cement mantle in a retrograde manner. An ultrasonic device also can be used to gain purchase on the

cement mantle and allow removal.

- However, the cement typically must be removed in pieces with the use of hand tools, burrs, drills, and/or ultrasonic devices.
- Metaphyseal cement mantles are often thick and can be debulked with the use of a high-speed burr.
- Hand tools such as splitters, T-shaped and V-shaped osteotomes, reverse hooks, and pituitary rongeurs are used methodically and carefully to break and remove metaphyseal and diaphyseal cement.
- To avoid iatrogenic fracture, a well-fixed and circumferentially intact cement mantle must be split before it is separated from the surrounding bone.
- Alternatively, motorized osteotomes can be used for cement removal. These tools often have a fluorescent headlight that facilitates removal of cement in the diaphysis, where visualization is poor.
- Removal of a well-fixed distal cement plug requires creation of a central hole in the plug with a burr, a drill, or an ultrasonic device. The surgeon should progressively enlarge this hole and use reverse hook curets to drive the cement fragment proximally. To avoid the risk of femoral fracture, care must be taken to create a central hole in the plug before instruments are inserted.
- If the distal cement plug expands past the isthmus of the femur, an ETO or cortical window may be necessary for safe extraction. In most patients, an ETO allows for more rapid cement removal with a decreased risk of perforation. This advantage must be weighed against the risks associated with ETO.
- Ultrasonic devices with specially designed probes can be used. These devices provide audible, visual, and tactile feedback to indicate the position of the probe, thereby minimizing the risk of damage to bone.
- An ultrasonic probe can be used to remove proximal cement by allowing the surgeon to cut longitudinal troughs in the cement and join them to facilitate removal of larger pieces of cement.
- Another probe is designed to scrape cement using a backward motion.
- Alternatively, a puller probe can be advanced partway through the cement column. The melted cement is allowed to harden around the tip of the probe. The handset is removed, and a slap hammer is attached and used to extract the distal cement column.

NONCEMENTED STEMS

- Noncemented stems are either proximally or extensively porous-coated. Removal of a loose, proximally coated, undersized stem is much easier than removal of a well-fixed, extensively porous-coated, canal-filling stem.
- As in the removal of a cemented stem, overhanging greater trochanteric bone must be removed to clear a trajectory for the shoulder of the prosthesis.

Removal of Proximally Coated Stems

- If the stem is determined to be loose on the basis of preoperative radiographs, the proximal extraction device is attached. Three to five firm, controlled disimpaction blows are administered.
- If these blows are not sufficient to disimpact the stem, the surgeon must disrupt the bone-prosthesis or fibrous tissue–prosthesis interface.
- Disruption of fibrous ingrowth may require the use of thin, flat, U-shaped osteotomes. Caution and constant vigilance must be maintained because osteotomes can easily result in femoral fracture by increasing hoop stresses or by veering off the implant surface and into the surrounding bone.
- The bone-implant interface of a proximally coated stem can be disrupted with the use of a pencil-tipped burr to divide the anterior, posterior, and lateral interfaces. Occasionally, the medial interface may be blocked by a collar. In patients in whom this occurs, a metal-cutting burr can be used to transect the collar to gain access to the medial aspect of the implant. To minimize the spread of metal debris, the patient's bone and soft tissues should be isolated with sponges or plastic drapes before a metal-cutting device is used. When burrs are used, care must be taken to work along the prosthesis at all times to avoid perforation of the cortices of the femur.
- After the surgeon has gained access to the medial calcar, a flexible osteotome or a Gigli saw can be used to disrupt the bone-implant interface.
- After the bone-implant the interface has been divided, the surgeon may again attempt to disimpact the prosthesis. If three to five blows are not sufficient to disimpact the prosthesis, the surgeon should determine whether further disruption of the bone-implant interface would result in unacceptable risk for fracture or perforation. If such disruption would be too risky, the surgeon may elect to use an ETO or Wagner osteotomy to facilitate removal of the prosthesis.
- In patients with a well-fixed and tapered stem, the surgeon should strongly consider use of an ETO. Even if the distal aspect of the stem is not coated, bony ongrowth may be present distally, especially on titanium stems.
- If an ETO is used for the removal of a proximally coated stem, the osteotomy is usually made just distal to the porous coating.
- However, some patients will have

bony ongrowth distal to the porous coating. In these patients, the osteotomy should be extended to near the tip of the stem. A pencil-tipped burr or a microsagittal saw is used to disrupt the bone-implant interface anteriorly and posteriorly.
- Alternatively, ultrasonic devices developed for the removal of noncemented stems can be used. These devices work in conjunction with curved serrated, or flat smooth or serrated osteotome probes that disrupt the interface.
- Next, the medial interface from the calcar to the cylindric aspect of the stem is disrupted. Because the use of a Gigli saw is effective in this step, the surgeon should have several Gigli saws available.
- The extraction device is attached, and three to five blows are applied. If these blows are not sufficient to remove the prosthesis, the stem is cut with metal-cutting burrs. The distal cylindric aspect of the stem is removed with the use of motorized trephines. Motorized trephines slightly larger than the stem diameter should be used to minimize bone loss.

Removal of Extensively Coated Stems
- An ETO is useful in facilitating the removal of extensively porous-coated stems (**Figure 3**).
- The distal margin of the osteotomy is determined on the basis of preoperative templating.
- In the removal of an extensively porous-coated implant, the osteotomy should be sufficiently distal to facilitate removal of the prosthesis and allow correction of any varus remodeling, while maintaining at least 4 to 6 cm of isthmic bone for reliable fixation of a revision stem.
- For the removal of a fully coated stem that is relatively short, the osteotomy can be made at the level of the stem tip if satisfactory fixation of the revision stem can be achieved below the level of the osteotomy.
- For removal of longer primary stems, the distal aspect of the osteotomy should be located just distal to the point at which the stem becomes cylindric (**Figure 4**).
- The stem is divided at this juncture, and the distal portion of the stem is removed with the use of trephines. Copious irrigation is necessary to avoid thermal damage from motorized trephines. The use of extra trephines and a patient approach may be needed.
- Care must be taken to avoid anterior perforation of the femur or substantial removal of anterior cortical bone.
- If a curved stem is being removed, the osteotomy must be sufficiently distal to allow a straight pathway below the bow of the stem.

Removal of Fluted Tapered Modular Stems
- The use of fluted tapered modular stems is becoming more common, particularly in patients with bone loss or Vancouver type B3 periprosthetic femur fractures.
- For removal of these stems, an ETO is performed at or distal to the modular junction.
- The proximal bone-prosthesis interface is disrupted with the use of the techniques described previously.
- The proximal modular portion is disengaged from the Morse taper.
- The remaining portion of the stem is removed with trephines or with a technique that involves a long drill bit or a long Kirschner wire.
- The use of trephines does not allow the surgeon to account for the taper of the stem or anterior cortical abutment, and, therefore, can easily lead to eccentric reaming and cortical perforation.
- In the alternative technique, which may result in less bone loss, either a long drill bit or a long Kirschner wire is advanced along the concave channels between the splines to help disrupt the bone-prosthesis interface while following the taper of the stem. After the implant-bone interface is disrupted, a universal extraction device such as a vise grip is attached to the exposed Morse taper, and the taper is disimpacted with retrograde blows.

FRACTURED STEMS
- Fractured stems can be removed with a combination of techniques.
- An ETO allows the surgeon to place a trephine over the distal stem fragment and remove it, as described for the removal of the distal segment of an extensively porous-coated stem.
- Alternatively, the surgeon can use the Moreland punch technique, in which a narrow, longitudinal cortical slot is cut in the anterior femur over the proximal aspect of the distal segment. A carbide punch is driven into the stem at a 45° angle, and the stem is pushed proximally. The carbide punch is then placed more distally on the stem through the same cortical slot, and force is applied to drive the stem more proximally. This process is repeated until the stem is sufficiently loose to be removed.

Wound Closure
- The wound is closed in a standard manner.

Postoperative Regimen

In the absence of hip instability, postoperative use of an abduction orthosis is not necessary. If an ETO was used,

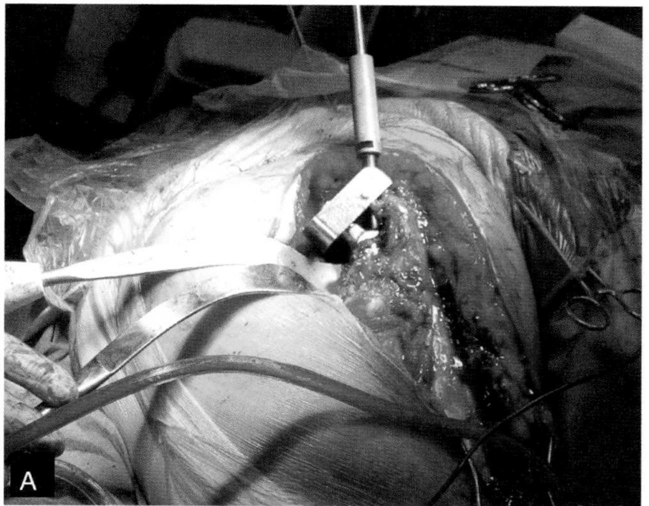

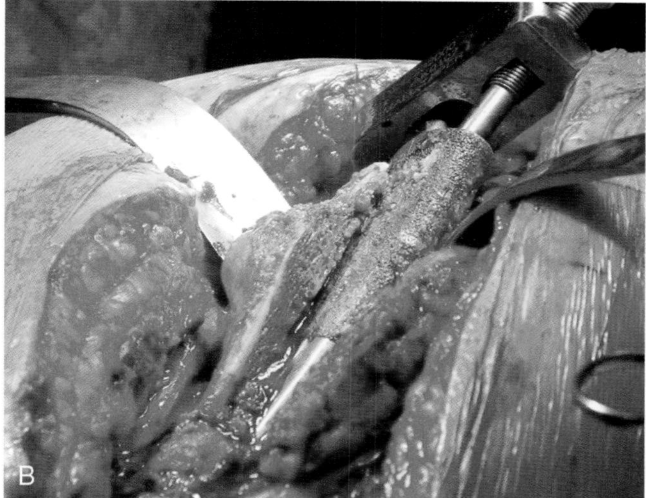

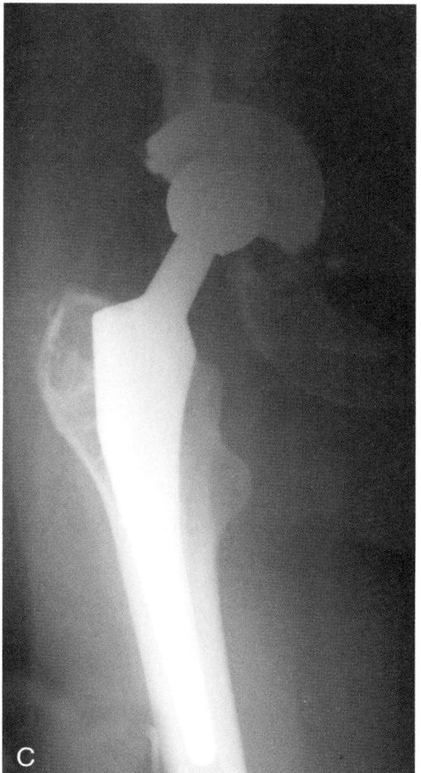

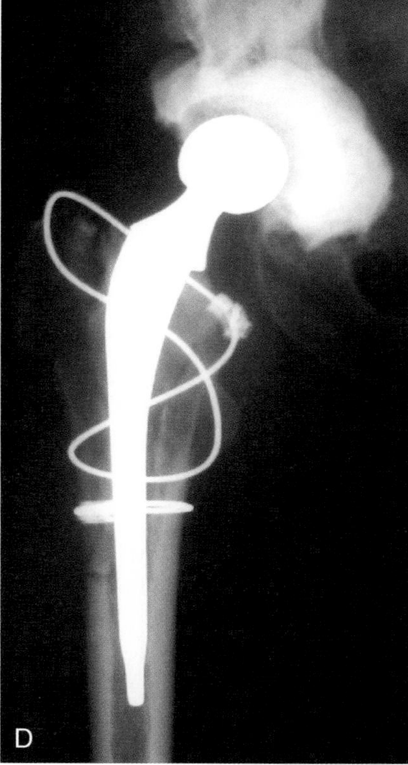

Figure 3 **A,** Intraoperative photograph shows a universal femoral extraction device attached to the femoral trunnion. **B,** Intraoperative photograph shows an extended trochanteric osteotomy. **C,** Preoperative AP radiograph demonstrates an infected total hip arthroplasty with a well-fixed noncemented femoral implant. **D,** Postoperative AP radiograph demonstrates placement of an articulated antibiotic-loaded spacer after removal of the femoral and acetabular implants. Extended trochanteric osteotomy was necessary to facilitate removal of the well-fixed femoral implant. (Reproduced from Nelson CL: Femoral revision: Component removal, in Lieberman JR, Berry DJ, eds: *Advanced Reconstruction: Hip*. Rosemont, IL, American Academy of Orthopaedic Surgeons, 2005, pp 395-400.)

protected weight bearing and avoidance of active abduction for 6 weeks postoperatively may be beneficial. Weight bearing is at the discretion of the surgeon, and any restrictions are determined according to the surgeon's preference and experience.

Avoiding Pitfalls and Complications

A wide exposure and generous release of soft tissue around the femur will allow for less forceful femoral rotation and manipulation, thereby decreasing the risk of spiral fractures, especially in patients with osteopenic bone. Avoidance of the use of osteotomes in the space between the prosthesis and the cement or host bone also can reduce the risk of fracture. When an ETO is created, the use of a burr to create a rounded distal

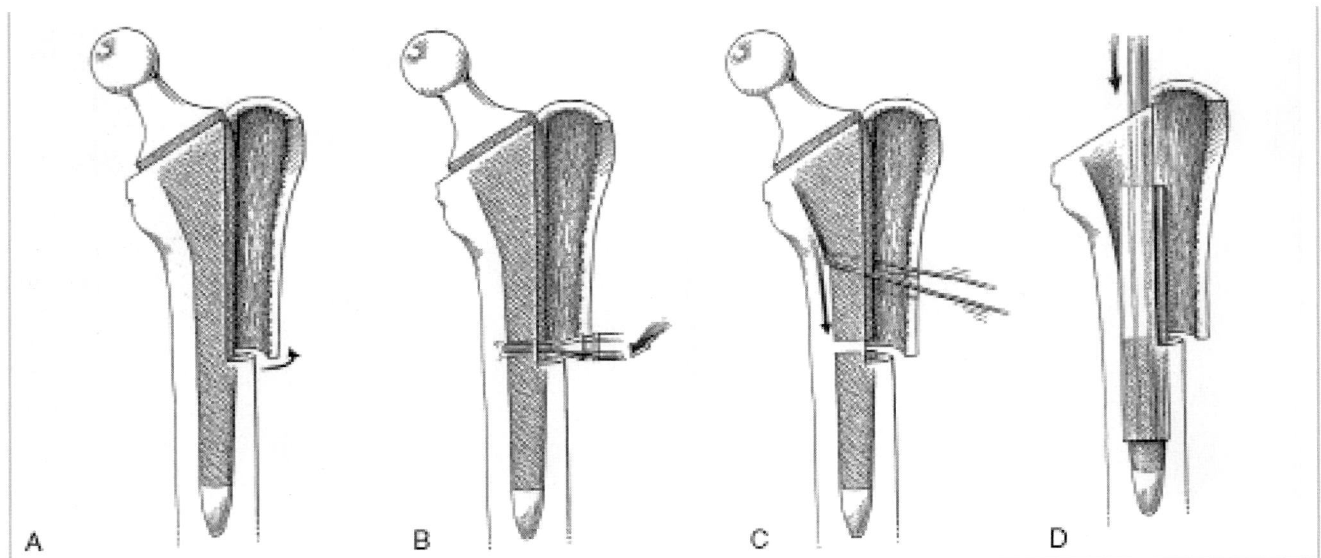

Figure 4 Illustrations depict the use of extended trochanteric osteotomy for the removal of an extensively porous-coated stem. **A,** An extended greater trochanteric osteotomy provides access to the stem. **B,** A high-speed, metal-cutting instrument is used to divide the implant below the metaphyseal flare. **C,** A Gigli saw is used to cut the medial areas of bony ingrowth into the proximal stem. **D,** A trephine is used to free the distal stem from the diaphysis. (Reproduced with permission from the Mayo Foundation for Medical Education and Research, Rochester, MN.)

osteotomy may result in a lesser stress riser than would result from the creation of a transverse osteotomy with an oscillating saw. Compared with the use of a standard drill, the use of ultrasonic devices may decrease the likelihood of cortical perforation in the removal of a distal cement column. Finally, in most patients, careful extraction of the implant without excessive force will help avoid complications.

Bibliography

Aribindi R, Paprosky W, Nourbash P, Kronick J, Barba M: Extended proximal femoral osteotomy. *Instr Course Lect* 1999;48:19-26.

Berry DJ: Removal of cementless stems. *Instr Course Lect* 2003;52:331-336.

Duncan WW, Hubble MJ, Howell JR, Whitehouse SL, Timperley AJ, Gie GA: Revision of the cemented femoral stem using a cement-in-cement technique: A five- to 15-year review. *J Bone Joint Surg Br* 2009;91(5):577-582.

Glassman AH: Femoral component and cement removal, in Berry DJ, Trousdale RT, Dennis DA, Paprosky WG, eds: *Revision Total Hip and Knee Arthroplasty.* Philadelphia, PA, Lippincott Williams & Wilkins, 2012, pp 221-241.

Glassman AH: The removal of cementless total hip femoral components. *Instr Course Lect* 2002;51:93-101.

Glassman AH, Engh CA: The removal of porous-coated femoral hip stems. *Clin Orthop Relat Res* 1992;(285):164-180.

Hansen EN, Hozack WJ, Austin MS: Removal of well-fixed components, in Callaghan JJ, Rosenberg AG, Rubash HE, eds: *The Adult Hip*, ed 3. Philadelphia, PA, Wolters Kluwer, 2016, pp 1283-1298, vol 2.

Lieberman JR, Moeckel BH, Evans BG, Salvati EA, Ranawat CS: Cement-within-cement revision hip arthroplasty. *J Bone Joint Surg Br* 1993;75(6):869-871.

Masri BA, Mitchell PA, Duncan CP: Removal of solidly fixed implants during revision hip and knee arthroplasty. *J Am Acad Orthop Surg* 2005;13(1):18-27.

Moskal JT, Shen FH, Brown TE: The fate of stable femoral components retained during isolated acetabular revision: A six- to twelve-year follow-up study. *J Bone Joint Surg Am* 2002;84(2):250-255.

Paprosky WG, Weeden SH, Bowling JW Jr: Component removal in revision total hip arthroplasty. *Clin Orthop Relat Res* 2001;393:181-193.

Chapter 57
Femoral Revision With Cemented Stems

Rami Madanat, MD, PhD, FEBOT
Ola Rolfson, MD, PhD
Henrik Malchau, MD, PhD
A. J. Timperley, MBChB, FRCS, DPhil (Oxon)

Indications

Aseptic loosening is the most common reason for revision of total hip arthroplasty (THA), followed by deep infection, periprosthetic fracture, recurrent dislocation, osteolysis, polyethylene wear, and implant failure. The main goal of revision hip arthroplasty is to achieve a durable construct with stable implant fixation, joint stability, and, if possible, restoration of bone stock. Opinions differ markedly concerning the ideal method of implant fixation for femoral revision. The optimal method for each patient depends on the type of implant previously inserted, the reason for surgical intervention, and the condition of the host bone. Although the results of noncemented fixation are encouraging, these techniques usually require extension of the zone of fixation distally and can cause further proximal bone loss as a result of unloading and consequent stress shielding, making future revision even more challenging. The femoral revision technique should be chosen on the basis of the specific patient's needs in an effort to achieve the lowest possible short- and longer-term morbidity, high patient satisfaction, and a good functional outcome. Benefits of the use of cement in femoral revision include the possibility of immediate fixation, enhancement of proximal bone stock, the ability to bypass defects, and elution of antibiotics. The most important factors to consider in the choice of femoral fixation are the indication for revision surgery, the mechanism of failure of the existing implant, bone stock and quality, and femoral anatomy.

The primary indication for the use of cement in revision surgery is in revision of a previously cemented femoral implant in a patient in whom the cement mantle remains intact and fixed to bone. Cement-in-cement revision may be sufficient in these patients. Cemented revision has a major role in two-stage revision for the management of infected THA because polymethyl methacrylate (PMMA) acts as a carrier for appropriate antibiotics, allowing local elution of antibiotics into the tissues at high concentration. Studies have demonstrated good long-term results of femoral revision with or without the use of cement in patients requiring revision for aseptic loosening. Therefore, patient age and activity demands are not substantial factors in the decision-making process, provided that appropriate techniques are used.

An algorithmic approach may facilitate the decision-making process (**Figure 1**). In combination with the cement-in-cement technique or femoral impaction grafting, revision of a cemented stem may be considered in patients of any age. To ensure the best clinical outcomes, surgeons performing

Dr. Rolfson or an immediate family member serves as a board member, owner, officer, or committee member of the International Society of Arthroplasty Registries and the Swedish Hip Arthroplasty Register. Dr. Malchau or an immediate family member has received royalties from Stryker; serves as a paid consultant to or is an employee of CeramTec; serves as an unpaid consultant to Zimmer Biomet; has stock or stock options held in RSA Biomedical; has received research or institutional support from DePuy Synthes, Smith & Nephew, Stryker, and Zimmer Biomet; and serves as a board member, owner, officer, or committee member of the International Hip Society, the International Society of Arthroplasty Registries, and RSA Biomedical. Dr. Timperley or an immediate family member has received royalties and research or institutional support from Stryker, and serves as a board member, owner, officer, or committee member of the British Orthopaedic Association and the British Hip Society. Neither Dr. Madanat nor any immediate family member has received anything of value from or has stock or stock options held in a commercial company or institution related directly or indirectly to the subject of this chapter.

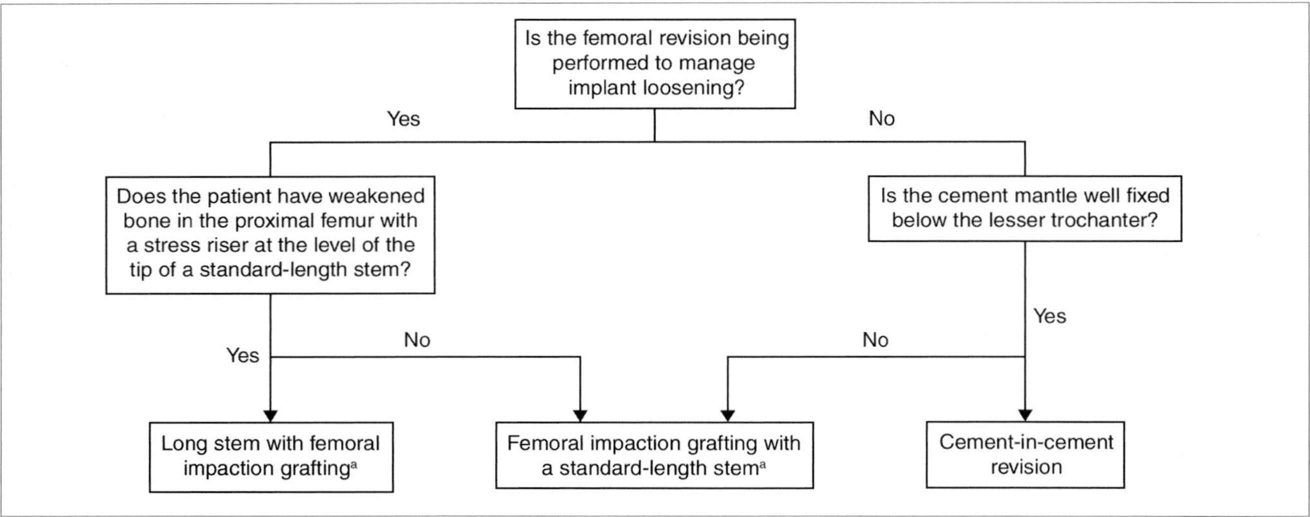

Figure 1 Algorithm depicts the decision-making process in revision of a cemented femoral implant. [a]Recementing an implant into a damaged femur should be reserved for elderly patients or patients with substantial comorbidities in whom impaction grafting or noncemented fixation would be inappropriate (because of factors such as unacceptably long surgical time or lack of distal fixation for noncemented options).

femoral revision arthroplasty must be proficient in all available techniques for femoral reconstruction, both cemented and noncemented.

Cement-in-Cement Revision

Revision THA is associated with a multitude of challenges. In patients with a well-fixed cemented implant that must be revised, removing the complete cement mantle before implanting a new prosthesis often is not recommended. The cement-in-cement technique was first described in 1978 and involves cementing a new femoral implant into an intact cement mantle. In this technique, the inside of the existing cement mantle is burred, if necessary, to accommodate a new implant, and cement is introduced into the cavity to bond to the existing cement. Excellent long-term results of this technique have been reported. Leaving the cement mantle intact avoids potential complications of cement removal, such as bleeding, cortex perforation, and fracture. The technique is indicated in a variety of revision arthroplasty situations (**Figures 2** and **3**). The technique can be used after removal of a femoral implant to improve exposure of the acetabulum, in patients with limb-length inequality requiring femoral length adjustment, for the management of recurrent dislocation secondary to implant malposition (change of femoral anteversion), in patients undergoing revision for the management of a broken implant with an intact distal mantle, for the conversion of a cemented hemiarthroplasty to THA, and for the management of select Vancouver type B2 periprosthetic femur fractures.

Impaction Grafting

Historically, cemented femoral revision was indicated only in elderly patients with low activity demands as well as an intact diaphysis and minimal bone loss in the metaphyseal region. However, the technique of impacting morcellized allograft chips into the canal, introduced in 1987, has widened the spectrum of indications for the use of cemented stems in revision in patients of all age groups. Failure of a femoral implant often results in loss of cancellous bone and/or cortical bone; therefore, the host bone is often inadequate for fixation of a revision stem. In combination with a cemented stem, impaction grafting facilitates restoration of femoral bone stock through incorporation and subsequent remodeling of the impacted morcellized bone graft by the host bone. Impaction allografting has been widely used in both acetabular and femoral revisions for the restoration of bone stock.

Femoral impaction grafting is particularly useful in patients in whom proximal bone stock is deficient because fixation can often be achieved without extending the zone of fixation distally. Additionally, the impacted bone has been shown to incorporate with the host bone and subsequently remodel along lines of stress as predicted by Wolff's law, resulting in proximal loading of the femoral bone. Impaction grafting is useful in patients with a damaged or expanded diaphysis in whom a long, large-diameter noncemented femoral stem would otherwise be required. In addition, angular deformities of the residual femur can be more easily accommodated with a cemented stem than with a noncemented stem. The use of structural allograft and a long cemented stem can be used as an alternative to a tumor-type implant in patients with more complex bone stock deficiencies,

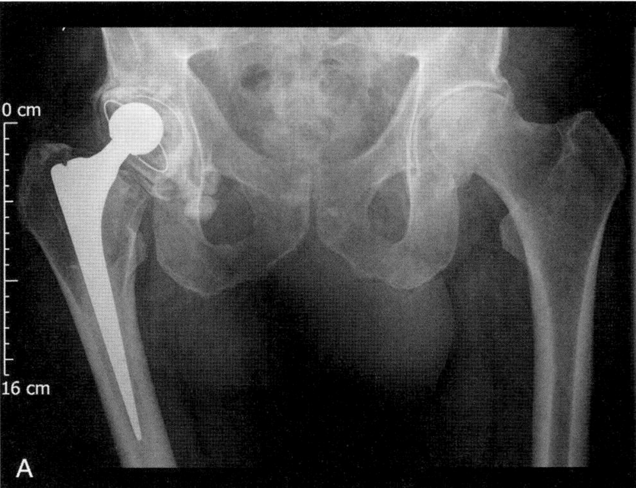

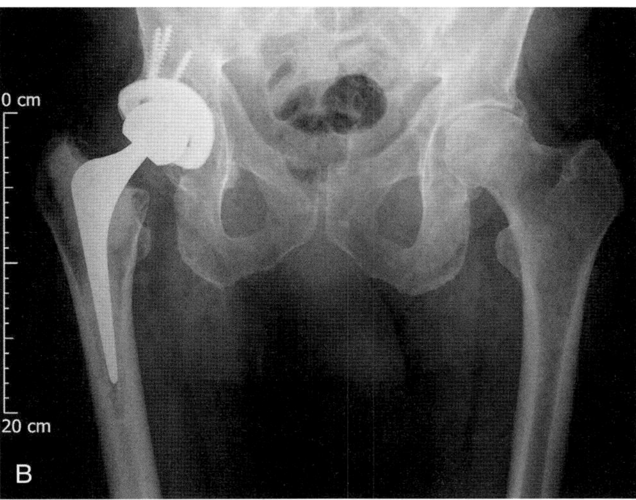

Figure 2 AP pelvic radiographs demonstrate cement-in-cement revision of a femoral implant in the right hip performed to address loosening of a cemented acetabular implant. **A,** Preoperative radiograph demonstrates a well-fixed stem and lysis in the proximal femur. The cement below the level of the lesser trochanter is osseointegrated. Good trabecular bone was exposed after removal of the stem. **B,** Postoperative radiograph demonstrates cement-in-cement revision with a short stem of the same offset as the previous stem.

such as a severely damaged proximal femur.

The ideal scenario for impaction bone grafting is in patients with cavitary bone defects affecting the metaphysis and diaphysis and resulting in a wide femoral canal. In patients who have small to medium cortical defects, a contained cavity can be constructed using wire mesh and wires or cables. A long stem is indicated in patients who exhibit loss of cortical bone stock at a level that would be reached by the tip of a standard-length stem; in patients who have periprosthetic fracture; and in patients who have substantially expanded internal dimensions of the diaphysis (**Figure 4**). Impaction grafting is indicated in the presence of poor proximal bone stock; in patients in whom the endosteal surface of the femur is sclerotic and therefore not suitable for fixation; in patients in whom diaphyseal fixation with a noncemented prosthesis would be difficult or impossible because of the dimensions of the femur; in patients who have periprosthetic fracture and in whom proximal femoral bone stock is deficient; and in patients undergoing femoral reconstruction procedures in which an extended trochanteric osteotomy has been done. Impaction grafting also can be used in the second stage of a two-stage revision for the management of infection.

Contraindications

Cement-in-cement revision is contraindicated in patients in whom failure has occurred at the cement-bone interface below the level of the lesser trochanter. It also is contraindicated in patients with radiolucent lines or endosteal bone lysis around the cement mantle. Impaction grafting is contraindicated in very elderly or infirm patients in whom distal fixation can be achieved, especially if the use of circumferential wire mesh would be required to address the bone deficiency.

Alternative Treatments

A noncemented stem can be used if the bone quality is sufficient. Most implant manufacturers offer modular and nonmodular proximally and extensively porous-coated implant systems that can be used, depending on the quality of the residual bone. Tapered or scratch-fit stems can be used to achieve distal fixation. These noncemented implants are useful in the revision of noncemented stems in patients in whom aggressive reaming of the femoral canal has resulted in a lack of cancellous bone in the proximal femur but in whom impaction grafting is not indicated.

Results

The use of cemented stems that use the taper slip principle (no bond between cement and the stem) has increased, and this technique often results in well-fixed, osseointegrated cement mantles that function well into the third and fourth decades after insertion. In practices in which these stems have been used for long periods, cement-in-cement revision is commonly performed when indicated. Cement-in-cement revision can be extremely useful because of its low risk of complications and associated morbidity. In patients who have a

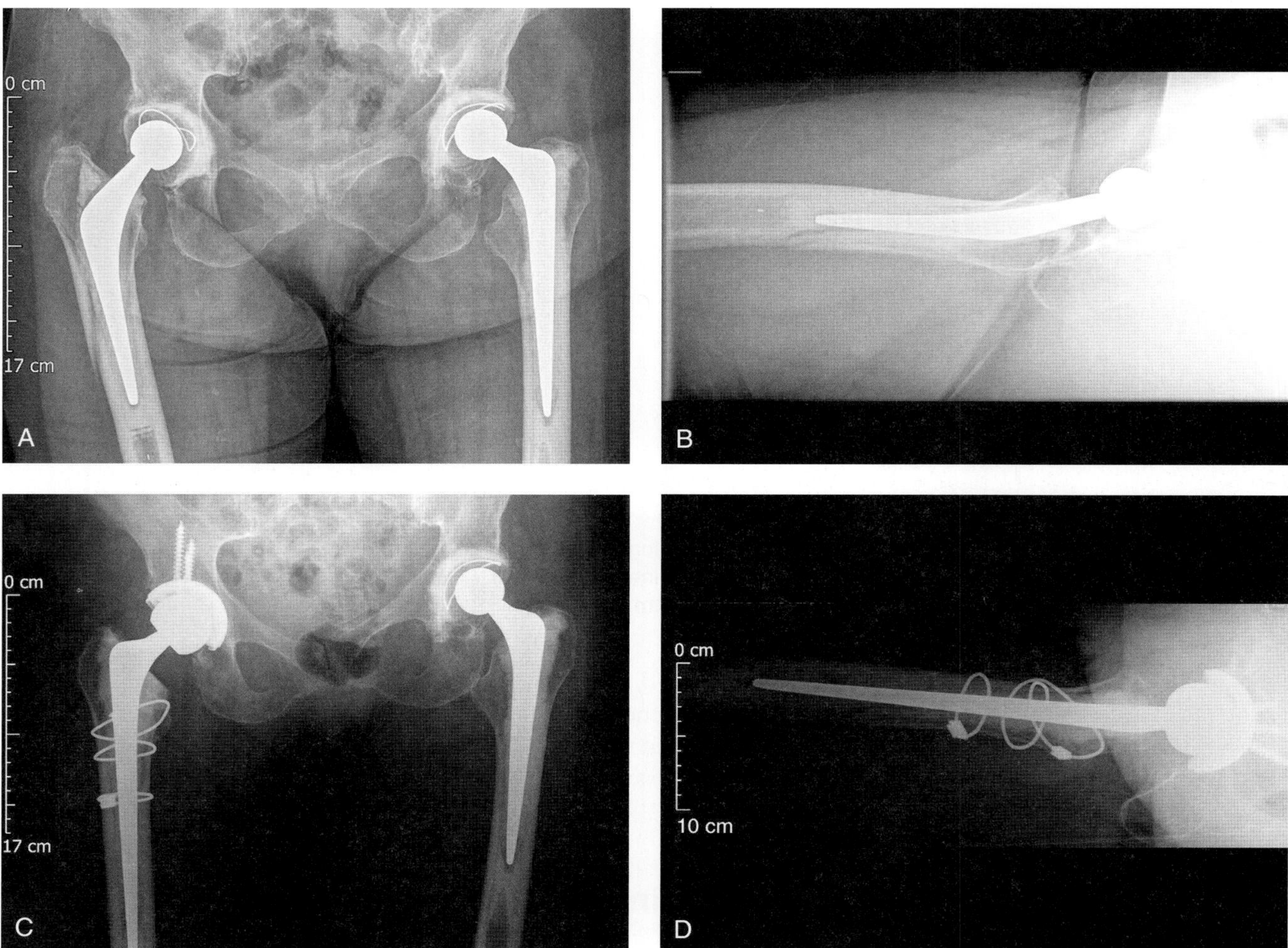

Figure 3 AP pelvic (**A**) and lateral hip (**B**) radiographs demonstrate Vancouver type B1 periprosthetic fracture around a well-fixed cemented stem in a right hip. Postoperative AP pelvic (**C**) and lateral hip (**D**) radiographs demonstrate fracture reduction and cement-in-cement revision. The well-fixed cement in the femoral canal was burred to allow insertion of a longer stem.

stable cement mantle, the cement-in-cement technique has demonstrated good to excellent results (**Table 1**). Recent studies have demonstrated encouraging short-term to midterm results of cement-in-cement revision in the management of Vancouver type B2 periprosthetic fractures in patients in whom the cement-bone interface is well fixed and the fracture is reducible.

Early reports in the 1970s and 1980s of revision THA procedures in which implants were simply recemented into damaged femurs were discouraging. Revision performed using primary arthroplasty techniques and implants had high failure rates resulting from loosening, fracture, infection, and dislocation. The reported incidence of fractures and perforations was as high as 21% in some series. Data from the Swedish Hip Arthroplasty Register and recent publications have shown that cemented femoral revision with appropriate patient selection and meticulous surgical technique can result in satisfactory fixation between the cement and bone (**Table 2**). Studies using contemporary cementing techniques have generally reported femoral revision rates of less than 10% at follow-up of 10 to 13 years. The authors of a recent study with a minimum 20-year follow-up reported radiologic femoral loosening, including rerevision for aseptic loosening, in 13.8% of hips. However, these results are inferior to those obtained with primary cemented stems. This difference can be attributed partly to the condition of the femoral canal, which in these patients often is inadequate to allow the necessary mechanical interlock of cement and bone, leading to a higher prevalence of progressive radiolucent lines and subsequent loosening.

Results of cemented femoral revision do not seem to be as durable as those of noncemented femoral revision, with reported combined rates of radiographic

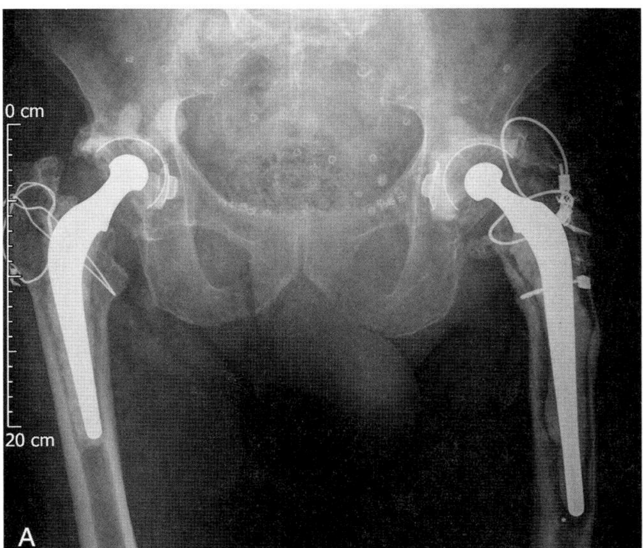

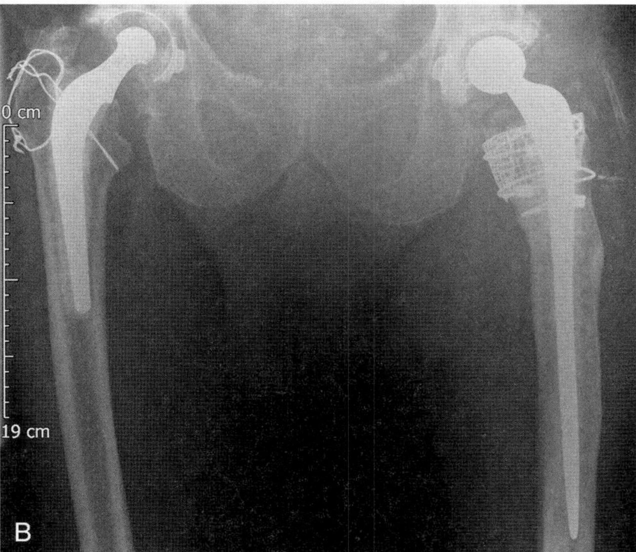

Figure 4 **A,** AP pelvic radiograph demonstrates a loose long cemented stem with lysis and substantial loss of bone stock in a left hip. **B,** Postoperative AP pelvic radiograph demonstrates revision to a long stem with femoral impaction grafting. A mesh was used in the calcar area to contain the allograft chips during impaction.

loosening and revision of 3% to 5% at follow-up of 9 to 14 years. However, comparison of results obtained with the two methods is difficult because of the paucity of prospective, randomized studies in which cemented and noncemented revisions are directly compared. In addition, some studies report results of clinical evaluation, whereas others report radiographic observations or a combination of the two criteria. No standardized evaluation methods have been defined, and differences in surgical technique can confound comparisons. Because of the inconsistent and often unsatisfactory long-term results of femoral revision with cement alone, most specialists have largely abandoned this technique in favor of impaction grafting and insertion of a cemented implant.

Several studies of the use of impaction grafting in femoral revision have demonstrated greater than 90% survivorship of any femoral revisions and greater than 98% survivorship of revisions performed to manage aseptic loosening (**Table 2**). Similarly, a long-term study of more than 1,180 patients in the Swedish Hip Arthroplasty Register demonstrated a cumulative survival rate of 94% at 15 years postoperatively. Complications associated with impaction grafting mainly include intraoperative fractures resulting from the force required to impact the allograft. These fractures can be avoided with careful technique and, as necessary, reinforcement of the proximal femur with cables and occasionally wire mesh. Several millimeters of subsidence of tapered, polished stems within the cement mantle can be expected as a result of so-called cold flow or creep of PMMA. However, subsidence of greater than 3 mm typically is related to inadequate impaction of the allograft before cementing and can be avoided with meticulous surgical technique. Inadequate femoral reconstruction in patients who have poor host bone quality increases the risk of postoperative periprosthetic fracture. In patients who have poor bone quality and a stress riser at the level of a standard-length stem, the use of a longer stem and the modified impaction grafting technique described for these implants is recommended.

Techniques

Setup/Exposure

- Any surgical approach may be used for cemented stem revision. The choice of approach is often at the surgeon's discretion.
- The approach used in the previous surgical procedure and the soft-tissue quality may be useful in determining whether to use a posterior or direct lateral approach.
- The posterior approach may provide better visualization and access to the femoral canal.
- Both the posterior and direct lateral approaches allow the use of extended trochanteric osteotomies if necessary.
- The authors of this chapter advise against the use of the direct anterior and anterolateral (Watson-Jones) approaches in revision THA.

Procedure

REMOVAL OF A CEMENTED STEM

- Before the stem is extracted, the proximal cement around the

Table 1 Results of Femoral Revision With the Cement-in-Cement Technique

Authors (Year)	Number of Hips (Patients)	Implant Type	Reason for Revision	Mean Patient Age in Years (Range)	Mean Follow-up in Years (Range)	Success Rate (%)[a]	Results
Quinlan et al (2006)	54 (42)	53 Exeter (Stryker Howmedica Osteonics), 1 Howse (Johnson & Johnson)	Cup loosening (80%), loose/fractured femoral implant (6%), dislocation (6%), infection (6%), other (2%)	70 (45-85)	2 (0.5-4)	100	No revisions or complications No radiographically loose stems Mean scores: HHS, 85.2; OHS, 19.6; UCLA activity profile, 5.9; SF-36, 78
Mandziak et al (2007)	23 (23)	13 Exeter, 10 CPT (Zimmer)	Dislocation (57%), cup loosening (35%), limb length discrepancy (4%), infection (4%)	75[b] (34-93)	5[b] (1-12)	91.3	1 secondary surgery for periprosthetic fracture 1 revision for cup loosening No radiographically loose stems (14 hips reviewed)
Goto et al (2008)	44 (38)	33 PHS, 7 KC, 4 HS-3 (all implants made by Japan Medical Materials)	Cup loosening	66 (48-78)	5 (2-10)	97.7	1 revision for loosening/fracture 9 perioperative proximal femoral fractures and 1 perforation 3 dislocations Mean Japanese Orthopaedic Association score was 77.8 at 2 yr postoperatively
Duncan et al (2009)	136 (134)	133 Exeter, 1 Charnley (DePuy), 1 McKee-Arden (Deloro Surgical), 1 Müller (Zimmer)	Cup failure (75%), dislocation (15%), infection (6%), fracture (2%), other (2%)	71 (42-91)	8 (5 to 15)	92 (all stem failures), 100 (aseptic stem loosening)	35 revisions (26 for acetabular failure, 4 for infection, 3 for instability, 1 for fracture, 1 for stem fracture) No radiographically loose stems Mean scores: HHS (pain subscale), 40; HHS (function subscale), 28; OHS 33.5
Marcos et al (2009)	37 (35)	3 Charnley, 6 Exeter, 28 C-Stem (DePuy)	Cup failure (54%), dislocation (35%), stem fracture (6%), hemiarthroplasty failure (5%)	68 (29-68)	4 (1-12)	91.8	4 revisions (2 for acetabular failure, 1 for superficial infection, 1 for dislocation) No radiographically loose stems Mean Merle d'Aubigné hip score, 16.6
Stefanovich-Lawbuary et al (2014)	44 (44)	C-Stem AMT (DePuy)	Cup loosening (64%), dislocation (23%), hemiarthroplasty failure (5%), infection (5%), fracture (3%)	72 (42-90)	5 (2-12)	95.2	2 revisions (1 for pelvic discontinuity, 1 for infection) No radiographically loose stems Mean scores: OHS, 34; EQ-5D, 0.814: Self-Administered Patient Satisfaction Scale, 94

HHS = Harris hip score, OHS = Oxford Hip Score, SF-36 = Medical Outcomes Study 36-Item Short Form, UCLA = University of California Los Angeles.
[a] Success is defined as implant survival, with revision as the end point.
[b] Median time reported.

shoulder of the stem is removed with the use of a high-speed burr.
- Polished, tapered, collarless stems are relatively easy to remove with the use of a punch or an in-line slap hammer.
- Matte, collared, and/or curved stems may pose greater difficulties.
- Removal of more of the proximal cement facilitates stem extraction and helps prevent iatrogenic trochanteric fractures.
- The following steps in the surgical technique depend on the stem revision method that will be used.

CEMENT-IN-CEMENT TECHNIQUE

- After the stem is removed, the calcar region is trimmed 2 to 3 mm to allow inspection of the cement-bone interface.
- Cement-in-cement revision requires an integrated, intact cement mantle as assessed by means of preoperative anterolateral and lateral radiographs and intraoperative examination of the proximal cement-bone interface. At a minimum, the cement mantle must be intact below the level of the lesser trochanter. Other revision methods should be used if the patient has soft tissue in the cement-bone interface below this level, proximal bone loss, or an insufficient cement mantle.
- The superficial cement surface is roughened with a burr or an ultrasonic probe to improve integration of the new cement.
- In patients who have a previously malpositioned implant, the remaining cement mantle can similarly be burred from within to allow correct positioning of the new stem.
- Collarless, polished revision stems smaller than the original stem can be used for cement-in-cement revision.
- Limb length and stability are assessed with the use of a trial prosthesis to determine the position of the final implant in terms of depth of insertion (to obtain the desired limb length) and anteversion.
- The original cement mantle is thoroughly irrigated and dried.
- The cement is injected in a liquid phase in retrograde fashion with the use of a narrow nozzle and is pressurized with a cement gun and proximal seal to improve the application of the new PMMA onto the old cement and facilitate chemical bonding.
- In the management of select Vancouver type B2 periprosthetic femur fractures, the use of the cement-in-cement technique, with careful preoperative and intraoperative assessment, is rapid and less technically demanding than complete cement removal. This technique involves removing the implant, which is no longer fixed to the cement mantle, and reducing and fixing the fractured segments that are still attached to the cement. Leaving the well-fixed cement on the bony fragments facilitates strong, accurate reduction.
- In the cement-in-cement technique, the surgeon should apply the standard principles of fracture fixation. Some patients may require application of a long plate in addition to the use of wires and cable. If necessary, a burr is used to expand parts of the cement mantle from within to accommodate the new stem. A new implant is cemented into the reduced cement mantle. Accurate reduction and fixation of the fragments is necessary to prevent substantial leakage of cement through the fracture lines.
- In patients with short oblique or transverse distal fractures, the surgeon should bypass the fracture with a long cemented stem instead of relying on a plate for fixation. In these patients, cement is burred from the inside of the mantle to allow a long stem to pass into the distal canal. A distal cement plug is placed. After cement is inserted in retrograde fashion with a gun, the long stem is inserted into the prepared femur. This method results in a cement-in-cement reconstruction in the proximal femur; distally, the stem will be cemented into host bone.

REMOVAL OF CEMENT

- If the quality of the host bone or the cement mantle is insufficient to allow cement-in-cement revision, the cement must be removed.
- Removal of well-fixed cement can be technically demanding and time-consuming unless dedicated instruments are used. Care must be taken to avoid fracture or perforation.
- Cement removal typically is performed with the use of a combination of tools, such as a high-speed burr, hand chisels, cement osteotomes, cement drills, reverse hooks, and an ultrasonic cement-removal instrument.
- The authors of this chapter recommend the use of a headlight or a canal light to improve visualization of the femoral canal.
- A crucial step in the removal of distal cement is to pierce the cement plug in the center of the femoral canal. This step is far more easily and safely achieved with an ultrasonic perforating device than with other instruments. Intraoperative fluoroscopy can be helpful before the ultrasonic perforator or drill is advanced into the distal cement plug. A conical cement tap attached to a slap hammer is used to remove the cement plug. If this technique is unsuccessful, the distal plug can be removed with the use of an ultrasonic probe advanced centrally through the plug

Table 2 Results of Cemented Femoral Revision

Authors (Year)	Number of Hips (Patients)	Implant Type	Reason for Revision	Bone Grafting
Haydon et al (2004)	97	27 Mallory-Head (Biomet), 15 HNR (Stryker/Howmedica), 13 Harris Design-2 (Stryker/Howmedica), 9 Endurance (DePuy), 5 Iowa (Zimmer), 28 other	Aseptic loosening (66%), infection (11%), fracture (10%), stem fracture (6%), pain (3%), other (4%)	Strut (71%), cancellous (29%)
Sierra et al (2008)	42 (40)	18 Exeter 220 mm, 14 Exeter 240 mm, 10 Exeter 260 mm (Stryker)	Aseptic loosening (55%), periprosthetic fracture (19%), fracture nonunion (21%), infection (5%)	Impaction
ten Have et al (2012)	31 (29)	Exeter standard	Aseptic loosening (80%), loosening and fracture (10%), conversion from Girdlestone procedure (7%), pain (3%)	Impaction
Trumm et al (2014)	80 (74)	34 Charnley (DePuy), 39 Iowa, 7 other	Aseptic loosening (58%), dislocation (20%), stem fracture (10%), other (12%)	None
Solomon et al (2015)	219 (211)	188 Exeter, 31 CPT (Zimmer); 137 long stems, 82 standard stems	Aseptic loosening (75%), periprosthetic fracture (12%), dislocation (3%), infection (4%), other (6%)	Morcellized (21%), strut and morcellized (7%)
te Stroet et al (2015)	208 (202)	185 standard Exeter (150 mm), 23 long Exeter (205 to 260 mm)	Aseptic loosening (76%), septic loosening (17%), pain (3%), other (4%)	Impaction

HHS = Harris hip score, HNR = Head and Neck Replacement.

[a] Success is defined as femoral implant survival with the specified end points.

and followed by the use of ultrasonic scrapers.

- After removal of the cement, any membranes or fibrous tissue adhering to bone must be removed with techniques such as backward curettage and brushing.

CEMENTED FEMORAL REVISION

- Cemented femoral revision is rarely indicated. Alternative methods of revision should be considered except in very elderly or ill patients in whom an expeditious surgical procedure is required.
- Thorough preparation of the femoral canal is required. Preparation includes meticulous removal of fibrous tissue, careful roughening of sclerotic areas to expose cancellous bone, assessment of the presence of defects or perforations, and cautious reaming to allow distal passage of the revision stem.
- The length of the revision stem should exceed the length of the replaced stem, and the revision stem should extend two femoral shaft diameters distal to any perforation or defect.
- Implant sizing should allow for a cement mantle of at least 2 mm.
- If a collared device is used, the authors of this chapter recommend the use of a trial prosthesis with different calcar length options to allow attainment of the optimal implant positioning to achieve stability.
- A distal femoral plug is created with an appropriately sized polyethylene cement restrictor or with a cement plug inserted at the proper depth.
- Cementing is performed with the use of modern techniques, including brushing, thorough irrigation, drying, vacuum mixing, and pressurization of the cement before the stem is introduced.
- The authors of this chapter typically recommend the use of a suction technique and the mixing of three

Table 2 Results of Cemented Femoral Revision (*continued*)

Mean Patient Age in Years (Range)	Mean Follow-up in Years (Range)	Success Rate (%)[a]	Results
68 (39-86)	10.3 (5-23)	Repeat revision for any reason: 87 Aseptic loosening: 91	6% fracture 3% dislocation 2% perforation Mean HHS, 71 (range, 15-100)
74 (49-89)	7.5	Repeat revision for any reason: 90 Failure for any reason: 64	7.1% fracture 4.7% dislocation 7.1% infection Mean Oxford Hip Score, 30
65 (35-82)	12.6 (10-14.7)	Repeat revision for any reason: 100 Revision surgery and subsidence ≥15 mm: 77	12.9% fracture 3.2% dislocation Mean HHS, 76 (range, 22-98)
62 (23-89)	13 (0.2-27)	Repeat revision for any reason: 73.5 Aseptic loosening: 92.5	3.6% implant fracture 1.2% dislocation 91% of patients had no or mild pain All patients were satisfied
72 (30-90)	13 (8-20)	Repeat revision for aseptic loosening (long stems): 97 Repeat revision for aseptic loosening (standard stems): 91	Long stems: 6% fracture, 8% perforation, 14% dislocation, 2% infection Standard stems: 7% fracture, 4% perforation, 13% dislocation, 1% infection Mean HHS (pain subscale) was 40 for long stems and 33 for standard stems
65 (31-95)	10.6 (5-21)	Repeat revision for aseptic loosening: 99 Repeat revision for any reason: 95	7.2% fracture 5.8% dislocation 5.8% infection Mean HHS, 80 (range, 22-100)

HHS = Harris hip score, HNR = Head and Neck Replacement.

[a] Success is defined as femoral implant survival with the specified end points.

batches of cement to ensure that enough material is available to fill the canal.

IMPACTION GRAFTING

- The cemented revision technique with impaction allografting of cancellous bone is intended to reconstitute bone deficiencies in the proximal femur while providing stable fixation of the stem.
- The femur must be meticulously assessed for bone deficiencies and appropriately reinforced with the use of metal mesh, cables or wires, and strut allografts.
- The authors of this chapter recommend fresh-frozen cancellous bone graft morcellized into chips of 2 to 4 mm in size for use in the distal canal.
- Warm irrigation fluid is used to wash osseous fat out of the bone chips to allow more stable compaction of chips and penetration of the cement into the material.
- The distal restrictor is placed 2 cm distal to the anticipated location of the tip of the stem. Most surgeons prefer to use cannulated tamps to create a symmetric neo-endosteum and avoid valgus malalignment.
- A 2-cm layer of graft is impacted distally against the restrictor.
- Additional graft is gradually added and impacted with the use of cannulated tamps of progressively larger diameters until the diameter of the impactor reaches the shape of the proximal stem. The size of this impaction instrument should correspond with the size of the stem that will be implanted.
- To allow for an adequate cement mantle, the dimensions of the proximal packers are deliberately oversized. The challenge is to impact the graft firmly and homogeneously enough to provide stability but avoid femoral fractures.
- Because of the risk of fracture

resulting from the high forces applied during impaction, reinforcement of the proximal femur is extremely important.
- The aim is to create a neoendosteum of 5 to 6 mm in thickness in the proximal femur. In this area, bone chips of 8 to 10 mm in size should be used to improve torsional stability. These larger chips can be packed proximally around the final impactor, which in most systems is designed to allow for trial reduction.
- The reconstruction is evaluated for rotational stability.
- The packed femoral canal is filled distally with cement in retrograde fashion with the use of a suction catheter.
- After the catheter is removed, the column of cement is pressurized with the use of the cement gun and a proximal seal.
- When the cement reaches a doughlike consistency, the stem is slowly introduced, taking care to place the implant in the previously determined position.

Wound Closure

- Meticulous reattachment of detached tendons around the greater trochanter is recommended.
- Wound closure is done in a standard manner.

Postoperative Regimen

Cemented prostheses provide immediate implant stability and allow early mobilization. Postoperative radiographs are useful in assessing the quality of the cement mantle. Patients are usually allowed immediate full weight bearing postoperatively with the use of crutches for 6 to 8 weeks. Partial weight bearing may be more appropriate in patients who have undergone impaction grafting of large defects or who have sustained an intraoperative fracture. For patients who undergo impaction grafting, most authors suggest touch-down weight bearing for 6 to 8 weeks postoperatively, followed by 4 to 6 weeks of gradually increased weight bearing, for a total of 12 weeks on crutches. Permanent restrictions are similar to those specified after a primary THA. Patients are seen for routine postoperative follow-up at 6 weeks, 6 months, and yearly thereafter, and radiographs are obtained at these intervals.

Avoiding Pitfalls and Complications

Use of the cement-in-cement technique requires careful surface preparation because fat or blood on the cement surface can compromise bonding. A thin layer of blood or marrow can cause up to an 85% reduction in shear strength and an 80% reduction in tensile strength of the cement-to-cement interface. Preparation of the femoral canal with a burr or an ultrasonic device will allow for a larger cement mantle and thereby increase the surface area of contact between the old and new cement. Some surgeons recommend that the new cement be placed into the femoral canal before it reaches a doughlike consistency to improve the interface between the new and old cement. To do so, the surgeon pressurizes the cement with the use of a proximal seal and gun. It is important to perform preoperative templating of several different implants with different offsets and have them available intraoperatively. If a collared implant is used, extended femoral neck lengths may be especially useful in restoring offset.

Revision of a failed femoral implant can be technically challenging. A successful procedure requires careful and detailed preoperative planning and templating, adequate exposure, and careful removal of the failed implant and cement to prevent additional damage to the greater trochanter and the cortical tube. Several technical tips may improve the results of cemented femoral revision. First, when cement is removed from the femoral canal, the cement must be split and chiseled away in a radial and longitudinal manner to avoid perforation of or damage to the cortex. Care must be taken to remove all accessible lateral cement from the stem shoulder to prevent fracture of the greater trochanter. Second, the neocortex that sometimes forms when a stem loosens should be removed to allow adequate interdigitation of the cement and bone. Third, the use of a stem that extends at least 2 to 3 femoral shaft diameters beyond the distal tip of the previous stem is recommended. Finally, a cement restrictor should be used to enhance cement fixation. If the stem will extend into the lower metaphyseal region where the femur flares, the surgeon can first inject a separate batch of cement with a long cement gun distal to where the tip of the prosthesis will be located and allow it to harden before injecting additional cement.

Intraoperative fractures usually are associated with cement removal or impaction grafting. The use of meticulous technique, careful planning, and dedicated equipment has substantially reduced the incidence of early failure and fracture in impaction allografting. Fluoroscopy can be used throughout the procedure to allow identification of an intraoperative fracture. If a femoral fracture occurs during the procedure, it must be reduced. Adequate reconstruction may involve the use of metal plating or a combination of metal plating and allograft bone struts. Usually, reconstruction is followed by impaction grafting of the reconstructed canal and placement of a cemented stem. If the fracture is well reduced and the impaction adequately executed, this technique will prevent extrusion of cement through the fractured areas.

Cortical defects should always be identified. If a simple cemented revision is to be performed, the defect should be manually obstructed during insertion of the cement to promote adequate pressurization and prevent extrusion of cement into the surrounding tissues. If extruded cement is identified, it can be removed easily after the cement has cured. If a cortical defect is identified during impaction grafting, the defect should be covered with a wire mesh held with cerclage wires to create a cavitary defect for impaction grafting. Finally, to maintain the stem in the proper position during insertion, the cement should be allowed to reach a doughlike consistency before the stem is introduced, and the stem should not be moved after it has been placed in the cement mantle in the correct position with regard to limb length and anteversion.

Bibliography

Briant-Evans TW, Veeramootoo D, Tsiridis E, Hubble MJ: Cement-in-cement stem revision for Vancouver type B periprosthetic femoral fractures after total hip arthroplasty: A 3-year follow-up of 23 cases. *Acta Orthop* 2009;80(5):548-552.

Duncan WW, Hubble MJ, Howell JR, Whitehouse SL, Timperley AJ, Gie GA: Revision of the cemented femoral stem using a cement-in-cement technique: A five- to 15-year review. *J Bone Joint Surg Br* 2009;91(5):577-582.

Gehrke T: Revision is not difficult, in Breusch S, Malchau H, eds: *The Well-Cemented Total Hip Arthroplasty*. Heidelberg, Germany, Springer Medizin Verlag, 2005, pp 348-358.

Gehrke T, Gebauer M, Kendoff D: Femoral stem impaction grafting: Extending the role of cement. *Bone Joint J* 2013;95-B(11 suppl A):92-94.

Gie GA, Linder L, Ling RS, Simon JP, Slooff TJ, Timperley AJ: Contained morselized allograft in revision total hip arthroplasty: Surgical technique. *Orthop Clin North Am* 1993;24(4):717-725.

Goto K, Kawanabe K, Akiyama H, Morimoto T, Nakamura T: Clinical and radiological evaluation of revision hip arthroplasty using the cement-in-cement technique. *J Bone Joint Surg Br* 2008;90(8):1013-1018.

Haydon CM, Burnett RS: Cemented femoral revision in total hip arthroplasty, in Scuderi GR, Tria AJ, Long WJ, Kang MN, eds: *Techniques in Revision Hip and Knee Arthroplasty*. Philadelphia, PA, Saunders, 2015, pp 466-474.

Haydon CM, Mehin R, Burnett S, et al: Revision total hip arthroplasty with use of a cemented femoral component: Results at a mean of ten years. *J Bone Joint Surg Am* 2004;86(6):1179-1185.

Holt G, Hook S, Hubble M: Revision total hip arthroplasty: The femoral side using cemented implants. *Int Orthop* 2011;35(2):267-273.

Lee AJ, Ling RS, Gheduzzi S, Simon JP, Renfro RJ: Factors affecting the mechanical and viscoelastic properties of acrylic bone cement. *J Mater Sci Mater Med* 2002;13(8):723-733.

Lieberman JR: Cemented femoral revision: Lest we forget. *J Arthroplasty* 2005;20(4 suppl 2):72-74.

Linder L: Cancellous impaction grafting in the human femur: Histological and radiographic observations in 6 autopsy femurs and 8 biopsies. *Acta Orthop Scand* 2000;71(6):543-552.

Ling RS, Charity J, Lee AJ, Whitehouse SL, Timperley AJ, Gie GA: The long-term results of the original Exeter polished cemented femoral component: A follow-up report. *J Arthroplasty* 2009;24(4):511-517.

Malchau H, Herberts P, Eisler T, Garellick G, Söderman P: The Swedish Total Hip Replacement Register. *J Bone Joint Surg Am* 2002;84(suppl 2):2-20.

Mandziak DG, Howie DW, Neale SD, McGee MA: Cement-within-cement stem exchange using the collarless polished double-taper stem. *J Arthroplasty* 2007;22(7):1000-1006.

Marcos L, Buttaro M, Comba F, Piccaluga F: Femoral cement within cement technique in carefully selected aseptic revision arthroplasties. *Int Orthop* 2009;33(3):633-637.

Maurer SG, Baitner AC, Di Cesare PE: Reconstruction of the failed femoral component and proximal femoral bone loss in revision hip surgery. *J Am Acad Orthop Surg* 2000;8(6):354-363.

Quinlan JF, O'Shea K, Doyle F, Brady OH: In-cement technique for revision hip arthroplasty. *J Bone Joint Surg Br* 2006;88(6):730-733.

Richards CJ, Duncan CP, Crawford RW: Cement-in-cement femoral revision for the treatment of highly selected Vancouver B2 periprosthetic fractures. *J Arthroplasty* 2011;26(2):335-337.

Schreurs BW, Arts JJ, Verdonschot N, Buma P, Slooff TJ, Gardeniers JW: Femoral component revision with use of impaction bone-grafting and a cemented polished stem: Surgical technique. *J Bone Joint Surg Am* 2006;88(suppl 1 pt 2):259-274.

Sierra RJ, Charity J, Tsiridis E, Timperley JA, Gie GA: The use of long cemented stems for femoral impaction grafting in revision total hip arthroplasty. *J Bone Joint Surg Am* 2008;90(6):1330-1336.

Solomon LB, Costi K, Kosuge D, Cordier T, McGee MA, Howie DW: Revision total hip arthroplasty using cemented collarless double-taper femoral components at a mean follow-up of 13 years (8 to 20): An update. *Bone Joint J* 2015;97-B(8):1038-1045.

Stefanovich-Lawbuary NS, Parry MC, Whitehouse MR, Blom AW: Cement in cement revision of the femoral component using a collarless triple taper: A midterm clinical and radiographic assessment. *J Arthroplasty* 2014;29(10):2002-2006.

Taylor JW, Rorabeck CH: Hip revision arthroplasty: Approach to the femoral side. *Clin Orthop Relat Res* 1999;369:208-222.

te Stroet MA, Rijnen WH, Gardeniers JW, van Kampen A, Schreurs BW: The outcome of femoral component revision arthroplasty with impaction allograft bone grafting and a cemented polished Exeter stem: A prospective cohort study of 208 revision arthroplasties with a mean follow-up of ten years. *Bone Joint J* 2015;97-B(6):771-779.

ten Have BL, Brouwer RW, van Biezen FC, Verhaar JA: Femoral revision surgery with impaction bone grafting: 31 hips followed prospectively for ten to 15 years. *J Bone Joint Surg Br* 2012;94(5):615-618.

Trumm BN, Callaghan JJ, George CA, Liu SS, Goetz DD, Johnston RC: Minimum 20-year follow-up results of revision total hip arthroplasty with improved cementing technique. *J Arthroplasty* 2014;29(1):236-241.

Chapter 58

Femoral Revision With Extensively Porous-Coated Stems

Neil Sheth, MD

Wayne G. Paprosky, MD

Indications

As the number of primary total hip arthroplasties performed increases, the revision burden also is expected to rise. Clinical scenarios that may require revision of the femoral implant include aseptic loosening, implant malposition, periprosthetic fracture, deep periprosthetic infection, femoral implant fracture, osteolysis, and poor implant track record. Regardless of the reason for femoral revision, adherence to certain reconstructive principles is necessary to achieve clinical success. Proper implant sizing reduces stem subsidence and helps to obtain initial fixation of the implant. Axial and rotational stability of the implant is critical and requires proper implant positioning with adequate interference fit to optimize the surface area available for biologic fixation.

The choice of femoral implant for the reconstruction is based on the location of bone loss (metaphyseal versus diaphyseal), the amount of residual bone stock (loss of cancellous bone support), and the amount of remaining femoral isthmus available for fixation of the femoral implant. The Paprosky classification has been validated for use in preoperative revision planning and assists in the selection of reconstruction options (**Figure 1**).

Paprosky type I bone loss refers to minimal metaphyseal bone loss with an absence of proximal femoral remodeling. Typically, these defects can be reconstructed with the use of a primary total hip arthroplasty implant, and proximal fixation within the femur can be achieved. Successful clinical results have been reported with the use of cemented stems and with noncemented proximal or diaphyseal-fitting stems.

Paprosky type II defects, the most common bone loss pattern, have more extensive proximal metaphyseal cancellous bone loss. Slight proximal femoral remodeling into varus and retroversion is commonly encountered. These defects require the use of a diaphyseally engaging stem such as an extensively porous-coated stem. Excellent clinical results have been reported with this type of reconstruction (**Figure 2**).

Paprosky type III defects are subclassified on the basis of the amount of residual femoral isthmus. Type IIIA bone loss is defined as severe metadiaphyseal bone loss with greater than 4 cm of isthmus remaining, whereas type IIIB defects are associated with less than 4 cm of residual isthmus remaining. The proximal femoral remodeling is typically more severe than in patients with type I or II defects. These patients may require the use of adjunctive measures for surgical exposure such as an extended trochanteric osteotomy (ETO). Type III defects are reconstructed with extensively porous-coated stems, which require 4 to 6 cm of isthmic fit (**Figure 3**), or with nonmodular tapered splined titanium stems, which require 1 to 2 cm of interference fit (**Figure 4**).

As with any surgical procedure, detailed preoperative planning is paramount in achieving clinical success. Femoral revision requires wide surgical exposure to perform the procedure and minimize the risk of inadvertent injury to adjacent structures. The posterior approach is most commonly used because it provides excellent exposure of both the acetabulum and femur and is the most extensile. Anteriorly based approaches have seen recent enthusiasm because they provide improved hip stability compared with the posterior approach, as well as excellent acetabular visualization. However, femoral exposure can be challenging with anteriorly based approaches.

Dr. Sheth or an immediate family member serves as a paid consultant to or is an employee of Zimmer Biomet. Dr. Paprosky or an immediate family member has received royalties from Stryker and Zimmer Biomet; serves as a paid consultant to or is an employee of Intellijoint Surgical, Medtronic, Stryker, and Zimmer Biomet; has stock or stock options held in Intellijoint Surgical, Ketai Medical, and Stryker; has received nonincome support (such as equipment or services), commercially derived honoraria, or other non–research-related funding (such as paid travel) from Northwestern Medicine; and serves as a board member, owner, officer, or committee member of The Hip Society.

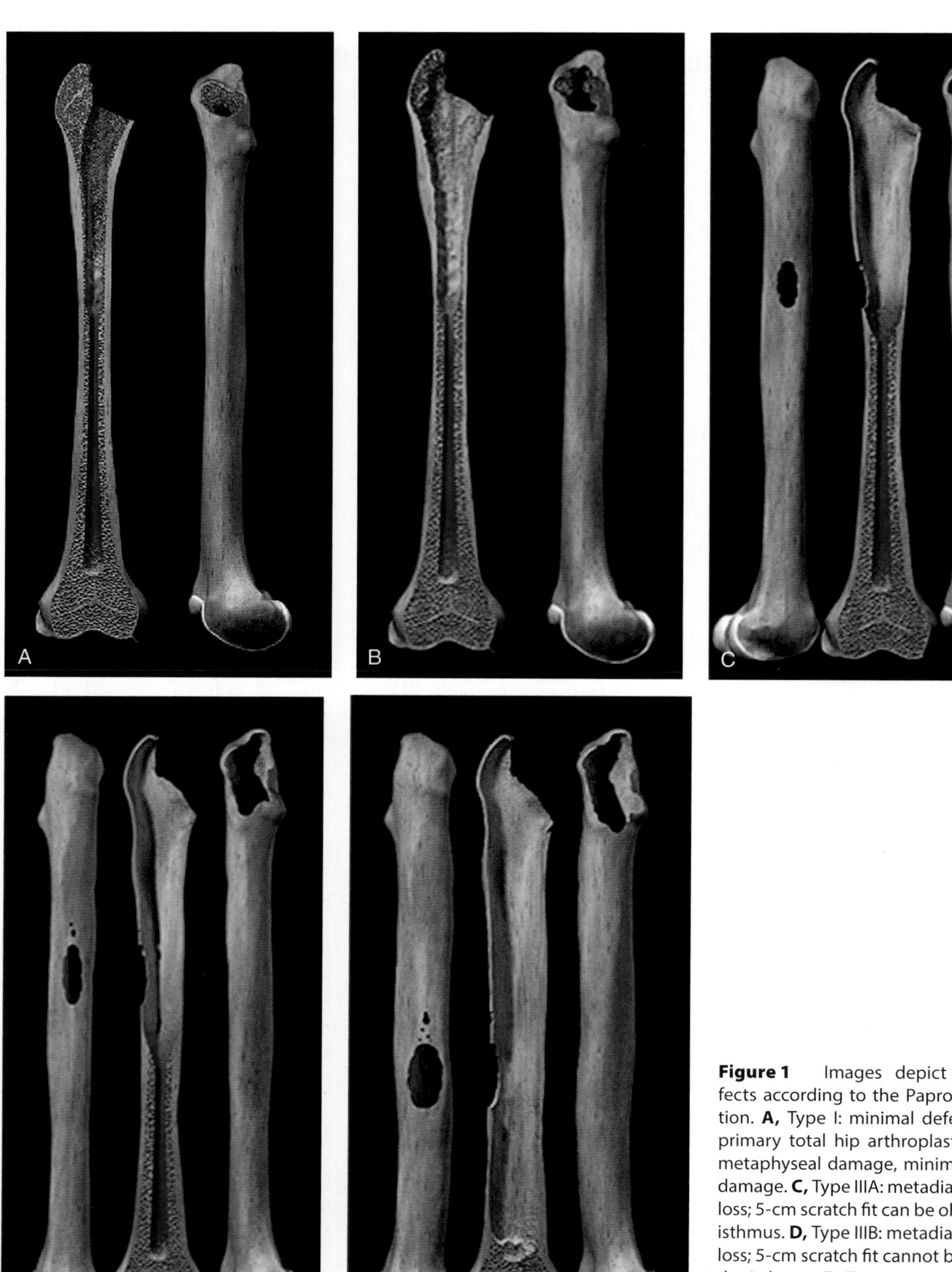

Figure 1 Images depict femoral defects according to the Paprosky classification. **A,** Type I: minimal defect; similar to primary total hip arthroplasty. **B,** Type II: metaphyseal damage, minimal diaphyseal damage. **C,** Type IIIA: metadiaphyseal bone loss; 5-cm scratch fit can be obtained at the isthmus. **D,** Type IIIB: metadiaphyseal bone loss; 5-cm scratch fit cannot be obtained at the isthmus. **E,** Type IV: extensive metadiaphyseal damage, thin cortices, widened canals. (Courtesy of DePuy Synthes, Warsaw, IN.)

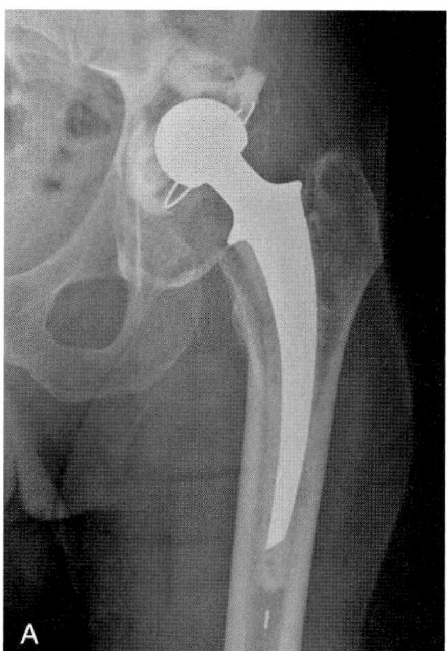

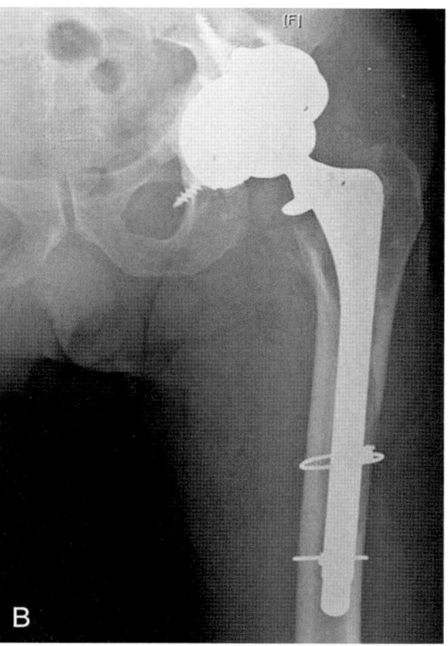

Figure 2 Preoperative (**A**) and 1-year postoperative (**B**) AP radiographs of a left hip demonstrate the use of an 8-inch, straight, extensively porous-coated stem for reconstruction in a patient with a loose cemented cup and stem with associated osteolysis. Cerclage cables were placed distally for protection of the femoral shaft even though an extended trochanteric osteotomy was not required.

Contraindications

Type III defects associated with a canal diameter greater than 19 mm should be reconstructed with the use of a tapered, splined titanium stem because extensively porous-coated stems with a large diameter are extremely stiff and would result in a substantial modulus mismatch with the surrounding bone stock. This differential in stiffness increases the likelihood of thigh pain, proximal femoral stress shielding, and periprosthetic fracture through the adjacent bone.

Patients with type IV defects have complete canal ectasia and severe metaphyseal and diaphyseal bone loss. The bone loss is so severe that minimal associated proximal femoral remodeling is present. Extensively porous-coated stems are not optimal in this clinical scenario. In these patients, reconstruction

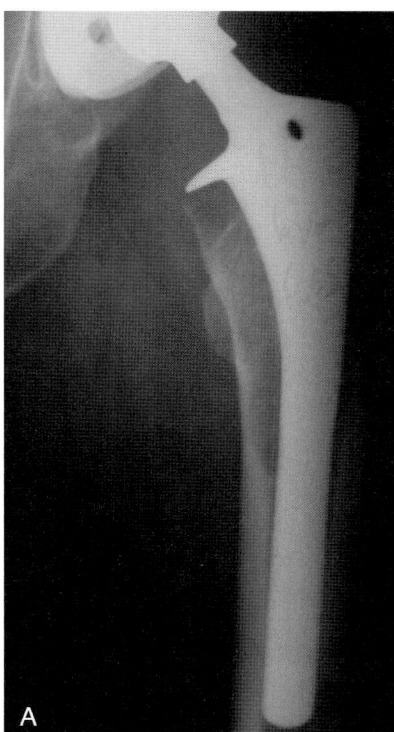

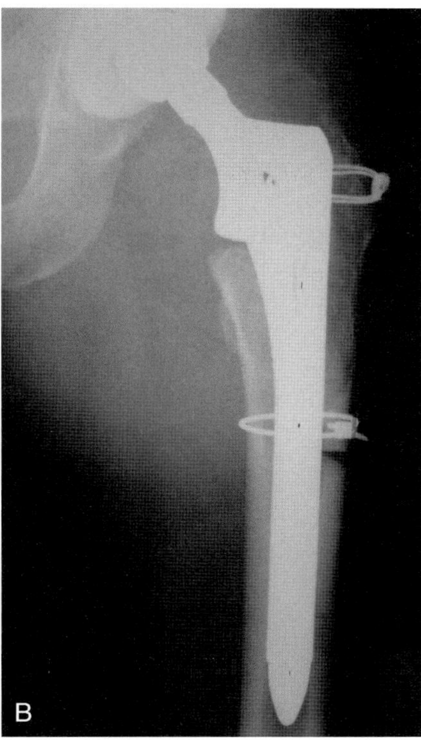

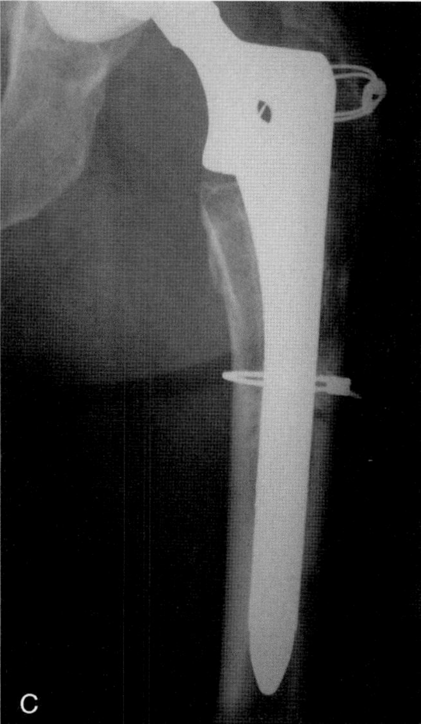

Figure 3 Preoperative (**A**), immediate postoperative (**B**), and 8-year postoperative (**C**) AP radiographs of a left hip demonstrate the use of an extensively porous-coated prosthesis in a 61-year-old patient with a loose cemented femoral implant. Note the healed trochanteric osteotomy. (Reproduced from Paprosky WG, Sporer SM: Femoral revision: Extensively porous-coated stems, in Lieberman JR, Berry DJ: *Advanced Reconstruction: Hip*. Rosemont, IL, American Academy of Orthopaedic Surgeons, 2005, pp 409-416.)

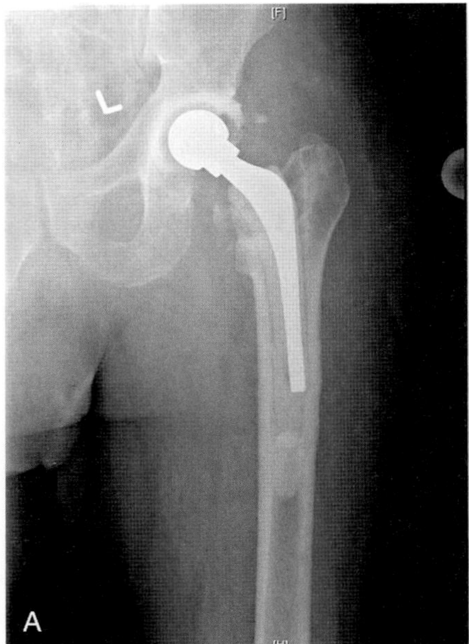

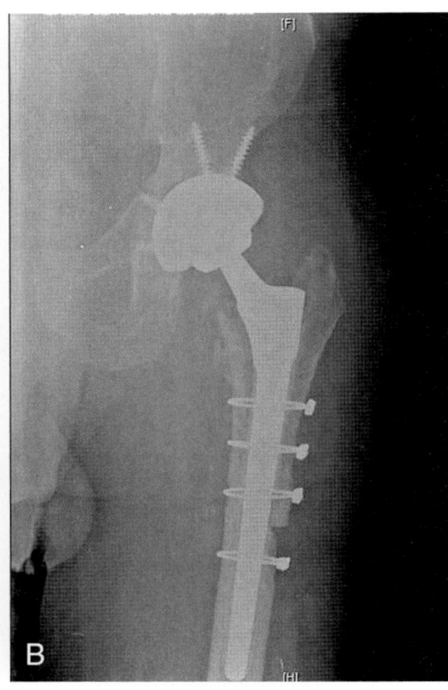

Figure 4 **A,** AP radiograph of a left hip demonstrates a Paprosky type III defect in a patient in whom periprosthetic infection developed after primary arthroplasty. **B,** AP radiograph of the hip obtained 18 months after revision surgery demonstrates a nonmodular splined tapered stem. A cerclage cable was placed distal to the extended trochanteric osteotomy to avoid distal propagation of the osteotomy.

is best performed with a long cemented stem, with or without concomitant impaction grafting of the canal; an allograft-prosthetic composite; a modular oncology prosthesis (proximal femoral replacement); or, in some patients, a noncemented fluted tapered modular stem.

Alternative Treatments

Extensively porous-coated implants were once considered the preferred method of revision femoral reconstruction. However, the increased versatility of modular tapered stems has made this stem design more attractive for femoral implant revision.

Results

Several studies have reported the use of extensively porous-coated stems in revision procedures with reliable long-term clinical outcomes (**Table 1**).

Techniques

Setup/Exposure

- A systematic approach to the surgical exposure is beneficial, especially when the procedure is performed by a surgeon with limited experience in revision procedures.
- The authors of this chapter prefer the posterior approach for hip revision procedures.
- The previous incision typically is incorporated into the surgical exposure.
- Previous incisions that are more anterior make femoral exposure more difficult, whereas previous incisions that are more posterior make acetabular exposure more difficult.
- If only a portion of the previous incision can be incorporated, a new incision can be made without concern for vascular compromise of the skin because the proximity of the hip to the central torso provides robust vascular anastamoses that allow the use of multiple incisions.
- Typically, a longitudinal incision that is in line with the posterior third of the femoral shaft is adequate to obtain visualization.
- After the fascial incision is made and the gluteus maximus is split in line with the muscle fibers, anatomic landmarks are identified.
- The posterior borders of the vastus lateralis and the gluteus medius are the most reproducible landmarks, even in patients with excessive scar tissue (**Figure 5**).
- The gluteus maximus insertion on the femur is recessed using electrocautery, taking care not to injure the sciatic nerve or the underlying branch of the inferior gluteal artery.

Procedure

- After the capsular approach and adequate release of surrounding scar tissue have been completed, the hip is dislocated in a controlled fashion with a bone hook.
- The affected leg is placed in a flexed, adducted, and internally rotated position to maximize visualization of the proximal femur. A proximal femoral elevator can help enhance visualization in this position.
- Before the stability of the femoral implant is checked, the shoulder of the prosthesis must be cleared of any bony overgrowth and fibrous tissue. If the femoral stem is loose and removal is not impeded by the greater trochanter, the stem can be removed safely.
- An ETO is extremely helpful in patients with well-fixed femoral implants (predominantly diaphyseally engaging stems), patients in whom removal of a long column of cement is required, or patients in

Table 1 Results of Revision With an Extensively Porous-Coated Femoral Implant

Authors (Year)	Number of Hips	Implant Type	Mean Patient Age in Years (Range)	Mean Follow-up in Years (Range)	Success Rate (%)[a]	Results[b]
Engh et al (2001)	211	AML (DePuy)	NR	12 (2-18)	94	39 hips required 44 component revisions; 26 of these underwent a first revision ≥10 yr after the index operation The overall femoral implant loosening rate was 5.4%
Moreland and Moreno (2001)	137	AML or Solution (DePuy)	63 (NA)	9.3 (5-16)	83	4% required repeat revision for aseptic femoral loosening 83% had radiographic evidence of bone ingrowth
Weeden and Paprosky (2002)	188	AML or Solution	61.2 (NA)	14.2 (11-16)	96	3.5% required repeat revision for aseptic femoral loosening 4.1% mechanical failure rate
Hamilton et al (2007)	905	AML or Solution	NR	5 and 10	98	20 hips (2.2%) required rerevision, 12 of which were for aseptic loosening 5-yr survivorship rate, 97.5% 10-yr survivorship rate, 95.9% Survivorship remained constant after 10 yr
Moon et al (2009)	35	Multiple implants	NR	6.5 (5-10)	100	No femoral stems required rerevision No radiographic evidence of implant loosening
Jayakumar et al (2011)	56	Multiple implants	NR	6 (NA)	100	No femoral stems required rerevision
Chung et al (2012)	96	Multiple implants	63 (23-89)	5.5 (2-11)	97	92 hips achieved bone ingrowth 1 hip (1%) was fibrous and stable 3 hips (3%) were in patients who died of unrelated causes
Thomsen et al (2013)	93	AML or Solution	69 (33-86)	14 (10-18)	94	94.4% cumulative survival rate without rerevision for any reason 97.6% cumulative survival rate without rerevision for aseptic loosening

AML = Anatomic Medullary Locking, NA = not available, NR = not reported.
[a] Success is defined based on femoral implants that did not require revision.
[b] Results data are based on hips.

whom the proximal femur has undergone substantial varus remodeling (**Figure 6**).

EXTENDED TROCHANTERIC OSTEOTOMY

- To initiate the ETO, the incision is extended distally, and the posterior margin of the vastus lateralis is identified.
- The gluteus maximus insertion is recessed in its entirety from the femur.
- The muscle belly of the vastus is mobilized anteriorly, taking care to minimize soft-tissue stripping from the anticipated femoral osteotomy fragment.
- The length of the osteotomy, which typically is measured radiographically during the preoperative planning phase, and the distal extent of the osteotomy are marked on the femur (**Figure 7**).
- The osteotomy is started proximally and proceeds in a posterolateral-to-anterolateral direction.
- With the affected leg held in an extended and internally rotated position, the osteotomy is progressed distally with the use of either an oscillating saw blade or a microsagittal saw.
- The osteotomy fragment should encompass one-third of the diameter

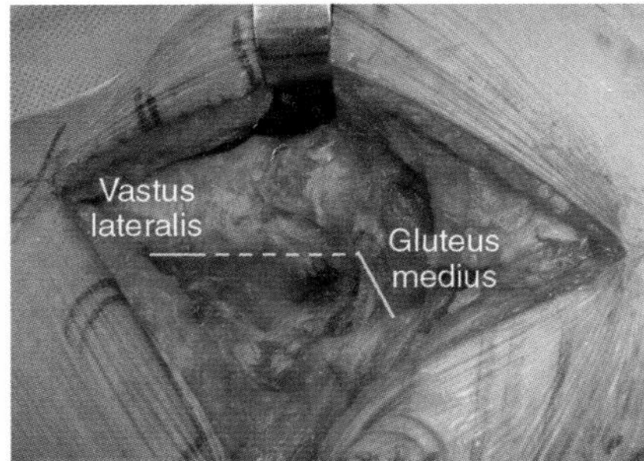

Figure 5 Intraoperative photograph shows the posterior border of the vastus lateralis and the posterior border of the gluteus medius, which are the two key landmarks when a posterior approach is used for surgical exposure in revision total hip arthroplasty. (Reproduced with permission from Sheth N, Courtney PM, Paprosky WG: Extended trochanteric osteotomy, in Berry DJ, Maloney M, eds: *Master Techniques in Orthopaedic Surgery: The Hip*, ed 3. Philadelphia, PA, Wolters Kluwer, 2016, pp 47-58.)

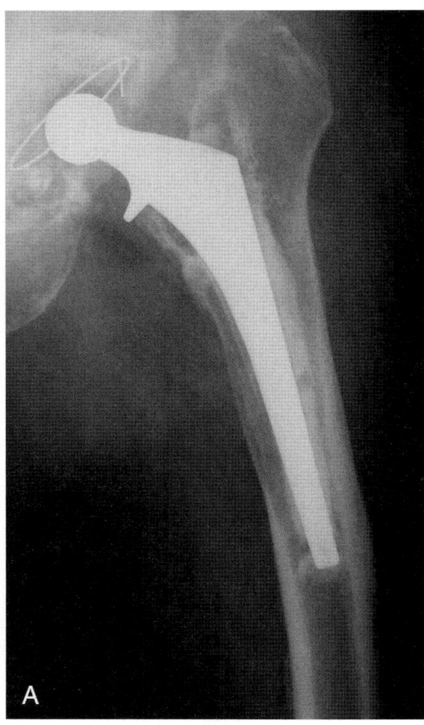

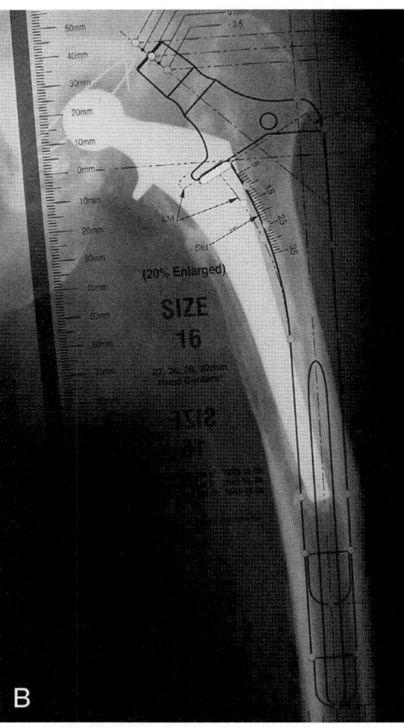

Figure 6 **A,** AP radiograph of a left hip in a patient with a well-fixed primary femoral implant in whom varus remodeling of the proximal femur has occurred. **B,** The same image with an overlaid template demonstrates the planned revision. An extended trochanteric osteotomy is required to avoid lateral cortical perforation during femoral preparation. (Reproduced from Paprosky WG, Sporer SM: Femoral revision: Extensively porous-coated stems, in Lieberman JR, Berry DJ: *Advanced Reconstruction: Hip*. Rosemont, IL, American Academy of Orthopaedic Surgeons, 2005, pp 409-416.)

of the femoral shaft and should be oriented perpendicular to the native femoral anteversion.

- At the distal extent, a pencil-tipped burr is used to make rounded edges as the osteotomy is extended transversely in the anterior direction. This method minimizes the risk of distal fracture propagation.
- The osteotomy is extended, starting proximally on the anterior cortex and proceeding approximately 1.5 cm distally.
- The osteotomy is then extended approximately 1.5 cm in a similar manner on the proximal femur, taking care to release the proximal anterior pseudocapsule.
- A series of wide osteotomes are used in a posterior-to-anterior direction to lever the fragment and complete the osteotomy.
- The greater trochanteric fragment, with the abductor complex and vastus lateralis attached, is retracted anteriorly, typically with the anterior blade of a Charnley bow. Anterolateral dissection on the osteotomy fragment should be avoided to minimize disruption of the anteriorly based blood supply to the fragment.
- With the osteotomy in this position, the femoral implant should be adequately visible for removal.

FEMORAL CANAL PREPARATION

- After the existing femoral implant has been removed, femoral canal preparation begins.
- The canal is débrided of all fibrous tissue to facilitate endosteal contact of the host bone with the new femoral implant.
- Concentric reaming of the canal is important to minimize the risk of cortical perforation.
- After ETO, direct visualization of the distal diaphyseal isthmus is possible, and decreases the risk of cortical perforation, especially in patients with proximal varus femoral remodeling.
- If ETO was performed, a circumferential femoral cerclage cable is placed just distal to the osteotomy site before the femur is reamed and broached to prevent femoral fracture during insertion of the implant.
- During the reaming process, the surgeon must pay attention to the distance over which reaming is performed. The distance of reaming should correlate to the length of the anticipated stem for reconstruction.
- At least 4 to 6 cm of interference fit is necessary when an extensively porous-coated stem is used. Alternative methods of reconstruction should be considered if adequate

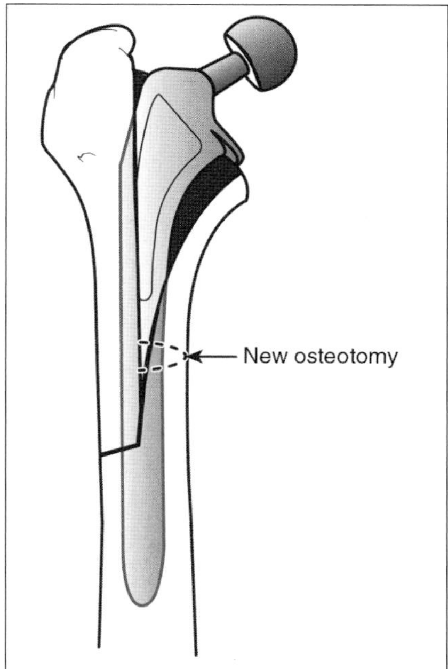

Figure 7 Illustration depicts an osteotomy of the remaining reduced bone that may be required to provide good bone apposition in patients with severe varus remodeling. Typically, the osteotomy is made with an oscillating saw blade or microsagittal saw 1 or 2 cm above the most distal aspect of the lateral osteotomy. (Reproduced from Paprosky WG, Sporer SM: Femoral revision: Extensively porous-coated stems, in Lieberman JR, Berry DJ: *Advanced Reconstruction: Hip.* Rosemont, IL, American Academy of Orthopaedic Surgeons, 2005, pp 409-416.)

fixation cannot be achieved.

- Sequential canal reaming is performed until endosteal contact is achieved. Straight cylindric reamers are used when a 6- or 8-inch straight, extensively porous-coated stem will be used. If the anterior femoral bow is encountered and the use of an 8- or 10-inch bowed stem is planned, flexible reamers are used to ream the femoral canal.
- In general, the femoral canal is reamed to a depth of 0.5 mm less than the intended stem size. For example, the canal should be reamed to a depth of 14.5 mm for a 15-mm stem.
- The final implant is placed by hand with 4 to 6 cm of the implant sitting proud, without the use of a mallet for impaction. If the implant cannot be placed to this level by hand, the canal should be reamed line to line to allow proper insertion of the implant.
- After a trial stem is placed, the hip is reduced and moved through a range of motion to assess stability.
- After the desired hip stability is achieved, the stem anteversion is marked on the femur.
- If a bowed stem is used, the surgeon cannot adjust the anteversion of the final implant because it is determined by the bow of the femur. If a stable hip cannot be achieved with a bowed stem, the use of a modular tapered splined stem should be considered.

FEMORAL STEM IMPLANTATION

- Implantation of an extensively porous-coated stem is best performed with the use of a hole gauge to determine if the tolerance specified by the implant manufacturer is appropriate for the distal portion of the stem. For example, a 16-mm stem should pass through the 16.25-mm hole, not the 16-mm hole.
- If the size of the stem does not match the corresponding hole-gauge size (for example, a 16-mm stem fits through the 16.5-mm hole and not through the 16.25-mm hole), a 0.75-mm reamer should be used if one is available, or the canal should be reamed line to line.
- A series of gentle blows with a mallet are used to seat the implant. The stem should advance with every mallet strike.

Wound Closure

- Meticulous wound closure is paramount to preventing wound complications and surgical site infection.
- The ETO fragment is secured, typically with two or three cables depending on the length of the osteotomy fragment.
- Release of the proximal anterior pseudocapsule at the start of the procedure allows proper reduction of the fragment without the need to place the affected limb in excessive abduction and internal rotation.
- The authors of this chapter prefer to repair the posterior capsule and short external rotators to the posterior aspect of the abductor complex in a soft-tissue repair.
- The gluteus maximus insertion does not require suture repair.
- The deep fascia and superficial soft tissues are closed in standard fashion.
- In patients who had substantial blood loss during the procedure, or in morbidly obese patients, a series of drains typically is used to minimize postoperative hematoma or seroma formation. The authors of this chapter prefer to place a 10-mm flat Jackson-Pratt drain deep to the fascia and a second drain superficial to the fascia. It is imperative to put sutures only in the tissue layers with good integrity: the deep fascia, Scarpa fascia, and dermis. Sutures placed in the adipose tissue will result in fat necrosis and increase the risk for seroma formation.
- In patients with substantial adipose tissue between the deep fascia and the epidermis, a second 10-mm flat Jackson-Pratt drain is placed over Scarpa fascia after it has been reapproximated.
- Typically, the skin is closed using nylon suture in a horizontal mattress formation.
- In morbidly obese patients, an incisional wound vacuum dressing typically is used for 72 hours postoperatively while the drains are in

place to decompress the deep dead space.

- The incisional wound vacuum dressing will create a negative pressure zone around the incision while it epithelializes in the first 36 to 72 hours postoperatively.

Postoperative Regimen

After femoral revision surgery, patients are placed on touch-down (20%) weight bearing for 6 weeks. In patients who underwent ETO, an abduction brace is used and active abduction is avoided for 6 weeks postoperatively. A crutch or walker is used during ambulation for the first 6 weeks postoperatively, with gradual advancement to ambulation with a cane after that time. If serial radiographs do not demonstrate implant migration, subsidence, or loosening at 6 weeks postoperatively, the patient is advanced to weight bearing as tolerated, and a strengthening program with physical therapy is begun.

Avoiding Pitfalls and Complications

Extensively porous-coated stems have demonstrated predictable results in patients who require revision femoral reconstruction. The nuances of these stems must be understood before they are used in revision surgery. These stems require 4 to 6 cm of interference fit to allow biologic fixation and immediate stability of the implant. Concentric reaming of the femoral canal is critical, and an ETO should be used for additional exposure to allow direct visualization of the femoral diaphysis when necessary.

When a longer (8- or 10-in) extensively porous-coated stem is used, a bowed implant can be used to address the bow of the native femur. The use of a bowed stem should be considered when use of a straight stem may result in anterior cortical perforation. However, bowed stems do not allow the surgeon to control the stem anteversion because the version is determined by the native bow of the femur when it is engaged by the diaphyseal portion of the implant.

If ETO is performed, a distal cerclage cable is used to prevent propagation of the fracture beyond the distal extent of the ETO. If a fracture of the femur is encountered, the stem should be removed and the fracture managed. If the stem is stable and a longitudinal femoral split occurs, the stem may be left in place and the fracture managed with supplemental cerclage cable fixation. To minimize the risk of fracture, line-to-line reaming of the femoral canal may be necessary when the stem cannot be brought down to 4 to 6 cm above the calcar before it is impacted with a mallet.

Bibliography

Berry DJ, Harmsen WS, Ilstrup D, Lewallen DG, Cabanela ME: Survivorship of uncemented proximally porous-coated femoral components. *Clin Orthop Relat Res* 1995;(319):168-177.

Chung LH, Wu PK, Chen CF, Chen WM, Chen TH, Liu CL: Extensively porous-coated stems for femoral revision: Reliable choice for stem revision in Paprosky femoral type III defects. *Orthopedics* 2012;35(7):e1017-e1021.

Engh CA Jr, Claus AM, Hopper RH Jr, Engh CA: Long-term results using the anatomic medullary locking hip prosthesis. *Clin Orthop Relat Res* 2001;(393):137-146.

Hamilton WG, Cashen DV, Ho H, Hopper RH Jr, Engh CA: Extensively porous-coated stems for femoral revision: A choice for all seasons. *J Arthroplasty* 2007;22(4 suppl 1):106-110.

Jayakumar P, Malik AK, Islam SU, Haddad FS: Revision hip arthroplasty using an extensively porous coated stem: Medium term results. *Hip Int* 2011;21(2):129-135.

Krishnamurthy AB, MacDonald SJ, Paprosky WG: 5- to 13-year follow-up study on cementless femoral components in revision surgery. *J Arthroplasty* 1997;12(8):839-847.

Lawrence JM, Engh CA, Macalino GE, Lauro GR: Outcome of revision hip arthroplasty done without cement. *J Bone Joint Surg Am* 1994;76(7):965-973.

Moon KH, Kang JS, Lee SH, Jung SR: Revision total hip arthroplasty using an extensively porous coated femoral stem. *Clin Orthop Surg* 2009;1(2):105-109.

Moreland JR, Bernstein ML: Femoral revision hip arthroplasty with uncemented, porous-coated stems. *Clin Orthop Relat Res* 1995;(319):141-150.

Moreland JR, Moreno MA: Cementless femoral revision arthroplasty of the hip: Minimum 5 years followup. *Clin Orthop Relat Res* 2001;(393):194-201.

Thomsen PB, Jensen NJ, Kampmann J, Bæk Hansen T: Revision hip arthroplasty with an extensively porous-coated stem: Excellent long-term results also in severe femoral bone stock loss. *Hip Int* 2013;23(4):352-358.

Weeden SH, Paprosky WG: Minimal 11-year follow-up of extensively porous-coated stems in femoral revision total hip arthroplasty. *J Arthroplasty* 2002;17(4 suppl 1):134-137.

Younger TI, Bradford MS, Magnus RE, Paprosky WG: Extended proximal femoral osteotomy: A new technique for femoral revision arthroplasty. *J Arthroplasty* 1995;10(3):329-338.

Chapter 59

Proximal Fixation Modular Porous-Coated Proximal Femoral Stems in Revision Hip Arthroplasty

Hugh U. Cameron, MBChB, FRCSC

Indications

In a patient who requires revision hip surgery, unless the implant to be revised is a resurfacing component, the native femur has suffered slight to severe damage. Slight damage may be noted in a patient who was initially treated with a neck-sparing stem, and severe damage may occur in a patient in whom a fully porous stem was used, resulting in osseointegration over its full length. Loading is required to return damaged bone to normal strength. The more proximal the level of loading after revision surgery, the more complete the recovery will be. Proximal loading is the goal of revision femoral stem insertion if it can be reliably achieved.

Types of femoral stem loosening include vertical sink, distal pivot, and medial midstem pivot, and each causes bone damage at a particular area of the femur. In vertical sink loosening, the femoral stem drifts into valgus, causing lateral erosion of the endosteal cortex distal to the greater trochanter, which results in trochanteric overhang. Distal pivot-type failure results in calcar erosion. Midstem pivot results in erosion-related damage to the distal-lateral shaft of the femur. Osteolysis resulting from particulate disease may be focal or confluent, as may occur with sepsis.

In most patients, the proximal femoral canal is much larger than the distal canal. Thus, to achieve proximal fixation (that is, at or above the lesser trochanter), the surgeon would require access intraoperatively to an infinite variety of stems with independent variation in proximal and distal diameters. This scenario is not economically feasible.

Revision using monoblock proximal fixation has been attempted. Attempts were made to achieve distal stability via distal canal fill (porous-coated anatomic and biologic ingrowth stems) or placement of distal locking screws, followed by placement of bone graft in the expanded proximal femur. One drawback to the use of bone graft is the development of a layer of fibrous tissue at the graft/stem interface before bone revascularization is achieved. Proximal fixation does not occur until fibrous tissue has transformed into bone via electromagnetic stimulation or the effects of bone morphogenetic protein in osteoinduction. In the long term, instability at the fibrous interface is likely to occur, which will eventually lead to micromotion and loosening.

Alternatively, reduction osteotomy can be performed to customize the proximal femur to fit the implant. The osteotomy is performed by removing a wedge of bone or using multiple vertical cuts, thereby compressing the femoral metaphysis around the implant. Drawbacks to reduction osteotomy include the time required for the procedure and the need for the use of multiple wires or cables with repeated sequential tightening. The author of this chapter has performed reduction osteotomy and achieved reasonably satisfactory outcomes. Collapsing the diaphysis is difficult even with a cable plate because of the stiffness of the diaphysis. Multiple cables are required.

Mismatch in metaphyseal and diaphyseal diameters can be addressed only with the use of a modular implant in which the proximal and distal diameters can be independently set. Previously, attempts were made to achieve distal modularity in primary surgeries by attaching an expanded distal sleeve or bullet to a monoblock stem. However, results with these stems were unsatisfactory, and they were withdrawn from the market. To achieve modularity in the midstem, the proximal component is attached to the distal stem by a Morse taper lock. In general, these tapered stems provide excellent fixation, and their use has rapidly increased within the past decade. Some problems have occurred with these stems, principally at the taper junction, and breakage has been reported. These tapered stems provide distal fixation, which is beyond the scope of this chapter. Proximal modularity can be achieved in a variety of ways. The original proximally porous-coated

Dr. Cameron or an immediate family member serves as an unpaid consultant to MicroPort Orthopedics.

modular stem was a monolithic stem to which a proximal porous-coated sleeve was attached by means of a Morse taper lock.

The author of this chapter has extensive experience with only one type of modular implant (S-ROM Modular Hip System; DePuy Synthes); however, factors to be considered in selecting and using modular implants are universally applicable (**Figure 1**). These factors include initial stem stability, femoral dilation, expansion or absence of bone proximally, and exclusion of the distal canal from the effective joint space.

The S-ROM stem is a 6 AL-4 Va titanium alloy. The primary stem is straight and circular and is canal filling. Canal fill over 2 cm means that the stem resists bending stresses in a manner similar to that of an intramedullary nail. Thin, sharp distal flutes measuring 0.6 mm in height are designed to engage the distal endosteal cortex to provide rotational stability. The monoblock stem is not degraded by the introduction of fixation elements. The sleeve is attached to the proximal femoral stem by a Morse taper lock. The metallurgy of the sleeve is degraded to some extent by porous coating. However, because of the softness of the titanium, after the sleeve welds to the stem, the hoop stress is frozen and does not cycle up and down, thereby rendering sleeve fracture unlikely.

The primary stem can be inserted in any version because it is circular and straight. The long stem is bowed at the 200-mm level to allow full distal canal fill. Because the implant is bowed to follow the femoral canal, the version is fixed. The proximal stem is set to 15° of anteversion, and left and right stems are available.

The sleeve can be fitted to the stem in any version, including 180° out of phase, which is important in a patient in whom the proximal femur is absent. The variety of sleeve sizes and shapes allows full canal fill at the distal end of the sleeve in most patients. The femoral canal is sealed at the point of canal fill, thus excluding the distal canal from the effective joint space. Because particulate debris from the bearing couple cannot enter the distal canal, distal femoral osteolysis is prevented. If distal osteolysis is present, however, a channel exists between the sleeve and bone interface allowing particulate debris to enter the distal canal.

The distal stem is polished to prevent bone ongrowth or osseointegration. A few of the early stems left grit blast and osseointegrated distally, leading to profound proximal stress shielding. The stem is split distally similar to a clothespin to reduce bending stiffness and end-stem pain. End-stem pain occurs either because the stem is loose or because of elastic modulus mismatch.

All bones are bent like a leaf-spring to allow them to deform under load. If a stiff metal canal filling stem occupies the medullary canal, then the femur cannot bend. As a result, bending is concentrated around the stem tip, and anterolateral pain may develop on femoral out-of-plane loading, such as standing up from a chair. By splitting the stem in the plane of bending, the femoral bending is distributed over a much larger surface. Therefore, end-stem pain is unusual with a primary stem and has seldom, if ever, been recorded with a long stem because of the long length of flexibility.

Contraindications

The only contraindication to use of a modular proximally porous-coated stem is failure to achieve initial stability. Even in a patient who has a Paprosky type III fracture, the author of this chapter almost always obtains initial stability. In one patient, the author of this chapter achieved stability by passing AO cortical fracture bone screws through the distal slot. The screws were removed as early as possible to avoid fretting and severe metallosis. Severe osteogenesis imperfecta is a contraindication to this type of implant, however. In one such patient treated by the author of this chapter, the patient was treated with a short femoral stem cemented into a long allograft, and osseointegration occurred. Modular stem insertion also is contraindicated in a patient in whom the proximal femur is absent and the distal one-half of the femur is filled with a long femoral stem originating at the knee joint. In one such patient treated by the author of this chapter, the patient was treated with staged reconstruction in which the proximal femur was stabilized with strut allografts and the construct allowed to heal, after which a short stem was cemented into the allograft complex.

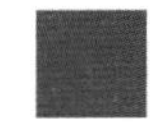

Alternative Treatments

The two alternative treatments to the use of a modular proximally porous-coated stem are impaction grafting and distal fixation. Good results have been achieved with impaction grafting. However, the cost of allograft bone makes impaction grafting an expensive option. The procedure also is time consuming and carries a steep learning curve. Distal fixation is successful in most patients. Reconstitution of the proximal femur remains imperfect because full loading is not possible, and most femoral revisions are managed with either tapered stems or porous-coated monoblock stems. The main disadvantage to distal fixation occurs if stem removal should become necessary. Removal of a well-integrated, distally fixed stem is challenging, especially if the stem is bowed.

Results

The author has performed several femoral stem insertions in patients undergoing revision hip arthroplasty and selects

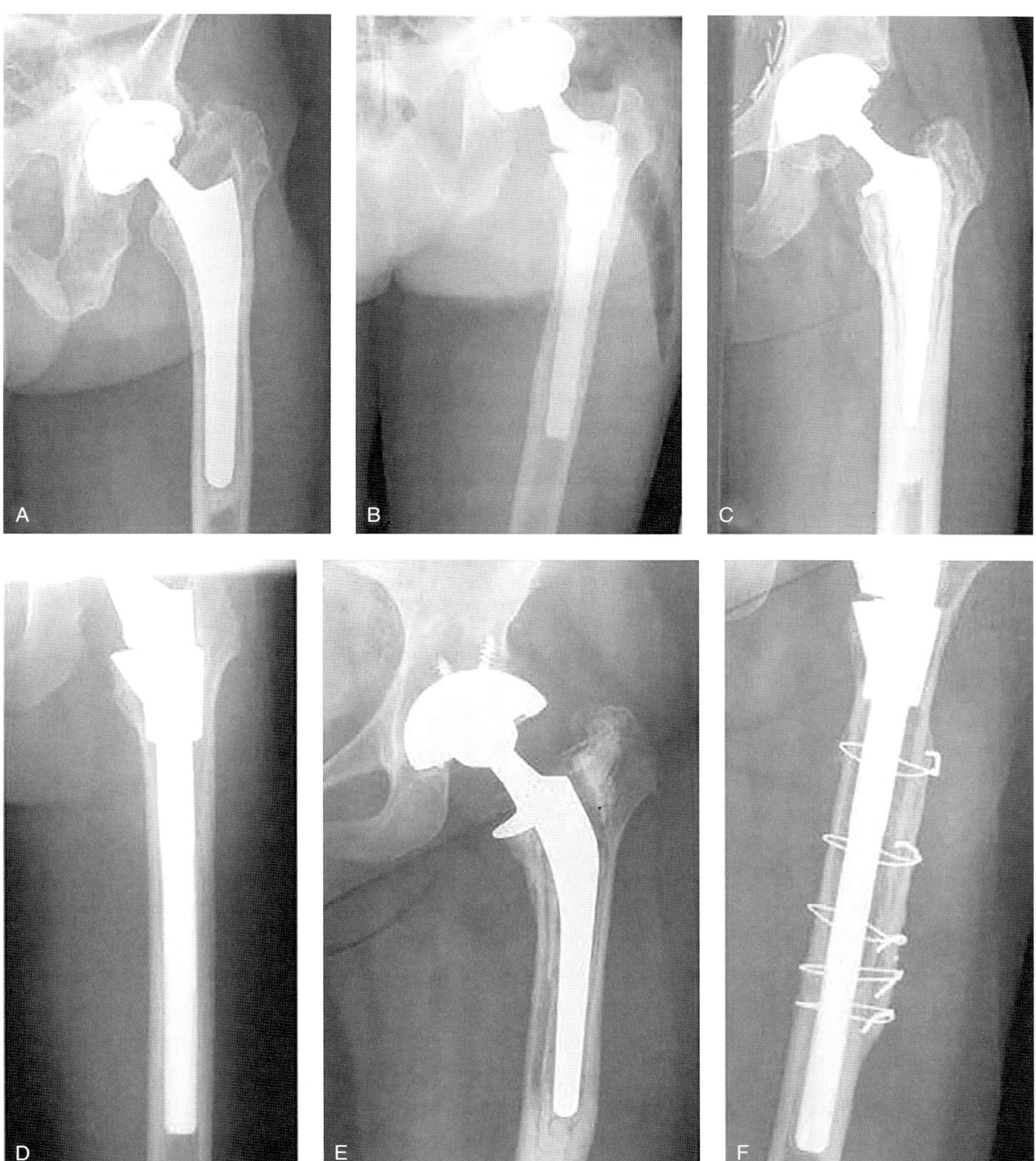

Figure 1 AP radiographs show the S-ROM (DePuy Synthes) modular proximally porous-coated stem in Paprosky type I (preoperative [**A**] and postoperative [**B**]), type II (preoperative [**C**] and postoperative [**D**]), and type III (preoperative [**E**] and postoperative [**F**]) defects. (Reproduced from Mattingly DA: Femoral revision: Modular proximally porous-coated stems, in Lieberman JR, Berry DJ, eds: *Advanced Reconstruction: Hip*. Rosemont, IL, American Academy of Orthopaedic Surgeons, 2005, pp 417-423.)

the modular stem type based on his own classification of femoral status. In type I femurs, the bone in the isthmus (that is, below the lesser trochanter) is intact, and a primary stem is used. In type II femurs, the bone distal to the isthmus is severely damaged, and a long bowed stem is necessary. A standard femoral neck is used in a patient in whom metaphyseal bone is present proximal to the lesser trochanter, but a calcar replacement neck is used if the metaphyseal bone is missing. Type III femurs are those in which 70 mm of bone is missing, and a structural allograft is used.

The author of this chapter has noted mostly good or excellent long-term results in patients with type I femurs managed with a short femoral stem. No patients in whom aseptic loosening developed required revision. Only five patients required intraoperative osteotomies as of 20-year follow-up. The incidence of low-grade lucency (fewer than three zones) was low, and rerevision was not necessary in the one patient who demonstrated high-grade lucency. Good to excellent results were achieved at 10- or 15-year follow-up in most patients with type II femurs treated with insertion of long femoral stems. This is notable because, with an unmodified rating system, few patients older than 75 years and with a normal hip will score better than fair. Most patients treated by the author required an osteotomy, whether femoral, transverse diaphyseal, extended trochanteric, or Wagner split. In a small number of patients, later stem removal was required for either sepsis or aseptic loosening. Four revisions were required in patients in whom only strut grafts were used; structural allografts should have been used instead. Few patients exhibited high-grade lucency, but low-grade lucency was apparent in nearly 25% of patients, mostly around the flexible distal legs of the split stem. Of the fewer than 10 patients treated with structural allograft to manage type III femurs, nearly one-half required rerevision surgery to switch to another allograft. Although the early structural allograft procedure likely was not performed well, even a well-done structural allograft likely has a finite life expectancy.

Technique

The following describes revision with the S-ROM prosthesis in particular.

Setup/Exposure

- AP and frog-leg lateral radiographs are obtained for preoperative templating. The lateral templates are especially important if use of a long-bowed stem is planned. Although diaphyseal templating is quite accurate, metaphyseal templating is not. A loose femoral component usually rotates posteriorly; thus, an AP radiograph alone of the femur or pelvis usually substantially underestimates the diameter of the metaphyseal canal.
- The area at which both the dorsalis pedis artery and the posterior tibial artery can be detected on Doppler ultrasonography are marked for use postoperatively in checking pedal pulses.
- No special surgical exposure is required. Proximal modularity does not affect the surgical approach. Anterior, anterolateral, or posterior approaches are equally applicable.
- A posterior approach affords enhanced visualization for a femoral revision because it allows the surgeon to look down the canal, whereas, with an anterior approach, the surgeon is looking up the canal. In addition, with a posterior approach, it is easier to determine version because the tibia, which is the guide to version, can be placed vertically. The author of this chapter prefers to use a posterior approach if a bowed stem is used because the ability to hold the tibia vertical during stem insertion facilitates determination of 15° of anteversion.
- An extended trochanteric osteotomy (ETO) can be performed if necessary. If a long osteotomy is necessary, a Wagner split is performed, retaining the attachment of the vastus lateralis to the anterior femur and, thus, the blood supply.
- If severe deformity is present, a transverse diaphyseal osteotomy can be performed. Before performing this osteotomy, a vertical groove is cut with a saw to allow anatomic rotational restoration. Simply creating a burr mark or using methylene blue is ineffective because these markings often are obliterated intraoperatively.

Instruments/Equipment/Implants Required

- A variety of stem extraction devices and cement removal tools should be available.
- Assuming that the original implant and cement have been removed, instruments necessary to insert the new stem are used, consisting of rigid reamers and flexible reamers.
- If a primary stem is to be used, then rigid reamers are adequate. If, however, a bowed stem is to be inserted, then flexible intramedullary reamers, such as intramedullary nail reamers, should be used over a guidewire.
- Cerclage wires, cable plates, and trochanteric claw plates should be available.
- In select patients, strut allografts or particulate allograft may be necessary. As surgeons become more experienced in the technique, the amount of graft used decreases accordingly.
- Particulate allograft has largely been replaced with bone graft substitutes because these off-the-shelf products

are easy to use and frequently are impregnated with antibiotic.

Procedure

- In preparation for implant insertion, the distal canal is reamed to allow canal fill of more than 2 to 3 cm.
- The optimal modular proximally porous-coated stem to use in a given patient is determined based on the femoral classification type developed by the author of this chapter. A primary stem is used in a type I femur, in which the bone in the isthmus (that is, below the lesser trochanter) is intact. In a type II femur, in which the bone distal to the isthmus is severely damaged, a long bowed stem should be used.
- If metaphyseal bone is present proximal to the lesser trochanter, a standard neck can be used. If the metaphyseal bone is missing, then a calcar replacement neck should be used.
- Rigid reamers are used for primary (short, straight) stems. These reamers intentionally are not self-advancing because the bone, especially in a revision, may be of poor quality.
- The reamer must be pushed. The canal is reamed to the minor diameter of the stem (that is, 13 mm for a 13-mm stem). The flutes add another 1.2 mm to the distal diameter, affording 1.2 mm of press fit. These flutes engage the endosteal cortex at least 2 to 3 cm before full insertion, which imparts rotational stability to the stem.
- If rotational stability is not achieved at this point in the procedure, then the stem is too small and a larger size is necessary.
- Reaming for a bowed stem is performed using flexible reamers such as the AO reamers over a 3.2-mm guidewire. Because a 3.2-mm guidewire will not ensure accurate canal reaming, the canal should be slightly overreamed (for example, to 13.5 mm for a 13-mm stem).
- The size of the diaphyseal reamer is determined based on preoperative templating. However, templating is not accurate for metaphyseal reaming because, frequently, the affected leg is in external rotation. Typically, the anterior-posterior measurement of the femoral metaphysis underestimates the actual canal diameter.
- After the diaphysis has been reamed, a canal-filling trial stem is inserted to ensure centralization of the metaphyseal reamers, which will ream out a cone.
- Metaphyseal fill has been achieved when the endosteum is felt to be smooth, usually at the anterior cortex at a depth of one fingerbreadth.
- The calcar is reamed with a side-cut drill or mill held in place by a guide, which gives proximal and distal canal fill. The drill is advanced until the endosteal cortex is reached.
- If failure of the original stem occurred because of proximal pivot or medial midstem pivot, then, typically, the calcar on which the proximal end of the original stem rested consists of dense eburnated bone.
- The calcar is ideal for load bearing because it is the site of strongest bone in the proximal femur. Reaming should stop at the level of the calcar and must not continue through it; instead, a sleeve is chosen to rest on that bone surface. Preferably, the sleeve hangs over the edge of the calcar to act as a collar should a stem sink and reorient into valgus. Even if valgus stem alignment occurs, the collar will be wide enough that the stem will remain outside the calcar, and vertical sink will be avoided.
- In a patient with a severely damaged or absent metaphysis, a calcar replacement neck can be used and the sleeve allowed to rest on the lesser trochanter, which is present in most patients. Sleeve and stem version are independent of each other; thus, the resting point of the sleeve is not important.
- In a patient with severely damaged, paper-thin metaphyseal bone, cerclage wires or cables can be used to reinforce the bone. The stem can sink only if the cerclage wires or cables break early, which is an unusual occurrence.
- The metaphyseal bone should be retained regardless of its quality. If the loose implant and debris (including the cement particles and granulomatous tissue) are removed and proximal loading occurs, then the metaphyseal bone will recover in strength and vitality remarkably quickly.
- Historically, strut grafts were used to reinforce the often paper-thin proximal femur. However, in the experience of the author of this chapter, although the strut grafts eventually unite, the struts are seldom necessary. If the proximal femur is fractured, then struts are useful. During the 9 months it takes for the strut to unite to the host bone, the strut acts as a fracture fixation plate. If struts are not available, then a fracture fixation plate can be secured with cerclage wire or cables or a cable plate construct.
- The combination of a large sleeve, calcar replacement neck and long head can be used to replace up to 70 mm of absent proximal femur.
- If more than 70 mm of proximal femur is absent, then a structural allograft is required. A proximal femoral allograft with a canal large enough to accept a revision stem may be difficult to find. Typically, use of a distal femoral allograft turned upside down to facilitate matching of the canal is easier.

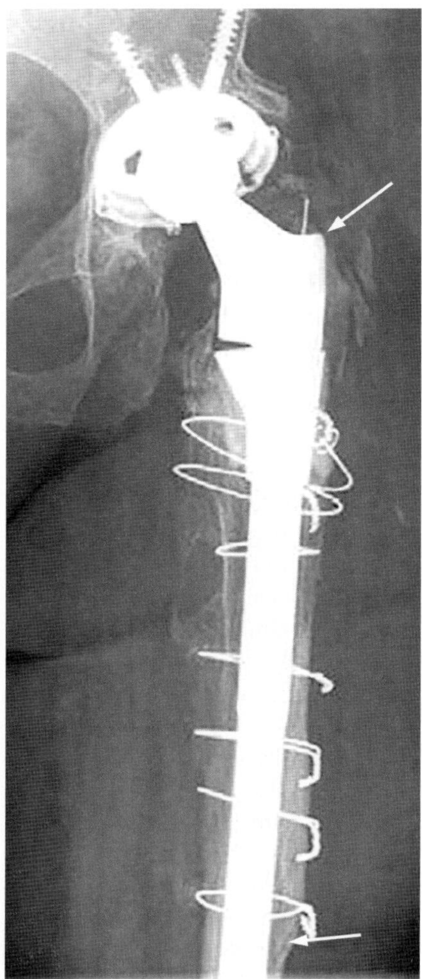

Figure 2 AP radiograph of a femur 5 years postoperatively shows an S-ROM sleeve (top arrow) cemented into a proximal allograft. The bottom arrow shows healing at the allograft–host bone junction. (Reproduced from Mattingly DA: Femoral revision: Modular proximally porous-coated stems, in Lieberman JR, Berry DJ, eds: *Advanced Reconstruction: Hip.* Rosemont, IL, American Academy of Orthopaedic Surgeons, 2005, pp 417-423.)

- Because the allograft is dead tissue, the sleeve is cemented to the allograft and the allograft-sleeve-stem component is used as a composite (**Figure 2**).
- If the surgeon has concerns regarding the strength of the construct, the allograft can be protected by a cerclage wire. A split allograft will not heal. If possible, the distal allograft should be fitted inside the remaining proximal host femur because, typically, this bone-in-bone configuration unites rapidly. If this is not possible, however, then a step-cut is made because it allows greater bone-on-bone healing area than a butt joint. During stem insertion, a cerclage wire is placed at or just distal to the stress point, which helps reduce the potential for split resulting from the hoop stress that occurs during stem insertion.
- If an ETO has been performed, the stem is inserted, and the osteotomy fragment is replaced. A high-speed burr can be used to sculpt the osteotomy fragment for proper fit. In a patient who had varus diaphyseal bowing of the proximal femur preoperatively, the greater trochanter will not close completely. The greater trochanter can be rotated to achieve anterior or posterior contact, depending on the optimum position, as well as lateralization of the gluteal muscles that remain attached to the trochanter. The residual gap is filled with bone graft or bone substitute.

Wound Closure

- Wound closure is routine. If the vastus lateralis has been elevated, it is tacked back in place.
- If the glutei were released during the procedure, then these muscles are carefully reattached with multiple sutures. Failure of the glutei to heal results in a permanent limp.
- If at the time of revision surgery gluteal pull-off or incomplete healing is discovered, then the smooth area to which the glutei should have been attached is roughened with the use of a saw. A long-standing avulsion of the glutei cannot simply be sewn and expected to heal. The bone is smooth and has lost its healing capacity, similar to an atrophic nonunion, and the gluteal tendons also are smooth and have lost their healing capacity. If the area is roughened with the use of a saw to produce bleeding bone, then healing usually can be achieved.
- The fascia lata is closed with interrupted sutures. Use of a running suture is not recommended because giving way of that suture would result in a fascial hernia. Although fascial hernias usually are not painful, they are unsightly.
- Drains are not used.

Postoperative Regimen

Pedal pulses are checked in the recovery room, using the area marked preoperatively for reference. In addition, plain radiographs are obtained in the recovery room to confirm alignment and ensure that dislocation has not occurred. Unless little or no damage to the proximal femur is present, the patient is advised to place reduced loading on the implant initially. Bone healing does not commence until 10 days postoperatively. For the first 6 weeks postoperatively, the patient is limited to toe-touch weight bearing to allow the commencement of osseointegration of the implant. Similarly, if the greater trochanter has been osteotomized, overload should be avoided for 6 weeks postoperatively (that is, no side leg lifting and limited hip flexion).

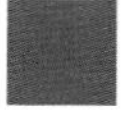

Avoiding Pitfalls and Complications

The surgeon must take care to avoid iatrogenic nerve injury. Although most surgeons advise dissection and protection of the sciatic nerve to protect it during the posterior approach, the author of this chapter thinks that this method actually increases the chance of nerve damage compared with staying clear of the nerve. Over-lengthening may put the nerve at risk of injury; however, the author of this chapter thinks that it is relatively safe to return the leg to its original length, including returning up to 5 cm. Vascular injury is always a risk. The most troublesome vascular structure in any approach is the ascending branch of the lateral circumflex femoral artery just below the acetabulum. This branch can retract down the leg and be difficult to access. In one patient in whom bleeding continued postoperatively, the author of this chapter enlisted the help of an interventional radiologist to isolate and embolize that artery. Although the risk of infection cannot be eradicated, it can be minimized by performing expeditious surgery and administration of intermittent irrigation with antibiotic solutions and/or diluted povidone-iodine solution.

The main complication in revision surgery is failure to achieve stability. The patient should not leave the operating room if stability has not been achieved. The exception to this rule is the rare patient with the paper-thin bone of a septic revision in whom the femur completely breaks up. To manage this condition, the author of this chapter performs what he has termed the bail and nail technique. In it, an intramedullary nail is inserted into what remains of the femur, and cerclage wire is used to secure the remaining bony fragments around the nail. The result is the same as with a Girdlestone resection. The presence of an intramedullary nail does not prevent eradication of infection. In the experience of the author of this chapter, bone healing occurs within 6 months postoperatively, making rerevision surgery relatively easy because the medullary canal is open and of uniform diameter after intraoperative removal of the nail.

Iatrogenic fracture cannot be avoided entirely given the quality of the bone. The severity can be minimized, however, with the use of prophylactic cerclage wires around stress risers. In theory, these wires can be taken off after implant insertion, but the author of this chapter prefers to leave them in place.

Greater trochanter fractures must be fixed. Contrary to some statements in the literature, the author of this chapter finds that trochanteric nonunions usually are symptomatic. A hook cable plate may be used, but it will often require later removal because it is bulky and can produce trochanteric bursitis. If the bone is adequate, two screws originating from the top of the greater trochanter and passing through both front and back of the prosthesis into the lesser trochanter provide substantial rotation and vertical stability. Alternatively, wiring and cabling may be used.

If a transverse diaphyseal osteotomy has been performed, the sleeve of the S-ROM stem typically provides rotational stability to the proximal femur and distal rotational stability to the endosteal flutes. If rotational stability is in doubt after stem insertion, then a strut allograft or a short semitubular plate with unicortical screws can be used.

Dislocation is always a risk after revision surgery, but the risk can be minimized by using increased offset components to increase tissue tension and ensuring accurate femoral version. Increased femoral head size may help reduce the risk of dislocation.

Aseptic loosening does not necessarily warrant rerevision. In a patient with very low activity demands who was treated with a long bowed stem, the symptoms may not be sufficient for rerevision. In general, if rerevision is required, the improved bone quality will be such that only the femoral component requires exchanging for one that is larger in diameter. If the bone has improved sufficiently, a long bowed stem may be replaced with a short primary stem. However, if sinkage has occurred, then the proximal stem shoulder may have moved laterally under the greater trochanter and it may be necessary to perform ETO for stem extraction.

Bibliography

Cameron HU: The 3-6-year results of a modular noncemented low-bending stiffness hip implant: A preliminary study. *J Arthroplasty* 1993;8(3):239-243.

Cameron HU: Bail and nail: Burst fracture of the femur during revision. *Seminars in Arthroplasty* 2013;24(2):124-125.

Cameron HU: The long-term success of modular proximal fixation stems in revision total hip arthroplasty. *J Arthroplasty* 2002;17(4 suppl 1):138-141.

Cameron HU: Management of femoral deformities during the total hip replacement. *Orthopedics* 1996;19(9):745-746.

Cameron HU: Modularity in primary total hip arthroplasty. *J Arthroplasty* 1996;11(3):332-334, discussion 337-338.

Cameron HU: Proximal femoral fixation when bone stock allows. *Seminars in Arthroplasty* 2011;22(2):110-111.

Cameron HU: Solution options: Modular hip stem design. *Orthopedics* 1995;18(9):824-826.

Cameron HU: The two- to six-year results with a proximally modular noncemented total hip replacement used in hip revisions. *Clin Orthop Relat Res* 1994;(298):47-53.

Cameron HU, Eren OT, Solomon M: Nerve injury in the prosthetic management of the dysplastic hip. *Orthopedics* 1998;21(9):980-981.

Ramaswamy R, Kosashvili Y, Cameron H: Bilateral total hip replacement in osteogenesis imperfecta with hyperplastic callus. *J Bone Joint Surg Br* 2009;91(6):812-814.

S-ROM Modular Hip System product manual. © DePuy Synthes Joint Reconstruction, Warsaw, IN, 2013. Available at: http://synthes.vo.llnwd.net/o16/LLNWMB8/US%20Mobile/Synthes%20North%20America/Product%20Support%20Materials/Technique%20Guides/S-ROM_Modular_Hip_System_Surgical_Technique_0601-36-050r8.pdf. Accessed August 18, 2016.

Chapter 60

Femoral Revision With Noncemented Tapered, Fluted Titanium Stems

Nemandra A. Sandiford, MSc, FRCS (Tr & Orth)
Clive P. Duncan, MD, MSc, FRCSC
Bassam A. Masri, MD, FRCSC
Donald S. Garbuz, MD, FRCSC

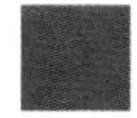

Indications

The use of revision total hip arthroplasty (THA) has steadily increased over the past decade as a result of an aging population; the increasing prevalence of hip arthroplasty; and the fact that increasingly younger, active, and more demanding patients are undergoing primary THA procedures. The challenge of revision THA is to produce a functional, pain-free, biomechanically sound hip in patients with suboptimal quantity and quality of bone and, in some patients, incompetent soft tissues around the hip.

A substantial number of tapered, fluted titanium stems are marketed for use in revision THA. Because no prospective studies have compared the currently available designs, no evidence is available to suggest the superiority of any one design. Encouraging clinical results have been reported with the use of modular and nonmodular designs. The senior authors of this chapter (D.S.G., C.P.D., B.A.M.) previously used tapered, fluted modular titanium stems in most patients and changed to the use of a nonmodular design after several junctional fractures were observed.

Modular noncemented tapered, fluted stems are ideal for use in patients with Paprosky type II and III bone defects. Several important design features contribute to their suitability for revision THA. The tapered geometry enables the stem to form a wedge within the femoral isthmus, allowing for axial stability. The cutting flutes in this design engage the endosteum to provide rotational stability. Modular proximal segments are provided in most systems, with variable offset and length options that allow the surgeon to achieve the optimal limb length, offset, femoral anteversion, and soft-tissue tension.

One advantage of modularity is the ability to independently size the proximal and distal segments of the femoral implant. This feature enables the surgeon to achieve optimal diaphyseal fixation and then independently size the metaphyseal segment, allowing for maximal stability and optimization of limb lengths and offset. This intraoperative versatility has made modular tapered stems an attractive option for use in revision THA.

Modular noncemented tapered, fluted revision stems have been used at the chapter authors' institution for more than 10 years. As noted, concerns with the use of modular stems arose after several junctional fractures were observed. As a result, use of a nonmodular stem for femoral revision has increased at the chapter authors' institution (**Figure 1**). The design used by the senior authors of this chapter (D.S.G., C.P.D., B.A.M.), although relatively new to North America, has been used in Europe since 1987. Early anecdotal evidence suggests that high levels of patient satisfaction and function and low dislocation rates have been achieved with this prosthesis.

Contraindications

Noncemented tapered, fluted stems have no specific contraindications.

Dr. Garbuz or an immediate family member serves as a paid consultant to Zimmer Biomet; has received research or institutional support from DePuy Synthes and Zimmer Biomet; and serves as a board member, owner, officer, or committee member of the M. E. Müller Foundation of North America. Dr. Duncan or an immediate family member is a member of a speakers' bureau or has made paid presentations on behalf of Zimmer Biomet. Dr. Masri or an immediate family member serves as a board member, owner, officer, or committee member of the Canadian Orthopaedic Association. Neither Dr. Sandiford nor any immediate family member has received anything of value from or has stock or stock options held in a commercial company or institution related directly or indirectly to the subject of this chapter.

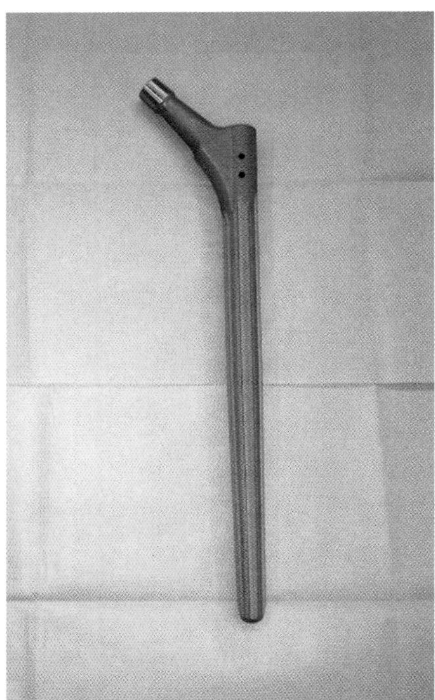

Figure 1 Photograph shows a nonmodular tapered, fluted titanium femoral stem (Wagner SL; Zimmer Biomet).

Alternative Treatments

Patients with Paprosky type I bone defects usually can be successfully treated with femoral implants that are used in primary THA. Achieving primary fixation in patients with Paprosky type IV defects can be challenging. These patients may require the use of a tumor prosthesis, an allograft-prosthetic composite, or impaction grafting with a cemented prosthesis. However, encouraging results have been reported with modular tapered, fluted stems even in select patients with type IV defects.

Results

Clinical outcomes of revision THA depend on multiple factors, including the quality of the intact femoral bone stock and the surrounding soft-tissue envelope. Results of studies of nonmodular and modular tapered, fluted stems are summarized in **Table 1**. Nonmodular tapered, fluted stems have been used in Europe since the 1980s. The Wagner SL (Zimmer Biomet) stem has the longest follow-up among nonmodular stems, with 96% survivorship reported at 15.8-year follow-up with aseptic loosening as the end point. Reconstitution of proximal femoral bone stock and high rates of union of extended trochanteric osteotomies (ETOs) have been reported with this prosthesis. The main problems reported with this design have been subsidence and dislocation. To address these issues, a design modification consisting of increased offset with increasing stem size was introduced. Subsidence was thought to be the result of three-point fixation, which can generally be avoided with careful surgical technique.

Modularity was introduced in an attempt to minimize these risks and improve the versatility of implants used in revision THA. Encouraging clinical and radiologic results have been reported with modular implants in patients with Paprosky type III and IV femoral defects. Substantial improvements in function and high levels of patient satisfaction were found in patients with advanced bone loss (Paprosky type IIIB and IV defects) and in patients with Vancouver type B2 and B3 periprosthetic fractures. Implant survivorship of 94% to 98%, with revision as the end point, has been reported at 2- to 7-year follow-up by several authors using different modular stem designs. Functional results have been similarly encouraging.

Subsidence has not been a substantial concern with noncemented modular tapered, fluted stems. However, fractures have been reported at the modular taper junction. These fractures typically occur in patients in whom stems <19 mm in diameter are used, patients in whom the proximal segment of the construct is unsupported, and patients with a body mass index >35 kg/m². The authors of this chapter are not aware of any reports of stem failure secondary to fracture of the second-generation nonmodular Wagner SL stems in patients with proximal bone deficiency in whom proximal structural support was not used, as has been reported with modular tapered, fluted titanium stems. Some current modular designs have a thickened proximal junction that allows their use without structural support in an attempt to reduce the risk of fractures.

Techniques

Preoperative Planning

MODULAR STEMS

- For preoperative planning, the authors of this chapter use radiographic images calibrated to the magnification of overlaid templates.
- The presence and extent of any limb-length discrepancy is determined on the basis of a transischial line drawn on the image.
- The acetabulum is templated to determine the center of rotation.
- Planning of the femoral implant should take into account the type of the existing implant, the type and quality of fixation, and the position of the implant relative to the center of the canal. An eccentric stem or cement mantle increases the risk of iatrogenic fracture during stem extraction, as does varus remodeling or trochanteric location over the medullary canal.
- The segment of the isthmus where maximal fixation will be achieved is marked.
- The need for an ETO is determined on the basis of templating on both the AP and lateral radiographs. Indications for an ETO include a well-fixed noncemented stem and proximal femoral remodeling in varus (coronal plane) and/or flexion (sagittal plane). A well-fixed cement mantle may also require an ETO.
- Several contemporary stem designs

Table 1 Results of Revision Total Hip Arthroplasty Using Modular or Nonmodular Tapered, Fluted Femoral Stems

Authors (Year)	Number of Patients (Hips)	Implant Type	Mean Patient Age in Years (Range)	Mean Follow-up in Months (Range)	Success Rate (%)[a]	Results[b]
Böhm and Bischel (2001)	123 (129)	Wagner SL nonmodular stem (Zimmer)	64.6 (36.7-86.3)	56 (2-133.2)	93.9	20% had subsidence >10 mm 5.4% dislocation rate
Gutiérrez del Alamo et al (2007)	77 (79)	Wagner SL nonmodular stem	72 (50-91)	100.8 (60-144)	92.3	1.3% had subsidence >10 mm 13.9% dislocation rate
Ovesen et al (2010)	125 hips	ZMR Hip System (Zimmer)	68 (33-92)	50 (24-86)	96.8	Mean subsidence, 2 mm 3.5% fracture rate
Richards et al (2010)	103	ZMR Hip System	70.2 (NR)	37 (24-83)	89.8	8.7% fracture rate
Regis et al (2011)	41 (41)	Wagner SL nonmodular stem	61 (29-80)	168 (124.8-189.6)	96.6	2.9% had subsidence >10 mm 1.5% dislocation rate
Restrepo et al (2011)	118 (122)	Modular stem	68 (34-88)	48 (24-84)	100	Mean subsidence, 1 mm No fractures
Weiss et al (2011)	87 (90)	Link MP (Waldemar Link)	72[c] (38-89)	72[c] (60-132)	98	Mean subsidence, 2.7 mm 1.0% fracture rate
Munro et al (2013)	47	ZMR Hip System or Revitan stem (Zimmer)	71.9 (44-93)	54 (24-143)	96	Mean subsidence, <12 mm No fractures
Palumbo et al (2013)	18	Restoration modular (Stryker)	69 (43-84)	54 (24-72)	94	Mean subsidence, 3.5 mm
Van Houwelingen et al (2013)	48	ZMR Hip System	70 (41-87)	84 (60-120)	94	Mean subsidence, 12.3 mm 16% fracture rate

NR = not reported.
[a] Success is defined as the absence of revision.
[b] Results based on number of hips.
[c] Median value.

have an anterior bevel or kink to minimize the risk of perforation of the anterior cortex (**Figure 2**). The bevel also guides the orientation of the stem during insertion. The extent of femoral bowing and the need for a beveled or kinked implant or a corrective osteotomy is determined with the use of templates overlaid on the lateral radiograph.

- After the region of optimal fixation is marked, the stem size is chosen. A cutout on the overlay allows the surgeon to mark the proximal extent of the stem. A bony landmark such as the greater or lesser trochanter is also used for reference. From that bony landmark, the proximal (body) segment of the implant is templated.
- The length and offset of the stem are chosen. The authors of this chapter prefer to use a large femoral head (36 or 40 mm) whenever possible to reduce the risk of instability. To optimize metaphyseal fit and fill, the authors of this chapter prefer to use the manufacturer's largest available body size at the modular junction.

NONMODULAR STEMS

- Preoperative planning for nonmodular stems is similar to that for modular stems.
- At least 4 cm of diaphyseal press fit is required. Choice of stem length is influenced by the location of this area in the femur.

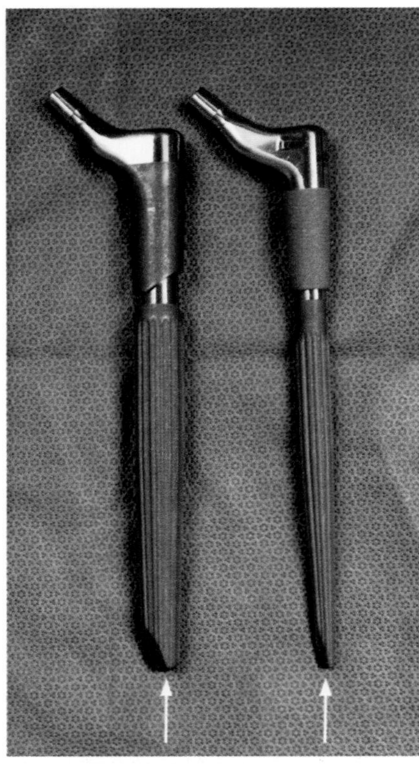

Figure 2 Photograph shows two modular tapered, fluted femoral stems, each with an anterior bevel (arrow) to minimize conflict with the femoral cortex.

- The caput-collum-diaphyseal angle is 135°.
- The tip of the greater trochanter is used as a reference for the center of rotation. Alternatively, if the greater trochanter is not in its anatomic location because of fracture or osteolysis, the lesser trochanter is used as a reference.

Setup/Exposure

- The patient is placed in the lateral decubitus position.
- If acetabular revision will be performed, the pelvis needs to be perpendicular to the surgical table. This position is achieved by centering the posterior support on the sacrum and the anterior support on the lateral third of the iliac crest.
- The anterior support is placed at the level of the umbilicus and angled distally to the iliac crest to allow >90° of hip flexion during the procedure.
- The entire limb is prepped to the level of the iliac crest and is draped free to allow access to the knee, if required.
- Old incisions are marked on the skin.
- An iodine-impregnated skin drape is placed.
- The authors of this chapter prefer to use a posterior approach incorporating the previous incision if possible. This approach enables exposure of the entire femur if necessary and allows visualization and protection of the sciatic nerve and the femur, facilitating the use of an ETO if necessary.

Instruments/Equipment/Implants Required

- Instruments required will depend on the prosthesis being removed; however, the following instruments should be available for removal of a cemented femoral stem.
- A high-speed burr is used to remove cement from the shoulder of the stem. This is particularly useful if a collarless polished tapered stem is in situ.
- Cement-cutting chisels are used.
- Cement reamers are used.
- A cement removal system is necessary to facilitate cement removal with minimal risk for injury to the bone.
- A headlamp is needed if removing a long cemented stem without an ETO.
- Power saws and drills are used.
- Cerclage cables are necessary if planning an ETO.
- An image intensifier should be on standby.
- If a specific stem extraction kit is not available, then a universal femoral stem extraction kit is required.
- Flexible osteotomes and Kirschner wires are used for development of the bone-prosthesis interface.
- A Gigli saw is effective for developing the bone-prosthesis interface of the calcar region if an ETO is used.

Procedure

- The existing implant is extracted.
- If acetabular revision is required, it is performed. Such revision is not described in this chapter.
- The femoral implant is inserted with or without the use of an ETO, according to the following techniques.
- When an endofemoral approach is used, nonmodular stems are ideal. When an ETO is used, both nonmodular and modular implants work well.

ENDOFEMORAL TECHNIQUE WITHOUT ETO

- All soft tissue and/or cement in the femoral canal is cleared with the use of reverse cutting hooks and cement-removal osteotomes.
- All soft tissue and debris at the medial aspect of the greater trochanter is removed with the use of rongeurs and curets.
- Intramedullary location of the femoral canal is confirmed by passing an olive-tipped guidewire down the canal.
- Conical hand reamers are used sequentially to prepare the diaphysis. Reaming continues until stability is demonstrated when axial and rotational loads are applied to the hand reamer and by tactile feedback obtained when the flutes of the reamer engage the endosteal bone. Care is taken to achieve excellent initial stability.
- In most modular implant systems, the handles of the reamers have marks that correspond to the desired center of rotation (**Figure 3**). The tip of the greater trochanter is usually used as a reference because

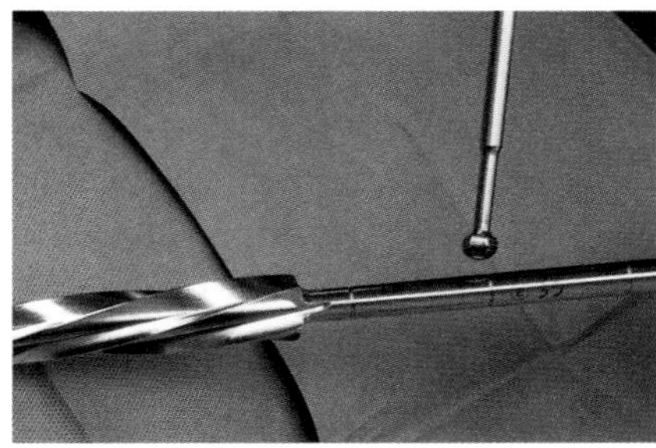

Figure 3 Photograph shows a conical reamer with etching corresponding with the center of rotation for each stem length. (Reproduced with permission from Sandiford NA, Duncan CP, Masri BA, Garbuz DS: Tapered fluted titanium stems in revision total hip arthroplasty, in Berry DJ, Maloney WJ, eds: *Master Techniques in Orthopaedic Surgery: The Hip*. Philadelphia, PA, Wolters Kluwer, 2016, pp 369-376.)

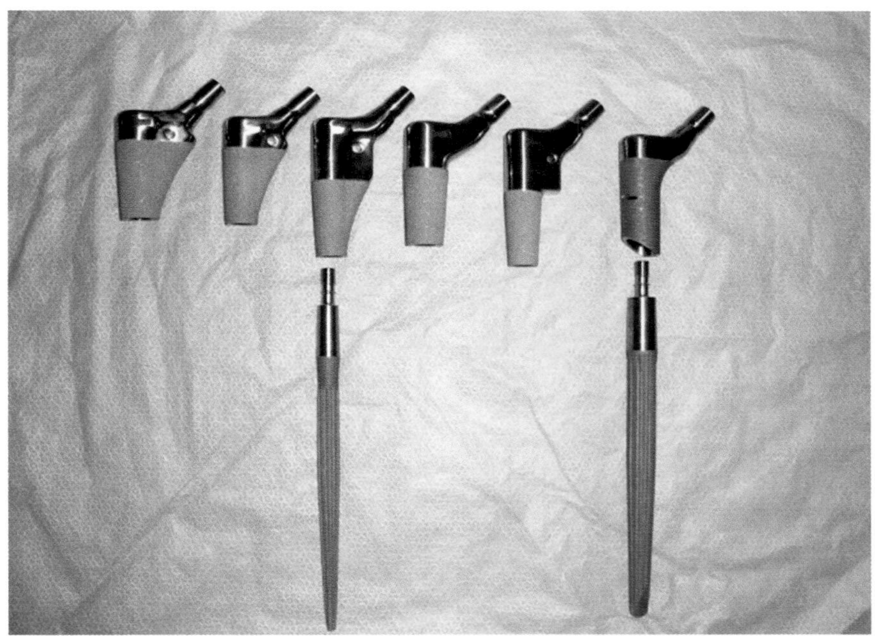

Figure 4 Photograph shows a contemporary modular femoral implant system with a variety of proximal (body) and distal (stem) shapes and sizes available.

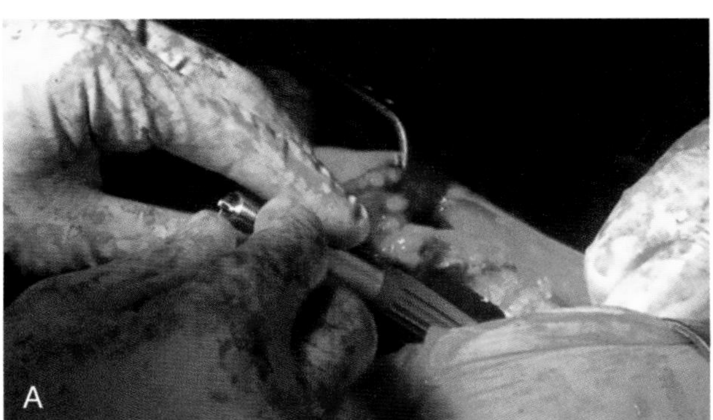

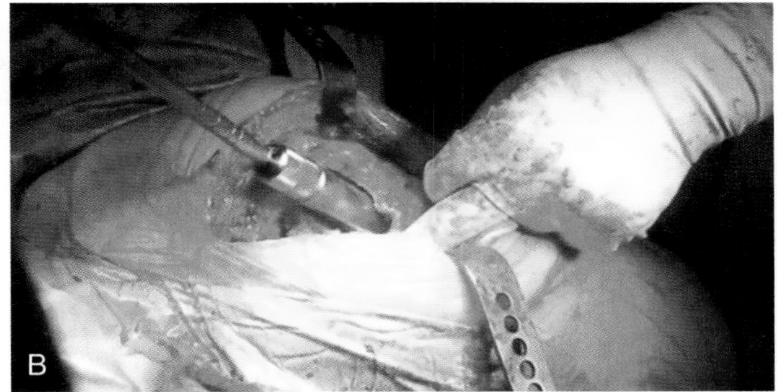

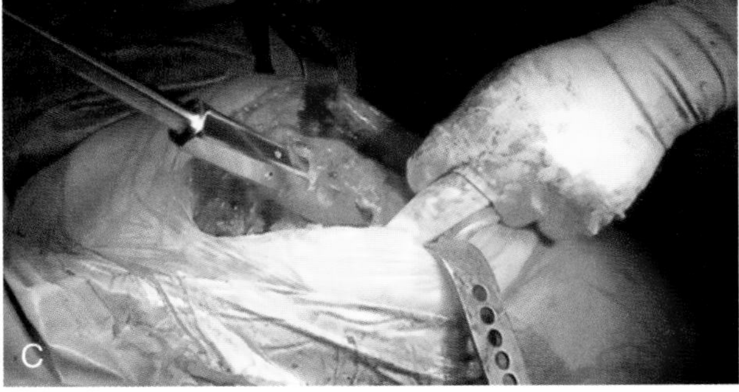

Figure 5 Intraoperative photographs of a right hip show insertion of a modular stem (**A**), application of a taper protector on the exposed trunnion (**B**), and reaming over the modular junction (**C**). (Panel C reproduced with permission from Sandiford NA, Duncan CP, Masri BA, Garbuz DS: Tapered fluted titanium stems in revision total hip arthroplasty, in Berry DJ, Maloney WJ, eds: *Master Techniques in Orthopaedic Surgery: The Hip*. Philadelphia, PA, Wolters Kluwer, 2016, pp 369-376.)

it corresponds in most patients to the desired center of rotation.

- Most modular systems offer several stem lengths (**Figure 4**). Reaming should be done to an intermediate length so that options remain available if the definitive stem sits proud or sinks below the desired level.
- The final distal stem is inserted and firmly seated (**Figure 5, A**).
- A taper protector is placed on the exposed trunnion (**Figure 5, B**).
- The proximal femur is prepared for placement of the body segment with the use of handheld reamers

over the taper protector (over the modular junction) (**Figure 5, C**). The distal stem that has been placed serves as a reference to ensure correct orientation of the proximal reamer.

- The taper protector is removed.
- A provisional body, determined on the basis of preoperative templating, is placed (**Figure 6**).
- A trial reduction is performed. Limb length, stability, abductor tension, and anteversion are assessed with the trial implant in place.
- If necessary, the choice of body shape, size, and offset are adjusted to achieve optimal biomechanics and accurately restore the center of rotation of the hip (**Figure 2**). The modularity of the implant allows the surgeon to achieve within 15° of the desired anteversion.
- The final prosthesis is opened.
- Reference points are marked on the bone or the skin using a sterile marker, with the tip of the greater trochanter used as a reference for limb length and the lesser trochanter used as a reference for anteversion.
- The final body is inserted over the trunnion of the stem and firmly affixed to it with a set screw. The desired anteversion is maintained with the use of a torque wrench and other instruments during this step (**Figure 7**).
- Alternatively, the prosthesis can be assembled on a separate back table before it is inserted. This technique is most easily accomplished in patients who have minimal bone loss and no substantial bowing or varus remodeling of the proximal femur.

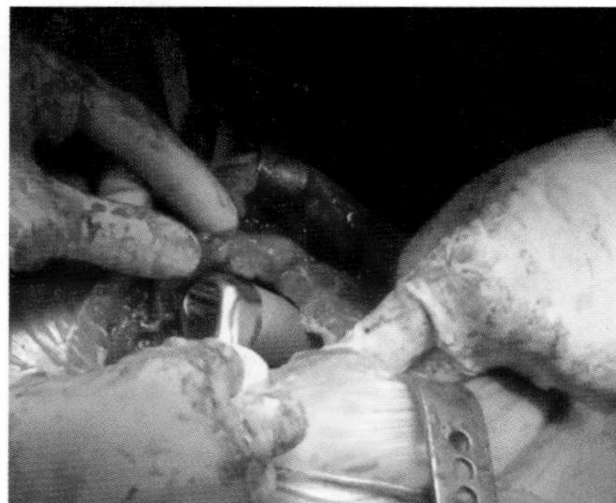

Figure 6 Intraoperative photograph of a right hip shows insertion of the proximal body segment. (Reproduced with permission from Sandiford NA, Duncan CP, Masri BA, Garbuz DS: Tapered fluted titanium stems in revision total hip arthroplasty, in Berry DJ, Maloney WJ, eds: *Master Techniques in Orthopaedic Surgery: The Hip.* Philadelphia, PA, Wolters Kluwer, 2016, pp 369-376.)

ETO

- The tip of the greater trochanter is used as a reference for the length of the ETO. The length of the ETO should allow 4 to 7 cm of close contact between the implant and the host bone distal to the osteotomy.
- The osteotomy is performed in the sagittal plane. A minimal amount of the vastus lateralis is elevated off the femur. The resulting muscular and bony flap is retracted anteriorly. In contrast to the Wagner osteotomy, in which the vastus lateralis is incised in midsubstance and a coronal femoral osteotomy bisects the greater trochanter and splits the hip abductors, this method preserves and protects the hip abductors.
- A prophylactic cerclage cable is placed 1 cm distal to the osteotomy site to reduce the risk of propagation of an iatrogenic fracture during reaming and insertion of the stem (**Figure 8**).
- The existing implant and cement are removed.
- Femoral preparation is performed with conical hand reamers. Reaming continues until excellent axial and rotational stability is achieved. Reaming is typically done to a level that will allow use of an intermediate body height.

INSERTION OF A MODULAR TAPERED, FLUTED STEM

- The first step is conical reaming similar to that described previously in the endofemoral technique. If an ETO is used, to ascertain the center of rotation, the length of the ETO fragment is measured, and a ruler is used to measure from the distal

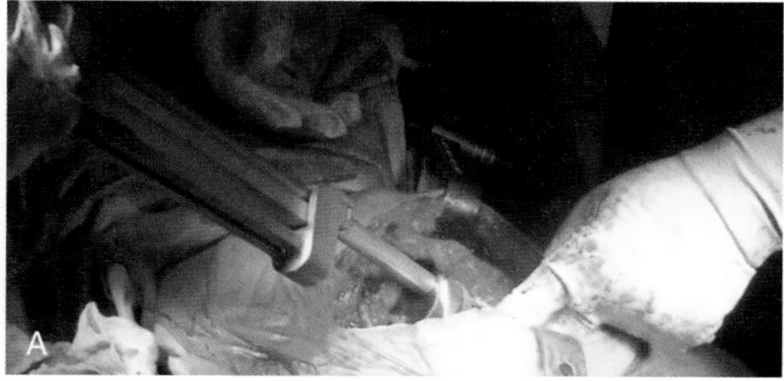

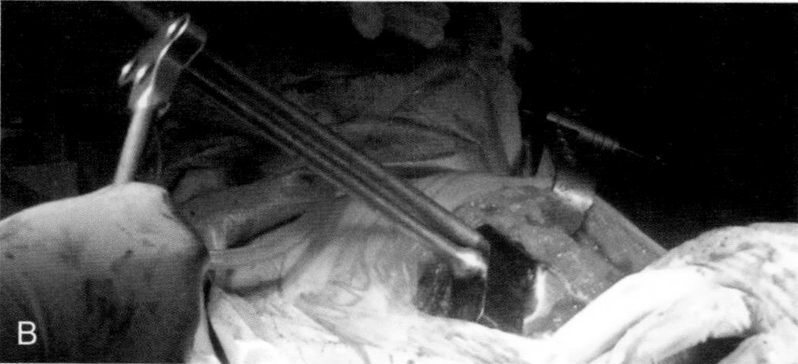

Figure 7 Intraoperative photographs of a right hip show placement of the implant body onto the definitive stem (**A**) and the use of a torque wrench to lock the modular segments together (**B**). The torque wrench also maintains the femoral neck version during this step.

end of the ETO fragment to the etch marks on the reamer.
- If a kinked or beveled stem will be used, the orientation is carefully assessed before insertion of the stem.
- The distal stem segment is inserted (**Figure 5, A**).
- The modular body options in revision implant systems allow adjustment of height and offset to maximize initial fixation. Etchings on the inserter handle guide the surgeon in selecting the optimal body height.
- Most systems offer a variety of sizes, shapes, lengths, and offsets, allowing the surgeon to achieve optimal fit and fill of the metaphysis and appropriate anteversion.
- Trial reductions are performed with different body options until optimal length and offset are achieved.
- After the appropriate body segment is selected, the trunnion of the stem is cleaned and the body is placed.
- The implant system preferred by the authors of this chapter includes an instrument for press fitting the body onto the stem trunnion.
- The two segments are affixed to each other with a locking screw applied with a torque wrench while the anteversion is maintained (**Figure 7**).
- The hip is reduced with a trial femoral head.
- After all parameters are reassessed (trial reduction is performed; length, offset, range of motion, and stability are evaluated), the final femoral head is applied.
- The reflected muscular and bony segment of the ETO is folded onto the prosthesis and fixed with cerclage cables or wires.
- The osteotomy fragment is contoured to the shape of the prosthesis with the use of a high-speed burr.
- Final fixation is achieved with the use of two or three cerclage cables or wires.

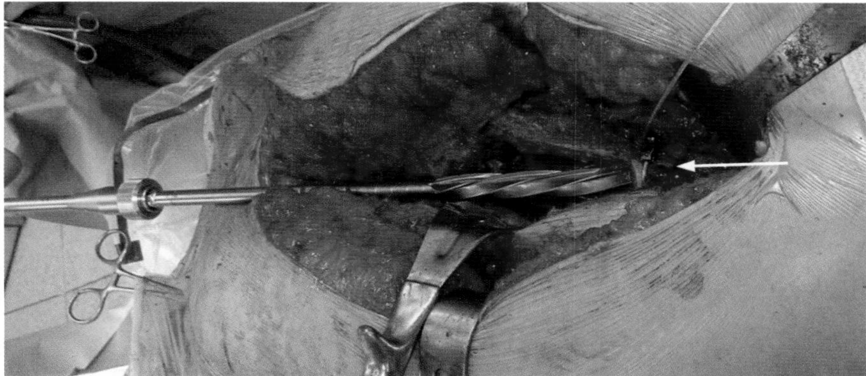

Figure 8 Intraoperative photograph of a right hip shows reaming after an extended trochanteric osteotomy was done. The arrow indicates a prophylactic cerclage wire that was applied 1 cm distal to the osteotomy site to reduce the risk of iatrogenic fracture. (Adapted with permission from Sandiford NA, Duncan CP, Masri BA, Garbuz DS: Tapered fluted titanium stems in revision total hip arthroplasty, in Berry DJ, Maloney WJ, eds: *Master Techniques in Orthopaedic Surgery: The Hip*. Philadelphia, PA, Wolters Kluwer, 2016, pp 369-376.)

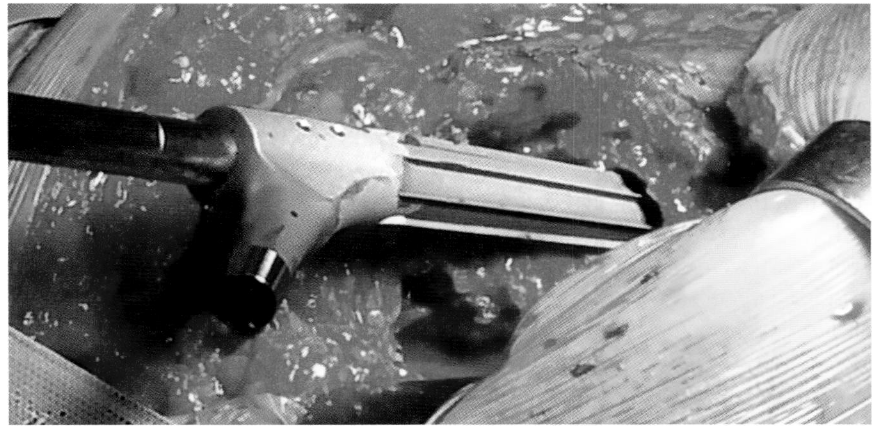

Figure 9 Intraoperative photograph shows insertion of a nonmodular stem.

INSERTION OF A NONMODULAR TAPERED, FLUTED STEM

- Reaming to achieve axial and rotational stability is a critical step in this technique.
- In general, the surgeon should aspire to use the shortest stem possible to achieve the desired fixation.
- After reaming, the trial implant is inserted. Anteversion is adjusted if necessary.
- After the trial implant is engaged, trial reduction is performed, and limb lengths and stability are assessed. Fine-tuning is accomplished with the use of trial femoral heads.
- If a limb-length discrepancy greater than 1 cm is present, a shorter or longer prosthesis can be used. To accommodate a longer stem, it may be necessary to seat the prosthesis slightly lower because the increments between stem sizes are 3 to 4 mm.
- Although the final stem is monoblock, the trials are modular, enabling the surgeon to fine-tune limb length during the trial reduction by changing proximal bodies on the stem (**Figures 1** and **9**).

Wound Closure

- Layered closure is performed to minimize formation of dead space.
- Transosseous sutures are placed through drill holes in the posterior aspect of the greater trochanter to reattach the short external rotators and posterior capsule to the greater trochanter.
- The skin is closed with staples.
- A sterile pressure dressing is applied.

Postoperative Regimen

Postoperative radiographs are routinely obtained in the postanesthesia care unit. The entire length of the prosthesis is imaged to confirm reduction, reveal occult fractures, and provide a baseline for future imaging studies. Antibiotic administration continues for 24 hours postoperatively. Most patients are instructed to maintain partial weight bearing for 6 weeks postoperatively. Toe-touch weight bearing is recommended if a complex reconstruction was performed, particularly on the acetabular side. Patients usually are discharged 3 to 5 days postoperatively. Clinical and radiologic follow-up examination occurs at 6 weeks postoperatively. If results of the follow-up examination are normal, weight bearing and rehabilitation are advanced.

Avoiding Pitfalls and Complications

Femoral fracture can occur during insertion of the stem segment, particularly in patients with poor bone quality and in those in whom an ETO is done. Placement of a prophylactic cerclage wire before reaming and stem insertion reduces the risk of femoral fracture. The surgeon should not hesitate to use intraoperative imaging if there is any concern regarding the integrity of the femur or in patients in whom unusually complex reconstruction is required. Fractures also can occur if a long stem is used without an ETO because of conflicting shapes of the femoral bow and the stem. For this reason, the authors of this chapter recommend the use of an ETO whenever the use of a long stem is considered. Postoperative radiographs should be obtained in the recovery room to facilitate early detection and management of fracture.

Subsidence is a concern with noncemented fluted, tapered nonmodular titanium stems. The risk of subsidence can be reduced with the use of careful preoperative planning, appropriate femoral preparation, selection of the most stable implant, and stable seating of the implant. Avoiding malpositioning of these stems in varus is critical. Surgeons who do not have extensive experience with these stems can use intraoperative radiography to ensure that the taper is well engaged and not in varus. This consideration is especially important when an endofemoral approach is used.

Junctional fractures can occur with modular stems. This complication occurs most often when a stem measuring less than 19 mm is used and the proximal segment is unsupported. The authors of this chapter recommend using stems greater than 19 mm and maximizing contact of the proximal segment with the existing metaphyseal bone. Newer implant systems have stronger junctions, which may decrease the rate of junctional fracture. Because of concerns of junctional fractures, nonmodular tapered stems are now used in most patients treated at the institution of the authors of this chapter.

Bibliography

Böhm P, Bischel O: Femoral revision with the Wagner SL revision stem: Evaluation of one hundred and twenty-nine revisions followed for a mean of 4.8 years. *J Bone Joint Surg Am* 2001;83(7):1023-1031.

Garbuz DS, Masri BA, Duncan CP, et al: Dislocation in revision THA: Do large heads (36 and 40 mm) result in reduced dislocation rates in a randomized clinical trial? *Clin Orthop Relat Res* 2012;470(2):351-356.

Gutiérrez del Alamo J, Garcia-Cimbrelo E, Castellanos V, Gil-Garay E: Radiographic bone regeneration and clinical outcome with the Wagner SL revision stem: A 5-year to 12-year follow-up study. *J Arthroplasty* 2007;22(4):515-524.

Isacson J, Stark A, Wallensten R: The Wagner revision prosthesis consistently restores femoral bone structure. *Int Orthop* 2000;24(3):139-142.

Lakstein D, Eliaz N, Levi O, et al: Fracture of cementless femoral stems at the mid-stem junction in modular revision hip arthroplasty systems. *J Bone Joint Surg Am* 2011;93(1):57-65.

Munro JT, Garbuz DS, Masri BA, Duncan CP: Tapered fluted titanium stems in the management of Vancouver B2 and B3 periprosthetic femoral fractures. *Clin Orthop Relat Res* 2014;472(2):590-598.

Munro JT, Masri BA, Garbuz DS, Duncan CP: Tapered fluted modular titanium stems in the management of Vancouver B2 and B3 peri-prosthetic fractures. *Bone Joint J* 2013;95-B(11 suppl A):17-20.

Ovesen O, Emmeluth C, Hofbauer C, Overgaard S: Revision total hip arthroplasty using a modular tapered stem with distal fixation: Good short-term results in 125 revisions. *J Arthroplasty* 2010;25(3):348-354.

Palumbo BT, Morrison KL, Baumgarten AS, Stein MI, Haidukewych GJ, Bernasek TL: Results of revision total hip arthroplasty with modular, titanium-tapered femoral stems in severe proximal metaphyseal and diaphyseal bone loss. *J Arthroplasty* 2013;28(4):690-694.

Regis D, Sandri A, Bonetti I, Braggion M, Bartolozzi P: Femoral revision with the Wagner tapered stem: A ten- to 15-year follow-up study. *J Bone Joint Surg Br* 2011;93(10):1320-1326.

Restrepo C, Mashadi M, Parvizi J, Austin MS, Hozack WJ: Modular femoral stems for revision total hip arthroplasty. *Clin Orthop Relat Res* 2011;469(2):476-482.

Richards CJ, Duncan CP, Masri BA, Garbuz DS: Femoral revision hip arthroplasty: A comparison of two stem designs. *Clin Orthop Relat Res* 2010;468(2):491-496.

Sandiford NA, Duncan CP, Masri BA, Garbuz DS: Tapered fluted titanium stems in revision total hip arthroplasty, in Berry DJ, Maloney WJ, eds: *Master Techniques in Orthopaedic Surgery: The Hip.* Philadelphia, PA, Wolters Kluwer, 2016, pp 369-376.

Schuh A, Werber S, Holzwarth U, Zeiler G: Cementless modular hip revision arthroplasty using the MRP Titan Revision Stem: Outcome of 79 hips after an average of 4 years' follow-up. *Arch Orthop Trauma Surg* 2004;124(5):306-309.

Van Houwelingen AP, Duncan CP, Masri BA, Greidanus NV, Garbuz DS: High survival of modular tapered stems for proximal femoral bone defects at 5 to 10 years followup. *Clin Orthop Relat Res* 2013;471(2):454-462.

Weeden SH, Paprosky WG: Minimal 11-year follow-up of extensively porous-coated stems in femoral revision total hip arthroplasty. *J Arthroplasty* 2002;17(4 suppl 1):134-137.

Weiss RJ, Beckman MO, Enocson A, Schmalholz A, Stark A: Minimum 5-year follow-up of a cementless, modular, tapered stem in hip revision arthroplasty. *J Arthroplasty* 2011;26(1):16-23.

Chapter 61
Femoral Revision With Impaction Bone Grafting and Cement

A. J. Timperley, MBChB, FRCS, DPhil (Oxon)
Jonathan R. Howell, MBBS, MSc, FRCS (Tr & Orth)

Indications

Femoral impaction grafting is a technique used to restore femoral bone stock in revision hip surgery. It involves the impaction of morcellized allograft bone into the femoral canal. The original technique, first used in the United Kingdom in 1987, requires introduction and pressurization of acrylic bone cement (polymethyl methacrylate) into a neomedullary canal formed by the compacted graft and the use of a polished tapered collarless femoral implant. The use of specially designed instruments allows tight compaction of the allograft chips with consistent alignment of the prosthesis in the medullary canal. Retrieval specimens and biopsies of impacted material have shown that the bone is often incorporated and remodeled, making good bone stock available for further revision procedures if required. Stainless steel wire meshes have been designed to constrain allograft chips in patients with uncontained defects in the proximal femur (**Figure 1**). Stability of the graft is achieved by vigorous impaction of allograft chips into the contained defect, allowing subsequent bony remodeling. Further reinforcement of the femur with strut allograft may be required. Long stems may be indicated in femurs that are deficient beyond the metaphyseal area. Specialized instruments allow impaction of the graft as far as 260 mm down the femur.

The impaction grafting technique is indicated in patients of any age in whom replenishment of proximal bone stock is important. It also is indicated in the following scenarios: when the endosteal surface of the femur is sclerotic and therefore not suitable for cement fixation; when a noncemented stem would achieve inadequate fixation; in revision procedures when the dimensions of the femur would make diaphyseal fixation of a noncemented prosthesis difficult or impossible; in patients with periprosthetic fracture who have deficient bone in the proximal femur; in the second stage of a two-stage revision for the management of infection in patients with femoral bone loss; and in femoral reconstruction procedures in which an extended trochanteric osteotomy has been performed. A long stem is indicated in patients who have cortical bone stock loss at the level that would be reached by the tip of a stem of conventional length, in patients with periprosthetic fracture, and in patients in whom the internal dimensions of the diaphysis are substantially expanded. Before the procedure is performed, active infection should be excluded. Adequate AP and lateral preoperative radiographs extending well below the tip of the implant requiring revision should be obtained and analyzed for the presence of endosteal and cortical femoral bone deficiencies. The radiographs should be templated to plan for an implant of the appropriate size, length, and offset. A stem long enough to bypass the defect by at least two cortical diameters should be used in patients with substantial distal cortical damage. Measurements are obtained to ensure that the implant will be seated to the correct level to accurately re-create leg length. An advantage of this technique compared with the use of noncemented implants is that it allows accurate re-creation of the hip biomechanics because stem size, offset, leg length, and version are all independently variable. Plain radiographs alone usually enable the surgeon to predict the need for allograft bone, femoral reconstruction meshes, strut allograft, and wires or cables and to estimate how many femoral heads will be required to obtain sufficient graft material.

Dr. Timperley or an immediate family member has received royalties and received research or institutional support from Stryker, and serves as a board member, owner, officer, or committee member of the British Orthopaedic Association and the British Hip Society. Dr. Howell or an immediate family member has received royalties from, serves as a paid consultant to, and has received research or institutional support from Stryker.

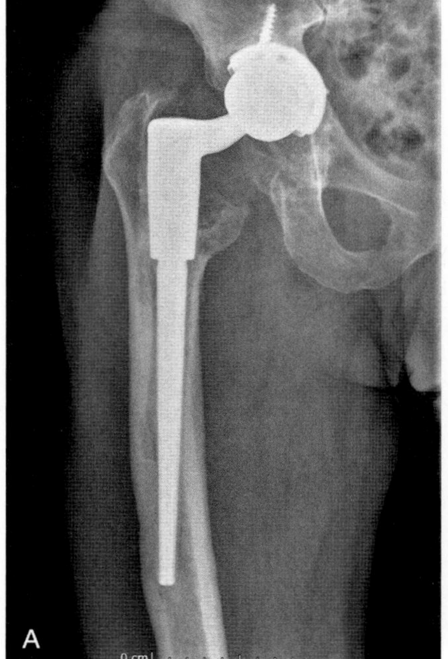

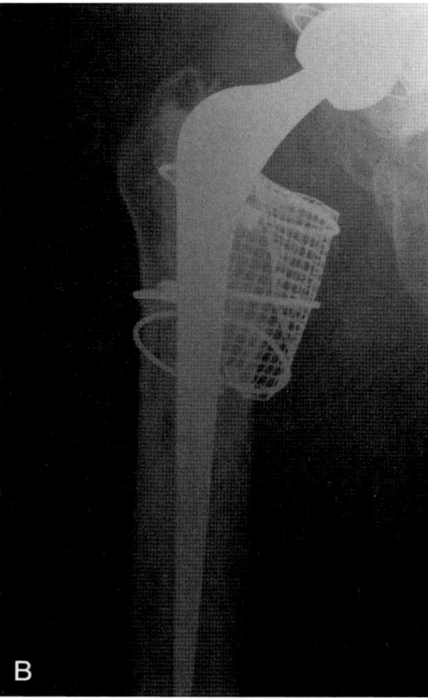

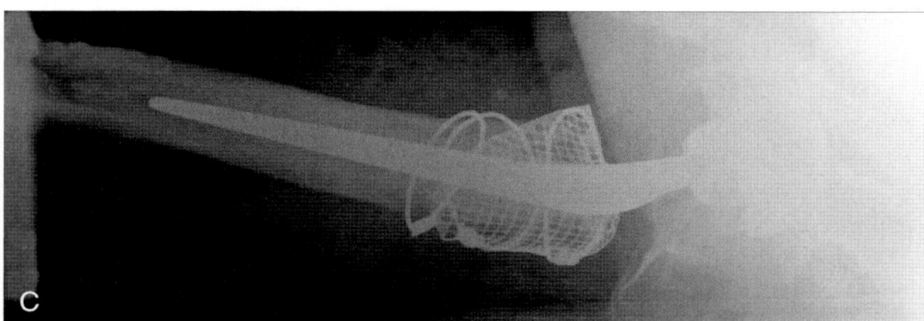

Figure 1 **A,** AP radiograph of a right hip demonstrates a failed noncemented femoral stem. The patient has cortical bone damage in zone 3/4 and at the calcar. Templating showed that a stem 205 mm long would be required to bypass the damaged area of cortical bone distally. **B,** Postoperative AP hip radiograph demonstrates a well-aligned 205-mm long, 44-mm offset stem. A mesh was placed around the proximal femur to constrain allograft chips. The mesh is held with three cables. **C,** Postoperative lateral hip radiograph demonstrates good alignment of the stem and satisfactory position of the wire mesh and cables.

Contraindications

Femoral impaction grafting is contraindicated in patients with extensive loss of bone stock in the proximal femur that would require circumferential wire mesh to address the bone deficiency. It probably is unnecessary when distal fixation can be achieved in very elderly patients or patients with substantial comorbidities and a reduced life expectancy.

Alternative Treatments

Noncemented implants with short or long stems are an alternative to the use of impacted allograft and a cemented implant. However, bone stock is more consistently augmented when the impaction grafting technique is used. Proximal loading of graft and host bone is achieved when a tapered, cemented implant subsides within the cement mantle by the mechanism of cement creep, thus encouraging proximal bone healing according to the Wolff law.

Results

Many midterm and long-term studies have shown excellent results after impaction grafting with the end point of aseptic loosening of the femoral implant (**Table 1**). In addition, a characteristic clinical feature of this technique is the excellent predictable level of pain relief it affords. Most studies have reported new bone formation in the proximal femur. Although notable complications of this technique were described in some early reports, the complications could usually be ascribed to inappropriate surgical technique.

Techniques

Setup/Exposure

- The technique is possible through any of the traditional approaches to the hip. The authors of this chapter prefer the posterior approach with the patient placed in the lateral position.
- The proximal femur is adequately exposed, and all existing implants and bone cement are removed.
- In patients in whom a single longitudinal osteotomy or an extended trochanteric osteotomy is performed to facilitate implant extraction, femoral impaction grafting can be performed after appropriate fixation of the femoral shaft with cables or wires. The site of the distal osteotomy must be bypassed by a longer stem. The entry point of the femoral

Table 1 Results of Impaction Grafting of the Femur

Authors (Year)	Number of Hips	Mean Patient Age in Years (Range)	Mean Follow-up in Years (Range)	Hip Survivorship Results
Wraighte and Howard (2008)	75	68 (35-87)	10.5 (6.3-13.1)	Survivorship at 10 yr was 92% with any femoral revision as the end point
Kerboull et al (2009)	129	64 (43-79)	8.2 (2-16)	Survivorship at 9 yr was 100% for the femoral implant with revision for any cause as the end point and 98% with radiologic loosening as the end point
Ornstein et al (2009)	1,305	71 (29-94)	8 (0.1-17.6)	Survivorship at 15 yr was 99.1% with aseptic loosening as the end point, 99.0% with subsidence as the end point, 98.6% with fracture as the end point, and 94% with failure for any reason as the end point
Garcia-Cimbrelo et al (2011)	81	64 (31-83)	10.4 (5-17)	Survivorship at 14 yr was 98.6% with aseptic loosening as the end point and 81.8% with revision for any reason as the end point
Lamberton et al (2011)	540	69.7 (31-95)	6.7 (2-15)	Survivorship at 10 yr was 98% with aseptic loosening as the end point, 90% with fracture but retention of stem as the end point, and 84% with revision for any reason as the end point
Iwase et al (2012)	99	66.3 (36-84)	5.2 (2-13)	Survivorship at 9 yr was 99% with aseptic loosening as the end point, 93.1% with any stem removal or exchange as the end point, and 94.8% with femoral fracture as the end point
te Stroet et al (2012)	33	63 (33-82)	17 (15-20)	Survivorship at 17 yr was 100% with revision for aseptic loosening as the end point and 83% with femoral revision for any reason as the end point
Garvin et al (2013)	78	67 (33-84)	10.6 (2-19)	Survivorship at 19 yr was 93% with revision for any reason as the end point and 98% with aseptic loosening as the end point
te Stroet et al (2014)	37	76 (39-93)	9 (5-18)	Survivorship at 9 yr was 96% with revision for any reason as the end point and 80.7% with any secondary surgery as the end point

canal is adequately opened laterally to facilitate preparation of the canal and insertion of a straight stem.

- A guidewire is inserted down the medullary canal in the mid-axis of the femur to ensure neutral alignment of the neomedullary canal (**Figure 2**).
- In patients with cortical deficiency, the deficiency is repaired with the use of wire meshes to create a contained cavity that will allow tight compaction of allograft chips.
- If the bone is of poor quality, prophylactic cerclage wiring of the proximal femur is recommended to reduce the risk for formation of a longitudinal split when the bone is impacted.

Procedure

PREPARATION OF THE BONE GRAFT AND SIZING ALLOGRAFT CHIPS

- Ideally, fresh-frozen femoral head graft, with all soft tissue, cartilage, and hard cortical bone removed, is used.
- For use in the distal femur up to the level of the lesser trochanter, allograft chips 2 to 3 mm in size are prepared by processing the prepared femoral head with a bone mill.
- In the proximal femur, impaction of larger bone chips 8 to 10 mm in size, made by hand with a large rongeur, will result in better stability with torsional loading. Later in the procedure, these large chips also will be packed tightly using dedicated hand-held instruments around the seated phantom stem that has been used for impaction.
- When a standard-length stem is used, two femoral heads will normally produce sufficient bone for the impaction grafting technique.

PLACEMENT OF THE DISTAL PLUG

- The diameter of the femoral canal is confirmed with canal size gauges

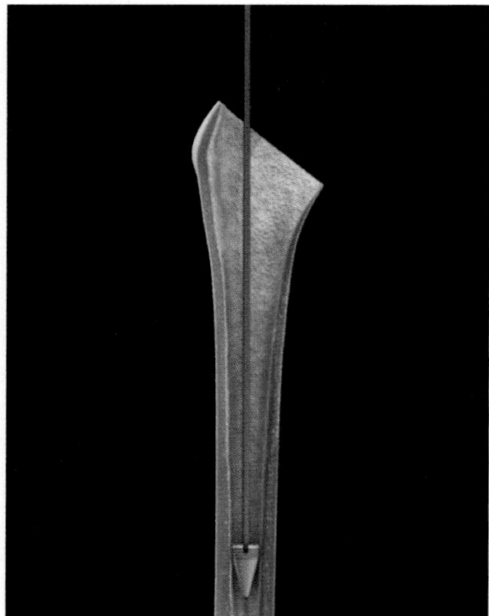

Figure 2 Illustration of a femur shows the use of a guidewire screwed to a distal polyethylene plug to align the impactors to create a neomedullary canal with impacted allograft bone.

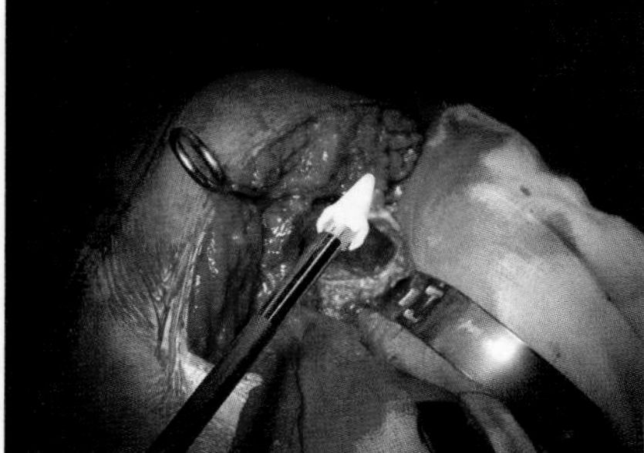

Figure 3 Intraoperative photograph shows a polyethylene plug attached to the guidewire and mounted on an introducer. The plug is inserted into the canal to a predetermined depth with the use of a slap hammer.

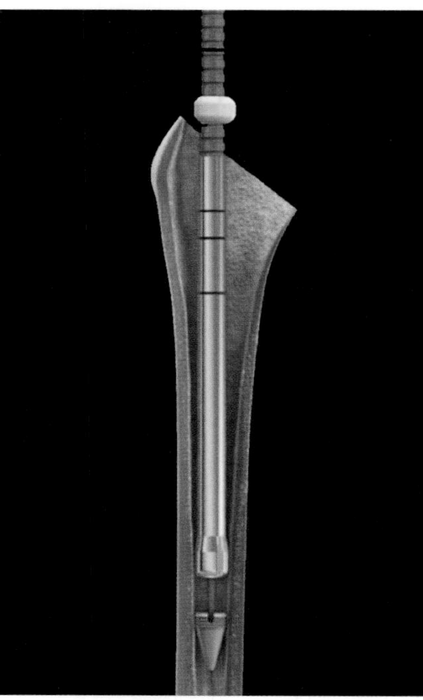

Figure 4 Illustration shows a marker attached to the shaft of a distal impactor to indicate the depth in the femoral canal to which the instrument can safely be used to impact bone without risk of splitting the femur.

2 cm distal to the planned location of the tip of the stem.

- A threaded polyethylene plug is screwed onto the intramedullary guidewire and inserted to this level with the use of a cannulated introducer sleeve coupled with a slap hammer (**Figure 3**).
- The guidewire is left in place to direct the cannulated instruments that will be used for the impaction grafting (**Figure 2**).
- If the plug is placed beyond the isthmus, the largest plug that fits through the isthmus is secured in the correct position with a 2-mm percutaneous Kirschner wire used as a skewer.

OVERVIEW: ALIGNMENT AND SIZE CHECK

- Before any bone is introduced, the proximal impactor of the templated size is passed over the guidewire to the level required to restore leg length.
- If the impactor does not pass easily in a neutral position, the proximal femoral canal is checked to ensure that it has been adequately opened laterally. If the impactor still catches within the canal, the use of a smaller femoral implant of the same offset may be necessary.
- Cannulated distal impactors are used over the guidewire to compact the graft material to the level of the tip of the stem.
- Above this level, proximal impactors designed to create a cavity with dimensions of a stem with cement mantle are used sequentially to impact the bone chips. A marker is placed on the stem of each distal impactor to show how far the anatomy will allow the impactor to pass down the canal (**Figure 4**). To avoid fracture during impaction, the impactor must not be driven beyond the marked depth.
- Sequentially larger distal impactors are passed over the guidewire and marked, starting with an impactor that is 2 mm smaller in diameter than the plug.

INTRODUCTION AND DISTAL PACKING OF THE GRAFT

- The small chips are introduced with an open-ended 10-mL syringe (**Figure 5**) and pushed down the canal with the impactors.

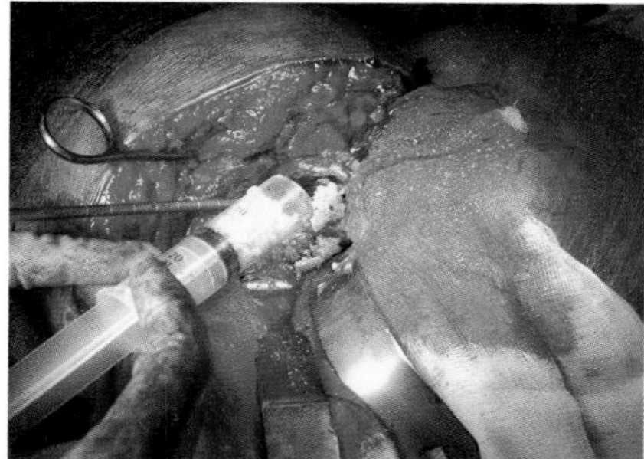

Figure 5 Intraoperative photograph shows introduction of allograft chips 2 to 4 mm in size with an open-ended 10-mL syringe. The chips are advanced down the femoral canal with the distal impactors.

- Starting with the smallest marked impactor, chips are introduced and impacted using progressively larger impactors passed down the guidewire (**Figure 6**). This process is continued until the canal is filled to the level where the stem tip will ultimately be positioned.

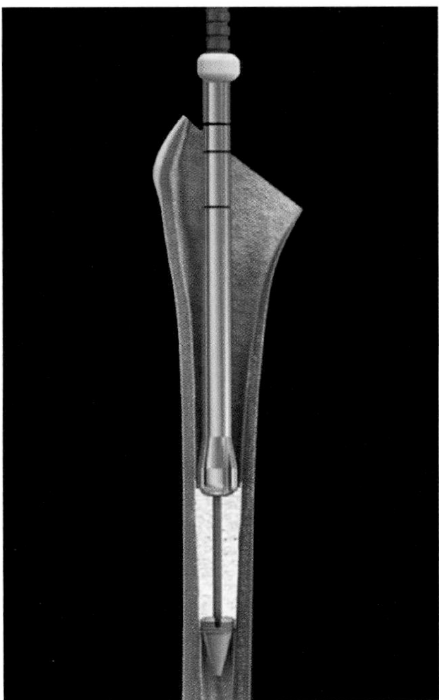

Figure 6 Illustration of a femur shows the use of a distal impactor. These impactors are used in sequence to fill the canal up to the distal impaction line. After the canal is filled to this depth, proximal impactors are used to create a cavity of impacted chips that allows space for both the stem and its cement mantle.

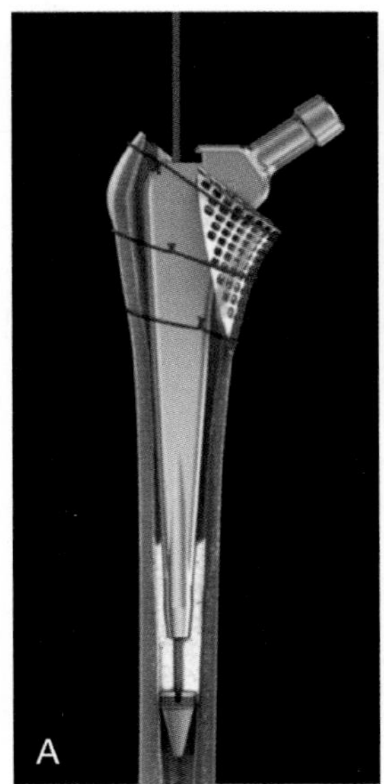

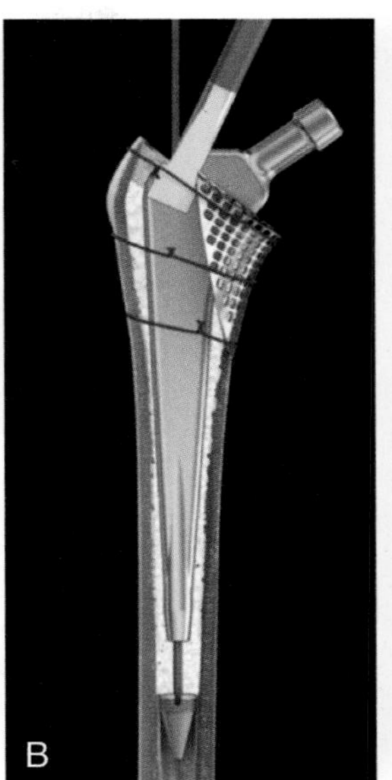

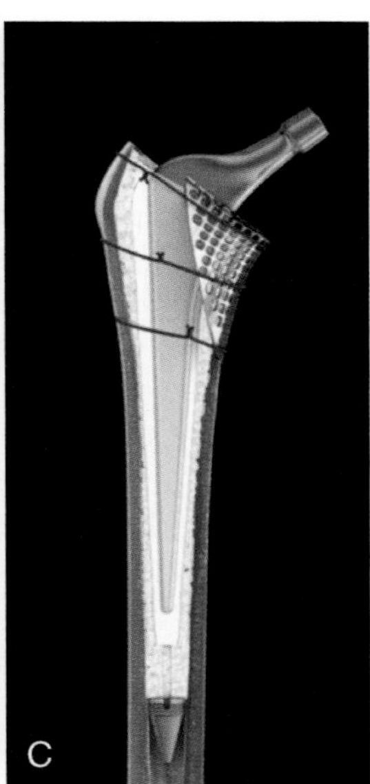

Figure 7 **A,** Illustration of a femur shows the proximal impactor introduced to the correct depth to establish appropriate leg length, which allows assessment of the need for a proximal mesh to constrain the bone chips. In this case, a mesh is used at the calcar to replace the lost host bone. The mesh is held in place with cerclage wires or cables. **B,** Illustration shows further packing of larger chips with proximal hand impactors and a mallet after the canal has been filled to the top with allograft bone. This step is important to establish torsional stability of the implant. **C,** Illustration shows the construct with the guidewire removed in preparation for cementing. The proximal impactor is left in place to compress the allograft chips until the last moment before cementing.

- From this level, termed the distal impaction line, proximal impactors are henceforth used to impact chips in the proximal canal, with the distal impactors only used by hand to guide the chips from the syringe down the canal.
- If the calibrations on the guidewire are seen to be migrating distally at any time, the plug should be held with a 2-mm Kirschner wire used as a skewer.

PROXIMAL PACKING OF THE GRAFT

- An appropriately sized proximal impactor is mounted on the slap hammer assembly and passed over the guidewire in the desired degree of version.
- Chips are inserted after each episode of impaction with the proximal impactor. The chips are pushed distally by hand with a distal impactor, and then the proximal impactor is reintroduced over the guidewire, progressively filling the canal and compacting the chips.
- Because the proximal impactor will be very stable within the impacted material, forceful use of the slap hammer is necessary to retrieve it from the canal.
- Larger chips can be used toward the proximal femur, starting just below the lesser trochanter.

PROXIMAL CANAL RECONSTRUCTION WITH WIRE MESH

- The graft can be compacted only if it is constrained by cortical bone or mesh. Any bony defect must be repaired with the use of stainless steel meshes.
- The most common deficiency is in the calcar area. Reconstruction of the calcar usually is easier after the bone impaction has commenced and the proximal impactor is stabilized in the allograft bed.
- With the proximal impactor seated to a level that restores appropriate leg length, a wire mesh that has been trimmed to cover the defect and overlap host bone is held in place with cerclage wires or cables (**Figure 7, A**).
- The proximal impactor is left in position to help orient correct position of the mesh. The mesh should extend to a level opposite the middle mark on the femoral implant and should not restrict appropriate version of the proximal impactor.

TRIAL REDUCTION

- A trial reduction is performed. The guidewire may be left in place

during trial reduction.
- Hip stability and leg length are assessed.
- Leg length can be adjusted by driving the impactor farther into the canal or by planning to position the femoral implant less far into the femur.
- The position of the mark on the proximal impactor in relation to the calcar and the position of the shoulder of the impactor in relation to the tip of the greater trochanter are marked to guide the depth to which the stem should be inserted.
- If the implant offset is not optimal, then a stem of larger or reduced offset may be used when appropriate. Leg length is determined solely by the depth of insertion of the stem and is independent of offset.

FURTHER PROXIMAL IMPACTION

- With the proximal impactor seated to the correct level, larger cancellous chips are packed with hand impactors and a mallet around the proximal femur (**Figure 7, B**). This step is important to ensure the torsional stability of the stem. In a capacious femur, substantially more bone can be introduced in this manner.
- After packing is completed, removal of the proximal impactor by hand should be impossible because of its stability in the construct.

CEMENTATION AND STEM INSERTION

- While the cement is being mixed, the slap hammer and guidewire are removed.
- The proximal impactor is left in place until the cement is ready to be injected (**Figure 7, C**).
- When the cement is ready for injection, the slap hammer is reattached and used to remove the proximal impactor (**Figure 8**) and introduce a 14-gauge suction catheter down to the distal end of the canal. The suction catheter will help clear blood and suck cement to the distal end of the cavity.
- The suction catheter is pulled out as the cement is injected in retrograde manner (**Figure 9**).
- After the canal is filled with cement, a proximal femoral seal is used to occlude the proximal end of the femur.
- Injection of cement into the closed cavity is continued, thus pressurizing the cement into the surface of the impacted chips.
- As the viscosity of the cement increases, the stem is inserted to the previously determined depth in the desired degree of anteversion.
- Leg length can be accurately restored by adjusting the depth of insertion of the stem into the bony cavity.
- If necessary for stability, the version of the stem can be altered by 15° to 20° within the cavity formed by the proximal impactor.
- The pressure within the canal is maintained with the use of a horse-collar–shaped proximal femoral seal held around the stem until polymerization is complete.
- A final trial reduction is performed.
- Offset and leg length can be fine-tuned simultaneously, if necessary, by changing the length of the femoral neck.

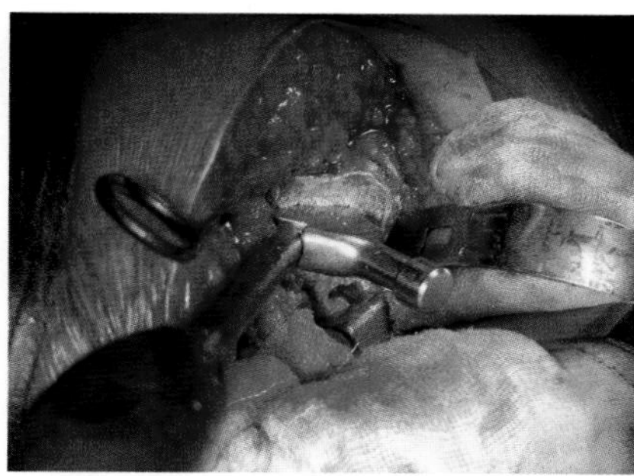

Figure 8 Intraoperative photograph of the proximal femur shows reattachment of the introducer handle to the proximal impactor. The proximal impactor is knocked out of the neomedullary canal when the cement is ready for injection.

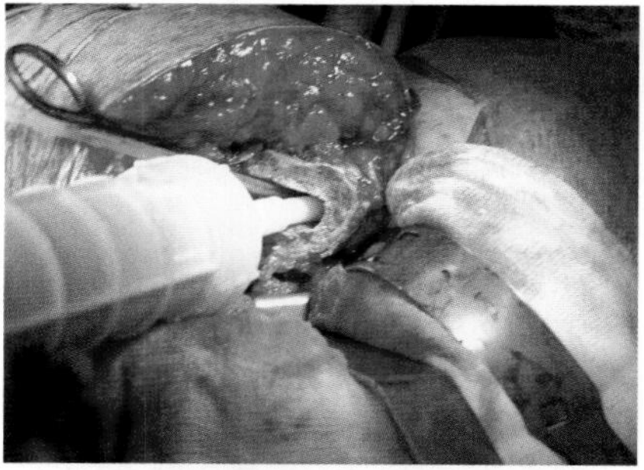

Figure 9 Intraoperative photograph shows injection of cement in retrograde manner initially over a distal suction catheter. The catheter is pulled out as soon as it blocks with cement. The entire femoral canal is filled from distal to proximal. Further pressurization is achieved by continued injection of polymethyl methacrylate through a proximal femoral seal. The stem is then inserted to the previously determined position to achieve the desired leg length and version. The offset is established by the geometry of the stem.

Wound Closure

- Routine closure of all layers is performed.

Postoperative Regimen

Patients are mobilized on the first postoperative day. Patients routinely are restricted to partial weight bearing for 6 weeks postoperatively. However, more elderly patients will need to proceed to full weight bearing immediately postoperatively. Patients are assessed radiographically and all are encouraged to progress to full weight bearing by 10 to 12 weeks postoperatively.

Avoiding Pitfalls and Complications

Although the principles of femoral impaction grafting are straightforward, many tips and tricks will help speed the procedure and reduce the surgical learning curve and consequent morbidity. Ideally, a surgeon should be trained by means of a fellowship at a center where this technique is routinely performed. Alternatively, the surgeon should attend workshops using cadavers and orthopaedic models for training and make multiple visits to reference centers to observe the procedure. Formal mentoring with an experienced surgeon is advised.

Adherence to the details of the technique can help reduce the risk of intraoperative and postoperative fractures. It is essential to adequately constrain the graft to allow vigorous compaction of the graft. Tight impaction, and thereby compaction, of the graft is necessary to prevent subsidence of greater than 2 to 3 mm. The construct must be stable enough to allow full weight bearing immediately after the procedure without the occurrence of substantial subsidence. Excellent torsional stability must be achieved at the completion of grafting. Intraoperative fractures can be prevented with appropriate augmentation of the proximal femur using mesh or prophylactic wires. The risk of postoperative fracture is reduced by bypassing damaged bone with a longer stem or with the use of a strut graft over stress risers near the tip of the implanted stem.

Bibliography

Bolder SB, Schreurs BW, Verdonschot N, Ling RS, Slooff TJ: The initial stability of an Exeter femoral stem after impaction bone grafting in combination with segmental defect reconstruction. *J Arthroplasty* 2004;19(5):598-604.

Fowler JL, Gie GA, Lee AJ, Ling RS: Experience with the Exeter total hip replacement since 1970. *Orthop Clin North Am* 1988;19(3):477-489.

Garcia-Cimbrelo E, Garcia-Rey E, Cruz-Pardos A: The extent of the bone defect affects the outcome of femoral reconstruction in revision surgery with impacted bone grafting: A five- to 17-year follow-up study. *J Bone Joint Surg Br* 2011;93(11):1457-1464.

Garvin KL, Konigsberg BS, Ommen ND, Lyden ER: What is the long-term survival of impaction allografting of the femur? *Clin Orthop Relat Res* 2013;471(12):3901-3911.

Gie GA, Linder L, Ling RS, Simon JP, Slooff TJ, Timperley AJ: Contained morselized allograft in revision total hip arthroplasty: Surgical technique. *Orthop Clin North Am* 1993;24(4):717-725.

Halliday BR, English HW, Timperley AJ, Gie GA, Ling RS: Femoral impaction grafting with cement in revision total hip replacement: Evolution of the technique and results. *J Bone Joint Surg Br* 2003;85(6):809-817.

Iwase T, Kouyama A, Matsushita N: Complete bone remodeling after calcar reconstruction with metal wire mesh and impaction bone grafting: A case report. *Nagoya J Med Sci* 2013;75(3-4):287-293.

Iwase T, Otsuka H, Katayama N, Fujita H: Impaction bone grafting for femoral revision hip arthroplasty with Exeter Universal stem in Japan. *Arch Orthop Trauma Surg* 2012;132(10):1487-1494.

Kerboull L, Hamadouche M, Kerboull M: Impaction grafting in association with the Charnley-Kerboull cemented femoral component: Operative technique and two- to 16-year follow-up results. *J Bone Joint Surg Br* 2009;91(3):304-309.

Lamberton TD, Kenny PJ, Whitehouse SL, Timperley AJ, Gie GA: Femoral impaction grafting in revision total hip arthroplasty: A follow-up of 540 hips. *J Arthroplasty* 2011;26(8):1154-1160.

Ling RS, Timperley AJ, Linder L: Histology of cancellous impaction grafting in the femur: A case report. *J Bone Joint Surg Br* 1993;75(5):693-696.

Ornstein E, Linder L, Ranstam J, Lewold S, Eisler T, Torper M: Femoral impaction bone grafting with the Exeter stem: The Swedish experience. Survivorship analysis of 1305 revisions performed between 1989 and 2002. *J Bone Joint Surg Br* 2009;91(4):441-446.

te Stroet MA, Bronsema E, Rijnen WH, Gardeniers JW, Schreurs BW: The use of a long stem cemented femoral component in revision total hip replacement: A follow-up study of five to 16 years. *Bone Joint J* 2014;96-B(9):1207-1213.

te Stroet MA, Gardeniers JW, Verdonschot N, Rijnen WH, Slooff TJ, Schreurs BW: Femoral component revision with use of impaction bone-grafting and a cemented polished stem: A concise follow-up, at fifteen to twenty years, of a previous report. *J Bone Joint Surg Am* 2012;94(23):e1731-e1734.

Ullmark G, Obrant KJ: Histology of impacted bone-graft incorporation. *J Arthroplasty* 2002;17(2):150-157.

Wraighte PJ, Howard PW: Femoral impaction bone allografting with an Exeter cemented collarless, polished, tapered stem in revision hip replacement: A mean follow-up of 10.5 years. *J Bone Joint Surg Br* 2008;90(8):1000-1004.

Chapter 62
Femoral Revision With Allograft Prosthetic Composite

Michael D. Ries, MD

Indications

An allograft prosthetic composite (APC) is indicated for patients in whom massive circumferential segmental proximal femoral bone loss precludes reconstruction with a more conventional proximally or distally fixed revision femoral stem. Proximal femoral bone loss can result from several causes, including osteolysis, periprosthetic fracture, and infection, usually in association with multiple prior total hip arthroplasty (THA) and revision procedures. The allograft is a circumferential structural replacement of the proximal femur. A long-stem femoral implant extends through the allograft and into the distal femoral host bone (**Figure 1**). Although revascularization of a cortical allograft is unlikely, the reconstruction provides sites for muscle attachment, may improve bone stock, and reduces femoral implant stresses.

Contraindications

The use of an APC is contraindicated in patients in whom bone stock is sufficient to permit reconstruction using other techniques. Active infection is a contraindication to use of an APC. Previous infection does not necessarily preclude the use of an APC if the infection has been adequately controlled. Successful reconstruction can be achieved after failure of an APC resulting from infection via two-stage débridement, insertion of an antibiotic cement spacer followed by a course of appropriate antibiotic therapy, and delayed second-stage reconstruction with another APC.

Typically, allografts are not tissue typed or matched to the patient; therefore, an immune response to the allograft can occur. Freezing the allograft reduces the host immune response. However, prior immune-mediated allograft rejection (which may result in an increased risk of allograft nonunion or resorption of another allograft) is a relative contraindication to use of an APC.

Poor soft-tissue coverage of the hip, such as after prior tumor irradiation or after multiple procedures, may be a relative contraindication to use of an APC. In patients with poor soft-tissue coverage, a separate soft-tissue flap coverage procedure may be necessary before or at the time of APC reconstruction.

Alternative Treatments

Circumferential bone loss of the proximal femur also can be managed with excision arthroplasty (Girdlestone procedure), proximal femoral replacement, or a distally fixed, tapered long-stem femoral implant. Excision arthroplasty is associated with considerable limb shortening and functional impairment in patients in whom bone loss extends distally beyond the subtrochanteric region. Ambulatory ability will be severely compromised after this procedure because of loss of hip mechanics and limb shortening. Therefore, excision arthroplasty should be reserved for nonambulatory patients who are not candidates for more extensive reconstructive procedures.

In proximal femoral replacement, the prosthesis consists of a large proximal metal body with dimensions similar to the proximal femur connected to a distal intramedullary stem (megaprosthesis). The distal stem, which usually is cemented into the host distal canal, provides the mechanical support for the implant (**Figure 2**). Proximal femoral replacement is mechanically similar to an APC that has not yet united with host bone at the host-allograft junction because the distal intramedullary portion of the long stem of either the APC or megaprosthesis provides the

Dr. Ries or an immediate family member has received royalties from Smith & Nephew; serves as a paid consultant to Smith & Nephew and Stryker; has stock or stock options held in OrthAlign; and serves as a board member, owner, officer, or committee member of the Foundation for the Advancement of Research in Medicine.

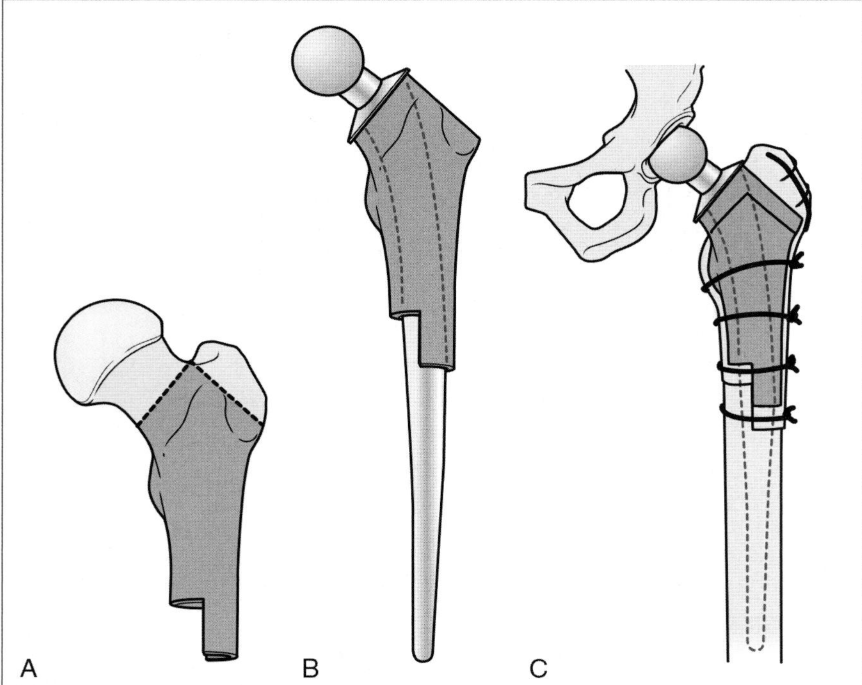

Figure 1 Illustrations depict steps in the implementation of an allograft prosthetic composite. **A,** A proximal femoral allograft is shaped to fit the area of bone loss. A distal step cut is made, and the femoral head and greater trochanter are marked for removal. **B,** A long-stem femoral implant is cemented into the bulk proximal femoral allograft. **C,** The allograft prosthetic composite is stabilized in the distal host bone via the intramedullary femoral stem. Residual proximal host bone remnants, including the patient's greater trochanter, are secured to the allograft with cables.

initial mechanical support for the reconstruction. However, after healing at the host-allograft junction, the proximal femoral allograft behaves mechanically as part of the femur, providing proximal support for the femoral stem. In an in vitro cadaver mechanical study of femoral cortical strain before and after APC reconstruction, proximal femoral bone strain was reduced substantially after an APC was performed compared with a simulated APC that had not healed at the host-allograft junction. The discontinuity between the proximal allograft and distal host bone eliminated absorption of bending stresses by the proximal allograft, which is similar to the function of a cemented proximal femoral replacement. However, after the host-allograft junction has healed, the proximal allograft and distal host bone reconstitute the cortical tube of the femur and weight-bearing bending stresses are transferred to the allograft. This load transfer reduces stresses on the intramedullary stem and the area of distal fixation in the host bone, which may reduce the risk of loosening with APC compared with a cemented proximal femoral replacement. However, use of a proximal femoral replacement also avoids the complications of allograft rejection and nonunion that can occur after an APC. A 1-year survivorship rate of 87% and a 5-year survivorship rate of 73% have been reported with use of a proximal femoral replacement in the management of nonneoplastic conditions.

Distally tapered noncemented modular stems often are used to manage failed THAs in patients with proximal femoral bone loss. Such reconstruction may be indicated to manage circumferential proximal femoral bone loss in patients in whom allograft is contraindicated (whether because of prior failed allograft reconstructions as a result of allograft rejection or infection) and those with inadequate distal host bone for reconstruction with a cemented distal femoral replacement (**Figure 3**). Although the use of distally tapered noncemented modular stems can reconstitute leg length and provide mechanical support for the lower limb, the modular junction between the proximal body and distal stem is subject to high bending and torsional stresses because of the absence of surrounding bone. These stresses can result in taper corrosion or catastrophic failure at the modular junction.

Results

Successful restoration of hip function has been reported in approximately 70% to 90% of hips at 4- to 16-year follow-up after APC reconstruction (**Table 1**). However, complications such as deep infection, host-allograft nonunion, allograft resorption, loosening, instability, and trochanteric nonunion also have been observed in most studies. Trochanteric nonunion has been reported in greater than 50% of hips. Although favorable long-term successful salvage of hip function can be expected after APC reconstruction, patients are at substantial risk for complications requiring rerevision surgery.

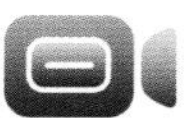

Video 62.1 Femoral Revision With Allograft Prosthetic Composite. Michael D. Ries, MD (4 min)

Technique

Setup/Exposure

- The patient is placed in the lateral decubitus position.

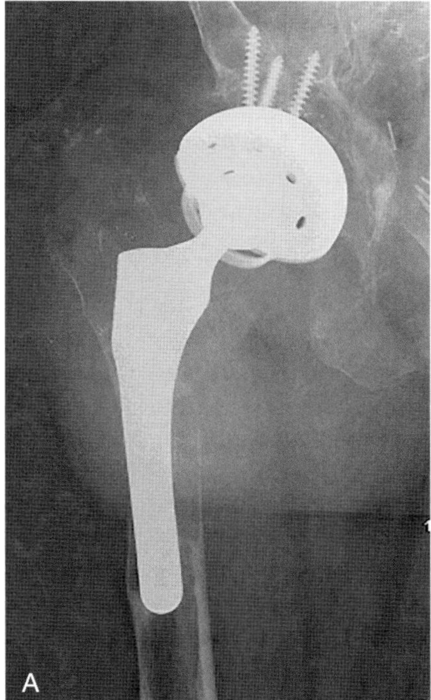

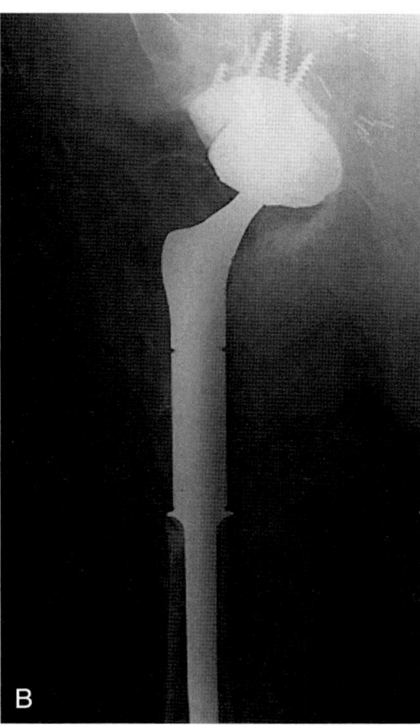

Figure 2 **A,** AP radiograph of the right hip from an 87-year-old man in whom severe osteolysis with segmental loss of proximal femoral bone stock developed 26 years after noncemented total hip arthroplasty with ultra-high–molecular-weight polyethylene sterilized with gamma irradiation in air. **B,** AP radiograph obtained 6 weeks after proximal femoral replacement with a cemented distal stem.

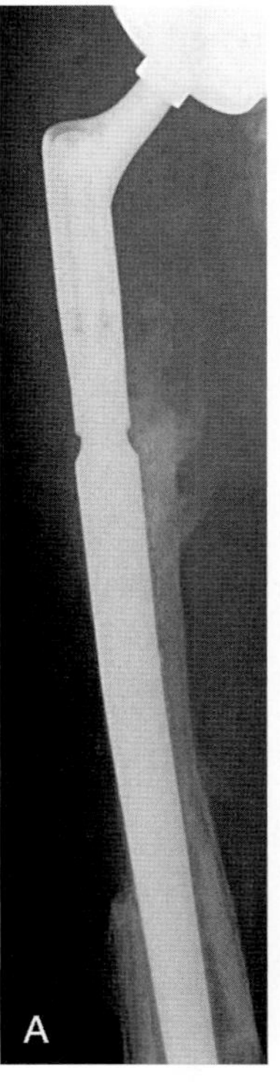

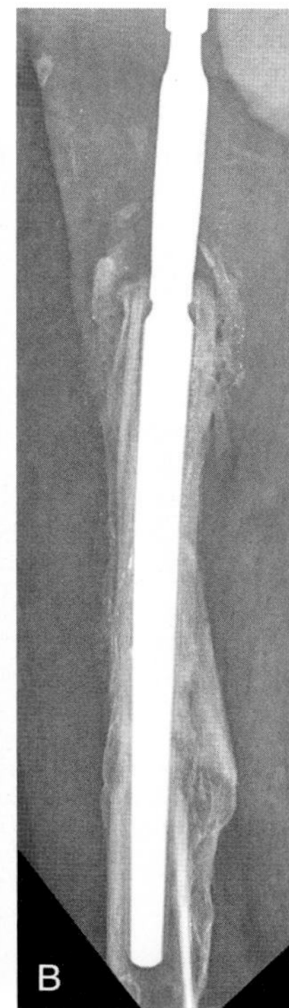

Figure 3 AP (**A**) and lateral (**B**) radiographs of a right hip after revision total hip arthroplasty to a distally fixed, modular tapered stem to manage segmental proximal femoral bone loss after two previous allograft prosthetic composite reconstructions failed due to allograft resorption and infection. This patient is at increased risk for taper corrosion or fracture at the modular junction because of the lack of proximal bony support for the implant.

- Previous lateral hip incisions should be used if possible.
- A long lateral incision is made, extending distally beyond the level of the host-allograft junction.
- A standard lateral incision is made in the tensor fascia lata, and the gluteus maximus muscle fibers are split proximally in line with their fibers to expose the deep muscle layer.
- A posterior approach to the hip and a lateral approach to the femur are preferred to maintain continuity of the gluteus medius and vastus lateralis muscles. The sciatic nerve is identified by means of palpation or direct visualization and is protected both from compression against retractors during the procedure and from excess lengthening during trial and final reduction of the implants.
- The greater trochanter (if present) and abductors are preserved and used for later reattachment to the proximal allograft.
- Often the vastus lateralis origin on the distal greater trochanter can be preserved, providing a soft-tissue sleeve of the gluteus medius, greater trochanter, and vastus lateralis (trochanteric slide) that can be used to augment soft-tissue stability of the hip and provide soft-tissue coverage over the proximal allograft.
- Vascularized thin osteolytic cortical bone fragments from the host proximal femur are preserved and secured to the outer surface of the allograft with cerclage cables or wires to promote host-allograft healing.
- Even if the abductors are not present, the remaining vastus lateralis is dissected posteriorly along the intermuscular septum and elevated in a posterior-to-anterior direction to expose the distal portion of the femur so that it can be closed over the distal allograft and host-allograft junction later in the procedure.

Instruments/Equipment/Implants Required

- An ipsilateral proximal femoral or whole femoral allograft must be obtained preoperatively.
- The desired level of the osteotomy is planned based on preoperative radiographs, and an allograft of appropriate size and length to bypass

Table 1 Results of Allograft Prosthetic Composite Reconstruction

Authors (Year)	Number of Hips	Mean Patient Age in Years (Range)	Mean Follow-up in Years (Range)	Success Rate (%)[a]	Complications
Blackley et al (2001)	63	62.5 (30.2-81.6)	11 (9.3-15)	77[b]	5 had an infection 3 had loosening 3 had a nonunion 2 had dislocation
Graham and Stockley (2004)	25	64 (28-86)	4.4 (1.3-8.4)	84[c]	2 had a nonunion 1 had an infection 2 had allograft resorption 9 had trochanteric nonunion
Wang and Wang (2004)	15	58.7 (41-68)	7.6 (4-11)	67	3 had an infection 2 had a nonunion 1 had a fracture 3 had allograft resorption 4 had trochanteric escape
Vastel et al (2007)	43	60.2 (25-79)	7 (2-15)	90	25 had a trochanteric nonunion 6 had dislocation 3 had loosening 1 had an infection
Lee et al (2009)	15	60.9 (32-84)	4.2 (2-9.8)	80	1 had a nonunion 1 had a nonunion and infection
Safir et al (2009)	50	63 (49-81)[d]	16.2 (15-22)	84	2 had an infection 6 had loosening 3 had a nonunion 4 had dislocation
Babis et al (2010)	72	59.9 (38-78)	12 (8-20)[e]	69[f]	2 had a nonunion 4 had loosening 3 had resorption 4 had an allograft fracture 1 had a stem fracture 5 had an infection 8 had dislocation 4 had a trochanteric nonunion

[a] Success is defined as construct retention and absence of deep infection.
[b] Success rate based on surviving 48 hips.
[c] Success rate based on lack of requirement for stem revision or surgical treatment of host-allograft nonunion and absence of deep infection.
[d] Patient age based on original cohort of 93 hips.
[e] Follow-up based on surviving 57 patients.
[f] Survivorship of allograft prosthetic construct at 10 years.

the area of proximal bone loss is selected.

- An oscillating saw is used to create the matching step cuts.
- Fresh-frozen allografts are preferred over fresh or freeze-dried allografts to provide adequate mechanical integrity of the graft while minimizing the risk of rejection. Often, the inner diameter of the host bone is larger than the inner diameter of the allograft, in which case press-fit stability of a long noncemented stem in the host bone is not feasible. A large allograft, typically from a male donor, allows use of a relatively large-diameter stem that fits inside both the allograft and distal host bone with press-fit distal stability (**Figure 4**).
- Fresh-frozen allografts typically are obtained from donors younger than 40 years because the cortical bone

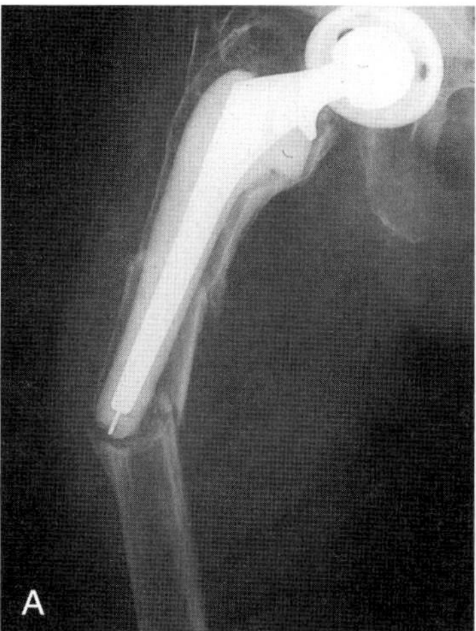

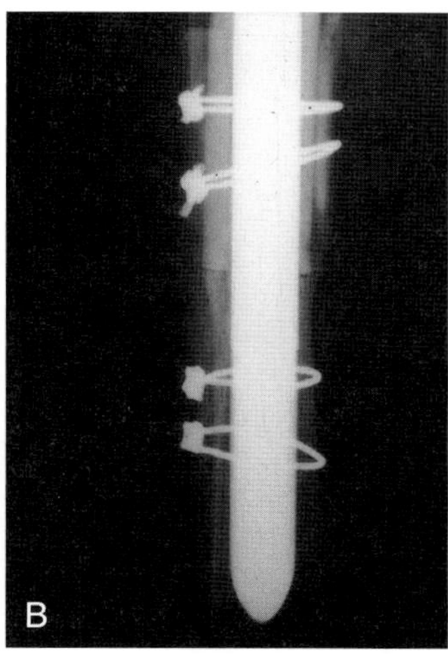

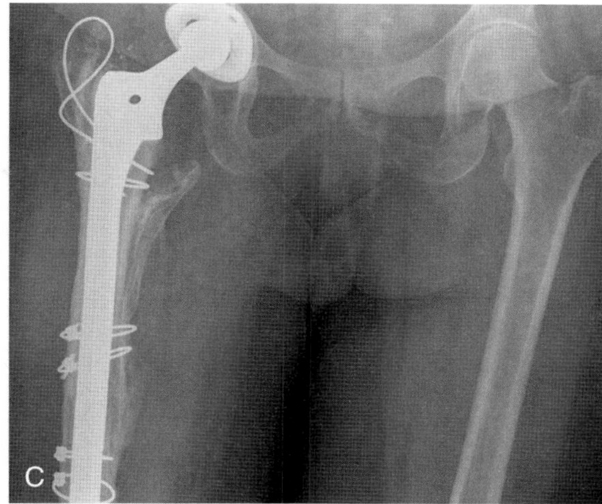

Figure 4 **A,** AP radiograph of the right hip from an 80-year-old woman with periprosthetic fracture around a loose cemented femoral stem and marked proximal femoral bone loss. **B,** AP femoral radiograph demonstrates reconstruction with an allograft prosthetic composite using a cylindrical, porous-coated long stem that was press fit into the distal host bone. The press-fit distal stem is seen extending into the intramedullary canal of the femur. **C,** AP pelvic radiograph obtained 2 years after reconstruction demonstrates that the allograft has united with the host bone, with evidence of bony remodeling. (Reproduced with permission from MacLachlan CE, Ries MD: Intramedullary step-cut osteotomy for revision total hip arthroplasty with allograft-host bone size mismatch. *J Arthroplasty* 2007;22[5]:657-662.)

is relatively thick and the inner diameter may be narrow.

- The proximal allograft can be prepared with broaches. However, a high-speed burr also is helpful to remove areas of dense bone and allow full seating of the stem into the allograft.
- A long-stem femoral implant that extends beyond the host-allograft junction into the distal host bone is used. Several implant lengths and diameters may be needed depending on the dimensions of the allograft and host bone as well as the location of the host-allograft junction. The location of the host-allograft junction and appropriate implant length to bypass the junction can be estimated based on preoperative radiographs. However, the inner diameters of the allograft and host bone are determined intraoperatively, so several implant diameters should be available.
- Modular implants provide more stem length and diameter options, and they help accommodate differences in the inner diameter between the allograft and host bone.
- A cortical allograft strut and cable plate should be available for use. Usually, one or both are needed to further stabilize the host-allograft junction.
- If the greater trochanter is viable and can be repaired to the proximal allograft, a trochanteric cable grip and cables will be needed.

Procedure

- On a back table, the interior of the allograft is reamed to accommodate the intramedullary revision stem.
- A clamp or vice can be helpful to secure the allograft to the back table during reaming because considerable torque may be generated when reaming into the hard distal allograft cortical bone.
- Sharp flexible and straight reamers usually are needed to expand the interior of the allograft.
- The interior of the allograft is overreamed to provide room for cement fixation of the prosthesis to the allograft and allow placement of a long stem that extends through the allograft.
- The acetabulum is reconstructed and the distal host bone transected or prepared with a step-cut osteotomy at a level appropriate to retain the maximum amount possible of viable, structurally intact, distal host bone.
- The minimum length of the APC is determined intraoperatively as the distance from the acetabular implant to the remaining distal host bone.
- If the inner diameters of the allograft and the distal host bone are reasonably close in size (within a few millimeters), the intramedullary stem can be press fit into the distal host bone for stability.
- Using an oscillating saw, matching step cuts are made on the proximal end of the remaining distal host bone and the distal allograft. The host bone step cut is prepared first, after which an initial matching step

cut is marked on the allograft with a pen to align with the host bone step cut. Care is taken to match the rotational alignment of the host bone and allograft so that the position of the proximal implant is aligned with the acetabular implant to minimize impingement during range of motion.

- An initial allograft distal step cut is made more distal than planned so that the APC is too long and cannot be reduced easily into the acetabular implant.
- A trial reduction is performed and soft-tissue tension is assessed to determine the amount of allograft shortening necessary to allow reduction of the hip.
- A second step cut is marked on the allograft to shorten it, and the trial reduction is repeated.
- After the appropriate length of allograft is determined, the distal allograft step cut is made to match the host bone step cut as closely as possible.
- If the inner diameter of the host bone is larger than the inner diameter of the allograft, then press-fit stability of a long noncemented stem in the host bone will not be feasible. In this case, a long step-cut osteotomy is made in the allograft and a transverse cut is made in the remaining distal host bone (**Figures 5** and **6**). A portion of the allograft step cut is inserted with the stem into the distal host bone for improved press-fit stability and a larger surface area for healing.
- The implant is cemented into the allograft on a back table.
- Antibiotic-impregnated cement is preferred because there will be a large nonvascularized APC in the wound.
- The cement is packed around the stem (with or without a cement gun), and the implant and cement are inserted together into the allograft.
- Excess cement is removed from the distal step cut to provide bone-to-bone contact at the host-allograft junction without cement interdigitation.
- After the cement has hardened, the APC is inserted into the distal host bone.
- If there is good press-fit stability of the distal stem into host bone, then cerclage cable fixation at the step-cut osteotomy may provide adequate stability and rotational control at the host-allograft junction. The addition of bone graft at the host-allograft junction should be considered to promote healing.
- Alternatively, a cable plate or allograft strut can be used to span the host-allograft junction for increased stability at the junction. If femoral hip and knee stems are in close proximity, reinforcing the host bone between the two stem tips (with an allograft strut or cable plate) at the time of APC reconstruction may help minimize the risk of periprosthetic fracture.
- Any bony remnants of the host proximal femur that have intact soft-tissue attachments should be applied to the outer surface of the allograft and secured with cables.

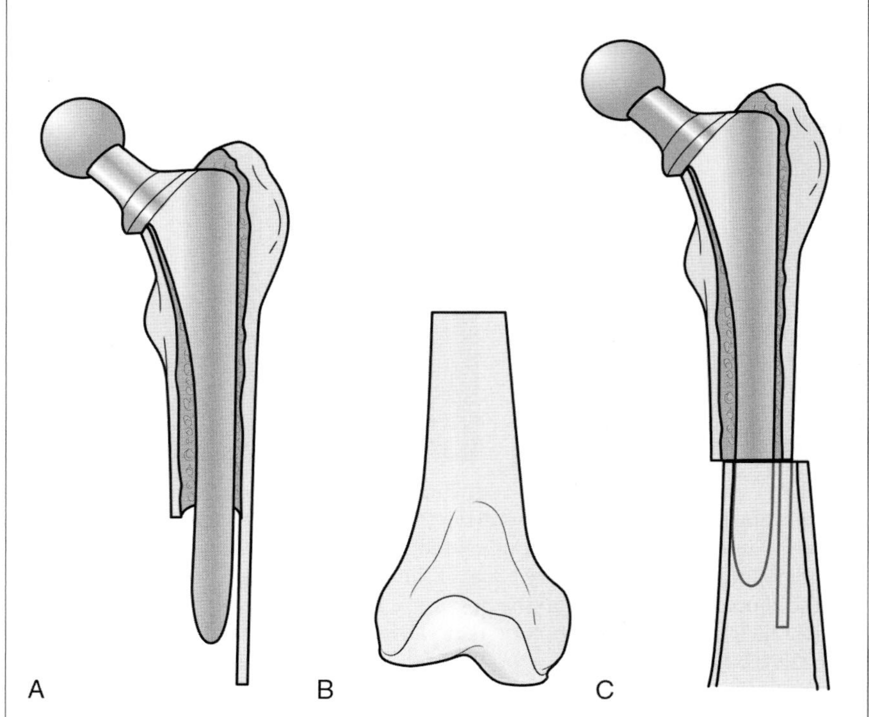

Figure 5 **A,** Illustration depicts an allograft prosthetic composite with a long distal step cut. **B,** Illustration depicts the transected host distal femur, which has a relatively wide inner diameter. **C,** Illustration depicts the allograft prosthetic composite inserted into the host bone. The long stem and the distal allograft cortical bone were press fit into the distal femoral canal.

Trochanteric Repair and Wound Closure

- The greater trochanter, if present and viable, can be attached to the allograft with cables or a cable grip. However, a high rate of trochanteric nonunion has been reported (**Table 1**); therefore, the viability and

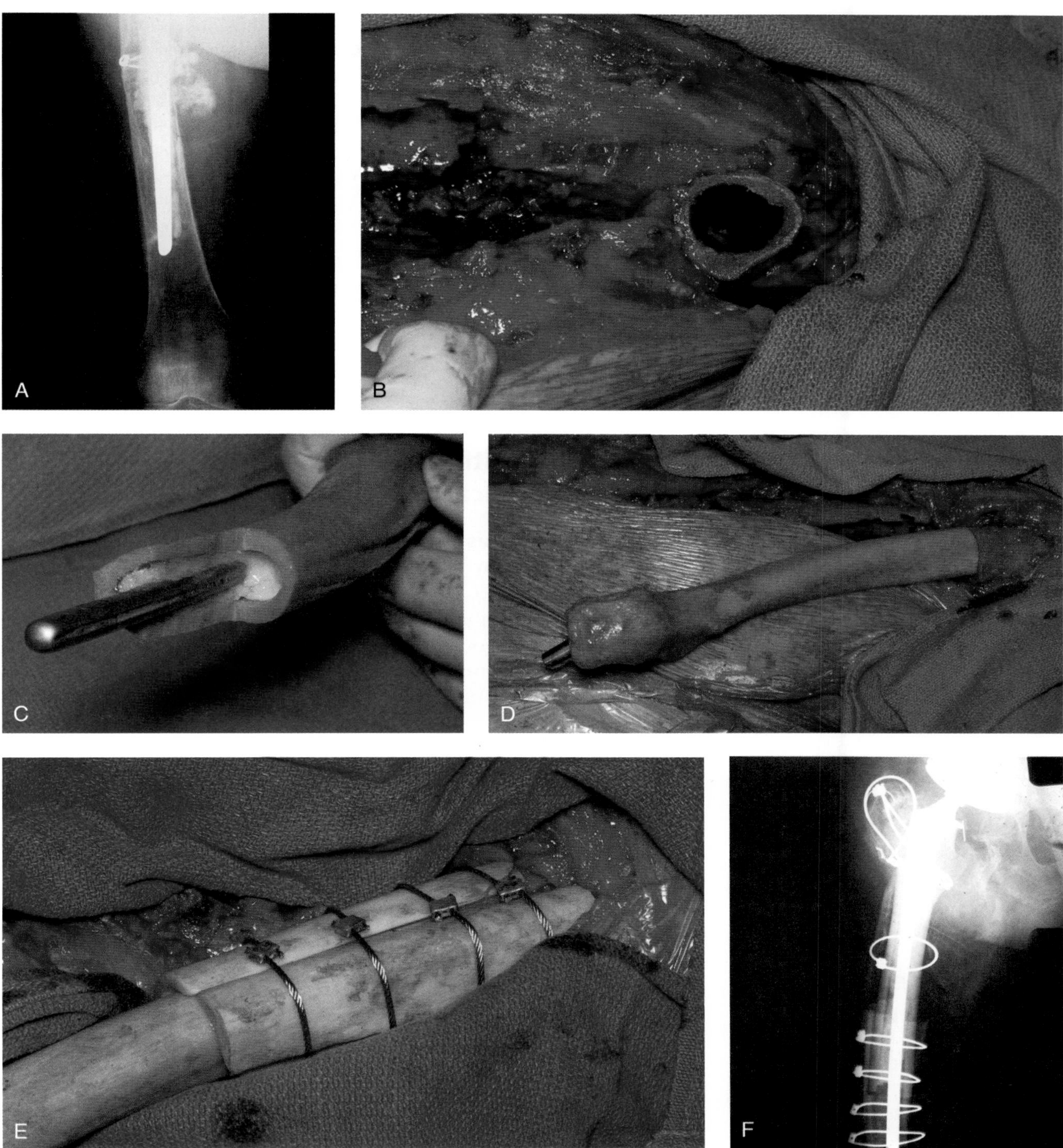

Figure 6 Images from a 64-year-old man who underwent femoral revision using allograft prosthetic composite (APC). **A,** AP radiograph of the right hip demonstrates a loose cemented femoral stem and segmental proximal bone loss to the mid-diaphysis of the femur. The patient has a relatively wide inner cortical diameter. **B,** Intraoperative photograph of the distal femur after transection just distal to the cement perforation shows the inner and outer cortical dimensions of the remaining host bone. **C,** Intraoperative photograph shows the distal allograft prepared with a distal step cut, with the long-stem revision femoral implant cemented into the APC. **D,** Intraoperative photograph shows the distal step cut of the APC press fit inside the host bone. **E,** Intraoperative photograph shows the addition of allograft struts and cerclage cables to further support the host-allograft junction. **F,** AP radiograph obtained 6 weeks postoperatively demonstrates overlap between the distal cortical bone of the allograft and host bone.

structural integrity of the trochanter should be carefully assessed to determine the feasibility of trochanteric union.

- If trochanteric reattachment is not feasible, the trochanter is thinned with a burr or excised.
- The soft-tissue sleeve of the abductors and vastus lateralis are sutured to the posterior capsule proximally and the intermuscular septum distally to cover as much of the allograft as possible with a deep layer of soft tissue.
- The fascial incision is repaired over a drain with nonabsorbable sutures. Because a large dead space usually is present between the fascia and APC, it may be necessary to leave the drain in place for several days to minimize the risk of hematoma formation.
- Intraoperative hemostasis can be augmented with tranexamic acid and techniques to ensure adequate coagulation of small vessels (such as management of muscle surfaces with a bipolar sealer). Subcutaneous closure is done in layers using absorbable sutures, and standard skin closure is performed. Negative-pressure wound therapy may help decrease edema in the superficial soft tissues and promote sealing of the skin incision.

Postoperative Regimen

The patient is restricted to toe-touch weight bearing on the affected limb for 6 weeks postoperatively, after which 50% weight bearing is allowed for the following 6 weeks. Weight-bearing activities can progress after radiographic evidence of healing is observed at the host-allograft junction.

Trochanteric precautions also should be followed, and active abduction and straight leg raising are avoided for 6 to 12 weeks postoperatively to protect the trochanteric or abductor muscle repair. A leg lifter device that supports the ipsilateral foot while getting in and out of bed also helps minimize active abduction activities.

The duration of postoperative antibiotic therapy to minimize infection risk in this patient population has not been clearly established. Postoperative intravenous antibiotic therapy for 2 weeks, followed by oral antibiotic therapy for 4 weeks, is used to maintain sterility of the dead space until soft-tissue healing has occurred.

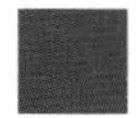

Avoiding Pitfalls and Complications

Deep Vein Thrombosis and Pulmonary Embolism

Typically, considerable soft-tissue dissection into the thigh is necessary during APC reconstruction. Postoperatively, the patient is considered to be at high risk for developing deep vein thrombosis or pulmonary embolism and should receive pharmacologic prophylaxis with adjusted-dose warfarin, low-molecular-weight heparin, or other similar agents. Use of aspirin combined with mechanical compression devices may not be adequate in this patient population.

Postoperative Hematoma and Infection

The presence of a proximal femoral allograft without soft-tissue attachments creates a potentially large dead space in the wound. The APC is in close proximity to muscle that may have a large surface area that can be a source of bleeding. The dead space can fill with blood, resulting in hematoma and possibly infection. Bleeding is an inherent risk, particularly because postoperative pharmacologic thromboembolic prophylaxis is indicated in patients undergoing APC.

If wound drainage persists resulting from hematoma, seroma, or infection, prompt aggressive management with irrigation and débridement is indicated in an effort to salvage the APC and avoid the development of chronic deep infection. Intravenous antibiotics for 6 weeks after irrigation and débridement also may be considered to manage suspected or confirmed bacterial contamination of a postoperative hematoma or seroma.

Deep infection of the APC that occurs either after failed postoperative irrigation and débridement with retention of the APC or as a result of late postoperative or hematogenous infection requires removal of the APC. The resulting bone defect can be managed with a large antibiotic cement spacer, followed by a course of antimicrobial therapy and delayed second-stage revision surgery. Although delayed two-stage reconstruction for management of an infected APC with another APC or proximal femoral replacement can be successful, the rate of successful salvage of a two-stage débridement and reimplantation of an infected APC is unknown and likely is considerably lower than the reported success rate of two-stage management of an infected primary THA.

Dislocation

The risk of dislocation after APC reconstruction is relatively high because proximal soft-tissue attachments to the APC are limited and abductor deficiency is common. Depending on the integrity of the abductors, a large-diameter femoral head or constrained liner should be considered to adequately stabilize the hip. Abduction bracing may be beneficial postoperatively to reduce the risk of instability. The need for an abduction brace or its relative benefit may depend on many factors, including the integrity of the abductor mechanism, femoral head size, intraoperative stability, patient compliance, and history of instability.

If postoperative dislocation occurs, then closed reduction with sedation or anesthesia is necessary. If recurrent dislocation develops, then surgery is necessary to correct any mechanical factors contributing to instability or for conversion to a constrained acetabular implant.

Neurovascular Injury

Injury to the sciatic or femoral nerve can occur from compression during acetabular retraction. Neurologic injury also may result from stretching caused by limb lengthening. Footdrop is a common manifestation of sciatic nerve injury; this weakness can be managed with an ankle-foot orthosis. Motor and sensory recovery often is slow and incomplete. Neurogenic pain, which is managed primarily with neuroleptic medications, is a poor prognostic indicator for recovery.

Nonunion

Lack of radiographic healing at the host-allograft junction can lead to fixation failure at or near the host-allograft junction. Nonunion, particularly painful nonunion, also can occur because of instability at the host-allograft junction, which may be difficult to detect clinically and radiographically. If secondary bone grafting of the nonunion site is planned and motion is detected intraoperatively at the host-allograft junction, then revision of the APC or additional fixation at the host-allograft junction is indicated, so appropriate implants and allograft materials should be available for surgery.

Periprosthetic Fracture

Periprosthetic fracture after APC reconstruction usually occurs at or near the stem tip and generally is associated with minor trauma. Risk factors for periprosthetic fracture include osteopenia, prior cortical screw holes, and, in patients with poor cognitive function or balance, an increased risk of falling. If a total knee femoral stem is present, the area between the distal end of the hip femoral implant and the proximal end of the femoral knee implant creates an area of stress concentration in the host bone, which can lead to fracture.

Limb-Length Inequality

Because proximal femoral bony landmarks are lacking in APC reconstruction, the selection of femoral allograft length is based primarily on the intraoperative assessment of soft-tissue tension, which may vary markedly. Clinical and radiographic evaluation of limb-length inequality preoperatively may help determine the degree of soft-tissue tension that is considered appropriate during trial and final reduction of the implants intraoperatively. Patients also should be counseled that some degree of limb-length inequality may exist postoperatively.

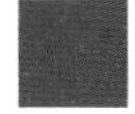

Bibliography

Babis GC, Sakellariou VI, O'Connor MI, Hanssen AD, Sim FH: Proximal femoral allograft-prosthesis composites in revision hip replacement: A 12-year follow-up study. *J Bone Joint Surg Br* 2010;92(3):349-355.

Blackley HR, Davis AM, Hutchison CR, Gross AE: Proximal femoral allografts for reconstruction of bone stock in revision arthroplasty of the hip: A nine to fifteen-year follow-up. *J Bone Joint Surg Am* 2001;83(3):346-354.

Graham NM, Stockley I: The use of structural proximal femoral allografts in complex revision hip arthroplasty. *J Bone Joint Surg Br* 2004;86(3):337-343.

Lakstein D, Eliaz N, Levi O, et al: Fracture of cementless femoral stems at the mid-stem junction in modular revision hip arthroplasty systems. *J Bone Joint Surg Am* 2011;93(1):57-65.

Lee SH, Ahn YJ, Chung SJ, Kim BK, Hwang JH: The use of allograft prosthetic composite for extensive proximal femoral bone deficiencies: A 2- to 9.8-year follow-up study. *J Arthroplasty* 2009;24(8):1241-1248.

MacLachlan CE, Ries MD: Intramedullary step-cut osteotomy for revision total hip arthroplasty with allograft-host bone size mismatch. *J Arthroplasty* 2007;22(5):657-662.

Parvizi J, Tarity TD, Slenker N, et al: Proximal femoral replacement in patients with non-neoplastic conditions. *J Bone Joint Surg Am* 2007;89(5):1036-1043.

Ries MD, Gomez MA, Eckhoff DG, Lewis DA, Brodie MR, Wiedel JD: An in vitro study of proximal femoral allograft strains in revision hip arthroplasty. *Med Eng Phys* 1994;16(4):292-296.

Safir O, Kellett CF, Flint M, Backstein D, Gross AE: Revision of the deficient proximal femur with a proximal femoral allograft. *Clin Orthop Relat Res* 2009;467(1):206-212.

Schmalzried TP, Noordin S, Amstutz HC: Update on nerve palsy associated with total hip replacement. *Clin Orthop Relat Res* 1997;(344):188-206.

Sternheim A, Drexler M, Kuzyk PR, Safir OA, Backstein DJ, Gross AE: Treatment of failed allograft prosthesis composites used for hip arthroplasty in the setting of severe proximal femoral bone defects. *J Arthroplasty* 2014;29(5):1058-1062.

Vastel L, Lemoine CT, Kerboull M, Courpied JP: Structural allograft and cemented long-stem prosthesis for complex revision hip arthroplasty: Use of a trochanteric claw plate improves final hip function. *Int Orthop* 2007;31(6):851-857.

Wang JW, Wang CJ: Proximal femoral allografts for bone deficiencies in revision hip arthroplasty: A medium-term follow-up study. *J Arthroplasty* 2004;19(7):845-852.

Video Reference

Ries MD: Video. *Femoral Revision With Allograft Prosthetic Composite*. Reno, NV, 2015.

Chapter 63
Conversion of Failed Hemiarthroplasty to Total Hip Arthroplasty

Michael Tanzer, MD, FRCSC
Dylan Tanzer, BSc

 Indications

Hemiarthroplasty of the hip is performed primarily for the management of femoral neck fractures. The implant can have a unipolar monoblock design or a modular femoral head-neck junction. A unipolar monoblock hemiarthroplasty implant, such as an Austin Moore or Thompson prosthesis, involves the use of a prosthetic femoral stem with a large, fixed head that replaces the natural femoral head. A hemiarthroplasty implant with a modular junction allows the use of either a unipolar or bipolar head. A unipolar modular hemiarthroplasty prosthesis has a femoral stem with an exchangeable large head that replaces the natural femoral head. A bipolar modular hemiarthroplasty involves the use of a femoral stem and standard head prosthesis that articulates with a mobile component that replaces the natural femoral head. Only the Australian and Swedish national joint registries specifically analyze the use of hemiarthroplasties. In the 2014 annual report of the Australian Orthopaedic Association National Joint Replacement Registry, the most common class of primary partial hip arthroplasty was the unipolar modular hemiarthroplasty, which accounted for 39.7% of all partial hip arthroplasty procedures. However, the registry report showed that the popularity of bipolar prostheses was increasing, whereas the use of unipolar hemiarthroplasty was starting to decrease. Unipolar monoblock prostheses were used mostly in patients 85 years and older. In the Swedish Hip Arthroplasty Register, the implant used for the management of a hip fracture was a unipolar hemiarthroplasty implant in 38% of procedures, a bipolar hemiarthroplasty implant in 34% of procedures, and a monoblock hemiarthroplasty implant in only 4% of the 45,362 procedures performed between 2005 and 2012.

Like any hip arthroplasty, hemiarthroplasties can fail and necessitate revision surgery. Failure rates primarily depend on the implant design and patient age. At 10 years after surgical management of a hip fracture, bipolar hemiarthroplasties have the lowest cumulative revision rate at 6.3%, followed by unipolar modular hemiarthroplasties at 9.6% and unipolar monoblock hemiarthroplasties at 8.4%.The failure rate is higher in patients younger than 75 years, with cumulative revision rates of 16.2%, 16.1%, and 9.4% for unipolar monoblock, unipolar modular, and bipolar implants, respectively.

The implant design of a failed hemiarthroplasty affects the options for revision arthroplasty. Failed unipolar monoblock implants always require revision of the stem, irrespective of the cause for revision, whereas failed unipolar or bipolar modular hemiarthroplasties can be managed with an isolated femoral head and acetabular revision, or revision of both the stem and the acetabulum. With any implant, failure of hemiarthroplasty is most commonly managed with conversion to total hip arthroplasty (THA). Conversion is most commonly performed for the management of chondrolysis with acetabular erosion, dislocation, fracture, infection, loosening and/or osteolysis, malposition, and pain. The relative incidence of the reasons for revision varies with hemiarthroplasty type (**Table 1**).

Preoperative assessment of a failed hemiarthroplasty is similar to the workup for a failed THA and should include evaluation for aseptic loosening and sepsis. A detailed history and physical examination, routine blood tests, careful review of the radiographs, and, if necessary, hip aspiration should be performed before revision surgery.

Dr. Michael Tanzer or an immediate family member serves as a paid consultant to Pipeline Biotechnology and Zimmer Biomet; has received research or institutional support from Johnson & Johnson and Zimmer Biomet; has received nonincome support (such as equipment or services), commercially derived honoraria, or other non–research-related funding (such as paid travel) from Zimmer Biomet; and serves as a board member, owner, officer, or committee member of the Hip Society. Mr. Dylan Tanzer has not received anything of value from and does not have stock or stock options held in a commercial company or institution related directly or indirectly to the subject of this chapter.

Table 1 Incidence of Indications for Revision by Type of Hemiarthroplasty

Reason for Revision	Unipolar Monoblock Hemiarthroplasty	Unipolar Modular Hemiarthroplasty	Bipolar Modular Hemiarthroplasty
Chondrolysis/acetabular erosion	3.9%	12.7%	7.7%
Dislocation	11.4%	19.9%	17.9%
Fracture	18.9%	15.5%	23.5%
Infection	9.6%	19.1%	18.6%
Loosening/lysis	46.7%	16.0%	20.5%
Malposition	1.0%	0.2%	0.4%
Pain	7.2%	12.7%	8.1%
Other	1.5%	3.9%	3.4%

Hemiarthroplasty is sometimes performed in younger patients, and over time, substantial bone loss may occur in association with the implant. A patient who has undergone hemiarthroplasty with a bipolar articulation is at risk for polyethylene wear and secondary osteolysis (**Figure 1**). Serial radiographs are important in determining the need for and timing of revision surgery in patients with asymptomatic osteolysis.

Pain secondary to acetabular erosion is common in patients with a hemiarthroplasty with a unipolar large-diameter femoral head and may be a cause for concern. In one study, researchers described the occurrence of severe metal-induced osteolysis and soft-tissue damage secondary to trunnion damage in two asymptomatic patients with contemporary endoprostheses and a unipolar head without an adaptor sleeve. In these two patients, trunnion damage occurred 10 and 13 years postoperatively and resulted in a severe reaction to metal debris with acetabular osteolysis, erosion of the greater trochanter, and loss of the abductor mechanism. The study authors noted that although erosion of the acetabulum with medial migration of a unipolar head is not uncommon in long-term follow-up after a hemiarthroplasty, the radiographic finding of superior migration of the implant and erosion of the greater trochanter should increase suspicion of trunnionosis. These radiographic changes may indicate the need for a complex revision with removal of a well-fixed stem and placement of a constrained liner or dual-mobility cup to manage the abductor deficiency rather

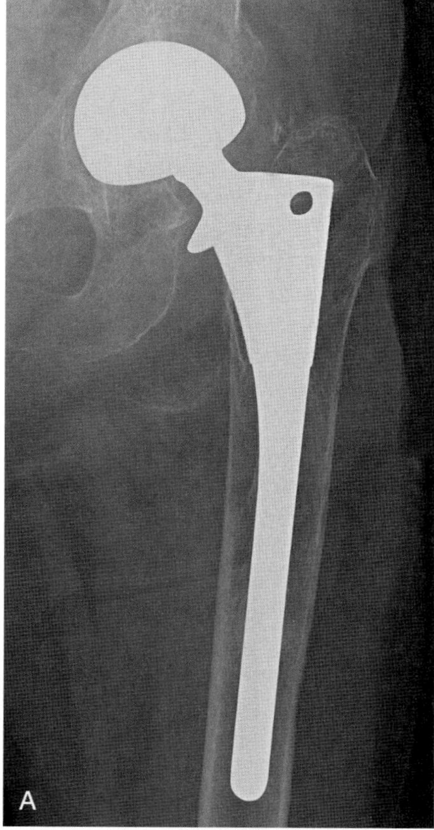

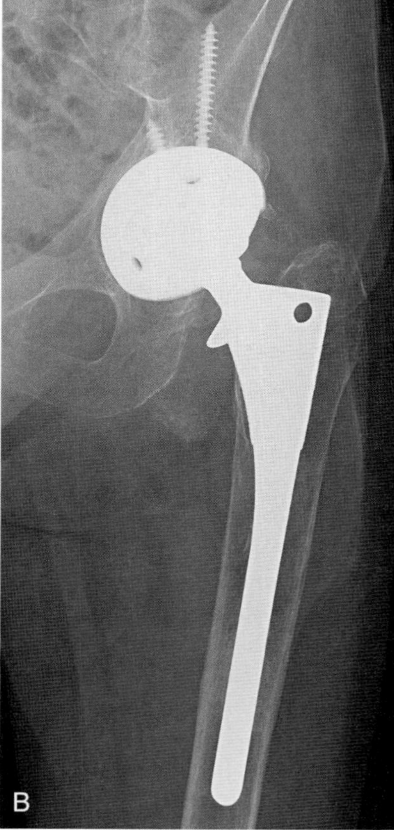

Figure 1 **A,** Preoperative AP radiograph of a left hip demonstrates a failed bipolar hemiarthroplasty in an 89-year-old woman. The patient has acetabular cartilage loss and bone loss with early acetabular osteolysis. The proximally porous-coated stem is not loose. The patient also has marked osteopenia of the proximal femur. **B,** AP radiograph obtained 2 years after an uncomplicated revision demonstrates a porous-coated acetabular implant with screws and a 36-mm femoral head.

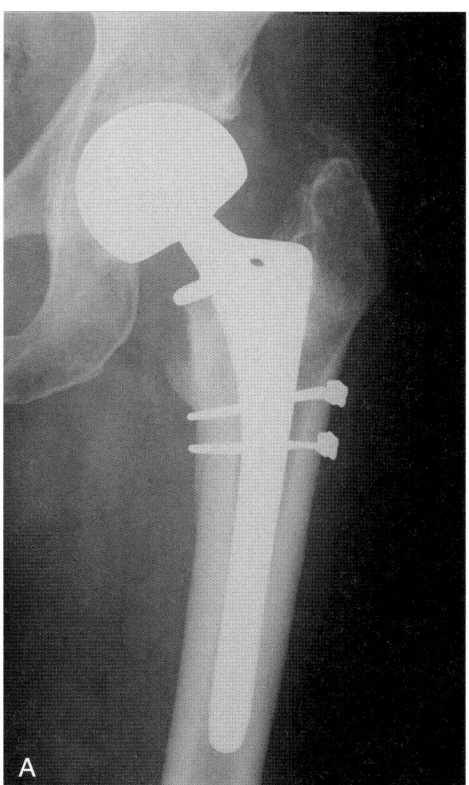

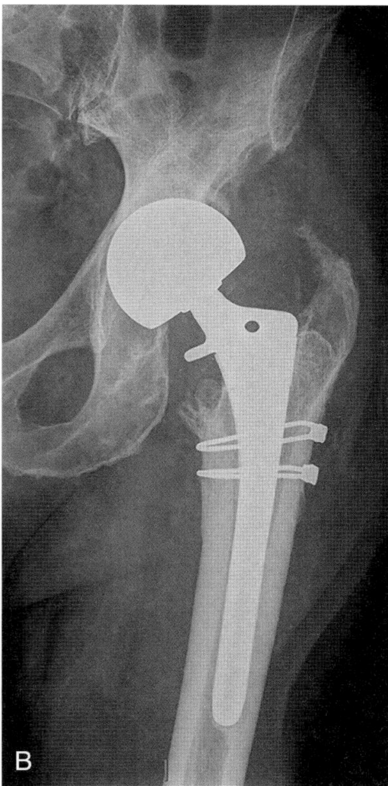

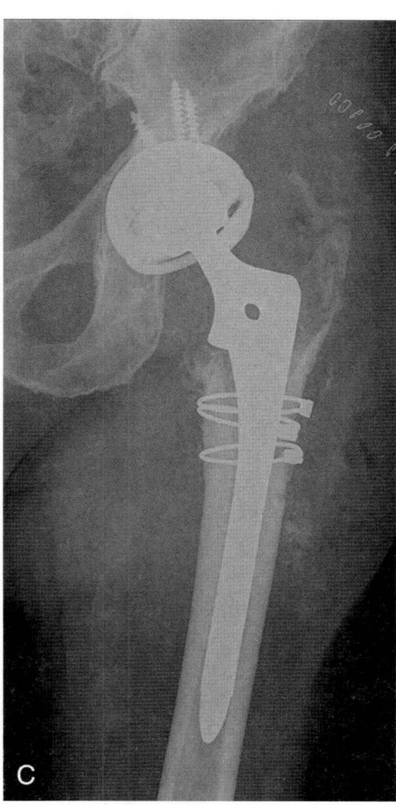

Figure 2 **A,** AP radiograph of a left hip demonstrates hemiarthroplasty with a unipolar head for the management of posttraumatic osteonecrosis. Cerclage wires were placed for the management of a nondisplaced calcar split. **B,** AP radiograph obtained before revision surgery demonstrates medial and superior migration of the unipolar head, osteolysis of the medial calcar, and thinning of the greater trochanter. **C,** AP radiograph obtained after complex revision surgery for the management of severe metallosis and osteolysis secondary to trunnionosis. The ingrown noncemented stem was removed via extended trochanteric osteotomy. The abductors were found to be severely compromised by the metallosis. Reconstruction was performed with the use of a long, extensively porous-coated calcar replacement stem and a porous-coated acetabular implant with screws and a constrained liner.

than merely placement of an acetabular cup and exchange of the femoral head (**Figure 2**). Additionally, two published case reports have described aggressive reactions to metal debris occurring in association with hemiarthroplasty with a unipolar head and a taper sleeve. In both patients, osteolysis and a pseudotumor developed as a reaction to the metal debris from the modular junction of the hemiarthroplasty. Unlike the long-term findings of the study mentioned previously, in which the patients did not have a taper sleeve between the unipolar head and the trunnion, these patients had symptoms only 2 years after the hemiarthroplasty. At the time of revision, the radiographs demonstrated focal acetabular osteolysis in one patient and more diffuse osteolysis with superior and medial migration of the head in the other patient. In both patients, the damage from the metal debris was limited to the acetabulum.

Early recognition and management of radiographic changes that elicit concern are required to avoid a potentially complex revision. The surgeon must have a high index of suspicion for associated bone and soft-tissue destruction when osteolytic changes are observed around modular stems with unipolar heads, or heads with a taper sleeve. Late recognition of osteolysis in these patients can necessitate extensive revision surgery with removal of a well-fixed stem and possibly the need for a constrained acetabular liner (**Figure 3**). Osteolysis secondary to wear of a bipolar articulation should be managed in a manner similar to a failing primary THA. Conversion must be performed before the patient sustains extensive bone loss that would compromise the outcome of the procedure.

The preoperative workup should indicate whether only the acetabulum needs to be reconstructed or whether both the stem and the acetabulum should be revised. After the underlying etiology of the patient's pain and/or radiographic failure is established, revision surgery can be planned. The strategies for revision of a failed hemiarthroplasty depend on the underlying reason for revision, the implant being revised, the patient's age and comorbidities, and the degree of host bone damage or loss. These strategies are generally the same as those used for revision of a failed THA. Reconstructive strategies can include acetabular reconstruction with or without bone graft, removal of a loose or well-fixed noncemented or cemented femoral implant, trochanteric osteotomy, femoral reconstruction with or without bone graft, repair of trunnion damage, and the potential use of large-diameter femoral heads or dual-mobility cups to manage recurrent dislocation.

Contraindications

In the unusual circumstance that the patient is too ill to undergo revision surgery or the patient has an infection of the implant that has not responded to appropriate management, the surgeon can consider leaving the hemiarthroplasty in place and providing supportive medical treatment or performing resection arthroplasty.

Alternative Treatments

There are no alternative treatments.

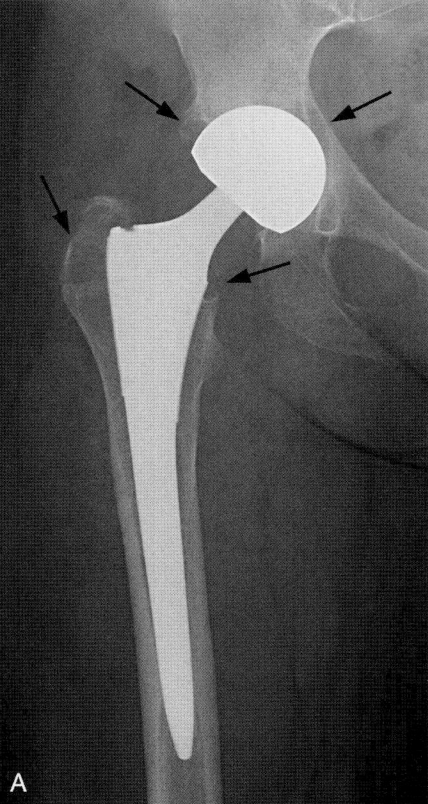

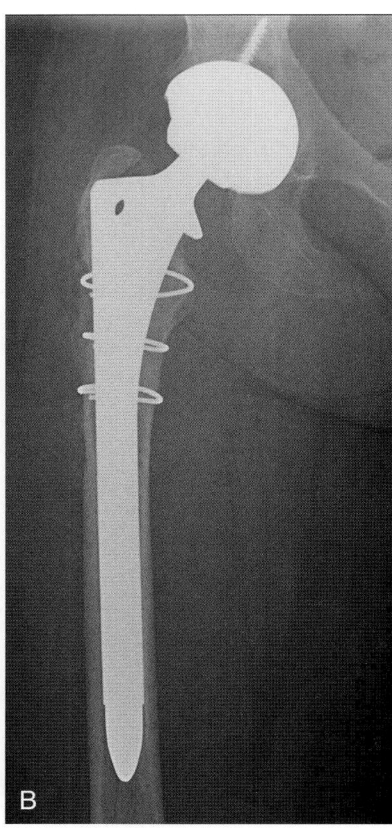

Figure 3 **A,** AP radiograph of a right hip demonstrates a proximally porous-coated stem with a unipolar head. The head has migrated medially through the ilioischial line. Osteolysis in the acetabulum, femoral calcar, and greater trochanter is evident (arrows). **B,** AP radiograph obtained 3 months after complex revision in which notable metallosis from the taper sleeve connecting the stem to the unipolar head was found. The sleeve was fixed to the trunnion and could not be removed. The ingrown noncemented stem was removed via extended trochanteric osteotomy. The hip was reconstructed with a porous noncemented cup with screws, a 36-mm femoral head, and a long, fully porous stem.

Results

Survivorship

The reported success rates of the conversion of a failed hemiarthroplasty depend on patient characteristics, the type of hemiarthroplasty being revised, the failure mechanism, whether the stem is revised, the revision implants used, and the length of follow-up. The long-term follow-up of converted hemiarthroplasties is limited considering that the Austin Moore prosthesis, in its present design, has been used since the late 1950s. Furthermore, many of these conversion studies have used revision THA principles that are now outdated. Nonetheless, the reported overall survivorship after conversion of a failed hemiarthroplasty is 80% to 100% at 2.7 to 7.4 years postoperatively (**Table 2**). Two more recent studies, in which modern techniques and implants were used, demonstrated 96% and 97% survivorship rates at a mean 7.2- and 6.4-year follow-up, respectively. No long-term studies have analyzed the outcomes of conversion of failed hemiarthroplasties.

Registry Results

Specific studies on the conversion of hemiarthroplasty to THA provide information on the results for an individual surgeon or institution. Although this type of study has the advantage of affording the opportunity to analyze numerous variables, the results may not be indicative of those of a larger number of procedures done by numerous surgeons. Registry data reflect information collected on a high volume of procedures, allowing markedly more accurate and valid evaluations of the outcomes of the procedure.

Table 2 Survivorship, Clinical Results, and Complications of Conversion of Hemiarthroplasty to Total Hip Arthroplasty (THA)

Authors (Year)	Number of Patients	Mean Patient Age in Years (Range)	Mean Follow-up in Years (Range)	Failure Rate (%)[a]	Results
Amstutz and Smith (1979)	41	63 (18-80)	3 (NR)	15	24% complication rate
Llinas et al (1991)	99	63 (NR)	7.4 (0.1-20)	6	Cemented acetabular implants of converted hemiarthroplasties had better radiologic survival rates than those in primary THA
Sharkey et al (1998)	45	65 (32-85)	2.9 (2-6.6)	4	Mean HHS improved from 37 to 87
Warwick et al (1998)	56	75 (45-90)	NR	7	48% complication rate
Bilgen et al (2000)	15	59 (30-75)	2.7 (1-4.5)	0	Mean HHS improved from 36 to 86
Sierra and Cabanela (2002)	132	73 (NR)	7.1 (5.1-15.3)	13	45% complication rate
Hammad and Abdel-Aal (2006)	47	64 (54-83)	3.7 (2.3-7)	0	Mean HHS improved from 41 to 86 6% complication rate
Diwanji et al (2008)	25	59 (25-82)	7.2 (3-16)	4	Mean HHS improved from 41 to 85 25% complication rate
Pankaj et al (2008)	44	62 (42-75)	6.4 (2-9)	2	Mean HHS improved from 38 to 86 23% complication rate

HHS = Harris hip score, NR = not reported.

[a] Failure is defined as definitive radiographic evidence of implant loosening or revision surgery for any reason.

The authors of one study identified 595 hips in the Norwegian Arthroplasty Register in which conversion to THA was performed between 1987 and 2004 for a failed hemiarthroplasty after femoral neck fracture. In 473 hips, the revision included exchange of the femoral stem, whereas in the remaining 122 hips, the femoral stem was not revised. Overall, the hips in which conversion to THA was performed with stem exchange had a significantly lower risk of failure (revision surgery for any reason) than did the hips in which conversion was performed with retention of the femoral stem (relative risk, 0.4). For the 473 conversion procedures in which the stem was revised, at a mean follow-up of 5.8 years there was no difference in the risk of failure compared with all revisions of stems in the registry, either for the complete prosthesis or the stem alone (relative risks, 0.8 and 0.9, respectively). However, in the 122 hips in which an acetabular implant was placed but the stem was retained, the authors of the study found a significantly increased risk of failure of both the acetabular cup and the complete prosthesis (relative risks, 4.8 and 4.6, respectively) at a mean follow-up of 3.6 years compared with the results of primary THA. The median time from the conversion procedure to the next revision was 3.6 years in the group with stem exchange and only 0.5 years in the group with retention of the femoral stem. The marked difference in the time intervals likely results from the predominant cause of revision, which was stem loosening in the group with stem exchange and dislocation in the group with stem retention. The results of the study suggest that converting a failed hemiarthroplasty to THA by implanting an acetabular cup may be more complex than previously thought.

Clinical Results

The clinical outcomes after conversion of a failed hemiarthroplasty to THA have generally been positive. Published studies demonstrate substantial improvements in Harris hip scores from a range of 36 to 41 preoperatively to a range of 85 to 87 postoperatively (**Table 2**). However, in the elimination of groin pain, the results of conversion surgery have been variable. The authors of one study found that groin or buttock pain was completely relieved in 80% of their patients and partially relieved in another 9% of patients. The 20% of patients in whom pain was not completely relieved continued to have groin or buttock pain, but no factor that would predict this outcome was identified. Similarly, the authors of a different study found that all patients treated surgically for groin pain reported significant improvement in their symptoms (the average preoperative Western Ontario and McMaster Universities Osteoarthritis Index improved from 16 preoperatively to 3 postoperatively on a 20-point scale; $P < 0.05$), but not all patients were pain free postoperatively.

Complications

Although the midterm survivorship and clinical results of conversion of failed hemiarthroplasty to THA are reasonable, the conversion procedure is associated with considerable intraoperative difficulties and postoperative complications. Complication rates of 6% to 48% have been reported for conversion of failed hemiarthroplasties, and in many studies, the complication rates are greater than 20% (**Table 2**). Complications most commonly include dislocation and fracture or perforation, and less frequently infection, trochanteric complications, and sciatic nerve injuries.

The authors of several studies have commented on the dislocation rate after conversion of a failed hemiarthroplasty to THA. However, only two studies have specifically addressed the rate of dislocation after conversion of a failed hemiarthroplasty to THA, and in both studies the dislocation rate was alarmingly high. The authors of one study reported on a series of nine elderly patients (mean age, 80 years [range, 62-87 years]) who underwent conversion of a hemiarthroplasty to THA. The revisions were performed through a Hardinge approach, an acetabular implant with a 28-mm articulation was used in all patients, and the stem was revised in all but one patient. Overall, four of the revised prostheses subsequently dislocated, for a dislocation rate of 50%. The authors of the study concluded that this group of patients should be treated differently from those who undergo other hip arthroplasties and that the capsule or pseudocapsule should be preserved whenever possible.

The authors of a study specifically comparing the dislocation rate after revision surgery for a failed hemiarthroplasty with that of revision surgery for a failed THA found that conversion of a failed hemiarthroplasty to THA was associated with a higher rate of dislocation than was revision of a failed THA. They reviewed 89 hemiarthroplasties that were converted to THA in 77 patients and compared the dislocation rate with that of 115 first-time revision THAs. Overall, significantly more dislocations occurred after the hemiarthroplasty conversion procedures than after the revision THA procedures (22% and 10%, respectively; $P < 0.018$). The acetabulum-only revisions and the revisions of both the acetabulum and the femoral implant were associated with similar dislocation rates. Additionally, the dislocation rates were the same for the modular and nonmodular femoral stems in both the conversion group and the THA revision group. The increased dislocation rate was thought to be related primarily to the compromised soft-tissue envelope, which is a particularly important risk factor for instability, and the substantial reduction of the femoral head size when revising a failed hemiarthroplasty to THA. The authors of the study concluded that at the time of conversion, the dislocation risk should be addressed with an emphasis on restoring the soft-tissue envelope, and a larger femoral head should be used to minimize downsizing of the femoral head. Currently, dual-mobility cups can be used to minimize the risk of postoperative dislocation in older patients.

Techniques

Setup/Exposure

- As in all hip revisions, preoperative templating is critical in identifying potential intraoperative difficulties and determining the appropriate surgical approach and implants required for successful reconstruction of a failed hemiarthroplasty.
- The surgical approach used to revise the hemiarthroplasty depends on the surgeon's preference, any previous incisions, and the exposure and reconstructive strategies required.
- In patients with a well-fixed stem, a trochanteric osteotomy is occasionally necessary to obtain adequate acetabular exposure or, in patients with recurrent dislocation, to adjust the soft-tissue tension of the abductors by advancing the trochanter.
- An extended trochanteric osteotomy (ETO) may be necessary in patients who have a well-fixed cemented or noncemented stem that needs to be removed, femoral cement that needs to be removed around a loose stem, or loosening of the femoral implant with varus remodeling of the proximal femur.
- An ETO also improves visualization of the acetabulum, and this factor may be accounted for in the intraoperative decision whether to perform an ETO.
- The technique for the ETO is the same as that used in a standard revision THA. The length of the osteotomy depends on the length of the medullary canal that needs to be exposed for the revision.
- The surgeon should consider placing a cerclage wire just distal to the ETO to minimize the risk of fracture in an osteoporotic femur.

Instruments/Equipment/ Implants Required

- As in all hip revision procedures, the surgeon must have all the necessary acetabular and femoral implants as well as revision instrumentation available to reconstruct the failed arthroplasty based on the preoperative planning.
- Because substantial intraoperative complications can occur, it is prudent to have revision implants, bone graft, and fracture fixation devices available.

Procedure

ACETABULAR RECONSTRUCTION

- Acetabular reconstruction typically is straightforward and should be performed using the same principles and techniques used in a primary THA procedure (**Figure 4**).
- However, in elderly patients, the acetabulum may be osteoporotic, and careful reaming is essential to avoid perforation or excessive removal of the acetabular bone stock.
- In some patients, the large femoral head articulating on the native acetabulum not only wears away the articular cartilage but also causes substantial acetabular bony erosion and protrusion. In these patients, the surgeon must decide whether the acetabular implant should be placed in the medial defect or reconstructed in its anatomic location. The reconstructive choice depends on the degree of erosion as well as the patient's age and functional status.
- In elderly patients with limited function, the acetabular implant may be placed in a nonanatomic, medialized position. If a noncemented acetabular implant is used, this method allows complete contact of the porous coating of the implant with the patient's host bone, thereby enhancing the probability of bone ingrowth. In these patients, the use of an offset liner may be necessary to place the femoral stem more laterally to avoid impingement of the femoral neck on the bony rim of the acetabulum.
- In younger and more active patients, placement of the acetabular implant in a more anatomic position is preferable. When a noncemented acetabular implant is used, the acetabulum should be underreamed so that the cup is inserted with press-fit fixation and is seated along the rim of the bony acetabulum. Care should be taken not to create a too-tight press fit, which can result in intraoperative fracture of an osteoporotic acetabulum. The medial defect between the acetabular floor and the cup should be filled with morcellized bone graft.
- Adjuvant screw fixation should be considered in patients in whom the bone quality is of concern.
- If a cemented cup is chosen for the reconstruction, the sclerotic acetabular subchondral bone must be addressed to obtain pressurization of the cement into the underlying host bone and an optimal bone-cement interface.

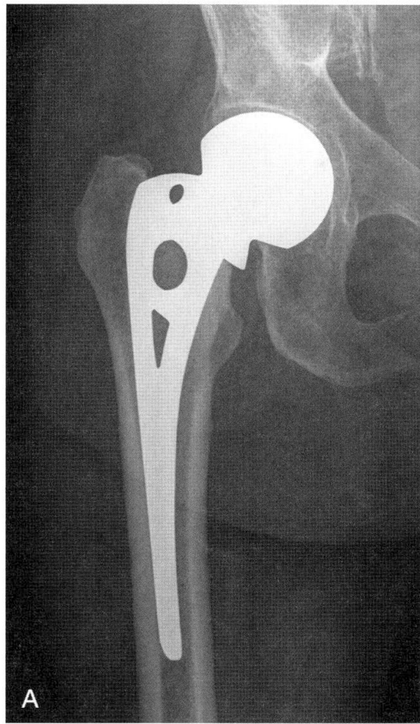

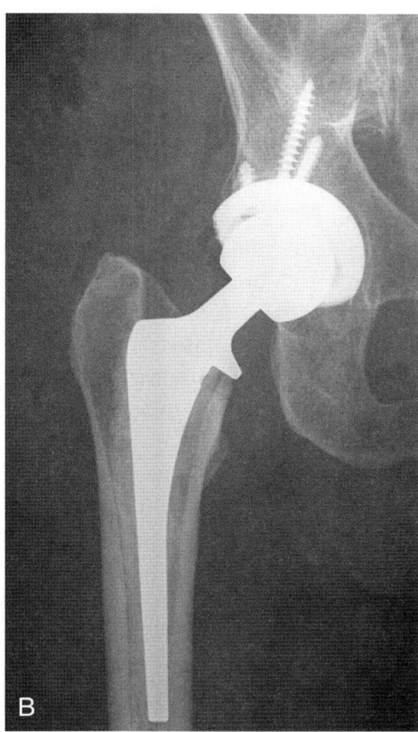

Figure 4 **A,** AP radiograph of a right hip demonstrates a failed monoblock Austin Moore prosthesis in a 73-year-old woman. Cartilage erosion is present, but the underlying acetabular bone is not eroded. **B,** AP radiograph demonstrates the hip after uncomplicated conversion to a hybrid total hip arthroplasty using primary hip arthroplasty implants.

FEMORAL REVISION

- Revision of the femoral stem is not always required during conversion of a failed hemiarthroplasty to THA. Stems that are well fixed, are in proper version, have appropriate offset, and have a modular neck allowing the limb length and soft-tissue balance to be restored can be retained (**Figure 1**).

- In these patients, exposure of the acetabulum usually can be obtained by removing the modular femoral unipolar or bipolar head, covering the trunnion to protect it from being scratched or damaged, and creating a so-called pocket by elevating the superior hip capsule from the bony pelvis and retracting the femoral neck-stem junction over the rim of the acetabulum so that the trunnion sits in the pocket, thereby allowing full access to the acetabulum.
- If the femoral stem needs to be removed, the same principles, strategies, techniques, reconstruction options, and implants that are used in a THA revision procedure should be used.
- A failed hemiarthroplasty in which the stem needs to be revised most commonly involves a loose noncemented femoral implant. Although the stem is loose, it is not always easily extracted without damaging or breaking the femur, especially in elderly patients. When a loose noncemented stem with a collar subsides, the collar frequently settles into the proximal femur and is enveloped by the patient's host bone. Similarly, the lateral aspect of the proximal portion of the femoral stem is commonly embedded into the greater trochanter.
- In these patients, even when the implant is grossly loose, the surgeon should avoid the temptation to simply remove the stem by striking it with an extractor. This method can result in fracture of the calcar and/or the greater trochanter.
- Instead, the entire proximal surface of the implant must be clearly visualized and any overlying bone removed before the implant is extracted.
- Laterally, this step can be accomplished with the use of a burr. The overhanging aspect of the greater trochanter is removed so that the lateral shoulder of the implant will not impinge on the trochanter when it is removed.
- Medially, the bone enveloping the collar can be removed with a burr, osteotome, or rongeur, or, more simply, the femoral neck can be resected at the level of the collar.
- Some implants, such as Austin Moore endoprostheses, have proximal fenestrations through which the intramedullary bone can grow (**Figure 5**). Using flexible osteotomes or a reciprocating saw, this bone must be transected anteriorly and posteriorly to safely remove the stem.
- After these steps have been completed, the loose stem can be extracted without risk of fracturing the proximal femur.
- Cemented revision of a failed noncemented endoprosthesis requires removal of the neocortex that typically surrounds the failed stem. This step can be accomplished with the use of osteotomes, curets, and/or a burr. In elderly patients with osteoporotic bone, prudence is required during this step because differentiation of the neocortex from the fragile femoral cortex can be difficult. This difficulty can result in inadvertent perforation of the cortex, resulting in subsequent extravasation of cement, and can increase the risk of a subsequent periprosthetic fracture (**Figure 5**). This difficulty is less problematic in revision to a noncemented stem because the reaming of the canal for the revision stem can include removal of the neocortex.

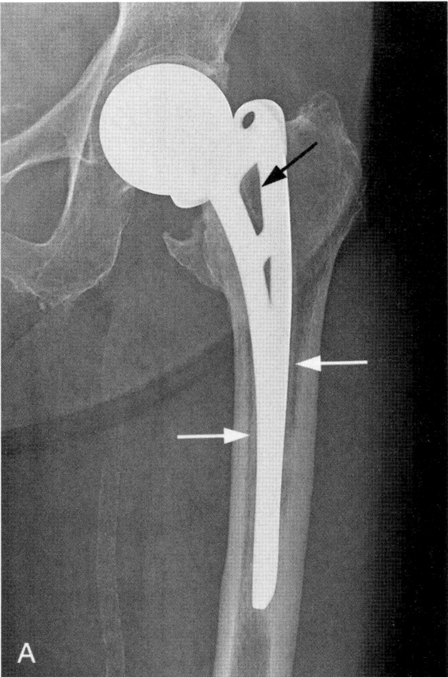

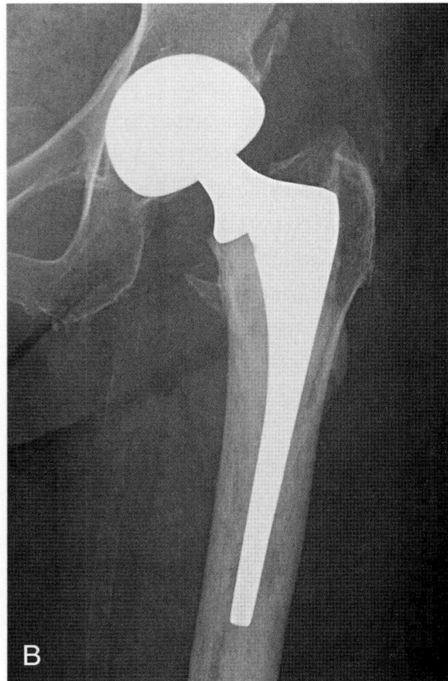

Figure 5 **A,** AP radiograph of a left hip demonstrates a failed Austin Moore hemiarthroplasty in an 88-year-old woman. Note the bone growing through the fenestration (black arrow) and the neocortex that has formed around the stem (white arrows). **B,** AP radiograph obtained after conversion to a hybrid total hip arthroplasty. The neocortex was removed to allow cement penetration to the femoral cortices. Inadvertent perforation of the proximal lateral cortex of the femur occurred during removal of the neocortex, resulting in some extravasation of cement laterally. The acetabular implant is a dual-mobility cup.

- Removal and revision of a well-fixed cemented or noncemented hemiarthroplasty stem follows the principles of revision of a THA (**Figure 6**). However, in patients with osteoporotic bone, the fragility of the femur increases the risk of intraoperative femoral fracture. Therefore, manipulation of the patient's leg should be done in a slow and cautious fashion. During exposure of the hip, preparation of the femur, and insertion of the revision stem, acute rotation and excessive torque on the femur should be avoided.
- In patients with a well-fixed cemented stem that requires revision, the use of an ETO should be considered to minimize the risk of femoral perforation during removal of cement adherent to the fragile femoral cortices. If an ETO is used in revision of the stem, placement of a prophylactic wire distal to the ETO should be considered to minimize the risk of a fracture extending distally from the ETO.
- Conversion of the large femoral head used in a hemiarthroplasty to the smaller femoral head used in revision THA increases the risk of dislocation. This risk is exacerbated in elderly patients with cognitive or neuromuscular issues. In these patients, careful consideration should be given to using the largest possible femoral head diameter or using a dual-mobility cup (**Figures 1**, **5**, and **6**).
- Restoration of the hip biomechanics is critical to minimize the risk of dislocation. Preoperative planning and intraoperative assessment are crucial to restore the patient's limb length and offset.
- When only the acetabulum is being revised, femoral offset can be adjusted with the use of an offset polyethylene acetabular liner (**Figure 7**).

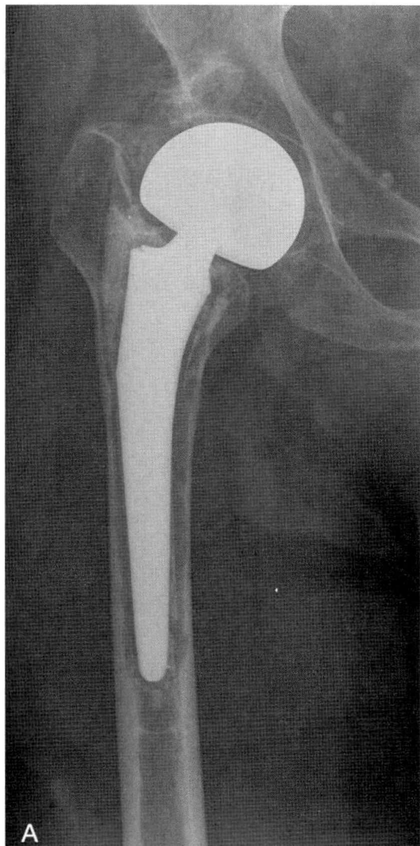

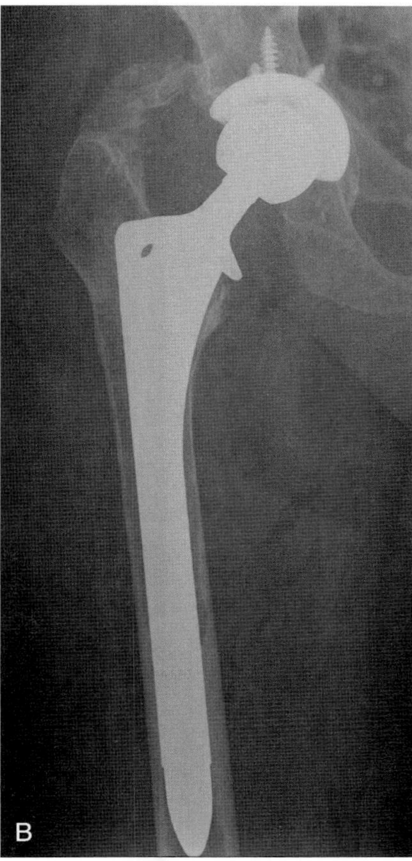

Figure 6 **A,** AP radiograph of a right hip demonstrates a failed cemented bipolar hemiarthroplasty in an 80-year-old woman. The stem has subsided underneath the calcar. Femoral osteolysis and acetabular erosion are present. **B,** Immediate postoperative AP radiograph demonstrates standard revision principles. The stem has been revised with a long, fully porous-coated stem that bypasses the previous cement mantle. The acetabular implant is a multihole, porous implant fixed with screws. A 36-mm femoral head was used.

Wound Closure

- Wound closure is the same as for any revision hip arthroplasty. However, when a posterior approach is used, the surgeon should make every effort to close the posterior capsule in order to decrease the risk of dislocation.

Postoperative Regimen

The postoperative care after revision of a failed hemiarthroplasty is similar to that after revision of a THA and depends on patient characteristics, the procedure that was done, the implants that were used, and the patient's bone stock. In elderly patients who may not be able to follow a restricted weight-bearing protocol, the choices of implant and surgical procedure should allow the patient to bear as much weight as possible. To avoid dislocation, postoperative activities should be limited until the soft tissues are well healed. These limitations depend on the surgical approach used.

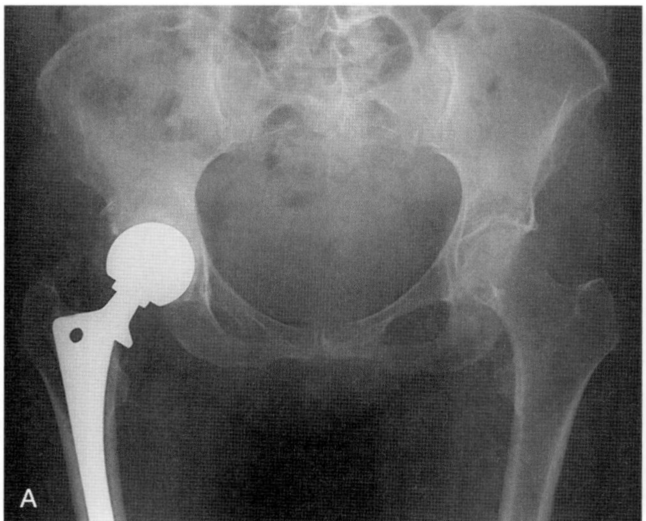

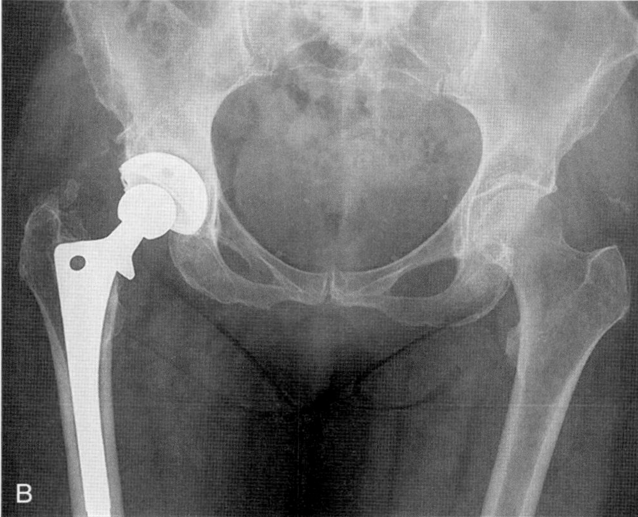

Figure 7 **A,** AP pelvic radiograph demonstrates acetabular erosion after a previous hemiarthroplasty with a unipolar head. **B,** AP pelvic radiograph obtained after revision surgery in which an offset polyethylene acetabular liner was used to restore femoral offset and limb length. The stem was not revised.

Avoiding Pitfalls and Complications

A failed hemiarthroplasty is most commonly converted to a THA. Although midterm survivorship rates are encouraging, the revision procedure can be technically challenging and is associated with a high rate of intraoperative complications. Careful preoperative workup and planning is required to determine whether the stem needs to be revised and to select a surgical technique that can be used to safely remove the implant without femoral perforation or fracture. Careful and gentle intraoperative preparation of the acetabulum and femur are required because many of these patients have osteoporotic bone. The selection of the revision implant should follow the modern principles of revision THA. With the use of the techniques described in this chapter to meticulously expose and prepare the femur and/or acetabulum, the surgeon can minimize the risk of fracture and perforation. Prevention of postoperative dislocation requires restoration of the soft-tissue envelope and biomechanics of the hip, as well as appropriate implant selection (**Figure 7**). To reduce the risk of postoperative dislocation, the normal hip biomechanics should be restored and the hip capsule repaired. The use of large-diameter femoral heads or dual-mobility cups, when possible, can also help prevent dislocation.

Bibliography

Amstutz HC, Smith RK: Total hip replacement following failed femoral hemiarthroplasty. *J Bone Joint Surg Am* 1979;61(8):1161-1166.

Australian Orthopaedic Association National Joint Replacement Registry: *Annual Report 2014.* Adelaide, SA, Australia, Australian Orthopaedic Association, 2014. Available at: https://aoanjrr.sahmri.com/documents/10180/172286/Annual%20Report%202014. Accessed September 6, 2016.

Bilgen O, Karaeminogullari O, Küleçioglu A: Results of conversion total hip prosthesis performed following painful hemiarthroplasty. *J Int Med Res* 2000;28(6):307-312.

Champion LM, McNally SA: Dislocation after revision of hemiarthroplasty to total hip replacement. *Injury* 2004;35(2):161-164.

Diwanji SR, Kim SK, Seon JK, Park SJ, Yoon TR: Clinical results of conversion total hip arthroplasty after failed bipolar hemiarthroplasty. *J Arthroplasty* 2008;23(7):1009-1015.

Figved W, Dybvik E, Frihagen F, et al: Conversion from failed hemiarthroplasty to total hip arthroplasty: A Norwegian Arthroplasty Register analysis of 595 hips with previous femoral neck fractures. *Acta Orthop* 2007;78(6):711-718.

Garellick G, Rogmark C, Kärrholm J, Rolfson O: *Swedish Hip Arthroplasty Register: Annual Report 2012*. Gothenburg, Sweden, Swedish Hip Arthroplasty Register, 2012. Available at: http://www.shpr.se/Libraries/Documents/AnnualReport_2012_Eng_WEB.sflb.ashx.

Hammad A, Abdel-Aal A: Conversion total hip arthroplasty: Functional outcome in Egyptian population. *Acta Orthop Belg* 2006;72(5):549-554.

Khair MM, Nam D, DiCarlo E, Su E: Aseptic lymphocyte dominated vasculitis-associated lesion resulting from trunnion corrosion in a cobalt-chrome unipolar hemiarthroplasty. *J Arthroplasty* 2013;28(1):196.e11-196.e14.

Llinas A, Sarmiento A, Ebramzadeh E, Gogan WJ, McKellop HA: Total hip replacement after failed hemiarthroplasty or mould arthroplasty: Comparison of results with those of primary replacements. *J Bone Joint Surg Br* 1991;73(6):902-907.

Mann MA, Tanzer D, Tanzer M: Severe metal-induced osteolysis many years after unipolar hip endoprosthesis. *Clin Orthop Relat Res* 2013;471(7):2078-2082.

Pankaj A, Malhotra R, Bhan S: Conversion of failed hemiarthroplasty to total hip arthroplasty: A short to mid-term follow-up study. *Indian J Orthop* 2008;42(3):294-300.

Sah AP, Estok DM II: Dislocation rate after conversion from hip hemiarthroplasty to total hip arthroplasty. *J Bone Joint Surg Am* 2008;90(3):506-516.

Sharkey PF, Rao R, Hozack WJ, Rothman RH, Carey C: Conversion of hemiarthroplasty to total hip arthroplasty: Can groin pain be eliminated? *J Arthroplasty* 1998;13(6):627-630.

Sierra RJ, Cabanela ME: Conversion of failed hip hemiarthroplasties after femoral neck fractures. *Clin Orthop Relat Res* 2002;(399):129-139.

Warwick D, Hubble M, Sarris I, Strange J: Revision of failed hemiarthroplasty for fractures at the hip. *Int Orthop* 1998;22(3):165-168.

Whitehouse MR, Endo M, Masri BA: Adverse local tissue reaction associated with a modular hip hemiarthroplasty. *Clin Orthop Relat Res* 2013;471(12):4082-4086.

SECTION 5
Alternative Reconstruction Procedures
Daniel J. Berry, MD

Chapter 64
Hip Arthroscopy for the Management of Structural Problems

Ryan A. Mlynarek, MD
James R. Ross, MD
Christopher M. Larson, MD
Bryan T. Kelly, MD
Asheesh Bedi, MD

Indications

Hip arthroscopy was first described in cadavers in 1931, although the difficulty of arthroscopic access to the hip joint was noted. The first reported clinical applications of hip arthroscopy were for the management of Charcot arthropathy, tuberculous arthritis, and septic arthritis. For much of the 20th century, hip arthroscopy was performed rarely because of the technical challenges associated with safe access to the hip joint and the limited applications of the technique. With recent advances in the understanding of hip pathology, improvements in surgical techniques, and the development of innovative technology and instrumentation, the indications for hip arthroscopy have expanded, and the procedure is performed more regularly. Hip arthroscopy is most commonly used to manage structural diseases of the hip, such as femoroacetabular impingement (FAI), labral tears, chondral defects, loose bodies, abductor injuries, and snapping hip disorders.

Femoroacetabular Impingement

FAI is a dynamic cause of hip pain resulting from the abnormal abutment of the femoral head-neck junction and the acetabular rim in terminal ranges of motion. FAI is classified as either cam type (characterized by asphericity and loss of offset at the femoral head-neck junction) or pincer type (characterized by overcoverage of the acetabular rim). Cam-type and pincer-type impingement can be a pathomorphologic cause of intra-articular disorders, such as labral or chondral injuries. Hip arthroscopy may be used to treat symptomatic patients in whom clinical and radiographic findings are consistent with FAI and in whom nonsurgical management has been unsuccessful. Arthroscopy is used to perform a femoral head-neck osteoplasty and/or acetabular rim resection to correct the underlying abnormalities and address the associated chondrolabral pathology in the prearthritic hip.

Labral Tears

The acetabular labrum is a triangle-shaped fibrocartilaginous structure that functions to deepen the acetabular socket and thus increase the acetabular surface area and volume. It acts as a gasket to maintain the articular synovial fluid seal, which is crucial for joint lubrication and cartilage preservation. Primary injuries to the labrum can result from acute trauma; however, most of these injuries are secondary to underlying structural pathology, such as developmental dysplasia of the hip, slipped capital femoral epiphysis, Legg-Calvé-Perthes disease, and FAI. FAI can result in damage to the anterosuperior labrum between the femoral head-neck junction and the acetabular rim with repetitive terminal hip flexion and internal rotation. Injuries to the posterior labrum are less common and typically result from a traumatic posterior dislocation or FAI-induced posterior instability. Capsular laxity, commonly seen in

Dr. Ross or an immediate family member serves as a paid consultant to Smith & Nephew. Dr. Larson or an immediate family member serves as a paid consultant to Smith & Nephew and A3 Surgical; has stock or stock options held in A3 Surgical; and has received research or institutional support from Smith & Nephew. Dr. Kelly or an immediate family member serves as an unpaid consultant to A3 Surgical and Arthrex and has stock or stock options held in A3 Surgical. Dr. Bedi or an immediate family member serves as a paid consultant to Arthrex; has stock or stock options held in A3 Surgical; and serves as a board member, owner, officer, or committee member of the American Orthopaedic Society for Sports Medicine. Neither Dr. Mlynarek nor any immediate family member has received anything of value from or has stock or stock options held in a commercial company or institution related directly or indirectly to the subject of this chapter.

patients with congenital disorders such as Down syndrome, Ehlers-Danlos syndrome, and Marfan syndrome, also can lead to rotational instability and result in damage to the anterosuperior labrum. The authors of one study reported that hips with a labral deficiency, regardless of the etiology of injury, undergo cartilage consolidation greater than 20% more rapidly than hips with an intact labrum do. In addition to its role in the maintenance of articular cartilage, hip kinetics, and stability, the labrum is involved in proprioceptive and nociceptive functions. Thus, patients with labral injuries may report mechanical symptoms, instability, and/or anterior groin pain. In patients who have persistent symptoms, clinical signs, and MRI findings consistent with labral injury, hip arthroscopy may be indicated to repair the labrum and/or reattach it to the acetabular rim and to address the underlying pathology responsible for the labral tear.

Chondral Defects

Hip chondral lesions can occur either in isolation or in conjunction with degenerative joint disease. These lesions may be traumatic in origin or secondary to other hip pathologies (eg, dysplasia, FAI, or osteonecrosis). In one study, these lesions tended to occur in the anterior (59%), posterior (25%), and superior (24%) acetabular quadrants. When associated with cam-type FAI, anterosuperior acetabular chondral delamination results from a repetitive inclusion-type injury caused by entry of the aspheric femoral head into the acetabulum. In pincer-type FAI, engagement of the overcovered acetabular rim and the femoral head-neck junction can result in an impaction-type injury to the labrum, leverage of the femoral head, and increased shear forces on the posteroinferior cartilage (contrecoup injury).

Because the articular cartilage is avascular and alymphatic, defects have little intrinsic healing potential. Cartilage restoration techniques that were originally used in the knee, such as microfracture, autologous chondrocyte implantation, and osteochondral autograft/allograft transplantation, have been adapted for the management of chondral defects in the hip. Patients with chondral lesions about the hip may have mechanical symptoms, anterior hip pain, and advanced imaging consistent with chondral pathology. Microfracture results in production of a marrow clot, creating an enriched environment for pluripotent marrow cells and mesenchymal stem cells to differentiate and facilitate fibrocartilage tissue formation. Indications for microfracture include focal and contained full-thickness lesions in the weight-bearing surface with an area less than or equal to 400 mm^2 and a stable edge. Microfracture is most commonly performed to address acetabular defects because femoral head defects are less common.

Loose Bodies

Loose bodies can be traumatic or atraumatic in origin. They may consist of foreign material or be cartilaginous, osseous, or osteocartilaginous in nature. Traumatic hip dislocation or acetabular wall fractures can result in intra-articular loose bodies. In a study of 151 fracture-dislocations of the hip, 91% of the hips had intra-articular loose bodies. The authors of a study of 36 patients noted loose bodies in 92% after dislocation or acetabular wall fracture, including 7 of 9 patients in whom no loose bodies were seen on plain radiographs or CT. Penetrating trauma, such as that caused by bullet fragments, also can result in intra-articular loose bodies. Additionally, degenerative joint disease often produces osteophytes that can become displaced, resulting in loose body formation. Benign synovial disorders of the hip, such as synovial chondromatosis, can result in shedding of pedunculated chondral bodies into the joint. Regardless of the source, intra-articular loose bodies can be removed at the time of open treatment of associated fractures or, if no open procedures are planned, with hip arthroscopy to prevent further damage to the articular cartilage. However, caution must be exercised when hip arthroscopy is performed in an acute posttraumatic scenario because of the increased risk of fluid extravasation and abdominal compartment syndrome.

Ligamentum Teres Rupture

The ligamentum teres originates from the posteroinferior acetabular fossa and inserts on the femoral fovea. Although some surgeons consider it to be a vestigial structure, others suggest that it serves as a secondary stabilizer of the hip and provides proprioceptive and nociceptive feedback. Thus, controversy exists among surgeons as to whether ligamentum teres tears are a potential cause of persistent anterior hip pain and/or instability, and, if so, whether the ligament should be repaired. According to the Gray classification, introduced in 1997, injuries to the ligamentum teres can be categorized as complete tears (type 1), partial-thickness tears (type 2), or degenerative tears (type 3). Since the introduction of that classification, injuries to the ligamentum teres have become more readily recognized because of the increased availability of advanced imaging and increased identification of these injuries at the time of hip arthroscopy. In a series of 271 patients undergoing hip arthroscopy, rupture of the ligamentum teres was the third most common pathology. In patients who experience persistent anterior groin pain reproducible in provocative testing and exhibit radiographic findings that elicit suspicion of a ligamentum teres tear, in whom an appropriate course of nonsurgical management has been unsuccessful, hip arthroscopy to address this pathology may be beneficial. Débridement is indicated to manage type 2 tears. Reconstruction has been performed rarely in patients with type

1 tears. The indications for and outcomes of reconstruction are not well defined.

Iliopsoas Tendinitis

Iliopsoas tendinitis, also called internal snapping hip syndrome, is a common source of dynamic anterior hip pain. A presenting symptom can be vague activity-related anterior hip pain that subsides with rest and worsens with rising from a seated position, ascending stairs, or walking up an incline. With worsening severity of the tendinitis, the underlying bursa may swell substantially and an audible snap may be heard as the iliopsoas tendon slides over the iliopectineal eminence or the anterior capsulolabral complex and femoral head. The diagnosis is made on the basis of the history and clinical examination and can be confirmed with dynamic ultrasonography and/or image-guided local anesthetic and corticosteroid injection. In patients who experience recurrent pain and mechanical symptoms in whom nonsurgical management has been unsuccessful, arthroscopic iliopsoas lengthening may be indicated. Transcapsular lengthening at the level of the joint or a release at the level of the lesser trochanter can be performed.

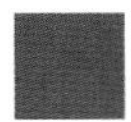

Contraindications

From 2003 through 2009, the number of hip arthroscopies performed in the United States increased 18-fold. Even as the surgical treatment pendulum has swung toward arthroscopic intervention, it is important to remember the limitations of this procedure. Absolute contraindications to hip arthroscopy include pathologic limitations that would prevent sufficient distraction to enable the surgeon to obtain adequate visualization and appropriately maneuver the surgical instrumentation. These limiting conditions include hip ankylosis, severe acetabular protrusion, and periarticular heterotopic ossification. Additionally, the presence of hip dysplasia or relative acetabular undercoverage is a contraindication to hip arthroscopy because further bony resection or attenuation of the capsulolabral complex can result in clinical instability. Relative contraindications include posterior femoral cam-type deformity and extra-articular trochanteric-pelvic impingement because these pathologies are difficult to safely access and thoroughly address via hip arthroscopy. In patients who have femoroacetabular joint space narrowing (Tönnis grade 2 or higher), hip arthroscopy has a limited role (if any). A study published in 2016 reported significantly higher rates of conversion to total hip arthroplasty in patients with Tönnis grade 2 or higher osteoarthritis compared with patients with Tönnis grade 0 or 1 osteoarthritis.

Alternative Treatments

Open and mini-open approaches have been described to address structural pathology of the hip. The surgical approach should be individualized to the patient on the basis of the pathology, the complexity of the disorder, and the surgeon's experience. Open surgical management includes surgical hip dislocation, whereas mini-open approaches often combine a direct anterior open approach with arthroscopy. Open and mini-open approaches allow the surgeon to obtain direct visualization of the intra-articular pathology and achieve comprehensive correction of the pathomorphology without the difficulty of viewing the region through multiple arthroscopic portals. They also allow the surgeon to access the posterior joint and correct extra-articular deformities that cannot be feasibly addressed via arthroscopy. However, open procedures can be technically challenging, and the numerous potential complications associated with open procedures must be considered.

Results

Arthroscopy enables the surgeon to address substantial structural pathologies of the hip with reliable outcomes while minimizing the potential complications that can result from the alternative surgical options. Because the field of hip arthroscopy is rapidly expanding and the indications are still being refined, critical evaluation of outcome studies is prudent (**Table 1**).

Techniques

Setup/Access

- Preoperative radiographs should include a well-centered AP pelvic radiograph and a lateral radiograph of the hip (frog-leg lateral view, 45° Dunn view, and/or 90° Dunn view). A false-profile radiograph may be necessary to allow the surgeon to evaluate anterior acetabular coverage and the morphology of the anterior inferior iliac spine.
- The patient is placed in the supine or lateral decubitus position. Currently, most surgeons perform hip arthroscopy with the patient in the supine position and use a standard fracture table or commercially available surgical table or device for distraction of the hip (**Figure 1**).
- Examination of the affected and unaffected hips is performed with the patient under anesthesia to evaluate the passive range of motion (ROM), with specific attention to hip flexion, internal rotation in 90° of flexion, and external rotation in 90° of flexion.
- Intraoperative fluoroscopy is performed and correlated with preoperative imaging to allow comparison of the bony resections with

Table 1 Results of Arthroscopic Management of Structural Disorders of the Hip

Authors (Year)	Number of Patients (Hips)	Procedure	Mean Patient Age in Years (Range)	Mean Follow-up in Months (Range)	Results
Mullis and Dahners (2006)	36 (39)	Loose body retrieval	NR	NR	Intra-articular loose body after hip dislocation or fracture of the acetabular wall was found in 33 patients Loose bodies were found in 7 of 9 patients with normal radiographs or CT
Philippon et al (2008)	9	Chondral microfracture	37.2 (21-47)	20 (10-36)	On second-look arthroscopy, 8 patients had >95% grade I or II repair product in chondral lesions, and 1 patient had diffuse osteoarthritis with grade IV repair product after 10 mo postoperatively
Bedi et al (2011)	10	Rim resection, cam osteoplasty	25.9 (19-31)	≥3	All patients had significant improvements in hip flexion ($P = 0.002$) and internal rotation ($P = 0.0002$)
Byrd and Jones (2011)	100	Rim resection, cam osteoplasty	34 (13-76)	24	79 patients had good or excellent outcomes Median improvement of 21.5 points on modified HHS
Fabricant et al (2012)	67	Iliopsoas lengthening	24.0 (NR)	12 (6-24)	Modified HHSs improved in 67 patients Postoperative modified HHSs were worse in patients who had increased femoral anteversion (>25°) than in patients who had low or normal femoral anteversion
Karthikeyan et al (2012)	20	Chondral microfracture	37 (17-54)	17 (5-47)	On second-look arthroscopy, 19 patients had fill of 96% ± 7% (mean ± SD) with macroscopic good-quality repair tissue, and 1 patient had <25% fill with poor-quality repair tissue
Lee et al (2012)	24	Loose body retrieval and synovectomy for the management of synovial chondromatosis	43 (32-63)	41 (12-133)	18 patients had good or excellent outcomes All loose bodies were successfully retrieved 4 patients experienced recurrence of disease 1 patient progressed to THA
Philippon et al (2012)	4	Ligamentum teres reconstruction	36 (30-41)	31 (6-60)	All patients had resolution of instability symptoms and returned to desired level of sport or activity 1 patient progressed to THA
Amenabar and O'Donnell (2013)	26 (27)	Ligamentum teres débridement	24.4 (12-45)	32 (23-49)	Modified HHSs and nonarthritic hip scores improved in all patients No patients required revision for recurrence of symptoms
Boykin et al (2013)	21 (23)	Labral reconstruction in elite athletes	28 (19-41)	41.4 (20-74)	18 patients returned to play 2 patients underwent revision because of lysis of capsulolabral adhesions 2 patients progressed to THA
Geyer et al (2013)	75 (76)	Labral reconstruction using iliotibial band autograft	38.5 (18-64)	49 (36-70)	Mean survivorship without arthroplasty was 56 mo 19 hips progressed to THA Patients who did not progress to THA had improvement in function and high satisfaction rates
El Bitar et al (2014)	55	Iliopsoas lengthening	28.2 (14.9-51.5)	27.6 (24-36)	45 patients had good or excellent satisfaction and resolution of symptoms

HHS = Harris hip score, NR = not reported, SD = standard deviation, THA = total hip arthroplasty.

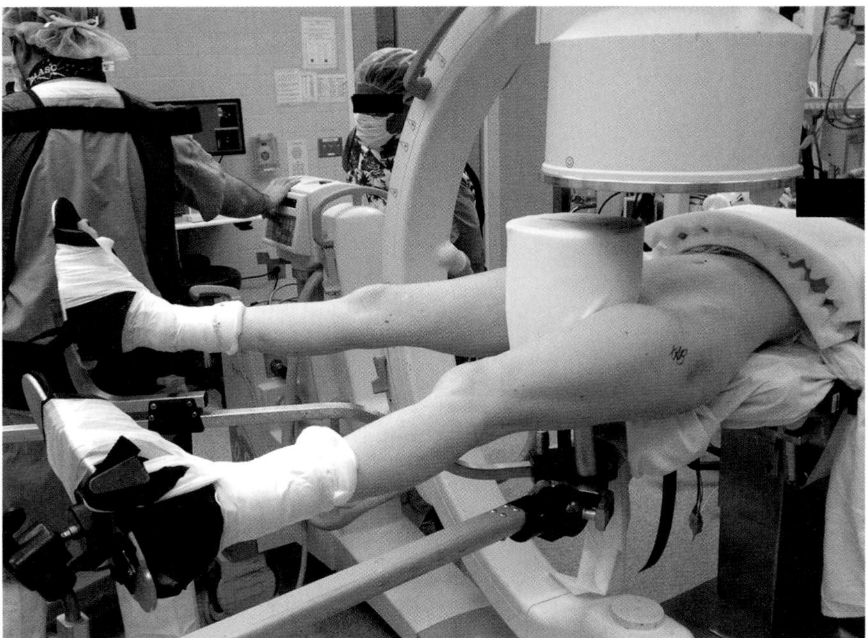

Figure 1 Photograph shows the setup for hip arthroscopy with the patient in the supine position. Note the careful padding of the perineal post and the use of secure, well-padded boots to avoid loss of traction and minimize the risk of traction-related neurapraxia. Often, the affected extremity is internally rotated to correct for femoral antetorsion and thereby facilitate placement of the initial proximal anterolateral portal.

the templated resections.

- The authors of this chapter typically obtain six intraoperative radiographs in which the patient's leg is placed in different positions, as described in a study published in 2014. These standard positions can assist in localization of the cam-type deformity to ensure appropriate resection and avoid excessive resection. The six fluoroscopic views correspond to specific clock-face positions on preoperative CT scans: AP internal rotation, 11:45; AP neutral rotation, 12:45; AP external rotation, 1:00; flexion and neutral rotation, 1:30; flexion and 40° external rotation, 2:15; and flexion and 60° external rotation, 2:30 (**Figure 2**).
- The patient's feet are well padded and adequately secured in surgical boots to avoid loss of traction during instrumentation of the central compartment.
- The perineal post is well padded and positioned just lateral to the midline in the direction of the affected extremity to avoid compression of the pudendal nerve and provide a vector of lateral force to assist in distraction of the joint.
- The affected hip is positioned in neutral abduction, 10° of flexion, and 15° of internal rotation.
- To minimize the risk of iatrogenic chondral injury, the minimal amount of traction necessary to distract the joint approximately 6 to 8 mm and allow for portal placement is applied.

ANTEROLATERAL PORTAL

- Typically, the anterolateral portal is established first to provide access to the hip under fluoroscopic guidance (**Figure 3**).
- This portal typically is located approximately 1 to 2 cm anterior and 1 to 2 cm proximal to the anterosuperior aspect of the greater trochanter. More recently, surgeons have placed the anterolateral portal more distally to allow a better trajectory for suture anchor placement and/or microfracture procedures.
- The authors of this chapter prefer to place the portal in the palpable interval between the gluteus medius muscle and the tensor fascia lata.
- A spinal needle is placed under fluoroscopic guidance. The surgeon should aim for the distal third of the distracted space and avoid labral penetration. It is often helpful to "vent" the joint by initially penetrating the joint capsule to allow for further joint distraction via release of intracapsular pressure. The spinal needle is withdrawn and redirected. Care is taken to avoid chondral injury to the femoral head.
- A nitinol wire is placed through the spinal needle until contact with the medial acetabular fossa is made.
- The spinal needle is withdrawn.
- A cannulated cannula is inserted over the nitinol wire, through the capsule, and into the joint.

MODIFIED ANTERIOR PORTAL

- The modified anterior portal is established under direct visualization (**Figure 4**).
- This portal is distal and lateral to the aforementioned anterolateral portal as well as the standard anterior portal, which is typically placed at the intersection of a line from the anterior superior iliac spine to the knee and a horizontal line at the level of the greater trochanter.
- The authors of this chapter prefer the modified anterior portal because it increases the distance from the lateral femoral cutaneous nerve, provides a better trajectory for instrumentation, and improves access to the labrum and the acetabular rim.

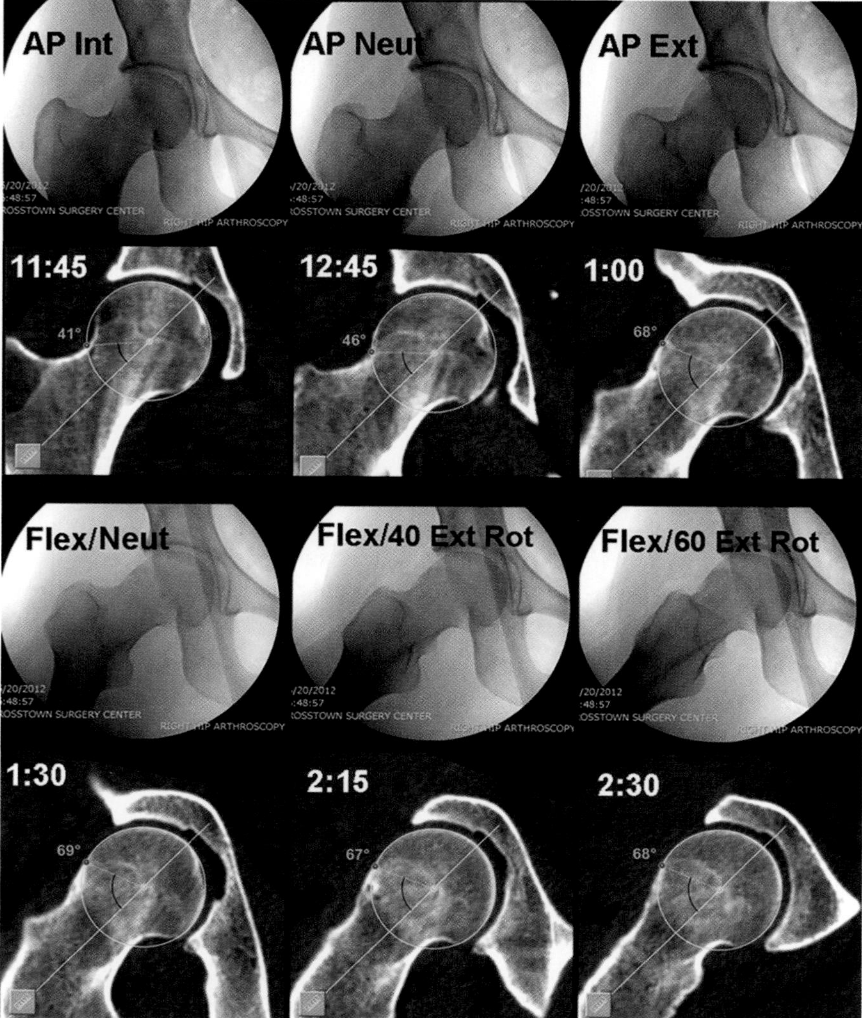

Figure 2 Examples of the six intraoperative fluoroscopic views from one patient, with corresponding clock-face positions as determined via alpha angle measurement on CT scans. Ext = external, Flex = flexion, Int = internal, Neut = neutral, Rot = rotation. (Reproduced with permission from Ross JR, Bedi A, Stone RM, et al: Intraoperative fluoroscopic imaging to treat cam deformities: Correlation with 3-dimensional computed tomography. *Am J Sports Med* 2014;42[6]:1370-1376.)

- An equilateral triangle can be drawn connecting the distal anterolateral, anterior, and proximal anterolateral portals. The authors of this chapter prefer to create the modified anterior portal 1 to 2 cm distal to the standard anterior portal. To establish this portal, a spinal needle is inserted carefully under direct visualization between the femoral head and the labrum (**Figure 4**). After the spinal needle is in place, a nitinol wire is inserted, and the spinal needle is withdrawn.
- Another cannula is inserted over the nitinol wire, with care taken to pull the wire back to avoid breakage.

INTERPORTAL CAPSULOTOMY

- The arthroscope is moved to the newly created modified anterior portal to visualize the previously placed anterolateral portal and confirm safe placement without labral penetration.
- A beaver blade is inserted through the cannula, and the cannula is withdrawn.
- The beaver blade is used to make a transverse interportal capsulotomy. Care is taken to preserve full-thickness capsular margins for later repair (**Figure 5**). The beaver blade is directed toward the arthroscope with care to avoid injury to the labrum and the femoral head.
- The arthroscope is moved back to the anterolateral portal.
- The beaver blade is inserted into the modified anterior portal and used to complete the interportal capsulotomy.

Instruments/Equipment/Implants Required

- A well-padded traction table with a perineal post is used.
- 30° and 70° arthroscopes are used.
- An 18-gauge spinal needle is used.
- A nitinol wire is used.
- A long beaver blade is used.
- Assorted motorized shavers and burrs measuring 4.0 and 5.5 mm in diameter are used.
- Assorted long cannulas measuring 8.5 mm in diameter are used.
- 30° and 45° suture lasso passers are used.
- A 90° radiofrequency ablation wand measuring 4.75 mm in diameter is used.
- Long suture/needle graspers are used.
- Assorted suture anchors are used.

Procedure for Central Compartment Pathology

ACETABULAR RIM RESECTION

- In patients with pincer-type FAI, the authors of this chapter prefer to address the acetabular rim pathomorphology first. A motorized shaver and radiofrequency ablation device is used to elevate the capsule and expose the extracapsular rim.

- The integrity of the labrum is evaluated. Preservation and repair is the preferred strategy. However, débridement may be necessary if ossification or intrasubstance cystic degeneration is present (**Figure 6**).
- If the labral morphology is relatively normal and the chondrolabral junction is intact, extracapsular exposure may allow for resection of the areas of bony overcoverage of the acetabular rim without formal detachment of the labrum.
- In patients with global or large focal overcoverage necessitating substantial rim resection, labral takedown and subsequent reattachment may be required. However, the authors of this chapter prefer to preserve the chondrolabral junction and transitional zone cartilage as much as possible.
- Rim resection is performed with the use of a motorized burr to contour the acetabular overcoverage and address any extracapsular deformity (below the level of the anterior inferior iliac spine) extending to or caudal to the margin of the acetabulum (**Figure 7**). To avoid excessive resection, intraoperative fluoroscopy is used to localize the area of the acetabular rim that is being addressed. Release of traction may be necessary to allow the surgeon to evaluate the relationship of the acetabular rim to the femoral head in patients requiring larger or global rim resection.
- The typical starting point for acetabular rim resection is either just inferior to the crossover sign or directly lateral to it, at the 12-o'clock position on intraoperative fluoroscopy.
- Pincer-type overcoverage often consists of harder bone with a yellow hue, whereas the normal, softer underlying cancellous bone has a pink hue.

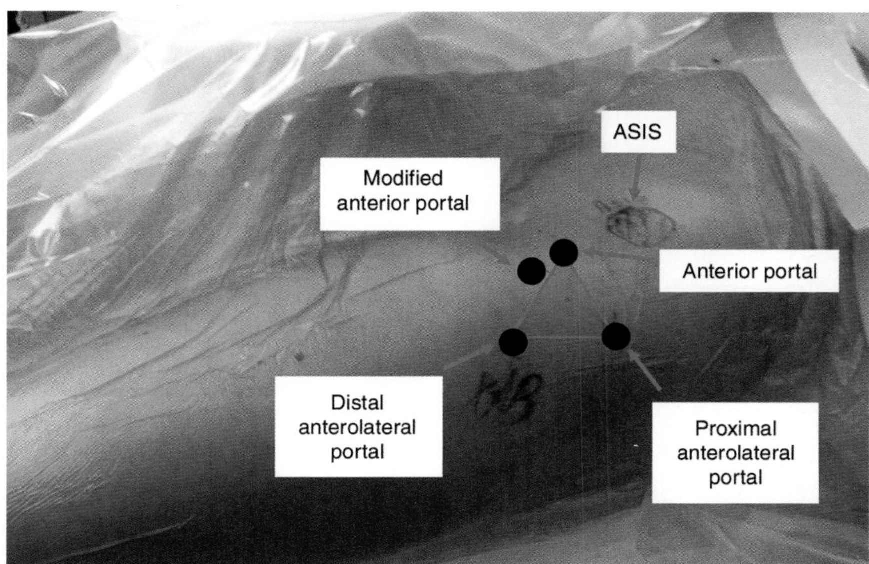

Figure 3 Photograph of a left hip shows the placement of the modified anterior portal, anterior portal, distal anterolateral portal, and proximal anterolateral portal for hip arthroscopy. ASIS = anterior superior iliac spine.

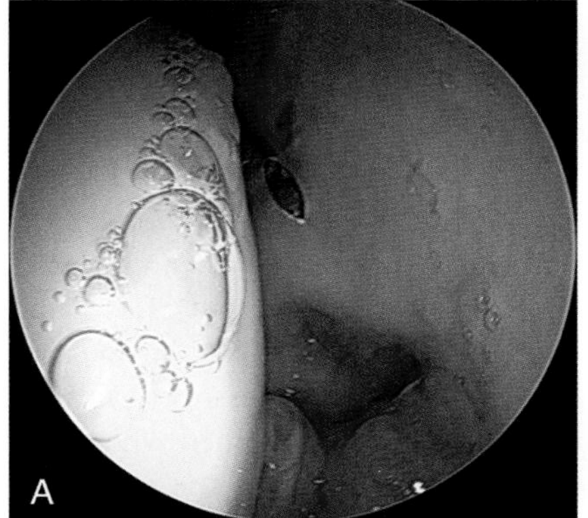

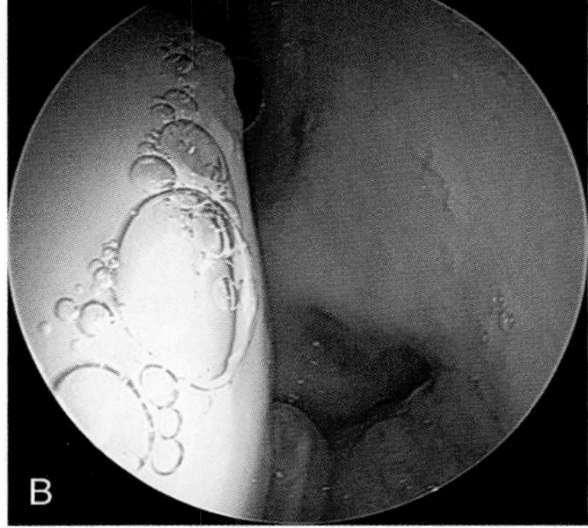

Figure 4 Arthroscopic images viewed through the distal anterolateral portal demonstrate establishment of the modified anterior portal under direct visualization with the use of a spinal needle (**A**) followed by insertion of a nitinol wire and a cannula (**B**).

- If a small os acetabuli or acetabular rim fracture is present, it is typically excised to resolve the impingement. However, if the patient has a larger fragment that is mobile when probed, or if the remaining acetabular rim is dysplastic, reduction and internal fixation may be performed with the use of one or two cannulated screws to avoid the risk of iatrogenic dysplasia and secondary instability.
- Intraoperative imaging and ROM are compared with preoperative planning to confirm the extent of rim resection. The resection is adjusted if necessary.
- If the patient has a posterior pincer-type lesion, a posterolateral portal may be established to address the posterior inferior acetabular rim.
- If any chondral delamination is observed, it is gently débrided to form a stable edge. Microfracture may be performed in patients with small, focal, and well-shouldered lesions.

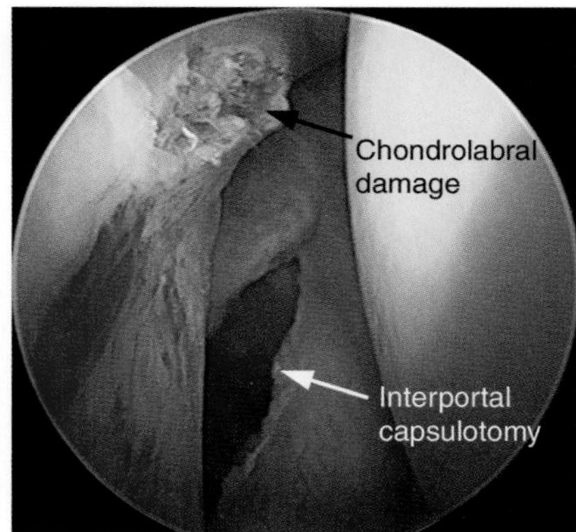

Figure 5 Arthroscopic image viewed through the modified anterior portal demonstrates visualization of the interportal capsulotomy. A beaver blade is inserted through the proximal anterolateral portal and is used to make the capsulotomy. The capsule adjacent to the labrum is preserved to allow later repair. The gluteus medius muscle is visualized and protected posteriorly.

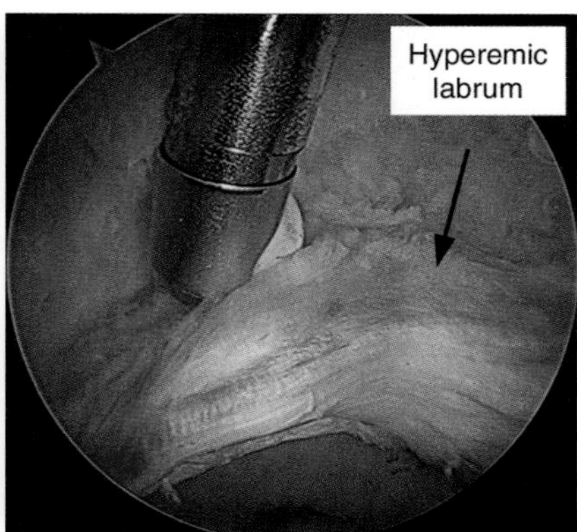

Figure 6 Arthroscopic image viewed through the distal anterolateral portal demonstrates labral takedown with the use of a radiofrequency ablation device for the resection of a large pincer-type lesion. This technique, followed by refixation after rim resection, may be required in patients with substantial pincer-type deformity.

LABRAL REPAIR

- The labrum is inspected to evaluate the tissue quality. Any fraying or nonviable fragments are resected with a motorized shaver, with care taken to preserve as much tissue as possible for later reattachment.
- In patients in whom an acetabular rim resection is not performed, the acetabulum is prepared with a motorized burr to remove the cortical bone, thus exposing the bleeding, cancellous bone. Care is taken to preserve the capsule during exposure of the extra-articular surface of the labrum for later repair, if planned.
- After the labrum and acetabulum are adequately prepared, suture anchors (bioabsorbable, polyetheretherketone, or all-suture) are placed approximately 2 to 4 mm from the edge of the acetabular rim to minimize the risk of iatrogenic chondral injury (**Figure 8**). Placement in close proximity to the acetabular margin minimizes the risk of labral eversion and loss of the suction seal.
- The suture anchors are placed in a distal-to-proximal trajectory under direct visualization to prevent intra-articular penetration. Additionally, fluoroscopy can be used to confirm placement of the drill superior to the acetabular sourcil.
- An additional, accessory distal portal may be established when necessary to improve the trajectory of drilling for suture anchors and prevent intra-articular injury and penetration into the central compartment (**Figure 3**).
- A suture-passing device is used to pass a single limb of the suture anchor through the chondrolabral junction and into the central compartment. This limb of the suture anchor is retrieved either around the outer edge of the labrum (circumferential configuration) or through the outer edge of the labrum (base configuration). The authors of this chapter prefer to use a base configuration stitch.
- The sutures are tied to reapproximate the labrum to the acetabular rim. Care is taken to minimize labral eversion to preserve an adequate articular synovial seal (**Figure 9**).

LABRAL RECONSTRUCTION

- If the labrum is inadequate for repair because of diminutive tissue, segmental loss, complete disruption of longitudinal fibers, complete ossification, or prior labral resection, labral reconstruction may be performed. Most surgeons reserve labral reconstruction primarily for use in revision hip procedures in patients who have a deficient labrum and loss of the synovial seal.
- Ipsilateral iliotibial band autograft may be used, and allograft tissues such as tibialis anterior or semitendinosus and hamstring autografts are secondary options. The authors of this chapter are not aware of any published studies that compare outcomes between autograft and allograft options for labral reconstruction.
- Irreparable tissue is débrided to create a stable edge of the remaining native labrum.
- The size of the defect is measured with the use of a probe and/or marked suture material.
- The acetabular rim is prepared with the use of a motorized burr, as described previously, to prepare the site of fixation and to address any pincer-type FAI.
- When an iliotibial band autograft is used, a rectangular graft is harvested from the ipsilateral leg with the use of a longitudinal incision made over the greater trochanter. The graft should be approximately 30% longer than the length of the labral defect and ideally 15 to 20 mm in width.
- The graft is tubularized with absorbable or nonabsorbable sutures and introduced to the hip joint through the modified anterior portal.

- A side-to-side repair is performed with the use of a suture-passing device to approximate the graft to the native labrum (**Figure 10**).
- Suture anchors are placed into the acetabular rim, as described previously, to further stabilize the graft and establish a sufficient labral seal.

MICROFRACTURE FOR THE MANAGEMENT OF CHONDRAL INJURIES

- The chondral defect is identified and probed. If any unstable cartilage is found, it is débrided with the use of a motorized shaver.
- A curet is used to clearly define the perpendicular margins of the defect to entrap the marrow clot. The curet is then used to remove the calcified cartilage layer and expose the subchondral bone. This step improves adherence of the resultant clot.
- Specialized, hip-specific microfracture awls are used to penetrate the subchondral bone in a perpendicular manner. The microfractures should be approximately 3 to 4 mm deep and spaced approximately 3 to 4 mm apart to preserve a subchondral bone bridge.
- Irrigation pump pressure is decreased to allow the surgeon to observe the release of marrow elements from the microfracture sites.

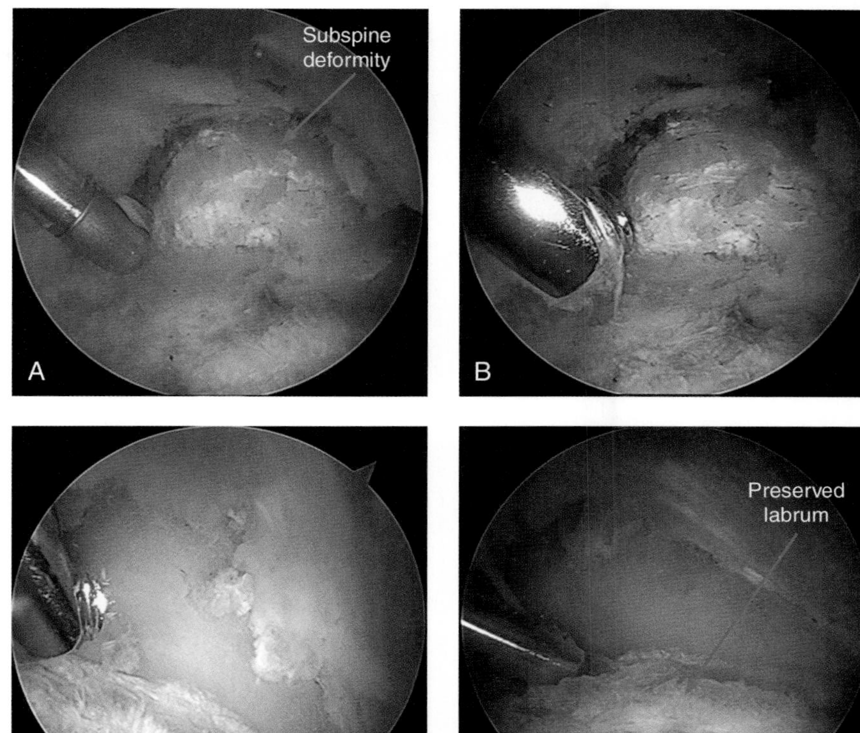

Figure 7 Arthroscopic images viewed through the distal anterolateral portal demonstrate acetabular rim resection. **A,** A radiofrequency ablation device is used to isolate a subspine, extra-articular pincer-type deformity. **B,** A motorized burr is used to resect the acetabular rim. **C,** The cartilage in the transition zone is preserved. **D,** The acetabular rim is prepared with the use of a motorized shaver.

REMOVAL OF LOOSE BODIES

- With proper portal placement and the use of 30° and 70° arthroscopes, the surgeon can visualize the entire central compartment for loose body retrieval.
- A thorough assessment of the intra-articular space begins with visualization through the anterolateral portal, followed by visualization through the modified anterior portal.
- A posterolateral portal may be used to remove any loose bodies in the posterior region.
- Most loose bodies can be removed with a simple grasper, a motorized shaver with suction, or simple lavage. In patients with large loose bodies, the portal can be dilated to allow the surgeon to use a long tonsil clamp or pituitary rongeur.

LIGAMENTUM TERES DÉBRIDEMENT

- All other central compartment pathology should be addressed before débridement is performed in the acetabular fossa because bleeding from this area may hinder visualization.
- The ligamentum teres is best viewed from the anterolateral portal with a 70° arthroscope and is best accessed with instruments via the modified anterior portal.
- The posterolateral portal may be used to access the posterior origin of the ligamentum teres.
- External rotation of the hip may facilitate visualization of the acetabular fossa.
- An arthroscopic biter or a motorized shaver with suction is used to débride the ruptured portion of the ligamentum teres.
- Care is taken to preserve stable portions of the ligament and avoid débridement of healthy tissue.

ILIOPSOAS LENGTHENING

- After the transverse interportal capsulotomy is made, the iliopsoas tendon can be visualized medially

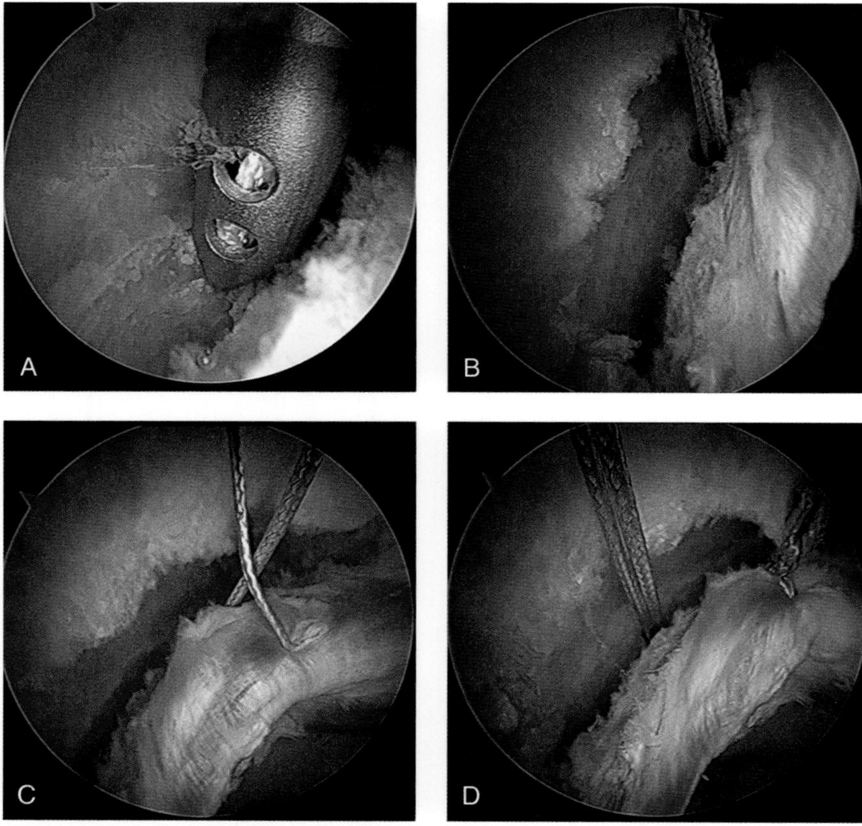

Figure 8 Arthroscopic images viewed through the distal anterolateral portal demonstrate labral repair. **A,** The acetabulum is prepared with the use of a motorized burr. **B,** Suture anchors are placed 2 to 4 mm from the edge of the acetabular rim. Placement of the suture anchors in proximity to the acetabular margin minimizes the risk of labral eversion. **C,** A base configuration stitch is used for refixation to preserve the suction seal. **D,** Two suture anchors are placed 3 to 4 mm apart.

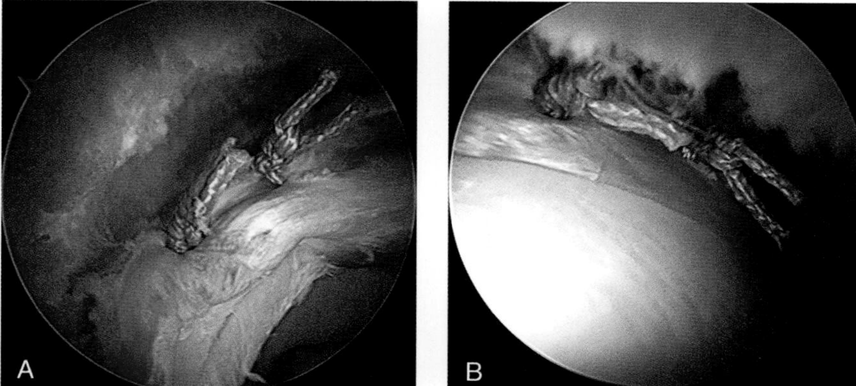

Figure 9 Arthroscopic images viewed through the distal anterolateral portal demonstrate the completion of the labral repair. **A,** The labral repair is completed with the use of two suture anchors and sutures in a base configuration. **B,** Traction is released to allow the surgeon to evaluate the suction seal and confirm that no knot impingement occurs.

through the capsular window.

- The presence of extracapsular synovitis and medial capsulolabral injury under the iliopsoas tendon can also confirm the pathology.
- The iliopsoas can be lengthened either at the level of the capsule or directly at the level of the lesser trochanter.
- The authors of this chapter typically prefer to use a transcapsular approach in which the lengthening is performed at the myotendinous junction because this method may preserve more hip flexor strength and secondary dynamic stability of the joint. However, in patients with psoas impingement and an oversized or retroverted total hip arthroplasty implant, release at the level of the lesser trochanter decreases the risk of capsular damage, instability, and iatrogenic infection.
- A radiofrequency ablation device can be used to perform a transcapsular iliopsoas lengthening. The iliopsoas tendon fibers are slowly divided under direct visualization, with care taken to avoid injury to the underlying muscle fibers (**Figure 11**). This step is best performed with the use of a 70° arthroscope in the anterolateral portal for visualization and the radiofrequency ablation device in the modified anterior portal.
- To perform the iliopsoas lengthening at the level of the lesser trochanter, the hip is flexed from 30° to 60° and externally rotated to allow fluoroscopic visualization of the lesser trochanter.
- An anterolateral inferior portal is established 2 to 3 cm distal and slightly anterior to the modified anterior portal. Blunt dissection down to the lesser trochanter and medial wall of the psoas bursa is performed with the use of a switching stick under fluoroscopic guidance. After

the switching stick is in position, a cannula is placed over it.

- A long spinal needle is used under fluoroscopic guidance and direct visualization to establish an additional working portal 3 to 4 cm distal to the anterolateral inferior portal.
- From this portal, a hook radiofrequency ablation probe is used to clear the psoas bursa so that the tendon can be directly visualized.
- The tendon is released from its insertion on the lesser trochanter.

Procedure for Peripheral Compartment Pathology

FEMORAL CAM OSTEOPLASTY

- A femoral cam-type deformity can be addressed through the modified anterior and proximal anterolateral portals when an interportal capsulotomy is performed.
- Flexion and external rotation of the leg can improve visualization of and access to the anterior aspect of the femoral head-neck junction.
- Extension and internal rotation of the leg can improve visualization of and access to the lateral and posterosuperior aspects of the femoral head-neck junction.
- Placing the leg into traction may facilitate access to the posterosuperior aspect of the femoral head-neck junction, which can be challenging.
- Additionally, a distal anterolateral accessory portal can be created to allow the surgeon to perform a T-shaped capsulotomy along the femoral neck, in line with the fibers of the iliofemoral ligament and between the muscle fibers of the gluteus minimus and iliocapsularis. When a T-shaped capsulotomy is performed, a switching stick can be placed in the anterolateral portal and behind the lateral femoral head-neck junction to retract the proximal lateral capsular flap. This method provides wide visualization to assist with correction of the deformity at the femoral head-neck junction (**Figure 12**).
- However, a T-shaped capsulotomy is not required. Alternatively, the capsular tissue can be retracted during resection with a motorized burr and careful positioning of the affected leg. Retraction of capsular tissue alone without capsulotomy may be particularly advisable in patients who have hypermobility or borderline dysplastic hip morphology.
- The most common zones of abnormality at the proximal femoral head-neck junction are evaluated with the use of the six fluoroscopic views described previously.
- The starting point and area of the planned resection are confirmed with fluoroscopy, and a motorized burr is used to restore the normal contour, concavity, and femoral head-neck offset (**Figure 13**).
- Care is taken not to resect greater than 30% of the femoral neck diameter because excessive resection has been shown to substantially decrease the energy required to cause femoral neck fracture.
- The area of resection is limited

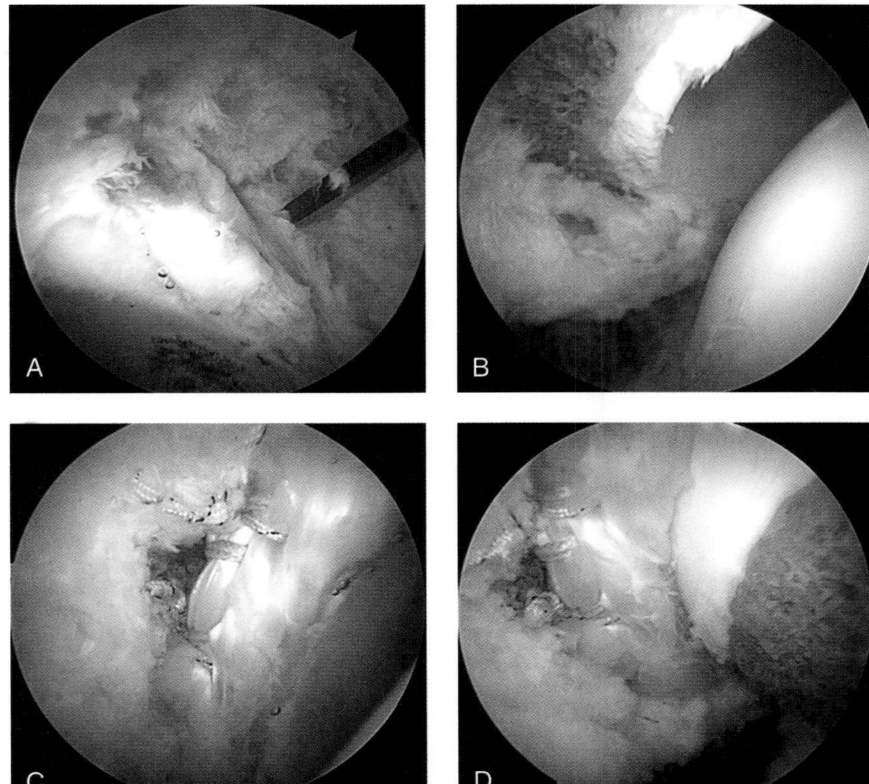

Figure 10 Arthroscopic views of steps in acetabular labral reconstruction. **A,** Revision right hip arthroscopy with the arthroscope in the distal anterolateral portal demonstrates a deficient anterosuperior labrum. **B,** Arthroscopic image viewed through the modified anterior portal demonstrates acetabular rim resection for the management of pincer-type femoroacetabular impingement and removal of the deficient labrum. **C,** Arthroscopic image viewed through the modified anterior portal demonstrates labral reconstruction with a tibialis anterior allograft. **D,** Arthroscopic image viewed through the modified anterior portal after release of traction demonstrates restoration of the labral synovial seal after labral reconstruction and femoral resection osteoplasty.

proximally and posteriorly by the perfusing superior and inferior retinacular vessels. The resection can be extended posteriorly and superiorly to the retinacular vessels if necessary; however, this must be done under direct visualization.

CAPSULAR REPAIR/PLICATION

- If a T-shaped capsulotomy was performed through the iliofemoral ligament, it is repaired with side-to-side nonabsorbable sutures, which are placed with the use of a combination of suture-shuttling and -passing devices (**Figure 14**).
- An interportal transverse capsulotomy can be repaired with the use of two to five side-to-side nonabsorbable sutures, which are placed in a similar manner. Care is taken to preserve the capsule on both the femoral and acetabular sides during instrumentation of the rim and labrum to ensure that sufficient tissue remains for later closure.
- Repair of the capsulotomy preserves the integrity of the iliofemoral ligament and minimizes the risk of postoperative instability.
- In patients with ligamentous laxity, arthroscopic capsular plication can be performed. An interportal and, in some patients, T-shaped capsulotomy is performed, and the edges of the capsule are resected to decrease the volume of the capsule when the edges are repaired together. The authors of this chapter prefer to use nonabsorbable sutures for capsular plication.

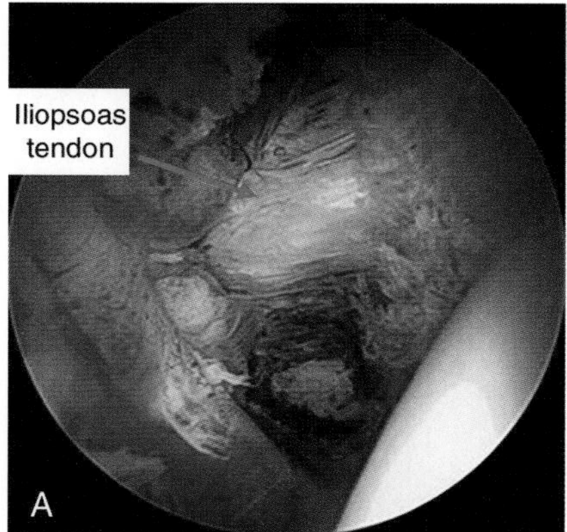

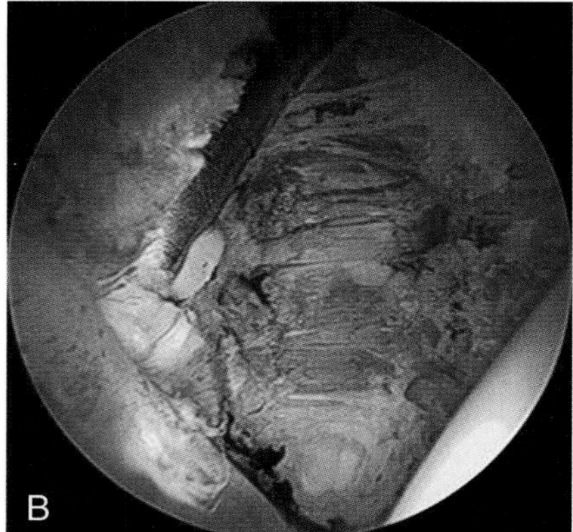

Figure 11 Arthroscopic images viewed with a 70° arthroscope in the anterolateral portal demonstrate the iliopsoas tendon (**A**) and the use of a radiofrequency ablation device placed in the modified anterior portal to release the tendon fibers under direct visualization (**B**) in a transcapsular approach.

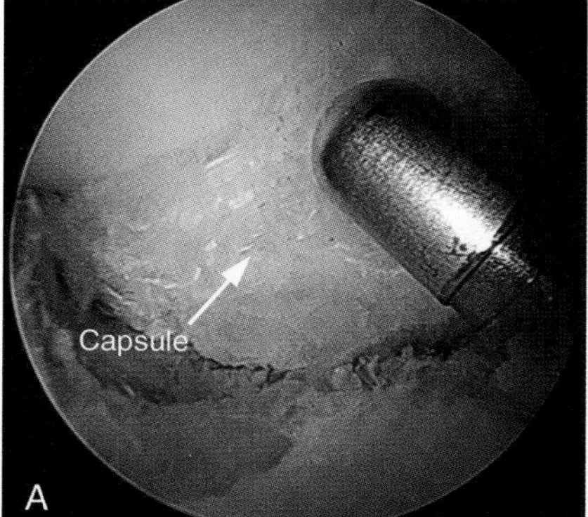

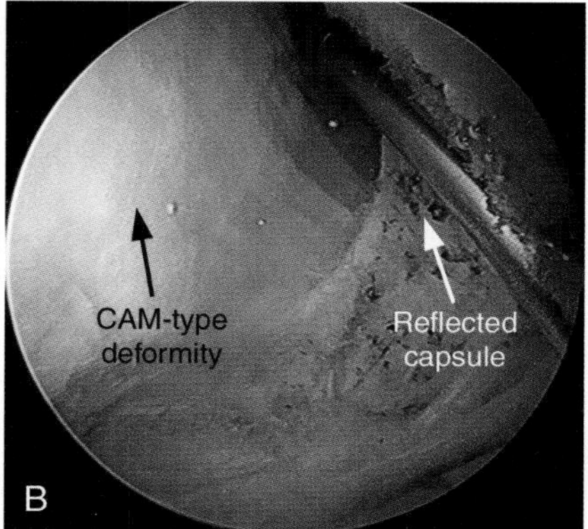

Figure 12 Arthroscopic image viewed through the distal anterolateral portal demonstrates the use of the intermuscular plane between the gluteus minimus and iliocapsularis muscles to prepare for the T-shaped capsulotomy. **B,** Arthroscopic image viewed through the distal anterolateral portal demonstrates exposure of a large and extensile cam-type deformity for circumferential resection.

Wound Closure

- The portal sites are reapproximated with the use of nylon suture in a simple, interrupted manner.
- Thin adhesive strips are applied to supplement the closure.
- A sterile dressing is placed.
- A continuous cold therapy unit is applied over the sterile dressing.
- The patient is placed in a hip flexion brace.

Postoperative Regimen

In the first 2 weeks postoperatively, the patient is allowed to perform full passive ROM hip flexion/extension as tolerated. Active hip flexion or external rotation greater than 20° is prohibited. Crutches are used. The patient is instructed to use a stationary bicycle for 20 minutes one or two times per day. In postoperative weeks 2 through 4, weight bearing is progressed, and the use of crutches is gradually discontinued. Hip ROM and strengthening of the core and hip are progressed in all directions except flexion (to avoid flexor tendinitis). In postoperative weeks 4 through 8, hip ROM and strengthening are progressed, including hip flexion. The patient is instructed to perform hip-hiking exercise on a stair climber. In postoperative weeks 8 through 12, hip and core strengthening are continued. Dynamic

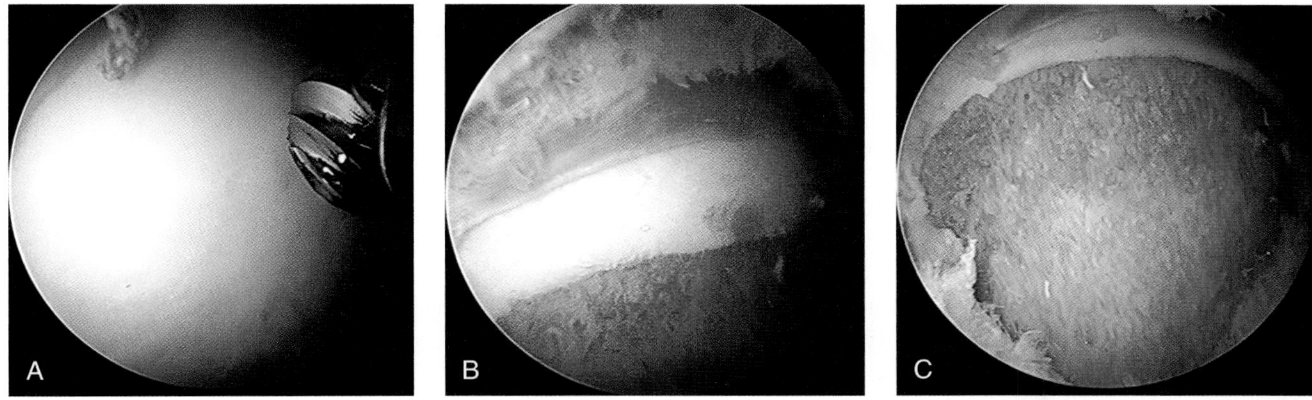

Figure 13 Arthroscopic images viewed through the distal anterolateral portal demonstrate resection of a large anterior and anterosuperior cam-type lesion via a T-shaped capsulotomy. A motorized burr (**A**) is used to identify the margins of the lesion (**B**). **C,** The cam-type lesion is resected, with care taken to preserve sphericity proximally and restore offset distally in all planes.

balance and endurance activities are performed. The patient begins a treadmill running program and sport-specific agility drills. The patient may return to sport after demonstrating satisfactory results on functional testing, including comparison with the contralateral side.

Avoiding Pitfalls and Complications

To reduce the risk of injury to the genitals and/or the pudendal nerve, a well-padded perineal post should be used and traction time minimized. To avoid injury to the sciatic nerve, hip flexion greater than 20° should be avoided when traction is applied. To minimize damage to the articular cartilage, 10 to 15 mm of radiographic joint distraction should be achieved before the joint is accessed. The capsulotomy should be performed under direct visualization to avoid iatrogenic injury. To avoid the risk of instrument breakage, the spinal needle, nitinol wire, and other instruments should be inspected for defects before use.

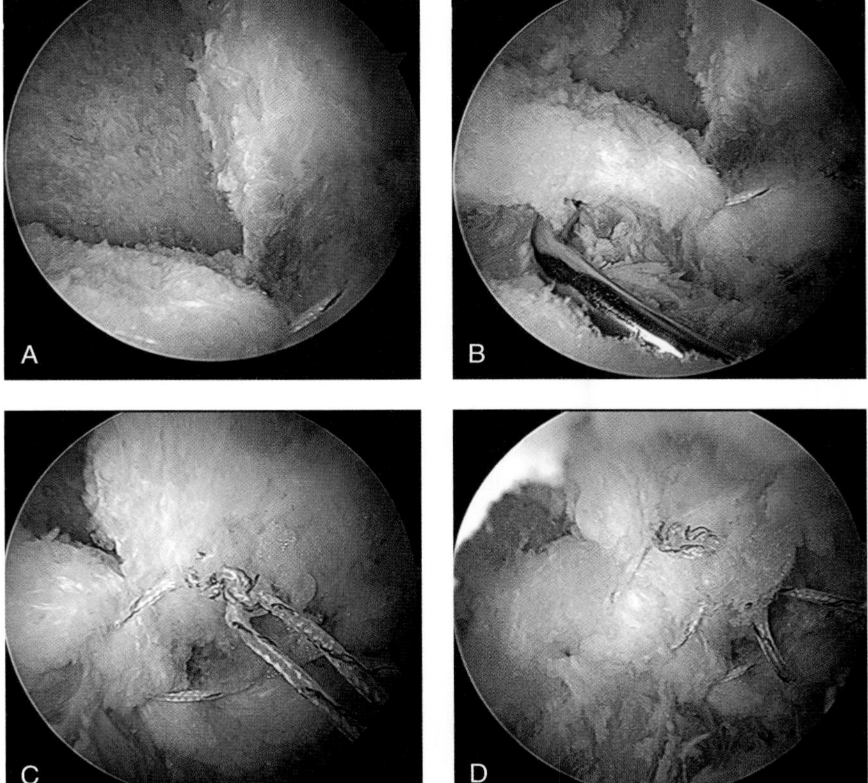

Figure 14 Arthroscopic images viewed through the distal anterolateral portal demonstrate capsular repair. **A,** The T-shaped capsulotomy is closed from distal to proximal. **B,** Horizontal mattress sutures are placed. **C,** Two or three sutures are used to reapproximate the capsule. **D,** The completed capsular repair is shown.

Bibliography

Adler RS, Buly R, Ambrose R, Sculco T: Diagnostic and therapeutic use of sonography-guided iliopsoas peritendinous injections. *AJR Am J Roentgenol* 2005;185(4):940-943.

Akimau P, Bhosale A, Harrison PE, et al: Autologous chondrocyte implantation with bone grafting for osteochondral defect due to posttraumatic osteonecrosis of the hip: A case report. *Acta Orthop* 2006;77(2):333-336.

Amenabar T, O'Donnell J: Successful treatment of isolated, partial thickness ligamentum teres (LT) tears with debridement and capsulorrhaphy. *Hip Int* 2013;23(6):576-582.

Bartlett CS, DiFelice GS, Buly RL, Quinn TJ, Green DS, Helfet DL: Cardiac arrest as a result of intraabdominal extravasation of fluid during arthroscopic removal of a loose body from the hip joint of a patient with an acetabular fracture. *J Orthop Trauma* 1998;12(4):294-299.

Bedi A, Dolan M, Hetsroni I, et al: Surgical treatment of femoroacetabular impingement improves hip kinematics: A computer-assisted model. *Am J Sports Med* 2011;39(suppl):43S-49S.

Bogunovic L, Gottlieb M, Pashos G, Baca G, Clohisy JC: Why do hip arthroscopy procedures fail? *Clin Orthop Relat Res* 2013;471(8):2523-2529.

Boykin RE, Patterson D, Briggs KK, Dee A, Philippon MJ: Results of arthroscopic labral reconstruction of the hip in elite athletes. *Am J Sports Med* 2013;41(10):2296-2301.

Buckwalter JA: Articular cartilage: Injuries and potential for healing. *J Orthop Sports Phys Ther* 1998;28(4):192-202.

Burman MS: Arthroscopy or the direct visualization of joints: An experimental cadaver study. 1931. *Clin Orthop Relat Res* 2001;(390):5-9.

Byrd JW: Hip arthroscopy utilizing the supine position. *Arthroscopy* 1994;10(3):275-280.

Byrd JW, Jones KS: Arthroscopic management of femoroacetabular impingement: Minimum 2-year follow-up. *Arthroscopy* 2011;27(10):1379-1388.

Byrd JW, Jones KS: Osteoarthritis caused by an inverted acetabular labrum: Radiographic diagnosis and arthroscopic treatment. *Arthroscopy* 2002;18(7):741-747.

Byrd JW, Jones KS: Prospective analysis of hip arthroscopy with 2-year follow-up. *Arthroscopy* 2000;16(6):578-587.

Byrd JW, Jones KS: Traumatic rupture of the ligamentum teres as a source of hip pain. *Arthroscopy* 2004;20(4):385-391.

Chandrasekaran S, Darwish N, Gui C, Lodhia P, Suarez-Ahedo C, Domb BG: Outcomes of hip arthroscopy in patients with Tönnis grade-2 osteoarthritis at a mean 2-year follow-up: Evaluation using a matched-pair analysis with Tönnis grade-0 and grade-1 cohorts. *J Bone Joint Surg Am* 2016;98(12):973-982.

Colvin AC, Harrast J, Harner C: Trends in hip arthroscopy. *J Bone Joint Surg Am* 2012;94(4):e23.

de SA D, Phillips M, Philippon MJ, Letkemann S, Simunovic N, Ayeni OR: Ligamentum teres injuries of the hip: A systematic review examining surgical indications, treatment options, and outcomes. *Arthroscopy* 2014;30(12):1634-1641.

Domb BG, Gui C, Lodhia P: How much arthritis is too much for hip arthroscopy: A systematic review. *Arthroscopy* 2015;31(3):520-529.

Ejnisman L, Philippon MJ, Lertwanich P: Acetabular labral tears: Diagnosis, repair, and a method for labral reconstruction. *Clin Sports Med* 2011;30(2):317-329.

El Bitar YF, Stake CE, Dunne KF, Botser IB, Domb BG: Arthroscopic iliopsoas fractional lengthening for internal snapping of the hip: Clinical outcomes with a minimum 2-year follow-up. *Am J Sports Med* 2014;42(7):1696-1703.

Epstein HC: Traumatic dislocations of the hip. *Clin Orthop Relat Res* 1973;(92):116-142.

Fabricant PD, Bedi A, De La Torre K, Kelly BT: Clinical outcomes after arthroscopic psoas lengthening: The effect of femoral version. *Arthroscopy* 2012;28(7):965-971.

Ferguson SJ, Bryant JT, Ganz R, Ito K: An in vitro investigation of the acetabular labral seal in hip joint mechanics. *J Biomech* 2003;36(2):171-178.

Geyer MR, Philippon MJ, Fagrelius TS, Briggs KK: Acetabular labral reconstruction with an iliotibial band autograft: Outcome and survivorship analysis at minimum 3-year follow-up. *Am J Sports Med* 2013;41(8):1750-1756.

Gray AJ, Villar RN: The ligamentum teres of the hip: An arthroscopic classification of its pathology. *Arthroscopy* 1997;13(5):575-578.

Ilizaliturri VM Jr, Villalobos FE Jr, Chaidez PA, Valero FS, Aguilera JM: Internal snapping hip syndrome: Treatment by endoscopic release of the iliopsoas tendon. *Arthroscopy* 2005;21(11):1375-1380.

Karthikeyan S, Roberts S, Griffin D: Microfracture for acetabular chondral defects in patients with femoroacetabular impingement: Results at second-look arthroscopic surgery. *Am J Sports Med* 2012;40(12):2725-2730.

Krych AJ, Lorich DG, Kelly BT: Treatment of focal osteochondral defects of the acetabulum with osteochondral allograft transplantation. *Orthopedics* 2011;34(7):e307-e311.

Lee JB, Kang C, Lee CH, Kim PS, Hwang DS: Arthroscopic treatment of synovial chondromatosis of the hip. *Am J Sports Med* 2012;40(6):1412-1418.

Mardones RM, Gonzalez C, Chen Q, Zobitz M, Kaufman KR, Trousdale RT: Surgical treatment of femoroacetabular impingement: Evaluation of the effect of the size of the resection. *J Bone Joint Surg Am* 2005;87(2):273-279.

McCarthy JC, Lee JA: Arthroscopic intervention in early hip disease. *Clin Orthop Relat Res* 2004;(429):157-162.

Mullis BH, Dahners LE: Hip arthroscopy to remove loose bodies after traumatic dislocation. *J Orthop Trauma* 2006;20(1):22-26.

O'Leary JA, Berend K, Vail TP: The relationship between diagnosis and outcome in arthroscopy of the hip. *Arthroscopy* 2001;17(2):181-188.

Philippon MJ: The role of arthroscopic thermal capsulorrhaphy in the hip. *Clin Sports Med* 2001;20(4):817-829.

Philippon MJ, Briggs KK, Hay CJ, Kuppersmith DA, Dewing CB, Huang MJ: Arthroscopic labral reconstruction in the hip using iliotibial band autograft: Technique and early outcomes. *Arthroscopy* 2010;26(6):750-756.

Philippon MJ, Briggs KK, Yen YM, Kuppersmith DA: Outcomes following hip arthroscopy for femoroacetabular impingement with associated chondrolabral dysfunction: Minimum two-year follow-up. *J Bone Joint Surg Br* 2009;91(1):16-23.

Philippon MJ, Pennock A, Gaskill TR: Arthroscopic reconstruction of the ligamentum teres: Technique and early outcomes. *J Bone Joint Surg Br* 2012;94(11):1494-1498.

Philippon MJ, Schenker ML: Arthroscopy for the treatment of femoroacetabular impingement in the athlete. *Clin Sports Med* 2006;25(2):299-308, ix.

Philippon MJ, Schenker ML, Briggs KK, Maxwell RB: Can microfracture produce repair tissue in acetabular chondral defects? *Arthroscopy* 2008;24(1):46-50.

Ross JR, Bedi A, Stone RM, et al: Intraoperative fluoroscopic imaging to treat cam deformities: Correlation with 3-dimensional computed tomography. *Am J Sports Med* 2014;42(6):1370-1376.

Santori N, Villar RN: Acetabular labral tears: Result of arthroscopic partial limbectomy. *Arthroscopy* 2000;16(1):11-15.

Steadman JR, Briggs KK, Rodrigo JJ, Kocher MS, Gill TJ, Rodkey WG: Outcomes of microfracture for traumatic chondral defects of the knee: Average 11-year follow-up. *Arthroscopy* 2003;19(5):477-484.

Takagi K: The classic: Arthroscope. Kenji Takagi. J. Jap. Orthop. Assoc., 1939. *Clin Orthop Relat Res* 1982;(167):6-8.

Chapter 65

Hip Arthroscopy for the Management of Nonstructural Problems

Christopher M. Larson, MD
Ryan A. Mlynarek, MD
Rebecca M. Stone, MS, ATC
Asheesh Bedi, MD

Indications

Capsular and Soft-Tissue Laxity

Hip pain often presents a diagnostic challenge. In the general population, the hip joint has both static and dynamic stability. Trauma or acute dislocation may disrupt this stability, resulting in fracture or injury to the labrum, the capsule, or the surrounding soft tissues. Additionally, surgeons have increasingly recognized that hypermobility and capsular and soft-tissue laxity can contribute to microinstability and resultant pain about the hip. Patients with these conditions are often athletes who participate in sports requiring deep flexion and repetitive twisting or pivoting of the hip. These increased rotational and translational forces may be combined with a subtle bony abnormality that adds to the stress of the dynamic stabilizers of the hip, resulting in capsulolabral strain, stretch, or tear. This condition seems to be more common in women than in men. Patients often have anterior groin pain, occasional subluxation, increased range of motion (ROM) of the hip, and reproducible pain with flexion, adduction, and internal rotation (FADIR) impingement testing. Generalized hypermobility can be assessed with the Beighton score. Less commonly, the patient may have an existing or suspected diagnosis of connective tissue disorder (Ehlers-Danlos or Marfan syndrome). Plain radiographs demonstrate normal acetabular morphology with subtle or no dysplastic features, or mild impingement with distal sclerosis of the femoral neck is observed on lateral femoral radiographs. These findings are consistent with slightly increased femoral anteversion and increased ROM and, therefore, elevated contact points between the femur and acetabulum. In select patients, an image-guided intra-articular anesthetic injection helps verify the hip joint as the source of pain. MRI may reveal evidence of capsular laxity, high capsular volume, and/or associated chondrolabral injury. If nonsurgical measures such as core stability exercises and reasonable activity modification do not improve a patient's symptoms, arthroscopic surgical management may be considered. Historically, thermal capsulorrhaphy was commonly performed to manage capsular laxity. Because of increasing evidence that use of capsulorrhaphy to address shoulder laxity results in chondrolysis, capsular plication has become the mainstay of surgical treatment.

Synovial Disorders

Synovial disorders, such as synovial chondromatosis, synovial osteochondromatosis, and pigmented villonodular synovitis (PVNS), can be managed via an arthroscopic approach. Synovial chondromatosis and osteochondromatosis represent a spectrum of intrasynovial metaplasia of pluripotent cells, resulting in the formation of both intra- and extra-articular loose bodies. These loose bodies may cause mechanical symptoms and progressive erosive changes at the articular or periarticular surfaces. Synovial chondromatosis and osteochondromatosis are most common in men aged 20 to 50 years and often cause an insidious onset of deep groin pain. PVNS is a benign but disabling proliferative disorder of the synovial lining. It is characterized by the deposition of

Dr. Larson or an immediate family member serves as a paid consultant to Smith & Nephew and A3 Surgical; has stock or stock options held in A3 Surgical; and has received research or institutional support from Smith & Nephew. Dr. Bedi or an immediate family member serves as a paid consultant to Arthrex; has stock or stock options held in A3 Surgical; and serves as a board member, owner, officer, or committee member of the American Orthopaedic Society for Sports Medicine. Neither of the following authors nor any immediate family member has received anything of value from or has stock or stock options held in a commercial company or institution related directly or indirectly to the subject of this chapter: Dr. Mlynarek and Ms. Stone.

hemosiderin-laden macrophages within the synovial membrane, leading to villi and nodular thickening and can be either focal or diffuse. Although the precise etiology of PVNS remains unclear, recent studies support the theory that the disease is a combination of a reactive inflammatory process and chromosomal translocation resulting in neoplastic proliferation of the synovium. PVNS occurs most frequently in patients aged 20 to 40 years and causes monoarticular stiffness and pain at rest. Mechanical symptoms are infrequent but can occur if a large, focal pedunculated mass is present. Diagnostic workup should begin with plain radiographs. However, radiographs often are insufficient to diagnose loose body formation because calcium deposition varies. Radiographs may demonstrate erosive changes in patients with progressive disease.

MRI is the imaging modality of choice to evaluate synovial disorders. In patients with synovial chondromatosis, ossified loose bodies exhibit low signal intensity on both T1- and T2-weighted images. Nonossified loose bodies demonstrate low signal intensity on T1-weighted images and high signal intensity on T2-weighted images. In patients with PVNS, the hemosiderin-laden macrophages within the synovial proliferation exhibit low signal intensity on both T1- and T2-weighted images. On gradient-recalled echo sequence imaging, a characteristic so-called blooming artifact, which is a result of the paramagnetic effects of the iron, is observed.

Synovial chondromatosis and PVNS can be predictably managed with hip arthroscopy if disease is limited to the foveal, medial femoral neck region, or the anterior hip joint. Patients with more diffuse PVNS or synovial chondromatosis with extensive posterior hip involvement may be more thoroughly treated with an open approach, such as surgical dislocation. Multiple short- and midterm clinical outcome studies have shown that the symptoms of diffuse PVNS and synovial chondromatosis with posterior hip involvement can be managed arthroscopically; however, this strategy can be technically challenging and time consuming.

Traumatic Labral Tears and Ligamentum Teres Injuries

Labral tears and ligamentum teres injuries can occasionally occur in the absence of substantial femoroacetabular impingement (FAI) or dysplasia as a result of twisting, hyperflexion injuries, lateral impact injuries, or traumatic subluxation or dislocation. Patients may experience pain, mechanical symptoms, and, less frequently, instability. If time, activity modification, and core stability exercises do not relieve symptoms, MRI may be performed to confirm a labral or ligamentum teres injury. However, ligamentum teres injuries can be difficult to detect on MRI. A diagnostic anesthetic injection is occasionally helpful to verify the hip joint as the source of pain before diagnostic and therapeutic arthroscopic hip procedures are considered. If nonsurgical management is unsuccessful and the diagnosis is confirmed via appropriate imaging, the use of arthroscopic labral repair and/or ligamentum teres débridement techniques may be considered. Historically, most labral tears were managed with débridement. However, in recent years surgeons have begun to perform labral repair to maintain the long-term integrity of the hip joint if the tear is amenable to repair.

Internal Snapping Hip Syndrome (Iliopsoas Impingement)

Internal snapping hip syndrome is caused by abrasion of the iliopsoas tendon over the iliopectineal eminence or the labrum and femoral head-neck junction. This abrasion can be asymptomatically reproduced in approximately 10% of the normal population when the hip is brought to full extension, adduction, and internal rotation from a 90° flexed, abducted, and externally rotated position. The snapping may be symptomatic, especially in athletes such as dancers and gymnasts who require exceptional flexibility with repetitive flexion and rotational moments. Most patients require only an explanation of the condition, avoidance of voluntary snapping, physical therapy, and, infrequently, a corticosteroid injection in the iliopsoas bursa. Uncommonly, a patient may experience recalcitrant, disabling internal snapping. In these patients, an endoscopic iliopsoas tenotomy may be considered. However, this treatment strategy should be avoided in patients who have substantial dysplastic morphologies or excessive femoral anteversion.

Endoscopic iliopsoas tenotomy also may be considered in patients with iliopsoas impingement after total hip arthroplasty (THA). The reported incidence of iliopsoas impingement after primary THA is approximately 4.3%. This impingement is most commonly associated with a prominent anteroinferior rim of the acetabular implant, which is either oversized or relatively less anteverted than normal (**Figure 1, A**). The impingement also can be caused by the presence of extruded cement, a reinforcement ring in a patient who has undergone revision surgery, or excessive offset or lengthening of the affected limb. Patients typically experience severe pain with active hip flexion, frequently noticed when entering or exiting a vehicle. Cross-table lateral radiographs may reveal the anterior prominence of the acetabular implant suggestive of the diagnosis, which can be confirmed with the use of dynamic ultrasonography combined with iliopsoas bursal corticosteroid injection. If a patient experiences temporary but short-lasting relief and continued disability after physical therapy, endoscopic release of the iliopsoas tendon at the level of the central compartment

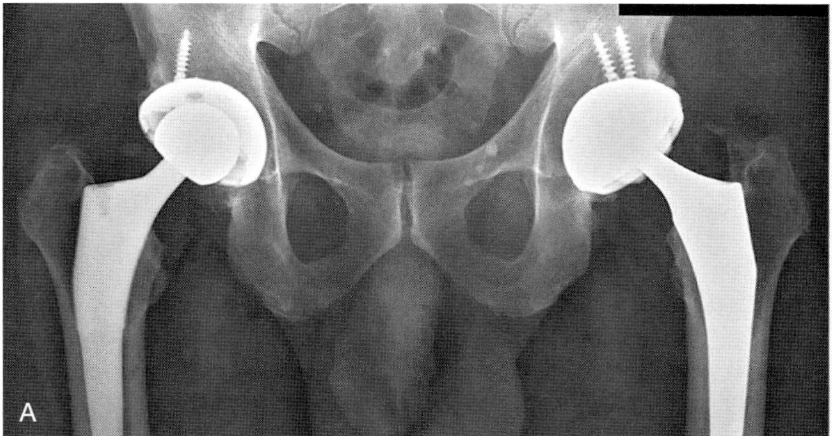

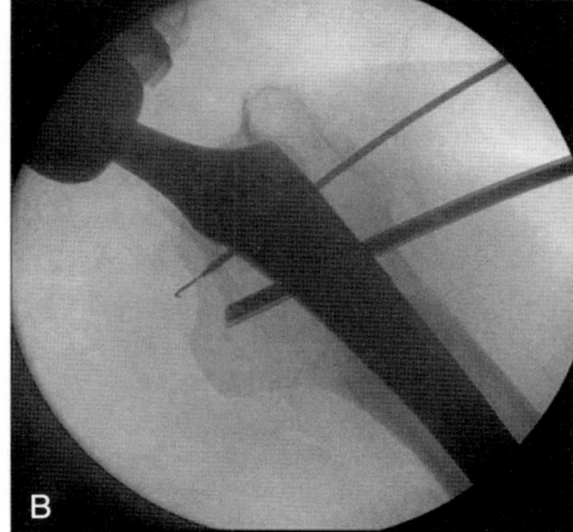

Figure 1 Images of a man who underwent bilateral total hip arthroplasty and has symptoms of iliopsoas tendinitis. **A,** AP pelvic radiograph demonstrates retroversion of the left acetabular implant. **B,** Intraoperative fluoroscopic image demonstrates endoscopic access to the left lesser trochanter in preparation for iliopsoas release.

or lesser trochanter may be considered (**Figure 1, B**).

Loose Bodies

Loose body formation can result from synovial disorders, Legg-Calvé-Perthes disease, osteoarthritis, bony avulsion of the ligamentum teres, the presence of foreign bodies from penetrating trauma such as a bullet or shrapnel, or traumatic subluxation or dislocation. The presence of loose bodies may cause mechanical symptoms and can lead to progressive damage of the articular cartilage. Arthroscopic retrieval of loose bodies is indicated in patients who have mechanical symptoms and minimal to no degenerative osteoarthritis.

Septic Arthritis of the Hip

Septic arthritis of the hip is a surgical emergency. Ramifications of the disease process can result in devastating complications such as systemic sepsis, chondrolysis, osteomyelitis, osteonecrosis of the femoral head, and osteoarthritis. Prompt diagnosis and treatment requires the clinician to assimilate clinical, radiographic, and laboratory data. Clinically, a patient with septic arthritis may have a history of fever, chills, increasing hip pain, inability to bear weight, or irritability with passive ROM of the hip. Plain radiographs often appear normal. Advanced imaging may demonstrate an effusion, early chondral destruction, or osteomyelitis. Laboratory studies often reveal leukocytosis, elevated inflammatory markers (erythrocyte sedimentation rate and C-reactive protein level), and, in samples obtained from image-guided aspiration of the hip, elevated synovial white blood cell count with left-shift differential and/or Gram stain consistent with bacterial infection. Open arthrotomy, the standard treatment for patients with septic arthritis, requires an extensive surgical approach and may require surgical dislocation, thus increasing the risk of osteonecrosis and postoperative instability. Arthroscopic irrigation and débridement has become an established and effective option for the management of septic arthritis of the hip.

Contraindications

Despite the expanding indications for hip arthroscopy, surgeons must recognize the limitations of this valuable tool. In a patient with capsular laxity and hypermobility, a predominance of bony dysplastic features (that is, lateral center-edge angle less than 20°, anterior center-edge angle less than15°, and Tönnis angle greater than13°) is a contraindication to arthroscopic treatment. The authors of this chapter also consider any lateral femoral subluxation or a break in the Shenton line a contraindication to hip arthroscopy.

In patients with synovial disorders of the hip, diffuse and posteriorly based pathology is extremely challenging to manage adequately; therefore, the authors of this chapter recommend open surgical management. Posteriorly located loose bodies, especially in patients with synovial chondromatosis, can be successfully retrieved with a combination of irrigation and suction via multiple portals. Moderate to severe osteoarthritis is a relative contraindication to the arthroscopic retrieval of loose bodies, especially in patients in whom aching nighttime pain, not mechanical symptoms, is the predominant symptom.

Iliopsoas tenotomy should be avoided in patients with instability, bony dysplastic morphologies, or excessive femoral anteversion. Likewise, iliopsoas tenotomy after THA should be performed only if all other possible diagnoses of persistent anterior hip pain after THA have been excluded. A thorough diagnostic workup should be performed to rule out aseptic loosening, implant malposition, and infection. Several diagnostic and therapeutic image-guided corticosteroid injections of the iliopsoas tendon may be performed to diagnose and temporarily manage iliopsoas impingement before surgical management is considered.

Other contraindications to hip arthroscopy include hip ankylosis, substantial soft-tissue contractures, and substantial heterotopic ossification or other limitations that may preclude adequate portal access.

Alternative Treatments

Alternatives to surgical treatment include a well-designed core stabilization rehabilitation program, reasonable activity modification based on a patient's profile and desires, NSAIDs, and the occasional use of intra-articular and iliopsoas bursal corticosteroid injections. Surgical alternatives for the management of capsular and soft-tissue laxity include hip arthroscopy and mini-open capsular plication, as well as surgical hip dislocation, which allows for complete management of chondrolabral injury, associated FAI, and capsular laxity. Surgical hip dislocation also is an effective alternative for the management of synovial disorders, especially in patients in whom pathology is diffuse or posteriorly based. Surgical hip dislocation is a reasonable alternative for the management of traumatic labral tears and ligamentum teres injuries and allows for the management of associated FAI and capsular injury in patients with prior subluxation or dislocation; however, surgical hip dislocation requires sacrifice of the already injured ligamentum teres. Iliopsoas impingement in the native hip and after THA can be managed with an open approach; however, arthroscopy or endoscopy offers potentially less morbidity and allows for additional evaluation of the hip joint if necessary. Loose bodies and septic arthritis of the hip can be surgically managed with mini-open or arthrotomy approaches. In some patients, posterior loose bodies and extensive synovial disease can be managed with surgical hip dislocation.

Results

Hip arthroscopy has continued to grow in popularity in the past decade. From 2003 to 2009, the number of hip arthroscopy procedures performed by candidates for American Board of Orthopaedic Surgery certification increased 18-fold. More importantly, advances in the understanding of pathologies about the hip, imaging technologies, and surgical techniques have resulted in good to excellent short- and midterm outcomes for patients who undergo arthroscopic hip procedures. As this field continues to expand, treating surgeons should evaluate the available outcome studies and practice evidence-based medicine (**Table 1**).

Techniques

Setup/Access

- Hip arthroscopy can be performed with the patient in the supine or lateral decubitus position. Most surgeons, including the authors of this chapter, prefer supine patient positioning.
- The authors of this chapter use either a standard fracture table or a commercially available surgical table that facilitates the use of traction and intraoperative dynamic manipulation of the hip.
- Preoperative examination of the affected and nonsurgical hips is performed with the patient under anesthesia to evaluate passive ROM, with specific attention to hip flexion, internal rotation in 90° of flexion, and external rotation in 90° of flexion.
- The patient's feet are well padded to prevent pedal neurapraxia and are placed in surgical traction boots, which facilitate adequate instrumentation of the central compartment.
- The perineal post is positioned slightly lateral to the midline and is well padded to help prevent pudendal and perineal neurapraxia. The position of the perineal post also provides a lateral force vector to facilitate joint distraction.
- The affected hip is positioned in neutral abduction, 10° of flexion, and 15° of internal rotation.
- The minimum amount of traction necessary to facilitate 6 to 8 mm of joint distraction for portal placement is applied.

PORTAL PLACEMENT

- The hip is first accessed via the anterolateral portal, which is established under fluoroscopic guidance.
- The interval between the gluteus medius and the tensor fascia lata is palpated. This interval lies approximately 1 to 2 cm anterior and 1 to 2 cm proximal to the anterosuperior corner of the greater trochanter. Portals based farther distally would allow a better angle for suture anchor placement and microfracture but less satisfactory access to the lunate fossae.
- A spinal needle is placed under fluoroscopic guidance. The surgeon should aim for the distal third of the distracted hip joint. Care is taken not to penetrate the capsule too close to the acetabular rim (to avoid injury to the labrum) or too close to the femoral head (to avoid chondral injury).
- It is helpful to vent the joint by penetrating the capsule to allow decompression, which facilitates further distraction without added

traction because the penetration of the needle releases the intracapsular pressure.

- After the spinal needle is in the appropriate position, a nitinol wire is placed through the spinal needle until it contacts the medial acetabular fossa. After the nitinol wire is in place, the spinal needle is removed.
- A cannula is inserted over the nitinol wire. The trajectory of the insertion often is confirmed via fluoroscopy because the nitinol wire is flexible and can bend or break if the cannula is not inserted coaxially to the wire.
- After the cannula is in place, the arthroscope is inserted through this portal.
- The mobility of the anterolateral portal is evaluated. Restricted motion may indicate that the portal was placed through the labrum; therefore, the surgeon must not sweep the cannula to gain mobility.
- The modified anterior portal is established under direct visualization with the arthroscope in the anterolateral portal.
- The modified anterior portal is placed approximately 1 to 2 cm lateral and 1 to 2 cm distal to the location of a standard anterior portal, which typically is placed at the intersection of a line from the anterior superior iliac spine to the lateral aspect of the knee and a horizontal line at the level of the greater trochanter. The position of the modified anterior portal increases the distance from the lateral femoral cutaneous nerve and improves the trajectory for instrumentation and suture anchor placement.
- Under direct visualization from the anterolateral portal, the modified anterior portal is established with the use of a spinal needle, followed by the use of a nitinol wire and cannula, as described previously.
- After the modified anterior portal is established, the arthroscope is switched from the anterolateral portal to the modified anterior portal to evaluate the placement of the cannula in the anterolateral portal. If the cannula was placed through the labrum, the cannula is removed and replaced under direct visualization with the use of a spinal needle, nitinol wire, and cannula.

INTERPORTAL CAPSULOTOMY

- A beaver blade is inserted through the anterolateral cannula to make the transverse interportal capsulotomy.
- After the blade is located in the central compartment, the cannula is backed out to maximize mobility of the instrument and allow for a complete capsulotomy. Care is taken to avoid injury to the labrum and femoral head and to preserve full-thickness margins for subsequent repair.
- The arthroscope is switched back to the anterolateral portal.
- The beaver blade is inserted through the modified anterior portal to complete the interportal capsulotomy under direct visualization.

Procedures

CAPSULAR AND SOFT-TISSUE LAXITY

- The patient is prepared and draped in the supine position as described previously in this chapter.
- The least amount of traction required for joint distraction is applied and confirmed with the use of fluoroscopy. Because of capsular laxity, less traction than usual may be necessary.
- The anterolateral portal is accessed first.
- The modified anterior portal is accessed under direct visualization.
- A thorough diagnostic arthroscopy is performed, with special attention paid to the capsulolabral structures.
- After diagnostic arthroscopy, any labral tears are addressed with a labral base configuration, as described later in this chapter, to restore the femoroacetabular suction seal and enhance stability.
- To begin the plication technique, an interportal capsulotomy is performed under direct visualization with the use of a beaver blade to expand the working space and mobilize the capsular tissues for plication (**Figure 2, A**).
- Traction is released, and the hip is flexed 20° to 30°.
- A working cannula is used in the anterolateral portal.
- A suture-passing device is used to penetrate the distal limb of the capsule and retrieve the suture through the proximal limb. A No. 2 absorbable or nonabsorbable suture is shuttled through the tissue (**Figure 2, B**).
- A knot pusher is used to approximate the plication to ensure adequate tissue tension. If necessary, multiple passes may be made to gather the redundant capsule, or more capsular tissue can be removed, resulting in greater degrees of plication (**Figure 2, C**).
- Typically, three to six sutures are placed to complete the capsular plication.
- To complete the closure of the anteromedial capsule, the anterolateral portal can be repositioned farther anteriorly. Alternatively, the working portal can be switched to complete the plication.
- A distal anterolateral accessory portal may be established under direct visualization to provide adequate access to the peripheral compartment.
- The authors of this chapter prefer to use a linear configuration of capsular sutures. However, several methods, including the multi-pleated capsular plication technique

Table 1 Results of Arthroscopic Procedures for the Management of Nonstructural Hip Pathology

Authors (Year)	Number of Patients	Procedure	Mean Patient Age in Years (Range)	Mean Follow-up in Months (Range)	Results[a]
Gédouin and Huten (2012)	10	Endoscopic tenotomy for the management of iliopsoas tendinopathy after THA	58 (45-80)	20 (12-60)	8 patients experienced complete relief of symptoms 2 patients experienced partial relief of symptoms Hip flexion muscle force returned to baseline function at a mean of 3.2 mo postoperatively Mean WOMAC score, 84 (range, 60-95) No reported complications
Larson et al (2012)	94	Arthroscopic labral débridement/ excision (44) or labral refixation (50) after correction of femoroacetabular impingement	Labral débridement group: 32 (16-57) Labral refixation group: 28 (16-52)	Labral débridement group: 44 (24-72) Labral refixation group: 41 (24-56)	At a mean 3.5-yr follow-up, subjective outcome scores showed significant improvement in both groups ($P < 0.01$) Postoperative HHS ($P = 0.001$), SF-12 ($P = 0.041$), and visual analog scale pain ($P = 0.004$) scores were all significantly better in the labral refixation group than in the labral débridement group Good to excellent results were reported in 68% of the labral débridement group and 92% of the labral refixation group
Lee et al (2012)	24	Loose body retrieval and synovectomy for the management of synovial chondromatosis	43 (32-63)	41 (12-133)	Significant improvement in clinical outcome scores (modified HHS [$P = 0.02$], UCLA activity scale [$P = 0.01$], visual analog scale [$P = 0.02$]) and ROM testing 18 patients reported good or excellent results Symptomatic disease recurred in 4 patients, 1 of whom required subsequent THA
Byrd et al (2013)	13	Arthroscopic partial synovectomy for the management of pigmented villonodular synovitis	27 (14-46)	63 (24-120)	Significant improvement in modified HHS scores ($P < 0.001$), with greatest improvement in patients with a diffuse pattern of pigmented villonodular synovitis 4 patients had concomitant grade IV articular cartilage lesions 1 patient underwent THA at 6 yr postoperatively Of the 7 patients who underwent follow-up MRI, 1 patient had evidence of residual but reduced synovial disease

HHS = Harris hip score, HOS-ADL = Hip Outcome score–activities of daily living, HOS-SSS = Hip Outcome score–sport-specific subscale, NA = not available, NAHS = Non-Arthritic Hip Score, ROM = range of motion, SF-12 = Medical Outcomes Study 12-Item Short Form, THA = total hip arthroplasty, UCLA = University of California–Los Angeles, WOMAC = Western Ontario and McMaster Universities Osteoarthritis Index.

[a] All reported outcome measures are mean values.

[b] 7.6% were lost to follow-up.

Table 1 Results of Arthroscopic Procedures for the Management of Nonstructural Hip Pathology (*continued*)

Authors (Year)	Number of Patients	Procedure	Mean Patient Age in Years (Range)	Mean Follow-up in Months (Range)	Results[a]
Domb et al (2013)	26	Capsular plication	20 (14-39)	27.5 (17-39)	Significant improvement in all clinical outcome scores (modified HHS, NAHS, HOS-SSS, HOS-ADL) and in visual analog scale scores ($P < 0.0001$ for each) Significant reduction in external rotation from 59° to 48° ($P = 0.007$) 17 patients reported good to excellent results 2 patients underwent revision arthroscopy for repeat capsular plication
de Sa et al (2014)	197[b]	Systematic review of arthroscopic management of synovial chondromatosis	42 (13-81)	NA (1-184)	Systematic review of 14 studies, with a pooled recurrence rate of 7.1% (14 of 197 patients) after removal of intra-articular osteochondral fragments and partial or complete synovectomy 1% rate of minor complications (transient perineal or pedal neurapraxia)
Jackson et al (2014)	54	Labral repair using base repair technique	29 (14-57)	28 (20-49)	Significant improvement in all clinical outcome scores (modified HHS, NAHS, HOS-ADL, HOS-SSS [$P < 0.0001$ for each]) 46 patients reported good to excellent results 3 patients underwent revision arthroscopy 2 patients underwent THA
Nelson and Keene (2014)	30	Arthroscopic iliopsoas tenotomy at the level of the central compartment	35 (15-57)	23 (12-37)	23 patients experienced complete resolution of their pain and hip snapping 3 patients experienced recurrent snapping of the tendon, 2 of whom underwent arthroscopic release at the level of the lesser trochanter to relieve their symptoms
de Sa et al (2015)	65	Systematic review of arthroscopic management of septic arthritis of the hip	24.5 (2.4-83)	19 (6-84)	All 11 studies demonstrated substantial improvements in pain and function Initial rate of infection eradication was 100% 1 hip required revision arthroscopy for recurrent methicillin-resistant *Staphylococcus aureus* infection

HHS = Harris hip score, HOS-ADL = Hip Outcome score–activities of daily living, HOS-SSS = Hip Outcome score–sport-specific subscale, NA = not available, NAHS = Non-Arthritic Hip Score, ROM = range of motion, SF-12 = Medical Outcomes Study 12-Item Short Form, THA = total hip arthroplasty, UCLA = University of California–Los Angeles, WOMAC = Western Ontario and McMaster Universities Osteoarthritis Index.

[a] All reported outcome measures are mean values.

[b] 7.6% were lost to follow-up.

frequently used in shoulder surgery, have been described. • Stability is evaluated via gentle

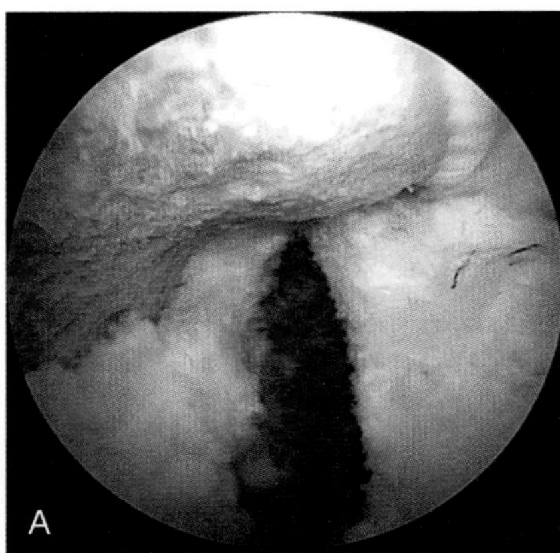

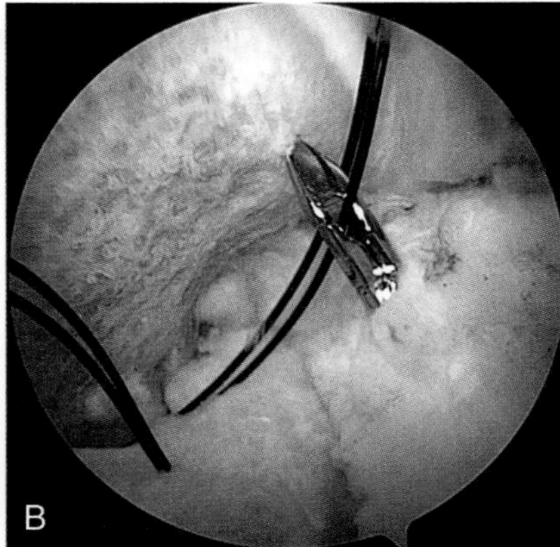

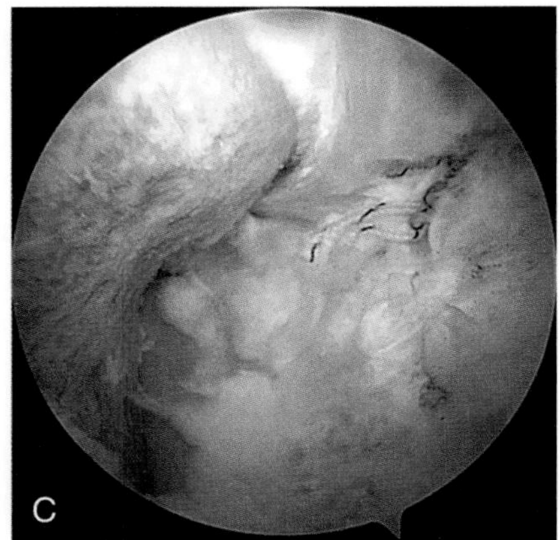

Figure 2 Arthroscopic images of a hip through the modified anterior portal show capsular plication. **A,** Under direct visualization, a beaver blade is used to perform a capsulotomy to expand the working space and mobilize the capsular tissues for plication. **B,** A suture-passing device is used to penetrate the distal limb of the capsule to shuttle a suture for plication. **C,** The capsulotomy is plicated to ensure adequate tissue tension.

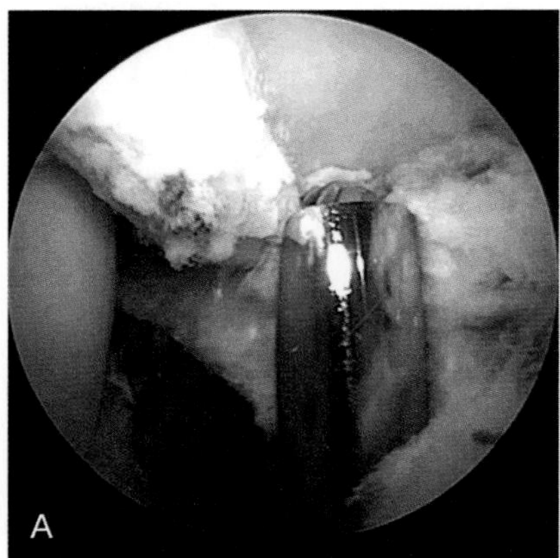

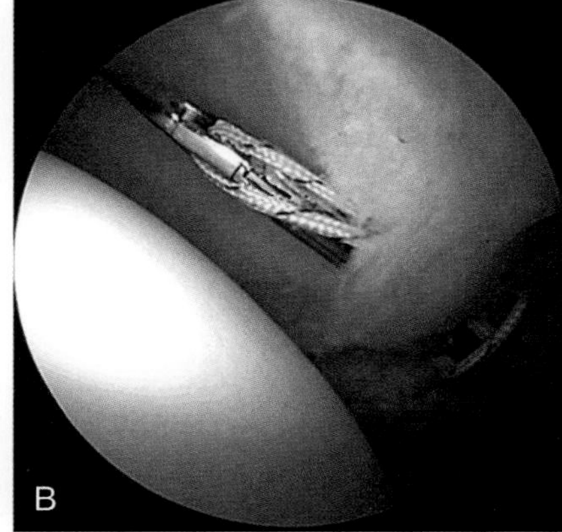

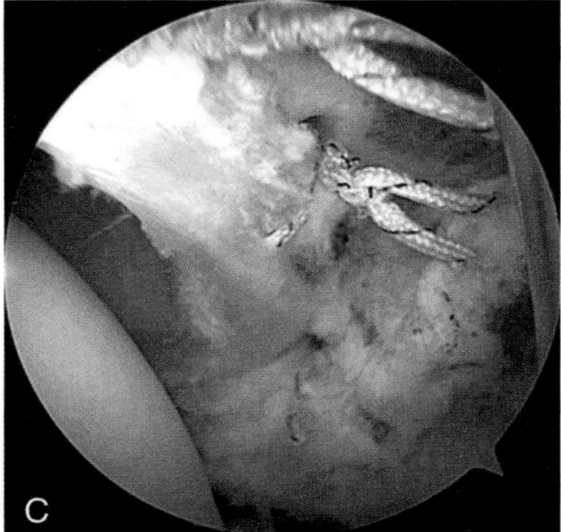

Figure 3 Arthroscopic images of a hip through the distal anterolateral portal show labral refixation. **A,** A motorized shaver is used to prepare the acetabular rim for suture anchor placement. **B,** A suture-passing device is used to pass a single suture limb through the chondrolabral junction. The suture limb is retrieved through the outer edge of the labrum. **C,** After suture passage, the labral base repair configuration is complete.

ROM of the hip, and rotational ROM is compared with preoperative assessments.

SYNOVIAL DISORDERS

- The central compartment is accessed via the anterolateral and modified anterior portals, with the use of minimal traction to gain safe access to the joint.
- Under direct visualization, an interportal capsulotomy is made with the use of a beaver blade to maximize maneuverability within the central compartment.
- Both 30° and 70° arthroscopes are used to assess the entire central compartment for loose body retrieval and systematically evaluate the synovium. The labrum, medial femoral head, acetabular fossa, and pulvinar are evaluated. Evaluation of the acetabular fossa is critical and is best done with the 30° arthroscope from the anterolateral portal because this location is commonly affected by synovial disorders.
- Loose bodies are removed with the use of graspers.
- Lesions entrapped by the synovium may be mobilized with the use of a motorized shaver.
- Management of both PVNS and synovial chondromatosis should include a thorough synovectomy of both the affected and normal-appearing synovium to minimize recurrence.
- Because PVNS lesions can be resistant to standard motorized shaving, the authors of this chapter recommend the use of an aggressive grasper for synovectomy. Biopsy samples of suspected lesions are

sent for pathologic analysis to confirm the diagnosis.

- Hemostasis is attained with the use of a radiofrequency ablation device.
- The anterior, superior, and posterior capsule is evaluated. Any suspected lesions are removed; however, the surgeon should use conservative judgment to avoid over-resection of capsular lesions, which may cause iatrogenic instability.
- Traction is released, and the hip is flexed to approximately 30° to allow the surgeon to evaluate the peripheral compartment.
- The distal anterolateral accessory portal is placed under direct visualization, as described previously in this chapter.
- The peripheral compartment is methodically evaluated for loose bodies and synovial lesions. Care is taken to inspect all areas of the compartment.

TRAUMATIC LABRAL TEARS AND LIGAMENTUM TERES INJURIES

- The standard anterolateral, modified anterior, and distal anterolateral accessory portals are used.
- A diagnostic arthroscopic examination is performed, and associated pathology is addressed.
- The labrum is evaluated systematically from anterior to posterior via the anterolateral and modified anterior portals.
- A radiofrequency ablation device may be used to clear any adjacent capsule and adjacent synovitis to clearly define the labrum.
- Frayed, nonviable tissue is débrided with the use of a motorized shaver, with care taken to maintain as much viable labrum as possible for repair.
- After the tear is identified and nonviable tissue is débrided, the labrum is mobilized, and a motorized shaver or thermal device is used to prepare the acetabular rim for refixation/repair of the labrum (**Figure 3, A**). To maximize healing potential, the cortex must be removed, and bleeding cancellous bone must be exposed.
- After the acetabular rim is prepared, suture anchors (bioabsorbable, polyetheretherketone, or all-suture) are placed, with the use of the modified anterior portal to access the 2- to 5-o'clock region (in a left hip) and the anterolateral portal to access the 12- to 2-o'clock region. If necessary, tears in the 10- to 12-o'clock region (left hip) are addressed via the posterolateral portal.
- The position of the anchors is critical to achieve adequate fixation and restoration of the femoroacetabular suction seal. Direct visualization and fluoroscopic guidance should be used to avoid intra-articular suture anchor penetration.
- The suture anchors are placed approximately 2 to 4 mm from the edge of the cartilage and 6 to 10 mm apart.
- After the suture anchors are placed, a suture-passing device is used to pass a single suture limb through the chondrolabral junction (**Figure 3, B**). The authors of this chapter prefer to pass the suture-passing device through the outer edge of the labrum to retrieve this suture and achieve a labral base repair configuration (**Figure 3, C**). If the tissue is not suitable for this passage, the suture limb is retrieved from around the outer edge of the labrum to achieve a circumferential repair configuration.
- The ligamentum teres is best evaluated with the use of a 30° or 70° arthroscope in the anterolateral portal, with the hip in maximal external rotation.
- An arthroscopic biter and a motorized shaver with suction may be used to débride the ligament as required to address mechanical pathology.

INTERNAL SNAPPING HIP SYNDROME (ILIOPSOAS IMPINGEMENT)

Iliopsoas Release at the Level of the Central Compartment

- In patients who have not undergone THA, the authors of this chapter prefer to use a central compartment transcapsular approach to release the iliopsoas tendon at the myotendinous junction. Compared with other techniques, this method requires fewer portals and may preserve more hip flexion strength and, therefore, provide more dynamic stability to the hip joint.
- The anterolateral and modified anterior portals are used.
- A transverse interportal capsulotomy is made.
- The iliopsoas tendon is visualized medially with the use of a 30° or 70° arthroscope through the anterolateral portal.
- A motorized shaver and radiofrequency ablation probe inserted through the modified anterior portal are used to isolate the iliopsoas tendon fibers from the underlying iliacus muscle.
- Under direct visualization, the tendon fibers are gradually divided with the use of the radiofrequency ablation probe.

Iliopsoas Release at the Level of the Lesser Trochanter

- In patients who have undergone THA, the authors of this chapter prefer to perform iliopsoas release at the level of the lesser trochanter because this method avoids violation of the capsule and, thus, minimizes the risk of instability and iatrogenic infection.
- The anterolateral, anteroinferior accessory, and distal anteroinferior working portals are used.
- The 30° arthroscope is positioned

in the iliopsoas bursa via the anterolateral portal.
- The hip is brought into approximately 30° of flexion and maximal external rotation, such that the lesser trochanter can be viewed fluoroscopically.
- Under direct visualization from the anterolateral portal, an anteroinferior accessory portal is established with the use of a spinal needle placed approximately 2 to 3 cm distal and slightly anterior to the anterolateral inferior portal.
- Under fluoroscopic guidance, a switching stick directed toward the lesser trochanter is used to bluntly dissect down to the medial wall of the iliopsoas bursa.
- A cannula is placed over the switching stick.
- Under direct visualization, an additional working portal is established approximately 2 to 3 cm distal to the anteroinferior accessory portal with the use of a long spinal needle.
- A hooked radiofrequency ablation device can be used within this working portal to clear the iliopsoas bursa and identify the longitudinal white tendon fibers.
- The tendon is released at the level of the lesser trochanter with the use of the radiofrequency ablation device (**Figure 1, B**).

LOOSE BODIES

- A systematic evaluation of the central compartment and a diagnostic arthroscopic examination are performed with 30° and 70° arthroscopes inserted through the anterolateral and modified anterior portals.
- Loose bodies are removed from the posterior region of the central compartment via a posterolateral portal.
- The use of a simple arthroscopic grasper or inflow through one portal and outflow through another, larger cannula may be sufficient to remove most loose bodies.
- Occasionally, the use of a long tonsil clamp or pituitary rongeur is necessary to remove large loose bodies.

SEPTIC ARTHRITIS OF THE HIP

- The anterolateral and modified anterior portals are established as described previously in this chapter.
- Initial penetration of the capsule under fluoroscopic guidance with the use of a spinal needle is confirmed via the backflow of purulent drainage, which is collected for culture.
- After the modified anterior portal has been established under direct visualization, systematic diagnostic arthroscopy is performed.
- Synovial biopsy samples are obtained for culture and histologic examination.
- Synovectomy is performed with the use of a motorized shaver and an arthroscopic biter.
- The joint is thoroughly irrigated with 9 to 12 L of physiologic saline.

Wound Closure

- The portal sites are reapproximated with the use of nylon suture in a simple, interrupted manner.
- Thin adhesive strips are applied to supplement the closure.
- A sterile dressing is placed.
- A continuous cold therapy unit is applied over the sterile dressing.
- The patient is placed in a hip flexion brace.

Postoperative Regimen

In the first 2 weeks postoperatively, the patient is allowed to perform full passive ROM hip flexion/extension as tolerated. Active hip flexion or external rotation greater than 20° is prohibited. Crutches are used. The patient is instructed to use a stationary bicycle for 20 minutes one or two times per day. In postoperative weeks 2 through 4, weight bearing is progressed, and the use of crutches is gradually discontinued. Hip ROM and strengthening of the core and hip are progressed in all directions except flexion (to avoid flexor tendinitis). In postoperative weeks 4 through 8, hip ROM and strengthening, including hip flexion, are progressed. The patient is instructed to perform hip-hiking exercise on a stair climber. In postoperative weeks 8 through 12, hip and core strengthening are continued. Dynamic balance and endurance activities are performed. The patient begins a treadmill running program and sport-specific agility drills. The patient may return to sport after demonstrating satisfactory results on functional testing, including comparison with the contralateral side.

Avoiding Pitfalls and Complications

To reduce the risk of injury to the genitals and/or the pudendal nerve, a well-padded perineal post should be used and traction time should be minimized. To avoid injury to the sciatic nerve, flexion of the hip greater than 20° should be avoided if traction is applied. To minimize damage to the articular cartilage, 10 to 15 mm of radiographic joint distraction should be achieved before the joint is accessed. The capsulotomy should be performed under direct visualization to avoid iatrogenic injury. To avoid the risk of instrument breakage, the spinal needle, nitinol wire, and other instruments should be inspected for defects before use.

Bibliography

Ala Eddine T, Remy F, Chantelot C, Giraud F, Migaud H, Duquennoy A: Anterior iliopsoas impingement after total hip arthroplasty: Diagnosis and conservative treatment in 9 cases [French]. *Rev Chir Orthop Reparatrice Appar Mot* 2001;87(8):815-819.

Bader R, Mittelmeier W, Zeiler G, Tokar I, Steinhauser E, Schuh A: Pitfalls in the use of acetabular reinforcement rings in total hip revision. *Arch Orthop Trauma Surg* 2005;125(8):558-563.

Beighton P, Solomon L, Soskolne CL: Articular mobility in an African population. *Ann Rheum Dis* 1973;32(5):413-418.

Ben Tov T, Amar E, Shapira A, Steinberg E, Atoun E, Rath E: Clinical and functional outcome after acetabular labral repair in patients aged older than 50 years. *Arthroscopy* 2014;30(3):305-310.

Bowman KF Jr, Fox J, Sekiya JK: A clinically relevant review of hip biomechanics. *Arthroscopy* 2010;26(8):1118-1129.

Byrd JW: Evaluation and management of the snapping iliopsoas tendon. *Instr Course Lect* 2006;55:347-355.

Byrd JW, Jones KS, Maiers GP II: Two to 10 years' follow-up of arthroscopic management of pigmented villonodular synovitis in the hip: A case series. *Arthroscopy* 2013;29(11):1783-1787.

Cardinal E, Buckwalter KA, Capello WN, Duval N: US of the snapping iliopsoas tendon. *Radiology* 1996;198(2):521-522.

Cheng XG, You YH, Liu W, Zhao T, Qu H: MRI features of pigmented villonodular synovitis (PVNS). *Clin Rheumatol* 2004;23(1):31-34.

Colvin AC, Harrast J, Harner C: Trends in hip arthroscopy. *J Bone Joint Surg Am* 2012;94(4):e23.

de Sa D, Cargnelli S, Catapano M, et al: Efficacy of hip arthroscopy for the management of septic arthritis: A systematic review. *Arthroscopy* 2015;31(7):1358-1370.

de Sa D, Horner NS, MacDonald A, et al: Arthroscopic surgery for synovial chondromatosis of the hip: A systematic review of rates and predisposing factors for recurrence. *Arthroscopy* 2014;30(11):1499-1504.e2.

Dienst M, Gödde S, Seil R, Hammer D, Kohn D: Hip arthroscopy without traction: In vivo anatomy of the peripheral hip joint cavity. *Arthroscopy* 2001;17(9):924-931.

Domb BG, Stake CE, Lindner D, El-Bitar Y, Jackson TJ: Arthroscopic capsular plication and labral preservation in borderline hip dysplasia: Two-year clinical outcomes of a surgical approach to a challenging problem. *Am J Sports Med* 2013;41(11):2591-2598.

Dy CJ, Thompson MT, Crawford MJ, Alexander JW, McCarthy JC, Noble PC: Tensile strain in the anterior part of the acetabular labrum during provocative maneuvering of the normal hip. *J Bone Joint Surg Am* 2008;90(7):1464-1472.

Fabricant PD, Bedi A, De La Torre K, Kelly BT: Clinical outcomes after arthroscopic psoas lengthening: The effect of femoral version. *Arthroscopy* 2012;28(7):965-971.

Gédouin JE, Huten D: Technique and results of endoscopic tenotomy in iliopsoas muscle tendinopathy secondary to total hip replacement: A series of 10 cases. *Orthop Traumatol Surg Res* 2012;98(suppl 4):S19-S25.

Good CR, Shindle MK, Kelly BT, Wanich T, Warren RF: Glenohumeral chondrolysis after shoulder arthroscopy with thermal capsulorrhaphy. *Arthroscopy* 2007;23(7):797.e1-797.e5.

Heaven S, de Sa D, Simunovic N, Williams DS, Naudie D, Ayeni OR: Hip arthroscopy in the setting of hip arthroplasty. *Knee Surg Sports Traumatol Arthrosc* 2016;24(1):287-294.

Hewitt JD, Glisson RR, Guilak F, Vail TP: The mechanical properties of the human hip capsule ligaments. *J Arthroplasty* 2002;17(1):82-89.

Jackson TJ, Hanypsiak B, Stake CE, Lindner D, El Bitar YF, Domb BG: Arthroscopic labral base repair in the hip: Clinical results of a described technique. *Arthroscopy* 2014;30(2):208-213.

Larson CM, Giveans MR, Stone RM: Arthroscopic debridement versus refixation of the acetabular labrum associated with femoroacetabular impingement: Mean 3.5-year follow-up. *Am J Sports Med* 2012;40(5):1015-1021.

Lee JB, Kang C, Lee CH, Kim PS, Hwang DS: Arthroscopic treatment of synovial chondromatosis of the hip. *Am J Sports Med* 2012;40(6):1412-1418.

Magerkurth O, Jacobson JA, Morag Y, Caoili E, Fessell D, Sekiya JK: Capsular laxity of the hip: Findings at magnetic resonance arthrography. *Arthroscopy* 2013;29(10):1615-1622.

Masih S, Antebi A: Imaging of pigmented villonodular synovitis. *Semin Musculoskelet Radiol* 2003;7(3):205-216.

Moorman CT III, Warren RF, Hershman EB, et al: Traumatic posterior hip subluxation in American football. *J Bone Joint Surg Am* 2003;85(7):1190-1196.

Nelson IR, Keene JS: Results of labral-level arthroscopic iliopsoas tenotomies for the treatment of labral impingement. *Arthroscopy* 2014;30(6):688-694.

Nilsson M, Höglund M, Panagopoulos I, et al: Molecular cytogenetic mapping of recurrent chromosomal breakpoints in tenosynovial giant cell tumors. *Virchows Arch* 2002;441(5):475-480.

Nusem I, Jabur MK, Playford EG: Arthroscopic treatment of septic arthritis of the hip. *Arthroscopy* 2006;22(8): 902.e1-902.e3.

Philippon MJ: The role of arthroscopic thermal capsulorrhaphy in the hip. *Clin Sports Med* 2001;20(4):817-829.

Polkowski GG, Clohisy JC: Hip biomechanics. *Sports Med Arthrosc* 2010;18(2):56-62.

Sekiya JK, Willobee JA, Miller MD, Hickman AJ, Willobee A: Arthroscopic multi-pleated capsular plication compared with open inferior capsular shift for reduction of shoulder volume in a cadaveric model. *Arthroscopy* 2007;23(11):1145-1151.

Shindle MK, Ranawat AS, Kelly BT: Diagnosis and management of traumatic and atraumatic hip instability in the athletic patient. *Clin Sports Med* 2006;25(2):309-326, ix-x.

Tibor LM, Sekiya JK: Differential diagnosis of pain around the hip joint. *Arthroscopy* 2008;24(12):1407-1421.

van der Heijden L, Gibbons CL, Dijkstra PD, et al: The management of diffuse-type giant cell tumour (pigmented villonodular synovitis) and giant cell tumour of tendon sheath (nodular tenosynovitis). *J Bone Joint Surg Br* 2012;94(7):882-888.

West RB, Rubin BP, Miller MA, et al: A landscape effect in tenosynovial giant-cell tumor from activation of CSF1 expression by a translocation in a minority of tumor cells. *Proc Natl Acad Sci U S A* 2006;103(3):690-695.

Chapter 66

Pelvic Osteotomies in Patients With Developmental Dysplasia of the Hip

Keith A. Fehring, MD
Peter K. Sculco, MD
Robert T. Trousdale, MD
Rafael J. Sierra, MD

Indications

Reorientation pelvic osteotomy may be performed in young patients (45 years or younger) with symptomatic hip dysplasia who do not have excessive proximal migration of the hip center and who have no more than mild degenerative changes of the articular surface. Severe secondary arthritic changes of the dysplastic hip portend a poor outcome after reorientation osteotomy. The primary abnormality in most patients with hip dysplasia is located on the acetabular side of the joint, although femoral-sided pathology is increasingly recognized. Pelvic osteotomy with reorientation of the acetabulum corrects the major anatomic abnormality that results in undercoverage of the femoral head and is present in most patients with hip dysplasia.

Single, double, triple, and other pelvic osteotomies have been described previously and aim to improve mechanics about the hip joint. Each of these osteotomies has advantages and disadvantages. The Bernese periacetabular osteotomy (PAO) has become the procedure of choice in many institutions for the treatment of young patients with symptomatic hip dysplasia in the absence of severe secondary arthritis (**Figure 1**). This osteotomy can be performed through one incision with a series of reproducible, extra-articular osteotomies and produces a freely mobile acetabular fragment that allows for large corrections in all necessary planes. Because the posterior column remains intact, the osteotomy is inherently stable, allowing relatively early weight bearing and faster recovery than can be achieved with other osteotomies. The shape of the pelvic ring is not markedly altered, allowing women to have normal vaginal child delivery after PAO. Furthermore, the surgical approach does not violate the abductor mechanism, which facilitates accelerated rehabilitation and functional recovery.

Dysplastic hips share a spectrum of anatomic abnormalities that vary depending on the severity of the dysplasia. On the pelvic side, the acetabulum is shallow, the hip center is lateralized, and the socket typically is excessively anteverted, resulting in anterior and superior acetabular deficiency (**Figure 2, A**). The socket is retroverted in approximately 18% to 40% of patients, and the acetabulum can be uncovered posteriorly (**Figure 2, B**). On the femoral side, the femoral neck often has excessive anteversion, and the femoral neck-shaft angle may be increased. Retroversion of the acetabulum or retrotorsion of the femur can lead to anterior impingement in flexion; however, in these patients

Dr. Fehring or an immediate family member has received royalties from, is a member of a speakers' bureau or has made paid presentations on behalf of, serves as a paid consultant to, has received research or institutional support from, and has received nonincome support (such as equipment or services), commercially derived honoraria, or other non–research-related funding (such as paid travel) from DePuy Synthes; and serves as a board member, owner, officer, or committee member of the American Association of Hip and Knee Surgeons and The Knee Society. Dr. Trousdale or an immediate family member has received royalties from and serves as a paid consultant to DePuy Synthes; and serves as a board member, owner, officer, or committee member of the American Association of Hip and Knee Surgeons, The Hip Society, and The Knee Society. Dr. Sierra or an immediate family member has received royalties from, is a member of a speakers' bureau or has made paid presentations on behalf of, and serves as a paid consultant to Zimmer Biomet; has received research or institutional support from DePuy Synthes, Stryker, and Zimmer Biomet; and serves as a board member, owner, officer, or committee member of the American Association of Hip and Knee Surgeons, the Mid-America Orthopaedic Association, and the M. E. Müller Foundation of North America. Neither Dr. Sculco nor any immediate family member has received anything of value from or has stock or stock options held in a commercial company or institution related directly or indirectly to the subject of this chapter.

the main source of pain is still the undercoverage of the femoral head. Overall, these anatomic abnormalities result in decreased contact area between the weight-bearing dome of the acetabulum and the femoral head.

Joint congruity is also an important factor to consider when evaluating a patient for reorientation osteotomy. A relatively round acetabulum that matches a relatively round femoral head produces a more reliable outcome after osteotomy than is likely to occur in less congruent joints. The lateralization of the hip center increases the body mass lever arm and creates higher forces during gait that are transmitted across a limited surface area. Because pressure equals force divided by area, the increased contact pressures likely accelerate degeneration of the articular cartilage. These biomechanical principles are reflected in longitudinal radiographic studies that clearly demonstrate the relationship of the risk of secondary osteoarthritis to the severity of hip dysplasia.

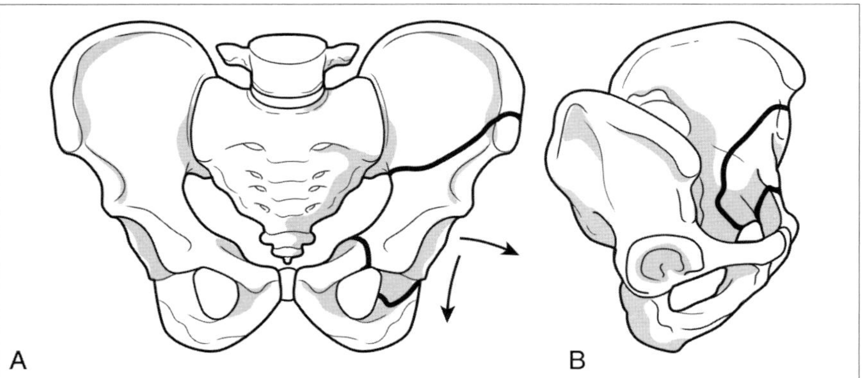

Figure 1 AP- (**A**) and lateral-view (**B**) pelvic illustrations depict the location of bone cuts for a Bernese periacetabular osteotomy. Arrows indicate the direction of rotation for the osteotomy.

Patients with hip dysplasia typically have activity-related groin pain that is, in part, related to instability of the femoral head and can sometimes be reproduced during clinical examination with hyperextension and external rotation of the hip. Catching, locking, or instability are frequently associated with labral and/or chondral pathology. Trochanteric or lateral hip pain is also common and is associated with abductor fatigue.

Radiographic evaluation begins with AP and lateral views of the pelvis and hip, as well as a false-profile view of the hip. MRI with or without gadolinium enhancement and CT are not routinely necessary to diagnose hip dysplasia but may be helpful in the evaluation of a painful hip in the absence of marked structural abnormalities. MRI and CT allow further evaluation of suspected intra-articular pathology such as labral tears, loose bodies, chondral defects, and synovial disease.

In symptomatic patients with hip dysplasia, increased joint congruity after reorientation of the osteotomized fragment allows more normal load transmission through a broader surface area

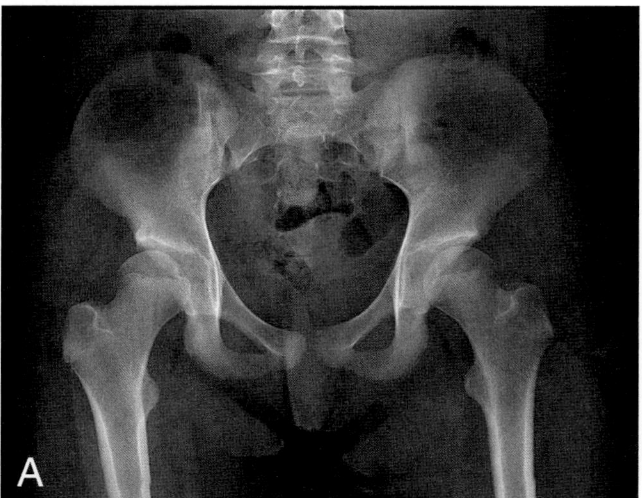

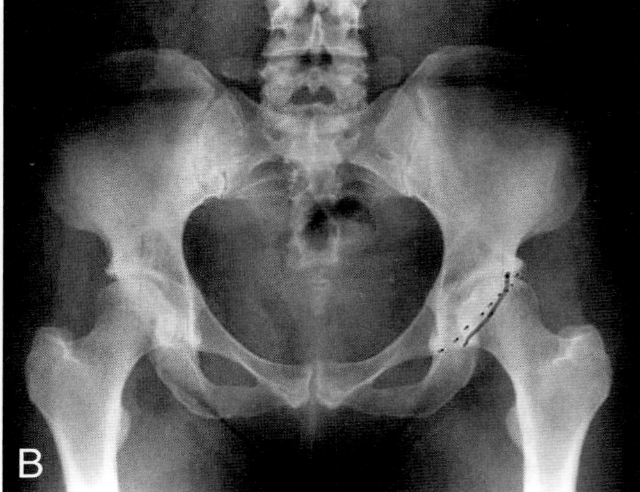

Figure 2 **A,** AP pelvic radiograph demonstrates classic dysplasia in both hips. The acetabulum is shallow, and the hip center is lateralized with anterior and superior deficiency. **B,** AP pelvic radiograph from a different patient demonstrates dysplasia of the left hip with a retroverted acetabulum. The posterior wall of the acetabulum (solid line) crosses over the anterior wall of the acetabulum (dotted line) before meeting the lateral edge of the sourcil. (Reproduced with permission from Trousdale R: Pelvic osteotomies for hip dysplasia, in Berry DJ, Lieberman JR: *Surgery of the Hip*. Philadelphia, PA, Elsevier, 2013, pp 717-721.)

subjected to less pressure. Some pelvic osteotomies also medialize the hip center of rotation, which lessens the reactive forces in the joint. These changes can be expected to reduce pain, improve function, and possibly protect the articular cartilage from further degeneration.

Contraindications

Contraindications to reorientation osteotomy include severe arthritis, marked incongruity of the hip joint, morbid obesity, patient age older than 45 years, and active infection of the hip joint.

Alternative Treatments

Patients who have dysplasia with no or minimal symptoms should initially be treated nonsurgically. The natural history of the dysplasia should be discussed with the patient, and radiographs should be obtained every few years to monitor for the development of arthritis. Reasonable initial recommendations include the use of NSAIDs and avoidance of high-impact activities. Surgical intervention should be reserved for patients with persistent symptoms and limitation of daily activities in the presence of marked structural abnormalities of the joint. Surgical options include arthroscopy, arthrodesis, resection arthroplasty, osteotomy, and total hip arthroplasty (THA). Pelvic realignment osteotomy is the procedure of choice in most young patients with symptomatic dysplasia and viable articular cartilage. THA should be reserved for patients who have marked articular cartilage loss or severe incongruency of the hip joint, or older patients (older than 45 years) with symptomatic hip disease with cartilage damage. Arthroscopy may be considered in select patients with mildly dysplastic hips with major mechanical symptoms related to either loose bodies or labral tears. However, the results of arthroscopy in patients with hip dysplasia have been inferior to the results in patients without hip dysplasia, and the procedure may even accelerate degenerative changes of the hip.

Before arthroscopy is offered to patients with symptomatic hip dysplasia, marked structural problems such as retroversion of the acetabulum and femoral offset issues should be ruled out. These problems may be subtle but can be detected with proper radiographic evaluation. In patients with these structural abnormalities, arthroscopy is unlikely to result in long-term relief of symptoms because the procedure does not address the underlying morphologic abnormalities causing labral pathology.

Arthrodesis and resection arthroplasty should be reserved for the rare patient with dysplasia (usually of neuromuscular origin for resection arthroplasty) who is not an appropriate candidate for osteotomy or THA.

Results

Studies of the long-term hip survivorship after PAO, defined as the lack of conversion to THA, ranges from 60% to 100% with maintenance of functional gains and range of motion (**Table 1**). Reverse PAOs for the management of acetabular retroversion have also demonstrated excellent long-term outcomes, with 100% survivorship at 10 years postoperatively in one study and no significant increase in the mean Tönnis osteoarthritis score. Several long-term outcome studies also have identified risk factors for failure after PAO: patient age older than 40 years, low preoperative Merle d'Aubigné and Postel score, preoperative Tönnis grade 2 or higher, malposition of the acetabular fragment (postoperative center-edge angle less than 30° or greater than 40°), hip incongruence, and a positive postoperative impingement sign. The authors of one study found that a positive postoperative impingement sign had the highest hazard ratio for failure and represented a residual structural deformity on either the acetabular or femoral side leading to iatrogenic femoroacetabular impingement (FAI). Other studies have supported proper acetabular orientation and the presence of a spheric femoral head as the two most important factors associated with long-term survivorship and the lowest risk of progression of osteoarthritis. Impingement could be secondary to untreated femoral deformity in patients with an isolated acetabular correction. The authors of one study reported that in patients undergoing an isolated PAO, a preoperative α angle greater than 55° was associated with worse patient-reported outcome scores. The effect of residual or untreated deformity was highlighted in a study of 2,263 PAOs in which residual structural deformity on either the femoral or acetabular side leading to FAI was found in 95% of patients who required secondary surgery.

In a recent radiographic study, the degree of femoral asphericity correlated with the severity of acetabular dysplasia and, more specifically, the Tönnis angle, suggesting that concomitant correction of femoral-sided deformity is more common in patients with more severe acetabular dysplasia. In a different study of intra-articular pathology identified at the time of PAO, decreased femoral head-neck offset was the most common contributor to the pathology (occurring in 129 of 151 patients). Management of intra-articular pathology with an arthrotomy at the time of the PAO was associated with a decreased rate of failure compared with not performing an arthrotomy (5.3% and 17.9%, respectively), perhaps related to the removal of the femoral-sided deformity. The safety of performing concomitant procedures was confirmed in a study comparing combined femoral osteochondroplasty and PAO with PAO alone. In that study, no difference was found in the rate of heterotopic

Table 1 Results of the Bernese Periacetabular Osteotomy in Patients With Hip Dysplasia

Authors (Year)	Number of Patients (Hips)	Mean Patient Age in Years (Range)	Mean Follow-up in Years (Range)	Success Rate (%)[a]	Results[b]
Trousdale et al (1995)	42 (42)	37 (11-56)	4 (2-8)	86	HHS improved by 24 points
Clohisy et al (2005)	13 (16)	17.6 (13.0-31.8)	4.2 (1.9-8.1)	100	Merle d'Aubigné hip score improved by 14.5 points
Cunningham et al (2006)	47 (52)	27.4 (NA)	2 (2-3.8)	90	HHS improved by 6.1 points
Peters et al (2006)	73 (83)	31	2.5	96	WOMAC improved by 33 points
Garras et al (2007)	52 (58)	37.6 (13-48)	5.6 (1.1-12.8)	95	Merle d'Aubigné hip score improved by 3.4 points
Steppacher et al (2008)	58 (68)	29 (13-56)	20.4 (19-23)	60	Merle d'Aubigné hip score improved by 0.6 points
Matheney et al (2009)	109 (135)	27	9	76	—
Troelsen et al (2009)	96 (116)	Median, 29.9 (NA)	6.8 (5.2-9.2)	82	—
Sucato et al (2010)	21 (24)	16 (NA)	1 (NA)	100	HHS improved by 10 points
Siebenrock et al (2014)	22 (29)	23 (14-41)	11 (9-12)	100	Merle d'Aubigné hip score improved by 2.9 points

HHS = Harris hip score, NA = not available, WOMAC = Western Ontario and McMaster Universities Osteoarthritis Index.

[a] Success is defined as procedures not requiring conversion to total hip arthroplasty.

[b] All results are mean values and indicate improvement from preoperatively to postoperatively.

ossification, infection, or fracture of the femoral neck, and reported functional outcomes were similar in the two groups at short-term follow-up. These findings support the concurrent management of both acetabular and femoral pathology with a comprehensive surgical plan as a way to improve long-term outcomes and reduce the need for revision surgery to address persistent structural deformity and impingement.

Recently, studies of intra-articular pathology, as assessed in either open or arthroscopic procedures, have emphasized labral tears and osteochondral lesions as potential causes of inferior outcomes after PAO. The role of arthroscopy before PAO is still under investigation. A recent report of 16 patients who underwent PAO and concomitant hip arthroscopy found substantial intra-articular pathology in all patients. In that study, the most common conditions were anterosuperior labral tears, femoral cam-type lesions, and articular chondral injury. Whether hip arthroscopy before PAO has a beneficial effect on clinical outcomes or survivorship remains unknown. Recent reports have shown no difference in Harris hip scores, complication rates, or revision rates in patients who undergo unsuccessful PAO and in whom the development of osteoarthritis necessitates THA, compared with patients who undergo THA without previous PAO.

In a prospective, multicenter study of complication rates in 205 PAOs performed by 10 experienced surgeons, major complications (Clavien-Dindo grade III or IV) occurred in 12 patients (5.9%), with 9 patients requiring revision surgery and 3 patients experiencing thromboembolic events. No vascular injuries, permanent nerve injuries, intra-articular osteotomies and/or fractures, or acetabular osteonecrosis occurred. This study, in which the procedures were performed by experienced surgeons who were beyond their learning curves, demonstrated the safety and efficacy of this procedure in a large cohort of patients despite the 5.9% risk of major complications.

Techniques

- The surgical technique for PAO has been extensively described in the literature but continues to evolve.
- The following is the authors' preferred technique.

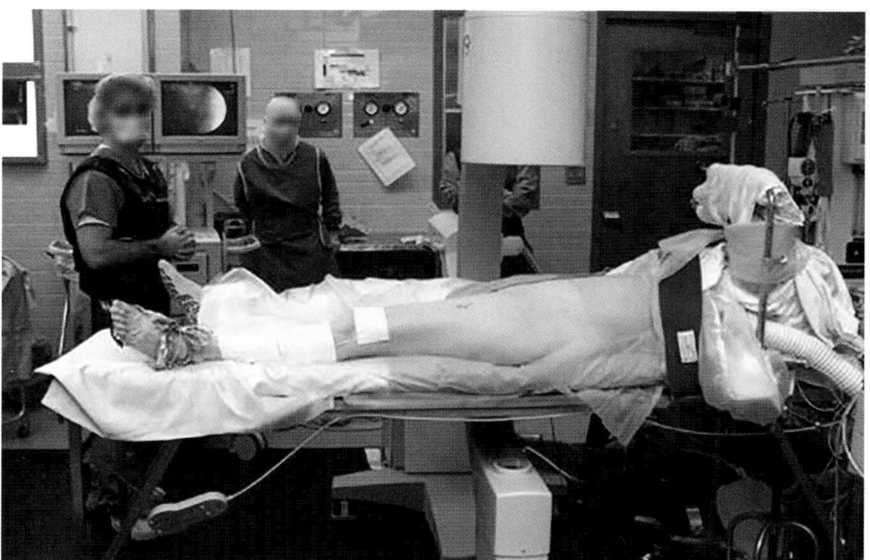

Figure 3 Intraoperative photograph shows preparation of a patient for pelvic osteotomy to manage hip dysplasia with fluoroscopic imaging and electromyographic monitoring equipment available. (Reproduced with permission from Trousdale R: Pelvic osteotomies for hip dysplasia, in Berry DJ, Lieberman JR: *Surgery of the Hip*. Philadelphia, PA, Elsevier, 2013, pp 717-721.)

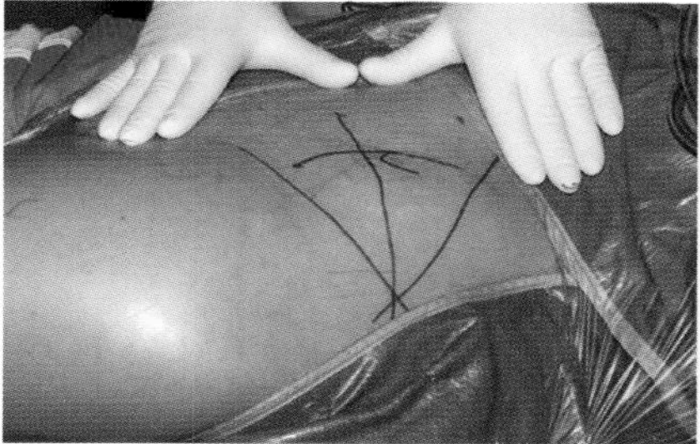

Figure 4 Intraoperative photograph shows the location of a skin incision on a left hip in preparation for pelvic osteotomy. (Reproduced with permission from Trousdale R: Pelvic osteotomies for hip dysplasia, in Berry DJ, Lieberman JR: *Surgery of the Hip*. Philadelphia, PA, Elsevier, 2013, pp 717-721.)

Setup/Exposure

- Regional epidural anesthesia is used in most patients.
- The patient is placed supine on an imaging table.
- The authors of this chapter no longer use preoperative autologous blood donation.
- An intraoperative cell saver is routinely used.
- Tranexamic acid is administered intravenously (1 g at the time of incision and 1 g at closure) to aid in blood conservation.
- The authors of this chapter use intraoperative electromyographic monitoring of the sciatic nerve and femoral nerve to aid in identification of intraoperative tension or pressure on these structures (**Figure 3**).
- Most surgeons use an anterior approach that spares the abductor muscles, performing the osteotomies through the inner aspect of the pelvis.
- The incision typically begins along the border of the iliac crest, proceeds along the anterior superior iliac spine, and continues distally, ending approximately 3 cm distal and anterior to the greater trochanter (**Figure 4**).
- The plane between the tensor fascia lata and the sartorius muscle is developed, and the deep fascia over the tensor fascia lata is incised to avoid direct injury to the lateral femoral cutaneous nerve.
- The sartorius origin is reflected from the anterior superior iliac spine.
- The hip is flexed and adducted, and the inner table of the pelvis is exposed to the sciatic notch.
- The iliopsoas tendon is retracted medially to expose the pubis.
- The direct head of the rectus femoris muscle can be reflected distally from the anterior inferior iliac spine to expose the anterior hip capsule. The hip joint may be opened at this time to allow evaluation for labral or chondral pathology.
- Many surgeons leave the direct head of the rectus femoris muscle intact, especially if they are not planning to perform an arthrotomy at the time of the PAO.
- Alternatively, arthroscopy may be performed before the open osteotomy procedure to address intra-articular pathology and alleviate the need for takedown of the direct head of the rectus femoris muscle.
- Blunt dissection proceeds distally and medially, with the use of an image intensifier for visualization.
- Scissors are used to palpate the ischium and the obturator foramen.

Procedure

- With the use of an image intensifier to prevent intra-articular extension of the osteotomy, the osteotomy procedure has become fairly predictable.
- The osteotomies include a partial osteotomy of the ischium, a complete osteotomy of the pubic bone, and a biplanar osteotomy of the ilium. The continuity of the posterior column is maintained.
- The authors of this chapter use the image intensifier at four critical points during the procedure: at the time of ischial osteotomy to ensure proper placement and orientation,

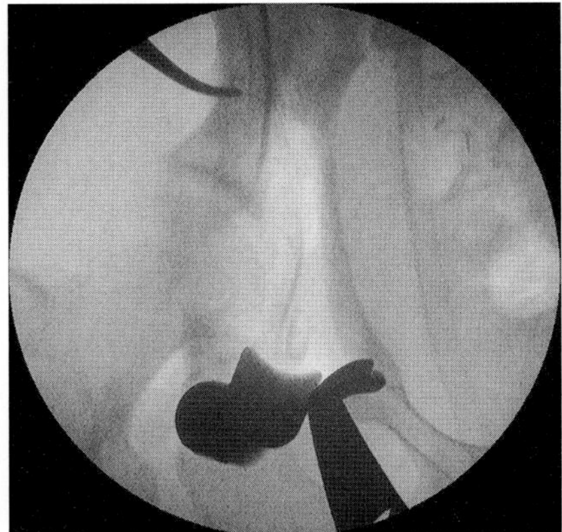

Figure 5 Intraoperative AP fluoroscopic image demonstrates placement of the ischial osteotome. A Hohmann retractor is in the lateral aspect of the pubis, and another osteotome is outlining the proposed iliac cut. (Reproduced with permission from Trousdale R: Pelvic osteotomies for hip dysplasia, in Berry DJ, Lieberman JR: *Surgery of the Hip*. Philadelphia, PA, Elsevier, 2013, pp 717-721.)

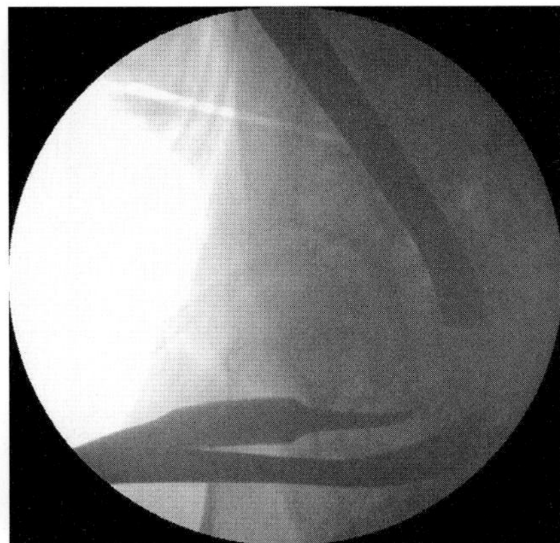

Figure 6 Intraoperative oblique fluoroscopic image demonstrates the posterior iliac cut as it joins the ischial cut. The cuts are extra-articular, and the posterior column is left intact.

during exposure of the pubic bone to ensure that it is sufficiently medial, for confirmation of correct placement of the iliac cut, and for proper extra-articular placement of the posterior osteotomy so as to avoid violating the posterior column of the pelvis.

- The ischial osteotomy is performed initially, with the use of an AP image to ensure that the osteotomy is sufficiently distal and medial and is oriented in the proper direction (**Figure 5**).
- The ischial osteotome is left in place to serve as a guide when the last osteotomy (the posterior iliac osteotomy) is performed. Often, the surgeon can palpate this osteotome medially and distally over the quadrilateral surface.
- The pubic bone is exposed with a Hohmann retractor, with the image intensifier used to ensure that the exposure is sufficiently medial to prevent entry of the osteotomy into the joint.
- The pubic osteotomy is performed in an oblique fashion, from proximal-medial to distal-lateral, which facilitates mobilization of the fragment.
- The iliac cut typically is performed at the level just distal to the anterior superior iliac spine. An AP image is obtained to ensure that the cut is high enough above the joint to allow satisfactory fixation of the distal fragment.
- It is often helpful to aim the iliac cut slightly distal to ensure that when the iliac cut is turned to connect with the ischial cut, the cuts meet at a level that is distal to the top of the sciatic notch.
- The image intensifier is particularly helpful for the last osteotomy. The authors of this chapter obtain a 55° to 65° oblique radiograph demonstrating the posterior column of the acetabulum to ensure that the posterior osteotomy is extra-articular and does not violate the posterior column of the pelvis (**Figure 6**).
- After all three osteotomies are completed in the proper location, the posterior column is left intact, and the acetabular fragment is mobilized.
- The acetabular fragment needs to move freely. The two most common sites at which motion of the fragment is restricted are the junctions of the posterior column with the ischial osteotomy and the pubic osteotomy.
- Obtaining the proper correction is the most challenging aspect of the procedure. The periacetabular segment typically is displaced medially, rotated anteriorly and laterally (with care taken to maintain proper anteversion or, if the hip has excessive version, appropriate retroversion), and provisionally fixed with two smooth pins.
- A true AP radiograph of the pelvis is obtained intraoperatively to assess the correction. Correction is considered satisfactory when the acetabular roof is horizontal; the femoral head is congruous; the anterior rim covers less of the femoral head than the posterior rim does, and the rims meet at the lateral edge of the sourcil, ensuring proper acetabular anteversion; the femoral head is medialized within 5 mm of the ilioischial line; and the Shenton line is near normal (**Figure 7**).
- Care must be taken to avoid elevation of the hip center, especially in hips in which a fair amount of medialization is required.
- The acetabular fragment is fixed with two or three long, fully threaded cortical screws.
- The authors of this chapter routinely evaluate intra-articular pathology by opening the hip joint capsule through the same approach used for the osteotomy or by means of arthroscopy performed before the osteotomy is done. Torn labral fragments are excised or repaired depending on the status of the labrum.
- The best approach to the management of intra-articular pathology, if it even needs to be addressed at the time of PAO, remains controversial.

Wound Closure

- The prominent anterior inferior iliac spine may be trimmed and inserted as bone graft in the gap created anteriorly by the transverse iliac osteotomy.
- The sartorius and rectus femoris muscle origins that were removed at the time of exposure are repaired.
- The deep fascia is closed with interrupted sutures.
- The skin closure is performed in routine fashion.
- A deep drain is placed and is used for 24 hours postoperatively.

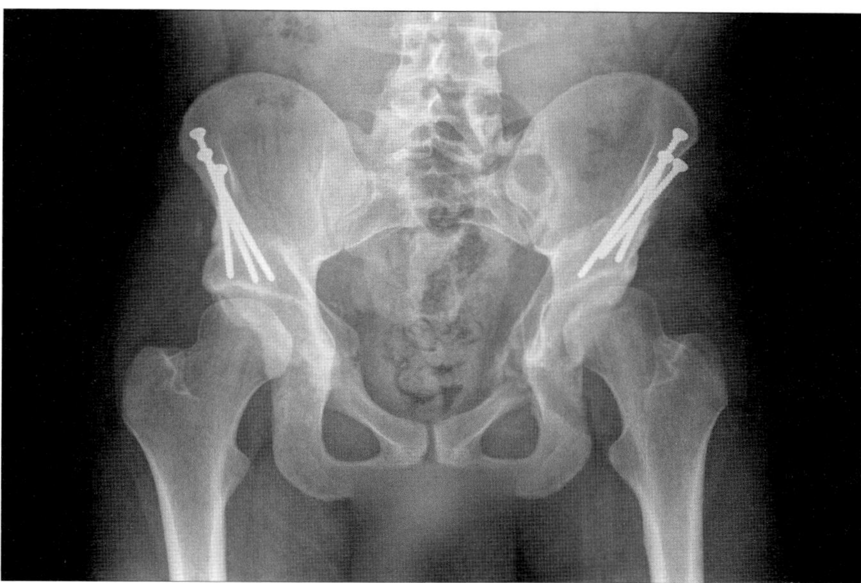

Figure 7 Postoperative AP pelvic radiograph demonstrates correction of bilateral classic hip dysplasia.

Postoperative Regimen

Postoperative epidural anesthesia is used for pain control for 48 hours. Most patients receive scheduled tramadol and acetaminophen, with low doses of narcotics as needed for the management of breakthrough pain. Aspirin is used for 6 weeks postoperatively for deep vein thrombosis prophylaxis. On the first postoperative day, the patient is mobilized with ambulatory aids. Weight bearing as tolerated, abduction exercises, water exercises, and stationary bike activities begin at 4 weeks postoperatively. A structured physical therapy program can be instituted after the second postoperative week.

Avoiding Pitfalls and Complications

Pelvic osteotomies are complex procedures. The overall experience and expertise of the surgeon are important factors affecting the incidence of complications. The learning curve of this procedure is steep, and the potential complication rate is high. The surgeon should obtain training in the technique from surgeons who routinely perform this procedure. In addition, practice in the anatomy laboratory before the surgeon independently performs this osteotomy is extremely helpful.

Complications after PAO include nerve injury, vascular injury, intra-articular extension of the osteotomy, nonunion, infection, and thromboembolic events. Obesity of the patient has been shown to be an independent risk factor for an increased complication rate after PAO, with a 22% rate of major complications in patients with body mass index greater than 30 kg/m^2 compared with 3% in nonobese patients undergoing acetabular fragment correction of similar accuracy. With the use of modified anterior approaches that do not violate the adductors, heterotopic ossification rarely occurs as a complication of this procedure.

Nerve dysfunction is a potential complication. Use of the anterior approach to the hip joint frequently results in injury to the lateral femoral cutaneous nerve or some of its branches. Up to 75% of patients report paresthesia in the lateral aspect of the thigh, but most of these patients do not require further treatment. Some surgeons use intraoperative electromyographic monitoring in an attempt to decrease the risk of intraoperative damage to the sciatic and femoral nerves; however, the effect of this strategy on the rate of neurapraxia remains unproven. In a study evaluating the incidence of major sciatic or femoral nerve injury in 1,760 PAOs, a complication rate of 2.1% was reported (with the femoral nerve more commonly injured), and 47% of the patients with complications had complete recovery at a mean of 5.5 months postoperatively. No patient-related or surgical risk factors were identified.

Inadvertent extension of the osteotomy into an undesired location can occur. Intra-articular extension of the ischial osteotomy has been reported, especially in hips with marked proximal femoral head migration and a lax inferior capsule. Such extension does not cause articular incongruity but can interrupt the blood supply to the acetabulum and contribute to necrosis of the osteotomized fragment. Intra-articular extension of the vertical limb of the iliac osteotomy can create an incongruent joint after correction and lead to secondary arthrosis. The iliac osteotomy also can be extended inadvertently through the posterior column into the sciatic notch, destabilizing the pelvic ring. The use of intraoperative fluoroscopy minimizes the risk of this serious complication.

The incidence of stress fracture after PAO was previously reported to be only 2% to 3%, but in a recent report the rate was found to be 18.4%. Although most (91%) of these stress fractures healed, nonunion of the pubic osteotomy occurred in 62.5% of these patients, compared with 7% of patients without a stress fracture. Other potential causes of nonunion of the pubis, or less commonly nonunion of the ischial osteotomy, include large interfragmentary gaps, insufficient position of the osteotomy fragment, and interposition of the iliopsoas tendon in the pubic osteotomy. Fortunately, almost all pubic nonunions are asymptomatic radiologic findings and do not require active management. Likewise, bone grafting or plate fixation are rarely required for iliac or ischial nonunions.

The most common complication after PAO remains poor positioning of the fragment. Overcorrection of the osteotomized fragment can lead to anterior or lateral impingement symptoms or posterior subluxation of the femoral head. Femoral head subluxation also can result from uncorrected associated marked femoral deformity. Anterior FAI can be a sign of excessive anterior correction or retroversion of the acetabular fragment, but it can also complicate appropriate correction. If this problem is recognized intraoperatively, it can be addressed by means of repositioning of the fragment or judicial trimming of the anterior femoral neck just inferior to the femoral head articular surface.

Bibliography

Albers CE, Steppacher SD, Ganz R, Tannast M, Siebenrock KA: Impingement adversely affects 10-year survivorship after periacetabular osteotomy for DDH. *Clin Orthop Relat Res* 2013;471(5):1602-1614.

Amanatullah DF, Stryker L, Schoenecker P, et al: Similar clinical outcomes for THAs with and without prior periacetabular osteotomy. *Clin Orthop Relat Res* 2015;473(2):685-691.

Beaulé PE, Dowding C, Parker G, Ryu JJ: What factors predict improvements in outcomes scores and reoperations after the Bernese periacetabular osteotomy? *Clin Orthop Relat Res* 2015;473(2):615-622.

Clohisy JC, Barrett SE, Gordon JE, Delgado ED, Schoenecker PL: Periacetabular osteotomy for the treatment of severe acetabular dysplasia. *J Bone Joint Surg Am* 2005;87(2):254-259.

Clohisy JC, Nepple JJ, Larson CM, Zaltz I, Millis M; Academic Network of Conservation Hip Outcome Research (ANCHOR) Members: Persistent structural disease is the most common cause of repeat hip preservation surgery. *Clin Orthop Relat Res* 2013;471(12):3788-3794.

Cunningham T, Jessel R, Zurakowski D, Millis MB, Kim YJ: Delayed gadolinium-enhanced magnetic resonance imaging of cartilage to predict early failure of Bernese periacetabular osteotomy for hip dysplasia. *J Bone Joint Surg Am* 2006;88(7):1540-1548.

Domb BG, Lareau JM, Baydoun H, Botser I, Millis MB, Yen YM: Is intraarticular pathology common in patients with hip dysplasia undergoing periacetabular osteotomy? *Clin Orthop Relat Res* 2014;472(2):674-680.

Garras DN, Crowder TT, Olson SA: Medium-term results of the Bernese periacetabular osteotomy in the treatment of symptomatic developmental dysplasia of the hip. *J Bone Joint Surg Br* 2007;89(6):721-724.

Ginnetti JG, Pelt CE, Erickson JA, Van Dine C, Peters CL: Prevalence and treatment of intraarticular pathology recognized at the time of periacetabular osteotomy for the dysplastic hip. *Clin Orthop Relat Res* 2013;471(2):498-503.

Malviya A, Dandachli W, Beech Z, Bankes MJ, Witt JD: The incidence of stress fracture following peri-acetabular osteotomy: An under-reported complication. *Bone Joint J* 2015;97-B(1):24-28.

Matheney T, Kim YJ, Zurakowski D, Matero C, Millis M: Intermediate to long-term results following the Bernese periacetabular osteotomy and predictors of clinical outcome. *J Bone Joint Surg Am* 2009;91(9):2113-2123.

Nassif NA, Schoenecker PL, Thorsness R, Clohisy JC: Periacetabular osteotomy and combined femoral head-neck junction osteochondroplasty: A minimum two-year follow-up cohort study. *J Bone Joint Surg Am* 2012;94(21):1959-1966.

Novais EN, Potter GD, Clohisy JC, et al: Obesity is a major risk factor for the development of complications after peri-acetabular osteotomy. *Bone Joint J* 2015;97-B(1):29-34.

Okano K, Yamaguchi K, Ninomiya Y, Matsubayashi S, Osaki M, Takahashi K: Femoral head deformity and severity of acetabular dysplasia of the hip. *Bone Joint J* 2013;95-B(9):1192-1196.

Peters CL, Erickson JA, Hines JL: Early results of the Bernese periacetabular osteotomy: The learning curve at an academic medical center. *J Bone Joint Surg Am* 2006;88(9):1920-1926.

Siebenrock KA, Schaller C, Tannast M, Keel M, Büchler L: Anteverting periacetabular osteotomy for symptomatic acetabular retroversion: Results at ten years. *J Bone Joint Surg Am* 2014;96(21):1785-1792.

Sierra RJ, Beaule P, Zaltz I, Millis MB, Clohisy JC, Trousdale RT; ANCHOR group: Prevention of nerve injury after periacetabular osteotomy. *Clin Orthop Relat Res* 2012;470(8):2209-2219.

Steppacher SD, Tannast M, Ganz R, Siebenrock KA: Mean 20-year followup of Bernese periacetabular osteotomy. *Clin Orthop Relat Res* 2008;466(7):1633-1644.

Sucato DJ, Tulchin K, Shrader MW, DeLaRocha A, Gist T, Sheu G: Gait, hip strength and functional outcomes after a Ganz periacetabular osteotomy for adolescent hip dysplasia. *J Pediatr Orthop* 2010;30(4):344-350.

Troelsen A, Elmengaard B, Søballe K: Medium-term outcome of periacetabular osteotomy and predictors of conversion to total hip replacement. *J Bone Joint Surg Am* 2009;91(9):2169-2179.

Trousdale RT, Ekkernkamp A, Ganz R, Wallrichs SL: Periacetabular and intertrochanteric osteotomy for the treatment of osteoarthrosis in dysplastic hips. *J Bone Joint Surg Am* 1995;77(1):73-85.

Zaltz I, Baca G, Kim YJ, et al: Complications associated with the periacetabular osteotomy: A prospective multicenter study. *J Bone Joint Surg Am* 2014;96(23):1967-1974.

Chapter 67

Hip Arthrodesis

Stuart L. Weinstein, MD

Donald S. Garbuz, MD

Clive P. Duncan, MD, MSc, FRCSC

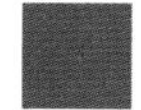

Indications

Hip arthrodesis was widely used to treat end-stage hip osteoarthritis before the development of total hip arthroplasty (THA). However, arthrodesis was largely abandoned in the 1930s in favor of motion-sparing procedures such as cup arthroplasty. Its popularity further eroded in the early 1970s as THA gained acceptance. Patients are aware of the success rates associated with THA, making hip arthrodesis a less attractive option. In addition, orthopaedic surgeons often have little experience with hip arthrodesis because of the limited number of surgeries performed each year.

Despite the high success rate of THA, concerns remain about its long-term durability in patients younger than 40 years of age. Revision rates as high as 45% have been reported in younger patients, but may be considerably less with uncemented implants and alternative bearing surfaces. Even with uncertainties about the long-term durability of THA, many young patients continue to choose THA because of its predictable pain relief, rapid recovery time, and excellent functional outcome.

Arthrodesis should be considered in selected symptomatic adolescents or adults younger than 40 years of age with monoarticular end-stage hip osteoarthritis and resultant pain. The ideal candidate is a manual laborer who wants to return to work. Patients should be free of low back pain, ipsilateral knee pain, and contralateral hip pain or pathology. Radiographs of these areas should be normal. Patients undergoing arthrodesis for osteonecrosis also should have MRI of the contralateral hip to rule out silent disease. Patients who do not meet all the indications for hip arthrodesis should be considered for alternative procedures such as resurfacing or THA.

Patients must have realistic expectations about the outcome of arthrodesis. Talking with other patients who have successfully undergone arthrodesis is helpful so that the patient can see that arthrodesis relieves hip pain, restores functional capacity, and allows for return to vigorous physical activity, including heavy manual labor. Should disabling low back pain, ipsilateral knee pain, or contralateral hip pain eventually develop, converting the arthrodesis to a THA may be an option. Patients must make an informed choice, with a clear realization of the limitations imposed by hip arthrodesis as well as the potential benefits and restrictions that may occur should it become necessary to convert the arthrodesis to a THA.

Contraindications

Hip arthrodesis is contraindicated in patients with contralateral hip pathology, symptoms in the lumbar spine, or evidence of knee pathology or instability on the ipsilateral side.

Nonambulatory children and some young adults with cerebral palsy, severe joint destruction, and degenerative joint disease are best treated with hip resection arthroplasty.

Alternative Treatments

Alternative treatments include nonsurgical measures, resection arthroplasty, osteotomy, hemiresurfacing, and THA.

Results

Most long-term studies report that patients are satisfied with the results of arthrodesis and lead active lives without hip pain. Several reports on the long-term durability of arthrodesis (**Table 1**) indicate that most patients return to manual labor for as long as 30 years. At long-term (approximately 20 years)

This chapter is reproduced from the first edition: Weinstein SL, Garbuz DS, Duncan CP: Hip arthrodesis, in Lieberman JR, Berry DJ, eds: Advanced Reconstruction: Hip. *Rosemont, IL, American Academy of Orthopaedic Surgeons, 2005, pp 495-501.*

Table 1 Long-Term Results of Hip Arthrodesis

Authors (Year)	Number of Hips	Mean Patient Age (Range)	Mean Follow-up (Range)	Results
Sponseller et al (1984)	53	14 yr (3–35 yr)	38 yr	57% low back pain 45% ipsilateral knee pain 17% contralateral knee pain
Callaghan et al (1985)	28	25 yr (10–58 yr)	37 yr (17–50 yr)	61% low back pain 57% ipsilateral knee pain 28% contralateral hip pain

Reproduced from Weinstein SL, Garbuz DS, Duncan CP: Hip arthrodesis, in Lieberman JR, Berry DJ, eds: *Advanced Reconstruction: Hip*. Rosemont, IL, American Academy of Orthopaedic Surgeons, 2005, pp 495-501.

follow-up, the most common complaints were low back pain and ipsilateral knee pain. However, 65% of these patients were uncertain whether they would choose the procedure again. Furthermore, patients are now rarely willing to accept the functional limitations that occur 10 to 15 years after hip fusion.

Both surgeon and patient must understand the functional and long-term limitations of a successful hip arthrodesis. Patients typically have a short leg and walk more slowly postoperatively. Most patients have a pain-free hip but still have more limitations on their activities than individuals who have not had arthrodesis. The most common complaints occur with activities that require hip flexion, such as sitting, bending, and putting on shoes and socks. Prolonged sitting in confined spaces such as theaters and airplanes is particularly troublesome, and some patients, especially women, have difficulty with sexual activity. Hip arthrodesis can be a successful and durable operation, but patients must anticipate its limitations.

Technique

Numerous surgical techniques are used to achieve hip fusion. Most modern techniques are designed to provide high fusion rates and minimize the need for postoperative immobilization. Another critical consideration is preservation of the hip abductors because future conversion to THA will be desired in a substantial number of patients.

One goal in performing hip arthrodesis is to ensure that as much normal hip architecture as possible is preserved in the event conversion to THA is necessary. Proper positioning of the leg in relation to the pelvis is important to prevent or delay the onset of back and knee symptoms. Gait analysis shows that increased transverse and sagittal rotation of the pelvis, increased knee flexion throughout the stance phase, and increased motion of the contralateral hip compensate for the loss of hip motion. The optimal position of fusion has not been established, but generally the hip should be fused in 20° to 30° of flexion, neutral to slight adduction, and 10° of external rotation. Abduction and internal rotation must be avoided. Some drift into adduction has been reported in fusions performed in younger patients; therefore, with these patients it is best to attempt a neutral position with reference to abduction and adduction.

Cobra Plating Technique (Iowa)

The goal of hip arthrodesis is to achieve a solid bony union sufficient to satisfy patients' high functional demands. This is accomplished through maximal bony contact and rigid internal fixation. It is also important to prevent shortening the limb in the event that conversion to THA becomes necessary. Patient positioning during surgery is critical so that the surgeon can assess the appropriate positioning of the limb in relation to the pelvis.

EXPOSURE

- The patient should be placed in a supine position with both hips properly prepared and draped. Bath blankets are placed under the middle of the patient's back to elevate the pelvis (**Figure 1**).
- Both lower extremities are prepared and draped free to allow visualization of the anterosuperior iliac spine on the contralateral side and to allow mobility of the opposite hip to check for appropriate limb positioning.
- A longitudinal 5- to 8-cm skin incision is made proximal and distal to the greater trochanter. Dissection is carried down to the interval between the tensor fasciae latae and the gluteus maximus.
- After the anterior and posterior borders of the gluteus medius are identified, a trochanteric osteotomy is performed, using either an osteotome or an oscillating saw, taking great care to prevent injury to the medial femoral circumflex vessels (**Figure 2**). Injury to the vessels may result in loss of blood supply to the femoral head.
- The hip joint capsule is incised in a T shape, with one limb along the

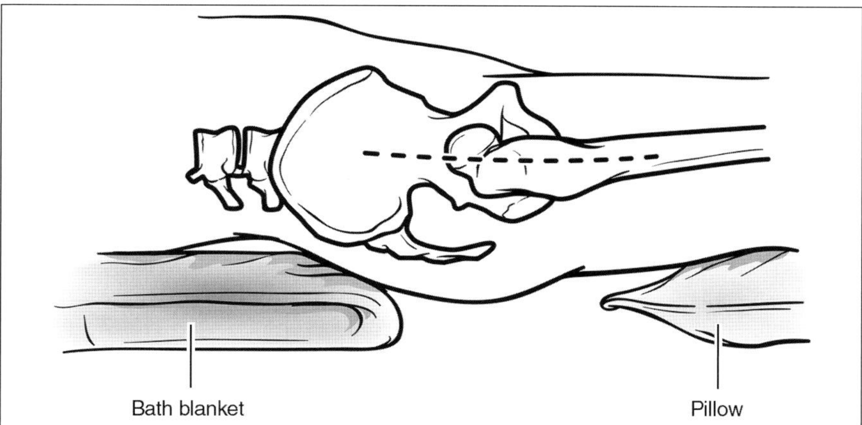

Figure 1 The patient is positioned on bath blankets from the shoulders to the pelvis to elevate the pelvis from the operating table. The patient's limbs are supported by pillows or bath blankets to maintain alignment and to ensure that they are the same level from the operating table. The incision extends 5 to 8 cm proximal and distal to the greater trochanter. (Reproduced from Weinstein SL, Garbuz DS, Duncan CP: Hip arthrodesis, in Lieberman JR, Berry DJ, eds: *Advanced Reconstruction: Hip*. Rosemont, IL, American Academy of Orthopaedic Surgeons, 2005, pp 495-501.)

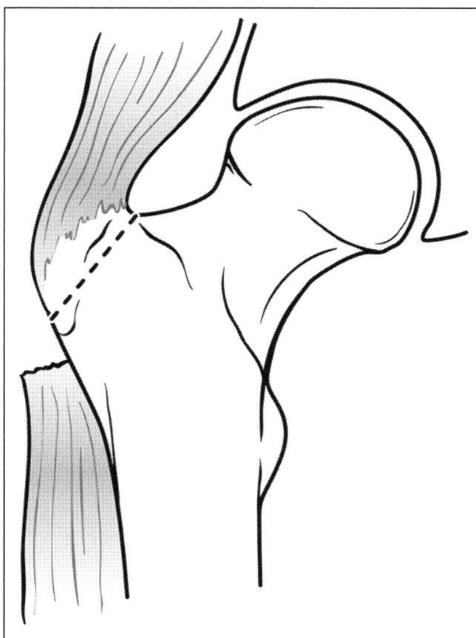

Figure 2 After identification of the anterior and posterior borders of the gluteus medius, retractors are inserted and a trochanteric osteotomy is performed using either an osteotome or an oscillating saw. It is important to prevent injury to the medial femoral circumflexed vessels. (Reproduced from Weinstein SL, Garbuz DS, Duncan CP: Hip arthrodesis, in Lieberman JR, Berry DJ, eds: *Advanced Reconstruction: Hip*. Rosemont, IL, American Academy of Orthopaedic Surgeons, 2005, pp 495-501.)

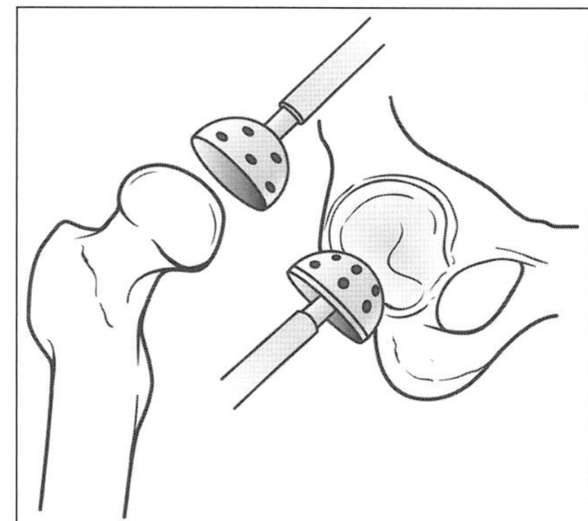

Figure 3 The femoral head is denuded of all cartilage and shaped to fit the acetabulum using a combination of straight and curved osteotomes and/or a concave hemispheric reamer. The acetabulum is prepared by removing all cartilage down to bleeding bone, usually by using a convex hemispheric reamer. (Reproduced from Weinstein SL, Garbuz DS, Duncan CP: Hip arthrodesis, in Lieberman JR, Berry DJ, eds: *Advanced Reconstruction: Hip*. Rosemont, IL, American Academy of Orthopaedic Surgeons, 2005, pp 495-501.)

acetabular margin anteriorly and a perpendicular incision toward the anterosuperior surface of the femoral head and neck. Again, care must be taken to avoid injury to the medial femoral circumflex vessels.

- Once the capsule has been incised, the femoral head can be dislocated anteriorly.

BONE PREPARATION

- The femoral head is denuded of all cartilage and shaped to fit the acetabulum. This can be done with a combination of straight and curved osteotomes and/or a concave hemispheric reamer (**Figure 3**). The extremity must not be shortened significantly; therefore, it is important to avoid shortening the proximal femur in patients with osteonecrosis or loss of femoral head height secondary to Legg-Calvé-Perthes disease or slipped capital femoral epiphysis. In patients with significant osteonecrosis, a power drill can be used to burr or fenestrate the femoral head.
- The acetabulum is prepared by removing all cartilage down to bleeding bone with a convex hemispheric reamer (**Figure 3**). A good bleeding surface on the acetabular side is extremely important to promote healing. Fenestrating the femoral head is preferred to the significant shortening that may be needed to reach bleeding bone, particularly in patients with osteonecrosis. Any marrow from the reaming should be saved for later use as supplemental graft.
- If the acetabulum is shallow and the hip has been subluxated, a pelvic osteotomy similar to the Chiari procedure is performed. The osteotomy extends from the sciatic notch to the anteroinferior spine just above the acetabulum (**Figure 4**), although the actual angle of the osteotomy is less important than it is in the Chiari procedure.
- The sciatic notch is carefully exposed, with subperiosteal dissection using a Cobb elevator and sponges.

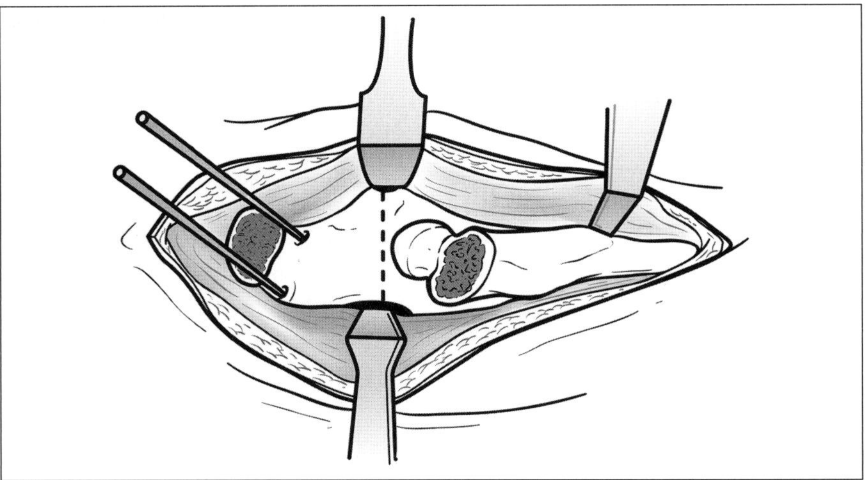

Figure 4 A pelvic osteotomy, similar to that of the Chiari procedure, is used when the acetabulum is shallow and the hip has been subluxated. The osteotomy extends from the sciatic notch to the anteroinferior spine just above the acetabulum. (Reproduced from Weinstein SL, Garbuz DS, Duncan CP: Hip arthrodesis, in Lieberman JR, Berry DJ, eds: *Advanced Reconstruction: Hip*. Rosemont, IL, American Academy of Orthopaedic Surgeons, 2005, pp 495-501.)

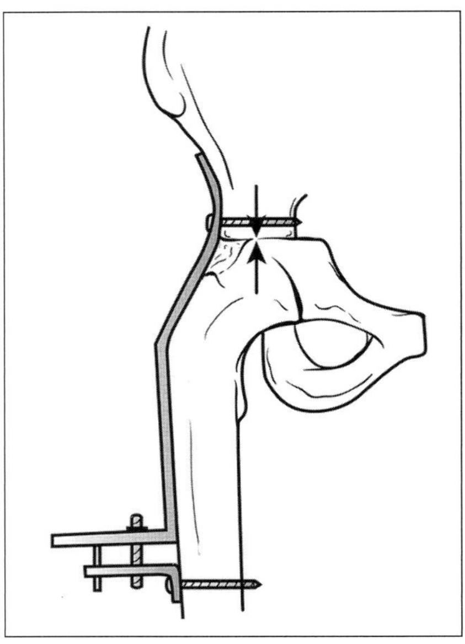

Figure 5 The cobra plate requires a distal bend so that the hip is not abducted when the plate is applied to the distal femur. The plate is subsequently attached to the distal ilium. (Reproduced from Weinstein SL, Garbuz DS, Duncan CP: Hip arthrodesis, in Lieberman JR, Berry DJ, eds: *Advanced Reconstruction: Hip*. Rosemont, IL, American Academy of Orthopaedic Surgeons, 2005, pp 495-501.)

- Once the notch is identified and a cobra retractor placed in it, the posterior cortex can be cut with a large right-angled Kerrison rongeur to ensure the osteotomy enters the notch at the appropriate point. The osteotomy is generally performed with osteotomes, although an oscillating saw may be used. The intrapelvic structures must be protected, and in some patients exposing the inner side of the pelvis subperiosteally may be helpful.
- The osteotomy should be displaced medially enough to provide adequate coverage superior to the femoral head and neck.
- After the femoral head and acetabulum are prepared and pelvic osteotomy (if necessary) is completed, the limb is placed into 25° to 30° of flexion, 5° to 10° of adduction, and 10° of external rotation; the limb is then held in position. A padded roll can be placed under the thigh to elevate the hip approximately 10° to 15°. This elevation, combined with the normal 15° of hip flexion present with normal lordosis, should place the hip in the appropriate degree of flexion. A long, sterile goniometer can be used to compare the position of the femur to the pelvis.
- With the opposite limb draped free, the hip can be hyperflexed to remove all lumbar lordosis and assess the degree of hip flexion in the operative hip. We suggest using fluoroscopy to assess abduction and adduction. The entire pelvis must be viewed, with the field encompassing both proximal femurs.

INTERNAL FIXATION

- A cobra plate is then appropriately contoured. A distal bend must be made in the cobra plate so that when it is applied to the distal femur it does not abduct the hip.
- The cobra plate is then attached to the distal ilium (above the osteotomy, if one has been made) and an AO tensioner is applied to the femur distal to the plate to apply appropriate compression (**Figure 5**). The remaining cortical screws are then drilled, tapped, and inserted.
- Finally, the greater trochanter is attached over the plate with a screw and washer.
- Any residual reaming materials are then packed into the gaps between the plate and the proximal femur (**Figure 6**).

WOUND CLOSURE

- A drain is placed, and the wound is closed.

POSTOPERATIVE REGIMEN

The patient can begin toe-touch weight bearing as tolerated beginning the first postoperative day. An orthotic can be used for the first 6 weeks after surgery if there is any question about the stability of fixation or patient compliance with postoperative instructions. Toe-touch weight bearing is maintained for approximately 6 weeks, and then the patient is reassessed clinically and

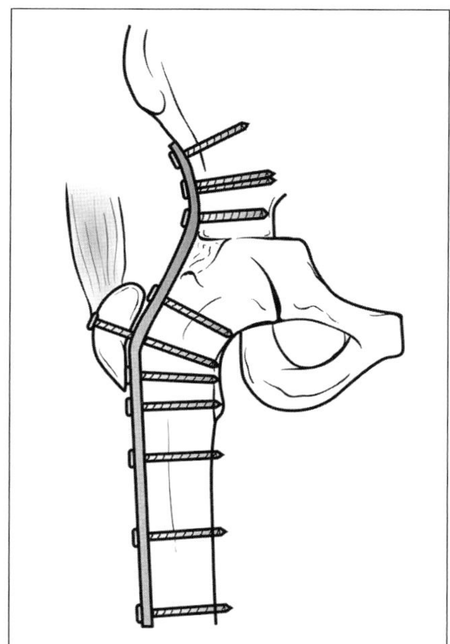

Figure 6 Cortical screws are drilled, tapped, and inserted. The greater trochanter is attached over the plate with a screw and washer. Any residual reamings are then packed in the gaps between the plate and the proximal femur. (Reproduced from Weinstein SL, Garbuz DS, Duncan CP: Hip arthrodesis, in Lieberman JR, Berry DJ, eds: *Advanced Reconstruction: Hip.* Rosemont, IL, American Academy of Orthopaedic Surgeons, 2005, pp 495-501.)

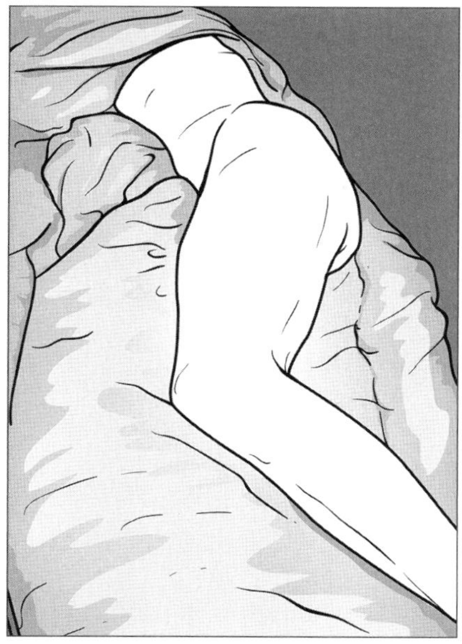

Figure 7 The patient is positioned in the lateral decubitus position with the affected hip facing up on a deflatable bean bag positioner. The lateral positioning needs to be precise; therefore, an AP radiograph is obtained to confirm alignment of the center of the sacrum with the symphysis pubis. (Reproduced from Weinstein SL, Garbuz DS, Duncan CP: Hip arthrodesis, in Lieberman JR, Berry DJ, eds: *Advanced Reconstruction: Hip.* Rosemont, IL, American Academy of Orthopaedic Surgeons, 2005, pp 495-501.)

radiographically. If satisfactory progress toward fusion is evident, weight bearing can be gradually increased over the next 6 to 10 weeks. Most patients do not require external walking aids by 4 to 5 months postoperatively.

Cobra Plating Technique (Vancouver)

The Vancouver technique is a modification of the original cobra plate compression technique described by Castle and Schneider. This technique avoids the need for pelvic osteotomy because the socket is medialized and the plate contoured to the pelvis and femur.

EXPOSURE

- The patient is placed in the lateral position with the affected hip facing up (**Figure 7**).
- The contralateral limb is flexed to help reduce spinal lordosis.
- An AP radiograph is obtained to confirm the position of the pelvis before the procedure begins.
- A straight lateral incision is centered over the greater trochanter and curved slightly posteriorly (**Figure 8, A**).

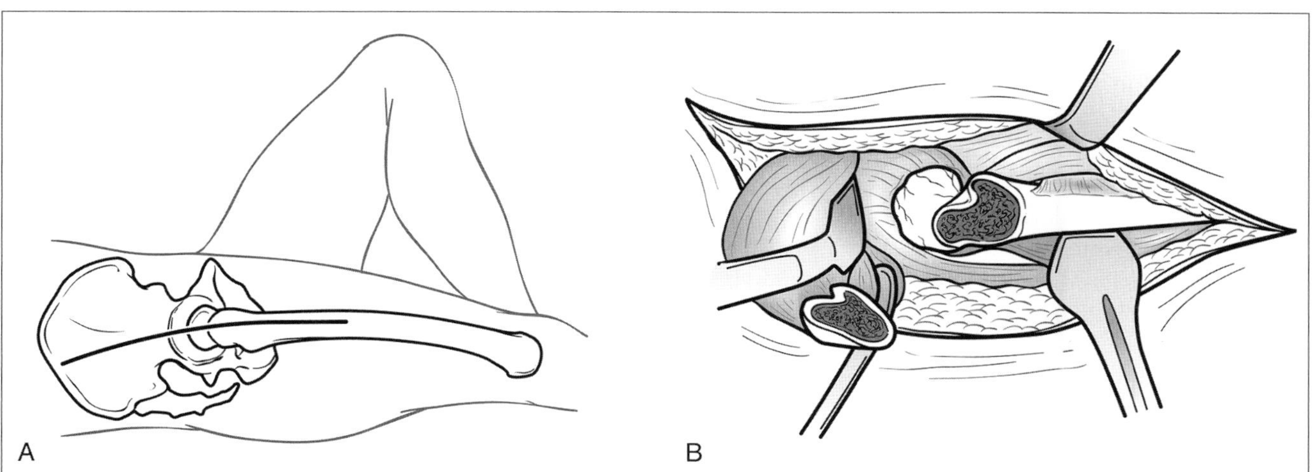

Figure 8 A slightly curved lateral incision is made (**A**), and the femur and capsule are exposed by elevation of the vastus lateralis and greater trochanter (**B**). (Reproduced from Weinstein SL, Garbuz DS, Duncan CP: Hip arthrodesis, in Lieberman JR, Berry DJ, eds: *Advanced Reconstruction: Hip.* Rosemont, IL, American Academy of Orthopaedic Surgeons, 2005, pp 495-501.)

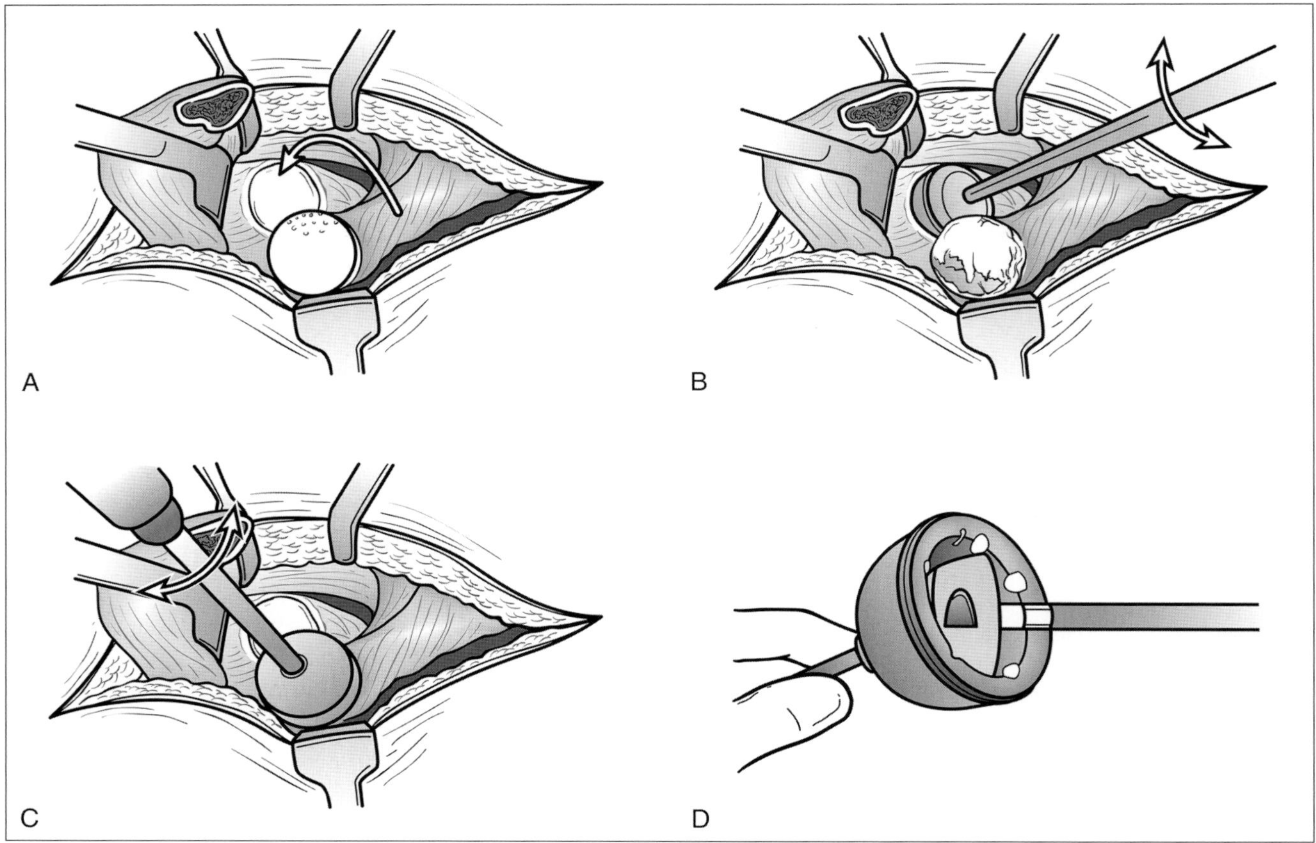

Figure 9 The hip is dislocated anteriorly (**A**) after which the acetabulum and femoral head are prepared with closely matching reamers (**B** and **C**). These reamers date from the first era of surface replacement (**D**). (Reproduced from Weinstein SL, Garbuz DS, Duncan CP: Hip arthrodesis, in Lieberman JR, Berry DJ, eds: *Advanced Reconstruction: Hip*. Rosemont, IL, American Academy of Orthopaedic Surgeons, 2005, pp 495-501.)

- The femoral shaft is exposed by elevating the vastus lateralis.
- A classic greater trochanteric osteotomy is then performed, and the trochanteric fragment is elevated and retracted proximally (**Figure 8, B**).
- An anterior capsulectomy is performed to ensure that the posterior capsule is preserved so that the extraosseous blood supply to the femoral head is not disrupted.

BONE PREPARATION

- The hip is dislocated anteriorly (**Figure 9, A**), and the acetabulum and femoral head are prepared.
- The acetabulum is reamed with hemispheric reamers and medialized to the level of the inner pelvis. The femoral head is reamed with an oversized female reamer. Matching reamers, formerly used for resurfacing THA, are used (**Figure 9, B** through **D**) so that a very tight cancellous bone to cancellous bone contact area is achieved.

INTERNAL FIXATION

- The limb is now positioned in 20° of flexion, 5° of external rotation, and 10° of adduction. Note that the adduction usually will be decreased by 10° once the outrigger compression device is applied.
- A cobra plate is selected, and benders are used to shape the plate to fit the outer table of the pelvis and the lateral aspect of the femur. The plate is initially fixed to the acetabulum with a central proximal screw. At this point, gentle compression is applied distally and an intraoperative radiograph is obtained to confirm the desired degree of adduction (femur relative to pelvis). At this point adduction should be 10° to 20° so that once compression is complete the limb will be in neutral adduction (ie, equivalent to 10° adduction of femoral shaft to pelvis).
- If the radiographs confirm appropriate positioning, the remaining proximal screws are inserted followed by compression with the AO compression device (**Figure 10, A**).
- Screws are then inserted through

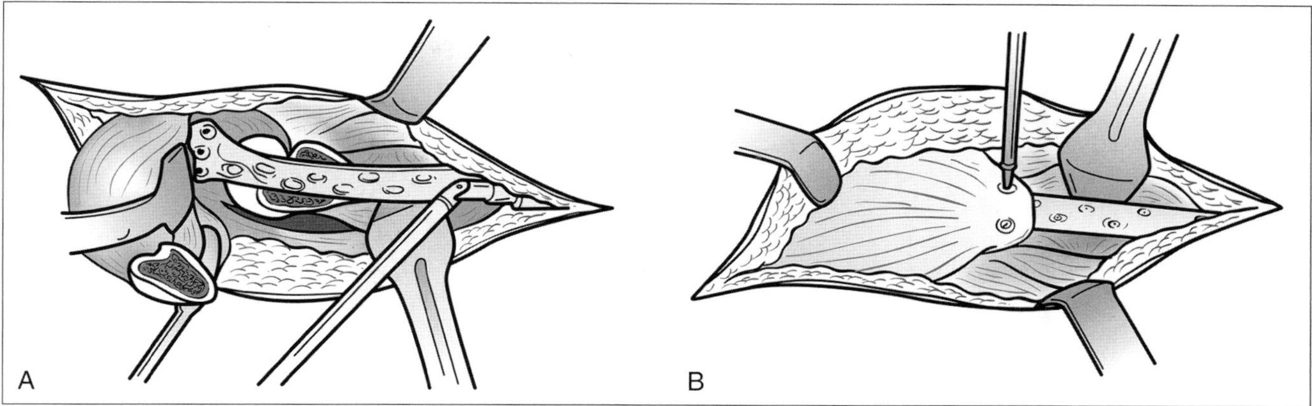

Figure 10 Initial fixation is with a proximal screw in the cobra head, and initial compression is with the distal outrigger (**A**) followed by radiographic confirmation of plate placement and limb alignment. The proximal screws are then inserted, compression is completed, the remaining screws inserted, and the greater trochanter accurately repositioned and fixed (**B**). (Reproduced from Weinstein SL, Garbuz DS, Duncan CP: Hip arthrodesis, in Lieberman JR, Berry DJ, eds: *Advanced Reconstruction: Hip*. Rosemont, IL, American Academy of Orthopaedic Surgeons, 2005, pp 495-501.)

the plate into the femoral shaft.

- The greater trochanter is then reattached in its anatomic position using cancellous screws with washers (**Figure 10, B**).

POSTOPERATIVE REGIMEN

The patient is placed on crutches for 3 months postoperatively, with toe-touch weight bearing during the first 6 weeks followed by progression to full weight bearing by 3 months postoperatively. Union is expected by 4 months postoperatively, and patients generally can expect to return to work by 6 to 12 months after surgery.

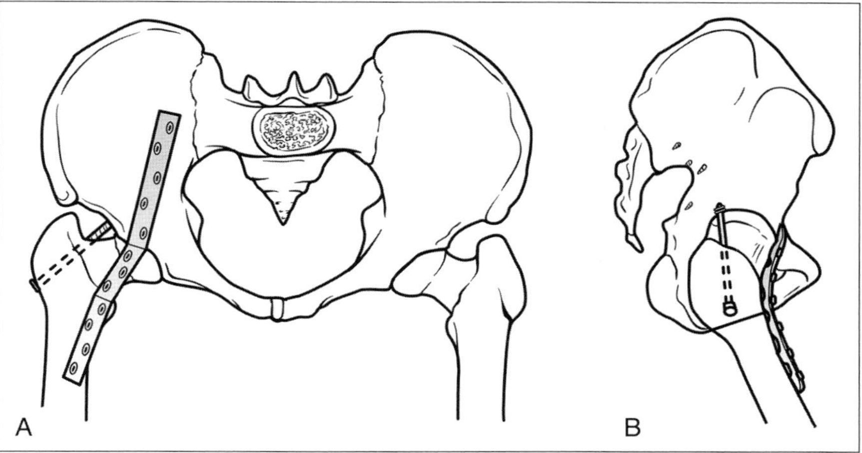

Figure 11 Anterior plating technique. AP (**A**) and lateral (**B**) views of the pelvis with optimal position of plate and lateral lag screw. (Reproduced from Beaulé PE, Matta JM, Mast JW: Hip arthrodesis: Current indications and techniques. *J Am Acad Orthop Surg* 2002;10[4]:249-258.)

Anterior Plating Technique

This technique, described by Beaulé and associates, has the same advantages as other modern hip arthrodesis techniques: rigid internal fixation, medialization of the construct, and maximal bone contact, but it also completely spares the abductors and minimizes deformity of the pelvis, both important technical considerations for patients who may later require conversion to THA.

EXPOSURE

- The patient is placed in the supine position, and a modified Smith-Peterson approach is used, including exposure of the inner aspect of the pelvis.
- The sartorius and two heads of the rectus are released from the origin.
- The vastus lateralis is elevated to expose the femur.

BONE PREPARATION AND PLATING

- After denuding the femoral head and acetabulum, a 6.5-mm lag screw is inserted from the lateral aspect of the greater trochanter into the supra-acetabular region.
- A 12- or 14-hole low-contact dynamic compression plate is molded to the anterior contour of the femur, pelvic brim, and proximal femur (**Figure 11**). The plate typically is fixed to the pelvis first.
- Compression is obtained by use of the tensioning device on the femur.
- The plate is then further secured to the femur with standard screws.

WOUND CLOSURE

- Routine wound closure in layers is performed.

POSTOPERATIVE REGIMEN

The patient is allowed weight bearing of approximately 30 lb for 10 weeks. After 12 weeks, if there is radiographic evidence of union, the patient is allowed full weight bearing. In the original series, the rate of union was 83%, and patient satisfaction was high.

Avoiding Pitfalls and Complications

A major pitfall of hip arthrodesis is malunion, but this can be avoided by strict adherence to surgical technique and the use of intraoperative radiographs. For surgeons with little prior experience with this procedure, supine positioning of the patient may assist in precise limb positioning.

Nonunion can occur but has decreased in incidence with use of modern techniques of internal fixation. Rates of union with modern techniques have been reported to be between 85% and 95%. If nonunion occurs, and infection has been ruled out, repeat arthrodesis with an iliac crest bone graft is the preferred treatment.

Patient satisfaction is the main goal of surgery. In the short term, a well-informed patient and a successful arthrodesis will usually result in a satisfied patient. A detailed discussion about outcomes and functional limitations should be part of the patient's informed consent process.

In the long term, difficulties are usually encountered in adjacent joints. Low back pain and ipsilateral knee pain are seen in more than half of all patients at long-term follow-up. In these patients, conversion to THA is appropriate. Conversion most predictably will relieve back pain and, to a lesser extent, relieve ipsilateral knee or contralateral hip pain. The outcome following THA will largely depend on the adequacy of the abductors, making it critically important to protect the abductors and the greater trochanter during the procedure.

Bibliography

Beaulé PE, Matta JM, Mast JW: Hip arthrodesis: Current indications and techniques. *J Am Acad Orthop Surg* 2002;10(4):249-258.

Callaghan JJ, Brand RA, Pedersen DR: Hip arthrodesis: A long-term follow-up. *J Bone Joint Surg Am* 1985;67(9):1328-1335.

Callaghan JJ, McBeath AA: Arthrodesis, in Callaghan JJ, Rosenberg AG, Rubash HE, eds: *The Adult Hip*. New York, NY, Lippincott-Raven, 1998, pp 749-759.

Duncan CP, Spangehl M, Beauchamp C, McGraw R: Hip arthrodesis: An important option for advanced disease in the young adult. *Can J Surg* 1995;38(suppl 1):S39-S45.

Fulkerson JP: Arthrodesis for disabling hip pain in children and adolescents. *Clin Orthop Relat Res* 1977;(128):296-302.

Karol LA, Halliday SE, Gourineni P: Gait and function after intra-articular arthrodesis of the hip in adolescents. *J Bone Joint Surg Am* 2000;82(4):561-569.

Kilgus DJ, Amstutz HC, Wolgin MA, Dorey FJ: Joint replacement for ankylosed hips. *J Bone Joint Surg Am* 1990;72(1):45-54.

Schneider R: Hip arthrodesis with the cobra head plate and pelvic osteotomy. *Reconstr Surg Traumatol* 1974;14(0):1-37.

Sponseller PD, McBeath AA, Perpich M: Hip arthrodesis in young patients: A long-term follow-up study. *J Bone Joint Surg Am* 1984;66(6):853-859.

Strathy GM, Fitzgerald RH Jr: Total hip arthroplasty in the ankylosed hip: A ten-year follow-up. *J Bone Joint Surg Am* 1988;70(7):963-966.

Chapter 68

Intertrochanteric Femoral Osteotomies for the Management of Developmental and Posttraumatic Conditions

Richard F. Santore, MD

Indications

Although contemporary total hip arthroplasty (THA) provides reliable and enduring results even in young patients, intertrochanteric osteotomy continues to have an important role in the armamentarium of the hip surgeon and is a valuable technique for hip preservation. In many patients, osteotomy is the best solution, especially when the patient does not have arthritis affecting the hip joint. Intertrochanteric osteotomy can be done as a stand-alone procedure or as an adjunct to a pelvic procedure such as a periacetabular or Chiari osteotomy. Intertrochanteric osteotomy offers substantial capacity for restoration of function, equalization of limb lengths (**Figures 1** and **2**), and correction of malrotation, excessive version, posttraumatic deformities, and developmental deformities. The function after an intertrochanteric osteotomy can approach, and even equal, that of a normal hip. Patient satisfaction after properly performed intertrochanteric osteotomies is high.

The blade plate and associated instruments, including 4.5-mm cortical screws, that are used for intertrochanteric osteotomy were designed in Switzerland in 1958 under the guidance of the founders of AO. The contribution of these surgeons, scientists, and engineers transformed the landscape of osteotomy procedures and fracture fixation by providing reliable instrumentation and implants. However, in the United States until the late 1970s, the use of plates and screws was considered too aggressive and too risky for use in patients with osteomyelitis, even after it was firmly established as the standard of care in Switzerland and much of Europe. Eventually, the Swiss methodology gained a solid footing in the United States.

Indications for osteotomy include collapse after internal fixation of a fracture or an iatrogenic deformity that results in limb-length inequality, malrotation of the limb, or the inability to insert a femoral stem. The goals of osteotomy include re-creation of normal or near-normal anatomy, limb length, and rotation. In patients with subtrochanteric deformity, the correction must be done at the site of the previous surgery.

Osteotomy can often be used in the management of femoral abnormalities, which are frequently seen in association with acetabular dysplasia. These morphologic variants include varus or valgus deformities of the upper femur in the frontal plane, excessive anteversion or retroversion of the femur in the sagittal plane, malrotation of the limb, and limb-length abnormalities. Dysplasia is more than an abnormality of the center-edge angle of Wiberg on a frontal plane radiograph of the hip. In addition to the femoral abnormalities, developmental dysplasia of the hip encompasses variation in the anatomy of the iliac wings and the position and shape of the anterior inferior iliac spine.

Pathology-Specific Indications

NONUNION OF FEMORAL NECK FRACTURE

The classic indication for intertrochanteric osteotomy is nonunion of a fracture of the femoral neck. A frontal plane valgus osteotomy using the AO blade plate can be performed to increase compression forces across the site of the nonunion. Osteotomies of less than or equal to 30° can be performed. Because pure valgus without wedge resection lengthens the limb, in most patients a corresponding wedge must be removed to prevent the lengthening. Placement of a threaded pin or a screw proximal to the chisel site before the seating chisel is inserted can prevent displacement of the nonunion. Because fractures of the femoral neck are associated with bone fragility, the surgeon must take care not to apply excessive axial compression on the osteotomy site and to leave a bony

Dr. Santore or an immediate family member serves as a paid consultant to Medacta; has stock or stock options held in Abbott, GlaxoSmithKline, Johnson & Johnson, Merck, Pfizer, Stryker, and Zimmer Biomet; and serves as a board member, owner, officer, or committee member of the Orthopaedic Research and Education Foundation and the Sharp HealthCare Foundation.

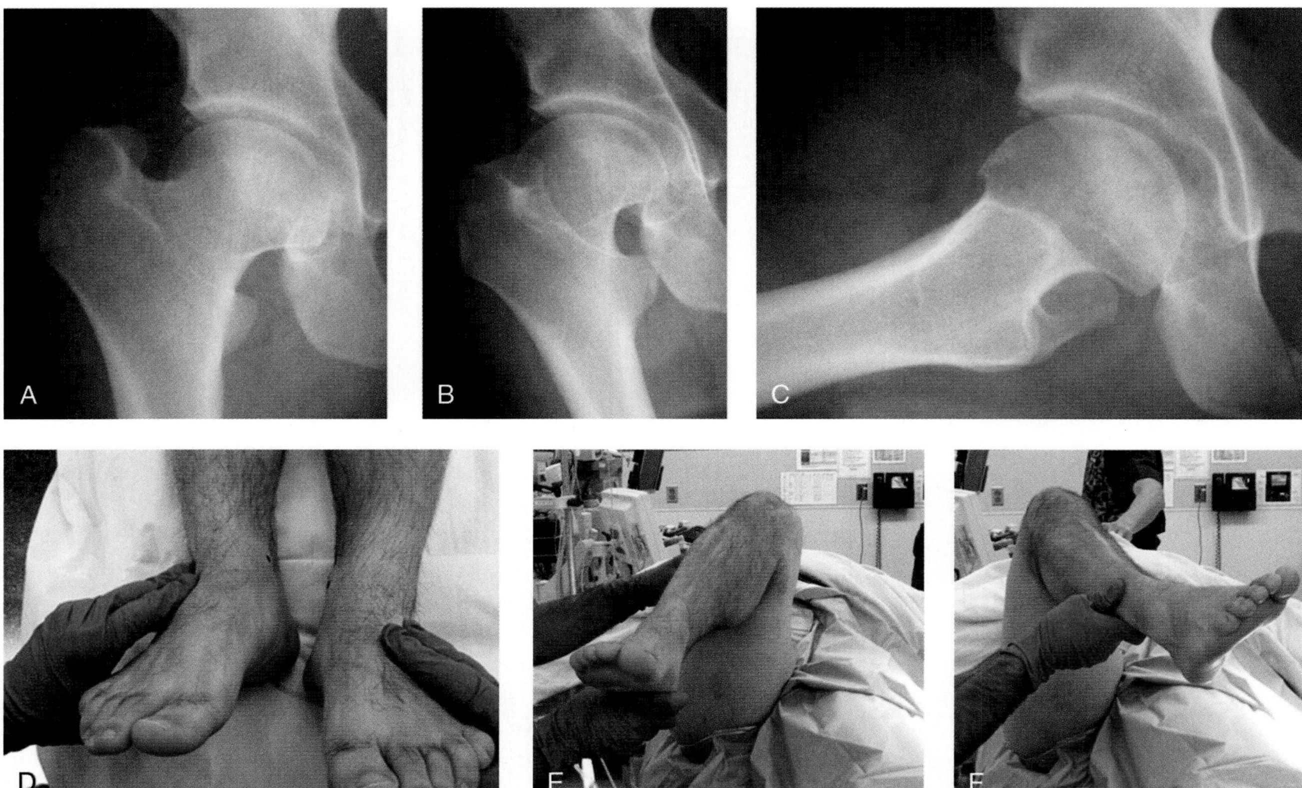

Figure 1 **A,** Preoperative AP radiograph of the right hip from a 28-year-old patient demonstrates a high-riding greater trochanter, acquired varus deformity, a short femoral neck, and a short limb. **B,** Preoperative AP radiograph obtained with the hip in adduction demonstrates good appearance of the joint and improved position of the greater trochanter. Importantly, the patient was comfortable in adduction, both when supine and when walking with the hip in an adducted position. **C,** Preoperative lateral radiograph demonstrates increased femoral head anteversion and poor anterior offset indicative of femoroacetabular impingement, as well as early arthritis. Preoperative photographs with the patient positioned supine show shortening of the right (affected) leg (**D**), the maximum passive internal rotation of the affected hip in the flexed position (**E**), and the maximum external rotation of the affected hip (**F**). Internal and external rotation were less than normal.

bridge of sufficient length between the chisel site and the osteotomy. Intertrochanteric osteotomy for the management of nonunion of the femoral neck usually consists of a simple frontal plane osteotomy. Concomitant bone grafting of the nonunion site is not routinely done and typically is not needed because of the high rate of success of the valgus osteotomy itself.

In contrast to the indications for THA, osteotomy is indicated if the hip joint is normal and not arthritic. However, studies have demonstrated that valgus osteotomies for the management of nonunion of the femoral neck are clinically effective even in patients who have osteonecrosis. A decade or more of good function can be achieved before THA becomes necessary. In patients with confirmed osteonecrosis, decision making should take into account the size of the necrotic sector because that factor is the primary determinant of success in all joint-preserving surgical procedures in patients with osteonecrosis. In patients with nonunion associated with large necrotic lesions, THA is the treatment of choice.

LIMB-LENGTH INEQUALITY

A short limb can be lengthened as much as 3 cm via valgus intertrochanteric osteotomy. In contrast to the gradual lengthening of Ilizarov and similar techniques, careful monitoring of the sciatic nerve is required when this procedure is done; for example, as when major lengthening occurs during THA for the management of developmental dysplasia of the hip or after resection arthroplasty. If lengthening is the principal or major objective, no wedges are removed, and the lateral edge of the upper segment articulates with the flat surface of the distal segment. Offset is controlled by the depth of insertion of the blade plate into the proximal segment.

A long limb can be shortened successfully by up to 7.5 cm via either a varus osteotomy or a segmental resection of

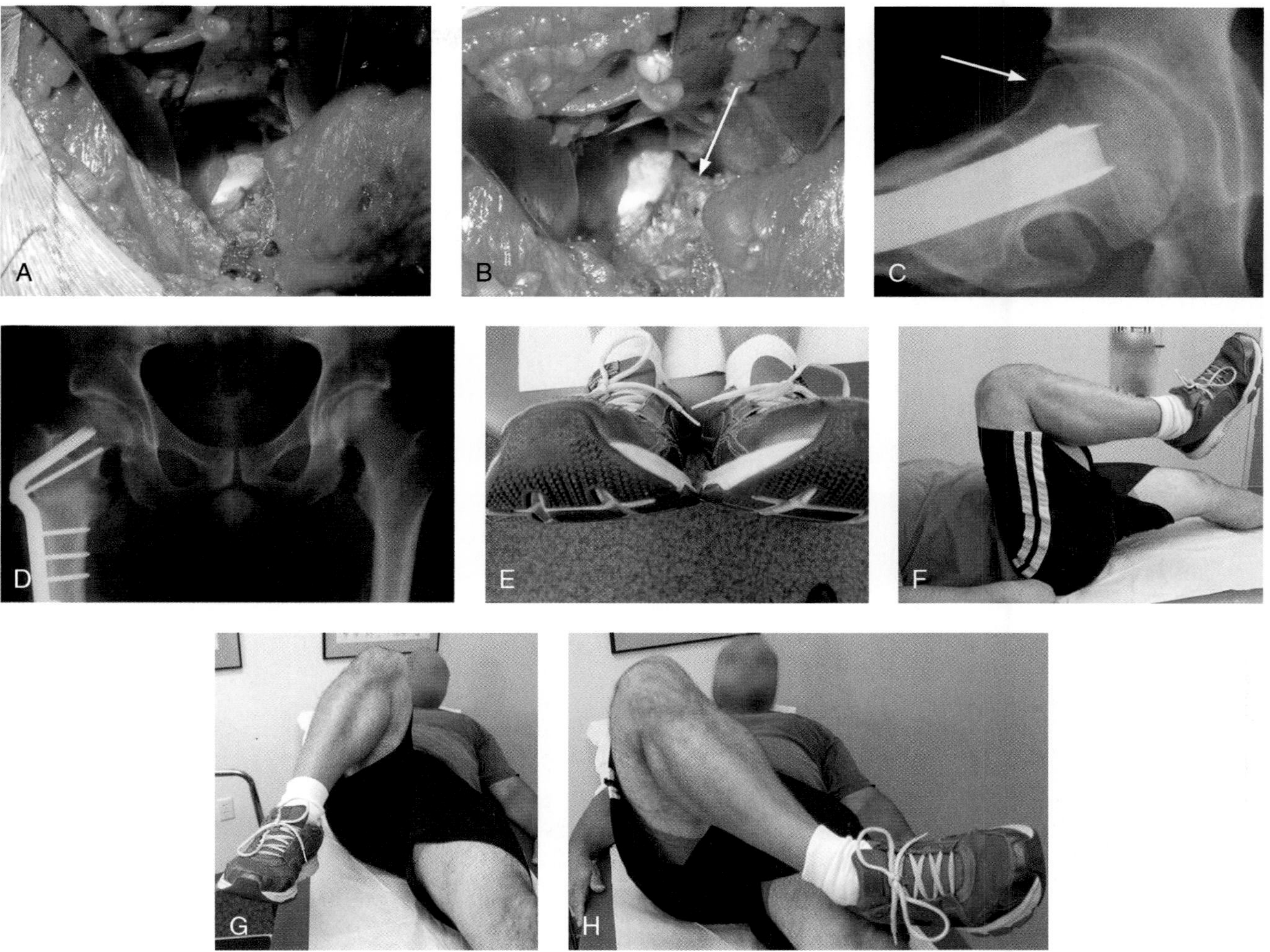

Figure 2 **A** and **B,** Intraoperative photographs of the same patient as Figure 1 show open femoral neck ostectomy through a Bombelli-type exposure for intertrochanteric osteotomy. The arrow in panel **B** indicates the area of femoral neck contouring. **C,** Lateral radiograph demonstrates extension osteotomy in the lateral plane and appearance after an open ostectomy (arrow). Note the intentionally decreased femoral anteversion and contouring of the femoral neck. **D,** Postoperative AP pelvic radiograph demonstrates the healed osteotomy in good alignment in the frontal plane, with normalization of the relationship of the tip of the greater trochanter to the femoral head. Appropriate alignment of the femoral shaft to the proximal fragment will allow easy insertion of a femoral prosthesis in the future, if necessary. **E,** A clinical photograph shows equal limb lengths after the osteotomy. This result highlights the utility of opening wedge valgus intertrochanteric osteotomy for lengthening a limb. Clinical photographs show improvement in all planes of motion: flexion (**F**), internal rotation in flexion (**G**), and external rotation in flexion (**H**). The patient returned to full duty as a firefighter and was able to complete his physical fitness tests and to lift weights. Additionally, he was able to sit cross-legged, which was not possible preoperatively.

a bone wedge without angular correction. If the femoral neck-shaft angle is normal and the patient has no acetabular dysplasia, a varus intertrochanteric osteotomy is contraindicated. In this circumstance, wedge resection is performed. Although 6 cm or less can be sacrificed, the author of this chapter has not resected more than 4 cm.

Valgus osteotomies result in lengthening and varus osteotomies result in shortening. When a valgus osteotomy is performed, the lengthening may be desirable and, in fact, may be a goal of the procedure. The lengthening is achieved via the displacement of the distal segment by the lateral edge of the femoral shaft when the side plate of the blade plate is reduced to the lateral cortex of the distal segment. The magnitude of lengthening increases as the valgus increases. That is, a 30° valgus osteotomy has greater capacity for lengthening compared with a 15° valgus osteotomy. The most the author of this chapter has done is a 40° valgus osteotomy (**Figure 3**). If lengthening is not desirable,

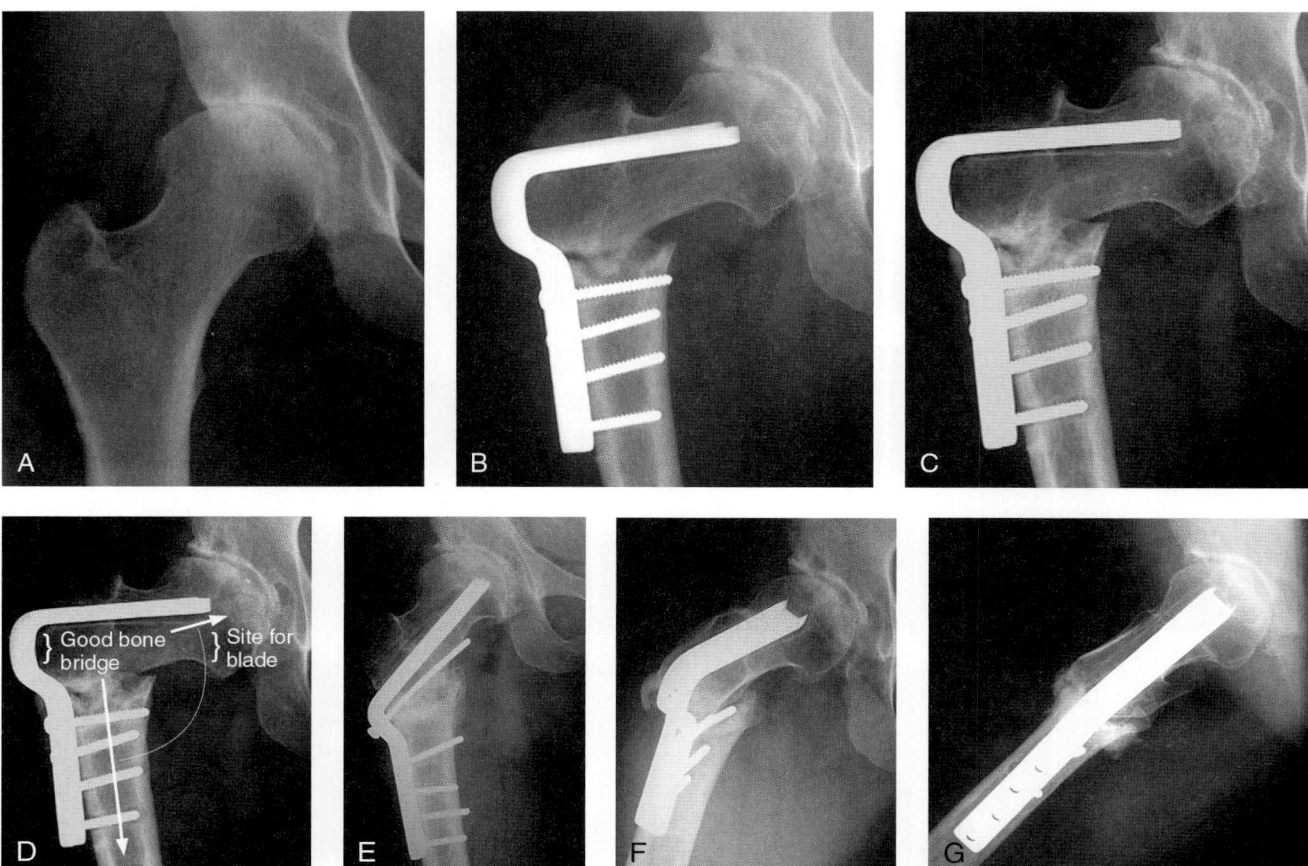

Figure 3 AP radiographs demonstrate the right hip of a 34-year-old woman before (**A**) and 6 months after (**B**) she underwent a salvage 40° varus intertrochanteric osteotomy at a different institution. **B,** The patient has a 90° femoral neck-shaft angle; excessive varus correction; nonunion; 3 cm shortening of the limb; and a severe limp resulting from the limb-length inequality, pain, and abductor weakness. Because the patient had severe arthritis, total hip arthroplasty (THA) should have been performed instead of the previous osteotomy. **C,** AP hip radiograph obtained 6 months after the initial osteotomy demonstrates nonunion and loose hardware. By the time the patient was referred to the author of this chapter, the loose hardware and collapse of the osteotomy site with further shortening of the limb would have made THA too complex, so opening wedge osteotomy was performed instead. **D,** The same AP radiograph as in panel **C** demonstrates sufficient good bone in the inferior femoral neck and head to allow a salvage intertrochanteric osteotomy. The arrows demarcate the 90° angle between the shaft and the femoral neck, and the bracket outlines the bone bridge, which is adequate for another osteotomy with a different device and place of insertion. Corrective valgus osteotomy was chosen to restore the anatomy, allow healing of the nonunion, achieve stable internal fixation, and restore abductor function in preparation for a safe and predictable THA in future. An opening-wedge 40° valgus osteotomy with a 130° AO blade plate was planned. **E,** AP hip radiograph obtained 2 years postoperatively demonstrates successful 40° valgus intertrochanteric osteotomy in the frontal plane, with restoration of physiologic offset between the proximal and distal segments. The procedure was executed to ensure ease of insertion of a THA stem in the future. Lateral radiographs obtained before (**F**) and 2 years after (**G**) the salvage valgus osteotomy demonstrate the results of the 20° flexion osteotomy and posterior shift of the proximal segment in the sagittal plane to prepare the femoral canal for the stem of a THA prosthesis. Unexpectedly, after the salvage osteotomy, the patient was free of pain and requested to indefinitely delay conversion to THA.

a wedge must be resected to avoid the lengthening that would otherwise occur. In fact, a full wedge resection may not be sufficient to offset all the lengthening. Palpation of the contralateral ankle may reveal the need for resection of an additional segmental wedge of several millimeters. The length effects can be anticipated in the preoperative planning but must be confirmed intraoperatively by direct palpation of the contralateral medial malleolus, which is easy to do because the procedure is always performed with the patient in the supine position.

Conversely, the shortening effect of a varus osteotomy is desirable if the ipsilateral leg is long preoperatively.

If a varus osteotomy is necessary but shortening is not desired, the shortening effect can be minimized by avoiding wedge resection and by performing the smallest varus osteotomy that will achieve the desired result. If a periacetabular osteotomy is performed, an adjunctive varus intertrochanteric osteotomy can be done if the limb is long preoperatively and the femoral neck and shaft are in valgus. Otherwise, shortening without varus can be accomplished via simple segmental resection to equalize the limb lengths. The equalization of preoperatively unequal limb lengths via an intertrochanteric osteotomy or combined periacetabular and intertrochanteric osteotomies typically results in substantial patient satisfaction.

MALROTATION

Malrotation of the lower extremity is frequently encountered in patients with dysplasia, posttraumatic deformities, slipped capital femoral epiphysis (SCFE), Legg-Calvé-Perthes disease, and otherwise undiagnosed knee pain. In some patients, derotation is the primary goal of an intertrochanteric osteotomy. A key principle of intertrochanteric osteotomy is that the osteotomy should almost always be made perpendicular to the long axis of the femur, and any needed derotation needs to be done and confirmed before wedges are resected. If derotation is done after wedge resection, complex deformities result. As is the case for most intertrochanteric osteotomies, the osteotomy is usually done at the upper border of the lesser trochanter so that any future surgical procedures will be in the context of normal anatomy distal to the osteotomy site and because healing at this level is highly reliable with low risk of nonunion.

COXA VALGA

Coxa valga, or the presence of a femoral neck-shaft angle greater than or equal to 140°, is common in patients who have dysplasia or malrotation. Before the advent of successful pelvic rotational osteotomies, varus osteotomy of the upper femur was the mainstay of surgical management of acetabular dysplasia. This varus osteotomy was particularly successful in patients with ipsilateral limb lengthening associated with dysplasia. A 15° to 20° varus osteotomy usually was ideal for equalization of limb lengths and improved coverage of the femoral head. More extreme varus, such as 30°, usually resulted in extreme shortening and persistent limp. Currently, periacetabular osteotomy alone is the procedure of choice. The exception is patients in whom the dysplasia is mild and correction of limb length is an important goal. In these patients, intertrochanteric osteotomy alone is the procedure of choice, and periacetabular osteotomy is not needed. In a study of the long-term outcomes of intertrochanteric osteotomy in patients with dysplasia in whom the femoral neck-shaft angle was greater than or equal to 144°, the success rate of intertrochanteric osteotomy at 10-year follow-up was 100%. Therefore, intertrochanteric osteotomy remains relevant for the management of coxa valga in certain clinical scenarios.

FEMORAL ANTEVERSION

Femoral anteversion can result from anterior displacement of the femoral head or malrotation of the limb. The two causes are not synonymous or interchangeable. Anterior displacement, as seen in patients with Legg-Calvé-Perthes disease and in patients with dysplasia, is managed with extension intertrochanteric osteotomy (**Figure 2**). Malrotation is managed with derotation at the time of intertrochanteric osteotomy to achieve balance in the range of motion (ROM). Anterior displacement and malrotation can occur simultaneously, requiring both extension and derotation in the same surgical procedure. If extension is done in the sagittal plane, the surgeon must take care to avoid overcorrection, which can result in iatrogenic impingement. The concept of extension osteotomy is based on the change in position of the segment distal to the osteotomy. An osteotomy is termed an extension osteotomy if the distal segment is moved posteriorly (that is, into extension) before osteosynthesis is achieved. Conversely, in a flexion osteotomy, the distal segment is flexed relative to the proximal segment. Flexion osteotomy is commonly used in intertrochanteric osteotomies performed for the management of osteonecrosis.

FEMORAL RETROVERSION

Although femoral retroversion is uncommon, it is a risk factor for anterior femoroacetabular impingement. Flexion intertrochanteric osteotomy can be performed to increase offset between the femoral head and neck.

HIGH-RIDING TROCHANTER AFTER LEGG-CALVÉ-PERTHES DISEASE

Patients who have been treated for Legg-Calvé-Perthes disease often have a high-riding greater trochanter, a short femoral neck, acetabular dysplasia, a short limb, and acetabular retroversion. Combined pelvic and femoral osteotomies commonly are indicated. If the limb is short, lengthening intertrochanteric osteotomy (valgus without wedge resection) and periacetabular osteotomy are performed concomitantly. If the patient does not have a short limb, lateral and distal advancement of the greater trochanter can be combined with a periacetabular osteotomy.

RESIDUAL DEFORMITY AFTER SCFE

Historically, the Imhäuser triplane osteotomy was used to manage deformities resulting from SCFE, including excessive external rotation, femoral head retroversion, relative varus of the femoral neck-shaft angle, and shortening of the limb. These deformities were amenable to improvement from the triplane osteotomy, which encompassed derotation (internal rotation of the distal segment), valgus, and flexion. With the advent of open surgical dislocation for the management of femoroacetabular impingement, the surgical procedure was modified to facilitate femoral neck osteotomy in a manner that preserved the blood supply to the femoral head, restored more normal anatomy, and permitted contouring of the femoral neck. This procedure is technically much more difficult than the triplane osteotomy at the intertrochanteric level. However, it involves some risk of osteonecrosis, as well as failure of fixation and nonunion of the greater trochanter. The effectiveness of the surgical dislocation approach makes it an appealing option for the management of new cases of SCFE as well, provided that a surgeon with the requisite training and experience performs the procedure. Nonetheless, triplane intertrochanteric osteotomy is a good option for the management of residual symptoms in patients with previous grade II SCFE that has healed. The key to triplane intertrochanteric osteotomy is the insertion of the seating chisel, which must take into account the need for appropriate valgus, flexion in the sagittal plane of less than or equal to 40°, and the appropriate amount of derotation after the osteotomy. Usually the amount of limb shortening is not substantial, so intraoperative adjustment of the limb length must be done using wedge resection or segmental resection of bone distal to the osteotomy site. Correction of the preoperative obligatory external rotation of the limb during hip flexion typically results in great patient satisfaction postoperatively.

ACQUIRED VARUS DEFORMITY

Planning and techniques for the management of acquired varus deformity in the frontal plane should follow the principles of management of nonunion of the femoral neck. In the sagittal plane, flexion or extension may be required, depending on the circumstances, such as associated femoral retroversion for femoral anteversion. A rotational osteotomy on the pelvic side also may be indicated. In some patients in whom limb lengths are equal, a distal/lateral transfer of the greater trochanter may be preferable.

Assessment and Evaluation

Several clinical factors should be considered in the decision-making process. Because many clinical assessments are specific to the patient's diagnosis, obtaining an accurate diagnosis is paramount. Assessment should include body weight, smoking status, age, and stiffness, as well as the patient's prior surgical treatment and goals of the surgical procedure under consideration. Specific tests include the position-of-comfort test and evaluation of leg length, hypermobility, muscle strength, limp, angular deformities of the knee, and rotation of the limb.

The patient's history of prior treatment and any prior surgical procedures must be determined. Malposition from a prior osteotomy can result in multiplane deformities that require osteotomy before or at the time of THA. The surgeon must ensure that the patient understands the philosophy of hip preservation and accepts the need for 3 months or longer of postoperative rehabilitation before normal walking is achieved. The surgeon also must understand the patient's goals. Some patients may want to return to high-demand sports and running, whereas others may want only to be pain free and able to walk more normally. Many patients assume that they will have normal function after the osteotomy procedure and not require hip arthroplasty in the future. The surgeon must actively counsel the patient preoperatively regarding realistic expectations of the function and longevity of the result. The author of this chapter advises all patients that the osteotomy is recommended for the management of a lifelong condition and that other appropriate interventions, including THA, may be necessary in the future. The goals of the procedure are to improve symptoms and function in the immediate postoperative period and delay the need for THA. Surgeons should not promise pain-free status or normal function after the osteotomy.

The author of this chapter has long used the position-of-comfort test. If a valgus osteotomy is chosen, such as for the management of SCFE, osteonecrosis, or dysplasia, the patient should be comfortable when the leg is placed in adduction, either supine or standing, in addition to having adequate passive adduction. The patient also should experience improved comfort with passive adduction on the examination table, as well as when standing with the ipsilateral leg adducted and walking with the leg in adduction.

Assessment of limb length is important because dysplasia, posttraumatic and postoperative deformities, and other diagnoses can be associated with limb-length abnormalities. A short ipsilateral limb may rule out varus intertrochanteric osteotomy because the varus osteotomy would further shorten the limb and likely result in an unacceptable outcome for the patient even if appropriate biomechanics and coverage of the hip were successfully achieved. If the ipsilateral limb is long, a varus osteotomy can facilitate equalization of the limb lengths and is a better option, even as an adjunct to periacetabular osteotomy. A primary goal of intertrochanteric osteotomy is to correct limb-length inequality while avoiding iatrogenic exacerbation of the inequality. An exception is when staged bilateral procedures of the same type are planned and the limb-length inequality will be present only after the first side has been done and before the second side is done.

Soft-tissue status should be assessed in all patients because hypermobility is a frequently associated condition, particularly in patients who have hip dysplasia. In patients who have hypermobility, enhancement of containment or coverage of the femoral head within the acetabulum is an important goal. Containment must be considered from a global perspective, not just in the frontal plane. Occasionally, a standard radiograph may demonstrate a near-normal appearance of the hip, whereas a true lateral, Dunn lateral, or false-profile radiograph or three-dimensional CT scan may show uncoverage of the femoral head anteriorly, resulting from focal anterior acetabular dysplasia or excessive anteversion of the upper femur, or both. In these patients, extension osteotomy in the sagittal plane can be effective.

Assessment of muscle strength is important, particularly in the abductors and flexors. Patients who underwent prior surgical procedures in childhood and those with neuromuscular dysplasia, posttraumatic muscle damage, and other muscular conditions require careful documentation of muscle strength, both to facilitate proper decision making and to ensure that any weakness is documented before the intertrochanteric osteotomy is performed so that the weakness is not incorrectly attributed to the osteotomy. Abductor weakness is commonly seen in patients with high-riding greater trochanters associated with coxa vara and in patients with the low-offset, coxa magna deformity and short femoral neck of Legg-Calvé-Perthes disease (combined low offset and high position). In these patients, the abductors can be strengthened with a trochanteric advancement osteotomy or valgus osteotomy. The decision is influenced by other factors, discussed later in this chapter. Weakness of hip flexion can result from tenotomies performed at the time of childhood pelvic osteotomy, such as Salter, Steel, Sutherland, or Eppright osteotomy, or after arthroscopic release. Adductor weakness can occur in the aftermath of surgical exposure for Steel osteotomies (direct damage to muscle) or can result from injury to the obturator nerve during intrapelvic surgical procedures, among other reasons. Gluteal weakness is less common but can occur in patients with postpolio syndrome and other neuromuscular conditions.

Any limp that is present must be analyzed to determine causation. Limp can result from abductor weakness (positive Trendelenburg gait); pain (antalgic gait); or limb-length inequality (uneven platform); as well as other causes, such as unrelated arthritis of the foot, pathology of the knee, or stress fracture. Most instances of limp can be attributed to at least one of the first three reasons. Frequently, more than one reason is present, such as in a patient with a high-riding trochanter associated with an ipsilateral short limb. Abductor muscle weakness can be iatrogenic, such as after major varus osteotomies performed in childhood or pelvic osteotomies with stripping of the abductor origin from the lateral side of the ileum. One author reported that approximately 30% of the varus osteotomies that he performed required subsequent trochanteric advancement, done at the time of blade plate removal, to restore normal gait.

Angular deformities of the knee must be taken into consideration because the mechanical axis of the limb is influenced by intertrochanteric osteotomy. A varus osteotomy will shift the mechanical axis medially, and a valgus osteotomy will shift the mechanical axis laterally. This shift can be offset by appropriate displacements of the shaft at the time of osteotomy (in general, a medial shift with a varus osteotomy and a lateral shift with a valgus osteotomy). However, this concern cannot override the more important consideration that the intertrochanteric osteotomy must result in the ability to insert a THA stem in the future.

Rotation of the hip must be assessed in flexion and in extension. Many patients with dysplasia have increased internal rotation, often associated with a history of sitting on their knees in childhood. Some patients have almost no external rotation and have internal rotation greater than or equal to 70°. When carefully questioned, these patients will describe substantial functional limitations in sitting, sports, and sexual function because of the deficit of external rotation. Turning and pivoting motions required in sports such as golf can be adversely affected. An intertrochanteric derotation osteotomy can result in substantial functional improvement and can be incorporated into the overall surgical plan. In a few patients, the author of this chapter has combined a periacetabular osteotomy with a pure derotation or derotation/extension intertrochanteric osteotomy. In some patients, derotation was the only indication for the osteotomy, and some of these patients required offsetting internal rotation of the limb because of external tibial torsion. Skeletally immature and young (younger than 30 years) female patients, who have a much higher prevalence of hip dysplasia and associated malrotation issues, and who present with anterior knee pain require careful examination for malrotation at the hip level and hypermobility before any stand-alone lateral releases or extensor mechanism realignment procedures of the knee are performed.

Timing of Periacetabular and Intertrochanteric Osteotomies

The timing of the osteotomies, that is, whether the periacetabular osteotomy should be performed before or after the intertrochanteric osteotomy, is controversial. The preference and longstanding practice of the author of this chapter is to perform the intertrochanteric osteotomy first, because doing so allows the surgeon to plan the intertrochanteric osteotomy more precisely on the basis of specific goals that are usually clearly identified in advance, such as derotation; limb-length correction; angular correction in one or more planes; or, most commonly, a combination of these reasons. The periacetabular osteotomy that follows is easily adjusted intraoperatively under fluoroscopic guidance. The intertrochanteric osteotomy is less forgiving and requires advance planning to avoid undesired displacements and undercorrection or overcorrection in one or more planes.

Preoperative Planning

Careful planning of an intertrochanteric osteotomy is as important as the surgical procedure itself. Among the most important goals is avoidance of displacement that would hinder insertion of a femoral stem during a future THA procedure. The Müller principles of precision drawings made by hand, two-plane computer programs, or CT-based planning of osteotomies in two or three dimensions, with or without three-dimensional printing, should be followed before any incision is made.

When planning an osteotomy, the surgeon must keep in mind that angular measurements, such as the starting femoral neck-shaft angle or the intended change to that angle, are independent of the magnification factor of the analog or digital radiograph. However, linear measurements such as the distance between the insertion site of a blade plate and the site of the osteotomy are influenced greatly by the size of the patient's bone and the magnification effect of the radiograph. For example, in planning for a tibial osteotomy of the knee historically it was thought that 1° of angular correction was equal to 1 mm of wedge resection in a closing wedge osteotomy. However, 1 mm of wedge resection height in a patient with very small bone size can lead to greater than 1° of correction and result in substantial overcorrection. Conversely, undercorrection would occur in a patient with large bone dimensions.

The use of digital radiographs has compounded the difficulty of accurate measurement. Assessment of linear dimensions on digital radiographs is not possible unless the original image was obtained with a magnification marker in the plane of the bone. Therefore, metal magnification markers must be used when radiographic images are acquired for the planning of osteotomies or fracture fixation, as well as for the templating of implants for THA.

Planning for the insertion of a classic AO blade plate depends on a few basic geometric principles (**Figure 4**). Supplementary angles are those that, when added together, form a straight line (180°). When two lines cross, two supplementary angles and two vertical angles are created. The vertical angles on either side of the point of intersection are equal to one another. Imagine inserting a 120° blade plate into a femoral head in neutral position, without any change in the angle of the bone when the side arm of the plate is affixed to the shaft of the femur. To determine the angle of insertion of the guidewires and seating chisel, relative to the lateral cortex of the femur, imagine the 120° plate superimposed on the femur, and imagine a line demarcated by the side arm of the blade plate extending indefinitely proximally and distally. Next, imagine a line extending from the blade portion of the plate indefinitely in both directions (medially and laterally). The angle from the shaft that corresponds to the 120° angle of the blade plate is 60° (because 120° and 60° are supplementary angles). That is, the 60° angle is subtended between the long axis of the lateral cortex of the femoral shaft and the imaginary line extending from the blade of the plate. Therefore, a 120° plate is inserted with no correction by inserting the chisel at a 60° angle from the shaft. Similarly, the chisel insertion angle for a 130° plate is 50° from the shaft, because 50° and 130° are supplementary angles (**Table 1**). With this concept taken into account, planning of an angular osteotomy is easy. For a 20° valgus osteotomy, 20° is added to 60° for an insertion angle of 80° to the shaft. After the seating chisel is inserted at an 80° angle and the osteotomy is made, the process of aligning the side of the plate to the shaft generates 20° of valgus in the upper fragment.

For high-angle blade plates of different geometry, such as 110° or 130°, the concepts are the same as for valgus corrections. For a 30° correction with a 130° plate, for example, recall that 130° and 50° are supplementary angles. To obtain 30° of valgus, 30° is added to 50°, for an insertion angle of the chisel of 80°. After the chisel is placed at 80° to the shaft, the 30° correction occurs automatically when the side arm of the plate is brought down to the lateral cortex. Thus, the same 80° angle of insertion of the blade plate that results in 30° correction with a 130° plate would result in 20° valgus correction with a 120° plate.

In a more advanced level of planning, the 120° plate can be used as the standard implant. If the intraoperative situation requires more valgus, the 120° plate can be exchanged for a 130° plate to achieve an extra 10° of valgus. Conversely, if 20° of valgus is found to be too extreme intraoperatively, the 120° plate can be exchanged for a 110° plate to decrease the valgus to 10°. Although the need for this flexibility is rare, its utility is self-evident.

For varus osteotomies, a 90° plate is customarily used. The supplementary angle of 90° is 90°. However, the intended direction of the angular change in the upper fragment is the reverse of that for valgus osteotomies. Therefore, the intended correction is subtracted from 90°. For example, in a 15° varus osteotomy, the angle of insertion of the chisel is 90° minus 15°, or 75°. When the blade of the blade plate is placed, 15° of varus is achieved. Some surgeons also have used the 90° plate in valgus osteotomies. In that scenario, the degree of valgus is added to the measurement of the plate. For example, 15° of valgus is added to 90° for an insertion angle of

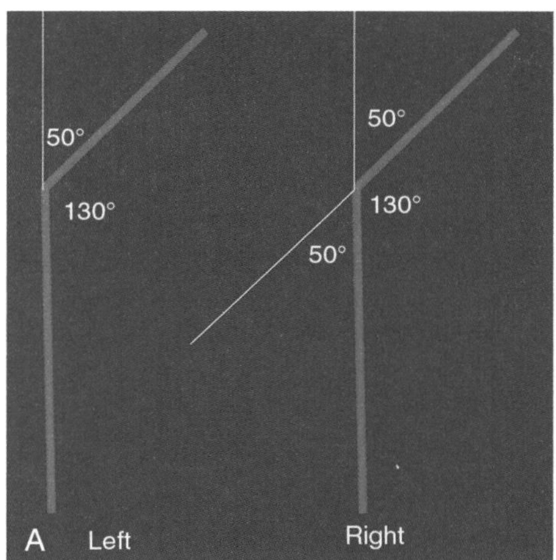

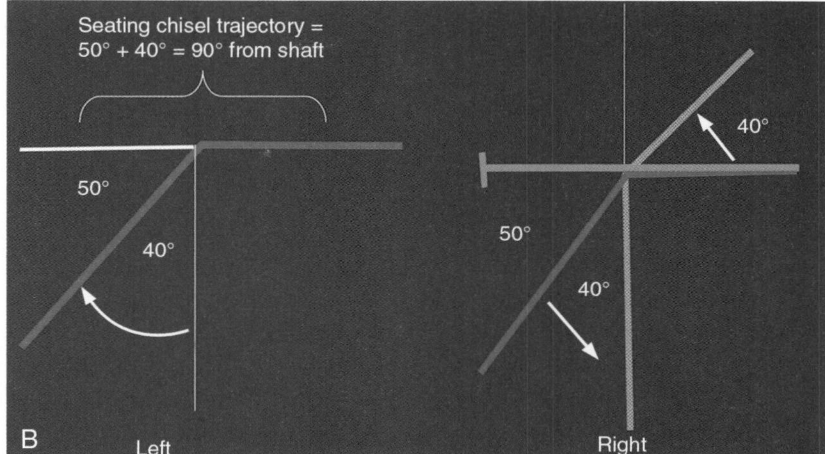

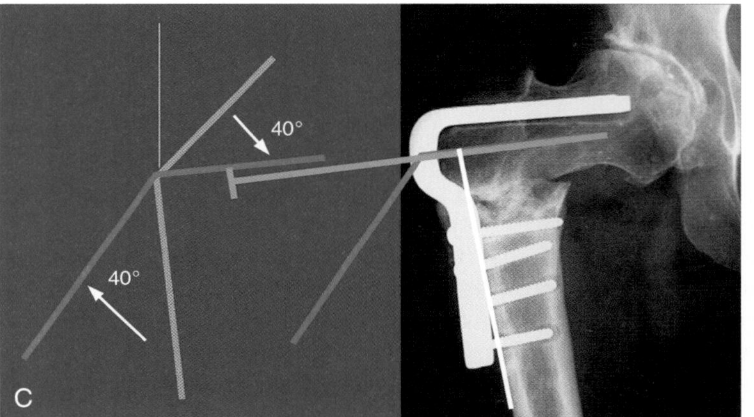

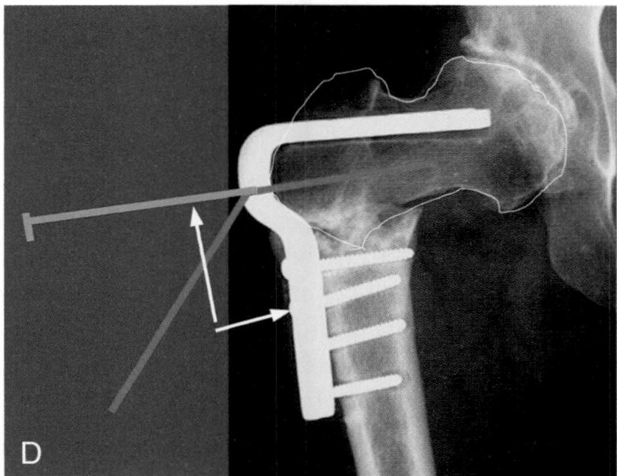

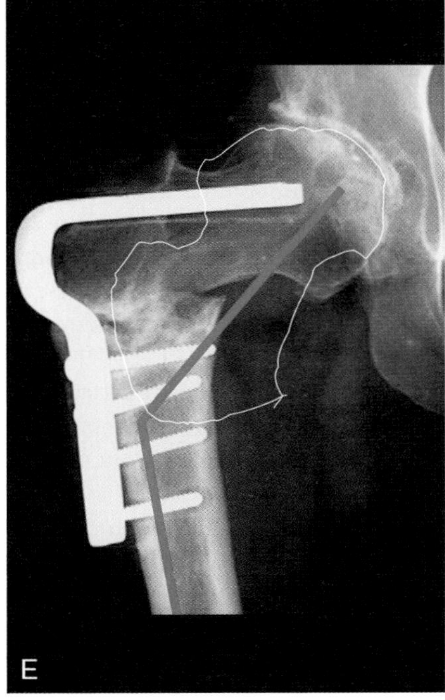

Figure 4 Diagrams and radiographs depict the basic geometry and appearance of a 130° blade plate placed in 40° for intertrochanteric osteotomy of the right hip. **A,** *Left,* The supplementary angle of 130° is 50°. *Right,* If the guidewire and plate were inserted at an angle of 50° to the shaft, no angular correction would result. This strategy is correct when a blade plate is used for fracture fixation with the goal of maintaining or restoring normal anatomy, but not for valgus or varus angular correction. **B,** *Left,* To achieve correction of 40°, 40° is added to 50°, resulting in a 90° angle to the shaft. *Right,* With the chisel (shown in green) inserted at a 90° angle, 40° of valgus will occur at the time of osteosynthesis of the side of the plate to the lateral cortex of the femoral shaft. When the blade plate is inserted at 90° to the shaft (red line parallel to green chisel line) and is cranked 40°, the correction occurs, with the red line (the blade plate) superimposed over the pink line (representing the plate in neutral position). **C** through **E,** Diagrams superimposed on Figure 3, B, show preoperative planning for insertion of the seating chisel (green) and the 130° blade plate (red). It is critically important to plan for a 15- to 24-mm bridge of good bone laterally between the site of insertion of the chisel and the site of the osteotomy. This patient had just enough good bone in the lower half of the femoral head and just enough good lateral cortex for a secure bone bridge to achieve the tension-band effect of the plate and to prevent fracture during reduction and compression. The white outline indicates the proximal segment in its preoperative position (**D**) and with the planned change in position by 40° (**E**), resulting in a marked improvement (decrease) in femoral offset, which was too great after the previous osteotomy. The final result will easily accommodate a standard cemented or noncemented total hip arthroplasty prosthesis in the future. The red line depicts the blade plate, and the white outline depicts the planned position of the femoral head and neck after the osteotomy. This planned positioning was achieved, as shown in Figure 3, E.

Table 1 Geometric Principles of 20° Valgus Intertrochanteric Osteotomy With High-Angle Blade Plates

Blade Plate Angle	Supplementary Angle	Chisel Insertion Angle
110°	180° – 110° = 70°	70° + 20° = 90°
120°	180° – 120° = 60°	60° + 20° = 80°
130°	180° – 130° = 50°	50° + 20° = 70°

105°. This method is technically more difficult than using the high-angle plates because the guidewire is farther from the lateral shaft, making the accuracy of the insertion more difficult.

Contraindications

Some issues are universal to decision making for any patient who is a potential candidate for a hip-preserving intertrochanteric osteotomy. Obese patients should be encouraged, and helped, to achieve a body mass index of less than 30 kg/m^2 via dietary changes and an appropriate exercise program. No published studies have reported the outcomes of osteotomy procedures after bariatric surgery, which may be associated with undesirable loss of muscle mass. Bariatric surgery should be considered with caution because it is unknown whether weight loss after bariatric surgery accrues from loss of adipose tissue only or loss of all tissues, including muscle, which would be undesirable.

Because smoking is associated with impaired bone and wound healing, no osteotomy should be performed on a patient who smokes. Patients should engage in a smoking cessation program and undergo a mandatory urine test to prove cessation preoperatively.

Patient age needs to be considered, but no absolute cutoff exists. In general, osteotomy can be performed safely in patients aged 35 years or younger. The author of this chapter has performed osteotomies on patients as old as 60 years in certain circumstances. Osteotomy should not be chosen on the basis of patient age alone. Depending on the circumstances, THA might be the treatment of choice even in patients as young as 16 years.

Other contraindications to intertrochanteric osteotomy include stiffness, inflammatory arthritis, infectious arthritis, and depression (the latter because recovery is arduous). For a varus intertrochanteric osteotomy, at least 15° of passive abduction is required, and for a valgus osteotomy, at least 15° of passive adduction is required. In a varus osteotomy, the femoral shaft is adducted relative to the osteotomy site, and passive abduction is necessary to return to neutral. In the absence of available passive abduction, a permanent deformity in adduction would ensue, which is analogous to the situation of excessive adduction after hip arthrodesis. The converse is true for the valgus osteotomy, which results in abduction of the segment distal to the osteotomy site.

Arthritis is not an absolute contraindication to intertrochanteric osteotomy, as it is for rotational pelvic osteotomy. Historically, salvage valgus intertrochanteric osteotomy was used in patients with superolateral arthritis secondary to dysplasia. Currently, those patients typically are treated with THA, which offers a superior quality of life, although intertrochanteric osteotomy may still be performed in appropriate circumstances. Varus intertrochanteric osteotomy also can be used as a salvage procedure when arthritis is present. These indications are rare.

Alternative Treatments

THA is the main surgical alternative to an osteotomy of the upper femur. In patients who have dysplasia, the principal alternative is a rotational pelvic osteotomy, which should be done whenever possible. Hip arthroscopy can be a reasonable alternative in patients with mechanical hip symptoms and mild dysplasia or mild impingement. Nonsurgical alternatives include activity modification to exclude vigorous and high-impact activities; weight loss to a body mass index of less than 30 if possible; use of impact-absorbing shoes and/or inserts, heel inserts, or shoe modification to lengthen the short side; change in occupation; the use of a cane or crutch on the contralateral side; and the use of nonnarcotic analgesics, glucosamine sulfate, or chondroitin sulfate. Long-term use of NSAIDs is controversial and requires caution. For patients who request an exercise program, the author of this chapter recommends swimming, including the use of floatation devices for the legs to avoid exercise-induced strain on the hip.

Results

Published results of intertrochanteric osteotomies are summarized in **Table 2**. The healing of valgus osteotomies for the management of nonunion of the femoral neck is nearly 100% for both the nonunion and the osteotomy site. The authors of one study reported a 94% rate of healing in 50 consecutive patients at a follow-up of 7 years. In patients in whom collapse was not present at the time of the index osteotomy, the rate of failure was independent of the presence of osteonecrosis. Conversion to arthroplasty was required in only seven patients. In a series of 13 patients treated with valgus osteotomy for failed internal fixation of fracture of the femoral neck, 12 patients

Table 2 Results of Intertrochanteric Osteotomy

Author(s) (Year)	Number Treated	Procedure or Approach	Mean Patient Age in Years (Range)	Mean Follow-up in Years (Range)	Success Rate (%)[a]	Results
Imhäuser (1977)	55 patients (68 hips)	Triplane osteotomy for the management of SCFE	—	(11-22)	78	—
Morscher (1980)	2,200 hips	Intertrochanteric osteotomies for the management of dysplasia and its sequelae	—	—	—	Long-term results were excellent in 30% and satisfactory in 30% of hips, with the remaining 40% requiring conversion to THA
Maistrelli et al (1988)	106 hips	Osteotomy for the management of osteonecrosis	47.5	8.2	58	—
Aronson et al (1989)	24 hips	Triplane osteotomy for the management of grade II SCFE	—	(2-10)	—	39% increase in total range of motion All hips were pain free
Marti et al (1989)	50 patients	Valgus osteotomy for the management of nonunion of the femoral neck	<70	7.1	94	7 patients required conversion to arthroplasty The failure rate was independent of the presence of osteonecrosis
Bartonícek et al (2003)	15 patients	Valgus osteotomy with a high-angle (120°) blade plate for the management of malunion or nonunion	(29-84)	5.5 (2-10)	—	Healing occurred in 14 patients

SCFE = slipped capital femoral epiphysis, THA = total hip arthroplasty.

[a] Success is defined as hips that were not converted to THA.

returned to full weight bearing without pain. Seven of eight patients who were working before injury returned to their original occupation after the osteotomy.

A study of triplane osteotomy for the management of SCFE in 55 patients (68 hips) demonstrated a 78% success rate at follow-up of 11 to 22 years. The authors of a different study of triplane osteotomy reported a 39% increase in total ROM and pain-free status in all 24 hips with grade II SCFE at follow-up of 2 to 10 years.

Intertrochanteric osteotomy for the management of malunion and nonunion at the intertrochanteric level had a high reported success rate in one series. In that study, healing occurred in 14 of 15 patients treated with valgus osteotomy with a high-angle (120°) blade plate. Osteotomy for the management of osteonecrosis has a less predictable outcome. The size of the lesion seems to be the most reliable predictor of success. Although the procedure was initially helpful, the authors of one study reported a good to excellent outcomes rate of only 58% at an average of 8.2 years after intertrochanteric osteotomy. The authors of a different study reported a steady rate of conversion to THA in the 10 years after intertrochanteric osteotomy for the management of osteonecrosis. Although 73% of patients were satisfied with the results at 5 years postoperatively, only 40% of hips had not been converted to THA by 8 years after the osteotomy. Small size of the necrotic segment has been shown to contribute favorably to the ultimate success of the osteotomy. One study demonstrated a 78% success rate in 474 hips managed with less than or equal to 180° of rotation via the Sugioka-type rotational intertrochanteric osteotomy. The authors of that study identified a correlation between the success rate and the size of the lesion and early Ficat stage of the osteonecrosis. For reasons not well understood, these results have not been replicated outside Japan, and the popularity of this approach has diminished in recent years.

In a Swiss multicenter study of 2,200 intertrochanteric osteotomies for the management of dysplasia and the sequellae of dysplasia, excellent long-term results were achieved in 30% of the hips and satisfactory results in another 30%. The remaining 40% of hips required conversion to THA. Varus osteotomy for the management of so-called coxa valga subluxans (moderate dysplasia associated with a congruent hip and a valgus neck-shaft angle greater than 144° of the upper femur) and valgus osteotomy for superolateral overload have demonstrated approximately a 70% likelihood of a good outcome at 10 years postoperatively.

In general, a good result of THA is superior in pain relief and restoration of near-normal function to that of a good result of an intertrochanteric osteotomy for the management of arthritis secondary to dysplasia. Almost all published series mix the results of varus- and valgus-producing osteotomies and do not distinguish between osteotomies performed to manage prearthritic pain and those performed as a salvage procedure in patients with established arthritis. Many of the procedures in the studies were performed before the advent of THA and represented the standard treatment of that era.

Techniques

Setup/Exposure

- The patient is placed on a radiolucent surgical table, such as a Jackson table, in the supine position with the ipsilateral thigh slightly off the edge of the table to facilitate frog lateral radiographs with the seating chisel in place later in the procedure.
- The opposite limb must be available for palpation to monitor limb-length status.
- Most intertrochanteric osteotomies are done at the upper border of the lesser trochanter. Because the anatomy of the upper femur below this level is normal, the insertion of a femoral stem in the future is straightforward.
- Subtrochanteric osteotomies, however, pose a serious problem for future THA on the femoral side.
- The incision is either entirely straight or initially straight with an anterior curve at the level of the greater trochanter, directed toward the anterior superior iliac spine (classic Bombelli incision; **Figure 2, A** and **B**).
- The Bombelli incision facilitates exposure of the anterior capsule in the interval between the abductor and tensor fascia lata muscles. With this incision, arthrotomy of the hip can be performed in a straightforward manner for the purpose of reduction of a fracture, resection of a cam lesion, or confirmation of safety of insertion of the chisel in the sagittal plane. The incision can be extended even more proximally to allow a pelvic osteotomy to be done.
- The author of this chapter prefers to make incisions for the intertrochanteric osteotomy and the periacetabular or Chiari osteotomy separately, keeping the intertrochanteric osteotomy incision straight whenever it is paired with a periacetabular osteotomy.
- If an arthrotomy is not needed in conjunction with a stand-alone intertrochanteric osteotomy, a straight incision works well.

Procedure

- The tensor fascia lata muscle is divided in line with the skin incision.
- The vastus lateralis muscle is elevated with careful ligation of the perforating vessels. When the perforating vessels are identified and ligated, bleeding can be reduced to several hundred milliliters at most for the standard intertrochanteric osteotomy.
- A Kirschner wire (K-wire) is inserted at the intended angle for the desired angular correction.
- The K-wire is inserted at the exact angle in the frontal plane, and the frog-lateral radiograph is used to ensure accurate insertion in the sagittal plane.
- The chisel should not be inserted until the position of the K-wire in both planes is perfect. The preoperative planning discussed previously addressed only the frontal plane. The addition of flexion (for the management of osteonecrosis or retroversion) is accomplished by rotating the chisel anteriorly (counterclockwise in a right hip) before insertion to achieve flexion of less than or equal to 40°.
- Conversely, extension (for the management of flexion contracture or anteversion) is achieved with posterior rotation (clockwise in a right hip).
- After the desired flexion or extension is achieved, a second K-wire is placed 10 mm proximal to the first to serve as a guide for chisel insertion in both planes.
- The chisel is inserted at the site established on the basis of the preoperative plan. The insertion site must be at least 15 mm and no more than 24 mm from the osteotomy level. During insertion of the chisel, care must be taken to move the chisel in and out incrementally to avoid incarceration of the chisel, which can make removal of the chisel after the osteotomy nearly impossible.
- After insertion of the chisel, the site of the osteotomy is established at the upper border of the lesser trochanter. These steps should follow the preoperative plan, with intraoperative fluoroscopic images obtained for confirmation.

- Minor adjustments of the insertion site of the chisel can be made to keep the osteotomy line at the upper border of the lesser trochanter. Encroachment into the lesser trochanter by several millimeters is acceptable.
- Typically, the osteotomy is made perpendicular to the long axis of the femur, which allows for derotation as necessary to correct malrotation.
- A longitudinal mark is typically made with the saw to control rotation before the osteotomy is done.
- After the osteotomy is done, the chisel is removed and replaced with the blade plate. The presence of the proximal K-wire helps ensure proper trajectory of this delicate maneuver.
- The author of this chapter recommends inserting a 4.5-mm cortical screw into the elbow hole of the plate and into the neck of the upper fragment after the blade plate is placed, before the angulation maneuver is performed. This method prevents stress on the bridge of bone between the chisel site and the osteotomy.
- If clinically indicated, release of the iliopsoas from the lesser trochanter can be done by placing the ipsilateral leg in the figure-of-4 position.
- Appropriate derotation is performed, if necessary.
- The side arm of the blade plate is secured to the femur with a large clamp.
- After limb lengths are checked, subtraction wedge osteotomies are performed, if necessary.
- An AO compression device is used to achieve axial compression.
- Radiographs are obtained, limb lengths are checked by palpating the medial malleoli side by side, and ROM is assessed.
- Additional bone can be resected if the affected limb is long.
- After all checks demonstrate satisfactory results, the screws are inserted into the side plate.
- After two screws are inserted, rotation is checked in a more vigorous manner to ensure it is correct.
- If adjustment of rotation is necessary, the screws are removed, the rotation is adjusted to accomplish the intended rotation, and new screws are inserted.

Wound Closure

- After all the screws are placed, final fluoroscopic images are obtained.
- The wound is closed. The author of this chapter prefers to use a 3-0 subcuticular monofilament absorbable suture, sealed with tissue adhesive and covered by a clear, breathable, waterproof dressing.

Postoperative Regimen

The author of this chapter uses a modified form of the multimodal pain protocol used after THA. Most patients experience no pain in the first 24 hours postoperatively. After that, pain is usually well controlled and typically does not rise to greater than 4 on a 10-point scale. Patients are encouraged to use the minimum amount of narcotics necessary and to avoid the use of narcotic medications after discharge, which usually occurs 3 to 5 days postoperatively. The breathable, waterproof wound dressing is left in place for 2 weeks postoperatively, during which time showers are permitted without restriction. No dressing changes are required. Ambulation with two crutches in a normal, heel-to-toe gait pattern is begun on the day of the procedure. Light weight bearing, approximating the weight of the leg, is encouraged. Weight bearing to tolerance is permitted after 4 weeks postoperatively, with progression to the use of a single crutch by approximately 10 weeks postoperatively. After 10 weeks, a single crutch or cane is used until the patient has no limp. Gait support is required for a longer period after opening wedge osteotomies than after closing wedge osteotomies. Water-based activities are encouraged as soon as the patient can get safely into and out of a swimming pool, usually at 4 weeks postoperatively.

Radiographs are obtained 6 weeks, 12 weeks, 6 months, and 1 year postoperatively. Hardware is removed any time after 1 year postoperatively in the presence of unequivocal evidence of mature bone healing and normal gait. Hardware removal is important for three reasons. First, bone strength is never normal under the plate. Second, the plate invariably causes hardware bursitis, and the patient's discomfort is relieved when the device is removed. Third, the risks of intraoperative fracture and postoperative infection related to a future THA procedure are lessened if the hardware is removed well before the THA procedure is performed. Although long-term patient satisfaction with a properly indicated and well-performed osteotomy is high, the patient must understand that the period of temporary disability is long. Return to work can occur at 3 weeks postoperatively for highly motivated patients in low-demand jobs. For high-demand occupations, such as military service, police work, or construction work, at least 6 months are required before the patient can return to work.

Avoiding Pitfalls and Complications

Intraoperative access to the contralateral ankle can help the surgeon assess the effect of the osteotomy on limb length. The entire affected leg should be prepped and draped free to allow evaluation of hip ROM and rotation of the osteosynthesis. Straight leg raising should be discouraged for the first few months postoperatively to minimize forces on the osteotomy site.

Bibliography

Aronson J, Bombelli R, Benedini A, Santore R: Slipped capital femoral epiphysis: A functional comparison of in situ pinning and primary osteotomy. *Techniques in Orthopedics* 1989;4:64.

Bartoníček J, Skála-Rosenbaum J, Dousa P: Valgus intertrochanteric osteotomy for malunion and nonunion of trochanteric fractures. *J Orthop Trauma* 2003;17(9):606-612.

Bombelli R: Therapy of superolateral types b) and c) and medial osteoarthritis, in *Osteoarthritis of the Hip: Classification and Pathogenesis. The Role of Osteotomy as a Consequent Therapy.* New York. NY, Springer-Verlag, 1983, pp 167-178.

Ferguson GM, Cabanela ME, Ilstrup DM: Total hip arthroplasty after failed intertrochanteric osteotomy. *J Bone Joint Surg Br* 1994;76(2):252-257.

Imhäuser G: Late results of Imhäuser's osteotomy for slipped capital femoral epiphysis [German]. *Z Orthop Ihre Grenzgeb* 1977;115(5):716-725.

Iwase T, Hasegawa Y, Kataoka Y, Matsuda T, Iwata H: Long-term results of intertrochanteric varus osteotomy for arthrosis of the dysplastic hip (over 10 years' follow-up). *Arch Orthop Trauma Surg* 1995;114(5):243-247.

Kerboul M, Thomine J, Postel M, Merle d'Aubigné R: The conservative surgical treatment of idiopathic aseptic necrosis of the femoral head. *J Bone Joint Surg Br* 1974;56(2):291-296.

Leunig M, Ganz R: The evolution and concepts of joint-preserving surgery of the hip. *Bone Joint J* 2014;96-B(1):5-18.

Maistrelli G, Fusco U, Avai A, Bombelli R: Osteonecrosis of the hip treated by intertrochanteric osteotomy: A four- to 15-year follow-up. *J Bone Joint Surg Br* 1988;70(5):761-766.

Marti RK, Schüller HM, Raaymakers EL: Intertrochanteric osteotomy for non-union of the femoral neck. *J Bone Joint Surg Br* 1989;71(5):782-787.

Millis MB, Poss R, Murphy SB: Osteotomies of the hip in the prevention and treatment of osteoarthritis. *Instr Course Lect* 1992;41:145-154.

Morscher E: Intertrochanteric osteotomy in osteoarthritis of the hip, in Riley L, ed: *The Hip: Proceedings of the Eighth Open Scientific Meeting of the Hip Society.* St. Louis, MO, Mosby, 1980, pp 24-46.

Mueller ME: The intertrochanteric osteotomy and pseudarthrosis of the femoral neck: 1957. *Clin Orthop Relat Res* 1999;363:5-8.

Nakagawa M, Iwata H, Sugiura S, Ida K, Hattori Y, Shido T: The evaluation of intertrochanteric osteotomy in relation to osteotomized angle and leg-length discrepancy for osteoarthritis of the hip. *Clin Orthop Relat Res* 1980;152:277-283.

Pauwels F: *Biomechanics of the Normal and Diseased Hip: Theoretical Foundation, Technique and Results of Treatment. An Atlas.* [German] Furlong RJ, Maquet P, trans. Berlin, Germany, Springer Verlag, 1976.

Santore RF: Intertrochanteric osteotomy for osteonecrosis. *Semin Arthroplasty* 1991;2(3):208-213.

Santore RF, Bombelli R: Long-term follow-up of the Bombelli experience with osteotomy for osteoarthritis: Results at 11 years. *Hip* 1983;106-128.

Trousdale RT, Ekkernkamp A, Ganz R, Wallrichs SL: Periacetabular and intertrochanteric osteotomy for the treatment of osteoarthrosis in dysplastic hips. *J Bone Joint Surg Am* 1995;77(1):73-85.

Wagner H, Zeiler G: Idiopathic necrosis of the femoral head: Result of intertrochanteric osteotomy and joint resurfacing, in Weil UH, ed: *Segmental Idiopathic Necrosis of the Femoral Head. Progress in Orthopaedic Surgery*, vol 5. Berlin, Germany, Springer-Verlag, 1981, pp 87-116.

Chapter 69
Open Management of Femoroacetabular Impingement

Joseph M. Schwab, MD
John C. Clohisy, MD

Indications

Femoroacetabular impingement (FAI) is a disease spectrum consisting of an abnormal functional relationship between the proximal femur and the acetabulum. The two major morphology types of FAI are cam type and pincer type. Cam-type impingement occurs when an aspheric femoral head-neck junction enters the acetabulum during motion. Pincer-type impingement occurs when acetabular overcoverage (resulting from either increased acetabular depth or acetabular retroversion) leads to abnormal contact of the acetabular rim and the femoral neck. Both types are believed to contribute to hip arthrosis. Despite some controversy, approximately 80% of patients with FAI are generally thought to have a mixed type of impingement that includes elements of both cam and pincer impingement. In addition, extra-articular FAI patterns (anterior inferior iliac spine, greater trochanter, ischiofemoral) are recognized as potential sources of symptomatic FAI.

Treatment is indicated in patients with cam-, pincer-, or mixed-type radiographic findings and pain attributable to the deformity. Pain typically is located in the groin but can occur in the buttock, over the greater trochanter, or along the lateral thigh. Patients typically have a positive anterior impingement test (symptoms reproduced with flexion, adduction, and internal rotation of the hip) or a positive posterior impingement test (symptoms reproduced with extension, adduction, and external rotation of the hip). Relief of symptoms with an intra-articular infiltration of corticosteroid or local anesthetic supports the diagnosis.

The choice of surgical procedure is based on the FAI pattern, patient and physician preferences, and the technical limitations of each procedure. Ideally, the chosen procedure should adequately address the deformity with the lowest risk of morbidity to the patient. Options include surgical hip dislocation, hip arthroscopy (not discussed in this chapter), limited open correction, and, in select patients, anteverting periacetabular osteotomy (not discussed in this chapter). Most FAI deformities are accessible with arthroscopic techniques. Patients with circumferential femoral deformity, extensive acetabular deformity, or complex FAI disease patterns, such as those resulting from residual slipped capital femoral epiphysis or Legg-Calvé-Perthes deformities, may be best treated with open surgical procedures (**Figure 1**).

The open surgical dislocation approach allows wide access to the acetabulum and proximal femur for the management of complex hip deformities. Surgical hip dislocation is a well-accepted strategy for the management of complex FAI disease patterns and is indicated for the correction of both cam- and pincer-type morphologies. Surgical hip dislocation is the procedure of choice if pathology exists in the posterior hip joint, a location in which arthroscopic access is difficult. Surgical hip dislocation cannot be used for the management of severe acetabular retroversion, which requires an anteverting periacetabular osteotomy.

Contraindications

Moderate to advanced osteoarthritis is a contraindication to joint-preserving surgery in patients with FAI. In addition, clinical imaging suggestive of FAI (that is, radiographic cam or pincer deformity) or decreased range of motion (ROM) in the absence of symptoms is a relative contraindication to surgical treatment. Asymptomatic FAI deformity should be managed with regular follow-up. In addition, although many patients with FAI experience pain with common activities

Dr. Clohisy or an immediate family member serves as a paid consultant to MicroPort Orthopedics and Smith & Nephew and has received research or institutional support from Pivot Medical, Smith & Nephew, and Zimmer Biomet. Neither Dr. Schwab nor any immediate family member has received anything of value from or has stock or stock options held in a commercial company or institution related directly or indirectly to the subject of this chapter.

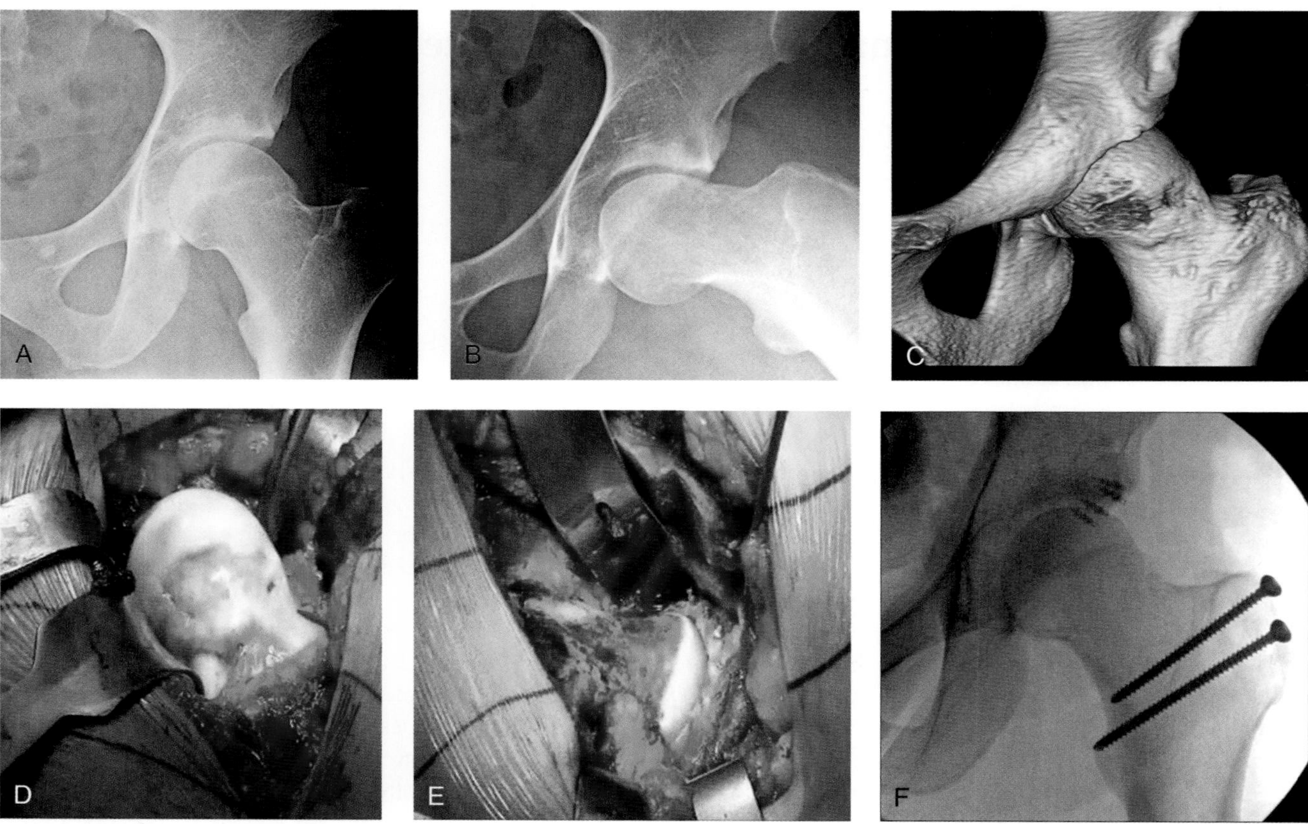

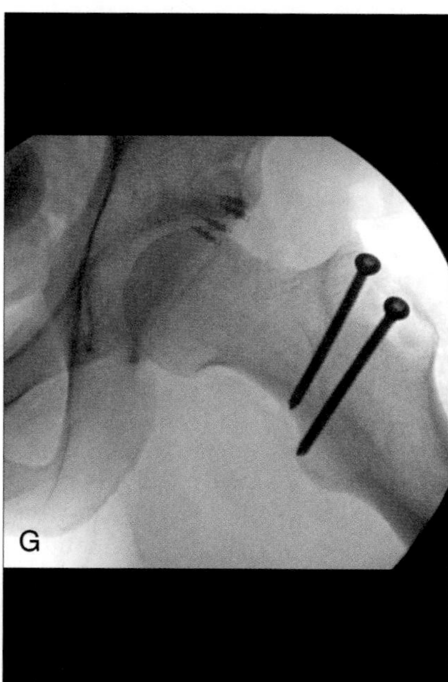

Figure 1 Images of the left hip of a 22-year-old patient who played recreational soccer and who previously underwent hip arthroscopy that was unsuccessful. **A,** AP radiograph demonstrates a crossover sign with anterosuperior overcoverage. The lateral femoral head-neck region demonstrates a prominence and insufficient lateral offset. Because the patient's symptoms did not improve with arthroscopy, revision hip impingement surgery was indicated. An open procedure was chosen because of concern for the posterolateral extent of the femoral head-neck junction deformity and for trochanteric pelvic impingement. **B,** Preoperative 45° Dunn radiograph demonstrates insufficient offset at the femoral head-neck junction and sclerosis of the acetabular rim with a subchondral cyst in the acetabulum. **C,** Preoperative three-dimensional CT scan demonstrates inadequate osteoplasty of the femoral head-neck junction with persistent prominence at the distal anterior head-neck region, the anterolateral head-neck junction, and the lateral head-neck junction. **D,** Intraoperative photograph demonstrates inadequate resection with residual femoral head-neck deformity both distal and lateral to the osteoplasty. **E,** Intraoperative photograph after extensive femoral head-neck osteoplasty, anterosuperior trochanteric osteoplasty, acetabular rim trimming, acetabular labral refixation, and inferior iliac spine decompression. Intraoperative dynamic examination demonstrated impingement-free functional range of motion. Intraoperative AP (**F**) and 45° Dunn lateral (**G**) fluoroscopic images demonstrate recontouring of the femoral head-neck junction, acetabular rim trimming, and anatomic reduction of the greater trochanter. The patient had an excellent result at 2-year follow-up. (Courtesy of John C. Clohisy, MD, St. Louis, MO.)

such as sitting, squatting, or walking, patients who can modify their activities to relieve symptoms do not necessarily require surgical intervention.

Alternative Treatments

Evidence regarding the results of nonsurgical management of symptomatic FAI is limited. Activity modification and a course of NSAIDs can help alleviate symptoms during early management of the disease. In patients with radiographically mild deformities, a course of structured physical therapy can be prescribed in an attempt to relieve symptoms. Physical therapy should focus on muscular balancing and proprioception while maintaining ROM within a pain-free zone. Attempts to increase ROM can exacerbate symptoms and should be avoided. In addition to physical therapy, patients with FAI who experience symptoms only with specific activities can undergo a trial of activity modification or avoidance to determine whether long-term relief is possible without surgical treatment.

Patients with symptomatic FAI and substantial degenerative radiographic changes could alternatively consider total hip arthroplasty (THA). Generally, THA should be reserved for patients 50 years and older with activity demands that can be accommodated with a prosthetic hip.

Results

In a systematic review of 11 studies (2 level III studies and 9 level IV studies) reporting results of both open and arthroscopic management of FAI with mean follow-up of 3.2 years (range, 2 to 5.2 years), hip pain was reduced and function was improved with both open and arthroscopic management in 68% to 96% of patients. Case series that reported both labral débridement and labral refixation demonstrated a higher percentage of favorable outcomes with labral refixation than with labral débridement. The reported rates of conversion to THA were zero to 26%. Major complications (osteonecrosis, femoral head-neck fracture, loss of fixation requiring revision surgery, trochanteric nonunion, failure of labral refixation, inadequate osteochondroplasty requiring surgical revision, deep infection, and clinically relevant heterotopic ossification) were reported in zero to 18% of the procedures. Single-center case series (**Table 1**) have also demonstrated favorable clinical results in most patients. More recent midterm studies demonstrate conversion to THA in zero to 7% of the patients, with high survivorship rates and improved pain and function scores.

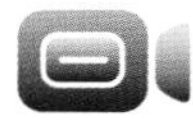

Video 69.1 Femoral Osteochondroplasty and Acetabular Labrum Re-fixation in Femoroacetabular Impingement. Alessandro Massè, MD; Alessandro Aprato, MD; Marco Favuto, MD; Alberto Nicodemo, MD; Reinhold Ganz, MD; Luigino Turchetto, MD; Guido Grappiolo, MD; Antonio Campacci, MD (18 min)

Techniques

Setup/Exposure

- The setup for surgical hip dislocation is similar to that used for a standard posterior-approach THA.
- The patient is placed in the lateral decubitus position with the entire affected extremity draped free.
- The patient is stabilized in this position to allow intraoperative hip flexion of greater than 90°.
- A tunnel cushion placed over the nonsurgical extremity protects it from injury and provides a supportive surface for the affected extremity during the procedure.
- A sterile leg bag, or pocket, is prepared on the anterior side of the patient to be used while the hip joint is dislocated.
- The skin incision is typically 20 to 25 cm long and is centered over the tip of the greater trochanter in line with the anterior third of the femur.
- The hip is approached through a Gibson interval, just anterior to the gluteus maximus muscle.
- The fascia overlying the gluteus medius muscle is incised at the anterior border of the gluteus maximus muscle.
- The gluteus maximus muscle is retracted posteriorly together with the overlying fascia of the gluteus medius. This technique helps protect the superior cluneal nerves and the branches of the superior gluteal artery, which may run in that fascia.
- The affected leg is internally rotated to expose the gluteus minimus, piriformis, and short external rotators. Care is taken to avoid disrupting these posterior structures because they protect the medial femoral circumflex artery (MFCA), which provides the major blood supply to the femoral head.

Instruments/Equipment/Implants Required

- Femoral head-neck offset correction can be performed with a curved osteotome, a burr, or a combination of both.
- Although hemispheric plastic templates of varying sizes can be used to assess the adequacy of cam resection, dynamic ROM testing is extremely important to confirm adequate decompression of FAI deformities.
- Trimming of the acetabular rim is accomplished with the use of either an osteotome or a burr.
- The labrum is refixed with the use

Table 1 Clinical Results of Open Hip Preservation Procedures

Authors (Year)	Number of Patients (Hips)	Procedure	Mean Patient Age in Years (Range)	Mean Follow-up in Years (Range)	Success Rate (%)[a]	Results
Beaulé et al (2007)	34 (37)	SHD	40.5 (19-54)	3.1 (2.1-5)	81	81% of patients had satisfactory outcomes No reported conversions to THA
Peters et al (2010)	94 (96)	SHD	28 (14-51)	2.17 (1.5-8)	94	94% of hips had good to excellent outcomes 6% of hips were converted to THA or had worsening Harris hip scores postoperatively
Naal et al (2012)	185 (233)	SHD	30 (14-55)	5 (2-10)	83	83% of patients rated hip function as normal or near normal 3% of hips were converted to THA
Siebenrock et al (2014)	22 (29)	Anteverting periacetabular osteotomy	23 (14-41)	11 (9-12)	92	Patients were treated for acetabular retroversion 92% of hips had good to excellent Merle d'Aubigné scores No conversion to THA 2 hips had radiographic progression of osteoarthritis
Steppacher et al (2014)	75 (97)	SHD	32 (15-52)	6 (5-7)	91	7% of hips had progression of osteoarthritis 7% of hips were converted to THA Kaplan-Meier analysis showed 91% survivorship at 5 yr postoperatively

SHD = surgical hip dislocation, THA = total hip arthroplasty.

[a] Success is defined as hips with good to excellent outcome scores, no conversion to THA or fusion, and no progression of osteoarthritis on most recent follow-up.

of small (2.0- to 3.0-mm) suture anchors.

- After correction of the impingement is accomplished, the greater trochanteric fragment is fixed with several standard 3.5- or 4.5-mm cortical screws.

Procedure

TROCHANTERIC OSTEOTOMY

- An osteotomy of the greater trochanter is performed. The osteotomy can be either a flat-cut or step-cut osteotomy, depending on the specific surgical goals.
- If trochanteric advancement or relative femoral neck lengthening is indicated, a flat-cut osteotomy is recommended.
- A step-cut osteotomy (**Figure 2**) provides greater resistance to superior migration secondary to pull from the gluteus medius and may allow for more accelerated rehabilitation.
- Before the osteotomy is performed, a line is marked from the tip of the greater trochanter to the posterior border of the vastus lateralis ridge with electrocautery. This step also cauterizes the trochanteric branch of the MFCA, which can otherwise cause bleeding when the osteotomy is performed.
- For the step-cut osteotomy, a narrow oscillating saw is passed from posterior to anterior, starting at the tip of the greater trochanter and extending approximately half of the length of the osteotomy. The blade is left in the osteotomy and used as a plane of reference. A broad oscillating saw is passed starting just distal to the vastus lateralis ridge and extending to a point approximately 6 mm medial to the distal end of the first cut. A 6-mm osteotome is passed to connect the two portions of the osteotomy. The trochanteric fragment is mobilized.
- For the flat-cut osteotomy, an

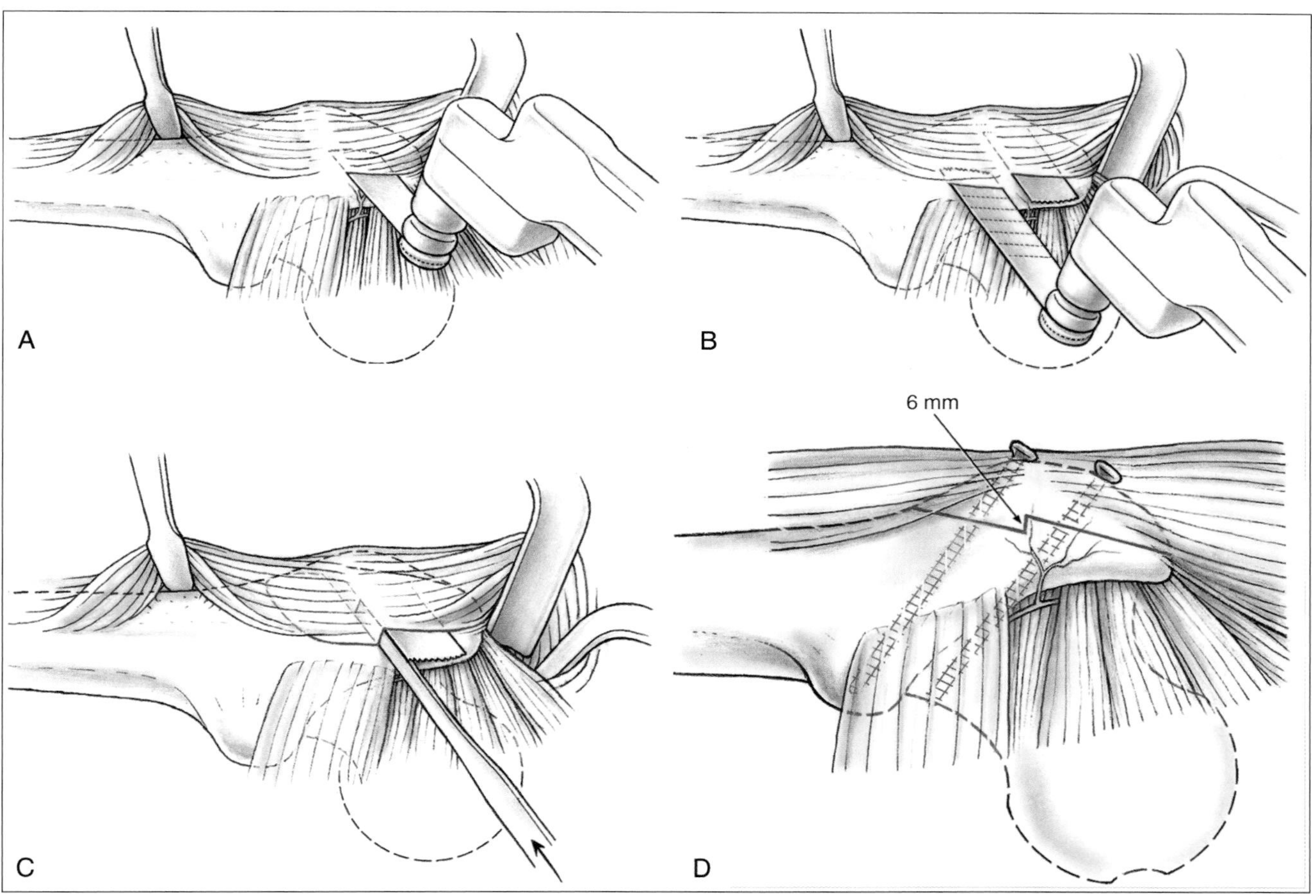

Figure 2 Illustrations depict the step-cut osteotomy (red lines) used in open management of femoroacetabular impingement. **A,** The osteotomy begins at the proximal greater trochanter and continues approximately one-half to three-fifths the length of the greater trochanter. **B,** The distal portion of the osteotomy begins just distal to the vastus lateralis ridge and is parallel to the proximal portion of the osteotomy but offset approximately 6 mm medially. **C,** An osteotome is used to connect the proximal and distal portions, completing the step-cut osteotomy. The arrow indicates the direction in which the osteotome is struck. **D,** Anatomic reduction and fixation of the osteotomy is done at the conclusion of the procedure. (Reproduced with permission from Bastian JD, Wolf AT, Wyss TF, Nötzli HP: Stepped osteotomy of the trochanter for stable, anatomic refixation. *Clin Orthop Relat Res* 2009;467[3]:732-738.)

oscillating saw is passed from posterior to anterior along the cauterized line. If anatomic fixation is desired, the anterior or anterosuperior portion of cortical bone can be left intact and fractured by prying the fragment up. This area is later used for fixation of the osteotomy. Otherwise, if mobility of the fragment is desired (as in the case of a trochanteric advancement), the osteotomy is completed with the saw. The thickness of the mobilized trochanteric fragment is approximately 1.5 cm.

CAPSULAR EXPOSURE

- After the trochanteric osteotomy is performed, the affected leg is taken out of internal rotation while the trochanteric fragment is mobilized anteriorly.
- Fibers of the vastus lateralis muscle are released from the femur down to the midpoint of the insertion of the gluteus maximus tendon to achieve mobilization of the fragment.
- Proximally, 1 to 2 mm of gluteus medius tendon remains on the stable portion of the greater trochanter and must be released to allow mobilization of the fragment anteriorly.
- Often, a few fibers of the piriformis tendon remain attached to the mobile fragment and must be carefully released to allow mobilization.
- Dissection is carried out between the gluteus minimus and piriformis muscles, which allows visualization of the joint capsule.
- To facilitate exposure of the capsule, the hip should be placed into slight flexion and external rotation while the gluteus medius and minimus are retracted superiorly.

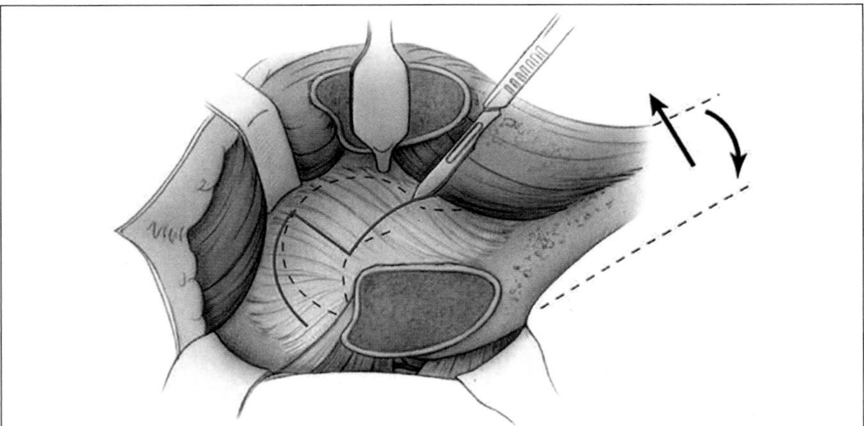

Figure 3 Illustration depicts a Z-shaped capsulotomy (red lines) used in open management of femoroacetabular impingement. The affected leg is positioned in flexion, abduction, and external rotation. Starting at the anterosuperior edge of the stable trochanter, an inside-out capsulotomy is performed in line with the femoral neck until the acetabular rim is reached. Care should be taken to visualize the labrum to avoid iatrogenic labral injury. The posterosuperior limb of the capsulotomy is then created along the acetabular rim to further expose the femoral head and labrum. Finally, the inferior limb of the capsulotomy is directed toward the anteroinferior rim of the acetabulum. The straight arrow indicates flexion, and the curved arrow indicates external rotation. The dashed lines indicate the position of the femur under the surrounding soft tissues. (Reproduced with permission from Espinosa N, Beck M, Rothenfluh DA, Ganz R, Leunig M: Treatment of femoro-acetabular impingement: Preliminary results of labral refixation. Surgical technique. *J Bone Joint Surg Am* 2007;89[suppl 2 pt 1]:36-53.)

CAPSULOTOMY

- Typically, a Z-shaped capsulotomy is performed, starting with the anterolateral capsule in line with the femoral neck (**Figure 3**).
- After initial penetration of the capsule with the scalpel, the capsulotomy is performed from inside out to help protect the cartilage and labrum from iatrogenic injury.
- The capsulotomy is extended to the rim of the acetabulum proximally and to the anterolateral tip of the stable trochanter distally.
- An anteroinferior limb of the capsulotomy is created, with care taken to stay anterior to the lesser trochanter to preserve the MFCA.
- The superior limb of the capsulotomy is developed along the rim of the acetabulum posteriorly until it reaches the retracted piriformis tendon.

DISLOCATION

- The hip is brought into flexion and external rotation to achieve dislocation.
- The authors of this chapter routinely place a bone hook around the inferior femoral neck to gently apply the appropriate force to the proximal femur to aid in dislocation.
- Curved scissors are used to transect the ligamentum teres, allowing full dislocation. However, in some patients, the ligamentum teres ruptures or may have already ruptured before dislocation.
- After the hip is dislocated, the affected leg is placed into the sterile bag that was prepared anterior to the patient.
- The proximal femur and acetabulum are circumferentially inspected.
- The remaining ligamentum teres is excised from the fovea capitis and can be used as a graft for the labrum if needed and if it would provide a graft of adequate size.

CORRECTION OF ACETABULAR PATHOLOGY

- With the hip joint dislocated, any acetabular pathomorphology is corrected.
- If trimming of the acetabular rim is to be performed, the labrum is reflected off the pathologic acetabular rim (as a bucket handle would be raised off the rim of a bucket) and protected.
- The acetabular rim is trimmed with the use of osteotomes or a burr until the pincer lesion is satisfactorily removed.
- Care is taken to avoid excessive excision of the acetabular rim, which can result in focal acetabular dysplasia.
- In patients with impingement involving the anterior inferior iliac spine, the posterior aspect of the direct head of the rectus femoris can be elevated from the spine to allow direct access for subspine decompression.
- After the acetabular rim is trimmed, the labrum is refixed with suture anchors and nonabsorbable sutures. If the labrum is insufficient to allow refixation, it can be reconstructed with graft tissue, including fascia lata, ligamentum teres, or any other readily available autograft.
- Delamination, or debonding of the cartilage from the subchondral bone, is common, especially in patients with predominantly cam-type FAI. Unstable cartilage lesions and focal full-thickness chondromalacia are less common but may be present.
- Controversy exists regarding the ideal management of cartilage lesions on the acetabulum. Options include microfracture, collagen

matrices, or allograft chondrocyte implantation.

CORRECTION OF FEMORAL PATHOLOGY

- Cam lesions are removed from the femoral head-neck junction.
- The extent of the lesion is easily demarcated with the use of a hemispheric plastic template sized to the femoral head.
- The size and location of the lesion, as well as its pathologic relationship with the acetabulum, also can be confirmed with ROM testing of the joint under direct visualization.
- The authors of this chapter routinely use a curved 10-mm osteotome to mark the border of the resection and remove the major portion of the cam lesion.
- After initial resection of the lesion is performed, the head is again tested with a template.
- The exposed femoral neck bone is contoured with a 5-mm round burr at half speed.
- After the contouring is completed, the hip is relocated, and the ROM is again visualized. The goal is 25° to 35° internal rotation at 90° of flexion.
- In patients with major femoral malalignment, a concurrent proximal femoral osteotomy (intertrochanteric or subtrochanteric) can be performed through the dislocation approach.
- Cartilage lesions on the femoral head are managed in a manner similar to the management of acetabular lesions.
- In addition, the use of allograft osteochondral plugs for larger lesions can be considered if an appropriately contoured graft is available.

Wound Closure

- The capsulotomy is closed anatomically with absorbable sutures.
- A watertight closure of the capsule is not necessary because efflux of the hemarthrosis may reduce the risk of iatrogenic osteonecrosis that can occur secondary to increased joint pressure.
- The mobile trochanteric fragment is reduced and fixed with two or three 3.5- or 4.5-mm cortical screws aimed toward the inferior femoral neck and lesser trochanter.
- The gluteus maximus fascia and the proximal iliotibial band are closed with a running absorbable suture.
- The subcutaneous tissue and skin are closed in routine fashion.
- Both deep and superficial drains can be used to reduce hematoma formation and allow more comfortable early passive motion.

Postoperative Regimen

Postoperatively, patients are placed in a continuous passive motion machine to minimize intra-articular adhesions. Mechanical and pharmacologic deep vein thrombosis prophylaxis is maintained while the patient is in the hospital, and pharmacologic prophylaxis is continued for at least 30 days postoperatively. Patients with a flat-cut trochanteric osteotomy are instructed to maintain touch-down weight bearing (approximately 15 kg) for 6 to 8 weeks postoperatively and then are advanced to full weight bearing. After full weight bearing is achieved, patients may begin abductor strengthening. Patients with a step-cut osteotomy are instructed to maintain partial weight bearing (50% body weight) for 3 to 6 weeks postoperatively, depending on the clinical situation and patient characteristics, and then are advanced to full weight bearing. Abductor strengthening begins after the patient is full weight bearing. All patients with a cam deformity correction are instructed to avoid high-impact activities such as running, jumping, cutting, or pivoting until 4 to 6 months postoperatively. This restriction helps prevent abnormally high stress across a weakened femoral neck, which can result in fracture of the femoral neck.

Patients are routinely seen for follow-up at 2 weeks, 6 weeks, 3 months, 1 year, and 2 years postoperatively and at appropriate intervals thereafter. This schedule provides adequate follow-up to evaluate activity and pain progression and gives the surgeon reasonable opportunity to examine the patient for complications such as trochanteric nonunion, radiographic progression of arthrosis, stress fracture of the femoral neck, and osteonecrosis.

Avoiding Pitfalls and Complications

Although management of FAI with open surgical hip dislocation is effective in reducing pain and increasing function, the surgeon must keep several key concepts in mind to achieve the best possible outcome. First, the health of the articular cartilage must be evaluated before surgical intervention is performed. Advanced imaging modalities are available to determine the composition of cartilage; however, clear guidelines for these modalities have not yet been established. The authors of this chapter recommend that a minimum of 2 to 3 mm of cartilage space be visible on plain radiographs. The authors of this chapter also recommend the use of MRI as an adjunct to evaluate the patient for pervasive chondromalacia, subchondral edema, and cystic degeneration.

Surgical dislocation is a safe approach to the hip, but osteonecrosis can occur if adequate attention is not paid to the location and course of the deep branch of the MFCA. This artery is particularly at risk during the initial approach, when the trochanteric osteotomy is prepared. In addition, the surgeon must take care when working over the retinacular vessels located on the posterosuperior femoral neck. These vessels are the terminal branches of the deep branch of the MFCA and provide the blood supply to the weight-bearing surface of the femoral head. The retinacular vessels can be disrupted if the cam lesion extends onto the posterosuperior femoral neck and care is not taken to protect them during decompression.

In patients with cam-type FAI with a labral tear and normal acetabular coverage, removing the acetabular rim can lead to iatrogenic dysplasia of the acetabulum. Likewise, if a planned acetabular rim resection is performed for the management of acetabular overcoverage, care should be taken to resect only the minimal amount needed to decompress the pincer lesion. If the patient has anterior overcoverage and posterior undercoverage (that is, a relatively retroverted acetabulum), the use of an anteverting periacetabular osteotomy can be considered.

Inadequate resection of all sources of impingement can lead to a poor postoperative outcome. Additional sources of impingement may become apparent after the primary impingement is removed. A comprehensive, dynamic intraoperative examination can help the surgeon identify the location and extent of additional intra- and extra-articular sources of impingement. The surgeon should maintain a high index of suspicion for additional sources of impingement in patients with complex FAI secondary to Legg-Calvé-Perthes disease and similar deformities. Three-dimensional CT can help identify potential extra-articular FAI preoperatively, but dynamic intraoperative assessment is necessary to determine clinical relevance. The hip should be tested for internal and external rotation at 90° of flexion and in full extension. In addition, abduction and adduction should be tested in both flexion and extension.

Bibliography

Bastian JD, Wolf AT, Wyss TF, Nötzli HP: Stepped osteotomy of the trochanter for stable, anatomic refixation. *Clin Orthop Relat Res* 2009;467(3):732-738.

Beaulé PE, Le Duff MJ, Zaragoza E: Quality of life following femoral head-neck osteochondroplasty for femoroacetabular impingement. *J Bone Joint Surg Am* 2007;89(4):773-779.

Beck M, Kalhor M, Leunig M, Ganz R: Hip morphology influences the pattern of damage to the acetabular cartilage: Femoroacetabular impingement as a cause of early osteoarthritis of the hip. *J Bone Joint Surg Br* 2005;87(7):1012-1018.

Clohisy JC, Knaus ER, Hunt DM, Lesher JM, Harris-Hayes M, Prather H: Clinical presentation of patients with symptomatic anterior hip impingement. *Clin Orthop Relat Res* 2009;467(3):638-644.

Clohisy JC, St John LC, Schutz AL: Surgical treatment of femoroacetabular impingement: A systematic review of the literature. *Clin Orthop Relat Res* 2010;468(2):555-564.

Espinosa N, Beck M, Rothenfluh DA, Ganz R, Leunig M: Treatment of femoro-acetabular impingement: Preliminary results of labral refixation. Surgical technique. *J Bone Joint Surg Am* 2007;89(suppl 2 pt 1):36-53.

Ganz R, Gill TJ, Gautier E, Ganz K, Krügel N, Berlemann U: Surgical dislocation of the adult hip: A technique with full access to the femoral head and acetabulum without the risk of avascular necrosis. *J Bone Joint Surg Br* 2001;83(8):1119-1124.

Ganz R, Parvizi J, Beck M, Leunig M, Nötzli H, Siebenrock KA: Femoroacetabular impingement: A cause for osteoarthritis of the hip. *Clin Orthop Relat Res* 2003;(417):112-120.

Gautier E, Ganz K, Krügel N, Gill T, Ganz R: Anatomy of the medial femoral circumflex artery and its surgical implications. *J Bone Joint Surg Br* 2000;82(5):679-683.

Hetsroni I, Poultsides L, Bedi A, Larson CM, Kelly BT: Anterior inferior iliac spine morphology correlates with hip range of motion: A classification system and dynamic model. *Clin Orthop Relat Res* 2013;471(8):2497-2503.

Naal FD, Miozzari HH, Schär M, Hesper T, Nötzli HP: Midterm results of surgical hip dislocation for the treatment of femoroacetabular impingement. *Am J Sports Med* 2012;40(7):1501-1510.

Nepple JJ, Byrd JW, Siebenrock KA, Prather H, Clohisy JC: Overview of treatment options, clinical results, and controversies in the management of femoroacetabular impingement. *J Am Acad Orthop Surg* 2013;21(suppl 1):S53-S58.

Peters CL, Schabel K, Anderson L, Erickson J: Open treatment of femoroacetabular impingement is associated with clinical improvement and low complication rate at short-term followup. *Clin Orthop Relat Res* 2010;468(2):504-510.

Ross JR, Schoenecker PL, Clohisy JC: Surgical dislocation of the hip: Evolving indications. *HSS J* 2013;9(1):60-69.

Siebenrock KA, Schaller C, Tannast M, Keel M, Büchler L: Anteverting periacetabular osteotomy for symptomatic acetabular retroversion: Results at ten years. *J Bone Joint Surg Am* 2014;96(21):1785-1792.

Sink EL, Beaulé PE, Sucato D, et al: Multicenter study of complications following surgical dislocation of the hip. *J Bone Joint Surg Am* 2011;93(12):1132-1136.

Steppacher SD, Huemmer C, Schwab JM, Tannast M, Siebenrock KA: Surgical hip dislocation for treatment of femoroacetabular impingement: Factors predicting 5-year survivorship. *Clin Orthop Relat Res* 2014;472(1):337-348.

Video Reference

Massè A, Aprato A, Favuto M, et al: Video. *Femoral Osteochondroplasty and Acetabular Labrum Re-fixation in Femoroacetabular Impingement*, Turin, Italy, 2012.

Chapter 70
Management of Early-Stage Osteonecrosis of the Femoral Head

Michael Mont, MD
Randa Elmallah, MD

Indications

In patients with early-stage osteonecrosis of the femoral head, surgical treatment options are aimed at preservation of the femoral head. Commonly used techniques include core decompression or percutaneous drilling, nonvascularized bone grafting, and vascularized bone grafting. Proximal femoral osteotomies can also be used for the management of early-stage osteonecrosis; however, this technique is not discussed in detail in this chapter.

Head-preserving techniques require healthy femoral and acetabular chondral surfaces. Therefore, the radiographic appearance of the femoral head is the major guide in determining the appropriate surgical strategy. Radiographic staging is performed with the use of AP and lateral radiographs as well as MRI. Numerous radiographic systems can be used for the classification of osteonecrosis. The most common classifications are the Ficat and Arlet, ARCO (Association Research Circulation Osseous), Japanese Investigation Committee, and University of Pennsylvania systems. For simplicity, assessment of osteonecrosis for treatment planning is often based on four factors determined in radiographic analysis: evaluation of precollapse or postcollapse status of the disease, lesion size, amount of femoral head depression, and acetabular involvement.

The femoral head is classified as precollapse or postcollapse on the basis of radiographic imaging. Precollapse disease is associated with the best prognosis of head-preserving strategies. Occasionally, a so-called crescent sign, resulting from a subchondral fracture, is observed in patients with precollapse disease (**Figure 1**). The presence of a crescent sign often indicates that the femoral head is at risk of biomechanical compromise. Precollapse disease with a crescent sign is associated with a prognosis worse than that of precollapse disease without this sign. If subchondral fracture or a collapse that is subtle or difficult to visualize is suspected, CT or radiographic tomography may aid in evaluation. Patients with evidence of femoral head collapse are considered to have advanced or postcollapse disease, which has the worst prognosis and often requires replacement of the femoral head.

Larger lesions correlate negatively with prognosis, and the size of the lesion often dictates the management strategy. The lesion size and amount of femoral head involvement can be classified by determining the Kerboull

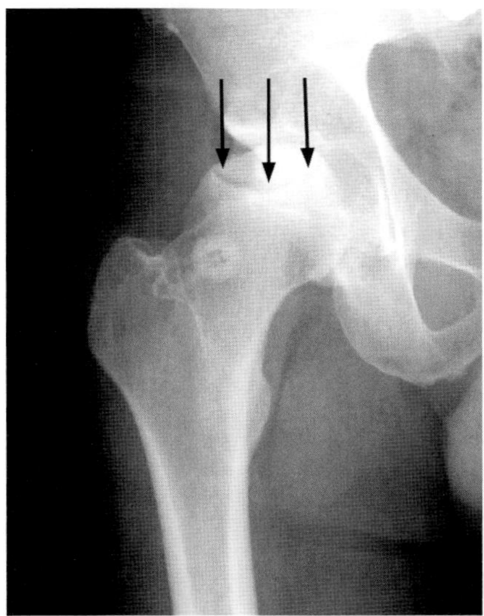

Figure 1 AP radiograph of a right hip demonstrates a Ficat and Arlet stage III lesion. A crescent sign (arrows) indicates subchondral fracture and collapse. (Reproduced from Mont MA, Ragland PS: Osteonecrosis of the femoral head: Early stage disease, in Lieberman JR, Berry DJ, eds: *Advanced Reconstruction: Hip*. Rosemont, IL, American Academy of Orthopaedic Surgeons, 2005, pp 517-525.)

Dr. Mont or an immediate family member has received royalties from Stryker; serves as a paid consultant to DJO, Medical Compression Systems, Sage Products, Stryker, and TissueGene; has received research or institutional support from DJO, the National Institutes of Health (the National Institute of Arthritis and Musculoskeletal and Skin Diseases and the Eunice Kennedy Shriver National Institute of Child Health and Human Development), Sage Products, Stryker, and TissueGene; and serves as a board member, owner, officer, or committee member of the American Academy of Orthopaedic Surgeons. Neither Dr. Elmallah nor any immediate family member has received anything of value from or has stock or stock options held in a commercial company or institution related directly or indirectly to the subject of this chapter.

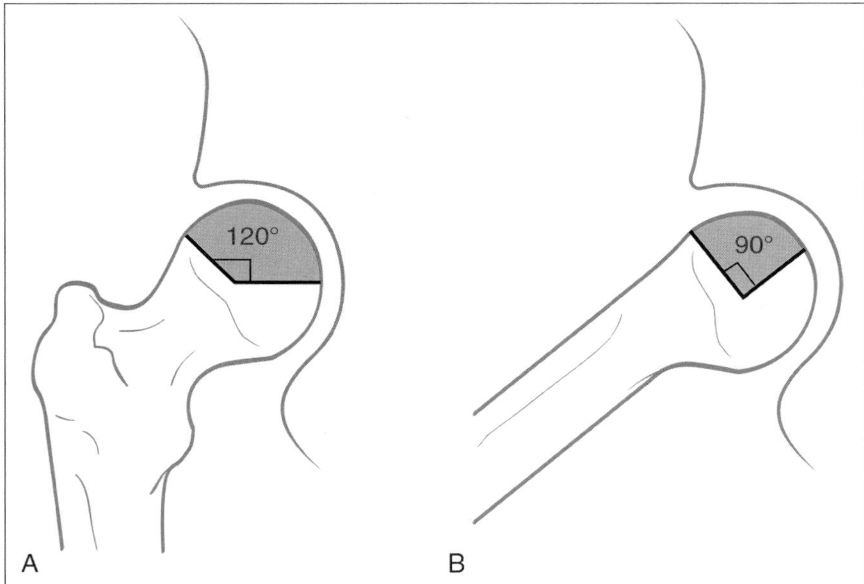

Figure 2 Illustrations depict determination of the extent of osteonecrosis of the femoral head. The arc of area involved is determined by drawing a line segment from the center of the femoral head to the joint line along the outer margins of the lesion in both the AP (**A**) and lateral (**B**) views. Patients with a total arc of involvement (that is, the sum of the angles in these two views) greater than 200° have a poor prognosis. In this figure, the total arc of involvement is 120° + 90° = 210°. (Reproduced from Mont MA, Ragland PS: Osteonecrosis of the femoral head: Early stage disease, in Lieberman JR, Berry DJ, eds: *Advanced Reconstruction: Hip*. Rosemont, IL, American Academy of Orthopaedic Surgeons, 2005, pp 517-525.)

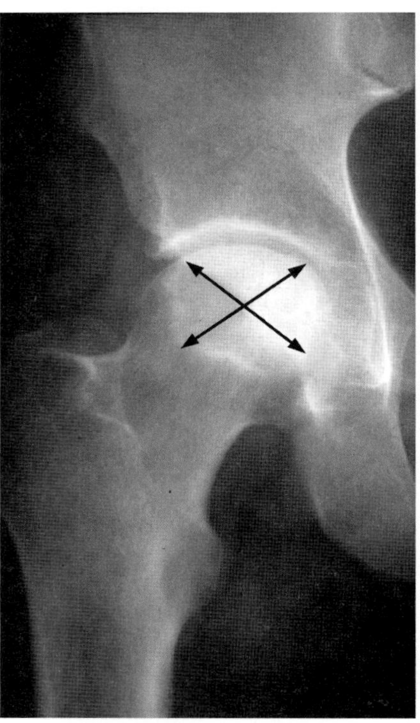

Figure 3 AP radiograph of a right hip demonstrates an easily identifiable large lesion (double-sided arrows) of the femoral head. (Reproduced from Mont MA, Ragland PS: Osteonecrosis of the femoral head: Early stage disease, in Lieberman JR, Berry DJ, eds: *Advanced Reconstruction: Hip*. Rosemont, IL, American Academy of Orthopaedic Surgeons, 2005, pp 517-525.)

angle, which is the angle of the necrotic area in the coronal and sagittal planes (**Figure 2**). Smaller lesions often have a combined necrotic angle less than 200° or less than 30% involvement of the femoral head. These lesions have a better prognosis and may be managed nonsurgically if the patient is asymptomatic, or surgically with a femoral head–preserving procedure, such as core decompression. Larger lesions with a necrotic angle greater than or equal to 200° or greater than or equal to 30% involvement of the femoral head have a poorer prognosis and higher risk of collapse. These lesions often require bone grafting or hip arthroplasty. Although the lesion size is often easily identifiable on plain radiographs, visualization may be difficult in patients with early-stage disease, in which case MRI may be used (**Figures 3** and **4**). Most MRI-based treatment algorithms can be used to determine the size of the lesion.

The amount of femoral head depression observed on radiographs also guides treatment. Femoral head depression of less than 2 mm is associated with a better prognosis of head-preserving surgery. Femoral head preservation occasionally is possible in a patient with depression of 2 to 4 mm. Depression of greater than 4 mm indicates disruption of the cartilage surface and is a poor prognostic indicator for head-preserving surgery.

The appearance of the acetabulum on radiographic imaging also aids in determining the appropriate treatment strategy. If the acetabulum has no disease involvement, head-preserving strategies may be appropriate. However, if loss of articular cartilage is observed or the patient has acetabular cysts or osteophytes (evidence of osteoarthritis), preservation of the femoral head is not recommended, and these patients will often require total hip arthroplasty (THA; **Figure 5**).

After these factors are considered, decisions can be made on which surgical techniques are most appropriate. The authors of this chapter follow the indications for surgical treatment presented in **Table 1**. In patients with symptomatic precollapse osteonecrosis and small lesions, core decompression, bone grafting, or osteotomies are appropriate. In patients with precollapse disease and larger lesions, bone grafting procedures may be appropriate. These procedures may involve the use of adjuncts such as bone morphogenetic proteins (BMPs) and stem cells. If patients have evidence of postcollapse disease and acetabular

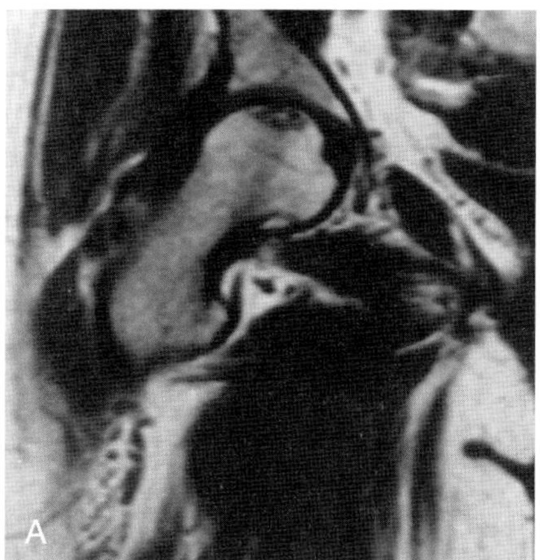

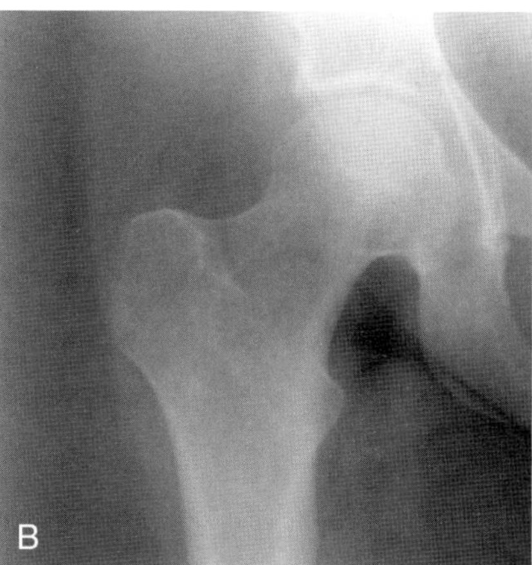

Figure 4 **A,** Coronal T1-weighted MRI of a right hip demonstrates Ficat and Arlet stage I osteonecrosis of the femoral head in a young symptomatic patient. **B,** The lesion is not visible on the plain AP hip radiograph. (Reproduced from Mont MA, Ragland PS: Osteonecrosis of the femoral head: Early stage disease, in Lieberman JR, Berry DJ, eds: *Advanced Reconstruction: Hip*. Rosemont, IL, American Academy of Orthopaedic Surgeons, 2005, pp 517-525.)

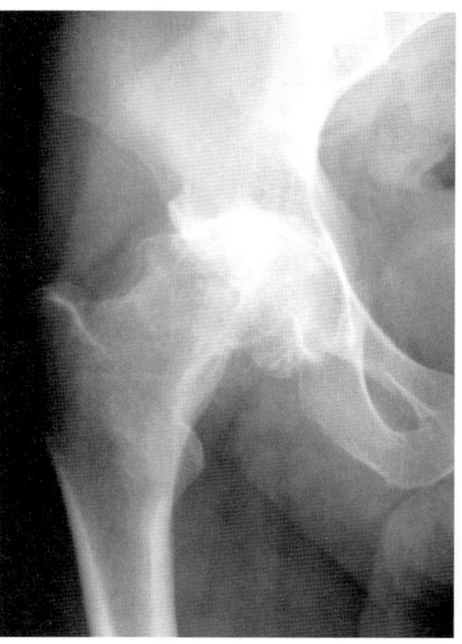

Figure 5 AP radiograph of a right hip demonstrates Ficat and Arlet stage IV osteonecrosis with acetabular involvement, femoral head collapse, and loss of joint interval. Standard total hip arthroplasty is the only option for surgical treatment of this patient. (Reproduced from Mont MA, Ragland PS: Osteonecrosis of the femoral head: Early stage disease, in Lieberman JR, Berry DJ, eds: *Advanced Reconstruction: Hip*. Rosemont, IL, American Academy of Orthopaedic Surgeons, 2005, pp 517-525.)

Table 1 Surgical Treatment Indications for Osteonecrosis of the Femoral Head

Osteonecrosis Stage	Description	Treatment Modalities
Precollapse	Asymptomatic	Nonsurgical management Consider core decompression or percutaneous drilling
	Symptomatic, small lesion	Core decompression, bone grafting, or osteotomies
	Large lesion	Consider bone grafting
Postcollapse	Large lesion with femoral head depression of >2 mm	Bone grafting or total hip arthroplasty
	Acetabular involvement/ osteoarthritis	Total hip arthroplasty

involvement, THA is often required. Occasionally, treatment decisions need to be made intraoperatively on the basis of visualization of bone viability, head depression, and cartilage damage.

Core Decompression and Percutaneous Drilling

Disruption of vascular blood supply is the main pathologic process behind osteonecrosis. Extravascular compression of blood vessels secondary to elevated intraosseous pressure within the femoral head has been postulated as one cause of poor blood flow. Core decompression is a technique to relieve intraosseous pressure. Typically, core decompression is done using 8- to 10-mm trephines for large-diameter drilling. Alternatively, percutaneous drilling can be performed with the use of 3- to 4-mm Steinmann pins to create multiple perforations in a manner similar to the core decompression technique (**Figure 6**). Core decompression or percutaneous drilling is indicated in patients who do not have advanced arthritis or subchondral collapse. These procedures are commonly performed in patients with precollapse disease and small lesions.

Nonvascularized Bone Grafting

In nonvascularized bone grafting, autograft or allograft material is implanted in the femoral head for structural support. This technique is used in patients with precollapse and early postcollapse lesions. Specifically, it has been successful in active patients typically younger than 40 years and often is used in patients in whom previous core decompression was unsuccessful.

Vascularized Bone Grafting

Vascularized bone grafting involves a vascularized pedicle of bone that is transplanted through a core track and anastomosed with the local blood supply to provide mechanical support and

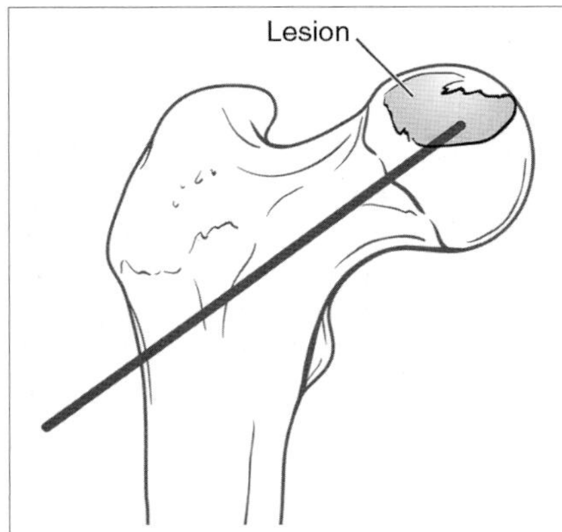

Figure 6 Illustration depicts the use of a 3.2-mm Steinmann pin to establish core tracks percutaneously through the femoral neck. This percutaneous drilling technique is performed through a lateral approach under fluoroscopic guidance. (Reproduced from Mont MA, Ragland PS: Osteonecrosis of the femoral head: Early stage disease, in Lieberman JR, Berry DJ, eds: *Advanced Reconstruction: Hip.* Rosemont, IL, American Academy of Orthopaedic Surgeons, 2005, pp 517-525.)

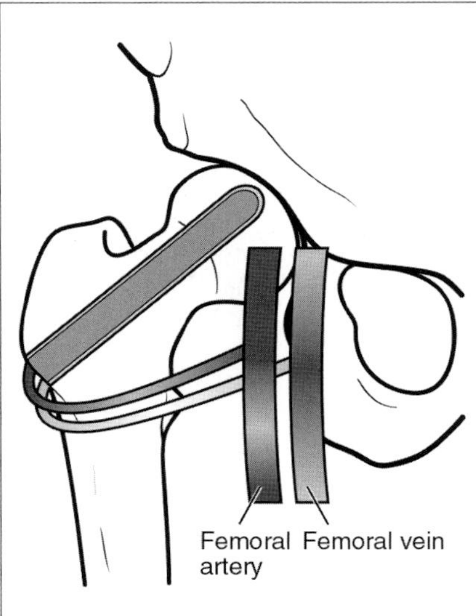

Figure 7 Illustration depicts the vascularized fibular grafting technique. The femoral artery supplies the femoral stem (Reproduced from Mont MA, Ragland PS: Osteonecrosis of the femoral head: Early stage disease, in Lieberman JR, Berry DJ, eds: *Advanced Reconstruction: Hip.* Rosemont, IL, American Academy of Orthopaedic Surgeons, 2005, pp 517-525.)

reintroduce vascular supply. Several grafting methods have been described, including muscle pedicle grafting, which involves one or more of four muscles—the quadratus femoris, sartorius, tensor fascia lata, and gluteus medius—and their pedicles. The choice of muscle graft or grafts depends on the location of the necrotic area in the femoral head. The chosen muscle is elevated from its bed and inserted into the defect, with its vascular supply maintained. In addition, a vascularized iliac bone graft may be used. This technique involves harvesting the bone graft with careful dissection of the deep circumflex iliac vessels to serve as the vascular pedicle. The graft is removed with its muscle sleeve and the vascular bundle attached and is transferred to the necrotic area. However, the most common technique is vascularized free fibular bone grafting, which is described later in this chapter (**Figure 7**).

The decision to perform vascularized bone grafting is made on a case-by-case basis and depends on a patient's age and activity level, the presence and number of risk factors for osteonecrosis, and the rate of disease progression. This technique is preferentially used in patients with symptomatic precollapse lesions, young and active patients (younger than 50 years), and patients in whom previous core decompression was unsuccessful.

Contraindications

Core decompression and percutaneous drilling are not recommended in patients with postcollapse lesions. Core decompression or percutaneous drilling techniques also should be avoided in patients with large lesions, patients who have acetabular involvement, and patients who are unable to comply with postoperative weight-bearing restrictions.

Nonvascularized bone grafting typically is not recommended in patients who have advanced, large lesions (total arc of involvement greater than or equal to 200° or greater than or equal to 30% involvement of the femoral head); articular depression of greater than 2 mm (advanced collapse); or acetabular involvement. Intraoperatively, this procedure should be aborted if delaminated cartilage is observed on the femoral head or if no viable bleeding bone is noted below the lesion (**Figure 8**). Patients are also considered unsuitable for this treatment if they may be unable to comply with postoperative precautions/protocols or are unable to tolerate the surgical procedure.

Vascularized bone grafting is not indicated in patients with asymptomatic precollapse lesions or advanced osteonecrosis. Early postcollapse disease is considered a relative contraindication for this procedure. This technique is often contraindicated in patients with femoral head articular depression of greater than 2 mm, large lesions, or acetabular involvement. Patients may be unsuitable candidates for this procedure if they are unable to comply with postoperative precautions/protocols. Patients with a history of thalassemia, hemoglobinopathy, or notable peripheral vascular disease usually are considered unsuitable candidates for vascularized bone grafting.

Alternative Treatments

THA may be the most appropriate and definitive treatment option in patients 40 years or older and patients who are medically compromised, as well as patients who have acetabular involvement. In addition, THA is an option for any patient who has persistent pain despite prior joint-preserving surgical treatment.

Occasionally, nonsurgical treatment is appropriate for asymptomatic patients who have small lesions, which

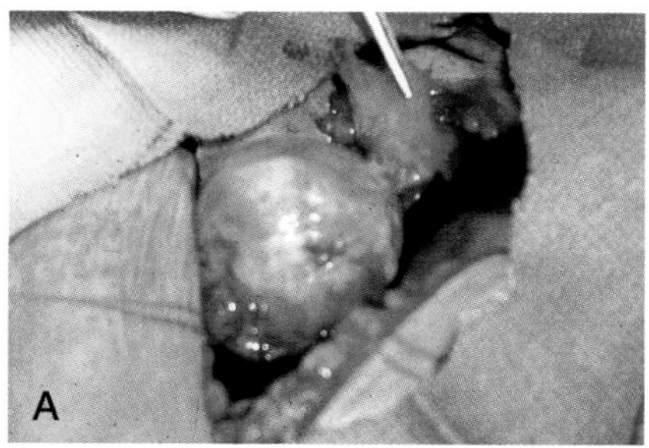

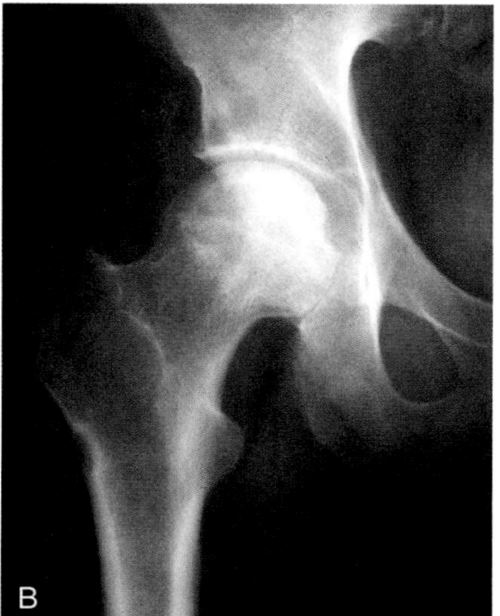

Figure 8 Intraoperative photograph (**A**) shows a femoral head with delaminated cartilage that was not apparent on the preoperative AP hip radiograph (**B**). (Reproduced from Mont MA, Ragland PS: Osteonecrosis of the femoral head: Early stage disease, in Lieberman JR, Berry DJ, eds: *Advanced Reconstruction: Hip.* Rosemont, IL, American Academy of Orthopaedic Surgeons, 2005, pp 517-525.)

often are diagnosed incidentally in the contralateral hip during evaluation of a symptomatic hip. However, recent evidence has demonstrated that asymptomatic osteonecrosis has a high prevalence of progression to symptomatic femoral head collapse. Protective weight bearing with the use of a cane or crutches has not been shown to be effective in preventing disease progression, and often it is used only to assist ambulation before surgical treatment.

Pharmacologic agents, such as diphosphonates, have been used with the aim of increasing bone mineral density and improving clinical function. Lipid-lowering agents such as statins have been hypothesized to target thrombosis and lipid deposition. Antiplatelet and anticoagulant drugs may improve blood flow and prevent progression of early osteonecrosis, particularly in patients with inherited coagulation disorders or genetic abnormalities leading to hypofibrinolysis or thrombophilia. Because results remain inconclusive, further prospective studies are needed to evaluate these modalities. Other nonsurgical modalities used in the management of osteonecrosis include extracorporeal shock wave therapy, which has demonstrated improvements in pain and functional scores, and hyperbaric oxygen. However, studies of these treatment modalities are limited, and insufficient evidence is available to support their use, which has been reported to be time consuming and sometimes expensive.

Results

Both core decompression and percutaneous drilling have demonstrated favorable results in the management of precollapse, smaller lesions, with success rates up to 100% (**Table 2**). In a study comparing multiple drilling with standard core decompression in 94 patients with sickle cell disease and osteonecrosis of the femoral head, no significant difference in outcomes was found between the two procedures; however, the author of the study noted that multiple drilling was considered safer and less invasive. The authors of a different study evaluated the outcomes of multiple percutaneous drillings in patients with precollapse osteonecrosis of the femoral head and reported that 80% of patients who had Ficat and Arlet stage I disease had successful outcomes, with minimal morbidity. To improve outcomes, core decompression has been combined with adjunctive therapies, such as the use of bone graft substitutes. The authors of a retrospective evaluation noted that core decompression with the use of human BMP in patients who had Ficat stage IIA osteonecrosis was successful in 14 of 15 hips (93%).

Multiple studies of nonvascularized bone grafting have been published (**Table 3**). In a study of nonvascularized bone grafting using the so-called trapdoor technique in 33 hips, 80% of the hips with Ficat stage II disease had not required further surgical management at minimum 2-year follow-up. The authors of the study concluded that the use of this technique may delay the need for THA. In a different study, researchers evaluated 76 precollapse hips and noted significantly improved functional outcomes (improvement in the mean Harris hip score from 63 points preoperatively to 82 points postoperatively; $P < 0.001$) and greater success in hips treated with core decompression and allograft compared with those treated with core decompression alone (91% and 55%, respectively). However, results have been variable in patients with higher stages of osteonecrosis. The authors of a retrospective study assessed tibial-source and fibular-source nonvascularized allografts in patients who had Ficat and Arlet stage 0 through IV osteonecrosis, of whom 44% had undergone revision at 4-year follow-up. The authors of the study also noted that tibial allografts had significantly better clinical and radiologic survivorship ($P = 0.002$). Success of this procedure relies on adequate decompression of the necrotic segment and the use of allograft for structural support to allow healing and remodeling. The authors of this chapter recommend that this technique be reserved for patients with earlier stages of osteonecrosis, but further higher-level studies are needed.

Several studies of the outcomes of vascularized bone grafting have demonstrated good clinical results, with success rates greater than 80% (**Table 4**). A systematic review published in

Table 2 Results of Core Decompression or Percutaneous Drilling to Manage Osteonecrosis of the Femoral Head

Author(s) (Year)	Number of Patients	Procedure or Approach	Mean Patient Age in Years (Range)	Mean Follow-up in Years (Range)	Success Rate (%)[a]	Results
Mont et al (2004)	35	Percutaneous drilling	42 (18-70)	2 (1.7-3.3)	Ficat and Arlet stage I: 80 Ficat and Arlet stage II: 57	No surgical complications Minimal morbidity
Neumayr et al (2006)	17	Core decompression and physical therapy	25 (NR)	3 (NR)	Steinberg stage I: 100 Steinberg stage II: 80	Improvement in functional scores was better with core decompression and physical therapy than in the 21 patients who underwent physical therapy alone
Kang et al (2012)	47	Percutaneous drilling with alendronate	44 (21-52)	5.3 (4-6.8)	Ficat and Arlet stage II: 91 Ficat and Arlet stage III: 62	46 other patients were treated with drilling alone Addition of alendronate demonstrated results superior to those of drilling alone, in terms of pain reduction and delay of progression of osteonecrosis
Zhao et al (2012)	50	Core decompression	34 (18-53)	5 (NR)	ARCO stage I: 100 ARCO stage II: 90	50 other patients were treated with mesenchymal stem cell implantation alone Study authors concluded that the use of mesenchymal stem cells may delay collapse of the femoral head
Abrisham et al (2013)	25	Core decompression	30 (25-35)	2 (NR)	Ficat and Arlet stage I: 100 Ficat and Arlet stage II: 82	Treatment yielded lower success rates in the 8 patients who used intravenous drugs than in the 17 patients who did not
Al Omran (2013)	94	Percutaneous drilling: standard core decompression (61), multiple drilling (33)	26 (15-33)	6 (3-10)	Ficat and Arlet stage IIA: 80 (standard), 78 (multiple drilling) Ficat and Arlet stage IIB: 52 (standard), 54 (multiple drilling)	No significant difference in outcomes between multiple drilling and standard core decompression Study author concluded that multiple drilling is safer and less invasive than standard core decompression

ARCO = Association Research Circulation Osseous classification, NR = not reported.

[a] Success in joint preservation and substantial improvement in pain and function.

Table 3 Results of Nonvascularized Bone Grafting in the Management of Osteonecrosis of the Femoral Head

Authors (Year)	Number of Patients	Mean Patient Age in Years (Range)	Follow-up in Years (Range)	Success Rate (%)[a]	Results
Keizer et al (2006)	65 (80 hips)	36 (23-49)	Mean, 4 (NR)	56	Cortical tibial autograft was used in 18 hips, and fibular allograft was used in 62 hips Tibial autograft had significantly better survivorship compared with fibular allograft ($P = 0.002$)
Seyler et al (2008)	33 (39 hips)	35 (18-52)	Mean, 3 (2-4.2)	67	The addition of growth factors to bone grafting effectively reduced donor site morbidity and may defer the need for joint arthroplasty
Yang et al (2010)	54	38 (25-49)	Minimum, 3 (3-6.5)	91	Bone grafting had encouraging success rates and early clinical results, with improvement in mean Harris hip score from 63 to 82

NR = not reported.
[a] Success in joint preservation and significant improvement in pain and function (% of patients).

2014 demonstrated that free vascularized fibular grafting may yield better results than core decompression or nonvascularized fibular grafting. In a study published in 2009, researchers evaluated the long-term results of muscle pedicle bone grafting in 152 patients who had Ficat and Arlet stages I through III osteonecrosis. At a mean follow-up of 17 years, 81% of hips with stage I osteonecrosis had radiologic improvement, compared with 70% of hips with stage III osteonecrosis. Hip survivorship was 92% in hips with stage II osteonecrosis and 82% in hips with stage III osteonecrosis. The authors of a different study reviewed 65 hips in which free vascularized fibular grafting was performed for the management of precollapse osteonecrosis. They noted that 75% of the hips had survival of at least 10 years, with pain and functional outcomes similar to those of hips that required conversion to THA. The authors of the study recommended the use of free vascularized fibular grafting in younger patients (mean age, 36 years) with symptomatic, precollapse osteonecrosis of the femoral head. More recently, novel techniques involving the use of mesenchymal stromal cells with vascularized bone grafts are undergoing exploratory clinical trials with promising demonstrations of bone regeneration. Vascularized bone grafting has shown promising results in patients with osteonecrosis of the femoral head, with better outcomes in patients with precollapse disease than in those with postcollapse disease.

Techniques

Core Decompression or Percutaneous Drilling

SETUP/EXPOSURE

- The patient is placed supine on a radiolucent surgical table or fracture table. The hip is prepped and draped in standard aseptic fashion.
- The affected limb is positioned with slight internal rotation to counteract the natural anteversion of the femoral neck.

PROCEDURE

- In standard core decompression, large-diameter drilling is performed. The tract is created above the superior level of the lesser trochanter to reduce the risk of stress fractures.
- With the use of a guidewire, an 8- to 10-mm–wide cannulated trephine is used to remove a core of bone from the lesion center.
- The necrotic bone is sent for pathologic analysis.
- Occasionally, cortical or cancellous strut grafting is performed to provide structural stability.
- BMPs and mesenchymal cells may be used to promote repair and aid bone growth.
- In percutaneous drilling, a Steinmann pin is inserted percutaneously, immediately inferior to the lateral cortical flare at the metaphyseal-diaphyseal junction in the center of the proximal femur.
- The pin is advanced under fluoroscopic guidance to the level of the proximal femoral neck.
- The trajectory is assessed with the use of AP and frog-lateral radiographs.
- After the trajectory is deemed acceptable, the pin is advanced through the femoral neck toward the lesion. Areas of sclerosis may be encountered during the drilling process.
- Two or three passes of the Steinmann pin may be required for larger lesions.
- After adequate decompression is

Table 4 Results of Vascularized Bone Grafting in the Management of Osteonecrosis of the Femoral Head

Authors (Year)	Number of Patients	Mean Patient Age in Years (Range)	Mean Follow-up in Years (Range)	Success Rate (%)[a]	Results
Baksi et al (2009)	152	36 (16-62)	17 (10-22)	85	Excellent Hospital for Special Surgery scores were obtained in 100% of hips with Ficat and Arlet stage I osteonecrosis, 92% of hips with stage II osteonecrosis, and 80% of hips with stage III osteonecrosis
Tetik et al (2011)	8	NR	1.8 (1-4.8)	100	13 other patients underwent nonvascularized grafting Patients treated with vascularized grafts had Harris hip and visual analog scale scores higher than those of patients treated with nonvascularized grafts
Zhao et al (2013)	52	39 (20-53)	5 (NR)	88	Greater success was noted in hips with earlier stages of osteonecrosis Mean Harris hip score improved from 50 to 91

NR = not reported.
[a] Success in joint preservation and significant improvement in pain and function (% of patients).

achieved, the pin is backed out while saline-soaked gauze is held at the junction of the pin and the skin.

WOUND CLOSURE

- Direct pressure is maintained at the site of the incision until hemostasis is achieved.
- An absorbable monofilament suture can be used for wound closure. However, a standard adhesive bandage is usually sufficient.

Nonvascularized Bone Grafting

SETUP/EXPOSURE

- The patient is counseled preoperatively that THA may be required if any contraindications are discovered intraoperatively.
- The patient is placed in the lateral decubitus position and secured with the pelvis perpendicular to the floor.
- A straight skin incision measuring approximately 10 cm is made.
- Subcutaneous dissection is performed to the level of the fascia lata.

PROCEDURE

- The abductors are retracted, and the anterior hip capsule is adequately exposed.
- An anterior capsulectomy is performed.
- The hip is evaluated for the presence of articular surface or subchondral collapse.
- After the femoral head is deemed appropriate, either the lightbulb procedure or the trapdoor procedure is performed, as follows.

Lightbulb Procedure

- A cortical window measuring approximately 2 cm × 2 cm is marked at the femoral head-neck junction with the use of electrocautery or methylene blue.
- A microsagittal saw is used to create the cortical window.
- The cortical window is raised with the use of a 0.25-in (6.35-mm) osteotome and placed in a saline-soaked gauze pad.
- Necrotic bone is débrided and excavated from the femoral head with the use of a combination of curved curets and a 4-mm round-tipped burr.
- The adequacy of débridement is visualized with the use of an arthroscope placed through the cortical window.
- After adequate débridement is completed, the defect is filled and packed with cancellous bone graft, allogeneic or autogenic cortical bone graft, or a combination of these grafts.
- The cortical window is returned to the defect and gently impacted with the use of a bone tamp and mallet.
- The fragment is secured with three 2-mm bioabsorbable pins. To maximize the strength of fixation, the pins are placed in divergent orientation.
- Electrocautery is used to weld the ends of the pins into place.
- The wound is irrigated with normal saline.

Trapdoor Procedure

- After exposure is obtained as described previously, the femoral head is dislocated anteriorly.

- A No. 15 scalpel and a 0.25-in (6.35-mm) osteotome are used to create an osteochondral window measuring 2 cm × 2 cm over the affected area of the femoral head.
- The flap is hinged back on its base.
- With the use of a 6-mm round-tipped burr and curved curets, necrotic segments of bone are débrided until a bleeding bed of viable bone is reached.
- After adequate débridement, the defect is packed and filled with bone chips, cancellous bone graft, autogenic or allogeneic cortical bone graft, or a combination of these graft types. The authors of this chapter typically use allograft enhanced with BMP.
- Bone chips are placed perpendicular to the articular surface to optimize structural support.
- The osteochondral flap is reattached with the use of two or three 2-mm bioabsorbable pins. To maximize the strength of the fixation, the pins are placed with divergent orientation.
- Extra care is taken to ensure that the pins are countersunk in the femoral head to avoid damage to the articular cartilage of the acetabulum. The pin ends are often welded with electrocautery.
- The hip is relocated.
- Excess capsular tissue is excised to prevent adhesive capsulitis or capsular hypertrophy.

WOUND CLOSURE

- Standard muscular repair is performed.
- The wound is closed in standard fashion.

Vascularized Bone Grafting

SETUP/EXPOSURE

- A microvascular surgeon should assist in the planning of the graft harvest and pedicle anastomosis for free vascularized fibular grafting.
- The ideal scenario is to have two surgical teams working simultaneously. One team harvests the graft, and the other is responsible for exposure and preparation of the hip.
- The patient is placed in the lateral decubitus position, with the affected side up and the pelvis perpendicular to the floor.
- The entire affected limb is prepped and draped.

PROCEDURE

- To begin the process of harvesting of the fibular graft, a tourniquet is applied above the knee.
- A straight lateral skin incision measuring 15 cm is made over the fibula. The incision should begin 10 cm distal to the head of the fibula and should end 10 cm proximal to the lateral malleolus.
- The subcutaneous tissue and peroneal muscles are dissected off the fibula.
- The fibular osteotomy is done with the use of an oscillating saw.
- The graft portion of the fibula is removed with at least 4 cm of peroneal pedicle available (ligated with hemostatic clips and divided from the posterior tibial artery).
- The tourniquet is released, and hemostasis is achieved.
- The wound is irrigated and packed.
- The diameter of the harvested fibula is measured to determine the diameter of the core tract.
- The vessels in the peroneal pedicle are assessed for leaks, adequately protected, and secured against the graft with absorbable braided 3-0 suture to prevent stripping of the pedicle and periosteum during graft insertion.
- After the proximal femur is adequately exposed, the entry point for the guide pin is determined under fluoroscopic guidance. The entry point should be approximately 2 cm distal to the vastus ridge and above the level of the lesser trochanter.
- After the entry point and trajectory are determined, the guide pin is advanced to the center of the osteonecrotic lesion under fluoroscopic guidance with AP and frog-lateral views.
- A core tract is opened with cannulated reamers. The tract should have a final diameter 1 to 2 mm larger than that of the fibular graft to allow the blood supply in the pedicle to flow freely.
- Cancellous autograft is packed into the débrided necrotic segment.
- After the graft is appropriately sized, it is inserted into the core tract within the packed autograft.
- After the graft is adequately seated, the pedicles of the peroneal artery and vein and the ascending lateral femoral circumflex artery and vein are anastomosed with the assistance of a microvascular surgeon.
- Vascularity is confirmed by the presence of back bleeding from the fibular endosteal bone.
- The graft is secured with a Kirschner wire extending from just above the distal end of the fibular graft to the medial cortex of the lesser trochanter.

WOUND CLOSURE

- The wound is closed in standard fashion.
- To prevent compression or tension on the pedicles, the origins of the vastus intermedius and lateralis muscle are not repaired after fibular grafting.

Postoperative Regimen

After core decompression and percutaneous drilling, the patient is discharged from the hospital on the day of the procedure. Deep vein thrombosis (DVT) prophylaxis is not routinely prescribed. Crutches are used for 6 weeks postoperatively to ensure 50% weight bearing on the affected leg. After 6 weeks postoperatively, the patient can progress to full weight bearing, and simple hip- and abductor-strengthening exercises are recommended.

After nonvascularized bone grafting, patients usually are admitted to the hospital for an average of 3 days. Mechanical and pharmacologic DVT prophylaxis is used. Early same-day mobilization with toe-touch weight bearing is encouraged. Toe-touch weight bearing is continued for 6 weeks postoperatively. At 6 weeks postoperatively, the patient can progress to 50% weight bearing. Physical therapy is often prescribed for abductor strengthening. Full weight bearing begins after 12 weeks postoperatively.

After vascularized bone grafting, the patient is admitted to the hospital; length of hospital stay is highly variable. Mechanical and pharmacologic DVT prophylaxis is used. Patients who have undergone fibular grafting are encouraged to perform simple toe and ankle range-of-motion exercises starting on postoperative day 1 because scarring of the flexor hallucis longus tendon may be present. A short leg posterior splint is used until the first dressing change on the second postoperative day. At 5 days postoperatively, the patency of the anastomosis is assessed by means of a digital subtraction angiogram. The patient is mobilized on the day of the procedure with physical therapy, and hip motion is encouraged. However, non–weight-bearing precautions are maintained for 6 weeks postoperatively, with the use of double crutches. At 6 weeks postoperatively, the patient begins toe-touch weight bearing. At 12 weeks postoperatively, 50% weight bearing is allowed. Full weight bearing is permitted at 6 months postoperatively, depending on graft incorporation and the initial size of the lesion.

After each of these procedures, patients are advised to avoid high-impact activity for 1 year postoperatively. The patient is seen for follow-up at 6 weeks, 12 weeks, 6 months, and 12 months postoperatively and yearly thereafter, with plain radiographs obtained at each visit.

Avoiding Pitfalls and Complications

During core decompression or percutaneous drilling, the patient is at risk of thermal skin necrosis from the percutaneous pin. Therefore, the use of saline-soaked gauze at the junction of the skin and the pin is advised. A starting point below the level of the lesser trochanter should be avoided to reduce risk for creating a stress riser or causing a subtrochanteric fracture of the femur. The use of larger amounts of force should be avoided in the process of drilling through areas of sclerosis because this step carries an increased risk of plunging through the femoral head into the hip joint. If the trajectory of the pin needs to be adjusted, the surgeon should use the same entry hole to avoid creating another stress riser with a new adjacent hole.

When performing nonvascularized bone grafting, the surgeon must take care to avoid damaging the acetabular labrum when performing the anterior capsulectomy because damage to the labrum can result in instability and pain. During the débridement of necrotic bone in the lightbulb procedure, the surgeon should take care to avoid penetration of the femoral head. If this complication occurs, the surgeon should consider converting the procedure to THA. During the lightbulb procedure, the use of an osteotome to establish the corners of the cortical window is recommended because propagation of the cortical window into the femoral neck may create a stress riser and result in fracture. During the trapdoor procedure, if bleeding bone is not encountered, the surgeon should consider conversion to THA. Meticulous repair of the abductor muscles after the procedure is necessary to ensure stability and re-create normal biomechanics. Because contraindications to nonvascularized bone grafting may be detected intraoperatively, the surgeon must be prepared and have the necessary equipment available to convert the procedure to THA.

In the vascularized bone grafting procedure, the fibular osteotomy must be done with care to protect the superficial peroneal nerve, which lies under the peroneus longus. An adequate length of fibular graft (approximately 13 cm) should be harvested, with care taken to leave at least 10 cm of fibula distal to the knee and at least 10 cm of fibula proximal to the ankle. When determining the entry site of the guide pin in the proximal femur, the surgeon must take care to stay above the level of the lesser trochanter to avoid creating a subtrochanteric stress riser. In addition, care must be taken to avoid penetration of the femoral head into the joint. To avoid compression that would hinder vascularity, the diameter of the core tract must be 1 to 2 mm larger than the diameter of the graft. At the conclusion of the procedure, the end of the Kirschner wire that was used to secure the graft should not be left prominent because prominence of the wire can result in pain, bursitis, and soft-tissue irritation. To avoid compromise of the pedicles, repair of the vastus intermedius and lateralis muscles should not be performed. After the procedure, simple ankle and toe range-of-motion exercises are recommended to avoid potential flexion contracture or clawing associated with scarring of the flexor hallucis longus tendon.

Bibliography

Abrisham SM, Hajiesmaeili MR, Soleimani H, Pahlavanhosseini H: Efficacy of core decompression of femoral head to treat avascular necrosis in intravenous drug users. *Acta Med Iran* 2013;51(4):250-253.

Agarwala S, Shah SB: Ten-year follow-up of avascular necrosis of femoral head treated with alendronate for 3 years. *J Arthroplasty* 2011;26(7):1128-1134.

Ali SA, Christy JM, Griesser MJ, Awan H, Pan X, Ellis TJ: Treatment of avascular necrosis of the femoral head utilising free vascularised fibular graft: A systematic review. *Hip Int* 2014;24(1):5-13.

Al Omran A: Multiple drilling compared with standard core decompression for avascular necrosis of the femoral head in sickle cell disease patients. *Arch Orthop Trauma Surg* 2013;133(5):609-613.

Aoyama T, Goto K, Kakinoki R, et al: An exploratory clinical trial for idiopathic osteonecrosis of femoral head by cultured autologous multipotent mesenchymal stromal cells augmented with vascularized bone grafts. *Tissue Eng Part B Rev* 2014;20(4):233-242.

Baksi DP, Pal AK, Baksi DD: Long-term results of decompression and muscle-pedicle bone grafting for osteonecrosis of the femoral head. *Int Orthop* 2009;33(1):41-47.

Eward WC, Rineer CA, Urbaniak JR, Richard MJ, Ruch DS: The vascularized fibular graft in precollapse osteonecrosis: Is long-term hip preservation possible? *Clin Orthop Relat Res* 2012;470(10):2819-2826.

Kang P, Pei F, Shen B, Zhou Z, Yang J: Are the results of multiple drilling and alendronate for osteonecrosis of the femoral head better than those of multiple drilling? A pilot study. *Joint Bone Spine* 2012;79(1):67-72.

Keizer SB, Kock NB, Dijkstra PD, Taminiau AH, Nelissen RG: Treatment of avascular necrosis of the hip by a non-vascularised cortical graft. *J Bone Joint Surg Br* 2006;88(4):460-466.

Lieberman JR, Conduah A, Urist MR: Treatment of osteonecrosis of the femoral head with core decompression and human bone morphogenetic protein. *Clin Orthop Relat Res* 2004;(429):139-145.

Mont MA, Ragland PS, Etienne G: Core decompression of the femoral head for osteonecrosis using percutaneous multiple small-diameter drilling. *Clin Orthop Relat Res* 2004;(429):131-138.

Mont MA, Zywiel MG, Marker DR, McGrath MS, Delanois RE: The natural history of untreated asymptomatic osteonecrosis of the femoral head: A systematic literature review. *J Bone Joint Surg Am* 2010;92(12):2165-2170.

Neumayr LD, Aguilar C, Earles AN, et al; National Osteonecrosis Trial in Sickle Cell Anemia Study Group: Physical therapy alone compared with core decompression and physical therapy for femoral head osteonecrosis in sickle cell disease: Results of a multicenter study at a mean of three years after treatment. *J Bone Joint Surg Am* 2006;88(12):2573-2582.

Seyler TM, Marker DR, Ulrich SD, Fatscher T, Mont MA: Nonvascularized bone grafting defers joint arthroplasty in hip osteonecrosis. *Clin Orthop Relat Res* 2008;466(5):1125-1132.

Tetik C, Başar H, Bezer M, Erol B, Ağir I, Esemenli T: Comparison of early results of vascularized and non-vascularized fibular grafting in the treatment of osteonecrosis of the femoral head. *Acta Orthop Traumatol Turc* 2011;45(5):326-334.

Yang S, Wu X, Xu W, Ye S, Liu X, Liu X: Structural augmentation with biomaterial-loaded allograft threaded cage for the treatment of femoral head osteonecrosis. *J Arthroplasty* 2010;25(8):1223-1230.

Zhao D, Cui D, Wang B, et al: Treatment of early stage osteonecrosis of the femoral head with autologous implantation of bone marrow-derived and cultured mesenchymal stem cells. *Bone* 2012;50(1):325-330.

Zhao D, Zhang Y, Wang W, et al: Tantalum rod implantation and vascularized iliac grafting for osteonecrosis of the femoral head. *Orthopedics* 2013;36(6):789-795.

Index

Page numbers with *f* indicate figures
Page numbers with *t* indicate tables

D

G

H

I

J

K

L

R

S

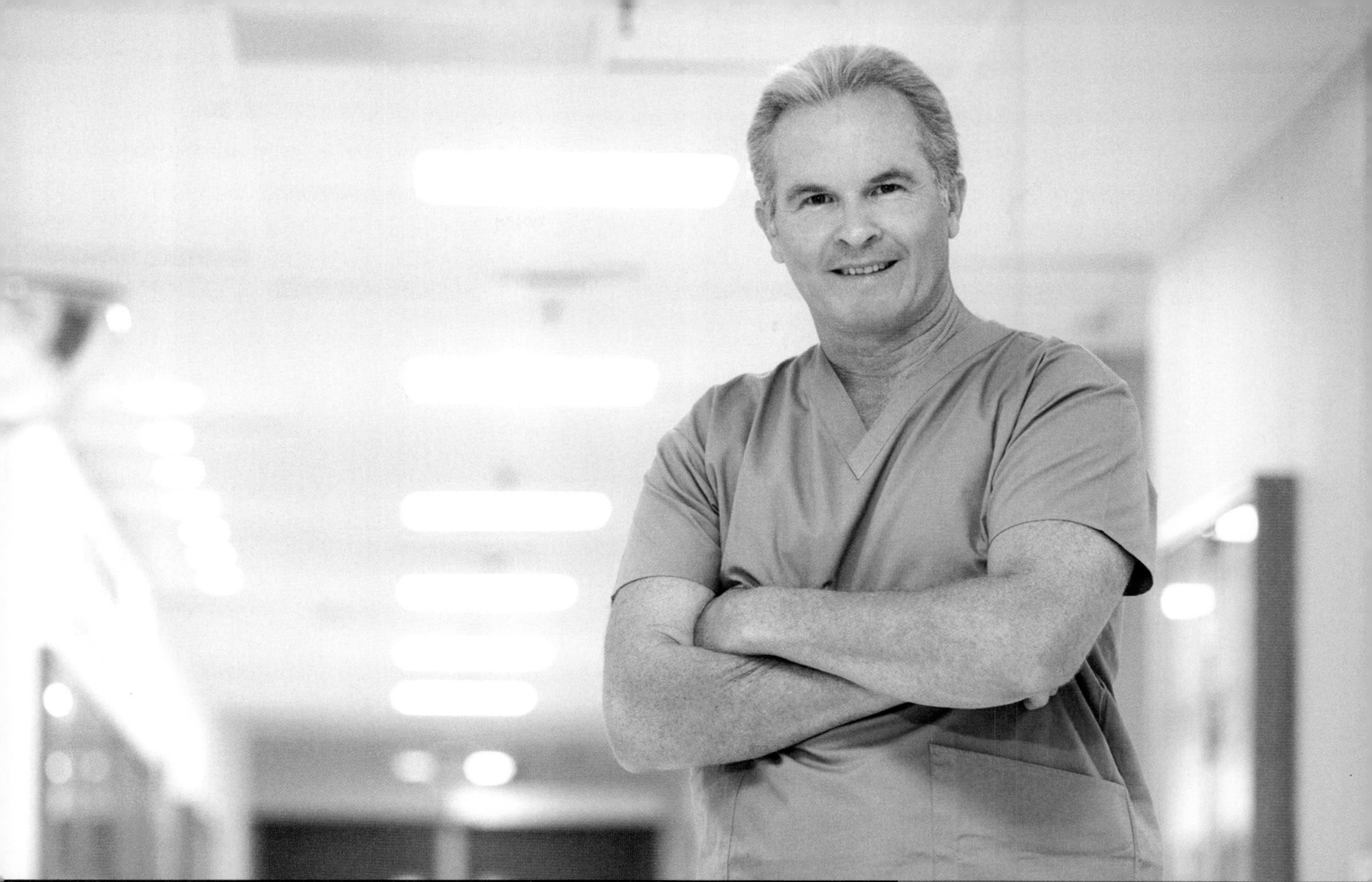

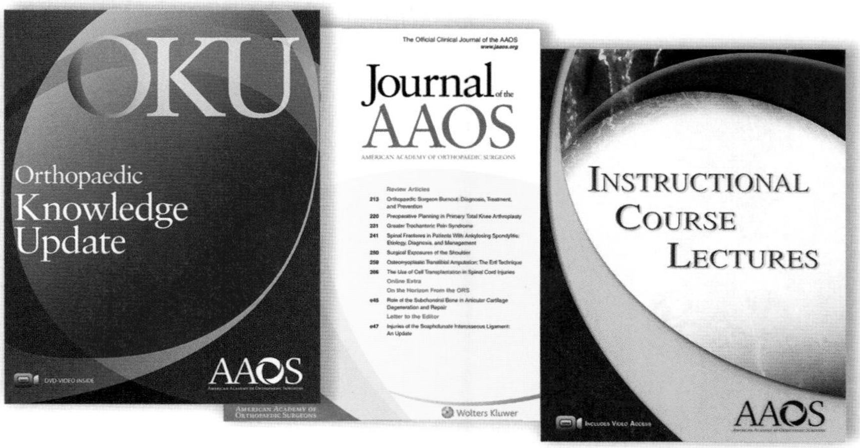